Cardiovascular Pathology

OTHER MONOGRAPHS IN THE SERIES MAJOR PROBLEMS IN PATHOLOGY

VIRGINIA A. LIVOLSI, M.D.
Series Editor

Published

Azzopardi: *Problems in Breast Pathology*

Frable: *Fine Needle Aspiration Biopsy*

Wigglesworth: *Perinatal Pathology, 2/ed*

Wirrels: *Surgical Pathology of Bone Marrow*

Katzenstein: *Katzenstein and Askin's Surgical Pathology of Non-Neoplastic Lung Disease, 3/ed*

Finegold: *Pathology of Neoplasia in Children and Adolescents*

Wolf and Neiman: *Disorders of the Spleen*

Fu and Regan: *Pathology of the Uterine Cervix, Vagina, and Vulva*

LiVolsi: *Surgical Pathology of the Thyroid*

Virmani, Atkinson, and Fenoglio: *Cardiovascular Pathology*

Whitehead: *Mucosal Biopsy of the Gastrointestinal Tract, 5/ed*

Mackay, Lukeman, and Ordonez: *Tumors of the Lung*

Ellis, Auclair, and Gnepp: *Surgical Pathology of the Salivary Glands*

Nash and Said: *Pathology of AIDS and HIV Infection*

Lloyd: *Surgical Pathology of the Pituitary Gland*

Henson and Albores-Saavedra: *Pathology of Incipient Neoplasia, 2/ed*

Taylor and Cote: *Immunomicroscopy, 2/ed*

Lack: *Pathology of Adrenal and Extra-Adrenal Paraganglia*

Kornstein: *Pathology of the Thymus and Mediastinum*

Jaffe: *Surgical Pathology of Lymph Nodes and Related Organs, 2/ed*

Striker, Striker, and d'Agati: *The Renal Biopsy, 3/ed*

Isaacs, Jr: *Tumors of the Fetus and Newborn*

Foster and Bostwick: *Pathology of the Prostate*

Neiman and Orazi: *Disorders of the Spleen, 2/ed*

Helliwell: *Pathology of Bone and Joint Neoplasms*

Owen and Kelly: *Pathology of the Gallbladder, Biliary Tract, and Pancreas*

Forthcoming

Fu: *Pathology of the Uterine Cervix, Vagina, and Vulva, 2/ed*

Weidner: *Surgical Pathology of the Breast*

LiVolsi: *Pathology of the Thyroid, 2/ed*

Foster and Ross: *Pathology of the Bladder*

Leonard: *Diagnostic Molecular Pathology*

Tomazewski: *Pathology of Renal Neoplasms*

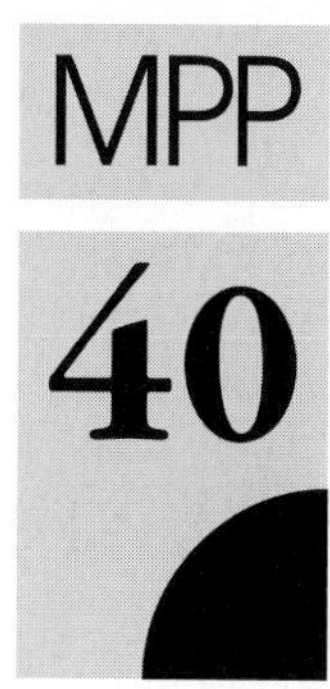

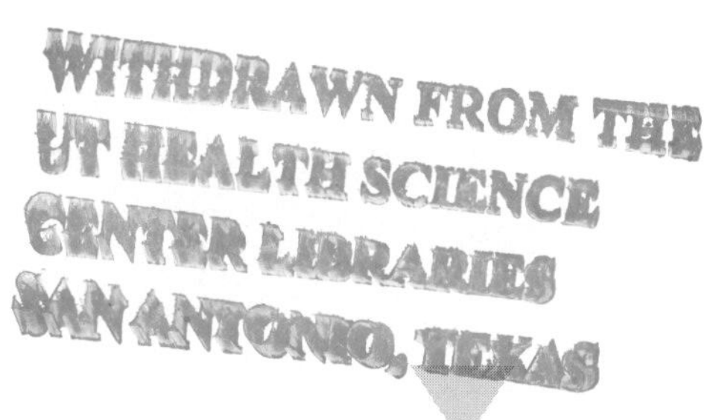

RENU VIRMANI, M.D.
Chairman
Department of Cardiovascular Pathology
Armed Forces Institute of Pathology
Washington, D.C.

ANDREW FARB, M.D.
Chief
Division of Cardiovascular Research
Armed Forces Institute of Pathology
Washington, D.C.

ALLEN BURKE, M.D.
Associate Chairman
Department of Cardiovascular Pathology
Armed Forces Institute of Pathology
Washington, D.C.

JAMES B. ATKINSON, M.D., Ph.D.
Professor of Pathology
Director, Surgical Pathology
Vanderbilt University Medical Center
Nashville, TN

Cardiovascular Pathology

Volume 40 in the Series

MAJOR PROBLEMS IN PATHOLOGY

second edition

W.B. SAUNDERS COMPANY
A Harcourt Health Sciences Company
PHILADELPHIA LONDON NEW YORK ST. LOUIS SYDNEY TORONTO

W.B. SAUNDERS COMPANY
A Harcourt Health Sciences Company

The Curtis Center
Independence Square West
Philadelphia, Pennsylvania 19106

Library of Congress Cataloging-in-Publication Data

Cardiovascular pathology / [edited by] Renu Virmani ...[et al.].—2nd ed.

p. ; cm.— (Major problems in pathology ; v. 40)

Includes bibliographical references and index.

ISBN 0–7216–8165–4

1. Cardiovascular system—Diseases. I. Virmani, Renu. II. Series.
[DNLM: 1. Cardiovascular Diseases—pathology. WG 142 C2645 2001]

RC669.9.C37 2001

616.1'07—dc21 2001020551

CARDIOVASCULAR PATHOLOGY ISBN 0–7216–8165–4

Printed in the United States of America

Last digit is the print number: 9 8 7 6 5 4 3 2 1

Foreword

The 2nd Edition of Cardiovascular Pathology by Dr. Virmani and colleagues is a worthy follow-up to the 1st Edition. The authors have expanded the discussion and description of cardiac and vascular diseases. They have included numerous tables with classification schemes, many of which have been elaborated by the authors. This extensively referenced and illustrative volume is a proud member of the Major Problems of Pathology series. It will certainly become a standard for a practicing pathologist who faces lesions of the heart and vascular systems.

VIRGINIA A. LIVOLSI, M.D.
UNIVERSITY OF PENNSYLVANIA
SERIES EDITOR

Preface to First Edition

This book highlights specific areas of cardiovascular pathology that are of particular importance to a practicing pathologist. It provides an update on recent developments in the field of cardiovascular pathology by addressing current topics in which recent developments have changed accepted concepts. Chapter 1, The Examination of the Heart, will serve as a baseline for pathologists and as a guide for the optimal method of evaluating different heart diseases. New developments in diagnostic imaging techniques, recent concepts of pathophysiology, and advances in experimental studies require close interaction between the cardiologist and the pathologist to incorporate innovative ways to correlate the pathologic anatomy with the clinical findings.

The ever-increasing diagnostic modalities being introduced in medical science require a close working relationship between the clinician and the pathologist in order for progress to continue. Chapter 2, The Cardiologist as Clinician and Pathologist: The Interactions of Both and the Limitations of Each, examines specifically how this relationship can be optimized to yield maximum information.

Overall the book deals with four important areas of cardiovascular pathology: ischemic heart disease, cardiomyopathies, the use of endomyocardial biopsy in diagnosing heart and combined heart–lung transplant rejection and underlying heart disease, and valvular heart disease and pathology of native and prosthetic valves.

RENU VIRMANI, M.D.
JAMES B. ATKINSON, PH.D.

Preface to Second Edition

This volume represents a major reorganization since the first edition. While keeping the focus on diagnostic autopsy and surgical pathology of the heart, the book has been consolidated and completely rewritten, with only three chapters (1, 8, and 9) retaining significant material from the previous work. In reducing the number of authors and chapters, our intent was to produce a readable, concise overview of the problems facing the practicing pathologist at the turn of the century.

In the 10 years since the appearance of the first addition of *Cardiovascular Pathology*, there have been several major developments that have made a significant impact on the diagnosis of cardiac disease. First, the application of molecular techniques to diagnosis, especially in cardiomyopathies and sudden death, have led to advances in understanding cardiovascular disease processes and changes in classification. Secondly, cardiologists are continually offering new imaging techniques and clinical interventions, resulting in the need for morphologic descriptions of tissue reactions and complications of these new therapies. Third, there has been an explosion of new information regarding the pathology and etiology of atherosclerosis, including the morphologic types of coronary thrombosis and classification of late coronary lesions. Finally, developments in the understanding and treatment of cardiac allografts have resulted in an extensive body of literature refining our approach to the vascular and myocardial alterations associated with transplant pathology. It is hoped that this volume adequately addresses these developments and will provide the general pathologist with a timely update in these areas, while continuing to offer a basic textbook on cardiac pathology.

Although endomyocardial biopsy remains the cornerstone for the evaluation of transplant rejection, the promises of endomyocardial biopsy in directing the treatment of patients with myocardial and cardiomyopathy has failed to materialize over the past decade. Although still critically important in the differential diagnosis of a select group of entities, we have not seen a steady increase in endomyocardial biopsy in the diagnosis of disease other than cardiac rejection. It remains to be seen if newer molecular diagnostic tools will be applied to heart biopsy tissue and, in the near future, fulfill our hopes that endomyocardial biopsy may assert itself as an integral part of the cardiologist's evaluation of patients. The chapters on endomyocardial biopsies in this volume will, we hope, provide the practitioner with the tools to generate meaningful reports to the requesting clinicians, and maintain the groundwork of morphologic alterations that will be necessary for future technologies.

The book continues to deal with the major areas of concern to the diagnostic pathologist: sudden death, ischemic heart disease, valve disease, interventional procedures, and endomyocardial biopsy. In addition, there are chapters on less common entities of tumors and nonatherosclerotic vascular diseases, and a comprehensive new chapter on pericardial diseases. Although diseases of peripheral vessels are not extensively covered, the final chapter on the aorta, pulmonary artery (including pulmonary embolism) and major veins, should provide an approach to the pathology of the vasculature in general. The introductory chapter on examination of the heart has retained classic material in the previous edition, while adding new information on the evaluation of specific heart diseases and cardiac devices.

We hope this text provides a useful resource for the practicing pathologists in their work with an expanding array of cardiovascular interventions and specimens.

RENU VIRMANI, M.D.
ALLEN BURKE, M.D.
ANDREW FARB, M.D
JAMES B. ATKINSON, M.D., PH.D.

Contents

Cardiovascular Pathology

Color Plates

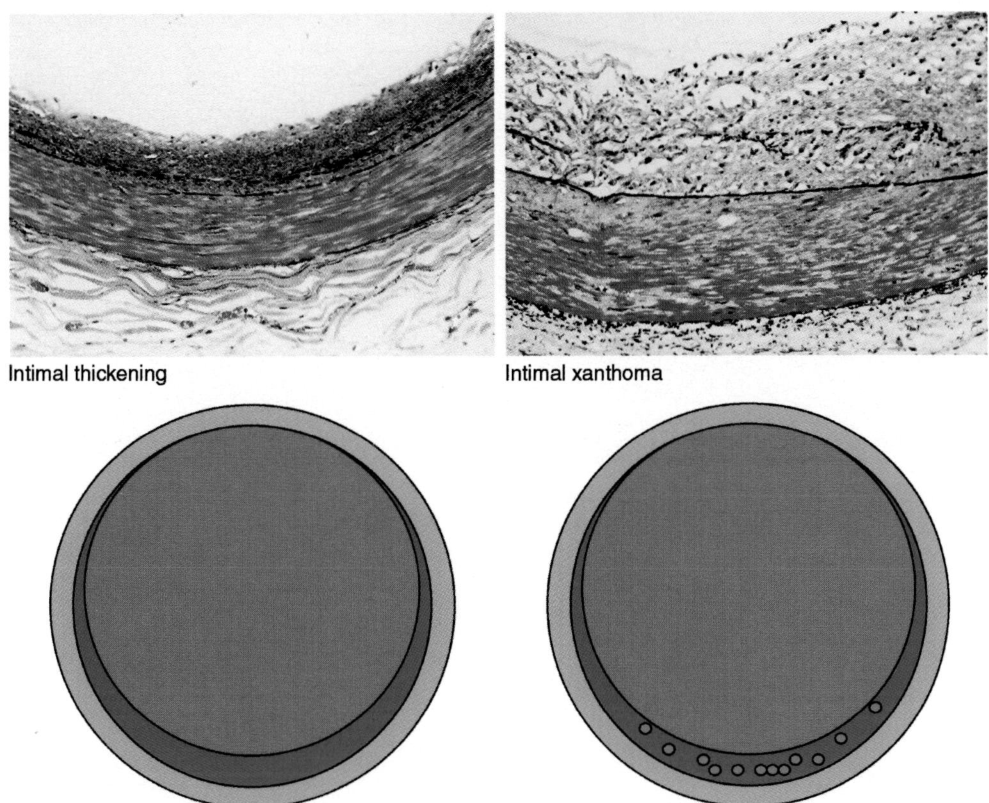

Color Plate 1. *(See Figure 2–2, page 31.)*

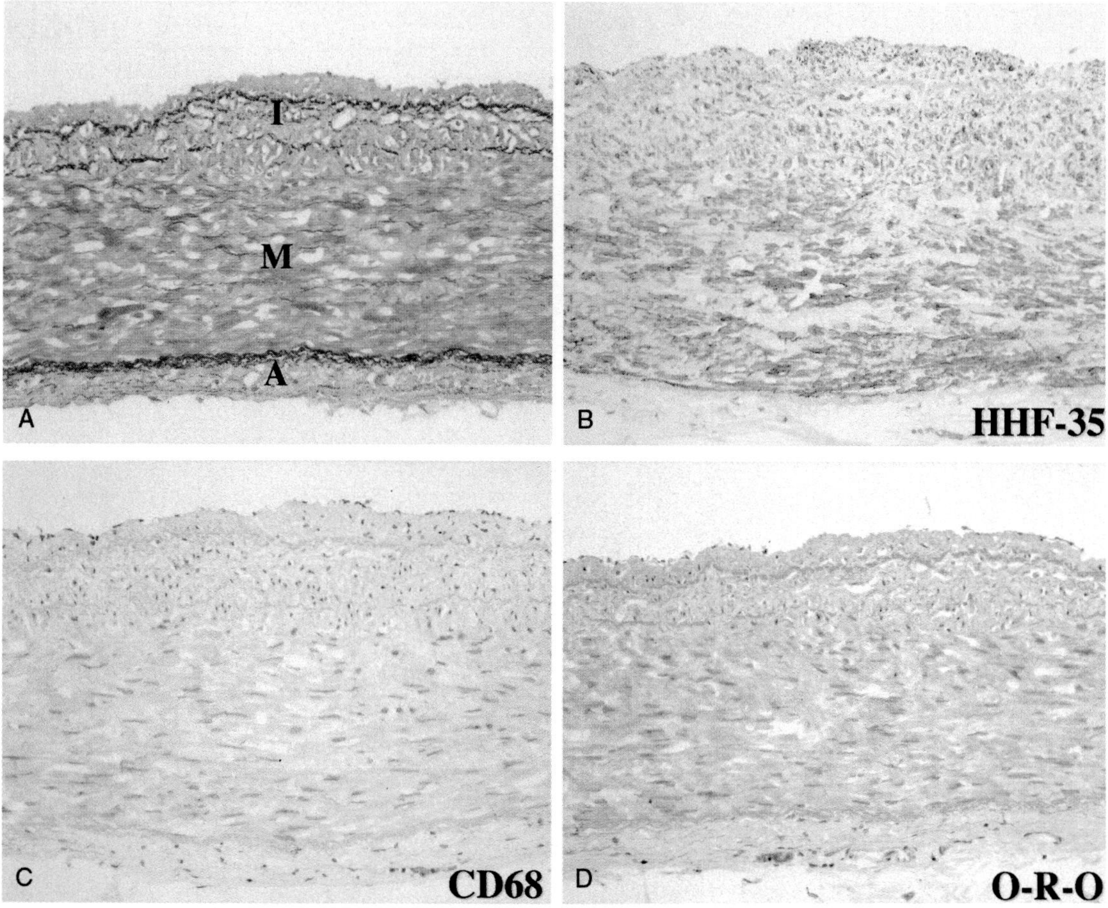

I
M
A
A

B
HHF-35

C
CD68

D
O-R-O

Color Plate 2. *(See Figure 2–3, page 32.)*

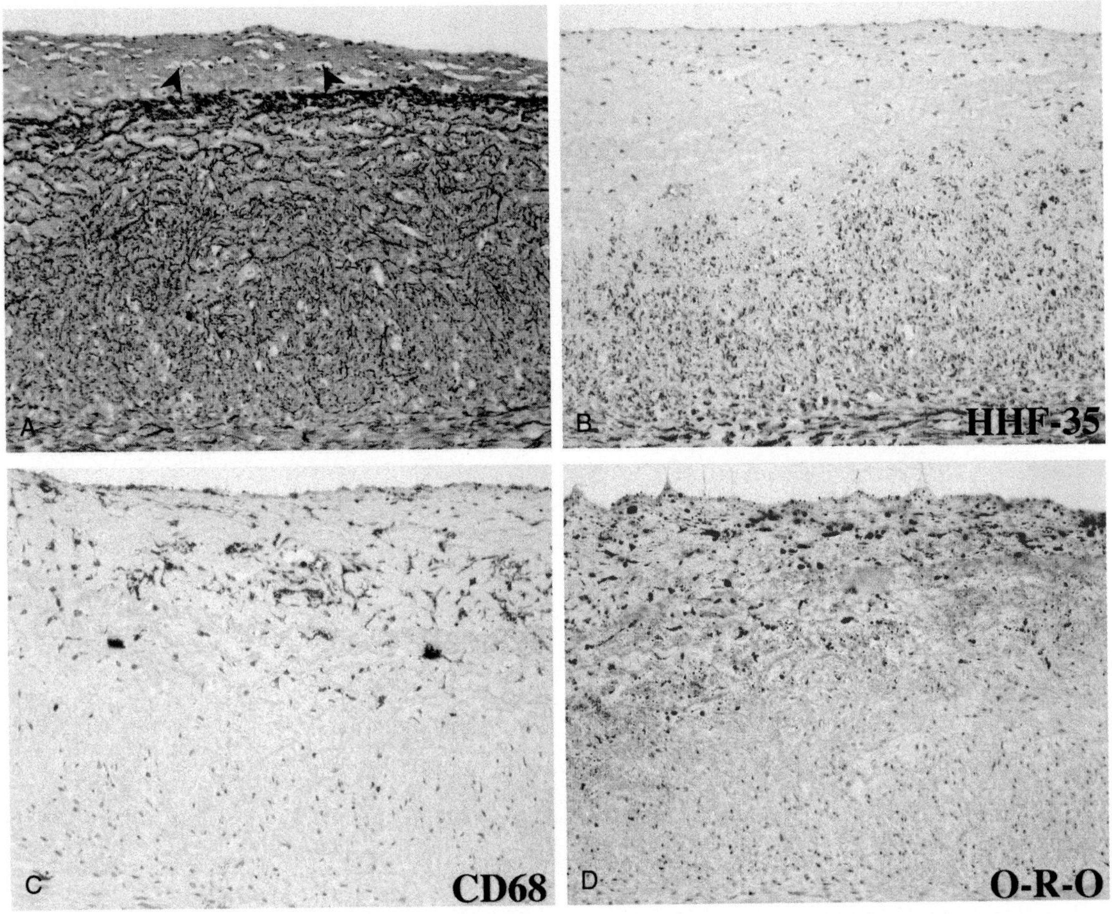

A
B
HHF-35
C
CD68
D
O-R-O

Color Plate 3. *(See Figure 2–4, page 33.)*

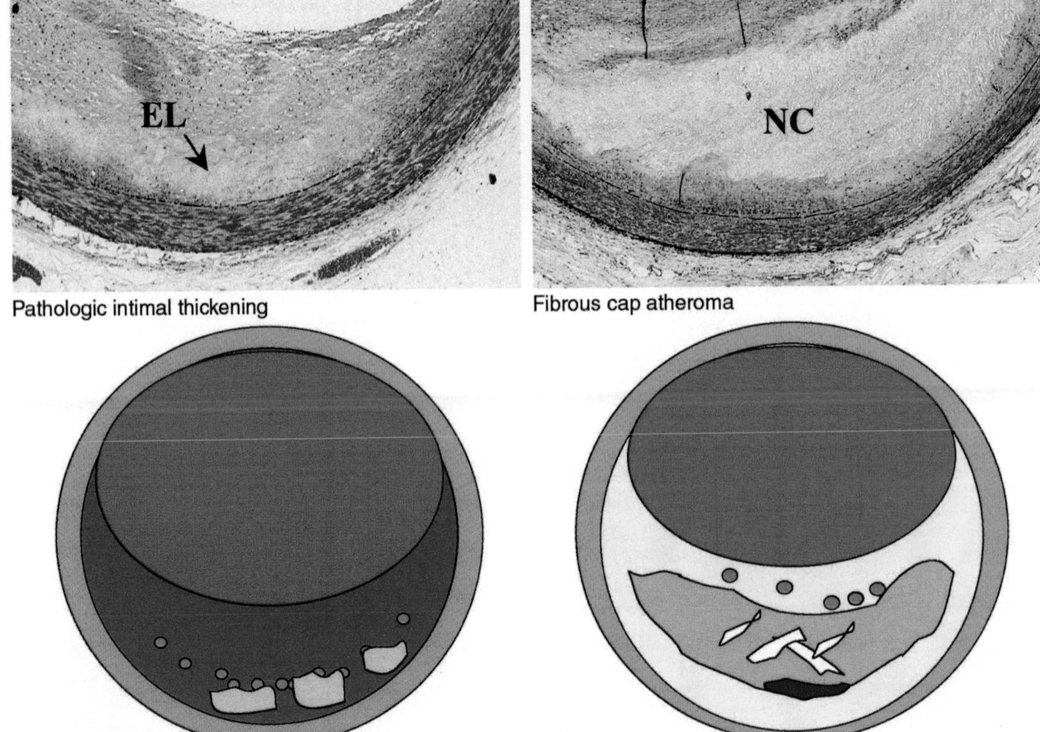

EL
NC
Pathologic intimal thickening
Fibrous cap atheroma

Color Plate 4. *(See Figure 2–5, page 34.)*

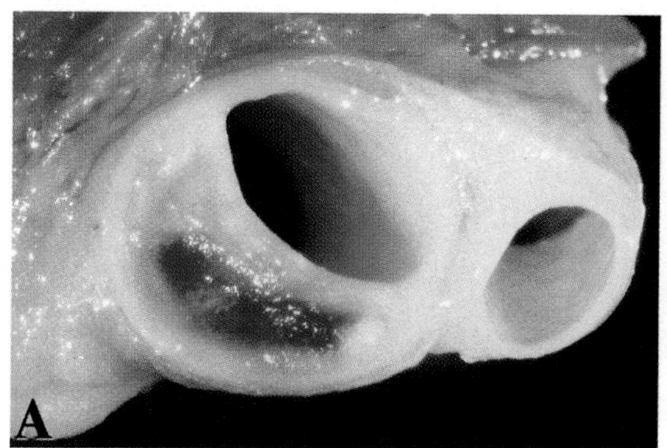

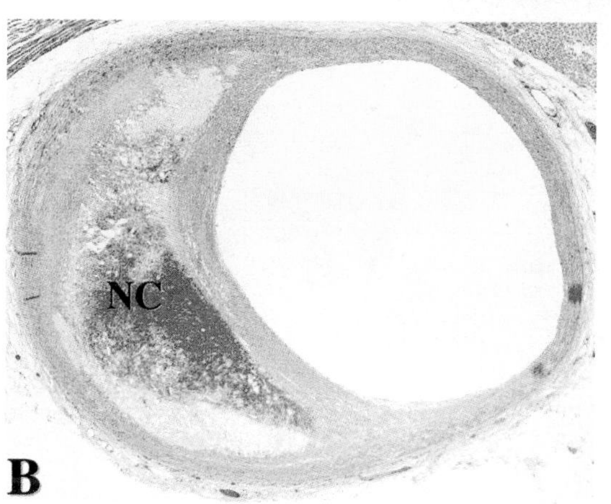

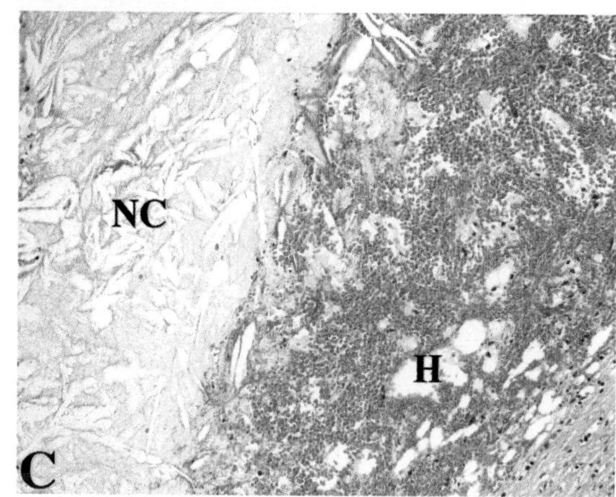

Color Plate 5. *(See Figure 2–6, page 35.)*

Fibrous cap atheroma with hemorrhage

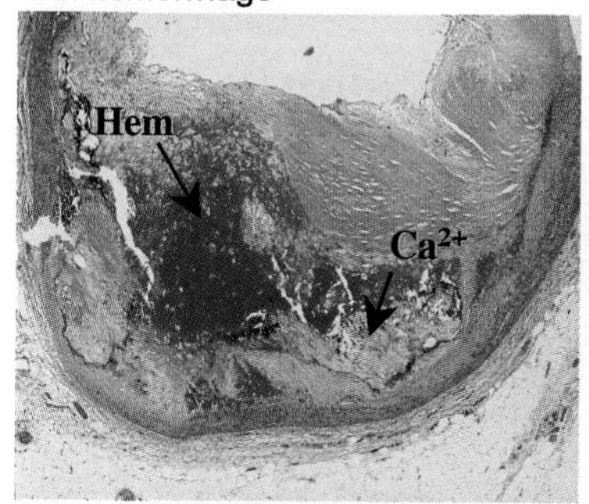

Thin fibrous cap atheroma

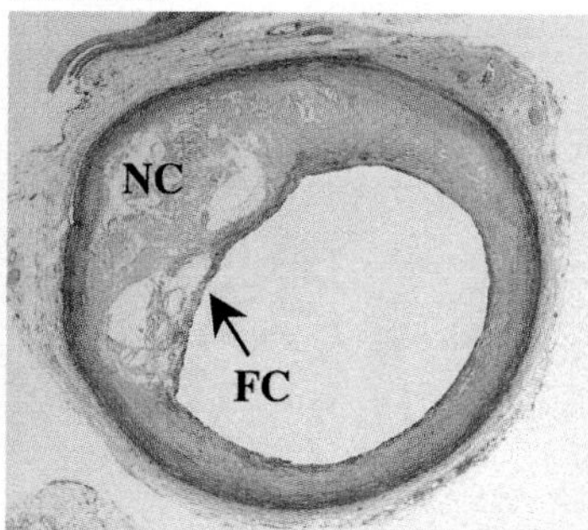

Fibrocalcific plaque

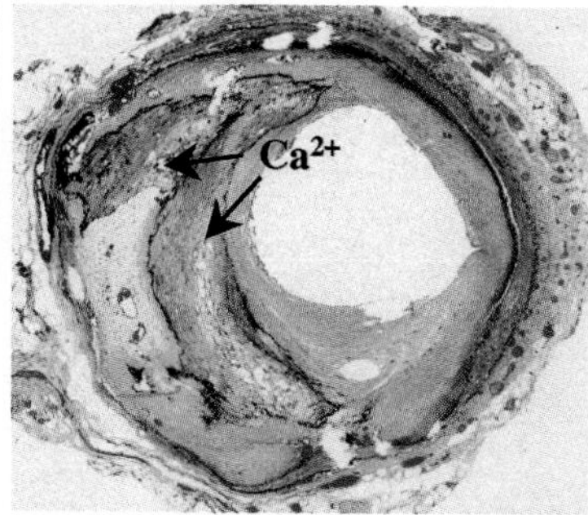

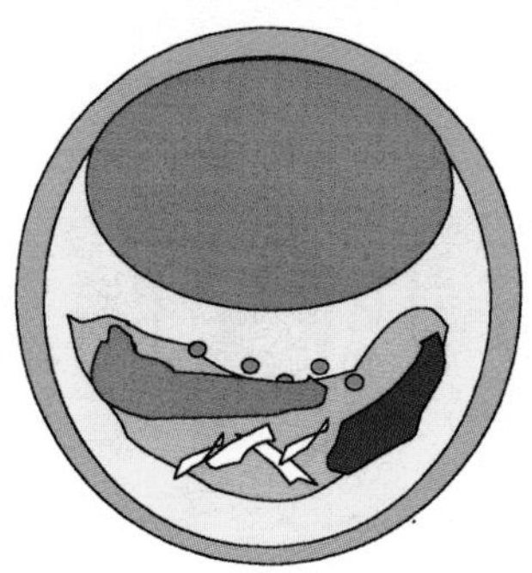

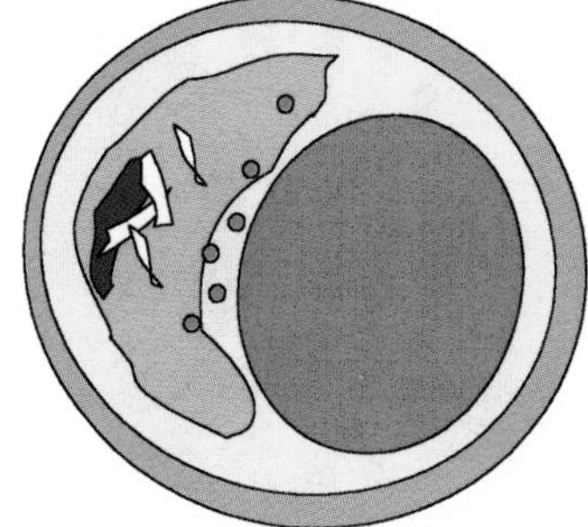

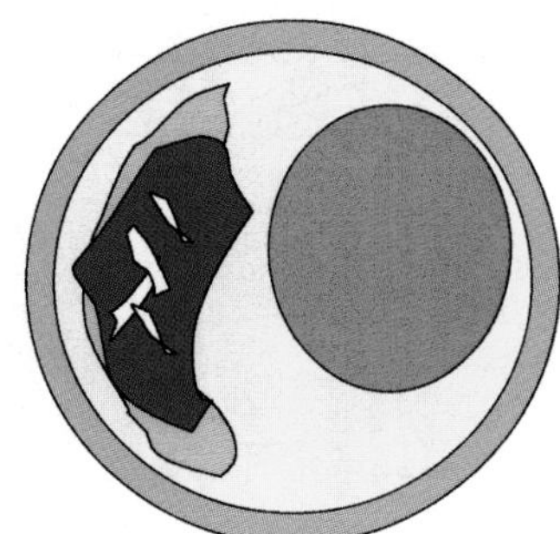

Color Plate 6. *(See Figure 2–7, page 36.)*

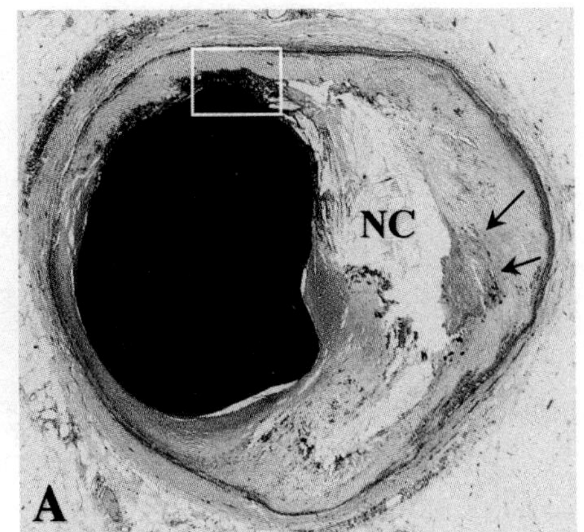

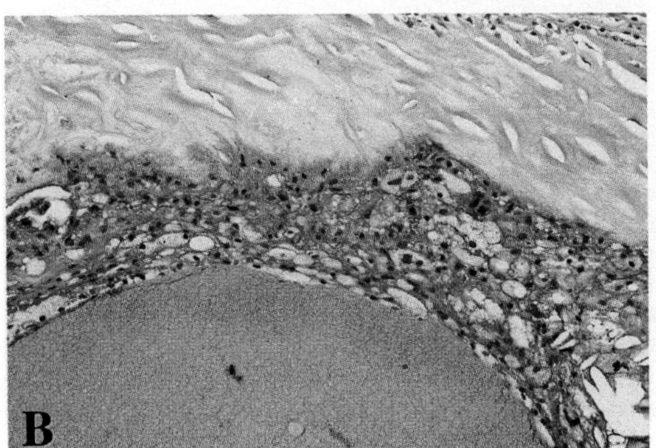

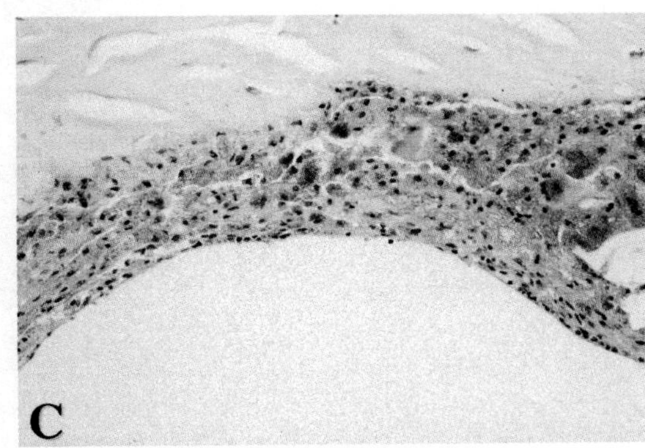

Color Plate 7. *(See Figure 2–8, page 37.)*

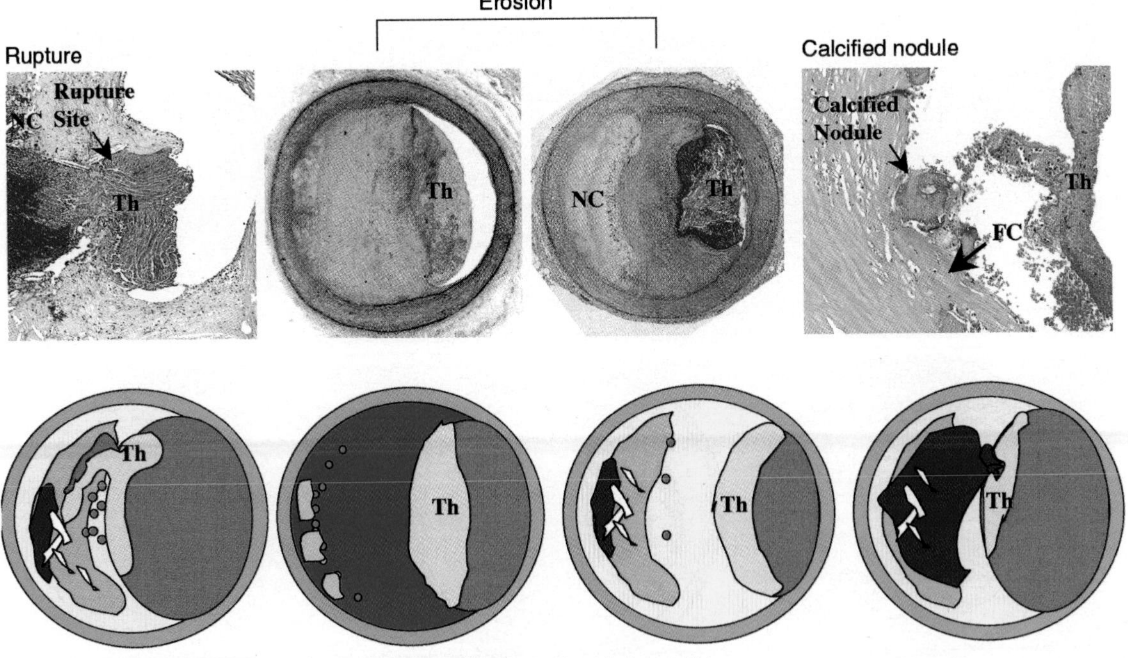

Color Plate 8. *(See Figure 2–9, page 38.)*

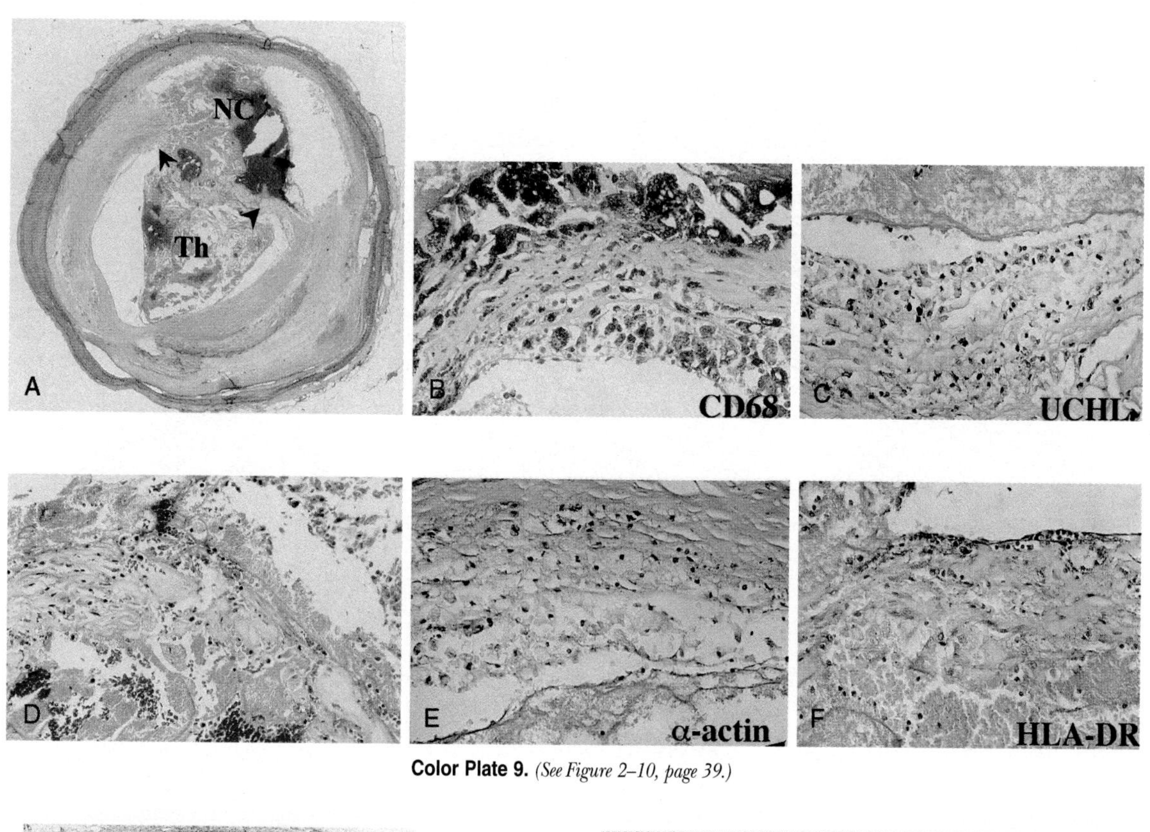

Color Plate 9. *(See Figure 2–10, page 39.)*

Color Plate 10. *(See Figure 2–11, page 40.)*

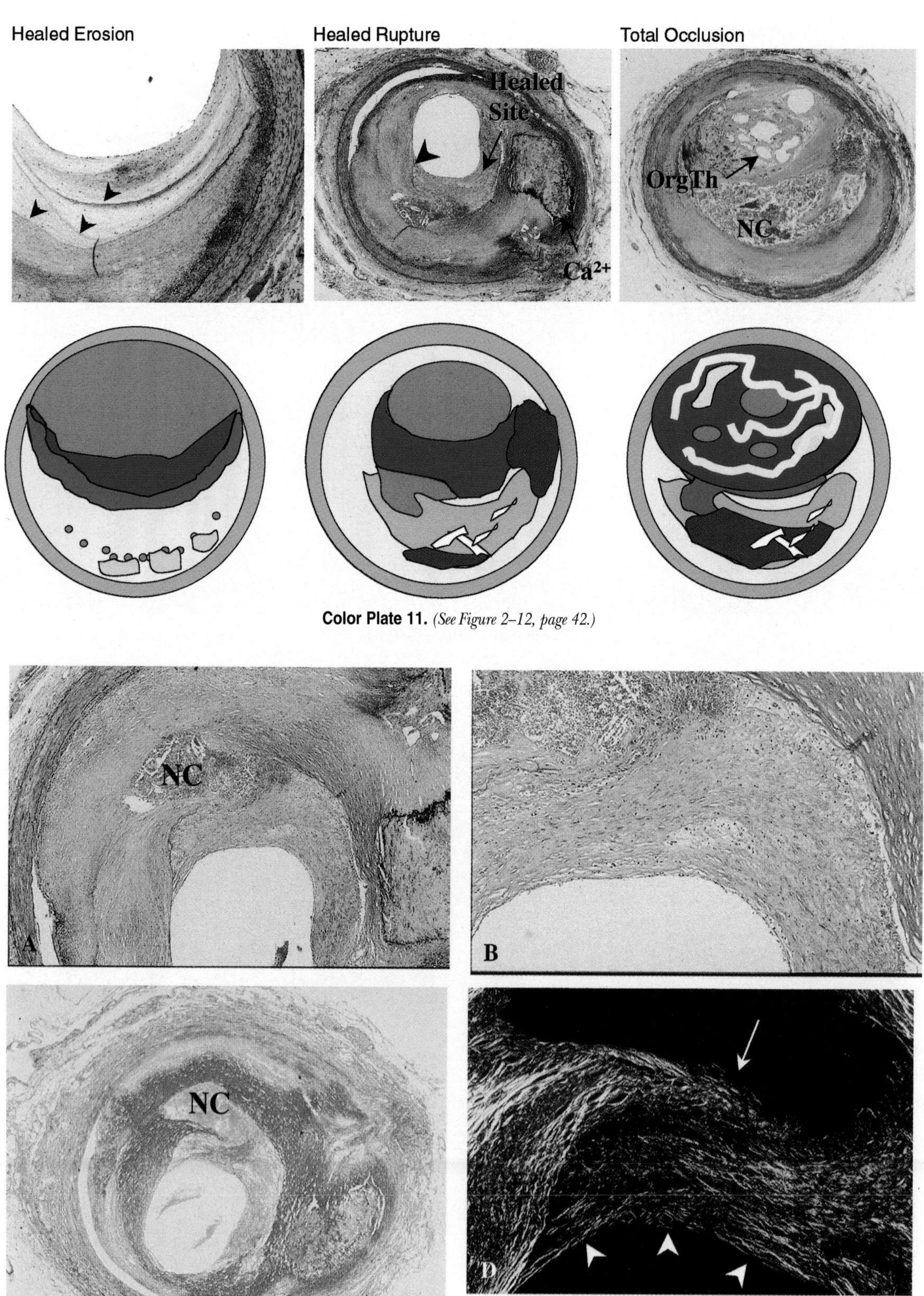

Color Plate 11. *(See Figure 2–12, page 42.)*

Color Plate 12. *(See Figure 2–13, page 43.)*

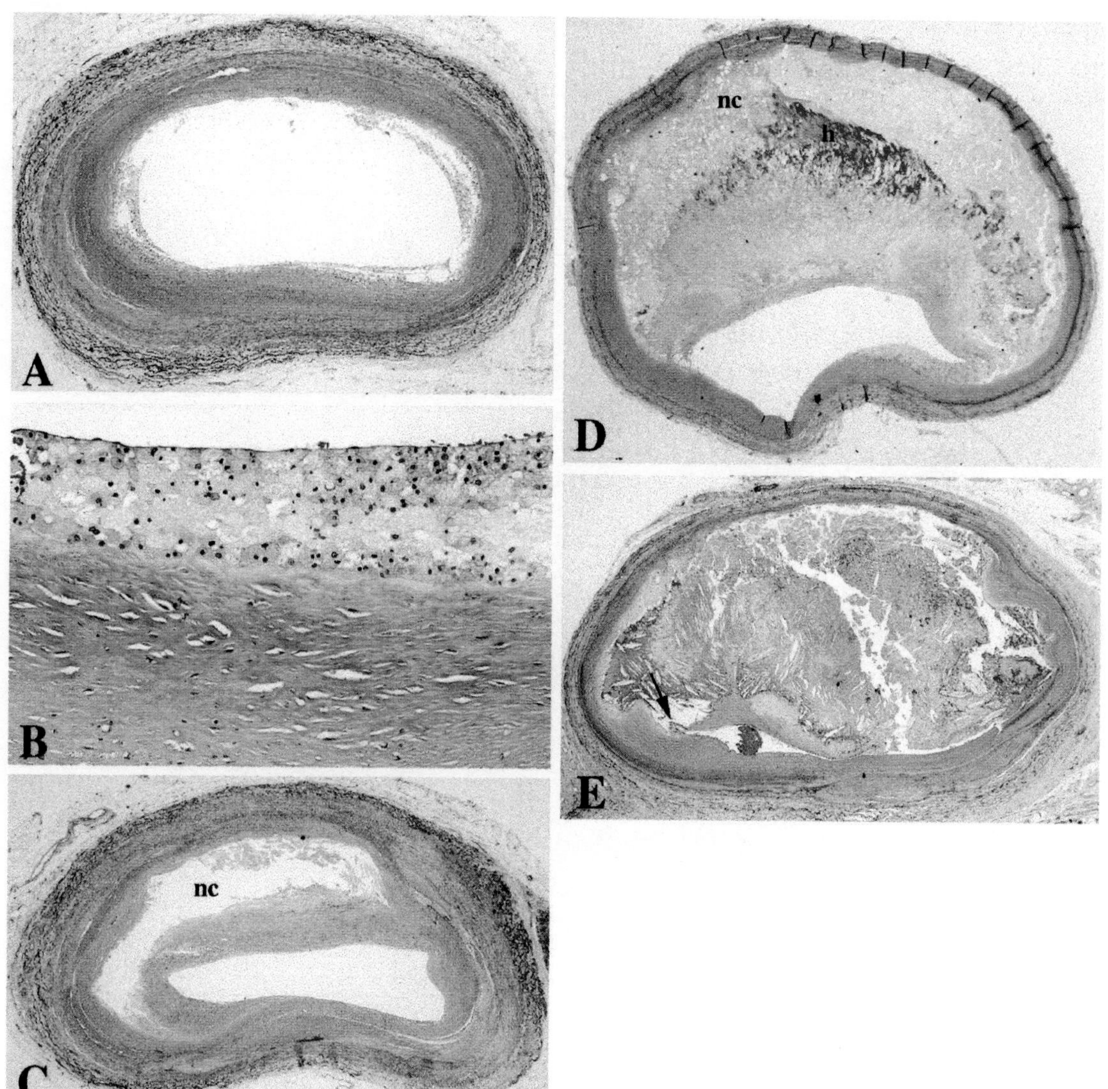

Color Plate 13. *(See Figure 3–7, page 63.)*

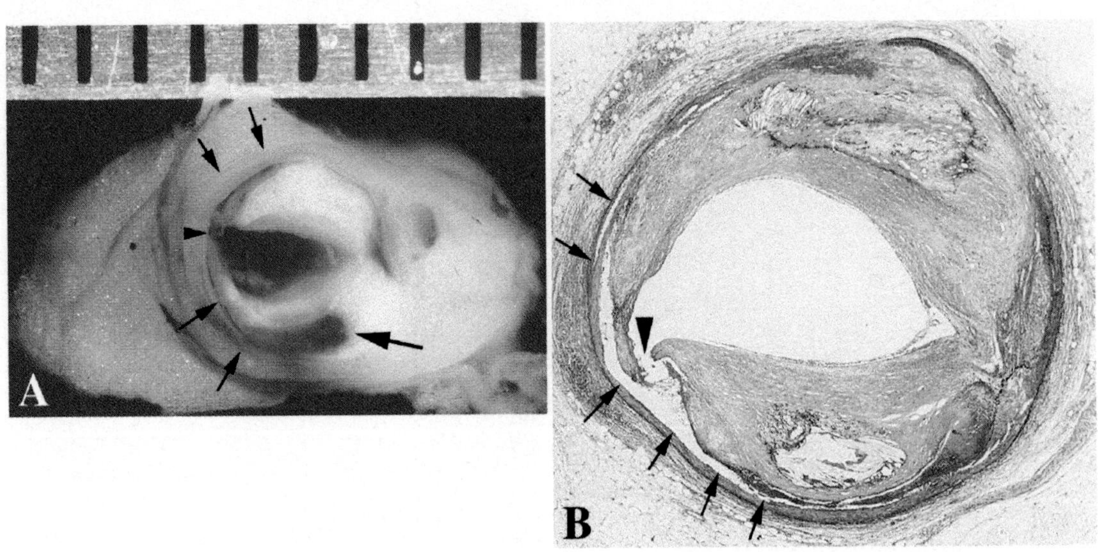

Color Plate 14. *(See Figure 3–10, page 67.)*

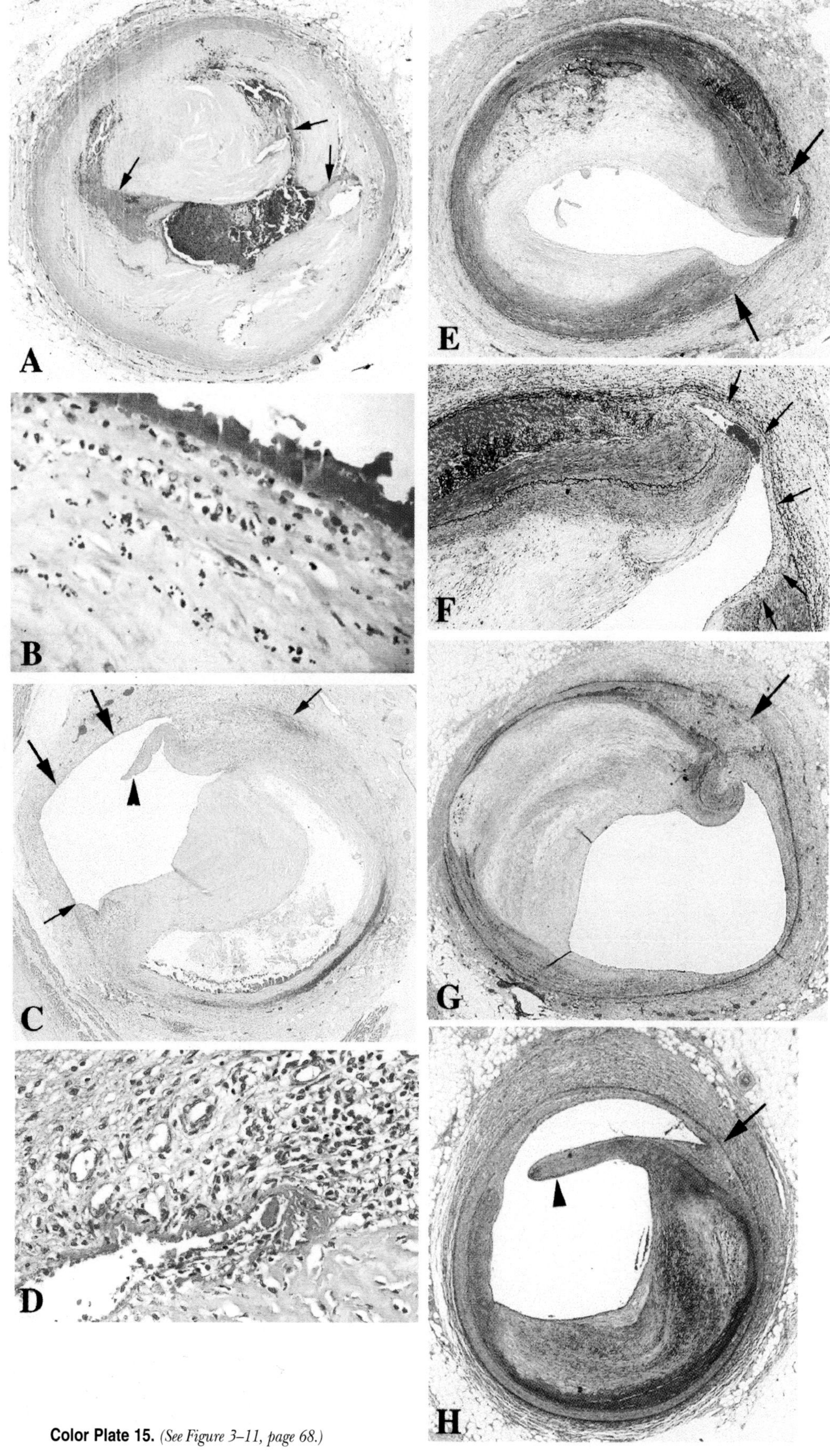

Color Plate 15. *(See Figure 3–11, page 68.)*

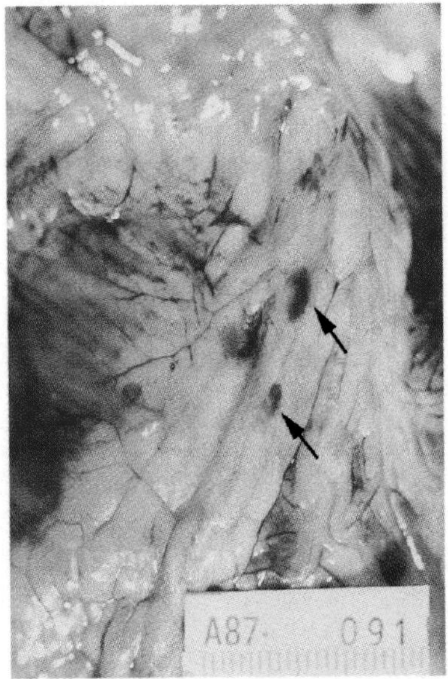

Color Plate 16. *(See Figure 3–13, page 73.)*

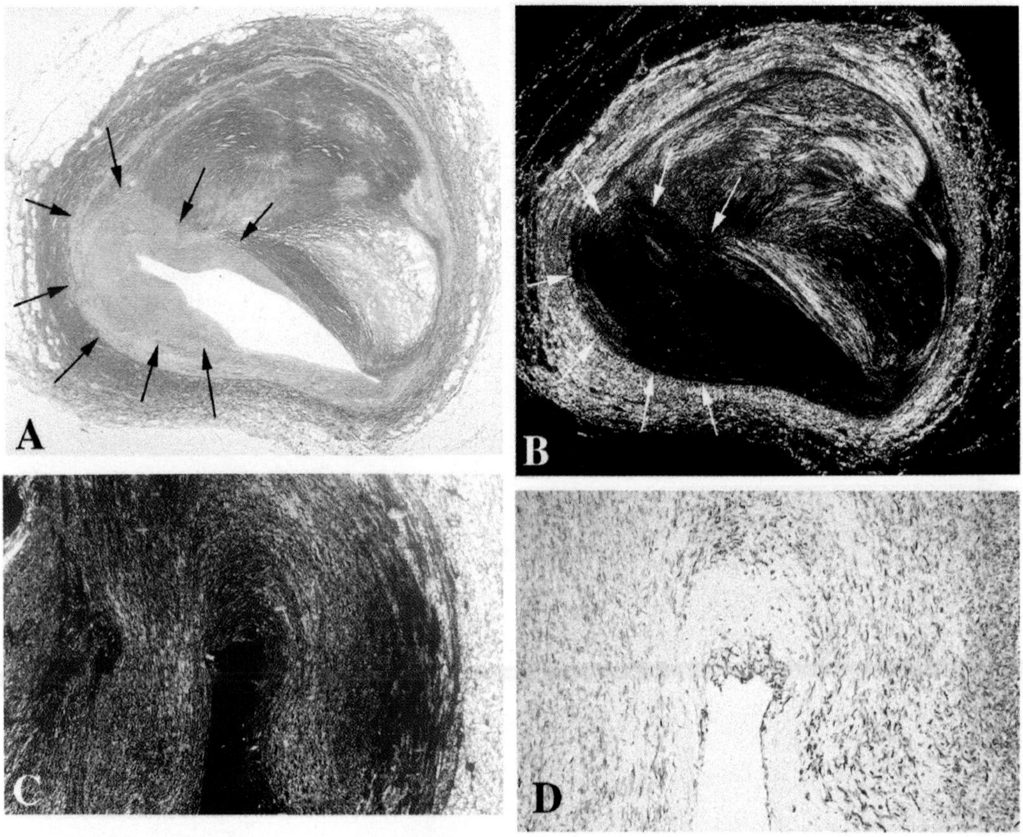

Color Plate 17. *(See Figure 3–14, page 74.)*

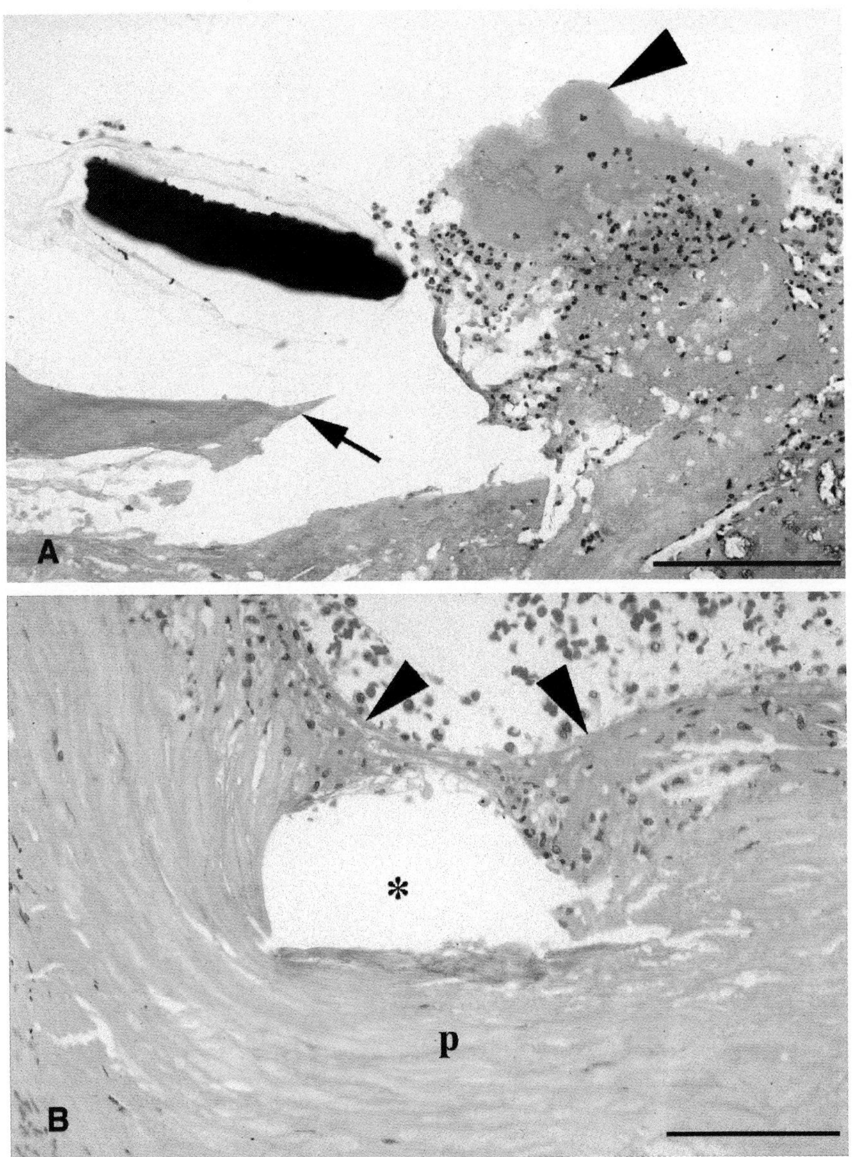

Color Plate 18. *(See Figure 3–18, page 81.)*

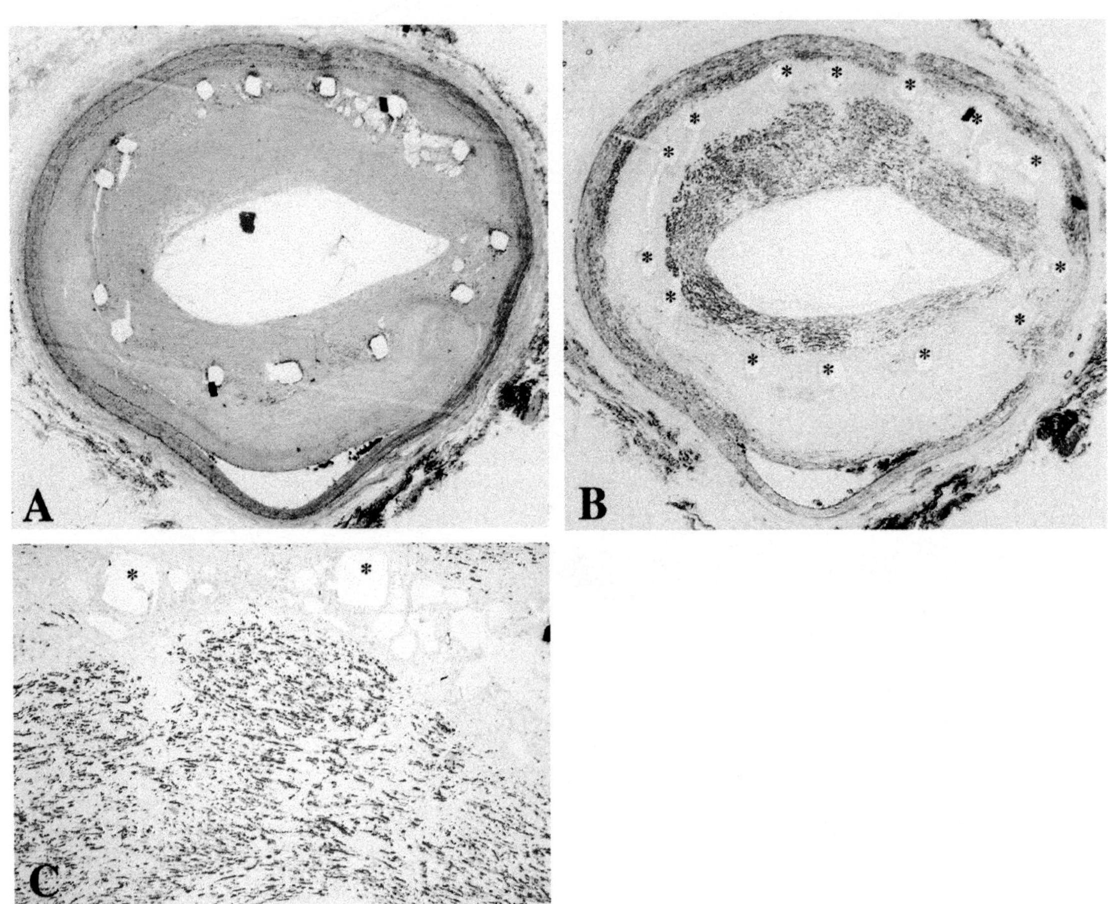

Color Plate 19. *(See Figure 3–21, page 83.)*

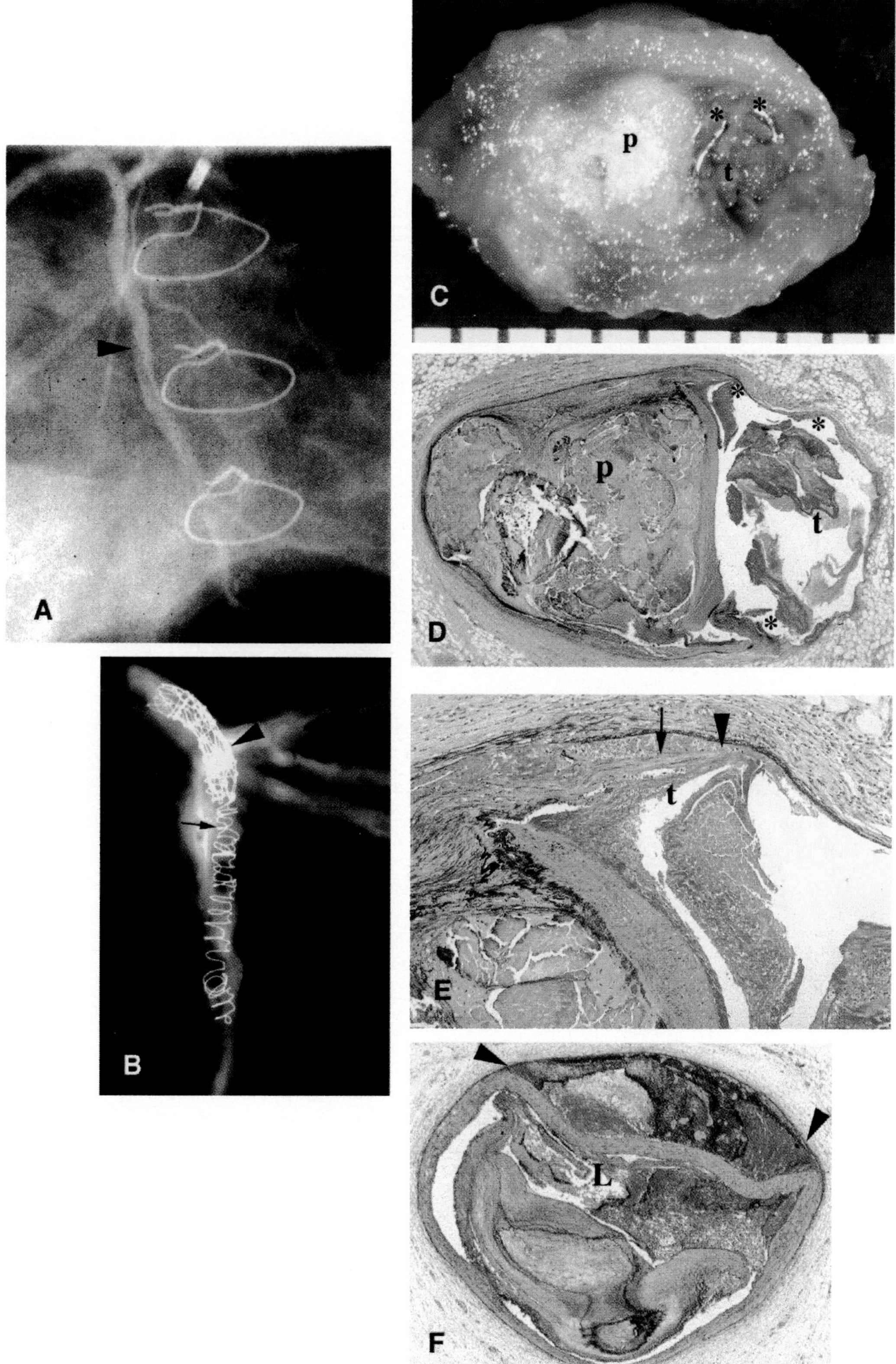

Color Plate 20. *(See Figure 3–24, page 86.)*

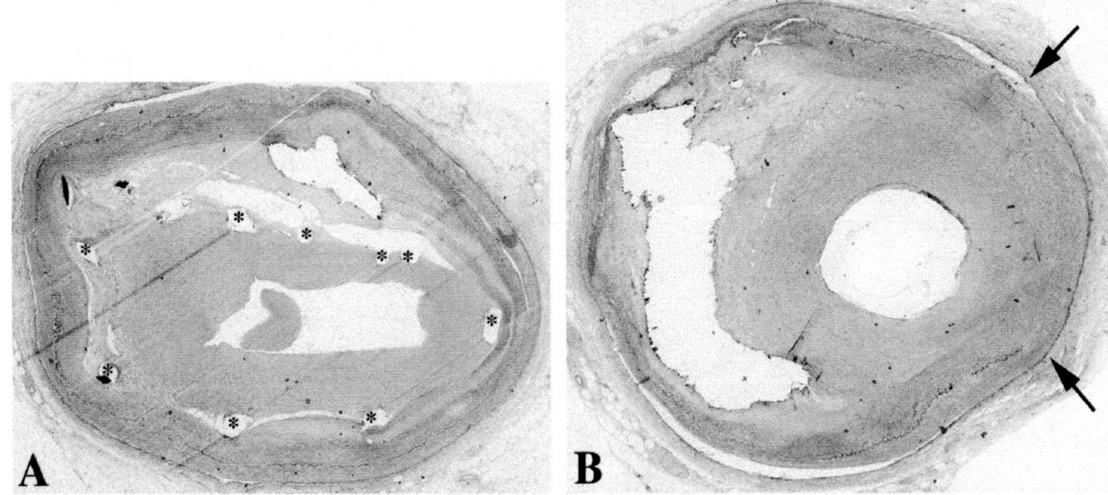

Color Plate 21. *(See Figure 3–27, page 90.)*

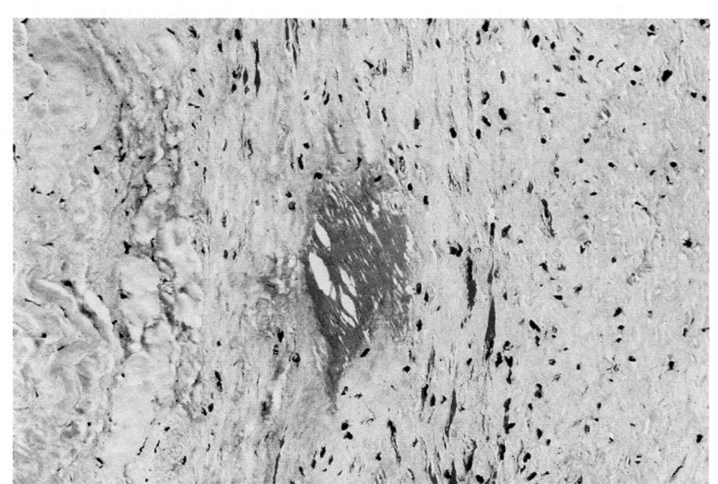

Color Plate 22. *(See Figure 4–9, page 117.)*

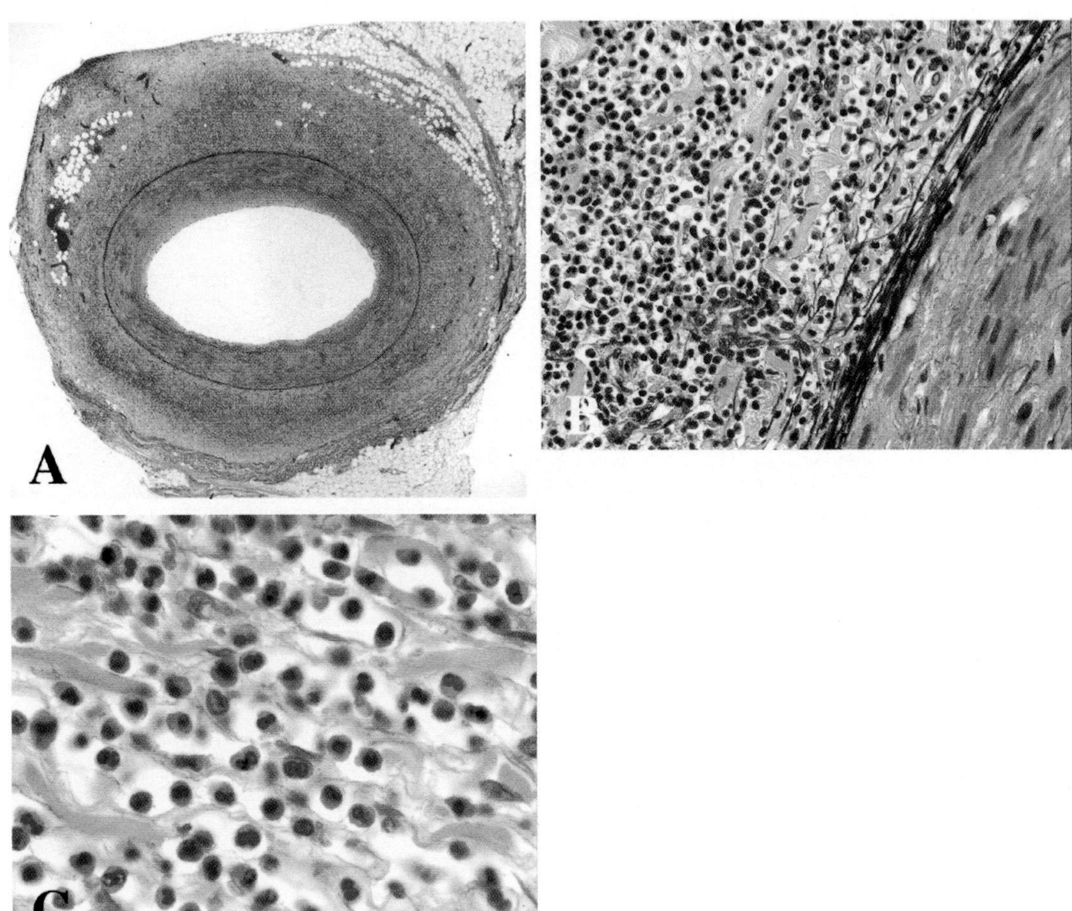

Color Plate 23. *(See Figure 4–22, page 134.)*

Chapter

1

EXAMINATION OF THE HEART

There is no single correct way of examining the heart at postmortem. Depending on the purpose of the autopsy examination, the available clinical history, and the likely cause of death, a variety of methods are appropriate. The purpose of this chapter is to guide the practicing pathologist to achieve the following goals in the cardiac dissection:

1. Establish, suggest, or rule out a likely cardiac cause of death.
2. Allow for optimal dissection techniques for photographing specimens.
3. Allow for optimal clinico-pathologic correlations (prior history, imaging studies).
4. Preserve the specimen in case further studies or further examination is necessary, for medical or legal reasons.

An established method of examination of the heart is to open the four chambers according to the direction of the flow of blood.[1,2] Briefly, the right atrium is opened from the inferior vena cavae to the tip of the atrial appendage; the right ventricle is opened along its lateral border through the tricuspid valve and annulus to the apex of the right ventricle with extension to the pulmonary outflow tract close to the ventricular septum. The left atrium is opened by cutting across the roof of the atrium between the left and right pulmonary veins; and the left ventricle is opened laterally between the anterior and posterior papillary muscles to the apex and then cut along the anterior wall adjacent to the ventricular septum through the aortic outflow tract. The classic method is a logical approach for congenital heart disease, in which preservation of the landmarks is useful. However, it is not optimal for evaluation of myocardial infarction, acute or healed, and for infiltrative diseases and cardiomyopathies. The flow-of-blood method does not readily allow for the assessment of ventricular cavity diameter and ventricular septal thickness, does not allow much visualization of the right or left ventricular myocardium, and misses pathologic changes not in the line of cutting of the myocardium.

TECHNIQUES FOR EXAMINATION OF THE HEART

Removal of the Heart

The examination of the adult heart begins after the anterior chest plate has been removed. A longitudinal cut through the anterior aspect of the pericardial sac is made. The amount of pericardial fluid is measured, and its character is noted. The surface of the visceral as well as parietal pericardium is also examined for exudates, adhesions, tumor nodules, or other lesions. A short longitudinal incision 2 cm above the pulmonary valve will enable a check for thromboemboli in the main pulmonary trunk *in situ*. The heart is removed by cutting the inferior vena cava just above the diaphragm and lifting the heart by the apex, reflecting it anteriorly and cephalad to facilitate exposure of the pulmonary veins at their pericardial re-

The opinions or assertions contained herein are the private views of the authors and are not to be construed as official or as reflecting the views of the Department of the Army or Navy or the Department of Defense.

flection. After it is confirmed that the pulmonary veins enter normally into the left atrium, the pulmonary veins are cut. The aorta and the pulmonary trunk, the last remaining connections, are cut transversely 2 cm above the semilunar valves. Following removal of the heart from the pericardial cavity and before weighing the specimen, postmortem blood clots should be removed manually and gently by flushing the heart with water from the left and right atria.

Examination of Native Coronary Arteries

A standardized and meticulous examination of the coronary arteries is especially important because there is a high likelihood of abnormalities and the majority of unexpected sudden deaths in adults will be caused by coronary disease. In the authors' experience in consultation, missed causes of sudden death are most commonly due to overlooking coronary lesions, either at the origin of the vessels or in their epicardial course.

In cases of suspected coronary disease, or in cases of sudden death in adults over 25 years of age, the ideal method of examining the coronary arteries is to first flush the coronary arteries with phosphate buffered saline, and then fusion fix the heart. The purpose of this procedure is threefold: to remove postmortem thrombi in the coronary circulation, to fix the sample adequately and quickly, and to fix the coronary arteries such that their histologic diameters and percent stenosis (if present) approximate *in vivo* dimensions. Injecting the coronary arteries with a barium-gelatin mixture after perfusion fixation and studying the vessels with radiographs is a tool to further characterize areas of narrowing and to determine patency of bypass grafts, but is time consuming and not essential for all cases of sudden death.[3, 4]

For coronary examination, the heart is perfusion fixed with 10% buffered formaldehyde retrograde from the ascending aorta at 100 mm Hg pressure (Fig. 1–1) for at least 30 minutes. A specially constructed Lucite plug or a rubber stopper with a central tubing is inserted into the aorta, taking care that the Lucite/rubber

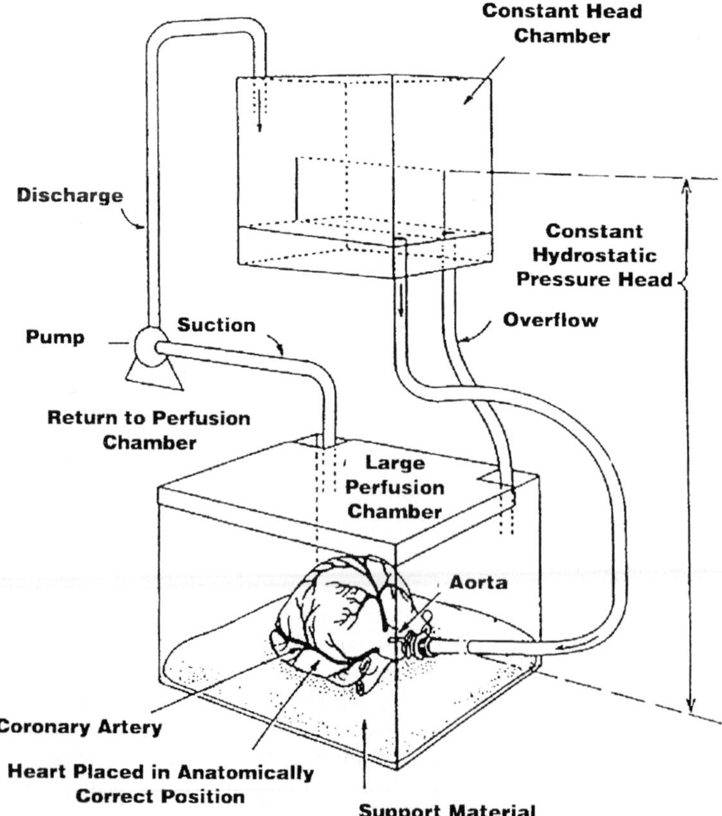

Figure 1–1. Diagram showing the method used for perfusion fixation of the heart. The constant head chamber is placed 135 cm above the perfusion chamber, and is connected via polyethylene tubing to the ascending aorta through the Lucite plug. The excess formaldehyde is suctioned back into the constant head chamber via a pump. Both chambers are covered in order to reduce formalin vapors. (Courtesy of Drs. J. Frederick Cornhill, D. Phil.)

plug does not touch the aortic valve. The Lucite plug is attached to tubing that is connected to the perfusion chamber.[5] The latter is placed 135 cm above the specimen, and this provides gravity perfusion pressure that is equivalent to 100 mm Hg. As a result, the coronary arteries are fixed in a distended state that approximate the dimensions observed in living patients. Myocardial fixation is also affected, but cardiac chambers are not fixed in a distended state, provided that the aortic valve is competent. If perfusion fixation is impractical, the heart should be fixed for 24 hours in 10% buffered formaldehyde before cutting, and postmortem clots within the atria and ventricles removed; for the latter, a section through the apex of the left ventricle may be necessary.

In cases of known or suspected coronary disease, radiography of the heart is recommended prior to sectioning. Postmortem radiographs aid in determining the extent of coronary calcification (heavily calcified arteries need to be removed and decalcified prior to sectioning); will show valvular calcification (aortic stenosis, mitral annular calcification); and will demonstrate coronary stents. Transluminal deployment of metal stents after angioplasty is now a standard of care, and these devices are currently a common finding at postmortem.

The ideal method for examining the coronary arterial tree is to perform postmortem angiography followed by X-ray of the heart in two different views. The coronary arteries are carefully dissected off the heart and X-rayed. If the arteries are heavily calcified, they are decalcified and then cut at 3- to 4-mm intervals and embedding in paraffin for histologic examination. Sections must be submitted from each of the arteries selecting the site of severest narrowing and/or the arteries with the thrombus. It is essential to state where the sections were taken, i.e., proximal, mid, or distal regions of the coronary arteries. Postmortem angiography may be performed either using barium-gelatin mixture or by polymer injection (MV-122; Canton Biomedical Products, Boulder, Colorado).

For the barium-gelatin mixture, we use polyethylene tubing (Clay Adams, Intramedic, PE 190 to 240, usually PE 205), the tip of which may be flared in a flame, to cannulate each ostium. The tubes are secured by a ligature at the origin of the coronary arteries, as close to the aorta as possible. The free end of each tube is attached to a hypodermic needle (usually 16 gauge) on the barrel of a disposable syringe (usually 30 mL). The pressure of injection is gradually increased to 100 to 120 mm Hg and maintained for 10 to 15 minutes. Following injection the cannulas are pulled out and the ligatures are tightened and knotted quickly. The heart is then fixed overnight in 10% buffered formaldehyde with attention paid to maintaining three-dimensional relationship. The quantity of formaldehyde should be ten times the volume of the heart in order for fixation to be optimal. The disadvantage to this method is that neither the ostium nor the left main coronary artery can be assessed. After washing the fixed specimen in water, radiographs are made in anteroposterior as well as left and right anterior oblique positions (Fig. 1–2). If the oblique positions are difficult to obtain, adequate information can be obtained with a superior view, that is, cephalad to caudal after the ventricles have been transversely sliced in a "bread loaf" manner.

The vessels that must be examined in all hearts include the four major epicardial coronary arteries: the left main, the left anterior descending, the left circumflex, and the right coronary arteries. In addition, it is not unusual to see severe luminal narrowing in smaller branches of the main coronary arteries; left diagonals, left obtuse marginal, ramus (intermediate) branch, and the posterior descending coronary arteries (Fig. 1–3). Following fixation and/or decalcification, the coronary arteries are cut transversely at 3 to 4 mm intervals with a sharp scalpel blade by a gentle sawing motion (not by firm pressure) to confirm sites of narrowing and to evaluate the pathologic process (e.g., atherosclerotic plaques, thrombi, dissections) directly.

If the coronary arteries are heavily calcified, it is desirable to remove the coronary arteries intact. Following dissection of the vessel from the epicardial surface, each coronary artery is carefully trimmed of excess fat and the intact arterial tree is placed in a container of formic acid if rapid decal over 12 to 18 hours is desired or in EDTA for slow decalcification. Decalcification of isolated segments of vessel may be sufficient for cases in which the coronary arteries are only focally calcified.

The areas of maximal narrowing are noted by specifying the degrees of reduction of the cross-sectional area of the lumen by visual inspection and further confirmed by histology (others prefer to divide the degree of narrowing into the following groups: 0–25%, 26–50%, 51–75%, 76–90%, 91–99%, and 100%). Most cardiologists agree that, in the absence of other car-

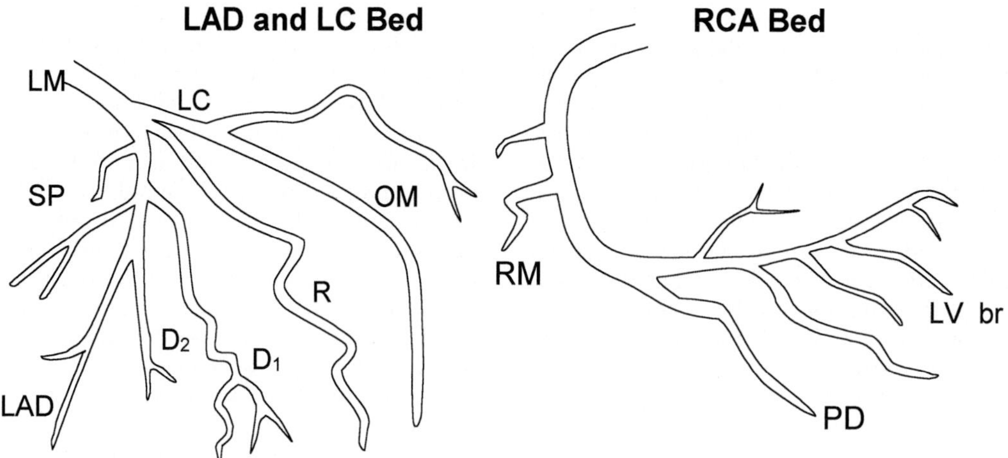

Figure 1–2. Diagram of the right and left epicardial coronary arteries as they arise from the aorta (right dominance). The four major arteries that must be described in detail are right (*RCA*), left main (*LM*), left anterior descending coronary (*LAD*), and the left circumflex (*LC*) coronary arteries. Not uncommonly, severe coronary (> 75% cross-sectional area luminal narrowing) artery disease may effect the smaller branches (*R* = Ramus intermediate, D_1 and D_2 = diagonals of LAD, *OM* = left obtuse marginal, *PD* = posterior descending artery, and *RM* = right marginal). The proximal LAD extends from the origin of LAD to the D_1, the mid LAD extends from 1 diagonal to 2.5 cm distally, and the remainder of the LAD is distal. The left circumflex is divided into proximal, region proximal to LOM, and the continuation of the LC is the distal segment. The right proximal is the first 2 cm of the artery, the mid extends up to the RM, and the distal extends up to the PDA. Occasionally, the right coronary can extend beyond the PD (so-called ''hyperdominant'' right) and provide left ventricular branches (*LV br*).

diac disease, significant or severe coronary artery narrowing is one that exceeds 75% cross-sectional luminal narrowing (equivalent to 50% diameter reduction). In a normal dog, it has been documented that resting blood flow is not compromised until arterial constriction reaches 80% of the diameter. However, maximal coronary blood flow begins to decrease when % diameter stenosis reaches 50%.[6,7] Blood flow is also dependent on the length of narrowing and the distensibility of the artery.

When reporting on the extent of coronary disease, particular attention should be paid to the left main coronary artery because disease in this vessel is very important clinically but frequently overlooked at autopsy.[8] Other sites frequently overlooked include the proximal left circumflex, which courses deep to the left atrial appendage, the obtuse marginal branch of the left circumflex, diagonal branches of the left anterior descending, and the distal right and posterior descending arteries. Cross sections from areas of maximal narrowing from each of the four major epicardial coronary arteries or their branches are selected for histologic examination. Sections of all coronary arteries containing thrombi are taken to aid in determining the type of underlying plaque morphology, i.e., plaque rupture or plaque erosion (ulceration) or calcified nodule. The site of maximal narrowing must be specified, i.e., proximal, middle, or distal coronary. Documenting the location of the severe narrowing may have medico-legal ramifications, as patients with severe distal disease, for example, may not have been good candidates for coronary artery bypass grafts if they had severe coronary disease that involved the distal coronary vessels. The final autopsy report must state the following:

1. Are the ostia of both the arteries and their location normal? (Both ectopic origin as well as high take-off above the sinotubular junction should be mentioned.)
2. Which is the dominant artery (the artery that supplies the posterior descending coronary artery)?
3. Is there severe (> 75% cross-sectional luminal narrowing) coronary artery disease present or absent?

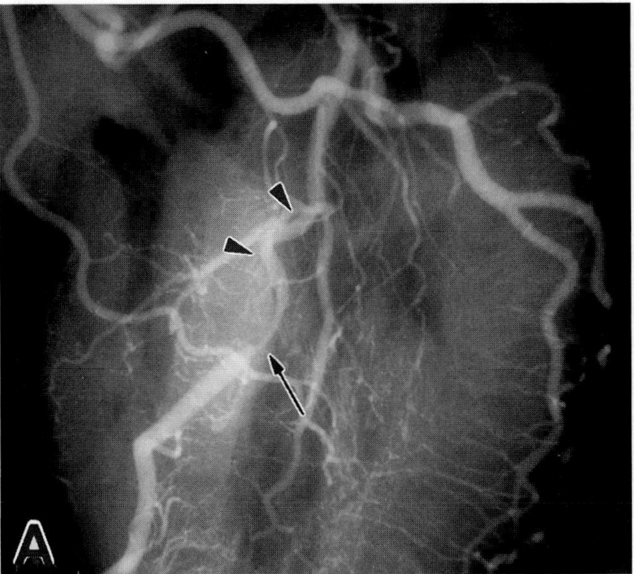

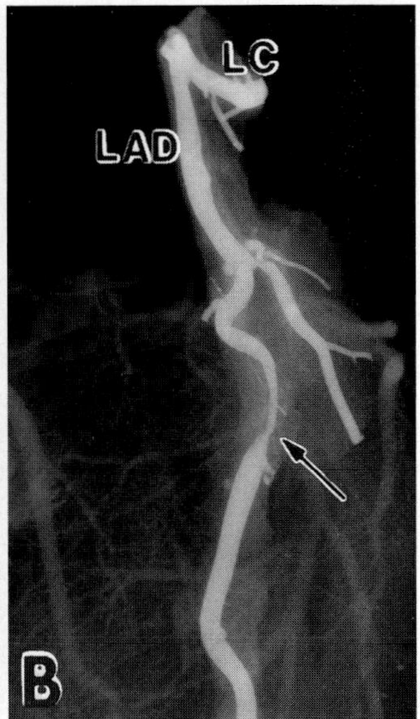

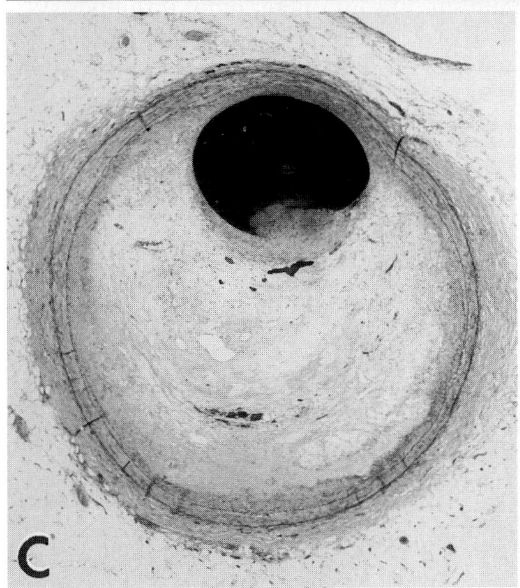

Figure 1–3. *A* shows a radiograph of the heart following injection of barium-gelatin dye into the coronary arteries. Note the left coronary artery (left anterior descending) is shown by the arrowhead and the area of severe narrowing (80% diameter reduction) is shown by the arrow. *B* shows the origin of the LAD and the left circumflex (*LC*) and the area of severe narrowing is easier to see at higher magnification and the angiography is helpful in sampling the appropriate area of narrowing. *C.* The coronary artery was sampled at the site of severe narrowing and shows presence of a thrombus (*arrowhead*) in the lumen which is filled with barium-gelatin mixture. The underlying plaque is eroded at the site of the thrombus.

4. If coronary artery disease is severe, state the extent of disease in left main coronary artery, left anterior descending (proximal, middle, or distal), left circumflex (proximal or distal), and right coronary artery (proximal, middle, or distal).
5. Are the main branches (left diagonals, left obtuse marginal, posterior descending) involved?

Examination of Bypass Grafts

When removing the heart at autopsy, care must be taken to avoid injury to the saphenous vein bypass grafts. A longer segment of the ascending aorta is left in continuity with the heart to enable examination of vein grafts from aortic orifice to distal anastomosis. Twists, as well as excessive tautness between aorta and distal anastomosis, are noted.[9] In cases of bypass grafts, it is certainly recommended to perfusion fix the specimen with formaldehyde from the aortic stump, taking care that the graft orifices are below the Lucite plug and the internal mammary artery is ligated near the site of severance from the chest wall. In cases where it is not possible to perfusion fix the heart, the heart may be immersion fixed in 10% buffered formaldehyde overnight and dissection of the grafts and native vessels is carried out the next morning. If possible, the full extent of the saphenous vein grafts is best visualized by barium-gelatin mixture followed by radiography.[3,4] It is best to inject all the vein grafts simultaneously and to obtain radiographs before injection of the coronary arteries. This enables more detailed study of the native coronary arteries distal to the graft as well as at the coronary graft anastomosis. Measurements of lumen diameters may be made from the radiographs. In those cases in which the internal mammary artery is anastomosed to the coronary system, the internal mammary artery is injected from where it has been severed during removal of the heart. The native coronary arteries are injected, fixed, and radiographed to evaluate the extent of disease in the remainder of the coronary arterial tree. The grafts and native arteries may then be removed from the heart, radiographed, and cut at 3- to 4-mm intervals to determine the extent of luminal narrowing, the presence or absence of thrombi, and/or the extent of atherosclerosis in vein grafts and coronary arteries.[10–13]

In cases of routine fixation, it is useful to radiograph and decalcify the arteries and grafts prior to sectioning, as calcification is common (Fig. 1–4). When there are no lesions identifiable grossly, random sections of the entire length of the grafts should be taken. Anastomotic sites are sectioned in different ways depending on whether the connection is end to end or end to side (Fig. 1–5); in general, the native artery should be cross-sectioned through the anastomotic site. The final autopsy report should contain the following information regarding bypass grafts:

1. Aortic ostium (location, patency) (saphenous vein bypass grafts only)
2. Graft course and length, jump graft and site if present, distal anastomotic site, areas of luminal narrowing and length (diffuse, focal disease), atherosclerosis, intimal thickening, aneurysm, fibrous obliteration, thrombosis
3. Distal anastomosis patency, amount of plaque or fibrointimal growth in native artery and in the vein, thrombosis (especially in cases of recent surgery)

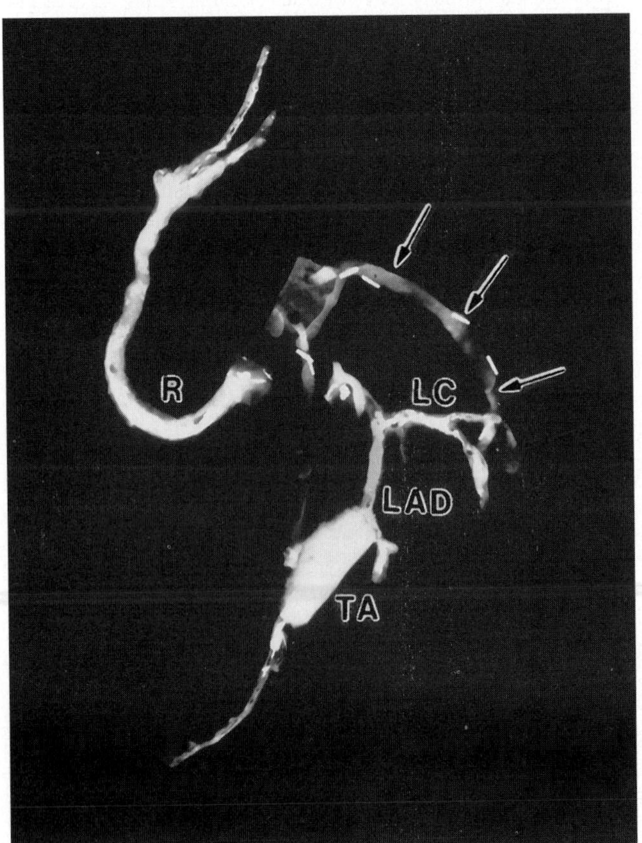

Figure 1–4. Radiograph of epicardial coronary arteries and saphenous vein bypass graft (*arrows*) to left circumflex (*LC*) removed at autopsy. Note focal calcification of the native arteries and absence of calcification of the vein graft. A portion of the left anterior coronary artery is surrounded by myocardium (bridged or tunneled coronary artery). Arteries are decalcified prior to sectioning and embedding in paraffin.

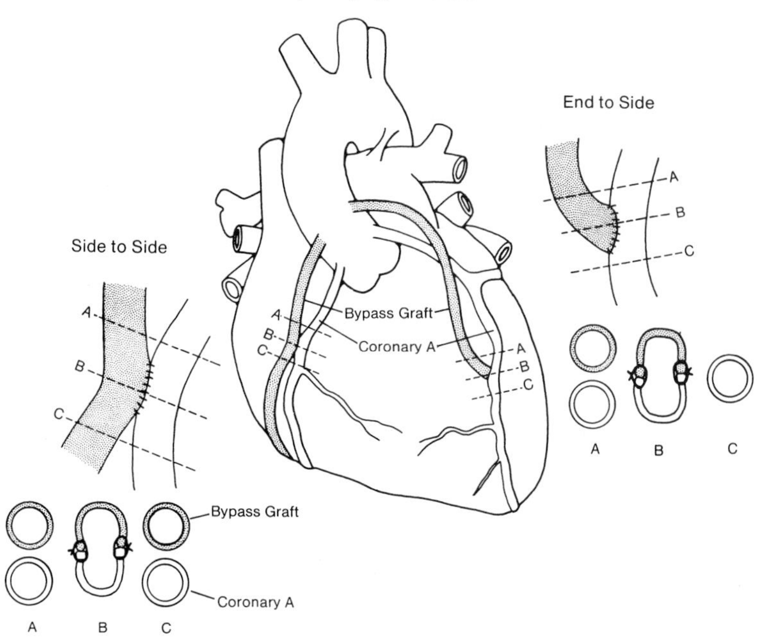

Figure 1–5. Diagram illustrating coronary artery bypass grafts that have end-to-side and side-to-side anastomoses in two separate grafts (*shaded area*) to left anterior descending and right coronary arteries, respectively. The figure illustrates the method used for sectioning of anastomotic site with end-to-side and side-to-side anastomoses to demonstrate if any of the three mechanisms for obstruction in the anastomotic site are present (i.e., compression or loss of arterial lumen, which may occur if the majority of the arterial wall has been used for anastomosis; thrombosis at the site of anastomosis; and dissection of the native coronary-artery at the site of anastomosis) and if the coronary artery has severe narrowing at the site of anastomosis due to severe atherosclerotic change. (Modified from Bulkley BH, Hutchins GM. Pathology of coronary artery bypass graft surgery. Arch Pathol 102:273, 1978, with permission.)

4. Run-off vessel (size; ≥ 1 mm is generally adequate; remember nonperfusion fixed specimens will underestimate vascular lumen size); areas of luminal narrowing (degree, distance from anastomotic site)
5. Extent and length of narrowing in the native artery proximal to the anastomosis (If the graft is occluded, could another intervention have been carried out?)

General Examination of the Myocardium (Bread-loafing)

The most common errors made by the practicing pathologist in sectioning the myocardium include longitudinal sections of myocardium; diagonal sections; sections of the ventricular septum that are not cross sections; and attempts at maintaining the specimen in a single piece. The method of sectioning the myocardium described below (cross-sectional method that is comparable to methods of cutting other organs, such as the brain) provides the following essential features:

1. Allows for measurements of the left ventricular cavity dimension, thickness of the ventricles at anterior, lateral, posterior sites; and thickness of the septum at various levels (basal, mid-ventricle, apical)
2. Allows for characterization of myocardial infarcts, transmural or subendocardial (involves the inner 2/3 of the left ventricle), and the wall of the ventricle involved, i.e., anterior, lateral, septum or inferior.
3. Allows for determination of infiltrative diseases, e.g., sarcoid, abscesses, tumor metastasis, etc.
4. Allows for proper sectioning of the myocardium (myofiber disarray, for example, can only be evaluated on sections taken at cross sections to the flow of blood)
5. Allows for echocardiographic correlation (short axis view)
6. Allows for preservation of other cardiac structures (valves, conduction system area)
7. Preserves the specimen for further study and photography, if necessary

Other possible methods of cross sections, such as long-axis or four-chamber echocardiographic views, are also appropriate in some patients with cardiomyopathy and are used for some photographs in this book. However, the short-axis cross sections are excellent for any form of adult heart disease, are simpler to perform, and do allow for easiest measurement and sectioning for histology.

The myocardium is sliced in a manner similar to that of cutting a loaf of bread. A series of short-axis cuts are made through the ventricles from apex to base (Fig. 1–6). This method is best accomplished using a long, sharp knife on the intact fixed specimen following examination of the coronary arteries. With the anterior aspect of the heart downward (against the cutting board), the cuts are made parallel to the posterior atrioventricular sulcus at 1- to 1.5-cm intervals from the apex of the heart to a point approximately 2.5 cm caudal to the sulcus or up to the mid-portion of the papillary muscles of the left ventricle. The result is a series of cross sections through the ventricles, including papillary muscles with the atrioventricular valve apparatus left intact in the remainder of the base of the heart.

Examination of the Myocardium in Cases of Ischemic Heart Disease

After bread-loafing the heart, the location and extent of the infarct is noted. Locations may be stated similar to clinical designations, such as anteroseptal or posterolateral (or inferolateral). The extent of infarction may be described in terms of circumference of the ventricle involved[14–16] and longitudinal portion of the ventricle involved (e.g., basal third, middle third, apical third) (Fig. 1–6*A* and *B*). The distribution within the wall is also described

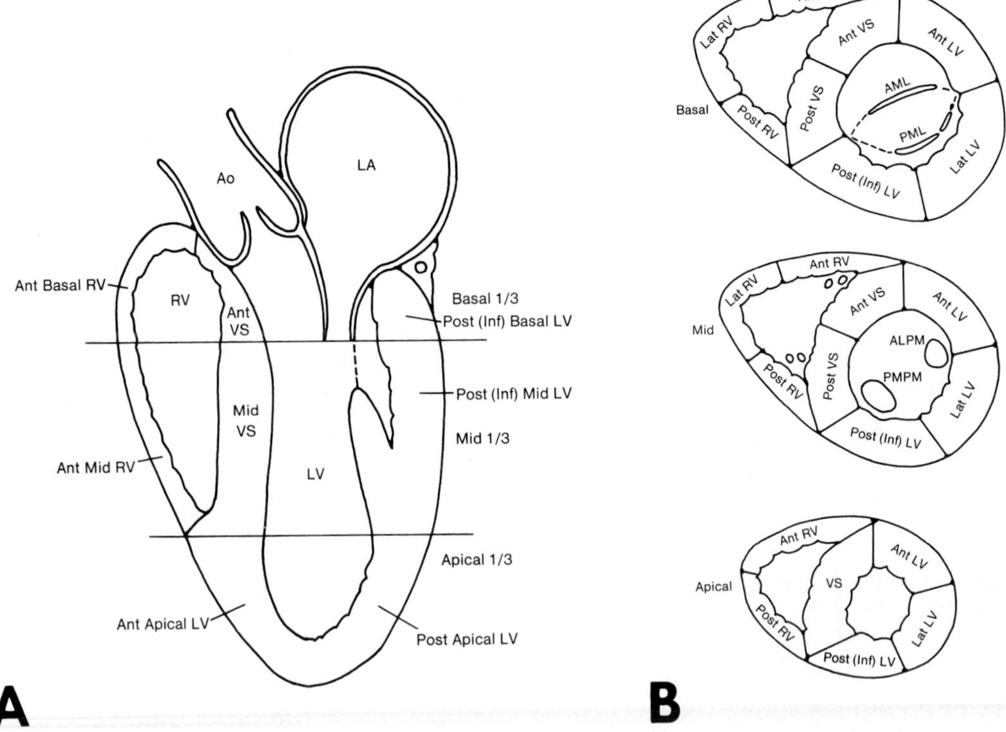

Figure 1–6. The location and extent of myocardial infarction must be indicated by the size, that is, how much of the base to apex is infarcted: basal one third, and/or middle one third, and/or apical one third or more than one third from base to apex. The diagram in *A* shows a long axis view of the heart with regional nomenclature. *B*. The location of the myocardial infarction in the left ventricle must also indicate the wall in which infarction occurred: anterior, posterior, lateral, septal, or any combination of these. This diagram illustrates a short-axis view through the basal, middle, and apical portions of the right and left ventricles. (*Ao*, aorta; *Ant*, anterior; *ALPM*, anterolateral papillary muscle; *AML*, anterior mitral leaflet; *Inf*, inferior, *LA*, left atrium; *LV*, left ventricle, *Mid*, middle; *PML*, posterior mitral leaflet; *PMPM*, posteromedial papillary muscle; *Post*, posterior, *RV*, right ventricle, *VS*, ventricular septum). (Modified from Edwards WD, Tajik AJ, Seward JB. Standardized nomenclature and anatomic basis for regional tomographic analysis of the heart. Mayo Clin Proc 56:479, 1981, with permission.)

(e.g., transmural or subendocardial; transmural when the infarct extends from the endocardium to the epicardium, and subendocardial when < 75% of the left ventricular wall is infarcted). The gross pathologic appearance of the myocardium serves as a relatively good index as to the age of the infarct but must be confirmed by histologic examination. Even if infarction cannot be identified grossly, it is important to section the myocardium in the distribution of the severely diseased coronary arteries more extensively. We normally submit five sections of the ventricle: one each from the anterior, lateral, and posterior wall of the left ventricle; septum (which may be two sections—the anterior half and the posterior half); and posterior wall of the right ventricle. Always take sections from the endocardium to the epicardium.

The essential points for description of the heart with an infarct are:

1. Location of the infarct (acute or healed) within the ventricles (anterior, anteroseptal, anterolateral, lateral, posterior, posterolateral, inferior, inferoseptal) (left and right ventricular walls [50% of inferior infarcts also have inferior right ventricular infarct], and rarely the atria may also be infarcted)
2. Transmural or subendocardial
3. Extent of the infarction base to apex, and circumferential involvement (% of the circumference of the left ventricle)

Examination of the Heart in Cardiomyopathy

The short-axis sectioning (bread loafing) method described above serves well for the examination of the cardiomyopathic heart. Cardiac hypertrophy and dilation may be demonstrated quite effectively by this method. If the left ventricular cavity measures > 4 cm, excluding the papillary muscles, it is considered that the patient was in congestive heart failure prior to death even if there is no history to corroborate the autopsy findings. In such cases, evidence of chronic congestion in the lungs (hemosiderin laden macrophages, and pulmonary edema) and liver should be sought. Left ventricular hypertrophy is said to be present if the left ventricular wall measures > 1.5 cm. On the other hand, if the left ventricular wall measures < 1.5 cm, the heart weight is increased, and the left ventricular cavity is enlarged, then there should be microscopic evidence of myocyte hypertrophy.

The heart may also be cut in four-chamber view by cutting the heart from the apex to base, along the acute margin of the right ventricle and the obtuse margin of the left ventricle and continuing the plane of section through the atria (Fig. 1–7). This four-chamber view is best for evaluating the atrial and ventricular chamber size. In cases of hypertrophic cardiomyopathy, the heart may be cut in the long-axis view of the left ventricular outflow tract, in order to demonstrate the left ventricular outflow tract obstruction present in over 50% of cases. For cutting the heart in the long-axis view, the plane of dissection of the aortic valve leaflet is through the right coronary and the posterior noncoronary leaflets, the anterior and the posterior mitral leaflets, the posterior and the anterior left atrial walls, ventricular septum, posterolateral wall of the left ventricle, and the anterior right ventricular wall (Fig. 1–8). If a heart with hypertrophic cardiomyopathy is cut in the long axis view, care must be taken to section the ventricular septum at cross sections.

Histologic examination of the myocardium is critical to determining the cause of the cardiomyopathy. In addition to sections of tissue with gross pathology, samples of the walls of all four cardiac chambers, the septum, and the papillary muscles should be taken. There are certain types of cardiomyopathy that warrant specific considerations for histologic sampling (see below). For this reason, and in order to document the absence of findings in unexpected sudden death in which the heart is not saved indefinitely, ample sampling of the right ventricle (specifically to rule out right ventricular dysplasia) and ventricular septum is warranted in all cases of sudden unexpected death without obvious cause.

Dilated Cardiomyopathy

The heart in dilated cardiomyopathy is traditionally examined by the four-chamber view, demonstrating the ventricular dilatation, which is usually greater than the atria. An equally acceptable method is the short axis (bread-loafing) method, which allows for measurement of the left ventricular cavity, and should be done at the level of the papillary muscles, excluding these from measurement. Occasional features include mural thrombi (especially in the atrial appendages), endocardial fibrosis, and ventricular scars. The diagnosis rests on histologic examination and exclusion of other cardiac causes of congestive failure (hy-

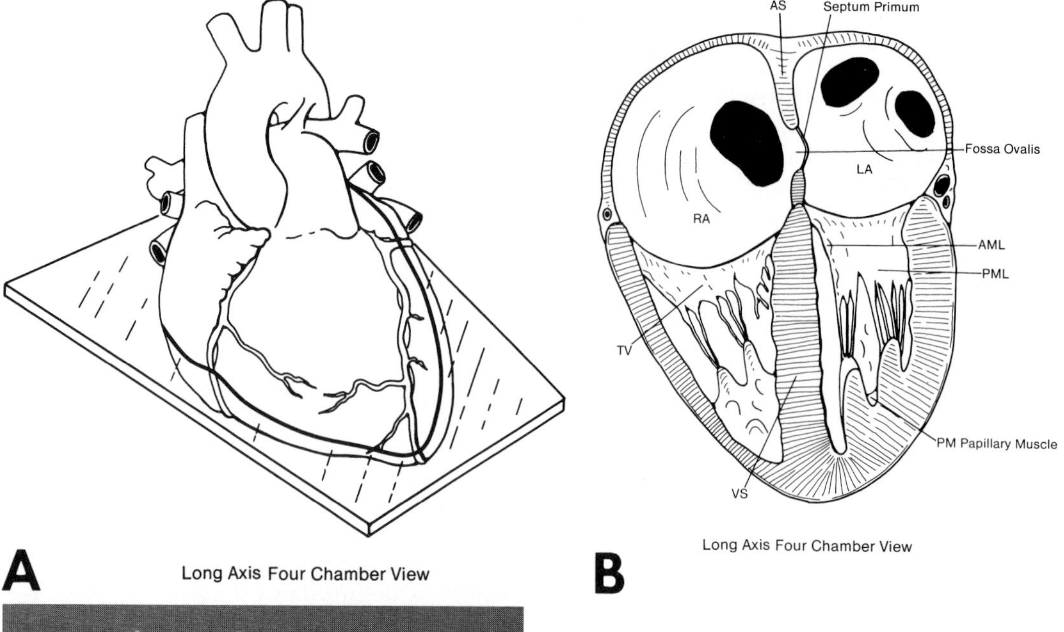

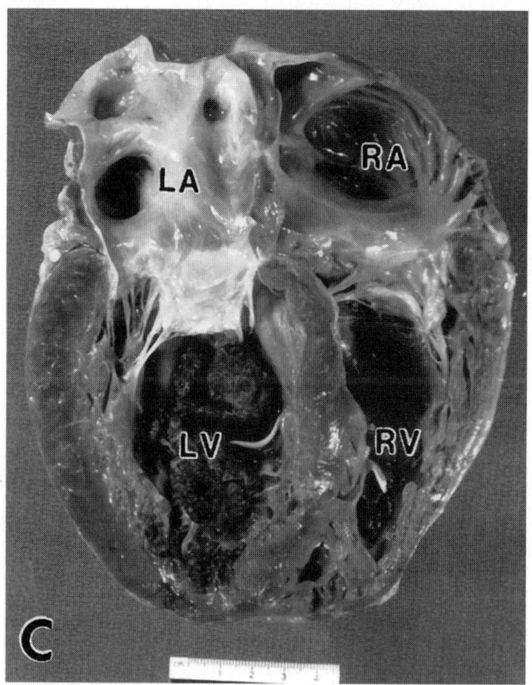

Figure 1–7. *A.* Diagram of the heart demonstrating the ultrasonic tomographic plane used for obtaining the long axis view of the heart. This four-chamber view is best used for evaluating the atrial and ventricular dimensions, intracavitary masses, ventricular and atrial septal defects, atrioventricular valve abnormalities, ventricular aneurysms, and the drainage of pulmonary veins. *B.* Diagram demonstrating the four-chamber view of the heart. This method involves sectioning the heart from apex to base, along the acute margin of the right ventricle and the obtuse margin of the left ventricle and continuing the plane of sectioning through the atria. The bisected specimen that is photographed should match with the antemortem cardiac image. *C.* Tomographic analysis of a heart from a 17-year-old boy who developed progressive heart failure over a course of 8 months showing four-chamber view with biventricular hypertrophy, four-chamber dilatation, and apical right and left ventricular thrombus. (*RA,* right atrium; *LA,* left atrium; *VS,* ventricular septum; *TV,* tricuspid valve; *AML,* anterior mitral leaflet; *PML,* posterior mitral leaflet). (*A* and *B* modified from Tajik AJ, Seward J, Hagler DJ, Muir DD, Lie JT. Two dimensional real-time ultrasonic imaging of the heart and great vessels: Technique, image orientation, structure notification and validation. Mayo Clin Proc 53:271,1978, with permission.)

pertensive heart disease, coronary disease, valve disease, pulmonary hypertension, and so on).

Hypertrophic Cardiomyopathy

Criteria established for myofiber disarray use sections of septum taken cross section. For this reason, sections to determine the presence of fibromuscular disarray are taken in the transverse plane, usually from the septal location with the largest dimension; it is easiest to take such sections if the heart is bread-loafed (short-axis view). In hearts with gross features of hypertrophic cardiomyopathy, or in hearts with concentric left ventricular hypertrophy of unknown cause, generous sampling of the septum (at least three sections) should be performed. In some cases, the septum is so thick that the cross section of septum needs to be bisected and placed in two cassettes. Rarely, hypertrophic

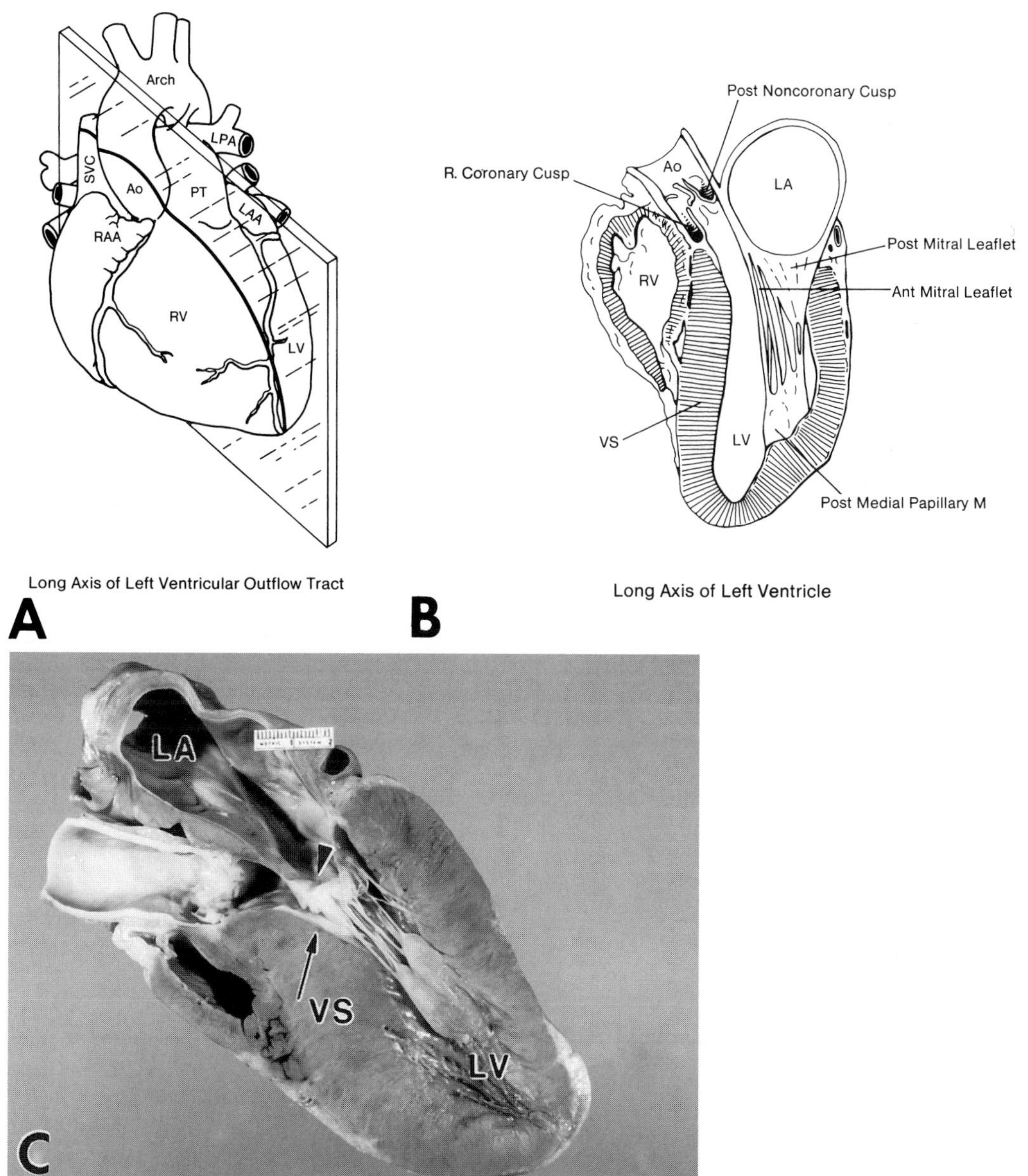

Figure 1–8. *A.* Diagram of the heart demonstrating the ultrasonic plane of the long axis view of the left ventricular outflow tract. The normal anatomic relationship of septal-aortic and mitral-aortic continuity are best shown by this plane of dissection. This method is used for aortic root pathology, including valvular, supravalvular, and intravalvular obstructions; left ventricular chamber size; posterior wall abnormalities; ventricular septal defects; mitral valve disease's and left atrial size. *B.* Anatomic landmarks seen with a long-axis view of the left ventricle. The plane of dissection of aortic valve leaflets is through the right coronary and posterior noncoronary leaflets. *C.* Left ventricular long-axis section in hypertrophic cardiomyopathy, showing asymmetric septal hypertrophy with a discrete left ventricular outflow tract plaque (*arrow*) and a thickened anterior mitral leaflet (*arrowhead*). (*Ao,* aorta; *LA,* left atrium; *LAA,* left-atrial appendage; *LPA,* left pulmonary artery; *LV,* left ventricle; *RAA,* right atrial appendage; *RV,* right ventricle; *SVC,* superior vena cave; *VS,* ventricular septum). (Modified from Tajik AJ, Seward JB, Hagler DJ, Muir DD, Lie JT. Two dimensional real-time ultrasonic imaging of the heart and great vessels: Technique, image orientation, structure identification and validation. Mayo Clin Proc 53:271, 1978. Reproduced with permission.)

cardiomyopathy may occur in the absence of cardiomegaly or other gross findings, the diagnosis resting on histologic examination of the ventricular septum.[17] For this reason, one could argue to sample generously the ventricular septum of all cases of unexpected sudden death.

Arrhythmogenic Right Ventricular Dysplasia-Cardiomyopathy

In the past, the right ventricle has been relatively ignored, but since the greater awareness of right ventricular infarction and right ventricular dysplasia/cardiomyopathy, it should be routine to examine the right ventricle carefully. In cases of sudden unexpected death without obvious cause, especially those that are exercise-related in young individuals, at least three sections of the right ventricle—lateral, anterior and posterior—should be taken. Right ventricular dysplasia can occasionally occur with minimal gross findings.[18]

When reporting case of cardiomyopathy it is important to report:

1. Presence of cardiomegaly (heart weight; should be reported in the context of body weight and height, see below)
2. Cavity dilatation, atrial or ventricular: left ventricular diameter at papillary muscles; right ventricular dilatation (best appreciated at apex); atrial dilatation (subjective assessment)
3. Presence of fibrosis, and its location in right or left ventricle
4. Type of cardiomyopathy: concentric left ventricular hypertrophy; asymmetric hypertrophy/hypertrophic cardiomyopathy; dilated cardiomyopathy; arrhythmogenic right ventricular dysplasia or cardiomyopathy; cardiomyopathy with restrictive features (large atria, normal-sized ventricular cavities, note presence of amyloid or endocardial disease); note that cardiomyopathy cannot always be classified

Evaluation of Cardiac Hypertrophy

The heart may not show any anatomic structural abnormality except that it is hypertrophied. Because cardiac hypertrophy may be a cause of death if severe, and physiologic in cases of chronic conditioning, the criteria for increased heart weight are important. We usually utilize the tables published from the Mayo Clinic giving the 95% confidence intervals for the height and weight of male and female individuals from birth to 99 years.[19, 20] If the hypertrophy is predominantly right-sided, evaluation of the lungs is important, as lung disease may result in pulmonary hypertension, right ventricular hypertrophy, and sudden death. Left ventricular hypertrophy is multifactorial, and includes cardiomyopathies, ischemic heart disease, idiopathic hypertrophy, and valvular heart disease.

Examination of the Heart Valves

Before cutting into the heart valves, the atrial and ventricular aspect of the atrioventricular valves and the ventricular and arterial aspects of the semilunar valves are examined (Fig. 1–9). Thus, the tricuspid valve is exposed by a lateral incision through the right atrium from the superior vena cave to 2 cm above the valve annulus. Similarly, the mitral valve may be studied following opening of the left atrium via an incision extending from one of the left pulmonary veins to one of the right pulmonary veins and another incision continuing through the atrium laterally to a point 2 cm above the annulus. If a valve abnormality requires closer inspection, the atria, including the interatrial septum, may be removed 1 to 2 cm above the atrioventricular valves (Fig. 1–9*A* and *B*). The ventricular aspects of the antrioventricular valves may be viewed following removal of the serial slices of ventricle as described previously. The semilunar valves are best studied after removal of the aorta (Fig. 1–9*C*) and the main pulmonary artery at a point just above the coronary ostia or valve annulus, respectively. If valvular abnormalities are identified grossly, the valve may be photographed prior to sectioning. Sectioning the valves occurs when the base of the heart is opened by flow of blood, after bread-loafing the apex and mid portion of the ventricles. The acute angle (right-sided lateral margin) and the obtuse angle (left-sided lateral margin) are opened, cutting through the tricuspid and mitral valves, respectively, and the pulmonary outflow tract opened by an incision along the anterior portion of the heart. If needed, the left ventricular outflow tract is opened, exposing the aortic valve and coronary ostia.

Measurement of the circumference of annuli, especially in valvular stenosis, is on the whole not very useful. In ectasia of the aorta, it is indeed a must to measure the aortic annulus as the valve will be normal in appearance but

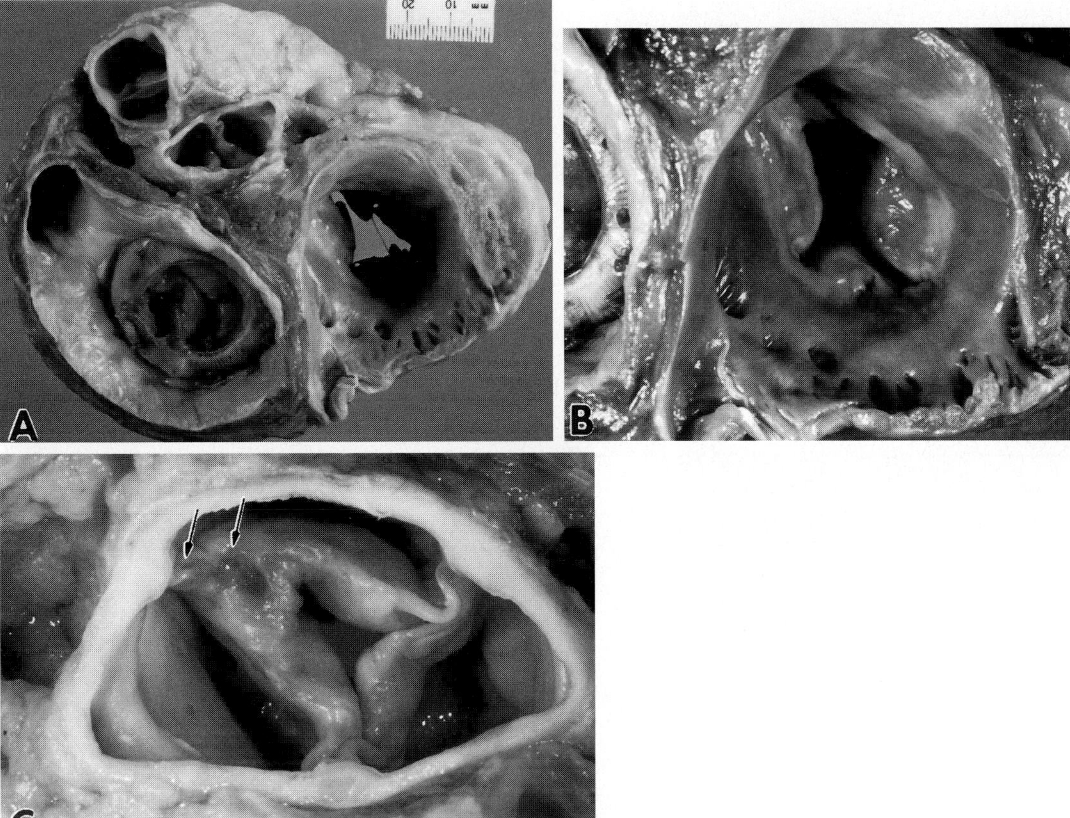

Figure 1–9. *A*. The appearance of the atrioventricular valves after removal of both the atria. The mitral valve has been replaced with a bioprosthetic porcine valve that shows a tear in the muscular leaflet close to the ring. *B*. The right atrium has been removed close to the tricuspid valve, note the valve margins are thickened, and the commissure between the posterior and the septal is fused secondary to chronic rheumatic valvulitis. *C*. The aortic valve is examined on removal of the aorta close to sinotubular junction. There is diffuse thickening of the valve, which is more marked at the free margins with one of the three commissures fused (*arrow*); these changes are consistent with chronic rheumatic valvulitis. (*AV*, aortic valve; *MV*, mitral valve; *PV*, pulmonary valve; and *TV*, tricuspid valve.)

the annulus will be dilated. Examination of the heart valves should document the type and severity of the valvular disease and its effect on the cardiac chambers and this includes microscopic evaluation. In selected cases the valvular pathology may be best visualized using a four-chamber cut[21–23] in the plane including both the acute and obtuse margins of the heart (refer to Fig. 1–7). The aortic valve may be demonstrated by a left ventricular long-axis cut passing from the apex through the outflow tract, ventricular septum, anterior mitral valve leaflet, and aortic valve (refer to Fig. 1–8).

In cases in which histology of a valve may be helpful, the leaflets are sectioned together with a portion of the adjacent chambers and/or vessel walls (Fig. 1–10). For example, the posterior leaflet of the mitral valve is sectioned including a portion of the left atrium and left ventricular free wall, while the anterior leaflet includes ventricular septum and noncoronary cusp of the aortic valve. In cases of rheumatic heart disease, sections of the atrial appendages are submitted for histologic examination, because the incidence of Aschoff nodules is highest in these structures.

Reporting of native valve disease should include the following:

1. The valve or valves involved, with a description of all valves
2. Does the valve demonstrate features suggesting that it was regurgitant (incompetent), stenotic, or both stenotic and incompetent?
3. In semilunar valves, numbers of cusps, and presence of fibrosis, raphes, calcification, or commissural fusion; vegetations—presence, size, shape, location on the valve; any destruction of the underlying valve

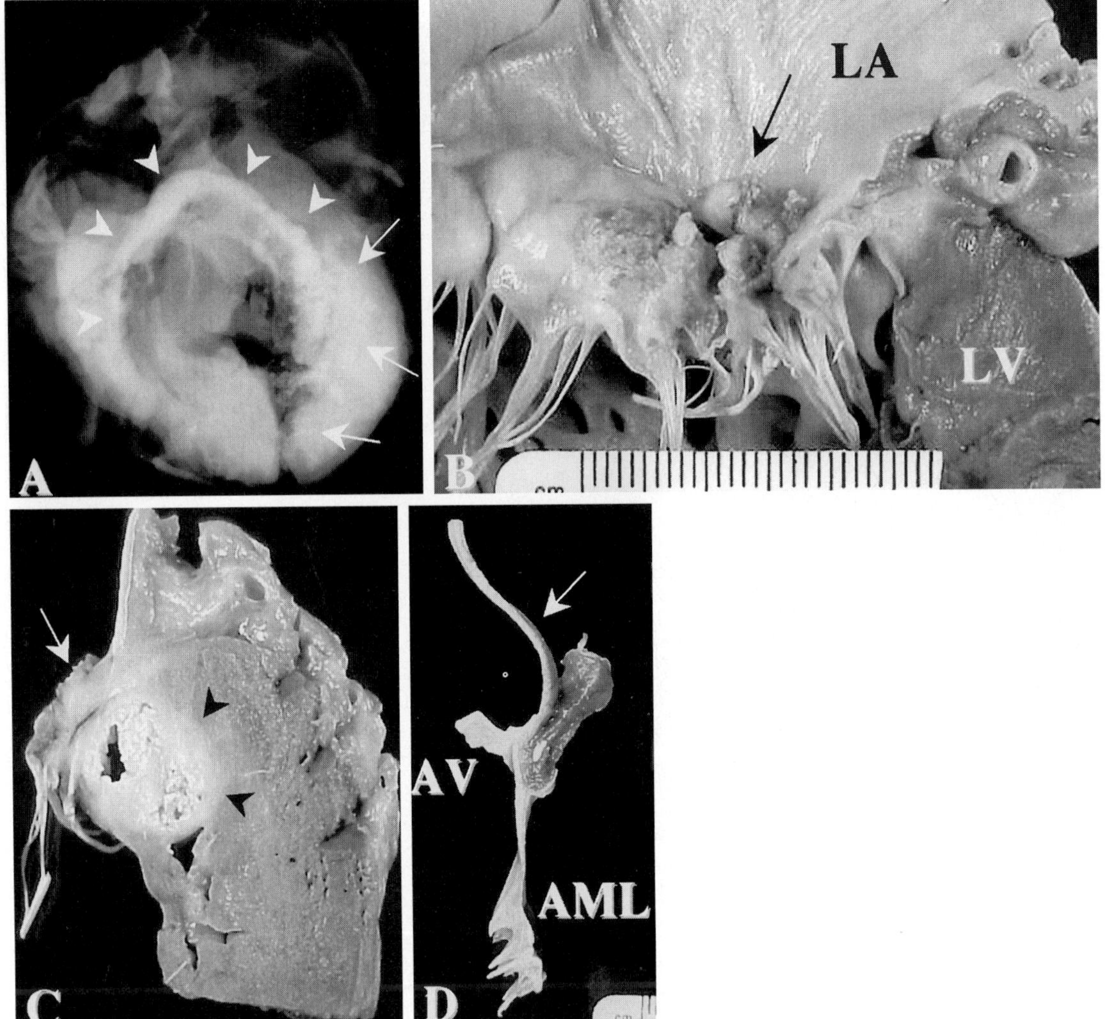

Figure 1–10. The extent of mitral annular calcification is best appreciated by radiography (*A*); this is a cranio-caudal view of the base of the heart. The area of the annulus showing calcification is outlined by arrowheads and three stents (*arrows*) had been deployed in left circumflex coronary artery. Stents are best appreciated in radiographs of the heart. *B*. The left side of the heart has been opened showing presence of friable vegetations (*arrow*) on the posterior mitral leaflet. *C* and *D* are sections taken for histologic processing to illustrate the manner in which sectioning of the posterior mitral leaflet and annulus should be taken. Note a portion of the left atrium and left ventricular wall are included; the arrow points to the friable vegetation on the atrial surface of the posterior valve leaflet and the arrowheads to the annular calcification. The anterior mitral leaflet (*AML*) section must include the posterior noncoronary cusp of the aortic valve (*AV*) and the sinus of Valsalva (*arrow*).

4. In atrioventricular valves, chordae tendineae—normal, thickened or fused, shortened; perforations fibrosis or calcified; commissural fusion; vegetations—presence, size, shape, location on the valve of any destruction of the underlying valve, perforations, or calcification
5. Do these features suggest a congenital or acquired process?
6. Circumference of the annulus, especially aortic (or diameter of aortic root at the level of the valve, as well as ascending aorta)
7. Ventricular and atrial cavity dilatation and extent; scarring, thrombi, localized endocardial lesions of regurgitation
8. In case of regurgitation of mitral valve from ischemic heart disease, describe the loca-

tion of the infarct, transmural or subendocardial, and involvement of the papillary muscle

Prosthetic Heart Valves

The objectives for examinations of valve implants include determination of (1) the type of implant (bioprosthesis or mechanical valve) and its size and position regarding annulus and chamber; (2) adequacy of movement of the valve apparatus; (3) presence of thrombi, vegetations, and paravalvular abscesses or leaks; and (4) evidence of valve degeneration. In particular, paravalvular abscesses may not be visible without careful inspection of the native annulus following removal of the implant. Demonstration of any pathology may be enhanced using short-axis cuts through the atrioventricular junction.

Examination of the Aorta

Because atherosclerosis is the most common lesion affecting the aorta, the aorta should be opened longitudinally along its posterior or dorsal aspect from the ascending aorta through the bifurcation and into both common iliac arteries. The extent of disease and the types of lesions may then be described. While this method enables inspection of the complete intimal surface, it may not be optimal for certain types of pathology, such as aortic aneurysms, which may best be demonstrated by cross-sectional slices 1 to 1.5 cm apart in the perfusion-fixed, distended specimen (Fig. 1–11). Aortic dissections may be examined by a longitudinal cut (long-axis cut) with the aorta cut into anterior and posterior halves (Fig. 1–12) or by transverse cut at 1- to 1.5-cm intervals after the aorta has been allowed to fix for 24 hours in a distended state or free floating in anatomic position in formaldehyde. The following points must be reported in case of atherosclerosis, aneurysms, and dissections:

1. Atherosclerotic disease must be reported as mild, moderate, or severe, and depends upon the type of plaques as well as the extent of involvement. The location of the severest le-

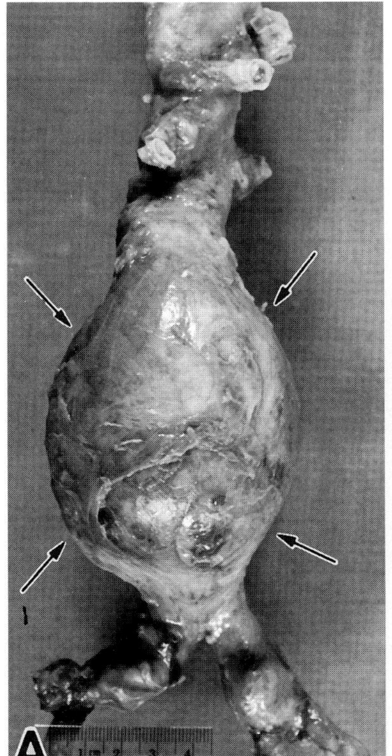

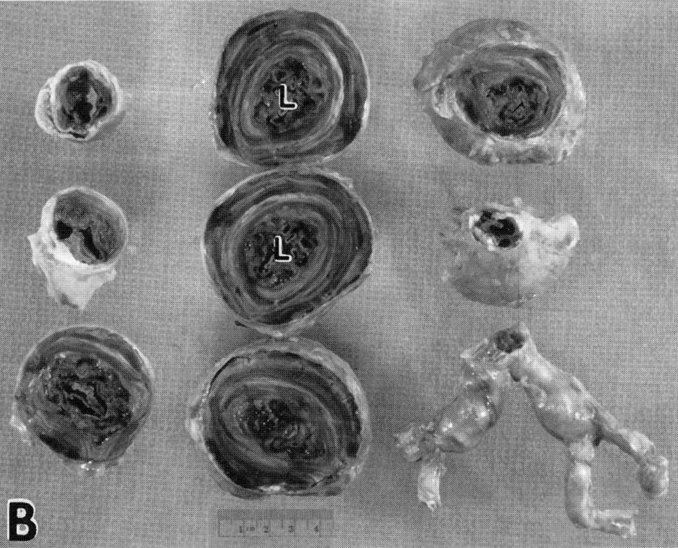

Figure 1–11. *A.* External view of the abdominal aorta with an infrarenal aneurysm (*arrows*). Note the size, which is best expressed as the largest diameter. In this case it is 7 cm. *B.* Same aneurysm cut transversely at 1.0 to 1.5 cm apart. Note the extent of lumina (*L*) narrowing secondary to an organizing thrombus.

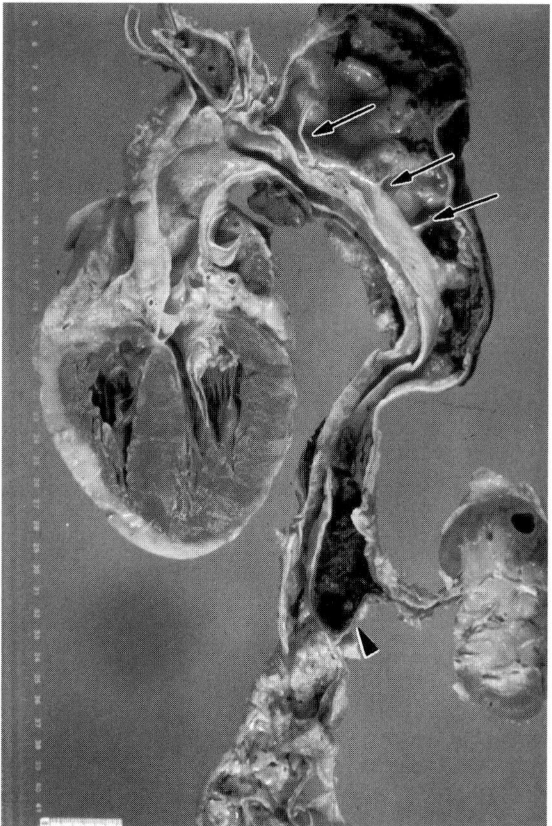

Figure 1–12. The heart has been cut in the long-axis plane, exposing the right and left ventricles and the aortic root and valve. The anterior wall of the aorta has been removed in this plane. Note the dissecting aneurysm that starts just distal to the subclavian artery and extends along the greater curvature of the aorta to just below the left renal artery (*arrowhead*). Within the false lumen there are fibrous strands (*arrows*) connecting the outer media and adventitia to the inner media and intima. Note also the organizing thrombus within a fusiform aneurysm distal to the subclavian and within the abdominal aorta of the false lumen.

sions must be mentioned especially if they are ulcerated.

2. For aneurysmal disease, state the site of the aneurysm (ascending aorta, arch, descending thoracic, abdominal aorta—suprarenal or infrarenal), the length and the width, if there is any leak or rupture of the wall and its location, luminal patency, and the type of underlying disease causing the aneurysm.

3. For dissections, the location of the entry tear (intimal tear) and the exit of the dissection (antegrade and retrograde from the tear) should be described. If there is a rupture of the false lumen (in most fatal cases), its location should be noted. If the entry of the dissection is identified (found in the vast majority), note if the tear is longitudinal or transverse, note the dimensions and the distance from the sinotubular junction, when located in the ascending aorta. If entry is in the descending aorta, give location in reference to ligamentum arteriosum.

Examination of the Conduction System

For cases in which conduction disturbances were suspected clinically (especially complete heart block), histologic examination of the cardiac conduction tissues is often rewarding in terms of documenting a structural basis for the problem. In other situations, especially unexpected sudden death, evaluation of the conduction system is rarely rewarding. It is much more common to identify an initially unsuspected cause of death upon reexamining the heart, than upon embarking on a conduction system study. However, after a thorough exclusion of noncardiac and evident cardiac causes of death has been performed, it is worthwhile for scientific as well as for medico-legal purposes to document that the structures of the specialized conduction system are intact.

Many pathologists are intimidated by the prospect of doing conduction system studies because the pertinent tissue cannot be visualized grossly. Yet, with practice and careful attention to anatomic landmarks, this part of the examination of the heart is really not so difficult.[24, 25]

In most humans the sinus node is a spindle-shaped structure located in the sulcus terminalis on the lateral aspect of the superior vena cava and the right atrium (Fig. 1–13). In some patients, it is a horseshoe-shaped structure wrapped across the superior aspect of this cavoatrial junction. Histologically, the sinus node consists of relatively small-diameter, haphazardly oriented atrial muscle cells admixed with connective tissue, collagen, and elastic fibers (Fig. 1–14). Often, the artery to the sinus node can be identified in or around the nodal tissue. Because the sinus node is not visible grossly, the entire block of tissue from the suspected area should be taken and serially sectioned, either in the plane perpendicular to the sulcus terminalis (parallel to the long axis of the superior vena cave) or in the plane containing the sulcus (perpendicular to the vessel). In small infants, serial sectioning of the entire cavoatrial junction is preferred.

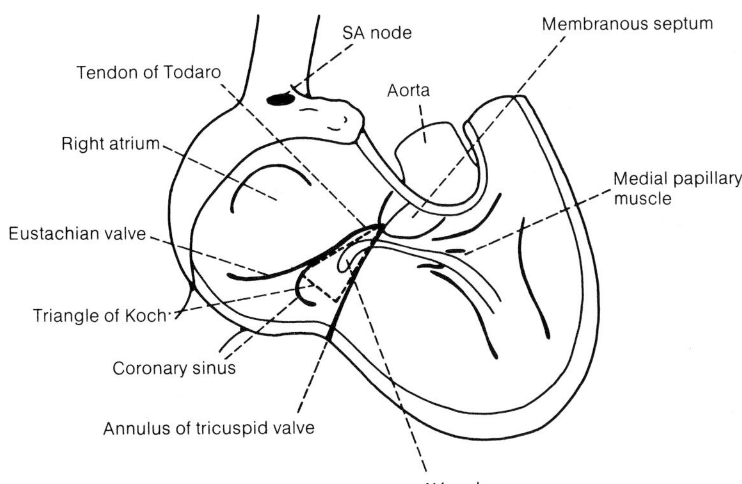

Figure 1–13. Diagram of location of the atrioventricular (*AL*) and sinoatrial (*SA*) nodes along with the landmarks that help in locating their positions during sectioning of the heart. (Modified from Davies MJ, Anderson RH, Becker AE. The Conduction System of the Heart. London: Butterworth & Co, 1983, with permission.)

There are no anatomically distinct muscle tracts for conduction through the atria. The impulse is collected in the atrioventricular node, which is located within the triangle of Koch in the floor of the right atrium. In the heart dissected in the traditional manner along the lines of blood flow, this region is delineated by the following landmarks: the tricuspid valve annulus inferiorly, the coronary sinus posteriorly, and the continuation of the valve guarding the coronary sinus (tendon of Todaro) superiorly (Fig. 1–15). The atrioventricular node lies within Koch's triangle (refer to Fig. 1–15), and the apex of the triangle anteriorly denotes the point at which the common bundle of His penetrates the fibrous annulus to reach the left ventricle. After penetrating the fibrous annulus at the crest of the ventricular septum, the bundle of His divides into left and right bundle branches. Thus, the tissue excised for study of the conduction system must include this area completely. From the opened right atrioventricular aspect (with the aortic outflow tract adjacent to the cutting surface), the block to be excised reaches from the anterior margin of the coronary sinus to the medial papillary muscle of the right ventricle, including 1 cm of atrium and ventricle on both sides of the valve. Alternatively, from the left ventricle outflow tract, the block can be cut perpendicular to the aortic valve from the margin of attachment of the anterior leaflet of the mitral valve to the left edge of the membranous septum. The block should include the noncoronary cusp of the

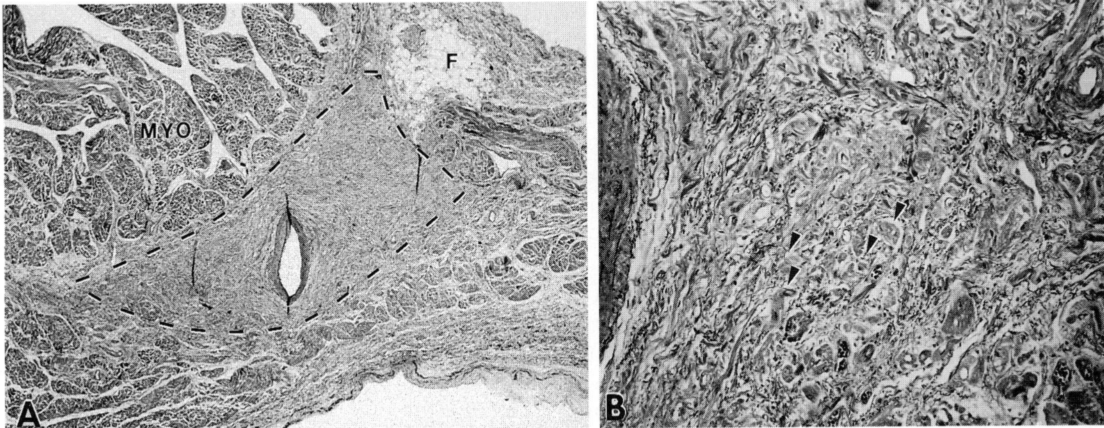

Figure 1–14. The sinus node (*outlined*) lies in the subepicardium. The superficial layer is surrounded by epicardial fat (*F*), and the deeper layers anastomose with the surrounding atrial myocardium (*MYO*). (Movat, × 25) *B.* High-power view of the SA node showing fibrous tissue, elastin fibers, and small SA node haphazardly arranged fibers.

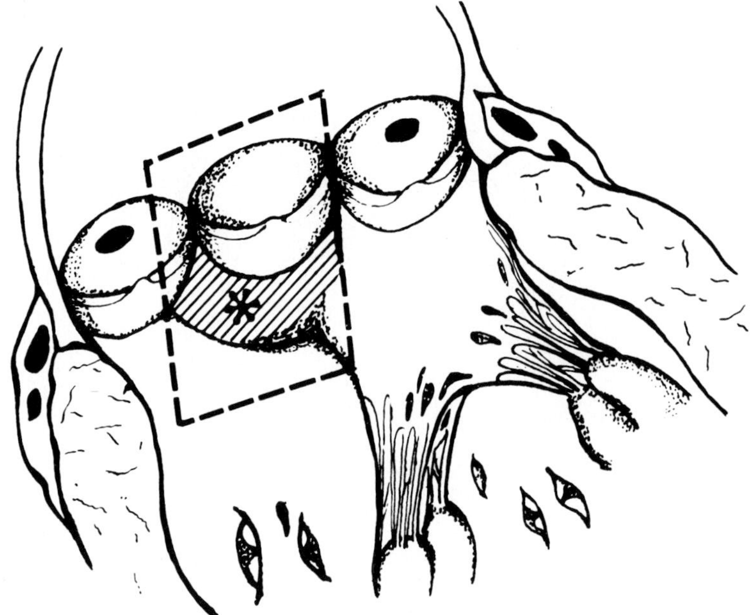

Figure 1–15. Diagram of landmarks for excising the major conduction from the left outflow tract. The membranous septum is marked by an asterisk.

aortic valve and the crest of the ventricular septum (refer to Fig. 1–15). In either case, the block of tissue removed should be divided in the plane perpendicular to the annulus, from posterior to anterior; the block to be sectioned should be marked with India ink so their orientation can be maintained throughout the embedding process. For infant hearts, the entire block of tissue should be step-sectioned with every fifth 10-μm thick section stained with Movat stain initially. In the adult heart, the entire tissue should be step-sectioned and every 25th or 50th section stained with Movat stain. Practically, the block of tissue is usually divided into five segments and one or two sections are cut from each segment.

The atrioventricular node, bundle, and bundle branches are histologically easily identifiable. The atrioventricular node consists of a network of muscle fibers that are smaller than the atrial and ventricular fibers. The cytoplasm is pale in comparison to the ventricular myocardium, but striations and intercalated disk are present. The nuclei are oval in longitudinal sections. The conduction tissue is markedly cellular due to the presence of a large number of endothelial cells and there is greater amount of elastic tissue than in the surrounding myocardium. As the node extends to penetrate the fibrous body and become the bundle of His, the fibers are less plexiform and more longitudinally oriented (Fig. 1–16).

Histologic Sampling

We recommend that at least four sections of the left ventricle be examined from the four walls of the heart and one section of the posterior wall of the right ventricle; sections should be taken from the mid ventricular slice. In the elderly we also like to take one section each from both the atria, as amyloidosis and drug reactions may be limited to the atria. As mentioned above, in sudden unexpected death in young individuals—especially those dying during exertion—right ventricular dysplasia and hypertrophic cardiomyopathy should be exhaustively ruled out, and samples of the right ventricle and ventricular septum taken for documentation, especially if the heart is not saved. If there are no obvious findings in sudden cardiac death, we recommend at least three sections of right ventricle and ventricular septum in such cases.

EVALUATION OF INTRACARDIAC DEVICES AT AUTOPSY

Types of Devices

The likelihood of the autopsy pathologist encountering a prosthetic device or implant in the heart is increasing. Currently, the types of devices implanted in the heart include pacemakers, defibrillators, prosthetic heart valves, prosthetic heart valve rings, conduits, and ven-

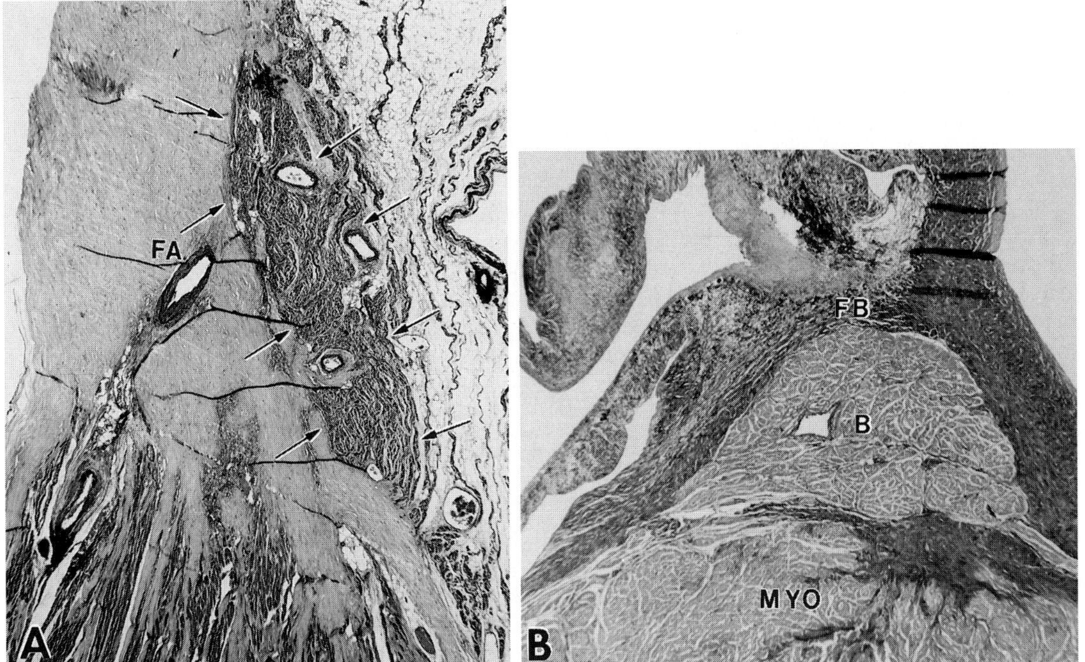

Figure 1–16. *A*. The atrioventricular node (*arrows*) is shown nested against the fibrous annulus (*FA*). *B*. The branching bundle (*BB*) is located above the septal myocardium (MYO). (Movat stain × 25).

tricular assist devices. Devices used primarily to treat congenital heart disease include occluder devices (atrial septal defect repair) and coils (to close fistulas and patent ductus arteriosus). Endoluminal stents are becoming more commonplace in the treatment of coronary, iliac, carotid, aortic, and peripheral arterial stenoses, and are described in detail in Chapter 3, along with left ventricular assist devices.

The components of implanted devices include polymers, metals and alloys, composites, ceramics, and biological materials. In the heart, polymers such as polyfluorocarbons are used for grafts, metals such as titanium and cobalt/chromium alloys for valve components and stents, ceramics such as pyrolytic carbon for valve occluders, and biologic materials for bioprosthetic valves. Biologic materials used in valves include porcine aortic valves; bovine pericardium, dura, and fascia lata; and homograft materials (human allografts and autografts). (See Chapter 7.)

Device Registries

There are no federal registries for archiving or enrolling explanted devices in the United States, as is the case in some European countries. However, there are mechanisms in place, albeit far from complete, for the tracking of cardiac implants.

The Federal Drug Administration (FDA) is involved in post-market assessment of devices by the FDA Medwatch program, which covers a wide variety of medical products. However, this program only covers malfunctions, and does not allow for the creation of a database of devices to include well-functioning implants. The Medical Device Reporting Database of the Medwatch program enlists approximately 100,000 malfunctioning devices yearly, largely through clinical data acquired from the manufacturers. Individuals, such as autopsy pathologists, are not required to report malfunctioning devices. However, through the hospital or other institution in which the autopsy was performed, certain requirements are set forth by the FDA. Hospitals are required to report all deaths related to device malfunction to the FDA and the device manufacturer within 10 days. All serious injuries due to device malfunction need to be reported to the manufacturer only (the manufacturer, in turn, is required to report all malfunctions to the FDA, even those that are relatively minor). The most common cardiac device reported to the FDA Medwatch program is the pacemaker, accounting for approximately

5,000 yearly.[26] To report to the FDA, a form must be sent in with the appropriate information; information is available from their toll-free number and Medwatch web site.

In addition to the FDA, there are a variety of registries tailored to specific devices. The National Cardiac Surgery database of the Society of Thoracic Surgeons tracks the majority of heart valves implanted in the United States.[27] Although there are no centralized registries for heart valve examination in the United States as there are in Europe,[28] many of the observations leading to the understanding of mechanical and bioprosthetic valve failure were made in the United States. In the case of mechanical valves, analysis of valve components by a variety of methods, including scanning electron microscopy, has demonstrated the presence of cracks and fractures in the pyrolytic carbon occluders and metal struts. Other signs of degeneration that have been made at explant and autopsy include ring leaks, cloth and Teflon wear, and silastic poppet swelling in earlier modes.[29] Despite the possibility of catastrophic failure of mechanical valves, they have proven remarkably durable, in contrast to bioprosthetic valves. The manufacturer of the St. Jude's valve has estimated only five noniatrogenic fractures in 7,000 valves implanted chronically in patients.[29] Examination of bioprosthetic valves at surgical explant and postmortem have shown consistent gradual degeneration characterized by calcification, lipid insudation, and tearing by a variety of techniques including routine histology, scanning and transmission electron microscopy, radiographic analysis, atomic absorption spectroscopy, and calcium analysis.[29]

There are a variety of pacemaker registries. In addition to that mandated by the FDA and the Health Care Financing Administration for Medicare patients between 1987 and 1997,[30] there are several pacemaker registries covering both the pulse generators and leads.[31] For specific types of ventricular assist devices, autopsy protocols providing guidelines for cultures, tissue sampling, time of autopsy, and preparation of the device have been devised for tracking infectious, thrombotic, and mechanical complications.[32] Standards for analysis of a wide variety of devices have been set by the National Institute of Standards and Technology, American Society for Testing and Materials.

Pathologist's Role in Evaluating Heart Devices

There are no clear-cut guidelines for the pathologist who performs autopsies on patients with heart devices. As stated above, any death related to a device malfunction should be reported to the FDA, and any serious injury to the manufacturer. This report is generally accomplished through the hospital quality-assurance mechanisms.

In cases of prosthetic valves, the pathologist should examine for degenerative changes, perivalvar leaks, thromboses, and ring abscesses. Fractures of struts with occluder escape are rare complications of mechanical valves, whereas degenerative calcific changes with infection and perforation are not uncommon in bioprosthetic valve leaflets (see Chapter 7). In cases of ventricular assist devices, thrombosis, infection, and device malfunction should be excluded, optimally in association with the manufacture,[32] in addition to chronic affects on the myocardium (see Chapter 3).

In cases of possible pacemaker malfunction, there are several options for interrogation of the pacemaker. The cardiology department in the hospital frequently can perform immediate interrogation of the device (see following), which requires the pulse generator. The manufacturer is best suited for evaluation of the leads, which are less likely to malfunction than the battery-powered generator. Although family concerns may result in sending the device to a site other than the manufacturer, the manufacturer is probably the most knowledgeable about the particular device, is mandated to report any malfunction to the FDA, and will post any defects on a variety of bulletins available on the World Wide Web. Ownership rights of an implanted device have not been established by law, nor has it been established if ownership confers the right to testing. Therefore, there are no legal guidelines to follow in choosing to test and where to test.[33]

Cardiac Pacing and Defibrillating Devices

Pacemakers

The indications for cardiac pacing include acquired atrioventricular block, bifascicular or trifascicular block, atrioventricular block after myocardial infarct, sick sinus syndrome (sinus node dysfunction), tachyarrhythmias, and neurally mediated syncope, Often, these arrhythmias exist with underlying cardiomyopathies (hypertrophic or dilated) or in patients with heart transplants (often sinus dysfunction).[34]

Pacemakers have two components: generators, which may be single or dual chamber, unipolar or bipolar, and may have a sensor for rate response; and the leads, which vary by polarity, type of insulation, and fixation mechanisms. There are a host of programming variables, including pacing mode, rate lowering, pulse width, amplitude, sensitivity and refractory, in addition to a maximum tracking rate and atrioventricular delay for dual chamber pacemakers.[34]

Pacemakers are described by a "NBE code" (NASPE/BPEG or North American Society for Pacing and Electrophysiology/British Pacing and Electrophysiology Group) of 3 to 5 letters. Position I signifies chambers paced (atrial, ventricular, or dual), and is notated by the letters "A, V or D." Position II signifies the chamber sensed, and uses the same letters as position I. Position III is tied to II, and indicates the mode of sensing response: "I" (inhibitory), withholding output in presence of sensed event (generally depolarization), or "D" (in dual chamber pacemakers), usually representing inhibition of atrial output and triggering ventricular output. "R" in position IV represents rate response (presence of sensor to regulate during periods of physical activity). The fifth position is reserved for antitachycardia features. In defibrillators (see following), "D" represents the ability to shock (dual shocks and paces). In a pacemaker only, "O" indicates no antitachycardia features, and "P" indicates pacing features.[35] An example of a simple pacemaker is VVI (lead only in right ventricle, which senses and paces in the ventricle, and ceases firing if a depolarization is sensed in the myocardium).

Complications of pacemaker insertion occur in 5 to 10% of patients, and include infection, inadequate capture, or sensing. Most occur within the first 3 months after the implantation.[36] It has been shown that the failure rate of pacemakers did not decline significantly in the 1990s, indicating the need for continued surveillance and registries for pacemakers.[31] Although most complications involve the pulse generator, degeneration of the polyurethane leads may also occur.[31, 37]

Interrogation of pacemakers, both in patients as well as autopsy, includes testing the battery, pacing threshold and pulse width, sensing function, and lead integrity. At autopsy, pathologic features associated with chronic indwelling pacemakers include entrapment of the pacing wire in the tricuspid valve, neointima formation around the lead adjacent to the valve and tip, and fibrous thickening at the tip encasing the lead within endocardial tissue (Fig. 1–17). These changes are not necessarily associated

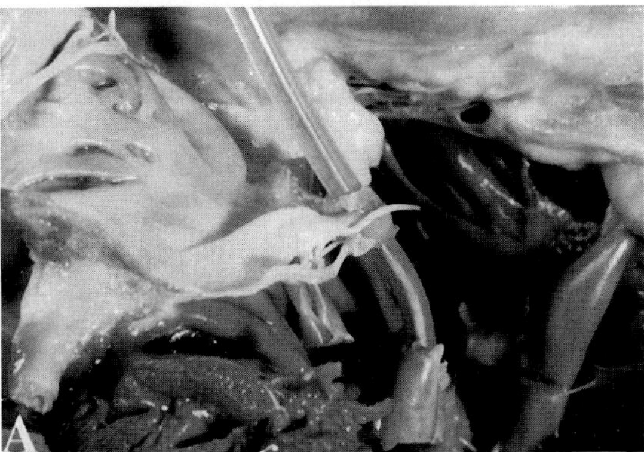

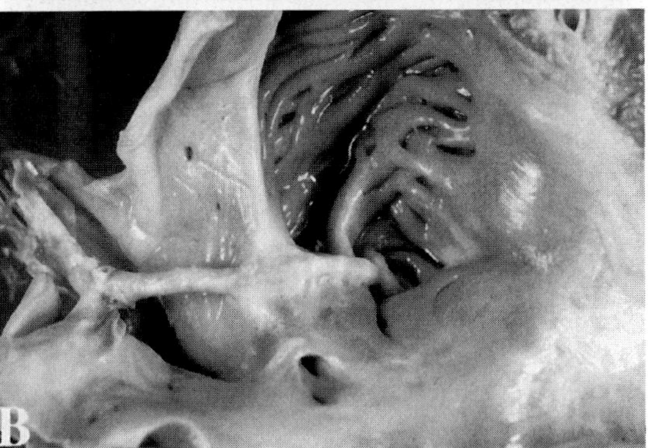

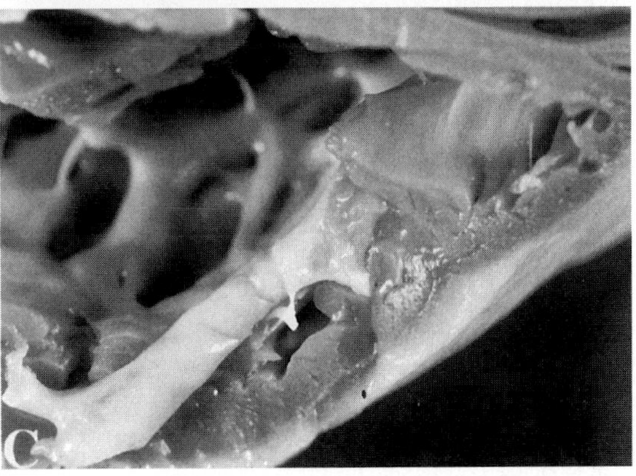

Figure 1–17. Pacemaker leads in the right heart. *A.* The patient was an 81-year-old black male with sick sinus syndrome. The VVI single chamber pacemaker lead in the right ventricle is seen coursing within the septal leaflet of the tricuspid valve. Perforation of the tricuspid valve is a common occurrence with chronic pacing and generally does not lead to significant insufficiency. *B* and *C.* The patient, a 73-year-old with chronic ischemic heart disease, had a dual chamber pacemaker. *B* demonstrates the atrial lead, which is encased in fibrous tissue (neointima). *C* demonstrates the ventricular lead, which has incited a fibrotic reaction in the apical endocardium of the right ventricle. The fibrous reaction, tricuspid valve encroachment, and sometimes extensive neointimal formation may make extraction of the pacemakers difficult without open heart surgery.

with duration of the pacemaker, and demonstrate the reasons for the difficulty in extracting pacemakers from living patients.[38, 39]

Defibrillators

Before the 1990s, implantation of a defibrillator (automatic implantable cardiac defibrillator, AICD) required thoracotomy and placement of an epicardial patch. These devices resulted in significant epicardial and pericardial fibrosis.[40] Since that time, defibrillators have become progressively smaller. They have evolved through a device consisting of a transvenous lead with a distal ring electrode coupled with subcutaneous defibrillator[41] to devices not much larger than standard pacemakers.[34] AICDs are often used in conjunction with antiarrhythmic therapy and ablative techniques, and have been shown prospectively to decrease the incidence of sudden death by as much as 39% at 1 year and 31% at 3 years compared with patients treated without AICDs.[34, 42] Indications for AICD include ischemic heart disease with decreased left ventricular function, long QT syndrome, idiopathic ventricular fibrillation, hypertrophic cardiomyopathy, arrhythmogenic right ventricular dysplasia, and syncope with inducible sustained ventricular tachycardia.

As with pacemakers, defibrillators would be evaluated for capabilities of sensing, pacing, defibrillation functions, battery status, lead system parameters, and replacement indicators. Associated pathologic findings include endocardial fibrosis, presumably caused by prior shocks, and epicardial fibrosis in the older AICDs. It has been postulated that endocardial fibrosis caused by defibrillation episodes could result in a new arrhythmia substrate, increase defibrillation and pacing thresholds, and deterioration of intracardiac electrograms.[41] Recently, it has been demonstrated that there is a risk for pathologists at autopsy to receive a potentially dangerous shock from active AICDs.[43] For this reason, it is imperative that autopsy pathologists have information prior to autopsy to prevent possible injury to him- or herself and autopsy assistants.

CARDIAC EXAMINATION FORM

Pericardium

Intact, congenital/acquired defect; fluid, amount and character (clear, fibrinous, hemorrhagic, chylous, etc.); adhesions (extent, location)

Coronary arteries

Coronary ostia
- Location in relationship to sinotubular junction and sinus of Valsalva
- Acute angle or ostial ridge present

Epicardial arteries
- Remove arteries from heart by blunt dissection
- Note dominance (right, left, combination)
- Postmortem X-ray (in patients > 45 years of age) to determine calcification
- Decalcification, 24 hours or more if needed
- Section at 3-mm intervals, noting:

Plaques (length, cross-sectional luminal narrowing, thrombus), dissections, etc.:
- Left main
- Proximal left anterior descending (LAD)
  - Note also presence of tunnel (myocardial bridge)
- Mid and distal LAD
- Left diagonal from LAD
- Proximal left circumflex and ramus intermedius, if present
- Distal left circumflex (if left dominant)
- Proximal right coronary
- Mid right coronary artery

Distal right coronary artery
Posterior descending coronary artery

Cardiac valves

Aortic valve
Trim ascending aorta 1 cm from aortic valve, and view from above
Aortic root diameter; numbers of aortic cusps; presence and location of raphe if present
Degree of stenosis and nodular calcification, if present
Commissural fusion (commissures involved and degree 1–3+);
Evidence of regurgitation (rolling and thickened valve leaflet edges)
Vegetations (size, location, evidence of valve destruction)
Fenestrations (size, location)

Mitral valve
Evidence of prolapse (mild, moderate, severe)
Degree of calcification of annulus (absent, mild, moderate, severe)
Valve leaflets: fibrotic thickening, calcific plaques, clefts
Vegetations; underlying valve destruction
Commissures: fusion and fibrosis, if present
Length of leaflet, annulus to free edge, anterior and posterior leaflets
Chordal disarray, thickening, shortening
Papillary muscles: fibrosis, malformations, fusion, rupture
Pulmonary valve: Number of leaflets, vegetations, fibrosis, dysplasia
Tricuspid valve: Prolapse/floppy changes; vegetations; underlying valve destruction; fibrosis, characteristics of chordae; evidence of annular dilatation
Prosthetic valve: Bioprosthetic (porcine, pericardial), mechanical (bileaflet, tilting disc, caged ball)

Left ventricle

Anterior wall: Thickness; scarring (patchy, subendocardial, transmural, subepicardial); acute infarction (subendocardial, transmural)
Lateral wall: Thickness; scarring, infarction (subendocardial, transmural)
Posterior wall: Thickness; scarring, acute infarction (subendocardial, transmural)
Interventricular septum: Thickness (anterior basal, posterior basal, apical); scarring (patchy, subendocardial, transmural, subepicardial); acute infarction
Cavity: Dimension at level of papillary muscles, not including muscles and trabeculae
Location of abnormality: Basal, mid or apical

Right ventricle

Anterior wall: Thickness, gross scarring, fat replacement
Lateral wall: Thickness, gross scarring, fat replacement
Posterior wall: Thickness, gross scarring, fat replacement, infarction (acute, healed)
Outflow region: Thickness, gross scarring; fat replacement
Cavity: Normal, mild, moderate severe dilatation (evaluate in apical slice, should not form apex)

Endocardium

Endocardial fibrosis (mild, moderate severe); mural thrombus (apical, inflow, involvement of mitral valve); relationship of thrombus to scarring or infarct

Atria

Dilatation, thrombus; foramen ovale: patent, closed; endocardial fibrosis: focal, diffuse; endocardial appearance: normal, waxy, suggestive of amyloid (patients > 70 or history suggestive of primary amyloidosis)

REFERENCES

1. Layman TE, Edwards JE. A method for dissection of the heart and major pulmonary vessels. Arch Pathol 82:314, 1966.
2. Ludwig J, Titus JL. Heart and vascular system. In: Ludwig J (ed): Current Method of Autopsy Practice. Philadelphia: WB Saunders, 1979.
3. Hutchins GM, Buckley BH, Ridolfi RL. Correlation of coronary arteriograms and left ventriculograms with postmortem studies. Circulation 56:32, 1977.
4. Hales MR, Carrington CB. A pigment gelatin mass for vascular injection. Yale J Biol Med 43:257, 1971.
5. Glagov S, Eckner FA, Lev M. Controlled pressure fixation approaches for hearts. Arch Pathol 76:640, 1963.
6. Gould KL, Lipscomb K, Hamilton GW. Physiologic basis for assessing critical coronary stenosis. Instantaneous flow response and regional distribution during coronary hyperemia as measures of coronary flow reserve. Am J Cardiol 33:87–94, 1974.
7. Lipscomb K, Gould KL. Mechanism of the effect of coronary artery stenosis on coronary flow in the dog. Am Heart J 89:60–67, 1975.
8. Isner JM, Kishel J, Kent KM. Accuracy of angiographic determination of the left main coronary arterial narrowing: Angiographic-histologic correlative analysis in 28 patients. Circulation 63:1056, 1981.
9. Roberts WC, Lachman AS, Virmani R. Twisting of an aortic-coronary bypass conduit: A complication of coronary surgery. J Thorac Cardiovasc Surg 75:722, 1978.
10. Atkinson JB, Forman MB, Perry JM, Virmani R. Correlation of saphenous vein bypass graft angiography with histologic changes at autopsy. Am J Cardiol 55:952, 1985.
11. Atkinson JB, Forman MB, Vaughn WK. Morphologic changes in long-term saphenous bypass grafts. Chest 88:341, 1985.
12. Buckley BH, Hutchins GM. Accelerated "atherosclerosis": A morphologic study of 97 saphenous vein coronary artery bypass grafts. Circulation 163, 1977.
13. Buckley BH, Hutchins GM. Pathology of coronary artery bypass graft surgery. Arch Pathol 102:273, 1978.
14. Lichtig C, Glagov S, Feldman S, Wissler RW. Myocardial ischemia in coronary artery atherosclerosis: A comprehensive approach to postmortem studies. Med Clin North Am 57:79, 1973.
15. Hackel BD, Ratliff NJ. A technique to estimate the quantity of infarcted myocardium post mortem. Am J Pathol 61:242, 1974.
16. Virmani R, Roberts WC. Quantification of coronary arterial narrowing and of left ventricular myocardial scarring in healed myocardial infarction with chronic, eventually fatal, congestive heart failure. Am J Med 68:831, 1980.
17. Maron BJ, Kragel AH, Roberts WC. Sudden death in hypertrophic cardiomyopathy with normal left ventricular mass. Br Heart J 63:308–310, 1990.
18. Burke AP, Robinson S, Radentz S, Smialek J, Virmani R. Sudden death in right ventricular dysplasia with minimal gross abnormalities. J Forensic Sci 44:438–443, 1999.
19. Kitzman DW, Scholz DG, Hagen PT, Ilstrup DM, Edwards WD. Age-related changes in normal human hearts during the first 10 decades of life. Part II (Maturity): A quantitative anatomic study of 765 specimens from subjects 20–99 years old. Mayo Clin Proc 63:137, 1988.
20. Scholz DG, Kitzman DW, Hagen PT, Ilstrup DM, Edwards WD. Age-related changes in normal human hearts during the first 10 decades of life. Part I (Growth): A quantitative anatomic study of 200 specimens from subjects from birth to 19 years old. Mayo Clin Proc 63:126, 1988.
21. Tajik AJ, Seward JB, Hagler DJ, Muir DD, Lie JT. Two dimensional real-time ultrasonic imaging of the heart and great vessels: Techniques, image orientation, structure identification and validation. Mayo Clin Proc 53:271, 1978.
22. Edwards WD. Anatomic basis for tomographic analysis of the heart at autopsy. Cardiology Clinics 2, 1984.
23. Roberts WC. Technique of opening the heart at autopsy. In: Hurst JW, Logue RB, Schlant RC, Wenger NK (eds): The Heart. New York: McGraw-Hill, 1982.
24. Davies MJ, Anderson RH, Becker AE. Anatomy of the conduction tissues. The Conduction System of the Heart. London: Butterworths, 9–70, 1983.
25. Rossi L. Histology of the conducting system and intrinsic nerves. Histopathology of Cardiac Arrhythmias. Milan: Casa Editrice Ambrosiana, 9–34, 1978.
26. Gross TP, Kessler LG. Medical device vigilance at FDA. In: Pallikarakis N, Anselmann N, Pernice A (eds): Information Exchange for Medical Devices. Vol. 28. Amsterdam: IOS Press, 17–24, 1996.
27. Jamieson WRE, Edwards FH, Schwartz M, Bero JW, Clark RE, Grover FL. Risk stratification for cardiac valve replacement. National Cardiac Surgery Database. Ann Thorac Surg 67:943–951, 1999.
28. Cromheecke ME, Overkamp PJB, de Mol BAJM, van Gaalen GL, Becker AE. Retrieval analysis of mechanical heart valves: Impact on design and clinical practice. Artif Organs 22:794–799, 1998.
29. Kaplan S. Biomaterial-host interactions: Consequences, determined by implant retrieval analysis. Med Prog Technol 20:209–230, 1994.
30. Cardiac pacemaker registry—FDA, HCFA. Final rule. Fed Regist 52:27756–27765, 1987.
31. Kawanishi DT, Song S, Furman S, et al. Failure rates of leads, pulse generators, and programmers have not diminished over the last 20 years: Formal monitoring of performance is still needed. BILITCH Registry and STIMAREC. Pacing Clin Electrophysiol 19:1819–1823, 1996.
32. Borovetz HS, Ramasamy N, Zerbe TR, Portner PM. Evaluation of an implantable ventricular assist system for humans with chronic refractory heart failure: Device explant protocol. ASAIO Journal 41:42–48, 1995.
33. Beyleveld D, Howells GG, Longley D. Heart valve ownership: Legal, ethical, and policy issues. J Heart Valve Dis 4:S2–S6, 1995.
34. Gregoratos G, Cheitlin MD, Conill A, et al. ACC/AHA guidelines for implantation of cardiac pacemakers and antiarrhythmia devices: A report of the American College of Cardiology/American Heart Association Task Force on Practice Guidelines (Committee on Pacemaker Implantation). J Am Coll Cardiol 31:1175–1209, 1998.
35. Bernstein AD, Camm AJ, Fletcher RD, et al. The NASPE/BPEG generic pacemaker code for antibradyarrhythmia and adaptive-rate pacing and antitachyarrhythmia devices. Pacing Clin Electrophysiol 10:794–799, 1987.
36. Kiviniemi MS, Pirnes MA, Eranen HJ, Kettunen RV, Hartikainen JE. Complications related to permanent

pacemaker therapy. Pacing Clin Electrophysiol 22:711–720, 1999.
37. Furman S, Benedek ZM. Survival of implantable pacemaker leads. The Implantable Lead Registry. Pacing Clin Electrophysiol 13:1910–1914, 1990.
38. Candinas R, Duru F, Schneider J, Luscher TF, Stokes K. Postmortem analysis of encapsulation around long-term ventricular endocardial pacing leads. Mayo Clin Proc 74:120–125, 1999.
39. Kozlowski D, Dubaniewicz A, Kozluk E, et al. The morphological conditions of the permanent pacemaker lead extraction. Folia Morphol 59:25–29, 2000.
40. Singer I, Hutchins GM, Mirowski M, et al. Pathologic findings related to the lead system and repeated defibrillations in patients with the automatic implantable cardioverter-defibrillator. J Am Coll Cardiol 10:382–388, 1987.
41. Epstein AE, Kay GN, Plumb VJ, Dailey SM, Anderson PG. Gross and microscopic pathological changes associated with nonthoracotomy implantable defibrillator leads. Circulation 98:1517–1524, 1998.
42. Pinski SL, Yao Q, Epstein AE, et al. Determinants of outcome in patients with sustained ventricular tachyarrhythmias: The antiarrhythmics versus implantable defibrillators (AVID) study registry. Am Heart J 139:804–814, 2000.
43. Prahlow JA, Guileyardo JM, Barnard JJ. The implantable cardioverter-defibrillator. A potential hazard for autopsy pathologists. Arch Pathol Lab Med 121:1076–1080, 1997.

Chapter

2

CORONARY HEART DISEASE AND ITS SYNDROMES

Despite the high prevalence of coronary artery disease, which remains the leading cause of death in the United States, there is often a reluctance among pathologists to take the time to describe the pathologic features of coronary artery plaques encountered at autopsy and in surgical specimens. The atherosclerotic plaque is heterogeneous, with a wide array of overt and subtle features that involve many of the basic processes in pathology. Morphologic features often correlate with clinical syndromes and risk-factor profiles. For these reasons, it is inadequate to simply make the diagnosis of atherosclerotic plaque; rather, the specific morphologic findings of an individual plaque should be studied, much like the various features of a neoplasm.

The most recognized forms of coronary heart disease are the acute syndromes: angina, unstable angina, myocardial infarction, and sudden death. The clinicopathologic correlates of these syndromes will be presented in this chapter. Coronary heart disease may also occur in the absence of typical chest pain or recognizable clinical ischemic syndromes. Presenting symptoms may also include variant (Prinzmetal) angina (see following), asymptomatic (silent) myocardial ischemia, congestive heart failure, and cardiac arrhythmias. The myocardial changes of acute and chronic ischemia are discussed in Chapter 5.

This chapter will focus first briefly on the epidemiology and clinical aspects of coronary artery disease, followed by a description of the morphologic lesions of atherosclerosis, from the early asymptomatic lesions to the late symptomatic plaques. Following a description of these lesions, lesions that typify each clinical syndrome, and the clinical and pathobiologic correlations of each type of plaque will be discussed. We hope that the reader will then understand the need and rationale for classification of acute and stable coronary plaques, and will gain a natural curiosity for a pathologic process encountered so frequently.

The opinions or assertions contained herein are the private views of the authors and are not to be construed as official or as reflecting the views of the Department of the Army or Navy or the Department of Defense.

EPIDEMIOLOGIC ASPECTS OF CORONARY HEART DISEASE

Prevalence and Risk Factors

Coronary heart disease remains the leading cause of death in the United States despite the recent decline in mortality rates from coronary heart disease in the latter part of this century.[1] More than 11 million Americans have coronary artery disease, which accounts for 44% of the mortality in the United States.[2] In a recent survey of the U.S. population aged ≥ 40 years, 11.8% report having angina pectoris or having had myocardial infarction or have electrocardiographic criteria consistent with previous myocardial infarction. Sudden cardiac death accounts for approximately 50% of all deaths due to coronary heart disease, and an even higher proportion in those dying before age 50 years.[3] Three hundred thousand individuals die suddenly in the United States every year, and a substantial proportion occur in individuals with no warning.[4]

There is a wide variation in the incidence of coronary artery disease worldwide. It is well known that there is a higher rate of coronary disease in the United States and/or developed Western societies, as compared with Asia and Africa and most of South America, due largely to environmental—specifically dietary—factors. The traditional risk factors for coronary atherosclerosis of elevated serum cholesterol, diabetes, cigarette smoking, and hypertension are associated with high rates of coronary disease when both countries or populations within individual countries are compared. Nations with a high rate of saturated fat intake, such as Scotland and Finland, have especially high rates of coronary disease, and areas with a diet rich in unsaturated fats, such as Crete, have very low rates. The Framingham and the more recent National Health and Nutrition Examination Survey cohorts have firmly established the association between traditional risk factors and coronary heart disease in the United States, which continues despite the recent decline in coronary deaths due to the modification of risk factors by the public.[5] However, a substantial proportion of coronary deaths occur in individuals without known traditional risk factors, and other dietary habits and genetic traits contribute to the development of coronary atherosclerosis.[6–8] Antioxidants present in vegetables and teas, and possibly dietary supplements, for example, may have an antiatherogenic effect. Genetic polymorphisms, modulated by diet, affect the serum level of homocysteine, which is associated with coronary artery disease.[9] Lipoprotein (a) levels, which are genetically determined,[10] may have an association with an increased risk for atherosclerosis independent of total or high-density lipoprotein cholesterol (HDL-C), as well as polymorphisms for apolipoprotein E.[11] A complete discussion of newer risk factors, including inflammatory markers, polymorphisms for platelet glycoprotein IIbIIIa,[12] fibrinogen, and angiotensin converting enzyme, is beyond the scope of this chapter. Some correlations between specific types of thrombus and traditional risk factors are discussed later in this chapter; for further information on risk factors and coronary disease, several recent reviews are available.[6, 8]

Gender Differences

The morbidity and mortality from coronary artery disease is higher in men than in women. One third of men in the United States will develop a major cardiovascular event before reaching the age of 60 years, whereas only one in ten women manifest the disease.[13] Coronary heart disease in women has classically been said to occur only following menopause and lags behind 10 years compared with men for total coronary heart disease and by 20 years for myocardial infarction and sudden death.[1] Epidemiologic, clinical, animal, and *in vitro* studies have supported the existence of a protective effect of estrogen, which is mediated in part by changes in LDL-cholesterol, HDL-cholesterol, Lp(a), fibrinogen, and homocysteine, and in part by direct effects on the vessels themselves. The stabilizing effects of estrogens on the atherosclerotic plaque are poorly understood. They may include an influence on vasomotor tone, inhibitory effects on smooth muscle cell proliferation, inhibition of the elaboration of growth factors and inflammatory cytokines, and effects on vascular cellular adhesion molecules. Morphologically, estrogen appears to inhibit the formation of large necrotic core, thin-capped atheroma and calcification, although there is no protection against the formation of erosive plaques[14, 15] (see following).

Racial Differences

Compared with that in white persons, the age-adjusted risk for coronary heart disease is lower in African-American men for all ages combined (25 to 74 years) (relative risk, 0.78), but higher in African-American women aged 25 to 54 years (relative risk, 1.76). However, there is an increase in the rate of sudden coronary death in African-American men as well as women as compared with whites (166/100,000 for white men, 209/100,000 for black men, 74/100,000 for white women, and 108/100,000 for black women[16]). The increased mortality in blacks, despite the lower prevalence of the disease, may be in part due to socioeconomic factors; increased risk factors such as hypertension, diabetes, and smoking; and access to health care. Among blacks hospitalized for acute coronary syndromes, left ventricular hypertrophy is a more important predictor of mortality than degree of coronary stenosis,[17] underscoring the importance of hypertension-induced hypertrophy in coronary disease in blacks. There are also racial differences in the fibrinolytic system, platelet survival time and levels of factor VIII, von Willebrand factor, and antithrombin; the contribution of these variations on mortality in African-Americans due to heart disease is unknown.

PATHOLOGIC CLASSIFICATION OF CORONARY PLAQUES

We have recently proposed[18] a comprehensive morphologic classification scheme, which is a modification of the American Heart Association classification,[19, 20] for symptomatic and asymptomatic atherosclerotic lesions (Tables 2–1 and 2–2, Fig. 2–1).

Intimal Thickening (Intimal Mass Lesion)

The intimal mass lesion consists of smooth muscle cells in a proteoglycan matrix, which may attain a thickness of the media or greater (Figs. 2–1 and 2–2). Although originally considered a form of fibroblast, it has been firmly established that intimal cells are variants of the smooth muscle cell.[21, 22] Important features lacking in intimal thickening is a significant amount of lipid, active proliferation, and inflammatory cells. While some human lesions may begin as intimal xanthomata, or fatty streaks, there is substantial evidence that most adult human lesions originate from preexisting intimal masses.[19, 20] Because intimal thickening occurs in children in similar locations as obstructive lesions in adults, intimal masses are thought to be a precursor to the majority of obstructive lesions. Unlike intimal xanthomas (fatty streaks), there is little evidence that the intimal mass lesion may regress, and atherosclerotic lesions in the hyperlipidemic swine model almost exclusively arise from these lesions.[23, 24]

Ikari et al. report that the intimal layer in the proximal left anterior descending coronary artery is rarely formed before 30 weeks of gestation; between 36 weeks gestation and birth, 35% of coronary arteries show intimal cells, and by 3 months after birth, all show intimal mass.[25] Therefore, the coronary artery intima may be a major determinant of the atherosclerotic process that will smolder for decades, and may eventually cause symptomatic disease. Thus, it appears that preexisting intimal cell masses possess and maintain unique properties that promote the focal accumulation of lipids and/or macrophages.

There is very little known about the initiation of the intimal mass lesion, other than that the process is clonal.[24, 26] The stimulus for the mono-

Table 2–1. Current AHA Classification

Terms for Atherosclerotic Lesions in Histological Classification		Other Terms for the Same Lesions Often Based on Appearance to the Unaided Eye	
Type I lesion	Initial lesion		
Type II lesion			
IIa	Progression-prone type II lesion	Fatty dot or streak	Early lesion
IIb	Progression-resistant type II lesion		
Type III lesion	Intermediate lesion (preatheroma)		
Type IV lesion	Atheroma	Atheromatous plaque, fibrolipid plaque, fibrous plaque, plaque	
Type V lesion			
Va	Fibroatheroma (type V lesion)		
Vb	Calcific lesion (type VII lesion)	Calcified plaque	Advanced lesions, raised lesions
Vc	Fibrotic lesion (type VIII)	Fibrous plaque	
Type VI lesion	Lesion with surface defect and/or hematoma/ hemorrhage and/or thrombotic deposit	Complicated lesion, complicated plaque	

From Virmani et al. Lessons from sudden coronary death. Arterioscler Thromb Vasc Biol 20:1265, 2000, with permission.

Table 2–2. Modified AHA Classification Based on Morphological Description

Lesion	*Description*	*Thrombus*
Nonatherosclerotic Intimal Lesions		
Intimal thickening	The normal accumulation of smooth muscle cells (SMCs) in the intima in the absence of lipid or macrophage foam cells	Absent
Intimal xanthoma (fatty streak)	Luminal accumulation of foam cells without a necrotic core or fibrous cap. Based on animal and human data, such lesions usually regress	Absent
Progressive atherosclerotic lesions		
Pathological intimal thickening	SMCs in a proteoglycan-rich matrix with areas of extracellular lipid accumulation without necrosis	Absent
Erosion	Luminal thrombosis; plaque same as above	Thrombus mostly mural and infrequently occlusive
Fibrous cap atheroma	Well-formed necrotic core with an overlying fibrous cap	Absent
Erosion	Luminal thrombosis; plaque same as above, no communication of thrombus with necrotic core	Thrombus mostly mural and infrequently occlusive
Thin fibrous cap atheromas	A thin fibrous cap infiltrated by macrophages and lymphocytes with rare SMCs and an underlying necrotic core	Absent; may contain intraplaque hemorrhage/fibrin
Plaque rupture	Fibroatheroma with ca disruption; luminal thrombus communicates with the underlying necrotic core	Thrombus often occlusive in fatal cases; nonocclusive if silent
Calcified nodule	Eruptive nodular calcification with underlying fibrocalcific plaque	Thrombus usually nonocclusive
Fibrocalcific plaque	Collagen-rich plaque with significant stenosis usually contains large areas of calcification with few inflammatory cells; a necrotic core may be resent	Absent

From Virmani et al. Lessons from sudden coronary death. Arterioscler Thromb Vasc Biol 20:1265, 2000, with permission.

clonal proliferation of smooth muscle cells is likely related to endothelial injury and accumulation of lipid within the intima.[27] The nature of endothelial injury is likely multifactorial, although contradictory to early studies it does not involve desquamation but is for the most part an intact dysfunctional endothelium. Significant numbers of inflammatory cells associated with preexisting intimal cell masses are uncommon and the relationship between the development and progression of this lesion and inflammation is unclear (Fig. 2–3).

Intimal Xanthoma

We have proposed the term "intimal xanthoma" instead of the type II, "fatty streak" in the American Heart Association (AHA) scheme. "Xanthoma" is a general term, which describes focal accumulations of fat-laden macrophages. Pathologically, this lesion is composed of accumulations of foamy macrophages within the intima containing smooth muscle cells within a proteoglycan-collagenous matrix (Figs. 2–2 and 2–4). There is no significant smooth muscle cell proliferation, calcification, accumulation of lipid pools, or necrotic core formation. Although T-lymphocytes have been identified in fatty streak lesions, they are not so prominent as macrophages. Mast cells have also been identified in intimal xanthomas both in the intima and adventitia. Most of the intimal xanthomas regress in humans, because the distribution of lesions in the third decade of life and beyond is different from the fatty streaks seen in children. The thoracic aorta[28, 29] is a lesion-resistant area, yet this is a site where there

(*Text continued on page 33.*)

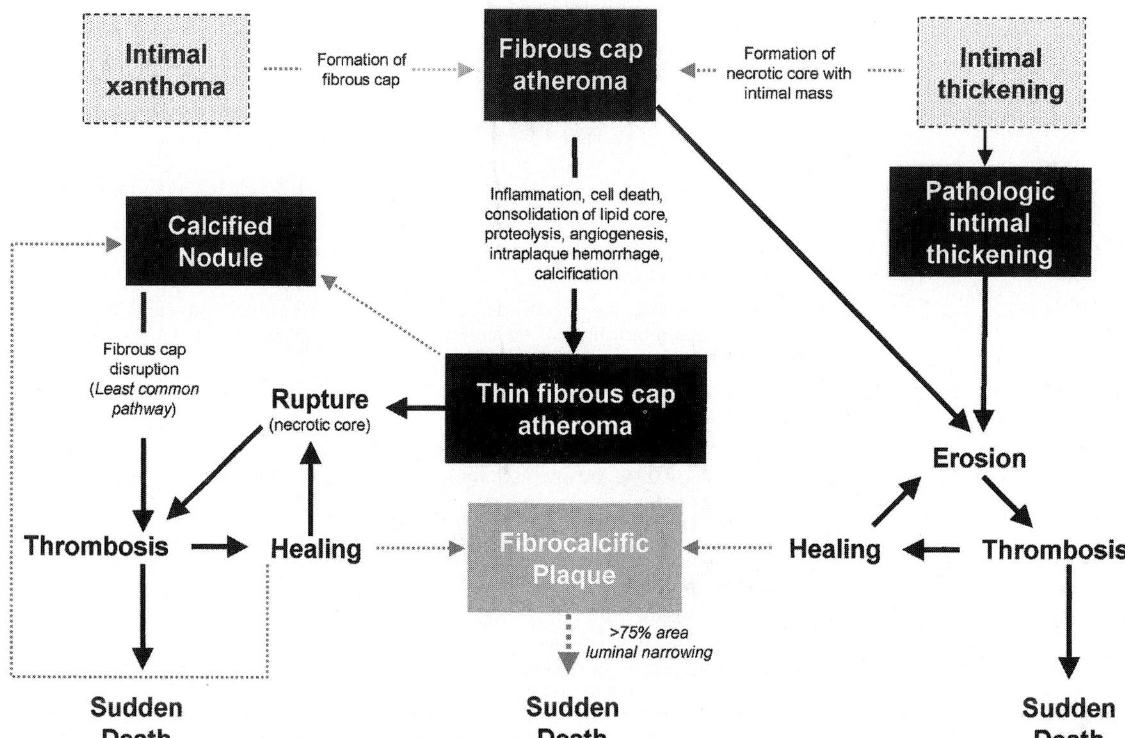

Figure 2–1. Our simplified scheme for classifying atherosclerotic lesions modified from the current American Heart Association recommendations. The boxed areas represent the seven categories of lesions. We have used dotted lines for two categories because there is controversy over the role each of them plays in the initial phase of lesion formation and both "lesions" can exist without progressing to a fibrous cap atheroma, (i.e., AHA type IV lesion). The processes leading to lesion progression are listed between categories. Lines (solid and dotted, the latter representing the least established processes) depict current concepts of how one category may progress to another with the thickness of the line representing the strength of the evidence that these events occur. (Virmani et al. Lessons from sudden coronary death. Arterioscler Thromb Vasc Biol 20:1265, 2000, with permission.)

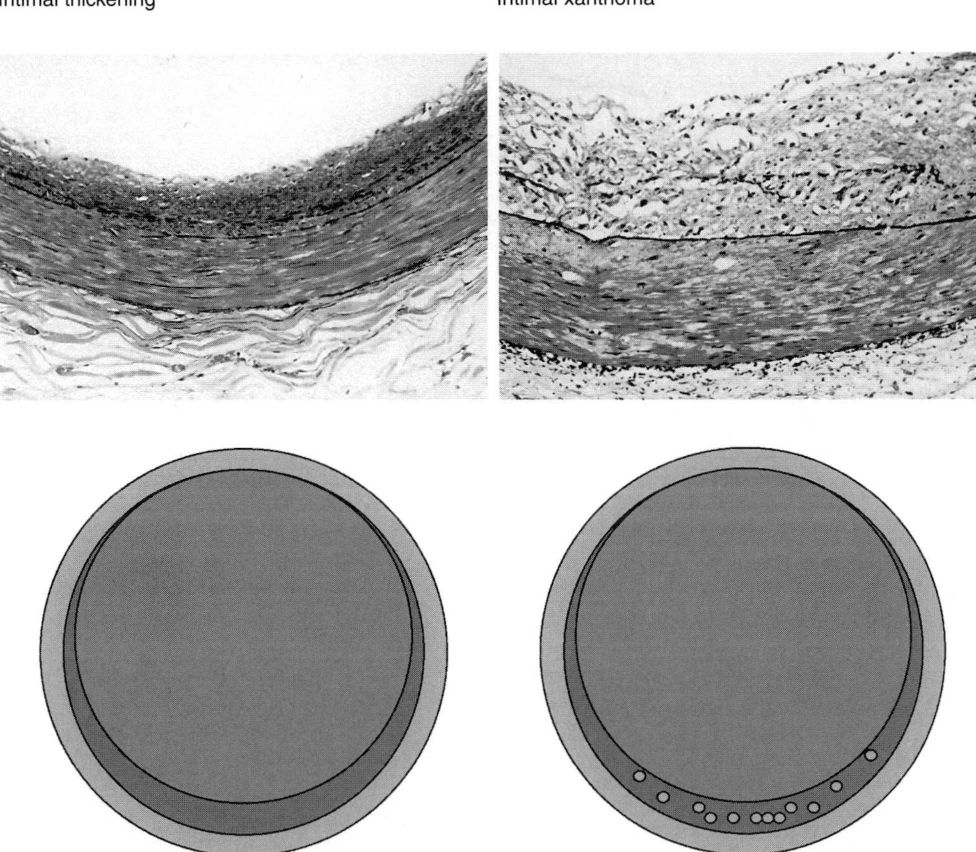

Figure 2–2. Pre-atherosclerotic coronary lesions. *Intimal thickening and intimal xanthoma*—Lesions uniformly present in all populations, although intimal xanthomas are more prevalent with exposure to a Western diet. *Intimal xanthomas* are commonly produced in animal models; however, they usually do not develop into progressive atherosclerotic lesions. Both lesions occur soon after birth; the intimal xanthoma (otherwise known as a fatty streak) is known to regress. *Intimal thickening* consists mainly of smooth muscle cells in a proteoglycan-rich matrix while *intimal xanthomas* primarily contain macrophage-derived foam cells, T-lymphocytes, and varying degrees of smooth muscle cells. (Virmani et al. Lessons from sudden coronary death. Arterioscler Thromb Vasc Biol 20:1266, 2000, with permission.)

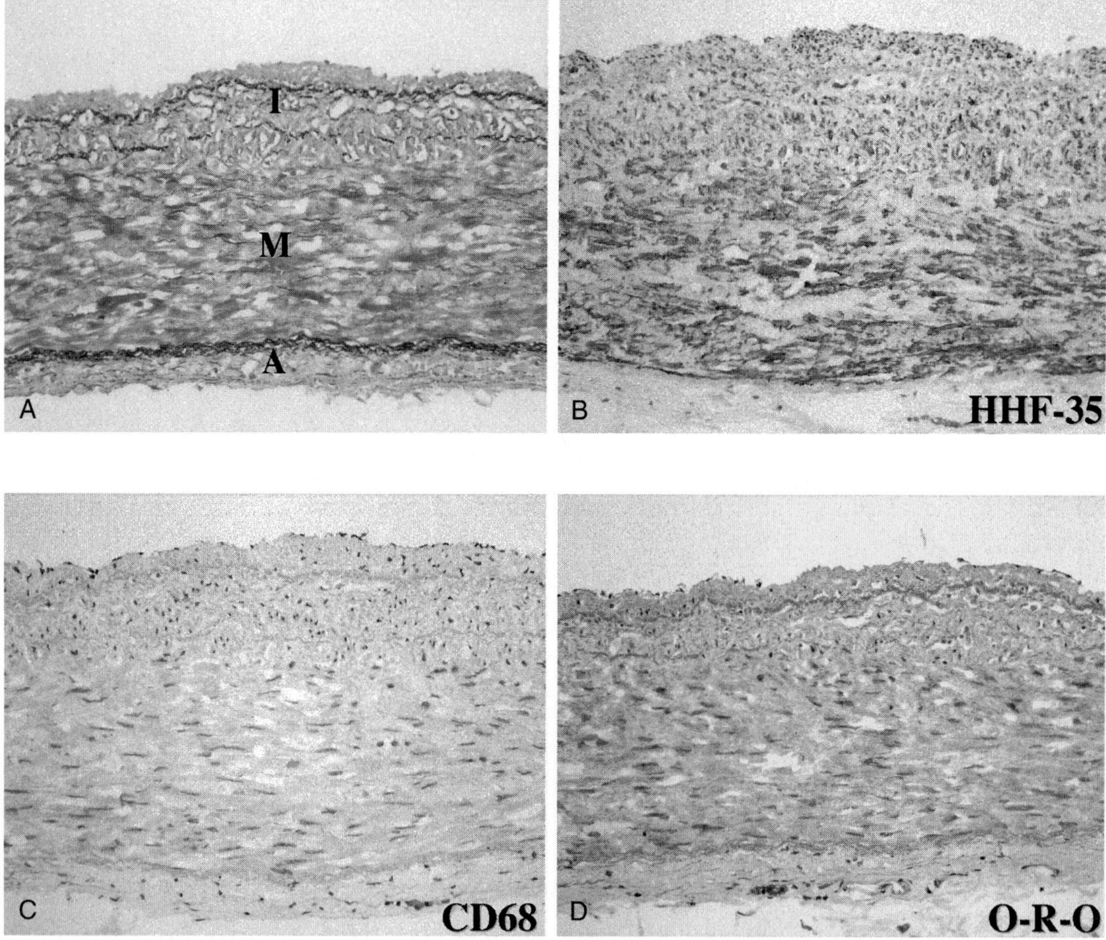

Figure 2–3. Intimal thickening. Coronary artery showing high-power view of the arterial wall consisting of media (*m*), intima (I), and adventitia (A). There is intimal thickening with splitting of the internal elastic lamina with smooth muscle cells interspersed in a proteoglycan rich matrix (green in *A*, Movat Stain). *B* shows HHF–35 staining of intimal and medial smooth muscle cells. No macrophages (CD-68) or oil-red-O positive areas identified (*C* and *D*, respectively).

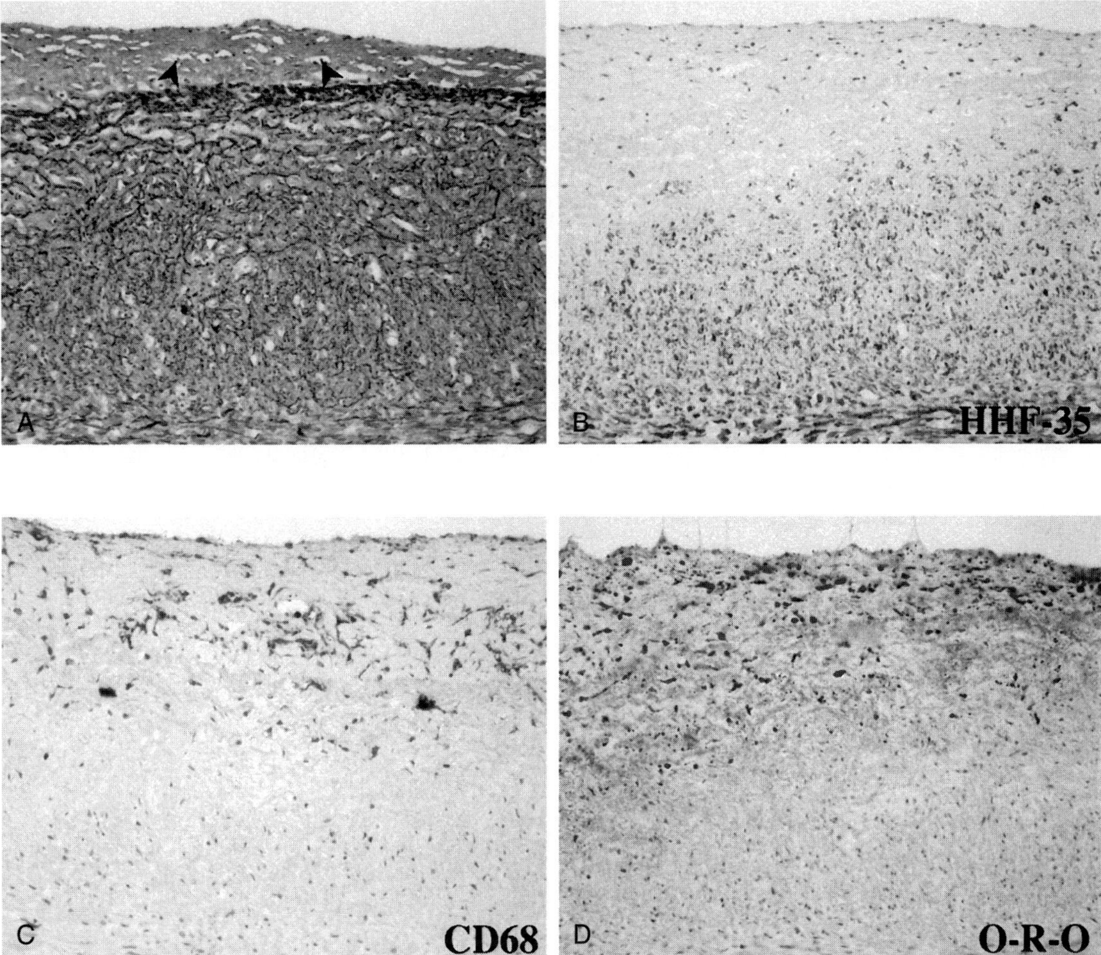

Figure 2–4. *A*. Early xanthomatous lesion with hard to discern macrophages (*arrowheads*) infiltrating the area of intimal thickening (Movat stain), which shows splitting of the internal elastic lamina. *B* shows HHF-35 staining of the intima. Note the most superficial layer does not stain for smooth muscle cells. *C* shows the most superficial area staining for macrophages (CD-68). The same area is oil-red-O positive (*D*), which is present both intra- and extracellularly.

are typically fatty streaks in children. In the right coronary artery, it is the first 2 cm, where fibroatheroma form, that is the lesion-prone area whereas fatty streaks extend into the proximal one half to two thirds of the vessel.[19, 20]

Fibroatheromas (Fibrous Cap Atheroma)

The transition between early lesions of atherosclerosis and the well-developed fibroatheroma is marked by an intermediate or preatheroma (type III) as referenced by the AHA classification.[19, 20] The preatheroma is characterized by the presence of extracellular lipid pools, which form between layers of smooth muscle cells. These pools tend to occur at sites of adaptive intimal thickening (Fig. 2–5). The lipid pools lie below the macrophage foam cell layers and are located in the proteoglycan matrix and among collagen fibers. No necrotic core is identified. These lesions by electron microscopy show large numbers of lipid droplets with or without peripheral laminated membranes and remnants of extracellular matrix components. The smooth muscle cells show lipid droplets in the cytoplasm. The composition of the preatheromas is richer in free cholesterol, fatty acids, sphingomyelin, lysolecithin, and triglyceride than the fatty streak lesion. The glycosaminogylcans with the highest affinity for plasma low-density lipoprotein is the dermatan sulfate, which consists of biglycan and decorin.[30] In addition to macrophages, the occurrence of intimal T-lymphocytes is not uncommon.

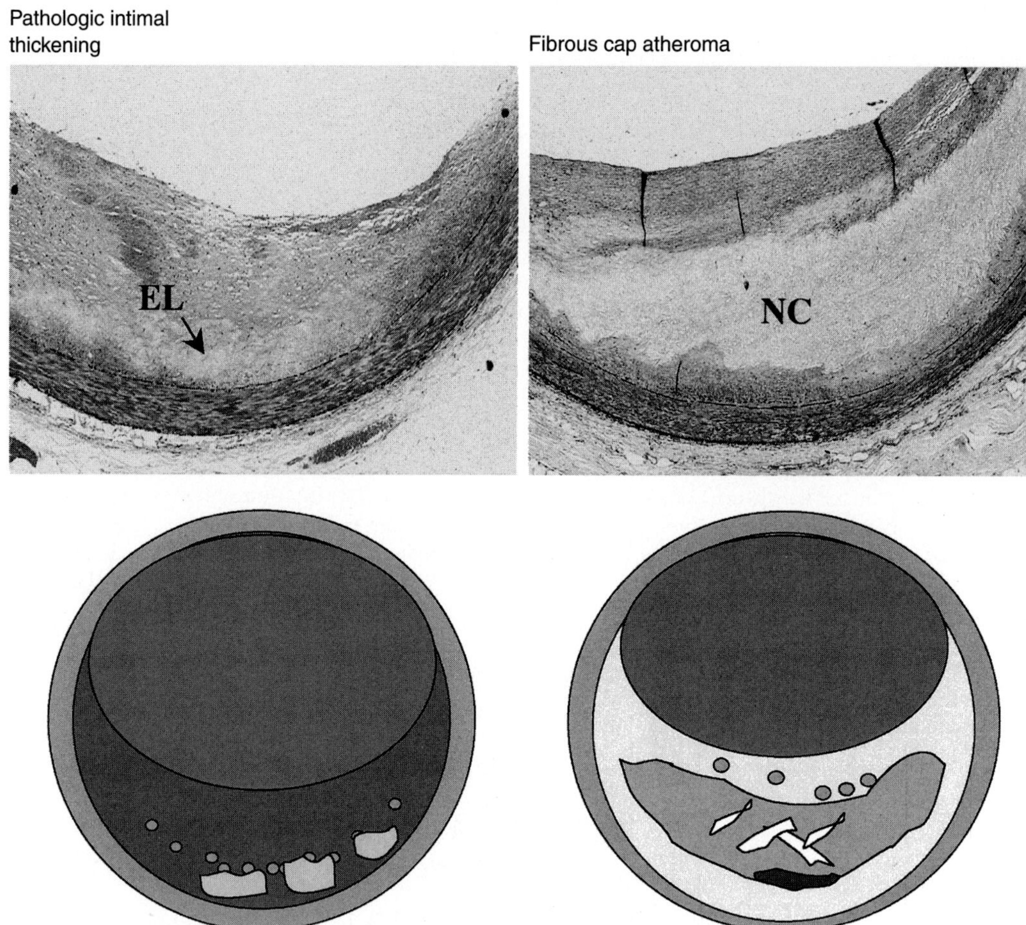

Figure 2–5. Pathological intimal thickening versus atheroma. *Pathologic intimal thickening* is a poorly defined entity sometimes referred to in the literature as an "intermediate lesion." True necrosis is not apparent and there is no evidence of cellular debris; some lipid may be present deep in the lesion but it is dispersed (*EL*, extracellular lipid). The fibrous cap overlying the areas of lipid is rich in smooth muscle cells and proteoglycans. Some scattered macrophages and lymphocytes may also be present, but are usually sparse. The more definitive lesion or *fibrous cap atheroma* classically shows a "true" necrotic core (*NC*) containing cholesterol esters, free cholesterol, phospholipids, and triglycerides. The fibrous cap consists of smooth muscle cells in a proteoglycan-collagenous matrix, with a variable number of macrophages and lymphocytes. The media underneath the plaque is often thin. (Virmani et al. Lessons from sudden coronary death. Arterioscler Thromb Vasc Biol 20:1267, 2000, with permission.)

The fibrous cap atheroma also called the type IV lesion by the AHA classification scheme is the first of the advanced lesions of coronary atherosclerosis (Fig. 2–5). Virchow likened this lesion as a dermal cyst (e.g., a sebaceous cyst, "Grutzbalg"), a fatty mass encapsulated by fibrous tissue. Thus, since the 1850s the defining feature of the "atheroma" has been the presence of a necrotic, fatty mass encapsulated by a fibrous tissue. This feature is analogous to the capsule containing an abscess and like an abscess the plaque can be ruptured.

The fibrous cap atheroma may result in significant luminal narrowing and is prone to complications of surface disruption, thrombosis, adventitial remodeling, and calcification. The relationship between inflammation and the development of the fibroatheroma is complex. The definition of fibroatheroma includes the presence of a lipid-rich core, and the origin and development of this core is key towards the understanding of the disease progression. As the atherosclerotic plaque enlarges, the lipid core becomes consolidated into one or more masses of extracellular lipid, cholesterol crystals, and necrotic debris. Only a few studies exist on the mechanisms of progression of a cellular xanthoma into a fibrous cap atheroma occupied by a necrotic core.[31]

Cholesterol in the fibrous cap atheroma occurs in intra- or extracellular droplets, liposomes, and crystals. Extracellular sources (i.e., plasma lipid) are especially important for accumulation of cholesteryl esters (predominantly cholesteryl linoleate) which predominate in later lesions and are similar to plasma low-density lipoprotein. The origin of the extracellular lipid, especially free cholesterol, has been long debated. Two theories have been suggested. One theory maintains that lipase mediated hydrolysis of phospholipids and cholesterol esters in the extracellular space leads to the production of free cholesterol, which, when concentrated, will crystallize.[32] The other theory suggests that cholesterol ester lipid droplets within macrophages form cholesterol crystals from hydrolysis within lysosomes.[33] Alternatively, we propose in advanced lesions with large necrotic cores that excessive free cholesterol also comes from the breakdown of erythrocyte cell membranes, contributing to the free cholesterol pool within the advanced plaque[34] (Fig. 2–6).

Thin Cap Fibroatheroma (A Vulnerable Plaque)

A common mechanism of disruption of the fibrous cap atheroma occurs via the thinning, or weakening, of the fibrous cap, resulting in fissures and ruptures. These breaks in the fibrous cap expose tissue factor to the lumen. The subsequent luminal thrombosis is the mechanism for increased luminal narrowing, vasospasm, and complications of embolization.

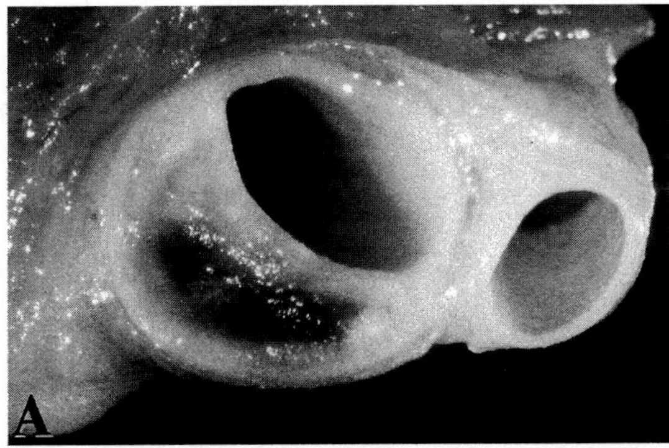

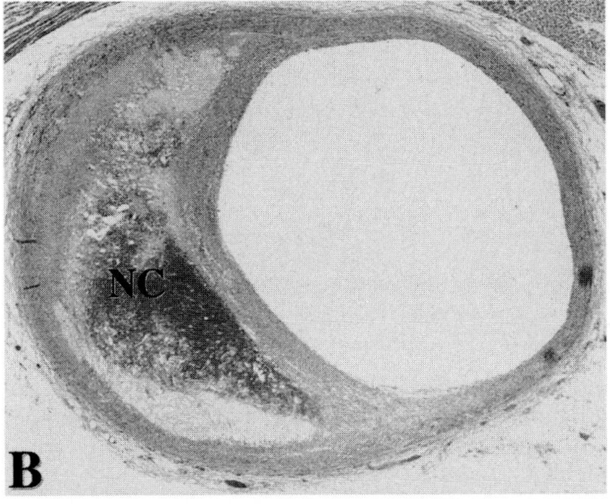

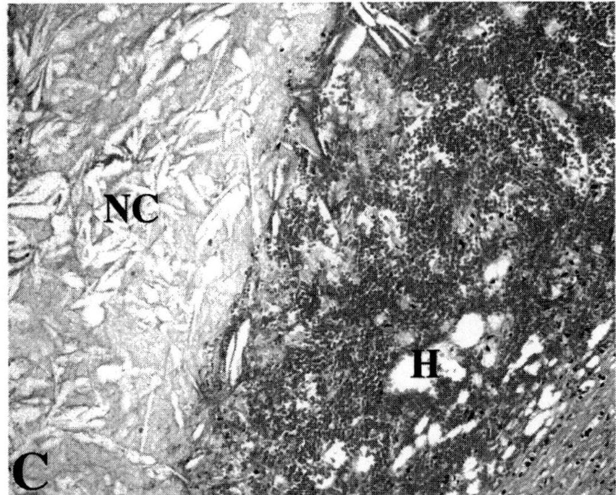

Figure 2–6. Hemorrhage into plaque. *A* demonstrates the left anterior descending artery and a diagonal branch with hemorrhage into a fibroatheromatous plaque. The deceased was a 33-year-old black male with a history of hypertension and chest pain; at autopsy, no cause of death was found other than a 70% fibroatheroma 3 cm distal to the illustrated segment. The heart weight was normal, at 330 grams. *B* demonstrates a hematoxylin eosin stain of the same artery, with a prominent necrotic core (*NC*). *C* demonstrates necrotic core (*NC*) with hemorrhage (*H*) and cholesterol clefts.

We have previously defined the thin-capped fibroatheroma as a lesion with a fibrous cap of 65 μm or less that is infiltrated by foam cells and T-lymphocytes[35] (Figs. 2–7 and 2–8). The thin-capped fibroatheroma typically contains a large necrotic core with cholesterol clefts and may also contain intraplaque hemorrhage and calcification. Prior areas of rupture may be evident, often resulting in multiple compartments of lipid-rich core and mild to moderate calcification. Coronary lesions also display variants of a thin-capped fibroatheromas; large collections of superficial macrophages overlying an intimal mass lesion, without significant lipid rich core. These lesions are commonly found in saphenous vein grafts and may represent processes important to the progression of atherosclerotic plaques.[36] Vein graft atherosclerotic disease is an accelerated form of native coronary atherosclerotic disease, frequently occurring within 10 years following implantation of veins.[37, 38] Morphologic features of vein graft disease suggests a larger role of foamy macrophages in plaque rupture and the origin of the necrotic core from breakdown of macrophages. However, because hemorrhage into a necrotic core is a frequent occurrence in vein graft (90% vs. 37% in all cause coronary atherosclerotic disease),[39, 40] it is not surprising that necrotic cores are larger in vein graft and richer in free cholesterol as they may originate from red cell membranes.

Although the macrophage is often considered the most important inflammatory cell in the progression of atherosclerosis, there has been increased attention to the role of T-lymphocytes. Because both macrophages and T-cells are present in the fibrous cap, antigen presentation with immune activation is likely to occur. Many T-cells in the developing atheroma bear interleukin-2 receptors and HLA-DR. The

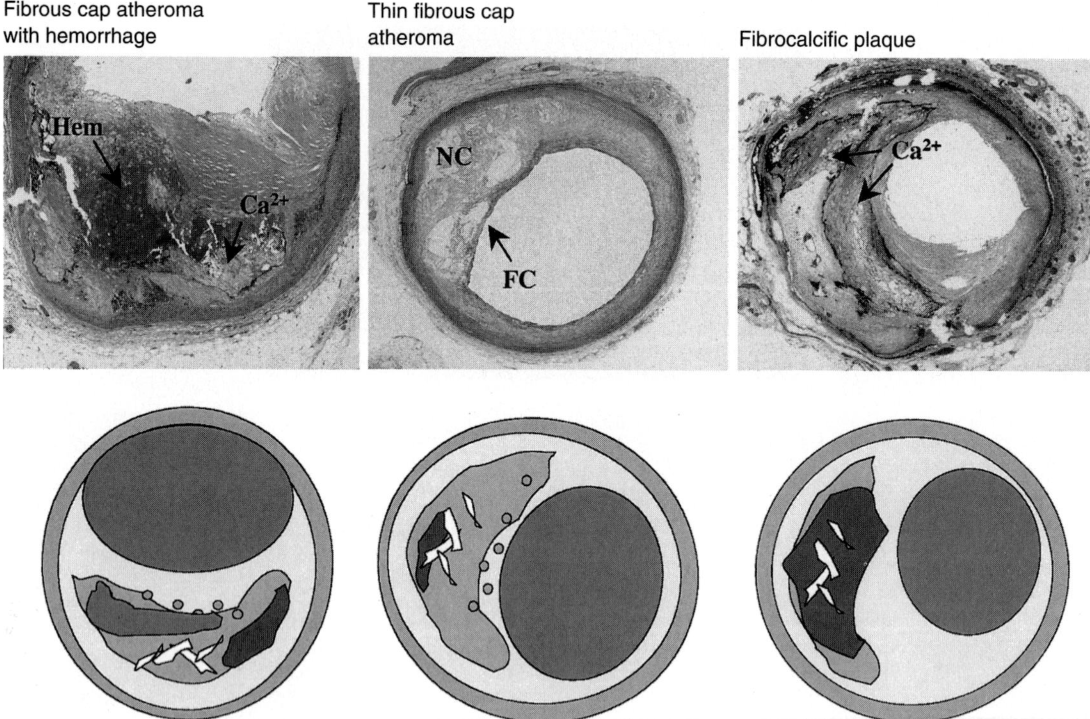

Figure 2–7. Variants of fibrous cap atheromas. *Fibroatheromas with intraplaque hemorrhage* are lesions with a necrotic core containing red blood cells and fibrin. The fibrous cap is mature and deep within the intima are areas of calcification. *Atrophic fibrous cap atheromas,* often referred to in the literature as "vulnerable plaques," are lesions with large necrotic cores containing numerous cholesterol clefts. The overlying atrophic fibrous cap (*FC*) is thin (< 65 mm) and is heavily infiltrated by macrophages; smooth muscle cells are rare and vasa vasorum are present within the adventitia and plaque. *Fibrocalcific plaques* are referred to as "stable" lesions in the literature. These lesions are predominantly comprised of dense collagen containing a few scattered smooth muscle cells and inflammatory cells; when present, the necrotic core is small. These lesions are often heavily calcified and it is difficult to determine previous hemorrhage and/or thrombosis that may be responsible for the plaque size. (Virmani et al. Lessons from sudden coronary death. Arterioscler Thromb Vasc Biol 20:1269, 2000, with permission.)

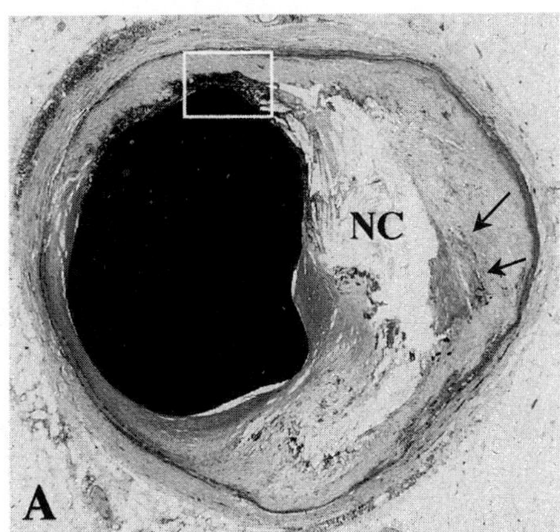

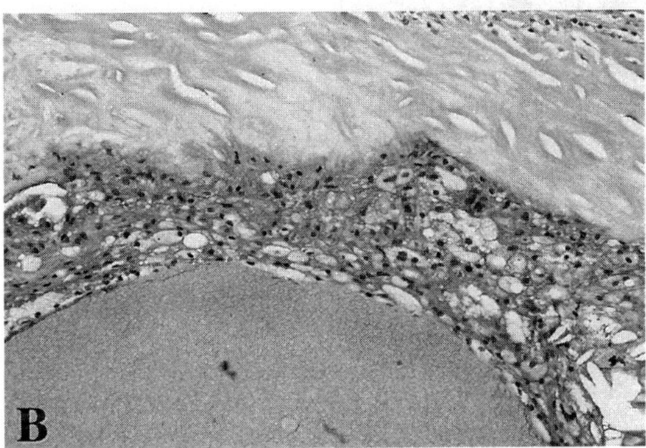

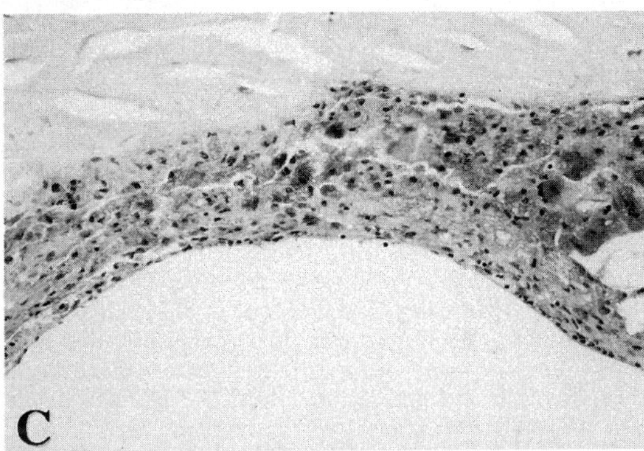

Figure 2–8. Vulnerable plaque (thin-capped atheroma). *A* (*top*) demonstrates a fibroatheroma with large necrotic core (*NC*) with focal calcification (*arrows*). The boxed area is at the shoulder region of the plaque. The black substance within the lumen is contrast material injected postmortem. *B* (*bottom left*) demonstrates a high magnification of a different thin-capped atheroma. The cap is infiltrated by macrophages, which are stained with anti-CD68 (*right*).

presence of the latter in plaques provides indirect evidence for local interferon-γ (INF-γ) secretion. In early lesions, macrophages outnumber lymphocytes by 10 to 50 times, and CD8 cells predominate over CD4 cells with a ratio of 2:1.[41, 42] However, in advanced plaques, there is a switch to a greater number of CD4 lymphocytes, with activation of HLA class II antigens.

The progression of a stable fibroatheroma into a rupture-prone thin-cap fibroatheroma is under intense investigation. Although a number of matrix metalloproteinases (MMPs) have been implicated in thinning of the fibrous cap, it is unclear when they become critical to lesion instability because they are present in abundance in early plaque.[43] However, one such MMP, stromelysin-3—a member of the serpin family—has been shown to colocalize with CD40 on endothelial cells, smooth muscle cells, and monocytes in advanced human atheroma. Activated T-lymphocytes express the CD40 ligand surface molecule, which, when activated, promotes the expression of adhesion molecules, cytokines, MMPs, and tissue factor.[44] Thus, the regulation of stromelysin-3 by ligand CD40 may be crucial to the progression of stable plaque to one prone to rupture and thrombosis.[45] Interruption of CD40L-CD40 signaling by administration of an anti-CD40L antibody has been demonstrated to limit atherosclerosis in mice lacking the receptor for low-density lipoprotein by inhibition of CD40 signaling (antibody directed against CD154 pathway).[44]

Coronary Thrombi

Plaque Rupture

Fibrous cap disruption resulting in continuity between the overlying thrombus and the necrotic core defines plaque rupture (Figs. 2–9 and 2–10). Ruptured lesions typically have a large necrotic core and a disrupted fibrous cap infiltrated by macrophages. The trigger for

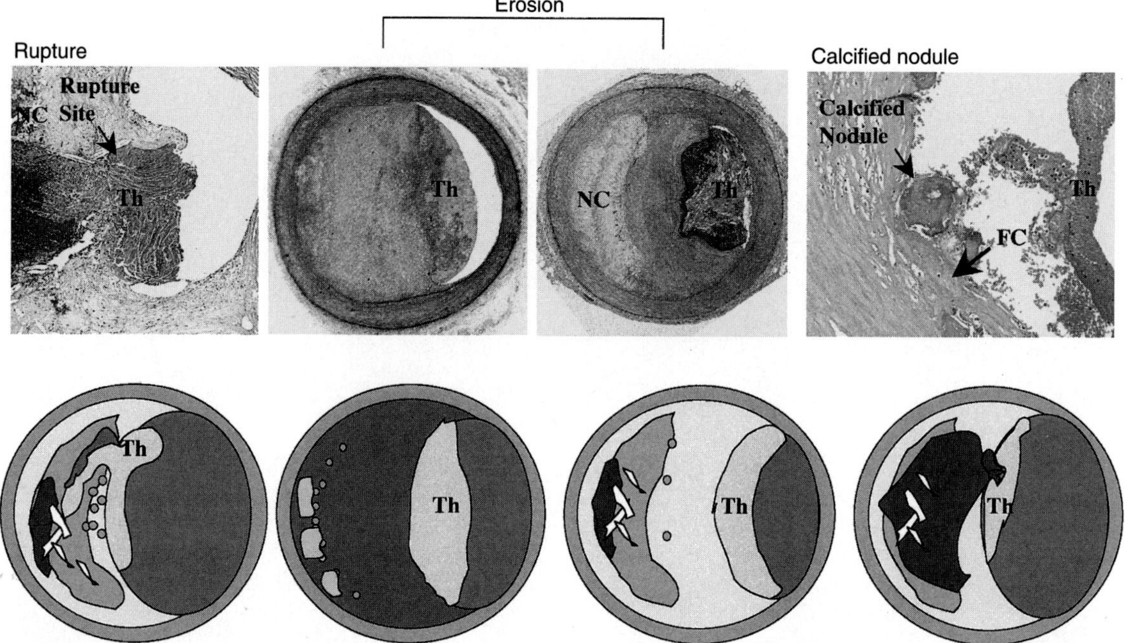

Figure 2–9. Atherosclerotic lesions with luminal thrombi. *Ruptured plaques* are atrophic fibrous cap atheromas with luminal thrombi (*Th*). These lesions usually have an extensive necrotic core containing large numbers of cholesterol crystals, and a thin fibrous cap (< 65 μm) infiltrated by foamy macrophages and a paucity of T-lymphocytes. The fibrous cap is thinnest at the site of rupture and consists of a few collagen bundles and rare smooth muscle cells. The luminal thrombus is in communication with the lipid rich necrotic core. *Erosions* occur over lesions rich in smooth muscle cells and proteoglycans. Luminal thrombi overly areas lacking surface endothelium. The deep intima of the eroded plaque often shows extracellular lipid pools, but necrotic cores are uncommon; when present, the necrotic core does not communicate with the luminal thrombus. Inflammatory infiltrate is usually absent; but, if present, is sparse and consists of macrophages and lymphocytes. A high-power view of the eroded surface indicated by a box is shown in Figure 2–8 for comparison with a similar eroded area of a thrombosed region adjacent to a ruptured plaque. *Calcified nodules* are plaques with luminal thrombi showing calcific nodules protruding into the lumen through a disrupted atrophic fibrous cap (*FC*). There is absence of endothelium at the site of the thrombus and inflammatory cells are absent (Virmani et al. Lessons from sudden coronary death. Arterioscler Thromb Vasc Biol 20:1268, 2000, with permission.)

plaque rupture is the object of intense study, and is likely related to those conditions that result in thinning of the fibroatheromatous cap (see preceding).

The density of macrophages at the site of rupture is typically very high, although in some cases, macrophages may be relatively sparse. In our experience, occasional neutrophils are not infrequently seen in plaque ruptures. In our own laboratory, we have shown that T-lymphocytes are present in 75% of ruptures.[46] Although macrophage density is maximal in plaque rupture, the number of T-lymphocytes do not vary among culprit lesions. The smooth muscle cell content within the fibrous cap at the rupture site is typically low. A majority of investigators have emphasized the importance of cytokine-mediated degradation of the fibrous cap. For example, Amento and colleagues in the laboratory of Peter Libby have shown the importance of interferon gamma (INF-γ), which markedly decreases the ability of human smooth muscle cells to express interstitial collagen genes.[47] Besides the inhibition of collagen synthesis, INF-γ may also inhibit proliferation and promote apoptosis of SMC.[48, 49] Moreover, INF-γ activates macrophages, which are rich in matrix metalloproteins (MMPs) that may promote the breakdown of collagen, proteoglycans, and elastins.[50, 51]

The MMPs consist of at least 16 zinc-dependent endopeptidases that possess catalytic activity against extracellular matrix.[52] *In vitro* studies have shown that several inflammatory mediators modulate the expression of MMPs.[51] Tumor necrosis factor-α and interleukin-1 increase MMP-1, MMP-3, and MMP-9 expression in SMCs and macrophages,[53–55] while interleukin-4, INF-γ, and interleukin-10 inhibit their synthesis.[56] MMPs

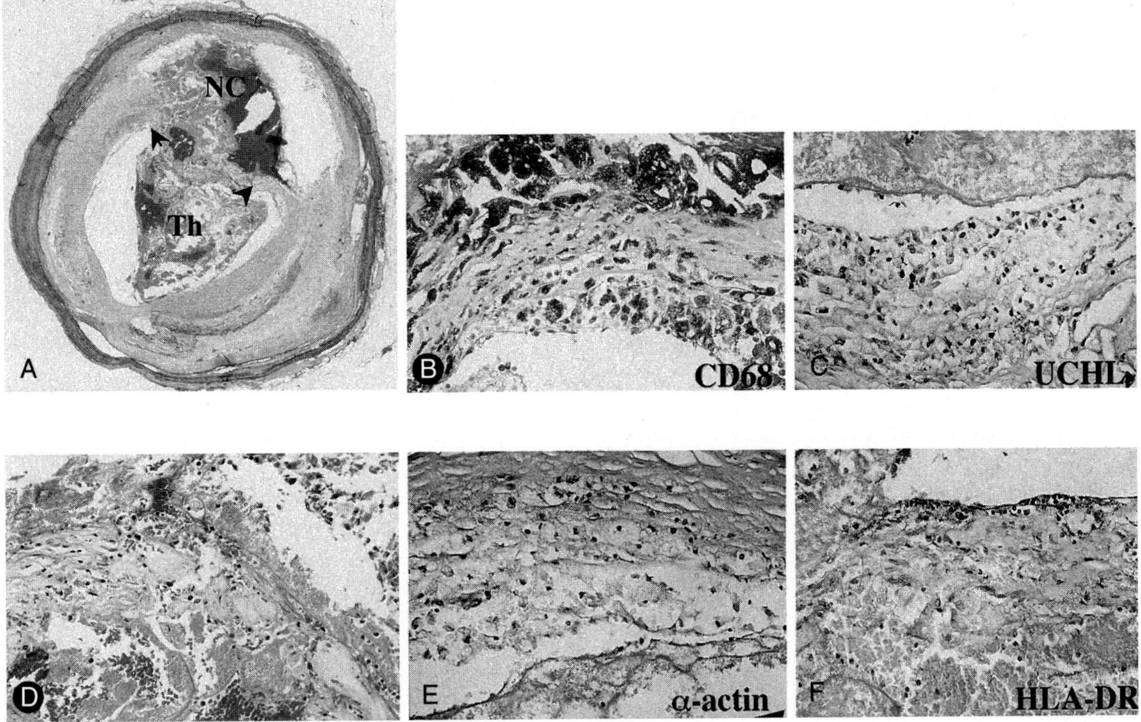

Figure 2–10. Acute thrombosis of the left anterior descending coronary artery was found in this 54-year-old man with witnessed cardiac arrest and death 2.5 hours after the onset of chest pain. A plaque with a large hemorrhagic lipid necrotic core (*NC*) and focal calcification is seen in *A* at low power; an occlusive thrombus (*Th*) is present. Arrowheads point to the edges of the ruptured cap. The edges of the rupture cap are illustrated at higher magnification (*D,* high power). Immunohistochemical staining demonstrates abundant macrophages (in *B*), an absence of smooth muscle cells (in *E*), and scattered T-cells (in *C*) with HLA-DR positive macrophages and T-cells (in *F*). (*A:* Movat pentachrome; *B:* Movat pentachrome; *C:* anti-KP-1; *D:* anti-smooth muscle actin; *E:* anti-UCHL-1; *F:* anti-HLA-DR). (Modified from Farb et al. Coronary plaque erosion without rupture into a lipid core. Circulation 93:1356, 1996, with permission.)

are also inhibited by endogenous tissue inhibitors of metalloproteinases (TIMPs).[57] Breakdown of fibrous cap collagen by MMPs released from monocyte-derived macrophages have been shown *in vitro* and lipid-laden macrophages from atherosclerotic plaques elaborate MMP-1 and MMP-3.[58] Although MMPs are a common finding in animal models of atherosclerosis, to our knowledge no one has been able to demonstrate plaque rupture in lesions where a necrotic core and fibrous cap are known to be present.[7] There is, however, direct evidence for collagenolysis within the fibrous cap from a study by Sukhova et al. in the laboratory of Peter Libby, which demonstrates collagenase-cleaved type I collagen by a novel cleavage-specific antibody.[59] Interestingly, type I collagen fragments were co-localized with MMP-1- and MMP-13-positive macrophages. Moreover, increased collagenolysis was found in atheromatous versus fibrous plaques and was associated with higher levels of proinflammatory cytokines, activators of MMPs.

Plaque Erosion

Erosion is a mechanism of plaque disruption that does not involve thinning of the fibrous cap (Figs. 2–9 and 2–11). The morphologic characteristics of plaque erosion include abundance of smooth muscle cells in a proteoglycan-rich matrix, and disruption of the surface endothelium without a prominent lipid core.[42, 46] The necrotic core is often absent in plaque erosion; when present, it is an insignificant part of the plaque, and on serial cuts does not communicate with the thrombus. Compared to rupture sites in thin-capped fibroatheroma, plaque erosion contains relatively few or no macrophages, and the numbers of T-lymphocytes are decreased compared with those found in ruptures[46] (Table 2–3). Erosions account for ap-

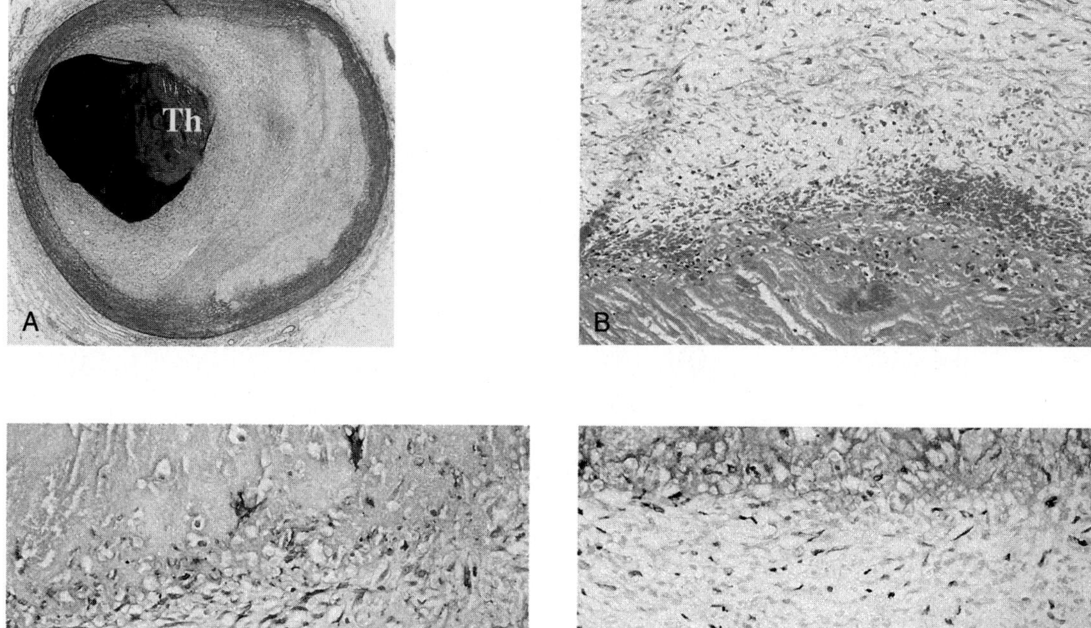

Figure 2–11. This 33-year-old woman had sudden collapse and witnessed cardiac arrest shortly after eating. Acute thrombosis of the left anterior descending coronary artery was found at autopsy, and the thrombosed segment is shown at low power in *A*. An eccentric plaque containing a nonocclusive thrombus (*Th*) is present, and the remainder of the lumen is filled with dark-gray barium gelatin. The eroded plaque surface is seen at high power in *B*, and numerous spindle-shaped cells are present in the plaque. The thrombus consists predominately of platelets, and the luminal plaque surface is cellular and rich in proteoglycans (green color by Movat staining in *A*). In *C*, actin immunohistochemical staining identifies the cells at the luminal surface in contact with the thrombus as smooth muscle cells. Occasional macrophages are present in the plaque and thrombus (in *D*). (*A:* Movat pentachrome × 5; *B:* hematoxylin-eosin ×150; *C:* anti-KP-1, × 300; *D:* anti-smooth muscle actin, × 300). (Modified from Farb et al. Coronary plaque erosion without rupture into a lipid core. Circulation 93:1358, 1996, with permission.)

proximately 35% of cases of thrombotic sudden coronary death, and are especially common in young women and men. These lesions are usually eccentric, rarely show calcification, and normally result in less severe narrowing than plaque rupture (Table 2–3). Currently, we have little understanding of the mechanisms of erosion. Besides the thrombus, the most striking aspects of this lesion are the absence of endothelium and the "activated" appearance of the underlying smooth muscle cells. Smooth muscle cells at the site of erosion are bizarre in shape and contain hyperchromatic nuclei with prominent nucleoli. It has been postulated that erosions result from vasospasm, and are often found in cigarette smokers.[14, 35] The role of inflammation in the pathogenesis of erosion, especially that of lymphocytic infiltrates has yet to be elucidated.

Calcified Nodule

A third lesion, albeit an infrequent cause of thrombotic occlusion without rupture, is referred to as a "calcified nodule" (Fig. 2–9). This term refers to a lesion with fibrous cap disruption and thrombi associated with eruptive, dense, calcified nodules.[18] The origin of this lesion is not precisely known, but appears to be associated with healed plaque ruptures. These lesions are found in the middle right coronary artery, where coronary torsion stress is maximal. It is unclear whether the fibrous cap wears down from physical forces exerted

Table 2–3. Coronary Thrombosis with Rupture into a Lipid Core (Plaque Rupture) Compared with Thrombosis Associated with Eroded Plaque without Lipid Pool Rupture (Plaque Erosion)

	Plaque Rupture (n = 28)	Plaque Erosion (n = 22)	p Value
Male : Female	23 : 5	11 : 11	0.03
Age (years)	53 ± 10	44 ± 7	<0.02
% Stenosis	78 ± 12	70 ± 11	<0.03
Calcified Plaque	19 (69%)	5 (23%)	0.002
Occlusive: Non-occlusive Thrombus	12 : 16	4 : 18	0.08
	(43%:57%)	(18%:82%)	
Concentric: Eccentric	13 : 15	4 : 18	0.07
	(46%:54%)	(18%:82%)	
Macrophages	28 (100%)	11 (50%)	<0.0001
T-cells	21 (75%)	7 (32%)	<0.004
Smooth muscle cells	11 (33%)	21 (95%)	<0.0001
HLA-DR positive	25 (89%)	8 (36%)	0.0002

Farb et al. Coronary plaque erosion without rupture into a lipid core. Circulation 93:1358, 1996, with permission.

by the nodules themselves, or proteases from the surrounding infiltrate, or both.

Healed Ruptures/Erosions

A disrupted fibrous cap where the thrombus is replaced by smooth muscle cells and proteoglycan, and collagen matrix characterize healed rupture (Figs. 2–12 and 2–13). Healed ruptures can be easily identified on Movat pentachrome staining (healed sites recognized by brilliant blue-green color), and may be further confirmed by picrosirius red staining and polarization microscopy.[60, 61] When viewed under polarized light, this special stain highlights collagen types III and I differentially, enabling visualization of interruptions in the fibrous cap. Healed sites consisted of breaks in collagen type I (yellow-red birefringence) overlying a necrotic core with superimposed layer of collagen type III (green birefringence). The matrix within the healed fibrous cap defect may consist of a proteoglycan-rich mass or a collagen-rich scar, depending on the phase of healing. Lesions with healed ruptures may exhibit multilayering of lipid and necrotic core, suggestive of previous episodes of thrombosis.

Thrombotic Total Occlusions and Thrombus Propagation and Embolism

Fresh occlusion is identified by a luminal thrombus containing platelet aggregates interspersed with inflammatory cells and a paucity of red cells (Fig. 2–9). The thrombus, however, often propagates from its original site and becomes fibrin-rich and contains interspersed red cells and leukocytes. In a fresh thrombus, there is no evidence of invasion by endothelial cells and/or smooth muscle cells. Little is known of the mechanism(s) involved in thrombus propagation and embolization. It has long been appreciated, however, that platelet aggregates within intramyocardial (mural) arteries may play a role in sudden ischemic death. It has been demonstrated that the majority of such aggregation occurs downstream from a thrombus within an epicardial artery.[62]

Old Occlusion

Old occlusions (chronic total occlusions) demonstrate luminal obstruction by dense collagen and/or proteoglycan with interspersed capillaries, arterioles, smooth muscle cells, and inflammatory cells (Fig. 2–12). These lesions may also demonstrate earlier phases of organizing thrombi containing fibrin, red blood cells, and granulation tissue, especially in the midportion of a long, occluded arterial segment. The significance of these lesions is primarily clinical, in that they may be difficult to successfully balloon percutaneously. At autopsy, total occlusions are typically associated with transmural infarcts in the region of the affected artery. Total occlusions often demonstrate shrinkage of the artery, perhaps due to the effect of collagen within the plaque and/or adventitia.

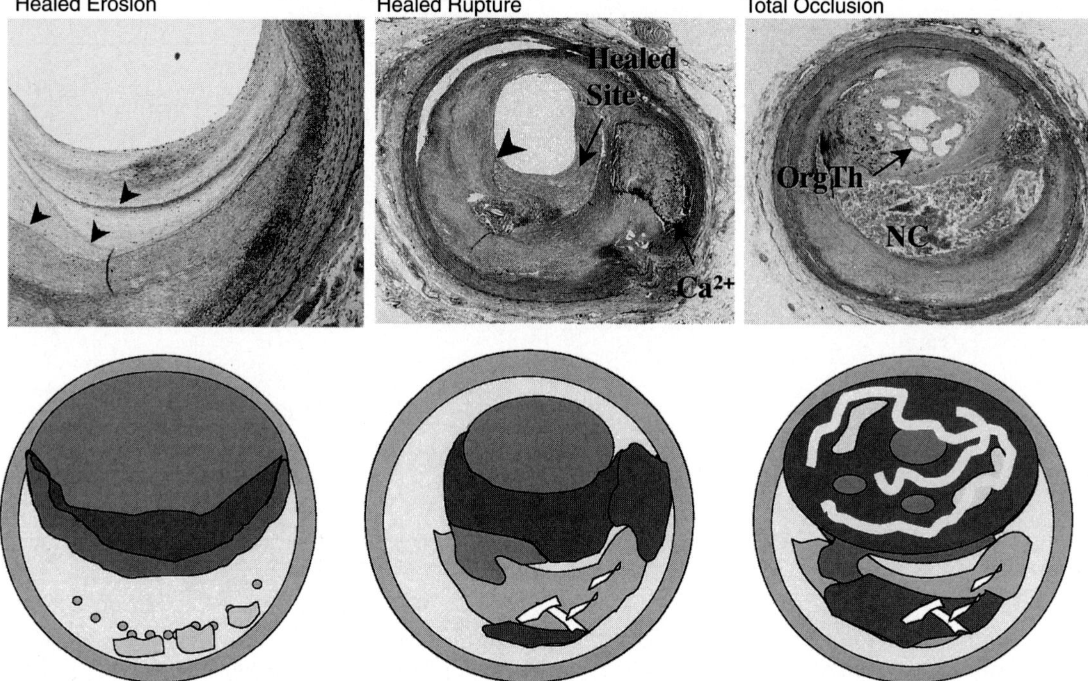

Figure 2–12. *Healed erosion* shows deep multilayering of collagen separated by elastin layers and a paucity of smooth muscle cells. The superficial plaque is rich in smooth muscle cells, collagen, and proteoglycans. *Healed ruptures* are lesions with rupture of the fibrous cap (*arrowhead*) over a necrotic core. The plaque overlying the disrupted cap (healed site) consists of smooth muscle cells and proteoglycan matrix and collagen (*arrow*). Plaques with *total occlusion* from prior thrombi contain mostly smooth muscle cells in a collagen-proteoglycan-rich matrix with capillaries and inflammatory cell infiltrate. This section shows a necrotic core (*NC*), although not always present, and the lumen is filled with an organized thrombus (*orgTh*) with multiple capillary channels. (Virmani et al. Lessons from sudden death. Arterioscler Thromb Vasc Biol 20:1271, 2000 with permission.)

Lesions Not Necessarily Associated with Thrombi

Fibrocalcific Lesions

Some plaques have thick fibrous caps overlying extensive accumulations of calcium in the intima close to the media. Because the lipid-laden necrotic core, if present, is usually small, we refer to this category of lesion as a fibrocalcific rather than an atheroma (Fig. 2–7). Of course, as shown in Figure 2–1, it is possible that the fibrocalcific lesion is the end stage of a process of atheromatous plaque rupture and/or erosion with healing and calcification.

Intraplaque Hemorrhage

Constantinides originally suggested that hemorrhage into a plaque occurs from cracks or fissures originating from the luminal surface.[63] Davies and Thomas later defined plaque fissure as an eccentric intraplaque hemorrhage with fibrin deposition within the necrotic core from "an entry into the plaque from the lumen."[64] The fissuring of the fibrous cap occurs at its thinnest portion, typically at the shoulder region allowing the entry of blood into the necrotic core. Although fissures lead to intraplaque hemorrhage, unless rupture occurs, it is unlikely that fissures cause death because hemorrhage is often found in the absence of luminal thrombi. However, as Davies suggested, plaque fissures may represent precursors or subtypes of plaque rupture.[65–68] Nonetheless, plaque fissures are often incidental findings in advanced plaques in deaths not attributed to cardiovascular causes.[69]

Alternatively, Paterson proposed that intraplaque hemorrhage is secondary to rupture of vasa-vasorum, a common feature of advanced lesions with plaque rupture and luminal thrombi.[70] In our series of sudden coronary death cases, hemorrhage into a plaque is most

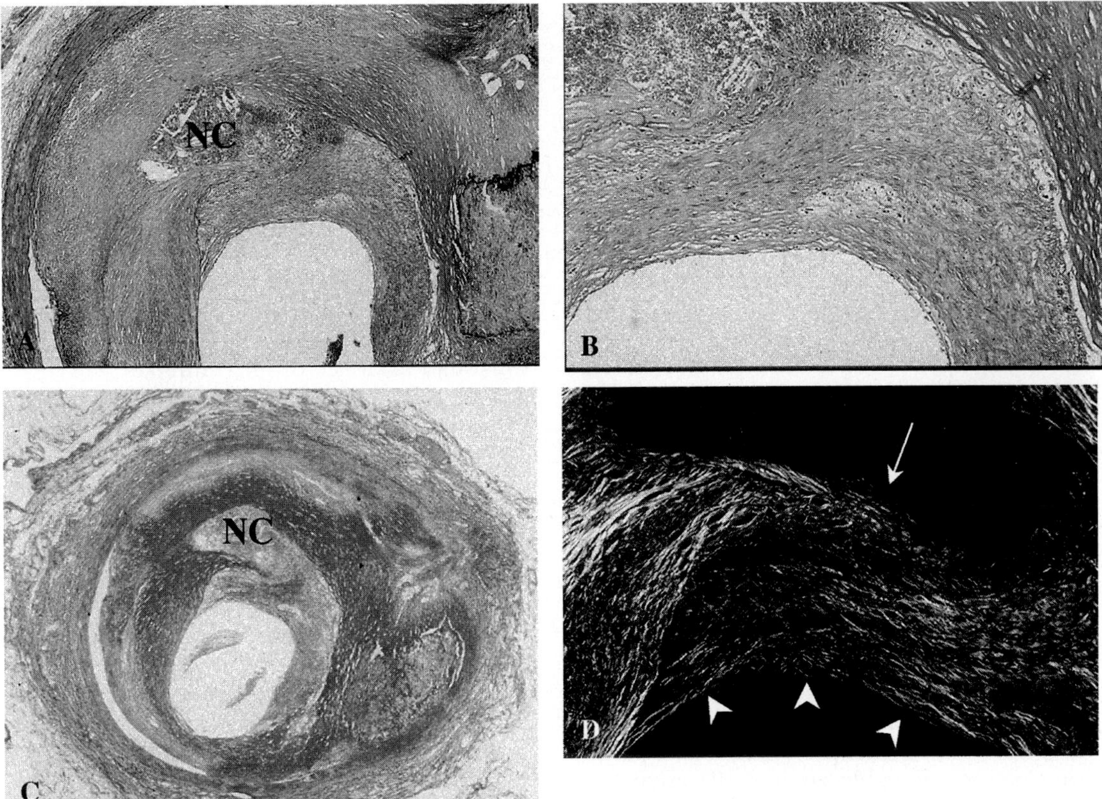

Figure 2–13. Healed plaque rupture. *A* demonstrates areas of intra-intimal lipid-rich core with hemorrhage and cholesterol clefts within the necrotic core (*NC*). *B* shows a higher magnification of the looser smooth muscle cell formation within a collagenous proteoglycan-rich neointima showing a clear demarcation with the more fibrous regions of the old plaque to the right. *C* and *D* demonstrate the layers of collagen by Sirius red staining. *C*, note the area of dense dark red collagen surrounding the lipid hemorrhagic cores seen in corresponding view in panel *A*. *D* demonstrates an image taken with polarized light. The dense collagen (type 1) which forms the fibrous cap is lighter reddish-yellow and is disrupted (*arrow*), with the newer greenish type III collagen on the right and above the rupture site. (*A* and *B*, Movat pentachrome).

frequent in ruptured plaques, but is also observed in lesions with only 40–50% cross-sectional luminal narrowing.

PATHOBIOLOGIC CORRELATES OF CORONARY ATHEROSCLEROSIS

Stable Angina

Clinical

Angina pectoris is a retrosternal chest discomfort or pain, which usually radiates to the arm and is caused by myocardial ischemia and is brought on by exertion. William Heberden (1772) is credited with the first description of stable angina.[71] William Osler in the 19th century associated the angina pectoris with obstruction and calcification of the coronary arteries.[72] The pathophysiologic explanation for the mechanism of chest pain is attributed to Gorlin, which was published in 1965, when the concept of myocardial oxygen supply and demand were articulated.[73] Typically, chest pain is relieved by rest or by nitroglycerin within minutes.

Pathologic Findings

The coronary arteries in patients with stable angina almost always show > 75% cross-sectional area luminal narrowing, equivalent to 50% diameter reduction. The associated plaque consists of either a calcified lipid-rich fibrous plaque (60%) or a predominantly pure fibrous lesion (40%).[74] The lumen may be either eccentric (when there is an associated arc of normal coronary artery wall) (76%) or concentric (when there is no arch of normal arterial wall)

(24%), and 40% are lipid rich with or without a hemorrhage and the others are fibrous plaque. There are usually no acute thrombi from either plaque rupture or plaque erosion identified in patients dying with stable angina. However, recanalized thrombi have been described in 79% of patients with isolated stable angina, and the iron deposition (a marker of plaque hemorrhage) within plaques is seen in 77% of cases.[74] From this high an incidence of recanalized thrombi in patients with stable angina, it can be inferred that plaque fissures and/or plaque hemorrhage and thrombosis culminate in stable angina with flow limiting lesion morphology. Sex differences in plaque morphology in patients with stable angina have not been reported.

Unstable Angina

Clinical

Unstable angina—also known as preinfarction angina, crescendo angina, or acute coronary insufficiency—is characterized by (1) crescendo angina superimposed on a preexisting pattern of stable angina, (2) angina of new onset (usually within 1 month) brought on by minimal exertion, or (3) angina at rest. The number of patients admitted to the hospital in the United States with unstable angina exceeds 570,000 per year.[75] It is reported that at least half the patients admitted with acute myocardial infarction have a prodrome of unstable angina.[76] Diagnosis of unstable angina requires absence of electrocardiographic (Q-wave or non-Q wave myocardial infarction) and cardiac enzyme changes (CK activity > 200 IU/L and CK-MB > 6.7 ng/mL) diagnostic of myocardial infarction.[77] At least 25% of patient with unstable angina have cardiac troponin I or T elevated; death and myocardial infarction is more frequent in those with elevated troponin I.[77] Clinically, all show at least one or more coronary arteries with > 50% diameter reduction and by angioscopy over 70% of patients show presence of luminal thrombi.[78] Platelet aggregation is believed to be the underlying mechanism of unstable angina but other factors may also play a role.[79, 80]

Pathologic Findings

Pathologic studies involving patients with unstable angina have shown significant variability in the incidence of acute thrombus. In two studies from the same laboratory, plaque hemorrhage was found in 64% of patients, plaque rupture in 36%, and acute luminal thrombi in 29%.[81, 82] In an earlier study, Guthrie et al.[83] found that 6 of 12 patients with unstable angina who had died during bypass had luminal coronary thrombosis. Falk et al. reported the highest incidence of thrombosis (81%) in patients who died within 24 hours of symptoms of progressing chest pain (unstable angina). In Falk et al.'s studies, no patient at autopsy had subendocardial or transmural infarction and about one third had evidence of microinfarcts.[84, 85]

The variability in the incidence of thrombosis at autopsy in patients with unstable angina probably reflects patient selection and the criteria used to diagnose unstable angina and myocardial infarction. However, because unstable angina often precedes acute myocardial infarction, it is not surprising that the incidence of thrombosis is high. Atherectomy specimens removed from patients with angina show a higher incidence of thrombosis in unstable angina than in stable angina; the incidence in unstable angina is equivalent to patients with acute myocardial infarction.[86, 87] In morphologic studies of autopsy patients dying with unstable angina, the atherosclerotic plaque often showed presence of a necrotic core, and are often calcified.

Prinzmetal's Angina or Variant Angina

The chest pain in Prinzmetal's angina occurs exclusively at rest, is usually not precipitated by exertion or emotional stress, and is associated with electrocardiographic ST-segment elevation.[88] Patients with variant angina are younger than patients with stable or unstable angina and usually do not have the classic risk-factor profile, except that they are often smokers. The mechanism has been convincingly shown to be secondary to coronary artery spasm: there is transient, abrupt, focal, marked reduction in the diameter of the epicardial artery. The site of vasospasm is usually adjacent to an atheromatous plaque. The mechanism is poorly understood and has been thought to involve hypercoagulability, endothelial injury, and hypercontractility of vascular medial smooth muscle cells due to liberation of vasoconstrictors like leukotrienes, serotonin, and histamine.[89] We have shown presence of noncritical stenosis from atherosclerosis at the site of vasospasm in a 33-year-old man with Prinzmetal's angina at autopsy who had excessive mast cells in the adventitia and only moderate atherosclerosis.[90]

Acute Myocardial Infarction

Clinical

Patients with acute myocardial infarction present with persistent, crushing, severe chest pain usually lasting > 30 minutes, often accompanied by a sensation of constriction and squeezing. Often the chest pain is retrosternal, radiating to the left arm and producing a tingling sensation in the hand and fingers. In 50% of patients there is accompanying nausea and vomiting. In the elderly, acute myocardial infarct may not present as chest pain, but as acute left ventricular failure.[91] World Health Organization criteria for the diagnosis of AMI requires that at least 2 of 3 elements be present: chest pain or discomfort, evolutionary changes on ECG (ST-segment elevation and Q waves), and a rise and a fall in serum cardiac markers (creatinine kinase and cardiac-specific isoenzymes, myoglobin, and cardiac-specific troponins [T or I]).

Pathologic Findings

There is a greater agreement between clinical and morphologic studies in acute myocardial infarction, as compared with unstable angina. Almost all myocardial infarctions occur from underlying atherosclerotic coronary disease with superimposed thrombus; in patients with electrocardiographic evidence of acute myocardial infarction, angiographically thrombi have been demonstrated to be present in 90%.[92] In necropsy studies the frequency of thrombi has varied from 50 to 98%.[113] This variability can partly be explained by the duration of symptoms to death.[64,93] Davies et al. reported rupture of a thin fibrous cap and an overlying thrombus in 75% of patients dying with acute myocardial infarction,[94] whereas Arbustini et al. demonstrate acute thrombi in 98% of patients, who had a mean age of 66, dying with myocardial infarction diagnosed by ECG and enzyme changes.[113] In Arbustini et al.'s series, 25% of thrombi were caused by plaque erosions, and 75% by plaque rupture; 37% of thrombi in women were erosions, as compared with 18% in men. Analysis of morphologic characteristics of atherosclerotic plaques from patients with acute myocardial infarction has suggested that plaques are rich in lipid and are often calcified, and plaque hemorrhage is seen in 90% of cases.[93] Plaque hemorrhage, calcification, and large necrotic cores are all features of plaque rupture, which is the morphologic substrate for a large proportion of patients dying with acute myocardial infarction.

It has been reported that at the site of thrombi in patients with acute myocardial infarction, the amount of underlying luminal narrowing is often < 50% diameter reduction.[95] Although thrombi are more likely to occur at sites of severe stenosis than in smaller plaques,[96] the number of sites for potential rupture with moderate narrowing is far greater. The characteristics, including luminal narrowing, of plaques that rupture are important to define in order to identify them before thrombosis occurs. Unfortunately, there is currently no method available, invasive or otherwise, that accurately pinpoints those plaques vulnerable to form thrombosis resulting in infarction.

Sudden Coronary Death

Definition

Sudden coronary death (SCD) (Table 2–4) signifies rapid death before evolution of symptoms that result in the diagnosis of a specific ischemic syndrome. It is important to have a uniform definition of SCD in order to better understand the pathogenetic mechanisms. The World Health Organization defines SD as death within 24 hours of symptoms, a time interval lengthy enough to result in inclusion of cases of acute myocardial infarction. We prefer the time limit of 6 hours (as histologic features of myocardial infarction will not develop within this time frame), although other definitions are even more strict, using a 1-hour cut off or instantaneous death.

Pathologic Findings

By definition, sudden death is considered coronary if at least one epicardial artery demonstrates greater than 75% cross-sectional area luminal narrowing by atherosclerotic plaque, or if there is an acute thrombus overlying a plaque of any severity. Because focally severe coronary disease may be found in noncoronary deaths, exclusion of other causes of deaths is essential before assigning a diagnosis of SCD (see Chapter 10). The incidence of various morphologic features in SCD varies by the definitions of SCD used and the patient population; these are dis-

Table 2–4. Distribution of Culprit Plaques by Sex and Age in 241 Cases of Sudden Coronary Death

	Acute Thrombi					
	Rupture	**Erosion**	**Calcified Nodule**	**Organized Thrombi**	**No Thrombi: Fibrocalcific Plaque**	**Totals**
Men						
< 50 years	46%	17%	2%	15%	20%	99
> 50 years	23%	10%	4%	33%	31%	83
Women						
< 50 years	3%	42%	0	15%	40%	33
> 50 years	35%	23%	4%	19%	19%	26
Totals	31%	19%	2%	22%*	26%¶	241

* 89% of these demonstrate healed myocardial infarct
¶ 50% of these have healed myocardial infarct
From Virmani et al. Lessons from sudden coronary death. Arterioscler Thromb Vasc Biol 20:1265, 2000, with permission.

cussed in Chapter 10. Briefly, the rate of acute thrombus ranges from 19% to 73%,[97, 98] with an intermediate frequency in our experience.[14,35,36] Healed myocardial infarction has been reported to be present in 75% of hearts in patients dying from SCD, whereas acute myocardial infarct is said to be present in 20 to 30% of cases.[99, 100] We have observed much lower incidence of healed myocardial infarction (40%) in patients with SCD but the incidence of acute myocardial infarction was similar (20%).[36]

Clinicopathologic Correlates of Plaque Rupture and Erosion

Until recently it was reported that symptomatic thrombotic coronary artery disease was caused solely from rupture of a thin fibrous cap.[84, 98] We have recently reported that thrombi in sudden coronary death may occur from three distinctly differently plaque morphologies.[18] The two most common lesions that account for 95% of all thrombi are plaque rupture and plaque erosion; least frequent is the ruptured calcified nodule. Plaque erosion is seen in younger individuals and is the most common form of thrombus in premenopausal women. In contrast to rupture, erosions are less often calcified, more often nonocclusive, and more often eccentric.[46]

As discussed earlier, the traditional risk factors for coronary disease include serum cholesterol, serum HDL-C, smoking hypertension, and diabetes mellitus. Elevated triglycerides are also a risk factor for coronary disease, but are often not an independent predictor in multivariate analysis when HDL-C is included, as triglycerides are inversely correlated with HDL-C. Obesity, as discussed earlier, is not considered a risk factor for coronary disease in many studies, although specific measurements of hip/waist or hip/height ratios are better correlated with atherosclerosis when compared to body mass index. We have correlated the association of traditional risk factors to plaque morphology in men and women dying suddenly with severe coronary disease.[14, 35] In 113 men, we determined the risk factors at autopsy by biochemical analysis of serum for total cholesterol (TC), HDL-C, TC/HDL ratio, and serum thiocyanate, a surrogate marker for smoking. Red cell glycosylated hemoglobin was used to determine presence of glucose intolerance. We observed that risk factors were present in 96.5% of sudden coronary death. Smoking was a predictor of acute thrombosis regardless of etiology, and plaque rupture correlated with high total cholesterol, low HDL-cholesterol, and a high TC/HDL-cholesterol ratio (Table 2–5). We also observed that as the cholesterol rose, so did the incidence of vulnerable plaque increase (Table 2–6).

We have observed in women that plaque erosion is highly correlated with smoking and is mostly seen in women < 50 years (Table 2–7). In contrast, plaque rupture is more frequent in women > 50 years and correlated with elevated total cholesterol.[14] Vulnerable plaques are more frequently seen in women > 50 years than < 50 years. Stable plaque with healed myocardial infarction is seen more frequently in women with ≥ 10% glycohemoglobin.[14]

The associations demonstrate that the morphologic heterogeneity of coronary atherothrombosis has an underlying pathogenetic basis. The fact that plaque erosion is not associated with elevated levels of cholesterol, in con-

Table 2–5. Risk Factors and Presence of Coronary Thrombosis in 113 Men Who Died Suddenly with Severe Coronary Artery Disease

Risk Factor	Acute Thrombus (n = 59)	Stable Plaque (n = 54)	P value (univariate)	P value (multivariate)†
Cigarette smokers (n, %)	44 (75%)	22 (41%)	< 0.001	0.004
Age, mean (years)	47.3 ± 8.9	52.7 ± 11.0	0.005	0.24
Hypertension (n, %)	11 (19%)	23 (43%)	0.008	0.22
Total cholesterol, mg/deciliter	249 ± 62	222 ± 100	0.08	> 0.4§
High density lipoprotein cholesterol, mg/deciliter	39 ± 15	45 ± 18	0.10	0.16
Black: White	11:48	16:38	0.19	0.38
Glycosylated hemoglobin, percent	7.6 ± 2.1	7.5 ± 2.5	0.90	> 0.4§

§ Dropped from analysis
† By logistic stepwise regression, P value to remove
Burke et al. Coronary risk factors and plaque morphology in patients with coronary disease dying suddenly. N Engl J Med 336:1276, 1997, with permission.

trast to rupture may explain why some individuals with normal lipid profiles suffer from severe coronary disease. The precise risk factor related to plaque erosion still remains elusive, but unpublished data suggest that thrombotic factors, in addition to vasospasm, may be important. Cigarette smoking appears to increase the likelihood of fatal thrombosis, regardless of etiology. It remains to be seen if newer risk factors, including homocysteine and polymorphisms for hemostatic factors, are associated specifically with one form of thrombosis or another.

Clinicopathologic Correlates of Healed Plaque Rupture

We have found healed ruptures are present in over 50% of patients dying with severe coronary disease. They are seen in three of four hearts that demonstrate an acute rupture site, but less than one of four hearts with an acute erosion, indicating that plaque ruptures tend to occur repeatedly in those patients with risk factors predisposing to the formation of thin-capped atheromas.[61] These risk factors include elevated total cholesterol and the ratio of total to high density lipoprotein cholesterol, elevated glycohemoglobin, a marker for glucose intolerance, and increased body mass index. We have also observed that layering of multiple prior rupture sites are present in areas of severe cross-sectional luminal narrowing. Therefore, healed ruptures are frequently observed in hypercholesterolemic, obese men with glucose intolerance, and may represent a mechanism of plaque progression. It is likely that the increased numbers of healed infarcts in patients with evidence of prior acute rupture indicate that nonlethal ruptures may, in some cases, result in silent myocardial infarction.

Mann and Davies report that healed plaque ruptures were a frequent finding in 31 men dying suddenly of coronary artery disease.[60] The incidence of healed plaque rupture increased with increasing stenosis: 16% of arteries with

Table 2–6. Mean Vulnerable Plaques and Serum Cholesterol Levels, 113 Men Dying Suddenly with Severe Coronary Disease

	All Cases	TC < 210 mg/dL and TC/HDL-C < 5	n	TC > 210 mg/dL or TC/HDL-C > 5	n	TC > 210 mg/dL and TC/HDL-C > 5	n
Totals	1.22 ± 1.44	0.17 ± 0.49	23	1.13 ± 1.43	32	1.69 ± 1.41§	58
Whites	1.41 ± 1.51	0.25 ± 0.58	16	1.45 ± 1.79	20	1.76 ± 1.44§	50
Blacks	0.65 ± 0.98¶	0.00 ± 0	7	0.64 ± 0.81	11	1.25 ± 1.3†	8

§ P < 0.001 vs. TC < 210 mg/dl and TC/HDL-C < 5
¶ P = 0.02 vs. whites
† P = 0.02 vs. TC < 210 mg/dl and TC/HDL-C < 5
Abbreviations: TC = total cholesterol; HDL-C = high density lipoprotein cholesterol
Burke AP, Farb A, Malcom GT, Liang Y-H, Smialek J, Virmani R. Coronary risk factors and plaque morphology in patients with coronary disease dying suddenly. N Engl J Med 336:1276, 1997, with permission.

Table 2–7. Risk Factors and Mechanism of Death, 51 Women with Severe Coronary Atherosclerosis

Risk Factor	Plaque Rupture (n = 8)	Plaque Erosion (n = 18)	Stable Plaque, Healed MI (n = 18)	Stable Plaque, no MI (n = 7)	P values (if < 0.05)
Age, years mean ± SD	58 ± 12	45 ± 8*	54 ± 13	43 ± 9	0.01 vs. rupture, 0.03 vs. stable, healed MI
Age > 50 years, n (%)	7 (87%)*	3 (17%)	9 (50%)	2 (29%)	0.001 vs. plaque erosion; 0.03 vs. stable plaque, no infarct
TC, mg/dL, mean ± SD	270 ± 55*	188 ± 48	203 ± 71	201 ± 57	0.007 vs. erosion; 0.007 vs. stable plaque, healed MI; 0.02 vs. stable plaque
HDL-C, mg/dL, mean ± SD	46 ± 12	39 ± 21	40 ± 23	48 ± 32	—
TC/HDL-C, mean ± SD	6.2 ± 1.8	6.0 ± 3.7	6.6 ± 3.9	5.2 ± 2.7	—
BMI, kg/m^2, mean ± SD	31 ± 4	27 ± 4	28 ± 9	30 ± 11	—
GlycoHgb, %, mean ± SD	8.8 ± 4.4	6.7 ± 0.7	10.2 ± 5.0*	8.0 ± 4.5	0.006 vs. erosion
Ht wt, g, mean ± SD	483 ± 108	372 ± 87*	460 ± 105	375 ± 129	0.02 vs. rupture and stable plaque, healed MI
Ht wt/BMI, mean ± SD	1.6 ± 0.5	1.4 ± 0.4	1.7 ± 0.4*	1.3 ± 0.2	0.02 vs. stable plaque; 0.04 vs. erosion
Smokers, n (%)	4 (50%)	14 (78%)	9 (50%)	2 (29%)	—
Htn, n (%)	3 (38%)	4 (22%)	9 (50%)	2 (29%)	—

Abbreviations: MI = myocardial infarct; TC = total cholesterol; HDL-C high density lipoprotein cholesterol; Ht wt = heart weight; BMI = body mass index; Htn = hypertension

Burke et al. Effect of risk factors on the mechanism of acute thrombosis and sudden coronary death in women. Circulation 97:2110, 1998, with permission.

0–20% narrowing demonstrated healed plaque ruptures, compared with 18% of arteries with 21–50% narrowing, and 73% of arteries with > 51% narrowing. The difference between the incidence of healed ruptures between arteries ≤ 50% and > 51% narrowing was highly significant ($p < 0.0001$).[60] These data support our findings that plaque growth is episodic, occurs suddenly, often silently, and is a major cause of plaque progression. Our data also suggest that, as a mechanism of plaque progression in women, healed ruptures are likely significant only in the postmenopausal age.

Coronary Calcification

Coronary calcification is a marker for atherosclerosis and has been used as a screening modality utilizing expensive noninvasive imaging by electron beam computed tomography (EBCT).[101–103] The extent of coronary calcification by EBCT shows a strong correlation with coronary plaque burden and the risk for future cardiovascular events. However, the presence of calcification is a poor predictor of the degree of coronary narrowing in an individual coronary segment,[104] and there is a broad range of calcification scores in patients without clinical coronary disease.[101] Autopsy studies have shown that the sensitivity of EBCT for the detection of severe coronary lesions is about 60%, compared with a specificity of 90%.[105] These values are highly affected by age, however; the sensitivity increases dramatically with age, as the specificity decreases.

We have examined sudden coronary death victims to determine if calcification is a marker of plaque instability, and have found that coronary calcification increases with age and progresses at a slower rate in women than men, being delayed by 5 to 10 years (Fig. 2–14). We have found in women a correlation of calcification with diabetes, body mass index, and hypertension. There are striking differences in the rates and degree of calcification when coronary

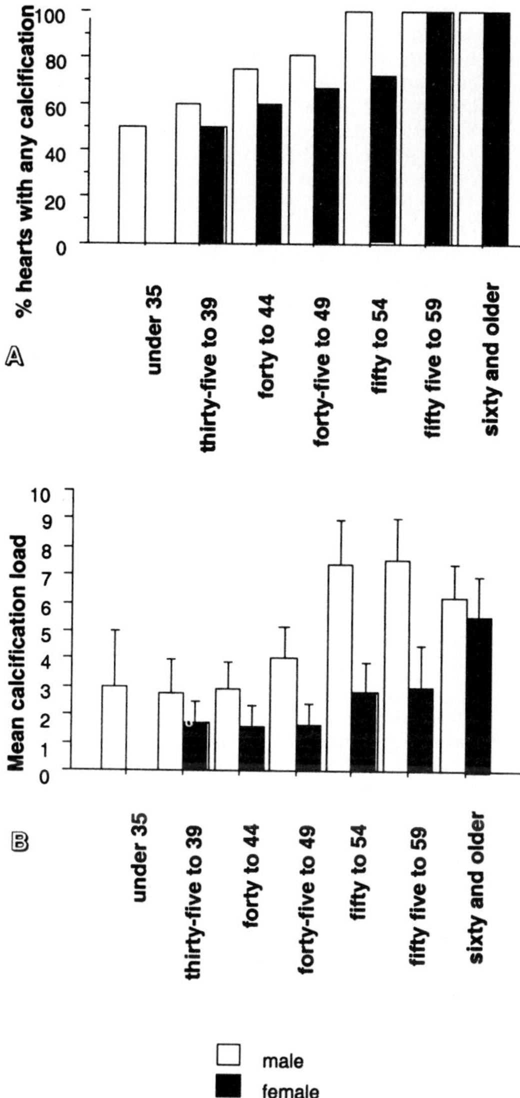

Figure 2–14. *A.* Incidence of coronary calcification in sudden coronary death, relation to age and gender. As age increases, there is an increase in the incidence of any calcification in the coronary arteries. This increase appears to demonstrate a delay of approximately one decade in women as compared with men. The incidence of calcification showed a statistically significant increase with age. The p value (student's T-test) between under 35 and 45–49 is p = 0.04; between 35–39 and 50–64, p = 0.03; and under 35 and 55–59 or > 60, p = 0.0003. *B.* Extent of coronary calcification in sudden coronary death, relation to age and gender. The peak degree of calcification in sudden coronary death appears to be in the 50's for men and in the 60's for women. The extent of calcification showed a statistically significant difference between younger and older ages; for example, the p value (student's T-test) between under 35 and 55–59 is p = 0.05; between 35–39 and 55–59, p = 0.01; and between 40–44 and 55–59, p = 0.01. (Burke et al. Coronary calcification. Z Kardiol 89:II/50, 2000, with permission.)

plaques are classified as described above. The highest frequency of coronary calcification is seen in acute plaque rupture, followed by healed ruptures, vulnerable plaque, stable plaque, and plaque erosion.[106] However, the mean calcification score is highest in healed plaque rupture, indicating that heavy calcification may actually impart a degree of plaque stability, and plaque erosions, which may result in infarction and death, are rarely calcified to a significant degree. Because of marked heterogeneity in coronary atherosclerotic plaques, it is simplistic to state that coronary calcification in itself is a marker of plaque instability; rather, the type of calcification must be considered in relationship to the morphology of the underlying plaque.

It is currently unclear if EBCT screening for the coronary disease should complement, or perhaps replace, established risk-factor profiles for coronary artery risk management. We have demonstrated that the predictors of sudden death using the Framingham risk index and measurement of calcification are distinct methods of assessing risk for sudden death.[107] Agreement in risk classification between histologic calcification score and the Framingham risk index occurs in 62% of cases. Either a focus of coronary artery calcification > 40 μm (62% of cases) or a Framingham risk score > average risk for age (62% of cases) were present in 66 of 79 (83.5%) cases. Excessive reliance on either method alone will produce errors in risk classification, particularly for patients at risk of plaque erosion, but this combination may be complementary.

Coronary Artery Remodeling

The autopsy description of atherosclerotic plaques in the coronary arteries has traditionally relied on measurements of cross-sectional luminal narrowing, as these measurements have reflected what is seen angiographically. However, it has been appreciated for over a decade that plaque size in itself is not the sole predictor of luminal narrowing, as there is marked compensatory enlargement of the coronary artery with plaque progression. The relationship between arterial expansion with increasing size of atherosclerotic plaque was initially studied by Glagov et al. in human coronary arteries.[108] Only when 40% or more cross-sectional luminal narrowing occurs is there a decrease in actual lumen diameter because of compensatory enlargement of the internal elastic lamina. Clarkson et al. demonstrated in a comparative study of human and nonhuman primates that lumen size is not correlated with plaque size or traditional risk factors, especially in patients without heart disease. Their study[109] emphasizes the need to consider true lumen size, and not percent cross-sectional luminal narrowing, when assessing the potential ischemic consequences of the atherosclerotic plaque.

Intracoronary ultrasound studies have shown that the site of the culprit lesion in unstable angina patients may undergo adaptive remodeling.[110] The absence of positive remodeling, or lack of compensatory arterial enlargement, may in large part be responsible for the development of symptomatic coronary disease. Positive remodeling has been associated with risk factors that may also explain the relationship of these risk factors with coronary plaque progression.[111, 112]

Currently, there is no simple method to estimate the degree of remodeling in the evaluation of routine autopsies. Morphometric measurements and comparison to reference points are necessary and generally restricted to investigational purposes. However, a subjective assessment of the degree of coronary ectasia in reporting cases of coronary artery disease is recommended for a thorough autopsy report. Coronary remodeling runs the gamut of slight shrinkage (negative remodeling) to marked ectasia of atherosclerotic segments. We are at the early stages of understanding the significance of the adaptive response of the adventitia and media to intimal disease, and autopsy studies are likely to contribute significantly to this understanding.

REFERENCES

1. Kannel WB. Incidence, prevalence, and mortality of coronary artery disease. In: Fuster V, Ross R, Topol EJ (eds): Atherosclerosis and Coronary Artery Disease. Philadelphia: Lippincott, 13–24, 1996.
2. National Center for Health Statistics, National Vital Statistics and the United States Bureau of the Census, Health, United States. Atlanta: Centers for Disease Control and Prevention, 1993.
3. Traven ND, Kuller LH, Ives DG, Rutan GH, Perper JA. Coronary heart disease mortality and sudden death among the 35–44-year age group in Allegheny County, Pennsylvania. Ann Epidemiol 6:130–136, 1996.
4. Annual Summary of Births, Marriages, Divorces and Deaths: United States, 1989. Washington, D.C.: National Center for Health Statistics, USDHHS, 1990.
5. Liao Y, McGee DL, Cooper RS, Sutkowski MB. How generalizable are coronary risk prediction models? Comparison of Framingham and two national cohorts. Am Heart J 137:837–845, 1999.
6. Kullo IJ, Gau GT, Tajik AJ. Novel risk factors for atherosclerosis. Mayo Clin Proc 75:369–380, 2000.
7. Dansky HM, Charlton SA, Sikes JL, Heath SC, Simantov R, Levin LF, Shu P, Moore KJ, Breslow JL, Smith JD. Genetic background determines the extent of atherosclerosis in ApoE-deficient mice. Arterioscler Thromb Vasc Biol 19:1960–1968, 1999.
8. Oparil S, Oberman A. Nontraditional cardiovascular risk factors. Am J Med Sci 317:193–207, 1999.
9. Mayer EL, Jacobsen DW, Robinson K. Homocysteine and coronary atherosclerosis. J Am Coll Cardiol 27:517–527, 1996.
10. Seman LJ, DeLuca C, Jenner JL, Cupples LA, McNamara JR, Wilson PW, Castelli WP, Ordovas JM, Schaefer EJ. Lipoprotein(a)-cholesterol and coronary heart disease in the Framingham Heart Study. Clin Chem 45:1039–1046, 1999.
11. Contois JH, Anamani DE, Tsongalis GJ. The underlying molecular mechanism of apolipoprotein E polymorphism: Relationships to lipid disorders, cardiovascular disease, and Alzheimer's disease. Clin Lab Med 16:105–123, 1996.
12. Weiss EJ, Bray PF, Tayback M, Schulman SP, Kickler TS, Becker LC, Weiss JL, Gerstenblith G, Goldschmidt-Clermont PJ. A polymorphism of a platelet glycoprotein receptor as an inherited risk factor for coronary thrombosis [see comments]. N Engl J Med 334:1090–1094, 1996.
13. Gordon T, Kannel WB. Premature mortality from coronary heart disease. The Framingham study. JAMA 215:1617–1625, 1971.
14. Burke AP, Farb A, Malcom GT, Liang Y, Smialek J, Virmani R. Effect of risk factors on the mechanism of acute thrombosis and sudden coronary death in women [see comments]. Circulation 97:2110–2106, 1998.
15. Burke A, Farb A, Malcom G, Virmani R. The effect of menopause on plaque morphology in coronary atherosclerosis. Am Heart J 2000; In press.
16. Gillum RF. Sudden cardiac death in Hispanic Americans and African Americans. Am J Public Health 87:1461–1466, 1997.
17. Liao Y, Cooper RS, McGee DL, Mensah GA, Ghali JK. The relative effects of left ventricular hypertrophy, coronary artery disease, and ventricular dysfunction on survival among black adults. JAMA 273:1592–1597, 1995.
18. Virmani R, Kolodgie FD, Burke AP, Farb A, Schwartz SM. Lessons from sudden coronary death: A comprehensive morphological classification scheme for atherosclerotic lesions [In Process Citation]. Arterioscler Thromb Vasc Biol 20:1262–1275, 2000.
19. Stary HC, Chandler AB, Glagov S, Guyton JR, Insull W, Jr., Rosenfeld ME, Schaffer SA, Schwartz CJ, Wagner WD, Wissler RW. A definition of initial, fatty streak, and intermediate lesions of atherosclerosis. A report from the Committee on Vascular Lesions of the Council on Arteriosclerosis, American Heart Association. Arterioscler Thromb 14:840–856, 1994.
20. Stary HC, Chandler AB, Dinsmore RE, Fuster V, Glagov S, Insull W, Jr., Rosenfeld ME, Schwartz CJ, Wagner WD, Wissler RW. A definition of advanced types of atherosclerotic lesions and a histological classification of atherosclerosis. A report from the Committee on Vascular Lesions of the Council on Arterio-

sclerosis, American Heart Association. Arterioscler Thromb Vasc Biol 15:1512–1531, 1995.
21. Haust MD. Myogenic foam cells in explants of fatty dots and streaks from rabbit aorta. Morphological studies. Atherosclerosis 441–464, 1977.
22. Geer JC, Haust MD. Smooth muscle cells in atherosclerosis. Monogr Athero 2:1–140, 1972.
23. Kim DN, Schmee J, Lee KT, Thomas WA. Atherosclerotic lesions in the coronary arteries of hyperlipidemic swine. Part 1. Cell increases, divisions, losses and cells of origin in first 90 days on diet. Atherosclerosis 64:231–242, 1987.
24. Schwartz SM, deBlois D, O'Brien ER. The intima. Soil for atherosclerosis and restenosis. Circ Res 77:445–465, 1995.
25. Ikari Y, McManus BM, Kenyon J, Schwartz SM. Neonatal intima formation in the human coronary artery. Arterioscler Thromb Vasc Biol 19:2036–2040, 1999.
26. McCaffrey TA, Du B, Consigli S, Szabo P, Bray PJ, Hartner L, Weksler BB, Sanborn TA, Bergman G, Bush HL, Jr. Genomic instability in the type II TGF-beta1 receptor gene in atherosclerotic and restenotic vascular cells. J Clin Invest 100:2182–2188, 1997.
27. Chatterjee SB, Dey S, Shi WY, Thomas K, Hutchins GM. Accumulation of glycosphingolipids in human atherosclerotic plaque and unaffected aorta tissues. Glycobiology 7:57–65, 1997.
28. Velican D, Velican C. Atherosclerotic involvement of the coronary arteries of adolescents and young adults. Atherosclerosis 36:449–460, 1980.
29. Strong JP, Malcom GT, McMahan CA, Tracy RE, Newman WP III, Herderick EE, Cornhill JF. Prevalence and extent of atherosclerosis in adolescents and young adults: Implications for prevention from the Pathobiological Determinants of Atherosclerosis in Youth Study. JAMA 281:727–735, 1999.
30. Evanko SP, Raines EW, Ross R, Gold LI, Wight TN. Proteoglycan distribution in lesions of atherosclerosis depends on lesion severity, structural characteristics, and the proximity of platelet-derived growth factor and transforming growth factor-beta. Am J Pathol 152:533–546, 1998.
31. Guyton JR, Klemp KF. Development of the lipid-rich core in human atherosclerosis. Arterioscler Thromb Vasc Biol 16:4–11, 1996.
32. Kruth HS. The fate of lipoprotein cholesterol entering the arterial wall. Curr Opin Lipidol 8:246–252, 1997.
33. Tangirala RK, Jerome WG, Jones NL, Small DM, Johnson WJ, Glick JM, Mahlberg FH, Rothblat GH. Formation of cholesterol monohydrate crystals in macrophage-derived foam cells. J Lipid Res 35:93–104, 1994.
34. Kruth HS. Localization of unesterified cholesterol in human atherosclerotic lesions. Am J Pathol 114:201–208, 1984.
35. Burke AP, Farb A, Malcom GT, Liang Y-H, Smialek J, Virmani R. Coronary risk factors and plaque morphology in patients with coronary disease dying suddenly. N Engl J Med 336:1276–1282, 1997.
36. Farb A, Tang AL, Burke AP, Sessums L, Liang Y, Virmani R. Sudden coronary death. Frequency of active coronary lesions, inactive coronary lesions, and myocardial infarction. Circulation 92:1701–1709, 1995.
37. Daida H, Yokoi H, Miyano H, Mokuno H, Satoh H, Kottke TE, Hosoda Y, Yamaguchi H. Relation of saphenous vein graft obstruction to serum cholesterol levels. J Am Coll Cardiol 25:193–197, 1995.
38. Bourassa MG, Enjalbert M, Campeau L, Lesperance J. Progression of atherosclerosis in coronary arteries and bypass grafts: Ten years later. Am J Cardiol 53:102C–107C, 1984.
39. Mautner SL, Mautner GC, Hunsberger SA, Roberts WC. Comparison of composition of atherosclerotic plaques in saphenous veins used as aortocoronary bypass conduits with plaques in native coronary arteries in the same men. Am J Cardiol 70:1380–1387, 1992.
40. Kalan JM, Roberts WC. Morphologic findings in saphenous veins used as coronary arterial bypass conduits for longer than 1 year: Necropsy analysis of 53 patients, 123 saphenous veins, and 1865 five-millimeter segments of veins. Am Heart J 119:1164–1184, 1990.
41. Hansson GK, Holm J, Jonasson L. Detection of activated T lymphocytes in the human atherosclerotic plaque. Am J Pathol 135:169–175, 1989.
42. van der Wal AC, Becker AE, van der Loos CM, Das PK. Site of intimal rupture or erosion of thrombosed coronary atherosclerotic plaques is characterized by an inflammatory process irrespective of the dominant plaque morphology. Circulation 89:36–44, 1994.
43. Schonbeck U, Sukhova GK, Graber P, Coulter S, Libby P. Augmented expression of cyclooxygenase-2 in human atherosclerotic lesions. Am J Pathol 155:1281–1291, 1999.
44. Mach F, Schonbeck U, Libby P. CD40 signaling in vascular cells: A key role in atherosclerosis? Atherosclerosis 137 Suppl:S89–95, 1998.
45. Mach F, Schonbeck U, Bonnefoy JY, Pober JS, Libby P. Activation of monocyte/macrophage functions related to acute atheroma complication by ligation of CD40: Induction of collagenase, stromelysin, and tissue factor. Circulation 96:396–399, 1997.
46. Farb A, Burke A, Tang A, Liang Y, Mannan P, Smialek J, Virmani R. Coronary plaque erosion without rupture into a lipid core: A frequent cause of coronary thrombosis in sudden coronary death. Circulation 93:1354–1363, 1996.
47. Amento EP, Ehsani N, Palmer H, Libby P. Cytokines and growth factors positively and negatively regulate interstitial collagen gene expression in human vascular smooth muscle cells. Arterioscler Thromb 11:1223–1230, 1991.
48. Geng YJ, Wu Q, Muszynski M, Hansson GK, Libby P. Apoptosis of vascular smooth muscle cells induced by in vitro stimulation with interferon-gamma, tumor necrosis factor-alpha, and interleukin-1 beta. Arterioscler Thromb Vasc Biol 16:19–27, 1996.
49. Hansson GK, Jonasson L, Holm J, Clowes MM, Clowes AW. Gamma-interferon regulates vascular smooth muscle proliferation and Ia antigen expression in vivo and in vitro. Circ Res 63:712–719, 1988.
50. Galis ZS, Muszynski M, Sukhova GK, Simon-Morrissey E, Libby P. Enhanced expression of vascular matrix metalloproteinases induced in vitro by cytokines and in regions of human atherosclerotic lesions. Ann N Y Acad Sci 748:501–507, 1995.
51. Galis ZS, Sukhova GK, Lark MW, Libby P. Increased expression of matrix metalloproteinases and matrix degrading activity in vulnerable regions of human atherosclerotic plaques. J Clin Invest 94:2493–2503, 1994.
52. George SJ. Tissue inhibitors of metalloproteinases and metalloproteinases in atherosclerosis. Curr Opin Lipidol 9:413–423, 1998.
53. Fabunmi RP, Baker AH, Murray EJ, Booth RF, Newby AC. Divergent regulation by growth factors and cytokines of 95 kDa and 72 kDa gelatinases and tissue inhibi-

tors or metalloproteinases-1, -2, and -3 in rabbit aortic smooth muscle cells. Biochem J 315:335–342, 1996.
54. Lee E, Grodzinsky AJ, Libby P, Clinton SK, Lark MW, Lee RT. Human vascular smooth muscle cell-monocyte interactions and metalloproteinase secretion in culture. Arterioscler Thromb Vasc Biol 15:2284–2289, 1995.
55. Shapiro SD, Campbell EJ, Kobayashi DK, Welgus HG. Immune modulation of metalloproteinase production in human macrophages. Selective pretranslational suppression of interstitial collagenase and stromelysin biosynthesis by interferon-gamma. J Clin Invest 86:1204–1210, 1990.
56. Sasaguri T, Arima N, Tanimoto A, Shimajiri S, Hamada T, Sasaguri Y. A role for interleukin 4 in production of matrix metalloproteinase 1 by human aortic smooth muscle cells. Atherosclerosis 138:247–253, 1998.
57. Ross R. Atherosclerosis—an inflammatory disease [see comments]. N Engl J Med 340:115–126, 1999.
58. Shah PK, Falk E, Badimon JJ, Fernandez-Ortiz A, Mailhac A, Villareal-Levy G, Fallon JT, Regnstrom J, Fuster V. Human monocyte-derived macrophages induce collagen breakdown in fibrous caps of atherosclerotic plaques. Potential role of matrix-degrading metalloproteinases and implications for plaque rupture. Circulation 92:1565–1569, 1995.
59. Sukhova GK, Schonbeck U, Rabkin E, Schoen FJ, Poole AR, Billinghurst RC, Libby P. Evidence for increased collagenolysis by interstitial collagenases-1 and 13 in vulnerable human atheromatous plaques. Circulation 99:2503–2509, 1999.
60. Mann J, Davies MJ. Mechanisms of progression in native coronary artery disease: Role of healed plaque disruption. Heart 82:265–268, 1999.
61. Burke AP, Farb A, Kolodgie FD, Malcom GT, Virmani R. Healed ruptured plaques are frequent in men with severe coronary disease and are associated with elevated total/high density lipoprotein (HDL) cholesterol. Circulation 96:I–235, 1997.
62. Davies MJ, Thomas AC, Knapman PA, Hangartner JR. Intramyocardial platelet aggregation in patients with unstable angina suffering sudden ischemic cardiac death. Circulation 73:418–427, 1986.
63. Constantinides P. Plaque fissuring in human coronary thrombosis. J Atheroscler Res 6:1–17, 1966.
64. Davies MJ, Thomas AC. Plaque fissuring—the cause of acute myocardial infarction, sudden ischaemic death, and crescendo angina. Br Heart J 53:363–373, 1985.
65. Davies MJ, Woolf N, Rowles PM, Pepper J. Morphology of the endothelium over atherosclerotic plaques in human coronary arteries. Br Heart J 60:459–464, 1988.
66. Davies MJ. A macro and micro view of coronary vascular insult in ischemic heart disease. Circulation 82:II38–46, 1990.
67. Davies MJ. Anatomic features in victims of sudden coronary death. Coronary artery pathology. Circulation 85:I19–24, 1992.
68. Davies MJ. Stability and instability: Two faces of coronary atherosclerosis. The Paul Dudley White Lecture 1995. Circulation 94:2013–2020, 1996.
69. Arbustini E, Grasso M, Diegoli M, Morbini P, Aguzzi A, Fasani R, Specchia G. Coronary thrombosis in non-cardiac death. Coron Artery Dis 4:751–759, 1993.
70. Paterson JC. Capillary rupture with intimal hemorrhage as a causative factor in coronary thrombosis. Arch Pathol 25:474–487, 1938.
71. Heberden W. Some account of a disorder of the breast. Med Trans Coll Physicians (Lond) 2:57, 1772.
72. Osler W. The Principles and Practice of Medicine. New York: Appleton, 655–659, 1892.
73. Gorlin R. Pathophysiology of cardiac pain. Circulation 32:138–148, 1965.
74. Hangartner JR, Charleston AJ, Davies MJ, Thomas AC. Morphological characteristics of clinically significant coronary artery stenosis in stable angina. Br Heart J 56:501–508, 1986.
75. Braunwald E, Jones RH, Mark DB, Brown J, Brown L, Cheitlin MD, Concannon CA, Cowan M, Edwards C, Fuster V, et al. Diagnosing and managing unstable angina. Agency for Health Care Policy and Research. Circulation 90:613–622, 1994.
76. Theroux P, Lidon RM. Unstable angina: Pathogenesis, diagnosis, and treatment. Curr Probl Cardiol 18:157–231, 1993.
77. Ottani F, Galvani M, Ferrini D, Nicolini FA. Clinical relevance of prodromal angina before acute myocardial infarction. Int J Cardiol 68 Suppl 1:S103–108, 1999.
78. Silva JA, Escobar A, Collins TJ, Ramee SR, White CJ. Unstable angina. A comparison of angioscopic findings between diabetic and nondiabetic patients. Circulation 92:1731–1736, 1995.
79. Willerson JT, Golino P, Eidt J, Campbell WB, Buja LM. Specific platelet mediators and unstable coronary artery lesions. Experimental evidence and potential clinical implications. Circulation 80:198–205, 1989.
80. Grande P, Grauholt AM, Madsen JK. Unstable angina pectoris. Platelet behavior and prognosis in progressive angina and intermediate coronary syndrome. Circulation 81:I16–19; discussion I22–23, 1990.
81. Virmani R, Roberts WC. Quantification of coronary arterial narrowing in clinically-isolated unstable angina pectoris. An analysis of 22 necropsy patients. Am J Med 67:792–799, 1979.
82. Roberts WC, Kragel AH, Gertz D, Roberts CS, Kalan JM. The heart in fatal unstable angina pectoris. Am J Cardiol 68:22B–27B, 1991.
83. Guthrie RB, Vlodaver Z, Nicoloff DM, Edwards JE. Pathology of stable and unstable angina pectoris. Circulation 51:1059–1063, 1975.
84. Falk E. Morphologic features of unstable atherothrombotic plaques underlying acute coronary syndromes. Am J Cardiol 63:114E–120E, 1989.
85. Falk E. Unstable angina with fatal outcome: Dynamic coronary thrombosis leading to infarction and/or sudden death. Circulation 71:699–708, 1985.
86. Depre C, Wijns W, Robert AM, Renkin JP, Havaux X. Pathology of unstable plaque: Correlation with the clinical severity of acute coronary syndromes. J Am Coll Cardiol 30:694–702, 1997.
87. Haft JI, Mariano DL, Goldstein J. Comparison of the histopathology of culprit lesions in chronic stable angina, unstable angina, and myocardial infarction. Clin Cardiol 20:651–655, 1997.
88. Prinzmetal M, Kennamer R, Merliss R. Variant form of angina pectoris. Am Med J 27:375–388, 1959.
89. McFadden EP, Clarke JG, Davies GJ, Kaski JC, Haider AW, Maseri A. Effect of intracoronary serotonin on coronary vessels in patients with stable angina and patients with variant angina [see comments]. N Engl J Med 324:648–654, 1991.
90. Forman MB, Oates JA, Robertson D, Robertson RM, Roberts LJd, Virmani R. Increased adventitial mast

cells in a patient with coronary spasm. N Engl J Med 313:1138–1141, 1985.
91. de Fockert JA. Clinical presentation of acute myocardial infarct in the elderly. Tijdschr Gerontol Geriatr 18:305–308, 1987.
92. DeWood MA, Spores J, Notske R, Mouser LT, Burroughs R, Golden MS, Lang HT. Prevalence of total coronary occlusion during the early hours of transmural myocardial infarction. N Engl J Med 303:897–902, 1980.
93. Kragel AH, Gertz SD, Roberts WC. Morphologic comparison of frequency and types of acute lesions in the major epicardial coronary arteries in unstable angina pectoris, sudden coronary death and acute mycoardial infarction. J Am Coll Cardiol 18:801–808, 1991.
94. Davies MJ, Woolf N, Robertson WB. Pathology of acute myocardial infarction with particular reference to occlusive coronary thrombi. Br Heart J 38:659–664, 1976.
95. Ambrose JA, Tannenbaum MA, Alexopoulos D, Hjemdahl-Monsen CE, Leavy J, Weiss M, Borrico S, Gorlin R, Fuster V. Angiographic progression of coronary artery disease and the development of myocardial infarction. J Am Coll Cardiol 12:56–62, 1988.
96. Qiao JH, Fishbein MC. The severity of coronary atherosclerosis at sites of plaque rupture with occlusive thrombosis. J Am Coll Cardiol 17:1138–1142, 1991.
97. Warnes CA, Roberts WC. Sudden coronary death: Comparison of patients with to those without coronary thrombus at necropsy. Am J Cardiol 54:1206–1211, 1984.
98. Davies MJ, Bland JM, Hangartner JR, Angelini A, Thomas AC. Factors influencing the presence or absence of acute coronary artery thrombi in sudden ischaemic death. Eur Heart J 10:203–208, 1989.
99. Reichenbach DD, Moss NS, Meyer E. Pathology of the heart in sudden cardiac death. Am J Cardiol 39:865–872, 1977.
100. Newman WPD, Tracy RE, Strong JP, Johnson WD, Oalmann MC. Pathology on sudden coronary death. Ann N Y Acad Sci 382:39–49, 1982.
101. Kennedy J, Shavelle R, Wang S, Budoff M, Detrano RC. Coronary calcium and standard risk factors in symptomatic patients referred for coronary angiography. Am Heart J 135:696–702, 1998.
102. Newman AB, Naydeck B, Sutton-Tyrrell K, Edmundowicz D, Gottdiener J, Kuller LH. Coronary artery calcification in older adults with minimal clinical or subclinical cardiovascular disease. J Am Geriatr Soc 48:256–263, 2000.
103. Detrano R, Hsiai T, Wang S, Puentes G, Fallavollita J, Shields P, Stanford W, Wolfkiel C, Georgiou D, Budoff M, Reed J. Prognostic value of coronary calcification and angiographic stenoses in patients undergoing coronary angiography. J Am Coll Cardiol 27:285–290, 1996.
104. Sangiorgi G, Rumberger JA, Severson A, Edwards WD, Gregoire J, Fitzpatrick LA, Schwartz RS. Arterial calcification and not lumen stenosis is highly correlated with atherosclerotic plaque burden in humans: A histologic study of 723 coronary artery segments using nondecalcifying methodology. J Am Coll Cardiol 31:126–133, 1998.
105. Simons DB, Schwartz RS, Edwards WD, Sheedy PF, Breen JF, Rumberger JA. Noninvasive definition of anatomic coronary artery disease by ultrafast computed tomographic scanning: A quantitative pathologic comparison study. J Am Coll Cardiol 20:1118–1126, 1992.
106. Burke AP, Taylor A, Farb A, Malcom G, Virmani R. Coronary calcification: Insights from sudden coronary death victims. Z Kardiol 89:(SII) 49–53, 2000.
107. Taylor AJ, Burke AP, O'Malley PG, Farb A, Malcom GT, Smialek J, Virmani R. A comparison of the Framingham risk index, coronary artery calcification, and culprit plaque morphology in sudden cardiac death. Circulation 101:1243–1248, 2000.
108. Glagov S, Weisenberg E, Zarins CK, Stankunavicius R, Kolettis GJ. Compensatory enlargement of human atherosclerotic coronary arteries. N Engl J Med 316:1371–1375, 1987.
109. Clarkson TB, Prichard RW, Morgan TM, Petrick GS, Klein KP. Remodeling of coronary arteries in human and nonhuman primates. JAMA 271:289–294, 1994.
110. Gyongyosi M, Yang P, Hassan A, Weidinger F, Domanovits H, Laggner A, Glogar D. Arterial remodelling of native human coronary arteries in patients with unstable angina pectoris: A prospective intravascular ultrasound study. Heart 82:68–74, 1999.
111. Gyongyosi M, Yang P, Hassan A, Weidinger F, Domanovits H, Laggner A, Glogar D. Coronary risk factors influence plaque morphology in patients with unstable angina. Coron Artery Dis 10:211–219, 1999.
112. Taylor AJ, Burke AP, Farb A, Yousefi P, Malcom GT, Smialek J, Virmani R. Arterial remodeling in the left coronary system: The role of high-density lipoprotein cholesterol. J Am Coll Cardiol 34:760–767, 1999.
113. Arbustini E, Dal Bello B, Morbini P, Burke AP, Bocciarelli M, Speechia G, Virmani R. Plaque erosion is a major substrate for coronary thrombosis in acute myocardial infarction. Heart 82:269–272, 1999.

Chapter

3

THE PATHOLOGY OF VASCULAR INTERVENTIONS

The last two decades have witnessed tremendous growth in the mechanical therapeutic approaches in the treatment of atherosclerotic coronary artery disease. Percutaneous revascularization procedures have become routine in the United States, initially with angioplasty balloons with subsequent development of new catheter-based devices to locally cut and/or remove atherosclerotic plaque. While clinical symptoms had been effectively treated with balloon angioplasty, restenosis emerged as its Achilles heel. The introduction of stents has been recognized as a significant clinical advance, especially in the treatment of acute complications following balloon angioplasty. Overall restenosis rates are reduced with stents, but in-stent restenosis remains a significant clinical problem, is more difficult to treat than restenosis following balloon angioplasty, and can be expected to increase in incidence as coronary stenting becomes more frequent and is utilized in less ideal lesions. Despite the advances in percutaneous approaches to coronary atherosclerosis, traditional coronary bypass surgery remains the treatment of choice for many patients with multivessel disease. Coronary bypass surgery has also evolved with less invasive approaches being utilized. Finally, there are now mechanical approaches that attempt to provide increased perfusion directly to the myocardium via the left ventricular cavity (transmyocardial revascularization) in patients in whom epicardial coronary revascularization is not feasible. In the peripheral arterial circulation, new graft devices have become available to treat aneurysms via a percutaneous approach.

Coronary and peripheral arterial interventions produce morphologic changes that are distinct from the pathology of the underlying atherosclerotic process and are heavily influenced by the procedure or device used and the duration of time from the procedure to pathologic analysis. In approaching cases of coronary revascularization, the pathologist's main role is to provide anatomic information into whether a particular surgical or catheter-based procedure was a success or failure. Most important, when the clinical outcome was poor or unexpected, the pathologist should offer insights into the mechanism of treatment failure as it relates to the patient's underlying disease, the coronary interventional procedure performed, and consequences and complications related to that treatment.

In this chapter, surgical coronary revascularization will be discussed first, followed by percutaneous approaches and direct myocardial revascularization. New percutaneous treatments for aortic aneurysmal disease will be presented. Finally, transmyocardial revascularization and ventricular assist devices will be discussed.

SURGICAL CORONARY ARTERY REVASCULARIZATION

Coronary artery bypass graft (CABG) surgery remains a cornerstone in the treatment of severe coronary artery atherosclerosis. Based on several large studies comparing medical therapy with CABG surgery, survival is improved with surgical treatment in patients with: (1) severe left main atherosclerotic disease; (2) left main equivalent disease (≥ 70% diameter stenosis of the proximal left anterior descending and proximal left circumflex arteries); (3) severe disease involving the three major coronary arteries, especially associated with severe ischemia involving a large area of myocardium; and (4) severe proximal left anterior descending coronary atherosclerosis with two- or three-vessel disease associated with left ventricular dysfunction.[1, 2] Further, CABG surgery is indicated in patients with disabling symptoms despite medical therapy.[2]

Despite the emergence of percutaneous procedures (balloon angioplasty, atherectomy, and stents), CABG surgery is especially useful in patients with multivessel (≥ 3 vessel) major epicardial coronary artery atherosclerosis and in patients with arterial anatomy in which percutaneous approaches are unlikely to afford long-term lumen patency (e.g., heavily calcified lesions and diffusely atherosclerotic arteries).

The clinical outcome of multivessel balloon angioplasty versus CABG has been compared in several trials including the Randomized Intervention Treatment of Angina (RITA) trial,[3] the Emory Angioplasty versus Surgery Trial (EAST),[4] the German Angioplasty Bypass Surgery Investigation (GABI),[5] and the Bypass Angioplasty Revascularization Investigation (BARI) study.[6] The consensus from these studies was that CABG surgery was associated with an increased incidence of short-term myocardial infarction (up to 10%), mortality (1–2%), cost, and hospital length of stay.[2] Over the long term, however, CABG surgery and angioplasty offered similar overall survival. At 10 years in the BARI trial, survival was 89.3% after CABG surgery and 86.3% with angioplasty.[1] There were no differences in the incidence of Q-wave myocardial infarction.[2] An important subgroup analysis in the BARI study showed improved survival in diabetic patients treated with CABG surgery which included placement of an internal mammary artery graft.[1] From a symptom standpoint, CABG surgery was associated with a greater freedom from angina, and there was a four- to tenfold increase in subsequent revascularization in angioplasty patients (as a result of restenosis following balloon angioplasty).[2] Because of the need for subsequent coronary interventions (e.g., repeat balloon angioplasty or crossover to CABG surgery), the reduced costs of balloon angioplasty that were present in the short-term were lost during a long-term follow-up.[2] Therefore, CABG surgery provides a generally more long-term definitive revascularization strategy than balloon angioplasty with slightly greater short-term complications and costs. It should be noted, however, these data are limited in their applicability to current practice, because they predate the widespread use of stent deployment in percutaneous coronary revascularization procedures.

Surgical Procedure

The goal of CABG surgery is to revascularize all arterial lesions with at least 50% diameter stenosis in the left main artery, three major epicardial arteries, and their main branches.[7] Because of its superior long-term patency (90% patency at 10 years),[8–10] the left internal mammary artery is used, most commonly, as a bypass graft to the left anterior descending coronary artery. The internal mammary artery is mobilized from the chest wall within its pedicle accompanied by the internal mammary vein, and a small amount of fat and skeletal muscle.[7] If the left internal mammary artery is of insufficient length to reach the left anterior descending artery, it may be used as a free graft with its proximal end implanted in the ascending aorta. Patency rates for free internal mammary grafts appear to be similar to mammary arteries used from their pedicles.[11] Occasionally, the right internal mammary, right gastroepiploic, and inferior epigastric arteries are used, especially in young individuals.[12] Recently, there has been greater use of radial arteries as bypass grafts with high patency rates.[13–15] Segments of the greater saphenous vein provide the vast majority of nonarterial bypass grafts. When revascularization requires more than five aortotomies, at least one graft will be anastomosed to more than one native coronary artery;[7] for example, an initial side-to-side anastomosis to the left diagonal artery followed by an end-to-side anastomosis to the left obtuse marginal artery. Proximal anastomoses are created in the right lateral side of the ascending aorta.

Traditional CABG surgery requires a mid-line thoracotomy, cross-clamping of the aorta, use of cardioplegia solution to arrest the heart, and placement of the patient on cardiopulmonary bypass. Newer, less-invasive surgical techniques include off bypass CABG surgery with a small median sternotomy, off bypass minimally invasive direct coronary bypass (MID-CAB) utilizing a small left thoracotomy, and video-assisted port-access CABG surgery utilizing femoral artery-femoral vein cardiopulmonary bypass, small incisions, and catheter-delivered cardioplegia. Most commonly in the MID-CAB procedure, an internal mammary artery is grafted to the left anterior descending artery with bypass of the left diagonal branches if necessary.[2] The use of multiple small incisions with the port-access procedure allows the surgeon to reach more areas of the heart, which offers the potential for more complete revascularization.[2] Early reports have suggested acceptable graft patency rates associated with these less-invasive surgical approaches.[16–23] While these less-invasive strategies result in less perioperative mortality, shorter hospital stays, and reduced costs, their superiority over traditional CABG surgery has not been established.

Pathologic Assessment of Coronary Bypass Grafts

Technical Considerations

The early patency of bypass grafts (arterial and vein conduits) is dependent on the adequacy of the anastomoses and avoidance of overstretch, twisting, and kinking of the grafts (Figs. 3–1 and 3–2).[24] More important, the severity of native coronary atherosclerosis plays a critical role in determining acute and long-term outcome. The coronary arterial anastomosis should be distal to all important flow-limiting stenoses. In patients with diffuse atherosclerosis, especially involving the distal arterial segments, it may be difficult to find a touchdown site that is free of significant atherosclerosis. Poor distal run-off leads to increasing the risk of vein graft thrombosis and augments bypass graft narrowing even if the surgical technique is flawless.[25] In coronary arteries $\leq$ 1.0 mm in diameter, the placement of sutures in the everted native artery wall in creating the vein anastomosis can compress the lumen area by up to 50%, increasing the risk of early graft occlusion.[25] Placement of a graft anastomosis into a native coronary artery that contains atherosclerotic plaque can precipitate the development of a focal arterial dissection.[26]

Internal Mammary Artery

The internal mammary artery (Fig. 3–3A and D) and arterial conduits in general (in contrast to arterialized saphenous veins) have multiple features that contribute to their high long-term patency as bypass grafts: dimensions similar to the coronary arteries, viable endothelial cells capable of secreting nitric oxide and prostacyclin, inherent resistance to atherosclerosis, and the large vascular run-off of the left anterior descending coronary bed.[7] When present, vasculopathy in internal mammary grafts most often takes the form of fibrointimal hyperplasia consisting of smooth muscle cells in a proteoglycan-rich extracellular matrix (Fig. 3–3E and F).[27] In technically well-placed internal mammary artery grafts, acute thrombosis is rare,[28] and chronic total occlusion (or organized thrombus [Fig. 3–3B]) most likely results from technical factors occurring during graft placement or poor distal arterial run-off. Internal mammary artery graft atherosclerosis is rare (Fig. 3–3C).[29, 30] In a study of 18 internal mammary grafts in place 12–118 months, atherosclerotic change, consisting of foam cell accumulation without lipid core formation, was present in only one graft, despite the fact that 83% of the patients had hyperlipidemia and 67% of the accompanying vein grafts had atherosclerotic lesions.[27] Pathologic changes affecting noninternal mammary arterial grafts are similar to internal mammary grafts.

Figure 3–1. Gross external views of coronary artery bypass graft (*CABG*) surgery hearts. In *A,* the internal mammary artery (*IMA, small arrows*), arising from the left subclavian artery, has been anastomosed to the distal left anterior descending (*LAD*) coronary artery. A saphenous vein bypass graft (*large arrows*) is anastomosed proximally to the ascending aorta (*Ao*) and distally to the left diagonal (*LD*) branch of the LAD. *B* shows the heart from 57-year-old man who underwent CABG surgery in 12 years antemortem, who presented with a non-Q-wave myocardial infarction. Cardiac catheterization demonstrated severe native coronary artery and bypass graft stenoses, which was treated with redo CABG surgery. The postoperative course was complicated by cardiogenic shock, renal failure, and death. The anterior surface of the heart shows two old grafts (*small arrows*) and three recent grafts, one to the left obtuse marginal (*arrowheads*), one to the left diagonal (*lower large arrow to LD*), and one to the left circumflex (*upper large arrow*). The native arteries have been dissected to show the anastomotic sites prior to sectioning of the grafts. *C* shows an unusual complication in a 51-year-old man who underwent CABG surgery following an acute myocardial infarction. Note the vein bypass graft from the aorta with side-to-side touchdown anastomosis to the left diagonal artery (*small arrow*) followed by a side-to-side touchdown anastomosis to first left obtuse marginal artery (*LOM, large arrow*) and a final end-to-side anastomosis to the second LOM artery (*not shown*). Note the nearly 90° angulation of the saphenous vein graft, which resulted in poor flow in the vein graft.

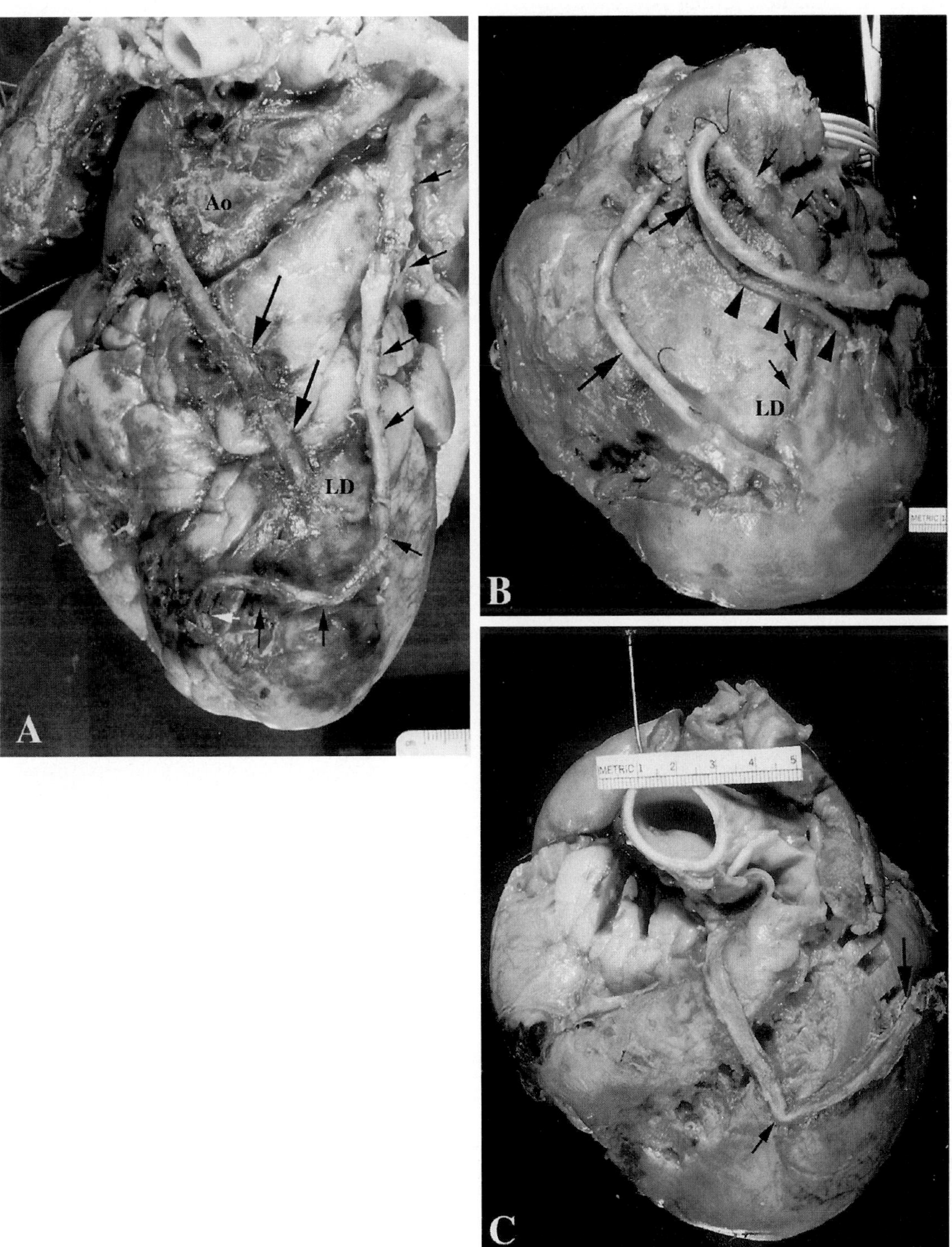

Figure 3–1. *See legend on opposite page*

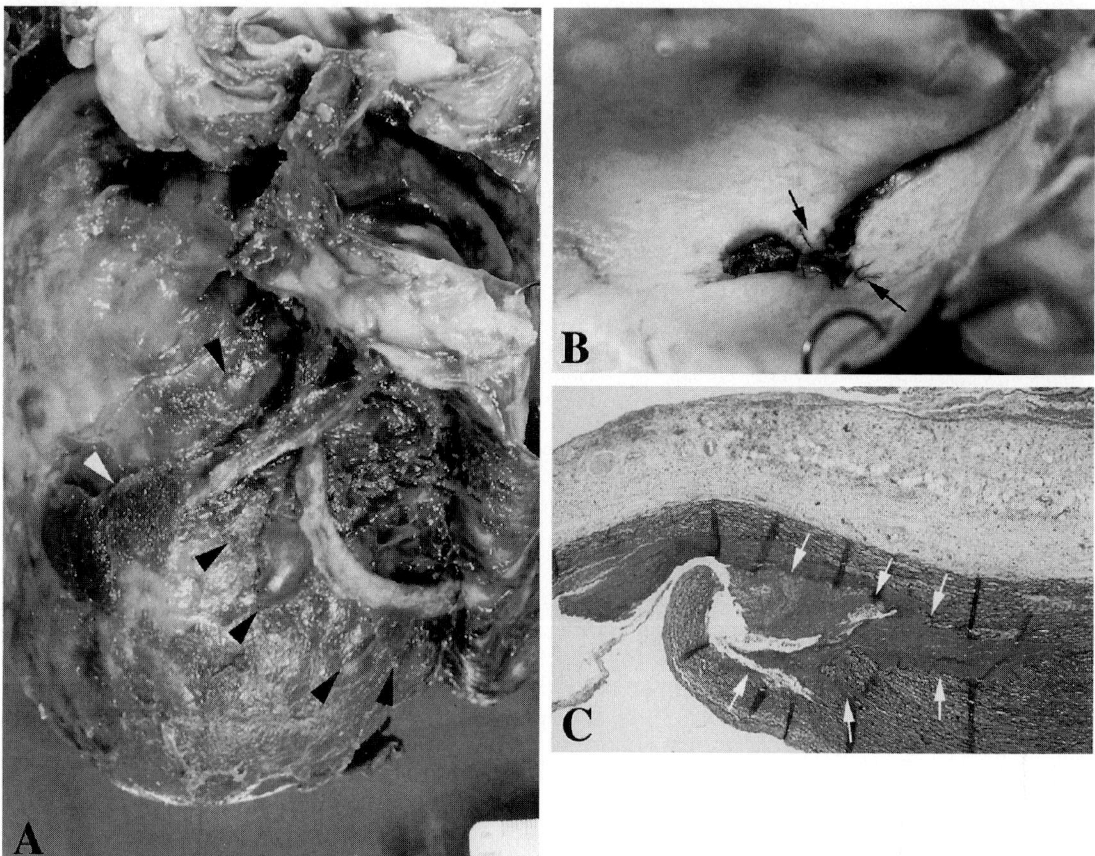

Figure 3–2. Gross photograph (*A*) of the heart from a patient who underwent bypass surgery 5 days antemortem complicated by hypotension on day of expiration. At autopsy, there was 250 ml of fresh blood in the pericardial sac. The surface of the heart demonstrated clotted blood associated with epicardial fat and fibrinous pericarditis (*area enclosed by arrowheads*). All anastomotic sites were intact, and no site of cardiac rupture was identified. It was felt that the epicardial hemorrhage occurred secondary to a postoperative coagulopathy. *B* shows a proximal aortic dissection with rupture at the site of a vein graft anastomosis (*arrows*) in a 69-year-old patient who died 3 days following CABG surgery. A histologic section (*C*) at the site of dissection shows the intimal tear and a dissecting hematoma (*arrows*) in the aortic wall.

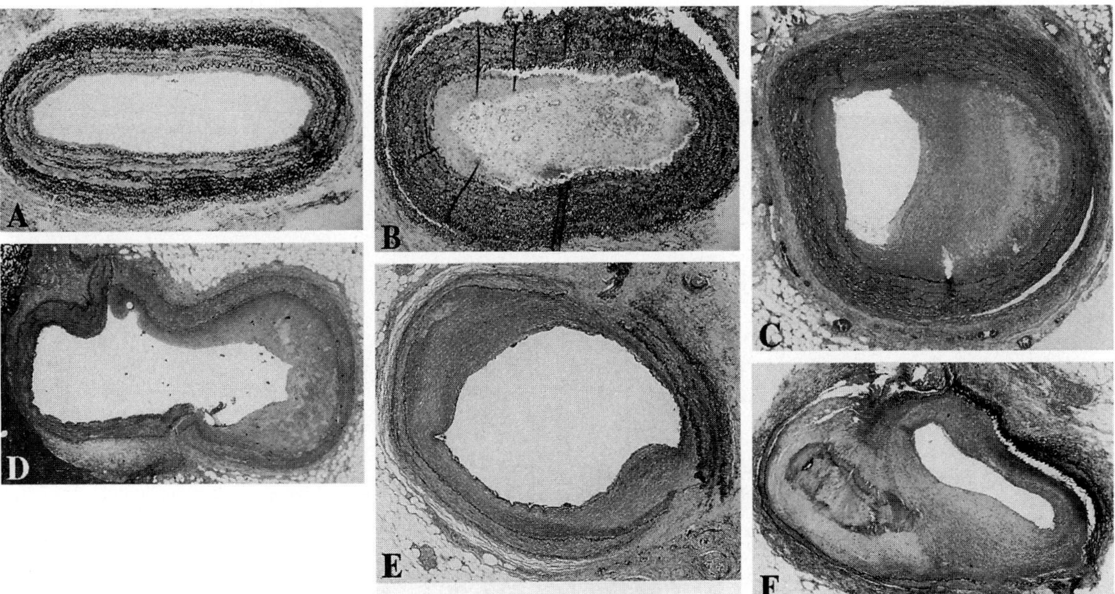

Figure 3–3. Internal mammary artery (*IMA*) histology. *A to C* show the spectrum of changes that may be seen following long-term placement of an IMA graft during CABG surgery. A normal IMA graft to the left anterior descending (*LAD*) artery, proximal to its anastomosis is shown in *A*. *B* shows chronic total occlusion of the IMA graft in a patient who died > 6 months post-bypass; an organized thrombus is present containing neoangiogenesis (small recanalization channels). In *C*, an IMA graft with atherosclerosis resulting in 75% lumen area narrowing is shown. Atherosclerosis is a rare complication of long-term IMA grafts. IMA-LAD artery anastomoses are shown in *D to F*. *D* shows a normal anastomosis in a patient who expired 3 days post-CABG surgery secondary to coagulopathy. No thrombus or neointimal formation is seen in the IMA graft (*to the left*), and mild atherosclerosis is present in the native coronary artery (*to the right*). In *E*, the IMA-LAD anastomosis 1 year post-CABG surgery shows mild intimal hyperplasia with minimal intimal thickening over the IMA (*right side of image*). *F* shows moderate intimal hyperplasia over the IMA graft (*to the right*) with relatively greater intimal thickening over the focally calcified atherosclerotic LAD (*to the left*).

Vein Bypass Grafts

Early Changes

Within the first 72 hours after placement, a thin layer of platelets and fibrin is deposited along the vein graft intimal surface (Fig. 3–4A and B). During this period, acute inflammatory cells are often present in the walls of the grafts (Fig. 3–4).[24] Diffuse intimal hyperplasia consisting of smooth muscle cells in a proteoglycan and collagen matrix is always observed in vein grafts in place > 1 month.[31–33] The mechanisms of this remodeling process[33] is believed to involve responses to endothelial injury and hemodynamic stress as the vein wall is subjected to the increased distending pressure of the arterial circulation. The initial extent of intimal thickening is inversely proportional to flow through the graft.[7] In vein grafts that demonstrate long-term patency, the vein lumen diameter approximates the lumen diameter of the native coronary artery to which it is anastomosed.[34] Over the course of a year after bypass surgery, medial smooth muscle cell loss with focal medial fibrosis and adventitial thickening are commonly seen.[24]

Vein Graft Thrombosis

Acute vein graft thrombosis may occur secondary to: (1) damage to the vein itself during harvest and insertion leading to excessive endothelial injury; (2) poor run-off due to plaque present at the anastomosis and/or severe distal native coronary atherosclerosis (Fig. 3–5A and B); or (3) technical factors (e.g., graft twisting or kinking or distal arterial dissection during creation of the anastomosis) (Figs. 3–1 and 3–5C and D).[24] Vein graft occlusion within the first postoperative month ranges from 3–12%, and is secondary to graft thrombosis in most cases.[12, 35, 36] Pathologically, the vein graft is obstructed and distended with thrombus for its entire course in patients who die in the early postoperative period. Additionally, acute myocardial infarction is seen in the territory supplied by the thrombosed graft (Fig. 3–4C–F). In patients who survive at least several months following CABG surgery

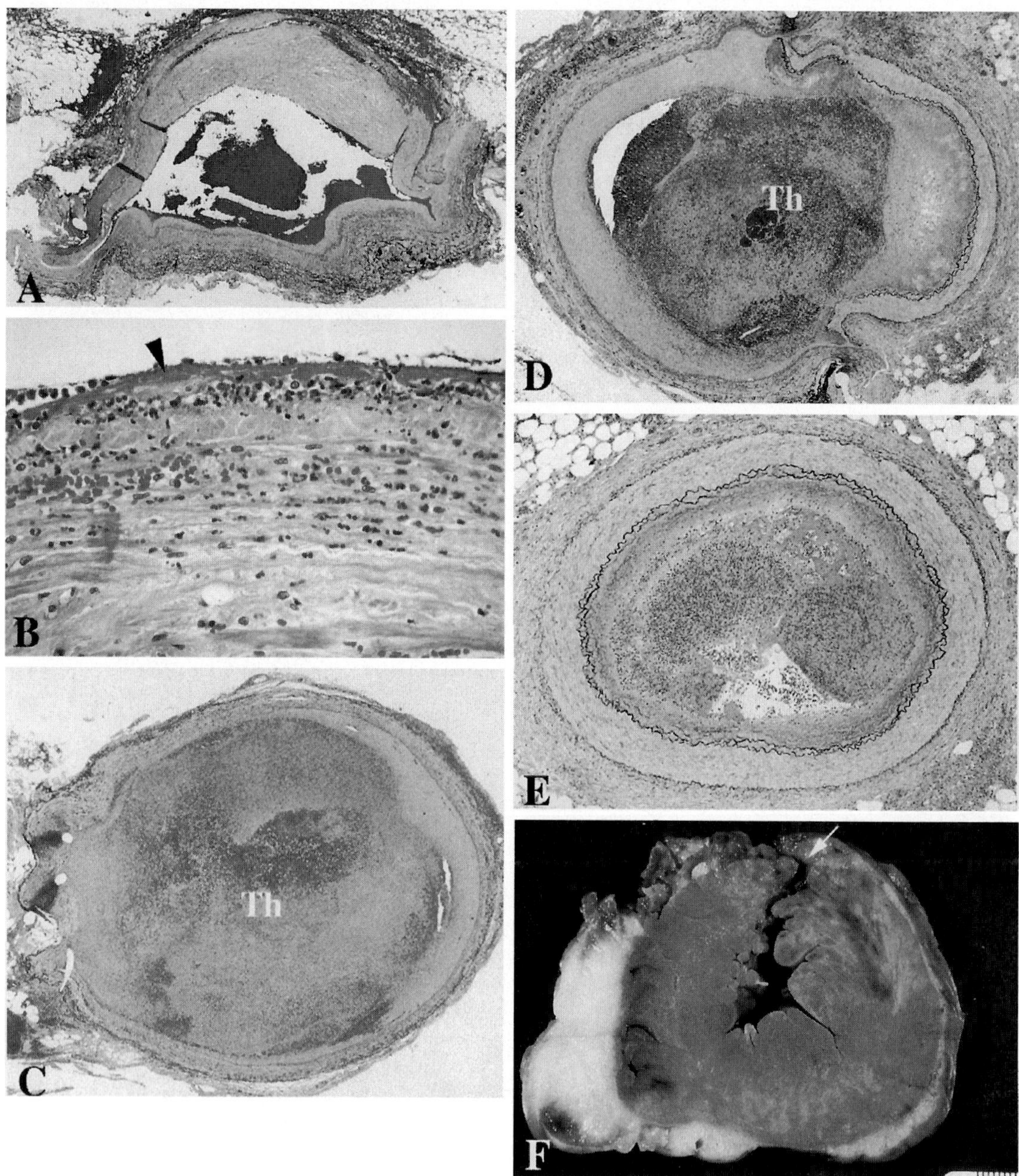

Figure 3–4. *A* and *B* are low- and high-power views, respectively, of the anastomosis between the native artery and the vein graft from a patient who died <1 day post-CABG surgery. The anastomotic site is intact; however, at high power (*B*), a thin layer of platelet deposition (*arrowhead*) is seen on the luminal surface, and there is an acute inflammatory cell infiltrate in the wall of the vein. *C to E* show vein graft, anastomotic site, and left diagonal coronary artery distal to the anastomosis, respectively, in a patient who died 3 days post-CABG surgery. Note that the vein graft proximal to the anastomosis (*C*), the anastomosis (*D*), and the left diagonal distal to the anastomosis (*E*) are occluded by a recent thrombus. Thrombosis of the vein graft and distal native vessel resulted in an acute transmural anterior myocardial infarction complicated by free wall rupture (*arrow* in *F*).

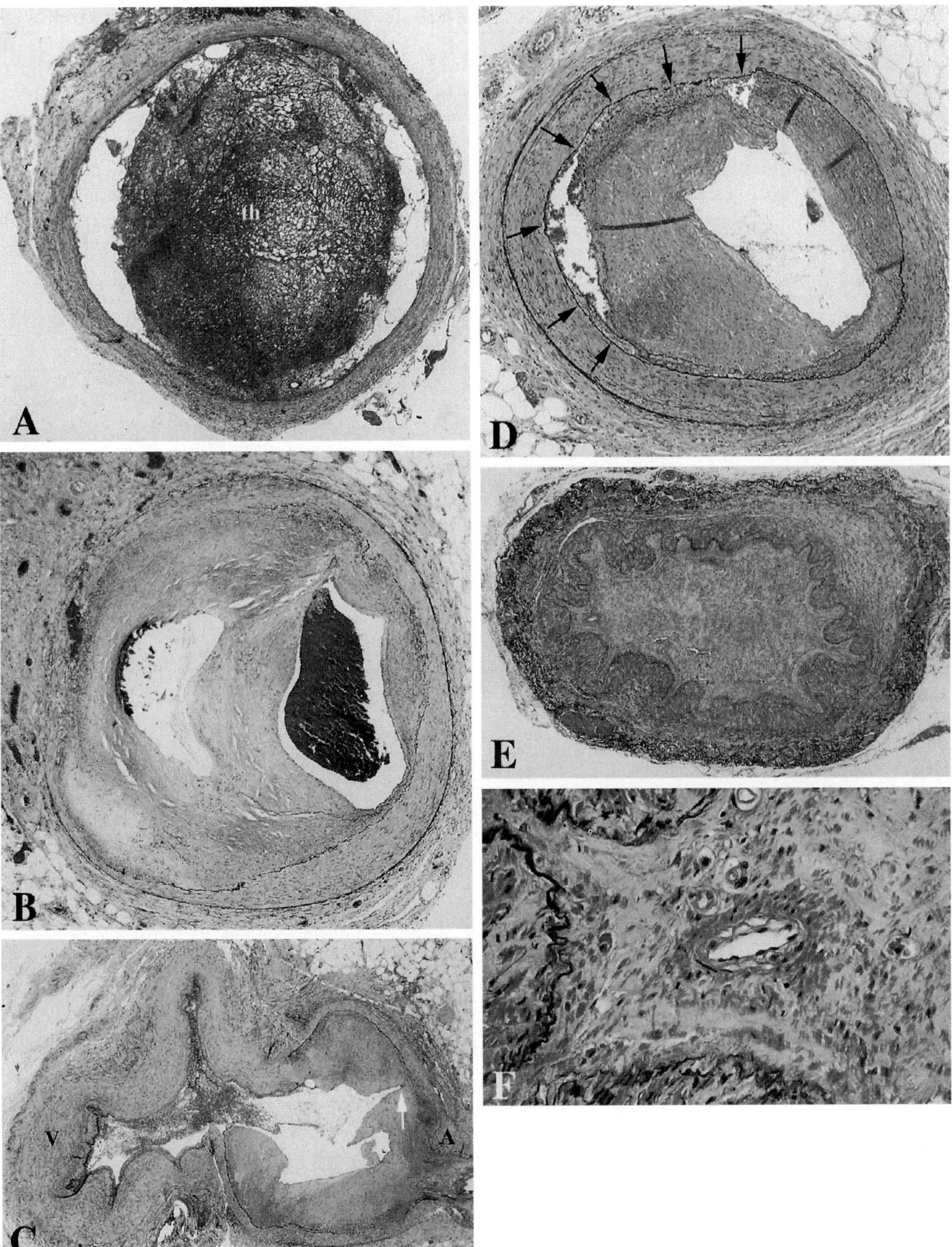

Figure 3–5. Acute complications of vein grafts. Histologic sections of vein graft (*A*) and native coronary artery distal to the anastomosis (*B*). Note total thrombotic (*th*) occlusion of the vein graft (in *A*) associated with poor distal run off as a result of severe distal coronary artery atherosclerosis (75% lumen area stenosis, in *B*). *C* shows the entry site (*arrow*) of an intimal dissection at the anastomosis of a bypass vein graft (*v*) to a native coronary artery (*a*). In *D,* a section of the native artery distal to the anastomosis in *C,* a deep intimal dissection is present involving > one third of the circumference of the artery (*arrows*). *E and F* are low- and high-power views, respectively, of cord-like chronically occluded vein graft containing an organized thrombus (*E*). The graft occluded shortly after placement. A high-power view of fibrous intima in the occluded vein is shown in *F;* there is focal recanalization of the thrombus.

in which acute vein graft thrombosis occurred, the graft appears as a thin fibrous cord throughout its length. Histologically, the vein wall is markedly contracted and the small lumen is occluded by organized thrombus characterized by a collagen and proteoglycan matrix containing smooth muscle cells and small recanalization channels (Fig. 3–5E and F).

Chronic Vein Graft Vasculopathy: Fibrointimal Hyperplasia and Atherosclerosis

For the majority of vein grafts, vasculopathy develops as an insidious lesion that is a major cause of morbidity and mortality. With the continued high volume of patients treated with CABG surgery and the aging of the population, the rates of repeat revascularization procedures (catheter-based and re-do CABG-surgery) are increasing. During the first 6 years post-CABG surgery, the rate of vein graft occlusion is 1–2%/year; from 6-10 years postoperatively, the occlusion rate increases to 4%/year. By 10 years post-CABG surgery, only 60% of vein grafts are patent, and only 50% of vein grafts are free of significant lumen stenosis.[12, 35–37]

The basic lesions of chronic vein graft vasculopathy are intimal hyperplasia (Fig. 3–6), atherosclerosis (Fig. 3–7), and combined atherosclerosis and fibrointimal proliferation.[38–42] In an autopsy study of 117 saphenous vein grafts in place 12–168 months antemortem, there were 25 atherosclerotic vessels, 66 with fibrointimal hyperplasia without atherosclerosis, and 26 fibrous cords (chronic total occlusions).[39] While the accumulation of fibrointimal hyperplasia did not cause severe graft narrowing in a majority of cases, it was associated with > 50% lumen area narrowing in 30% of grafts. Of grafts with atherosclerosis, 84% had > 50% lumen area narrowing (of which 64% had > 75% lumen area stenosis).[39]

Risk factors for native coronary artery atherosclerosis, particularly abnormal serum lipids, have also been correlated with atherosclerotic lesions in bypass vein grafts (Fig. 3–7).[34, 37–40] From clinical studies of the known atherosclerotic risk factors, elevated serum total cholesterol, LDL cholesterol, and triglycerides, and low serum HDL cholesterol levels appear to be important in the development of chronic vein graft lesions.[43–45] Reducing LAD-cholesterol levels to < 100 mg/dL with the lipid-lowering agent lovastatin (Mevacor) is associated with an increased frequency of vein graft patency.[46] Morphologic studies from autopsy hearts have

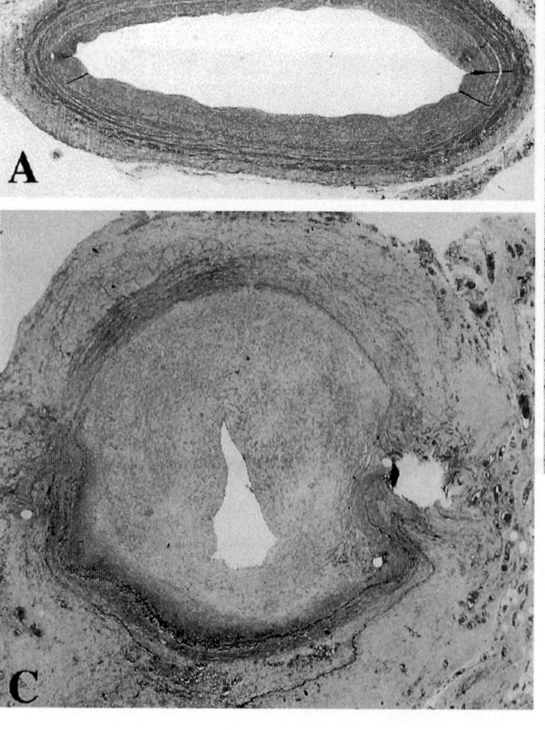

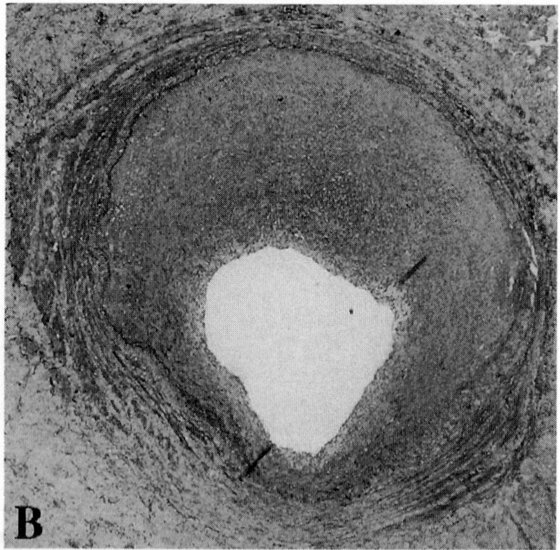

Figure 3–6. Vein graft intimal hyperplasia. *A to C* are histologic sections of vein grafts implanted ≥ 1 year antemortem. *A* shows mild fibrointimal thickening which is seen in all vein grafts that have been in place for > 3 months. More severe fibrointimal hyperplasia (*B*) is frequently seen in hypertensive individuals. Marked intimal thickening at the arterial anastomosis (*C*) can result in severe lumen stenosis and myocardial ischemia.

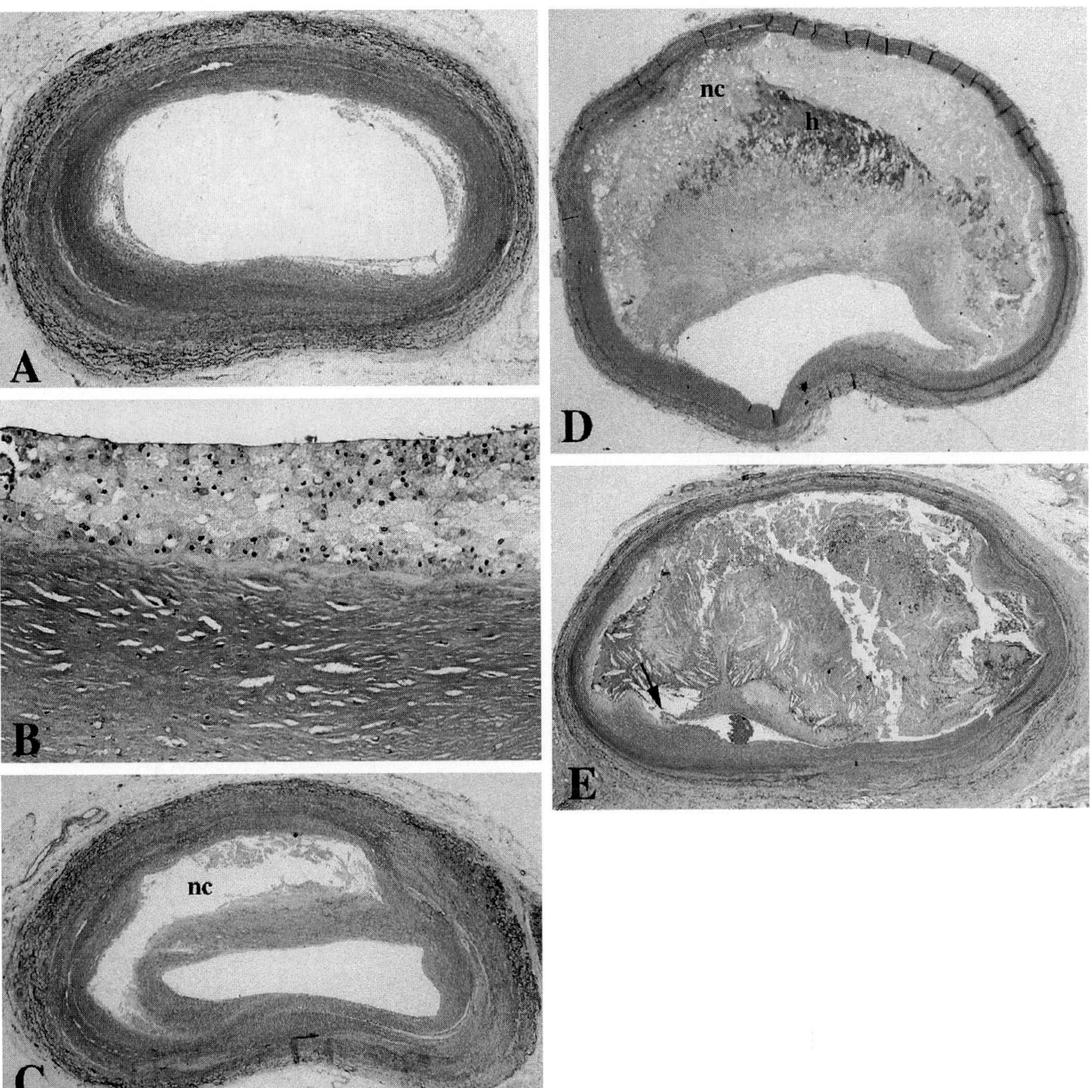

Figure 3–7. Vein graft atherosclerosis. *A* shows early atherosclerotic change characterized by luminal foam cells with underlying fibrointimal thickening. In *B* (high-power view of *A*), superficial foam cells accumulate over the fibrointima without a fibrous cap, a lesion rarely noted in native coronary artery atherosclerosis. A vein graft fibroatheroma with a well-developed necrotic core (*nc*) and an overlying thick fibrous cap is shown in *C*. Severe vein graft atherosclerosis (*D*) is characterized by a thin fibrous cap and a large necrotic core (*nc*) with hemorrhage (*h*). In advanced atherosclerotic vein graft lesions, rupture of a thin fibrous cap (*D, arrow*), at its thinnest portion, can precipitate lumen thrombus formation and acute myocardial infarction.

been generally supportive of the association of abnormal lipid levels and vein graft disease, and have provided histologic confirmation of the presence of atherosclerotic lesions (in contrast to fibrointimal hyperplasia).[38–40] In the above noted morphologic autopsy study of vein grafts, 68% of atherosclerotic vein grafts were associated with hypercholesterolemia compared with only 15% with fibrointimal hyperplasia.[39] Morphologic and angiography studies have shown that cigarette smoking is a risk factor for vein graft atherosclerosis.[40, 47] Studies of the relationship between diabetes mellitus and vein graft atherosclerosis have yielded inconsistent results.[12] There was a trend toward a higher mean serum glucose level in patients with vein graft atherosclerosis studied at autopsy versus those with fibrointimal hyperplasia.[39] In contrast to abnormal lipid levels and vein graft atherosclerosis, systemic hypertension appears to be associated with fibrointimal hyperplasia (Fig. 3–6); among autopsy vein grafts, 75% of grafts exhibiting fibrointimal hyperplasia (without atherosclerosis) were from patients with hypertension versus 25% of vein grafts with atherosclerosis.[39]

The histology of saphenous vein graft atherosclerosis (Fig. 3–7) differs somewhat from native coronary artery atherosclerosis and may reflect the relatively rapid evolution of its development. Typically, advanced atherosclerosis in vein grafts consists of a friable foam cell-rich lesion containing a large lipid (necrotic) core or several cores and a thin fibrous cap. Intraplaque hemorrhage within the large core is common (Fig. 3–7D), even in small plaques, but fibrocalcific lesions in vein grafts are rare. Just as in native coronary arteries, rupture of the fibrous cap can precipitate acute thrombus formation leading to acute myocardial infarction. (Fig. 3–7E).[43, 48] The friable, necrotic features of vein graft atherosclerotic plaques is probably responsible for the high incidence of distal embolization (resulting in non-Q-wave myocardial infarction and elevation of serum levels of cardiac enzymes) when these vessels are treated with catheter-based therapies (balloon angioplasty and stents).

In advanced atherosclerotic lesions, true vein graft aneurysms may form; these lesions may be multiple and are most often seen in grafts present ≥ 5 years (Fig. 3–8).[49–51] Vein graft aneurysms contain large poorly formed thrombi that occupy a large portion of the lumen. Another feature of degenerated atherosclerotic vein grafts is medial atrophy or complete disruption; in the latter instance, there may be extrusion of plaque contents into the adventitia associated with an adventitial inflammatory reaction (forming a pseudoaneurysm). At the aortic anastomosis, approximately two thirds of lesions consist of fibrointimal proliferation, with the remaining one third consisting of atherosclerotic plaque (with or without lipid core). Fibrointimal hyperplasia is present at > 90% of coronary artery anastomotic sites of long-term grafts.

To examine the progression of vein graft atherosclerotic lesions, we recently performed serial sectioning and morphologic assessment on 31 saphenous vein grafts from 16 patients in which vein grafts were in place ≥ 2 years (mean age of vein graft 8.5 ± 5.9 years, range 2–22 years).[52] There were 577 vein graft sections examined, of which 333 demonstrated fibrointimal hyperplasia and 242 showed atherosclerosis. Atherosclerotic lesions (Fig. 3–7) were classified as: (1) *superficial foam cell lesions,* characterized by surface foam cell accumulation without a fibrous cap or lipid core (present in 46% of atherosclerotic vein grafts); (2) *lipid core lesions* which had well-developed necrotic cores (29% of grafts); and (3) lesions with *hemorrhagic lipid cores* (25% of grafts).

In superficial foam cell lesions, there were accumulations of macrophages along the intimal surface; the vein graft intima consisted of proteoglycan and collagen and was largely devoid of smooth muscle cells.[52] In a previous study, vein graft intimal small muscle apoptosis has been observed at sites of foam cell accumulation, raising the possibility that a foam-cell derived factor(s) can induce smooth muscle cell death.[53] There was a continuous significant progression of lumen area percent stenosis from superficial foam cell lesions (37 ± 9% stenosis) to lipid core lesions (46 ± 17%) to hemorrhagic lipid core lesions (74 ± 19%).[52] Once a lipid core forms in a vein graft ath-

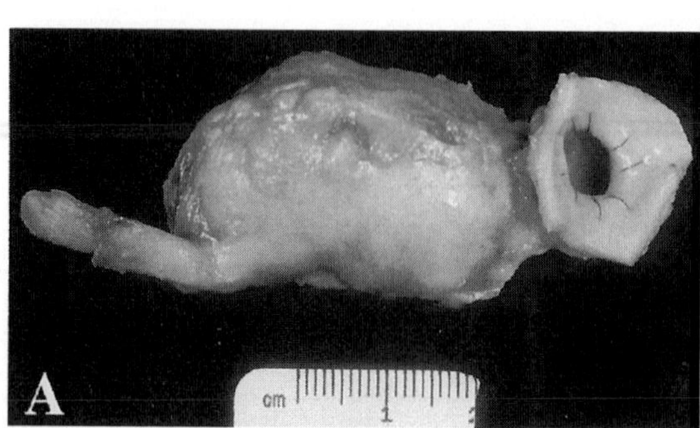

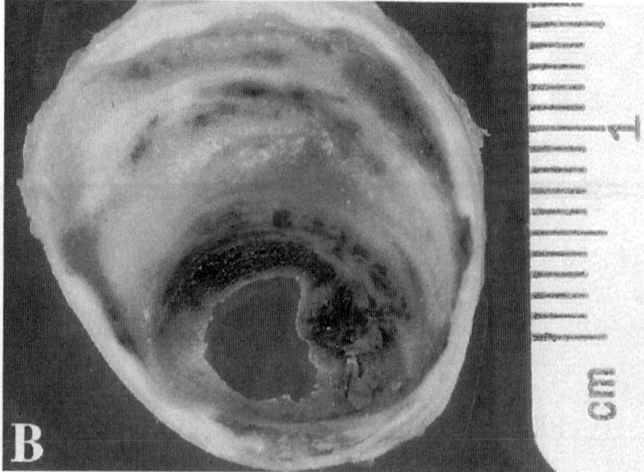

Figure 3–8. Vein graft aneurysm involving the proximal and mid portions of the graft (*A*). A cross section (*B*) shows laminated thrombus is present which was associated with intramyocardial emboli.

erosclerotic plaque, the risk of core hemorrhage increases as the lipid core size increases (8.6 ± 2.2 mm^2 with core hemorrhage vs. 1.5 ± 1.9 mm^2 without core hemorrhage) and as the percentage of the entire atherosclerotic plaque area that is occupied by the lipid core (59 ± 17% with core hemorrhage vs. 18 ± 19% without core hemorrhage). Therefore, vein graft atherosclerotic stenosis progression likely passes through phases of macrophage deposition on the vein graft intima followed by development of a lipid core; lipid core hemorrhage results in further lumen stenosis progression. These data suggest that inhibition of foam cell adherence is a potential therapeutic target for preventing SVG atherosclerosis and may be the mechanism for enhanced vein graft patency in lipid lowering trials.[46]

In patients with vein graft atherosclerosis, acute plaque rupture and lumen thrombosis is an important mechanism of morbidity and mortality.[43,48] In the study of atherosclerosis progression, plaque rupture and acute thrombosis were identified in 23% of sections with lipid cores present.[52] The mean lumen area stenosis in ruptured plaques was 75 ± 24%, which corresponds to a diameter stenosis of 55 ± 23% (95% confidence interval 42–67%). Similar to lipid core hemorrhage, the risk of plaque rupture increases as lipid core size increases and as the percentage of the entire atherosclerotic plaque area that is occupied by the lipid core. In vein graft atherosclerotic lesions, a diameter stenosis of ≥ 55% with a lipid core area of ≥ 5.1 mm^2 that occupies ≥ 44% of the total plaque area are morphologic predictors of plaque rupture and lumen thrombosis. Fibrous caps were 2.6-fold thinner in plaques with cap rupture compared with nonruptured plaques. Further, vein graft plaque rupture sites are frequently long (mean length 6.6 mm) and multifocal (3.2 rupture sites per vein graft) and are associated with long segments of plaque (2.1 cm) containing large, nonruptured lipid cores. This finding underscores the diffuse nature of vein graft atherosclerosis and the limited therapeutic benefit of percutaneous treatment that only addresses short focal lesions. Currently, there is an expanding use of interventional strategies (e.g., aspiration devices, covered stents) in which multiple areas are treated to reduce the incidence of necrotic core prolapse and embolization during stenting.[54]

Surgical Endarterectomy

In patients with diffuse coronary atherosclerosis undergoing CABG surgery, coronary endarterectomy can be performed, and is most often used in the distal right coronary artery.[55,56] Early reports indicated a high incidence of postoperative mortality and morbidity with reduced arterial patency rates in patients treated with surgical endarterectomy. More recent studies in selected patients demonstrate similar rates of survival and cardiovascular complications between CABG patients treated with or without coronary endarterectomy.[56–58]

Pathologically, the surgical coronary endarterectomy specimen shows the various types of plaque (fibrous plaque, lipid core, hemorrhagic plaque, and calcified plaque) present in advanced atherosclerotic disease. A portion of the arterial media may be present. In autopsy specimens evaluated early after endarterectomy, areas of plaque removal and partial medial resection are evident (Fig. 3–9). A layer of fibrin thrombus with associated inflammatory cells covers luminal surface of the residual plaque. Over the course of several weeks, a neointima forms composed of a collagen and proteoglycan matrix containing smooth muscle cells.

Role of the Pathologist

(See also Chapter 1). At autopsy, all bypass grafts should be identified based on their type (artery or vein) and by their native coronary target(s). Hearts with old grafts, and especially in patients with re-do CABG surgery, typically have dense pericardial fibrous adhesions which make dissection difficult. Twisted or taut grafts should be noted. Sectioning of the entire graft is necessary to locate focal lesions, and all significant lesions (> 50% lumen area stenosis) or possible thrombi should be submitted for histologic examination. Anastomotic sites should be carefully sectioned and examined histologically. The distal run-off native artery should be sectioned; not uncommonly, bypass graft failure can be explained by the presence of severe atherosclerosis distal to the graft anastomosis.

PERCUTANEOUS CORONARY REVASCULARIZATION

Percutaneous Transluminal Coronary Angioplasty

First introduced in 1977, percutaneous transluminal coronary angioplasty (PTCA) has

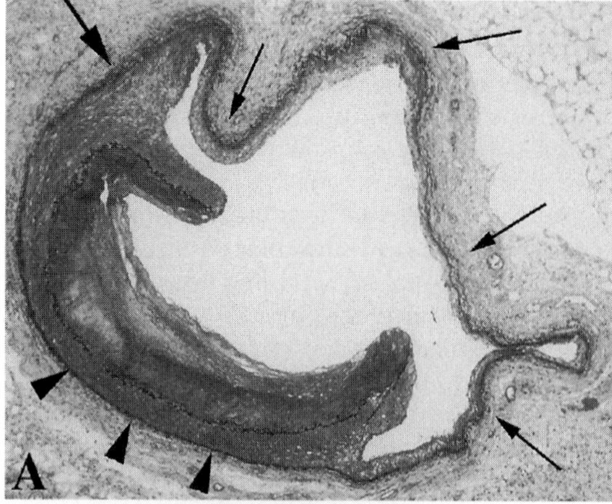

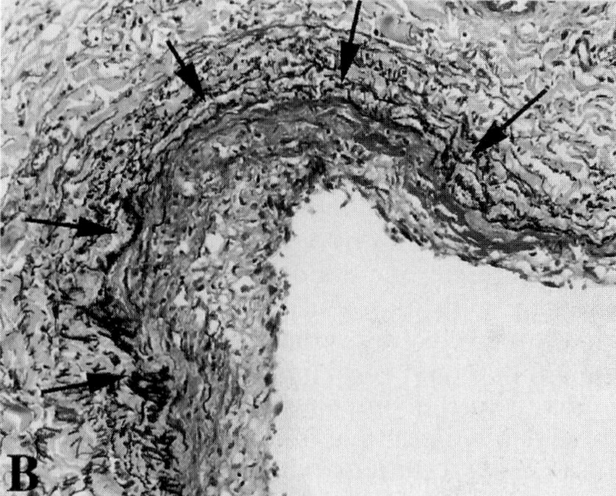

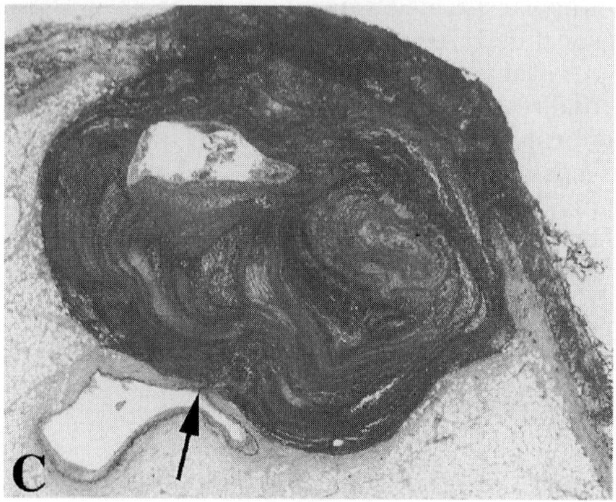

Figure 3–9. Surgical coronary atherectomy in a 70-year-old diabetic man with diffuse coronary atherosclerosis who died 14 days after CABG surgery. *A and B* are low- and high-power views of the right coronary artery that was treated with endarterectomy at the time of bypass grafting. Note that half of the coronary artery wall consists of only adventitia (*arrows, B*) and focal adjoining few layers of medial smooth muscle cells. At the edges of the plaque, a medial dissection (*large arrow, A*) is present associated with an early organizing thrombus. A normal media and overlying mild atherosclerotic plaque is seen (*arrowheads, A*). *C* shows a low-power view of a focal coronary artery rupture at an endarterectomy site; note the large overlying hematoma over the arterial rupture site (*arrow*).

become standard practice for percutaneous revascularization for significant coronary atherosclerosis.[59] In PTCA, catheters with balloons on their ends are passed into the coronary arteries under fluoroscopic guidance over steerable, flexible metallic guidewires to the lesion site. PTCA balloons are composed of varying types of polymers (e.g., polyethylene or polyvinyl chloride) and are manufactured in varying sizes (1.5–4.0 mm inflated diameter) to dilate lesions within small to large coronary arteries. The PTCA balloons are inflated to super-atmospheric pressures, (typically 4–12 ATM) to dilate the arterial lumen.

The efficacy of PTCA to increase lumen area and to provide relief of symptoms of atherosclerotic coronary disease is well-established.[60] In current practice, $\geq$ 90% of coronary lesions can be successfully dilated to increase lumen diameter by $\geq$ 20% and reduce lumen diameter stenosis to $<$ 50%.[60] However, in long-term studies, PTCA has not been shown to be clinically superior (reduction in cardiovascular mortality and morbidity) to: (1) CABG surgery in patients with multivessel coronary disease (see earlier); (2) medical therapy in patients with single-vessel disease;[61] or (3) aggressive lipid-lowering therapy in patients with stable angina.[62] Balloon angioplasty is being increasingly utilized to restore coronary patency in patients presenting with acute myocardial infarction and coronary thrombosis. Overall clinical results for direct-PTCA for acute myocardial infarction appear to be at least as good as thrombolytic therapy with a reduced incidence of coronary reocclusion and hemorrhagic stroke with angioplasty.[63–65]

The major acute coronary complications of PTCA involve abrupt renarrowing of the dilated artery. Elastic recoil can result in critical renarrowing of the artery within the first 24 hours after PTCA. The incidence of abrupt vessel closure after PTCA occurs in 4.4–8.3%,[66] and the mechanisms of abrupt occlusion include arterial dissection in which a dissecting hematoma compresses the true lumen, intraluminal thrombus, elastic recoil, vasospasm, and prolapse of plaque into the arterial lumen. Persistent arterial occlusion after PTCA is associated with frequent referral for emergency coronary bypass surgery, a 40% incidence of acute myocardial infarction, and a 4% incidence of death.[67] However, the need for emergency bypass has been greatly reduced by the use of intracoronary stents (see following). Stents are deployed routinely in current standard practice for acute coronary arterial closure, threatened arterial closure, inadequate lumen dilatation, and significant coronary dissection. Chronically, the benefit of PTCA is significantly compromised by restenosis (see following).

The Mechanism of Leumen Enlargement and Pathology of PTCA

Pathologic studies have been instrumental in understanding the mechanisms and clarifying the benefits and limitations of PTCA.[68–72] During balloon inflation within the coronary arteries, no plaque is removed; rather, high-pressure balloon inflation causes cracks in the atherosclerotic plaque at its thinnest, weakest point (Fig. 3–10). True lumen enlargement is produced when plaque disruption reaches the arterial media causing medial and adventitial stretch (Figs. 3–10 and 3–11). The expanded lumen produced by cracks in atherosclerotic plaque and medial stretch is referred to as the "acute lumen gain." Unless there is plastic deformation in the media and adventitia, resulting in an increase in the arterial outer circumference, there will be no significant net gain in the lumen area.[68] More often than not, medial stretch results in medial dissection (Fig. 3–12), which may precede anterograde and retrograde. Not uncommonly, and especially in eccentric arteries, PTCA causes full thickness medial rupture. Extensive dissection can cause critical luminal narrowing (Fig. 3–12). However, as long as there is no lumen compromise, the presence of medial dissection does not necessarily effect long-term outcome. Arterial perforation following PTCA fortunately is rare,[73] even in the setting of full thickness medial rupture, because of the strong collagenous adventitia. Acute arterial closure following PTCA (Fig. 3–12) is currently treated with bailout stenting (see following).

Restenosis

The most important complication that significantly limits the long-term clinical efficacy of PTCA is arterial restenosis. Clinical restenosis

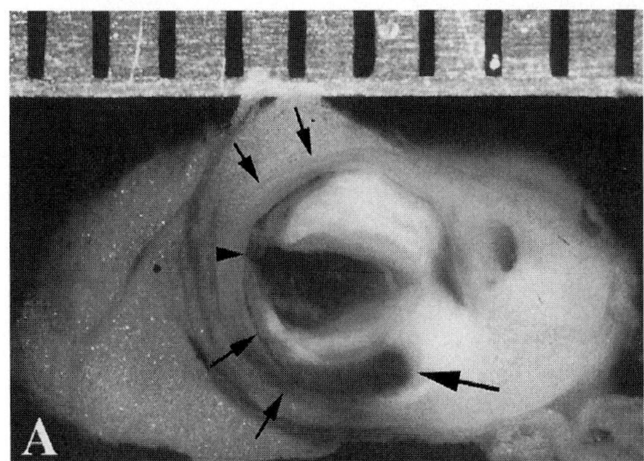

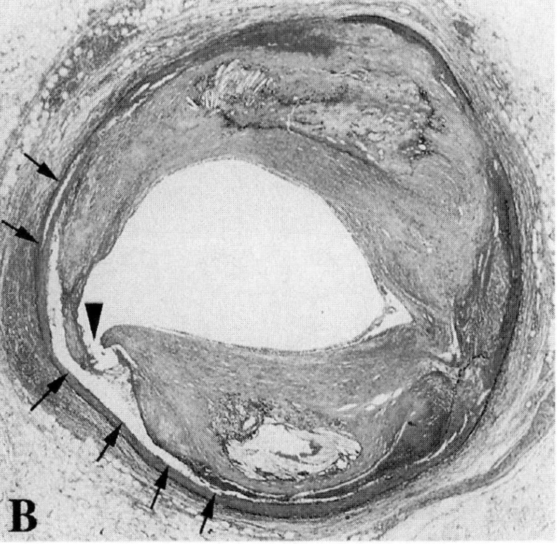

Figure 3–10. Pathology of acute angioplasty. Cross section of the left circumflex coronary artery at the balloon angioplasty site 12 hours after PTCA (*A*). Note hemorrhage at the media/plaque interface (*small arrows*) and hemorrhage within the necrotic core (*large arrow*). Angioplasty-induced plaque rupture occurs at the site of minimal plaque thickness (*arrowhead*). *B,* the corresponding histologic section of the artery in *A,* shows plaque disruption where the plaque is thinnest (*arrowhead*) and a dissection plane at the media/intimal plaque interface (*arrows*).

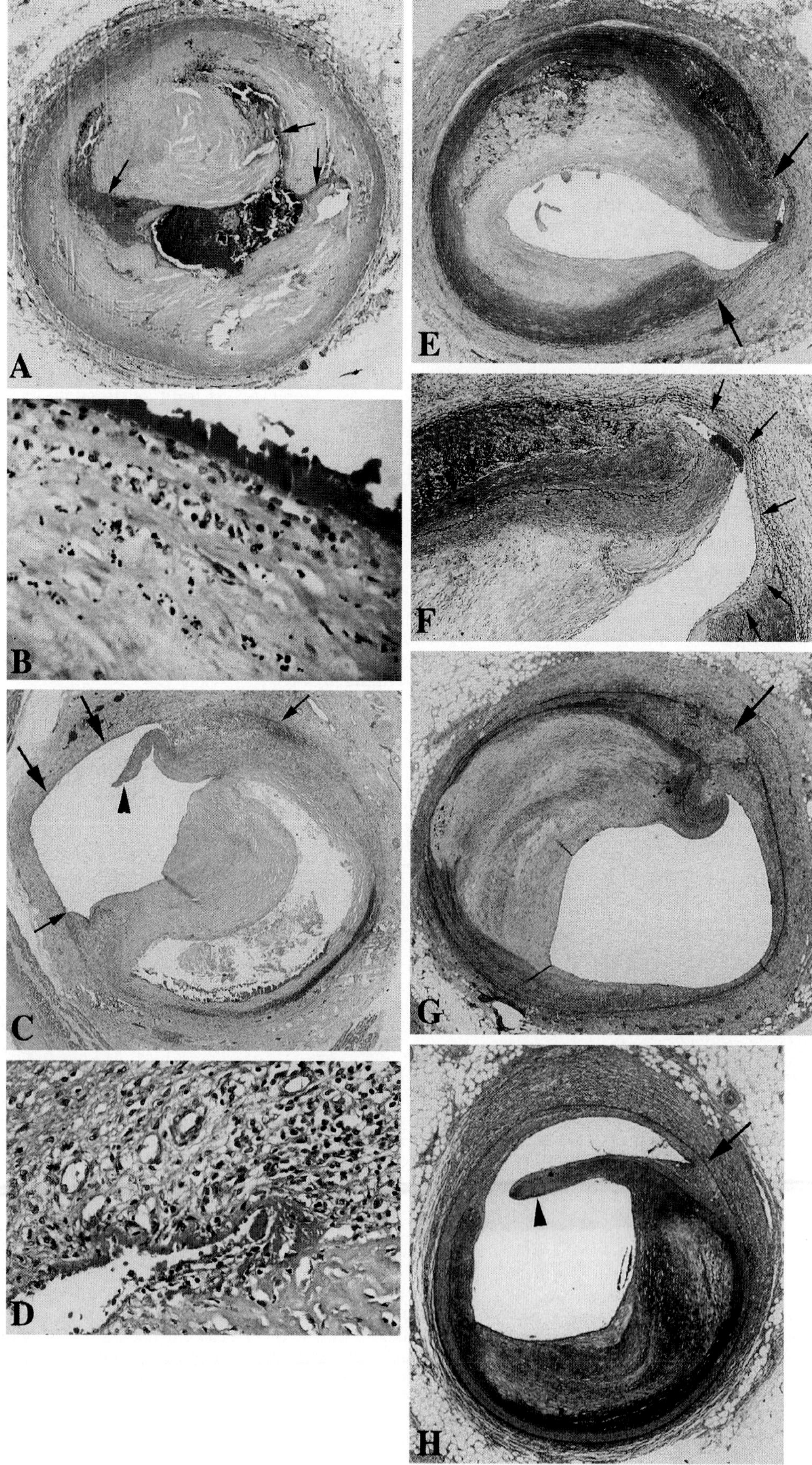

Figure 3–11. *See legend on opposite page*

after PTCA occur in 30–40% of patients and angiographic restenosis is seen in up to 50% of dilated arteries.[60] Clinically, restenosis is defined both as a dichotomous variable (> 50% diameter stenosis) or as a continuous variable (loss of ≥ 50% of the acute lumen gain). It should be noted that angiographic restenosis may not be associated with clinical signs or symptoms. Two pathophysiologic mechanisms are operative in the restenosis process ("late lumen loss"): (1) neointimal growth and (2) negative arterial remodeling. The pathophysiology of neointimal growth after PTCA leading to restenosis is incompletely understood and involves complex interactions among cellular elements (platelets and inflammatory cells), local noncellular elements (growth factors, adhesion molecules, and cytokines), and circulating proteins (coagulation factors).[74]

Neointimal growth post-PTCA essentially reflects an arterial response to injury. Immediately after PTCA and lasting several days, there is thrombus deposition associated with acute inflammation on the injured endothelial surface and within dissection planes in the plaque and media (Fig. 3–11A and B).[68] By 1–2 weeks, chronic inflammatory cells, especially macrophages, are seen (Fig. 3–11C and D). Experimental studies of endothelial balloon injury in normal animal arteries demonstrate migration of smooth muscle cells from the media to the intima followed by proliferation and synthesis of proteoglycan and collagen-rich extracellular matrix forming the neointima.[75] Smooth muscle cell proliferation appears to be maximal 3–7 days after arterial injury.[76, 77] For example, in the porcine coronary artery restenosis model, Carter et al. showed maximal cellular proliferation, assessed by proliferating cell nuclear antigen (PCNA) staining (a marker of cell proliferation), 7 days after stent placement (18.6 ± 3.5% of neointimal cells PCNA-positive) with declining proliferation at 14 days (9.6 ± 1.3% PCNA-positive) and 28 days (1.1 ± 1.0% PCNA-positive).[76] In experimental animals, the neointima is well-established by 1 month. In human atherosclerotic arteries treated with PTCA, a neointima containing smooth muscle cells and matrix, similar to animal experiments, can be recognized by 2 weeks and is well established by 3 months.[68]

While most experimental models of restenosis suggest that vascular smooth muscle cell proliferation is an important component of restenosis, the importance of smooth muscle cell proliferation in the development of restenosis in humans has not been settled. In a study of 37 atherectomy specimens (26 denovo plaques and 11 restenosis lesions), only 25% of restenotic atherectomy specimens demonstrated positive PCNA staining. Another study of restenotic tissue obtained by coronary atherectomy from stents in place 2.5–23 months showed a relatively hypocellular extracellular matrix; cellular proliferation (determined by Ki-67 staining) was rare.[78] In contrast, in a study of ten peripheral arterial lesions (six femoral arteries, three iliac arteries, and one subclavian artery) with stents implanted 4 to 25 months, lesions from the stented segments were hypercellular with actin positive cells demonstrating high proliferative activity (24.6 ± 2.3% PCNA-positive).[79] The reasons for the conflicting results among these atherectomy studies are uncertain and are probably due to variability and small size of the samples obtained by percutaneous atherectomy.

Inflammation and Growth Factors

Experimental and human studies suggest that inflammatory responses to PTCA play an important role in neointimal growth. The early thrombus formed within the first 1–3 days after

Figure 3–11. Stages of coronary artery repair following coronary balloon angioplasty (PTCA). *A* and *B* are low- and high-power photomicrographs from a 67-year-old man who died 3 days following PTCA. In *A,* note the cracks in the plaque (*arrows*) emanating from the lumen of a concentric atherosclerotic coronary artery. In *B,* a high-power view of the intimal surface shows a thin layer of platelet deposition and acute inflammation within the plaque. *C and D* are low- and high-power views of a coronary artery 1 week following PTCA. In *C,* an arterial dissection (*small arrow*) is present with focal medial rupture (*arrowhead*) and marked stretching of the adventitia (*large arrows*). At high power (*D*), the dissection site shows granulation tissue with organizing fibrin, neocapillary formation, smooth muscle cell infiltration, and chronic inflammation (lymphocytes and macrophages). *E and F* are low- and high-power views of a coronary artery 10 days post-balloon angioplasty. No luminal thrombus is present at the site of medial tear (*arrows, E*), and there is early neointima formation consisting of smooth muscle cells in a proteoglycan matrix (*arrows, F*). *G and H* are two cross sections of coronary arteries 14 days following PTCA; both show eccentric plaques and marked stretching of the media and adventitia with focal medial rupture. In *G,* there is a localized dissection, which is healing with granulation tissue (*arrow*). *H* shows a residual intimal flap with healing of the focal dissection (*arrow*).

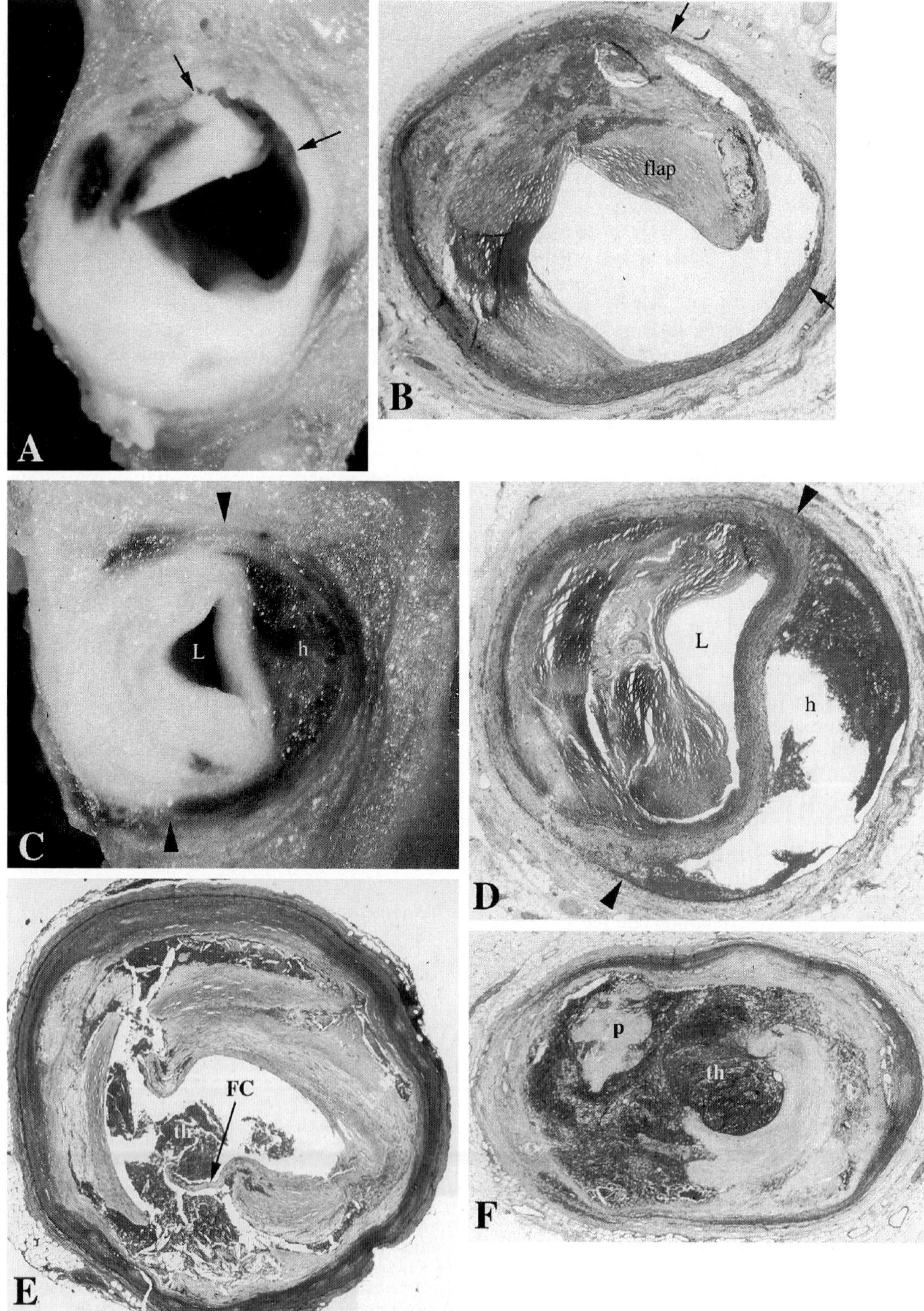

Figure 3–12. *See legend on opposite page*

PTCA in normal animal arteries typically contains neutrophils with few T-lymphocytes and monocytes.[76, 80] In balloon-injured and stented normal rabbit iliac arteries, neutrophils and monocytes adhere to the lumen surface at 3 days and infiltrate the vessel wall between 3 and 14 days.[80, 81] Arterial inflammation following PTCA (and stenting, see following) is also commonly seen in human atherosclerotic coronary arteries (Fig. 3–11). At early time points after PTCA, inflammation consists of neutrophils and mononuclear cells; from 1 to 3 weeks, mononuclear cells, granulation tissue, and neoangiogenesis predominate. For example, of 13 human coronary arteries treated with PTCA and examined $<$ 1 day to 5 days postprocedure, eight (62%) demonstrated acute inflammation.[68] Mononuclear cell infiltrates were seen most commonly between days 3 to 16, but were also present in some cases beyond 3 months post-PTCA.[68]

The contribution of inflammatory responses to the restenosis process is a topic of current investigation.[82] Activation of leukocytes occurs post-PTCA, and plasma levels of circulating granulocyte-derived elastase is increased with elevated generation of oxygen free radicals, indicative of cellular activation.[83] Increased granulocyte elastase release has also been associated with an increased incidence of restenosis after PTCA.[84] Further, activated neutrophils secrete multiple factors that can augment tissue injury (proteolytic enzymes and oxygen-derived free radicals), stimulate platelets (platelet activating factor), and attract monocytes.[85] Macrophages can also release reactive oxygen species[86] and proteins capable of stimulating smooth muscle cell migration and proliferation.[87–89]

In addition to cellular activation, arterial damage induced by PTCA also increases expression of leukocyte adhesion molecules. The β_2-integrin family of adhesion molecules are upregulated when granulocytes are stimulated and are responsible for neutrophil aggregation, firm adhesion of leukocytes to the endothelial surface, and transendothelial migration. Of the β_2-integrins, Mac-1 (expressed on granulocytes and monocytes) appears to be closely linked to the arterial healing and restenosis process postinjury.[90] Mac-1 is the primary fibrinogen receptor on leukocytes[91] and acts to permit leukocyte adhesion and transmigration at sites of platelet and fibrin deposition.[92] In patients, increased expression of Mac-1 on granulocyte and monocyte surfaces has been observed after PTCA.[90, 93–96] Importantly, the greater the increase in Mac-1 expression, the greater the likelihood of restenosis.[90, 94]

The selectin family of adhesion molecules (P, E, and L-selectin) mediate interactions between endothelial cells and leukocytes during leukocyte rolling, an action that precedes firm cellular adhesion.[92, 97, 98] In patients undergoing elective PTCA, circulating soluble L-selectin levels increase and are associated with increased expression of neutrophil Mac-1.[95, 96] Further, increased circulating L and P-selectin levels have been associated with postangioplasty restenosis.[99, 100] Intercellular adhesion molecule-1 (ICAM-1) is a member of the immunoglobulin gene superfamily. ICAM-1 is expressed on endothelial cells and on activated vascular smooth muscle cells, mediates leukocyte adhesion, and contains ligand binding sites for the β_2-integrins. An increased circulating level of ICAM-1 has been demonstrated in patients following coronary angioplasty (with or without accompanying acute myocardial infarction).[100, 101] An increase in ICAM-1 levels post-PTCA in patients was associated with increased frequency of coronary restenosis.[100, 101]

Inflammatory cytokines released by activated T-cells and macrophages [including TNF-α (tumor necrosis factor-α), interleukin-1β (IL-1β), interleukin-4 (IL-4), and IFN-γ (interferon-γ)] regulate complex interaction among smooth

Figure 3–12. Acute complications of balloon angioplasty. *A and B* are gross and corresponding histology of a coronary artery 3 days post-balloon angioplasty. Note a coronary dissection involving one fourth of the arterial circumference (*between arrows*) with lumen enlargement secondary to medial stretch and injury. As a result of the dissection (*arrow, B*), an intimal flap is formed by the atherosclerotic plaque, which has separated from the underlying media. *C and D* show gross and corresponding microscopic views of a coronary artery with extensive arterial dissection secondary to PTCA. In *C*, the dissection is indicated by arrowheads, and the false lumen contains the dissecting hematoma (*h*). The histologic view (*D*) of the artery shows the media lifted from the underlying adventitia, and the dissection plane is filled with a hematoma (*h*, most of hematoma has fallen off the section). Note that the dissection results in marked compromise of the lumen (*L*). *E* is a histologic section of a coronary artery from a patient who underwent angioplasty and died within hours of the procedure; there is hemorrhage within the necrotic core, rupture of a vulnerable plaque (*fc*, fibrous cap), and a luminal nonocclusive thrombus (*th*). *F* shows a coronary artery from a patient who underwent balloon angioplasty $<$ 48 hours antemortem. There is extensive plaque disruption, and a large occlusive thrombus (*th*) containing a fragment of plaque (*p*).

muscle cells, leukocytes, and adhesion molecules in the restenosis process. For example, IL-1β stimulates the proliferation of vascular smooth muscle cells *in vitro* and induces expression of ICAM-1 and VCAM-1.[102, 103] ICAM-1 and VCAM-1 on smooth muscle cells are also induced by TNF-α.[104, 105] In patients, IL-1β production by stimulated monocytes correlates with late lumen loss after PTCA.[106] Among the known growth factors, platelet-derived growth factor (derived from platelets) and basic fibroblast growth factor (derived from endothelial cell, macrophages, smooth muscle cells) are important mitogens for endothelial cells and smooth muscle cells.[107–109] Transforming growth factor-β secreted by platelets, endothelial cells, and macrophages promotes leukocyte chemotaxis, angiogenesis, and the secretion of extracellular matrix by smooth muscle cells.[72] Human restenotic coronary lesions demonstrate increased expression of transforming growth factor-β-inducible gene.[110]

The multiplicity of factors that are involved in the arterial restenosis process provide multiple targets for potential therapy. However, the complexity and overlap of the actions of the various inflammatory cells, adhesion molecules, cytokines, and growth factors on intimal growth make it unlikely that a single agent will be an effective antirestenosis therapy.

Histologic Predictors of Successful PTCA

Eccentric (rather than concentric) plaques are more likely to be successfully dilated because the angioplasty balloon is more likely to be able to split an arc of relatively thin plaque and stretch the subjacent arterial media (Fig. 3–11). In contrast, in concentric plaques, the PTCA balloon can only produce modest cracks in the surrounding plaque without an ability to stretch the media resulting in minimal acute lumen gain. In an autopsy study of human coronary arteries subjected to PTCA during life, long-term histologic success was seen in 48% of eccentric plaques versus 18% of concentric plaques.[68] Not surprisingly, plaques consisting of dense collagen are less likely to be successfully dilated than softer, fibropultaceous plaques. Cracks in concentric densely fibrotic plaques are typically small, do not extend to the media, and do not, therefore, result in an effective increase in lumen area. The effect of calcification on PTCA outcome is complex. Severely calcified plaques behave similarly to dense fibrous plaque and resist balloon dilatation. In contrast, mild to moderate calcification provides foci of regional differences in local stiffness between adjacent calcified and noncalcified regions.[111] It has been postulated that these differences in local stiffness allow for more effective arterial stretch secondary to longitudinal shearing with a reduced frequency of elastic recoil.[111]

Given these morphologic variables of the underlying atherosclerotic plaque, a critical determinate of late outcome after PTCA is the creation of a large acute lumen area. Angiographic studies have demonstrated that the greater the acute lumen gain after PTCA.[112–114] the greater the likelihood of a larger lumen being present chronically despite the fact that increased arterial injury correlates with increased neointimal growth.[70] This "bigger is better" hypothesis of improving long-term outcome by maximizing initial lumen expansion has been supported by pathologic analysis of coronary artery balloon angioplasty specimens. In a study of 28 postmortem coronary arteries subjected to PTCA an average of 71 weeks antemortem, the histologic acute lumen area was 34% greater ($4.1 \pm 1.9\ mm^2$ vs. $2.7 \pm 1.4\ mm^2$) in long-term successes than in long-term failures ($p < 0.0001$).[71] The acute lumen area as a percent of the area within the internal elastic lamina was 46 ± 10% in long-term successes vs. 27 ± 11% in failures. Because the amount of neointima growth was independent of vessel size, a larger acute lumen area reduces the chance that the neointimal growth that invariably occurs after PTCA will result in coronary restenosis.

Negative Remodeling

Arterial remodeling refers to changes in arterial dimensions in response to vascular disease. Glagov et al. observed an increase in arterial size during the early stages of atherosclerotic plaque growth so that there was no lumen compromise until plaque area approached approximately 40% of the area within the internal elastic lamina.[115] This increase in arterial size in which lumen area is maintained despite an increase in plaque size is referred to as "positive remodeling."

Following PTCA, in addition to neointimal growth, arterial constriction (negative remodeling) may augment late lumen loss and lead to restenosis. The mechanism of negative remodeling is believed to involve stretch-induced adventitial injury followed by adventitial fibrosis and contraction. Intravascular ultrasound studies suggest that up to 60% of the late lumen loss following PTCA is due to negative remodeling and the remaining 40% accounted by neointimal growth.[116] In morphologic studies, a reduction in the area within the external elastic lamina at the PTCA site relative to the proximal reference non-PTCA site (histologic negative remodeling) correlated with restenosis, and an increase in the area within the external elastic lamina correlated with a long-term histologic success.[117] Plaque size appears to be an important determinant of negative remodeling; a small plaque size allows for greater expansion of the external elastic lamina and greater arterial dilatation which mitigates against subsequent arterial constriction. Further, histologic studies suggest that arterial shrinkage induced by the underlying plaque may be relatively more important in the negative remodeling process than adventitial fibrosis.[117] Late negative arterial remodeling is prevented by stent deployment, an important advantage of stent use over angioplasty alone.

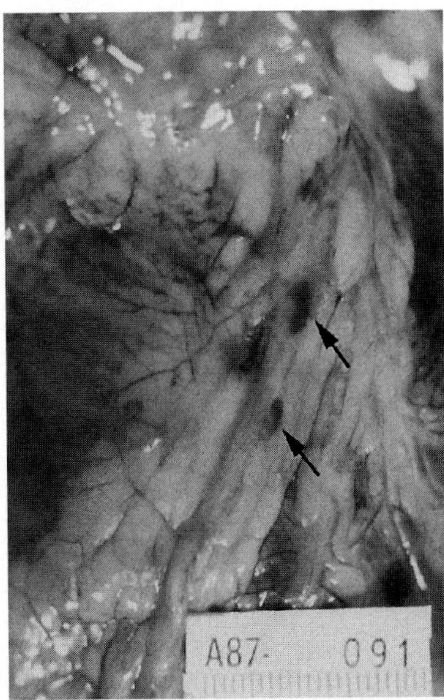

Figure 3–13. External view of the heart from a patient who died within 24 hours of percutaneous transluminal coronary angioplasty (PTCA). Focal areas of epicardial hemorrhage (*arrows*) in the area of PTCA are present on the adventitial surface of the left anterior descending coronary artery.

Role of the Pathologist in Assessing Coronary Arteries Subjected to PTCA

The clinical record and coronary angiogram report should be reviewed to establish which artery and the location within the artery (proximal, middle, or distal and/or arterial position relative to side branches) subjected to PTCA. In patients treated within 1 week antemortem, the epicardial surface of the dilated artery should be carefully inspected for evidence of adventitial hemorrhage (Fig. 3–13). The dilated artery should be cut transversely at 2- to 3-mm intervals following decalcification (if necessary). All arterial segments from the PTCA site should be processed for routine light microscopy and staining with hematoxylin and Movat pentachrome (or EVG). The coronary artery proximal and distal to the PTCA site should be sectioned at 2- to 3-mm intervals for evidence of propagated arterial dissection or severe coronary stenoses. Not uncommonly, significant atherosclerotic luminal narrowing is underestimated by coronary angiography and therefore not treated by percutaneous revascularization techniques.

The morphology of a coronary PTCA site is a function of the duration of time from the arterial balloon dilatation to death and follows a vascular response-to-injury model (Fig. 3–11).[68, 71] Early after PTCA (hours to several days), plaque disruption and medial dissection should be readily identified; these sites are lined by platelet/fibrin thrombus containing trapped erythrocytes and acute inflammatory cells. By 1 week after PTCA, there is organization of the thrombus with proliferating endothelial cells and inflammatory infiltrates (granulation tissue), and infiltrating smooth muscle cells become increasingly evident (Fig. 3–14). The early polyhedral-shaped smooth muscle cells have oval nuclei, abundant cytoplasm, few thin or intermediate filaments, abundant rough endoplasmic reticulum, and are arranged close to the underlying plaque.[72, 118] These features identify these early smooth muscle cells as maintaining a secretory phenotype. By 2 months, the smooth muscle cells assume their more typical spindle shape with elongated nuclei and reduced cytoplasm and are arranged parallel to the lumen. These cells stain strongly for α-actin and vimentin, consistent with a contractile phenotype.[119] It is the extent of smooth muscle cell accumulation and especially the synthesis of collagen and proteoglycan-rich matrix that define the restenosis lesion. The collagenous portion of the extracellular matrix consists of type III collagen (Fig. 3–14), and alcian blue stains demonstrate that the dominant proteoglycans in the extracellular matrix are chondroitin sul-

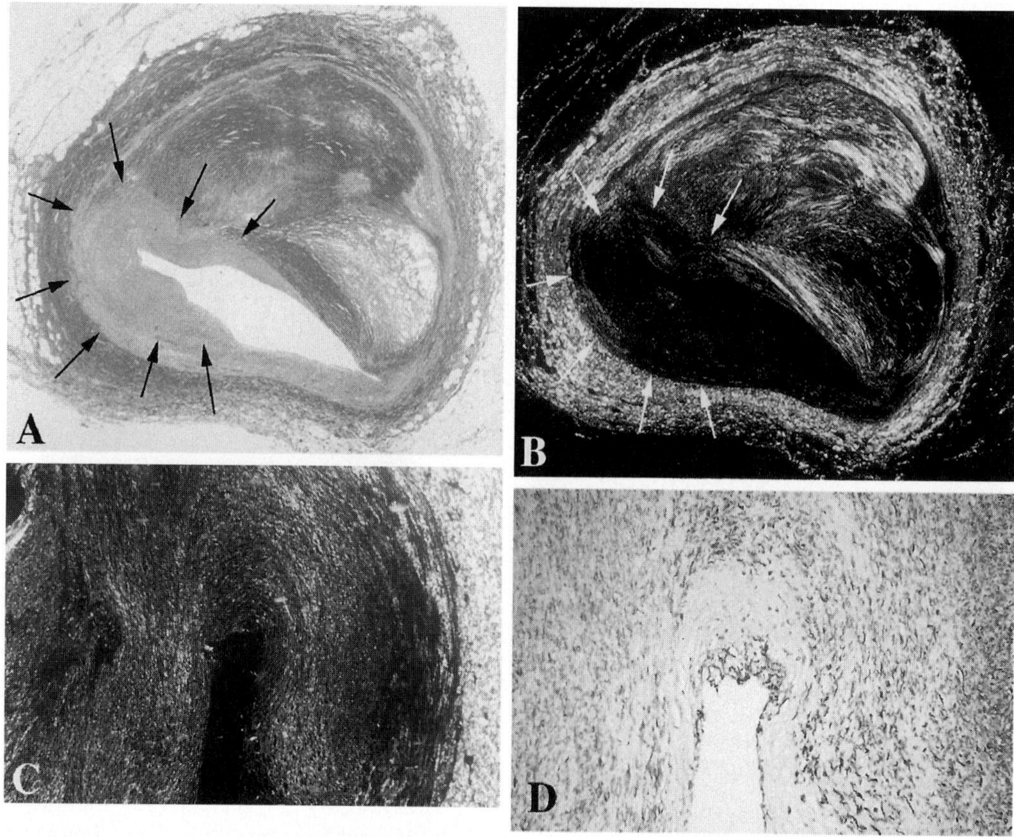

Figure 3–14. Post-balloon angioplasty healing. *A and B* are coronary sections from a 38-year-old man who had undergone PTCA 6 months antemortem. In *A,* Sirus red staining shows the PTCA site outlined by arrows with overlying neointimal formation. The same section viewed under polarized light is shown in *B* and *C;* the neointima is green (*within arrows*) indicating the presence of type III collagen, and the underlying plaque which is yellow-pink, indicative of type I collagen. Staining for α-actin (*D*) identifies smooth muscle cells within the neointima that is rich in type III collagen.

fate and hyaluronic acid.[120] With time, the proteoglycan and type III collagen are replaced by type I collagen resulting in retraction of the neointima.

Late (several years) after PTCA, it may be difficult to recognize the arterial PTCA site as cellular, collagen and proteoglycan-rich denovo plaque is similar in appearance to a restenosis lesion. Histologic evidence of previous balloon angioplasty is confirmed by the presence of a healed medial dissection or rupture site and interruption of collagen-rich plaque (yellow color on Movat pentachrome stain) by cellular proteoglycan-rich plaque (blue/green on Movat stain). In calcified atherosclerotic coronary arteries, plaque disruption occurs at the interface of calcified and noncalcified plaque.

In signing out coronary arteries treated with PTCA for pathology reports, the pathologist should comment on the presence (or absence) of lumen thrombus (acute, organizing, or organized), plaque disruption (acute, healing, or healed), and medial dissection or rupture (acute, healing, or healed; small or large). The presence of a mature neointima (compact smooth muscle cells in a collagen and proteoglycan matrix) defines post-PTCA healing. Extensive dissections that compromise the lumen should be specifically noted. We define restenosis as a lumen area stenosis of > 75%. These descriptions should also be utilized in arteries treated with atherectomy, laser catheters, and stents.

Rotational Atherectomy

Rotational coronary atherectomy is approved for percutaneous revascularization for coronary atherosclerosis. The rotoblator device consists of a stainless-steel elliptical-shaped burr coated with diamond microchips (30–50 μm in diameter) rotating at 160,000–180,000 rpm, which abrades atherosclerotic plaque as it spins.[121–123] Thus, the mechanism of action differs from balloon angioplasty, which induces plaque disruption and medial stretching with or without medial dissection and rupture. The rotoblator is particularly useful in heavily calcified lesions in which significant lumen expansion by balloon dilatation alone is unlikely to be successful.[124] More recently, the rotoblator is being used to treat in-stent restenosis.

Experimental *in vitro* and *in vivo* studies demonstrate that the vast majority of particulate debris generated by the rotoblator (average particle diameter $< 5\ \mu m$ and 98% of particles $< 10\ \mu m$) is sufficiently small to pass through intramyocardial capillaries without causing obstruction.[125, 126] However, elevation of serum cardiac enzymes and non-Q-wave myocardial infarction have been reported in 6–19% of patients[127] after rotoblator use, presumed to be secondary to capillary plugging by larger atherosclerotic particles.[121–124] These complications have been associated with an adverse clinical outcome. The extent of embolization of calcified plaque material may be a function of the severity and type of coronary calcification present. We have reported pathologic findings in two patients who died following rotational atherectomy.[128] In one patient with severe diffuse nodular coronary artery calcification, there were multiple calcific atheroemboli within intramyocardial arteries after rotoblator use (Fig. 3–15). In contrast, only one small atheroembolus was found in a patient with moderate coronary calcification consisting of calcified fibrous plaque.

Pathology of Rotational Atherectomy

In contrast to balloon angioplasty which splits plaque and stretches the media, rotational atherectomy abrades and removes plaque as it rotates at high speed. The rotating burr produces relatively smooth cuts in plaque in contrast to the irregular edges of the dissection planes produced by balloon angioplasty (Fig. 3–15).[128] It should be noted, however, that despite its name, rotational atherectomy does not selectively remove only plaque; the arterial media may also be resected if it is contacted by the spinning burr. Over time, arterial healing with the development of a smooth muscle-rich collagen and proteoglycan matrix occurs following rotational atherectomy.

Directional Atherectomy

Directional atherectomy catheters act as atherosclerotic plaque excision and retrieval systems. Plaque excision is accomplished by a rotating (2,000 rpm) cutter, which pushes the resected plaque into a nosecone-collecting chamber on the end of the catheter.[129] After an initial plaque excision, the entire catheter can rotate about its axis so that the cutter can resect more plaque at the lesion site. Initial procedural success rates with coronary directional atherectomy are in general similar to balloon angioplasty procedures,[129] with a 6% higher rate of acute complications and mortality at 1 year.[130, 131] The incidence of restenosis following directional atherectomy is approximately 40–50%,[130, 132, 133] and atherectomy has not proven to be more effective than PTCA alone.

Pathology of Directional Atherectomy

Atherectomy specimens consist of multiple thin fragments of tissue removed from the coronary artery wall (Fig. 3–16). The histologic appearance reflects whether the lesion treated is a denovo plaque or a restenosis specimen from a prior catheter-based intervention.[134] In denovo lesions, atherectomy specimens reflect the heterogeneity of features that are found in plaques: fibrous plaque, lipid core, thrombus, foam cells, lymphocytes, smooth muscle cells, and cholesterol clefts (Fig. 3–16). The directional atherectomy device is not capable of resecting heavily calcified plaque so that only small calcific plaque fragments are typically seen. Further, deep arterial wall excision is not uncommon; arterial media and adventitia are present in approximately 50% of atherectomy specimens (Fig. 3–16).[134] Deep arterial wall excision is not generally associated with an increased incidence of restenosis; however, the risk of coronary pseudoaneurysm is increased. In autopsy coronary arteries, it may be difficult to recognize the specific site of plaque removal, which may also be obscured by changes induced by adjunctive PTCA. Arteries examined within several days after atherectomy demonstrate focal areas of plaque resection associated with overlying thrombus and acute and chronic inflammatory cells. Healed postatherectomy lesions show the accumulation of restenosis tissue (proteoglycan/collagen extracellular matrix that is rich in smooth muscle cells) at sites of plaque excision (Fig. 3–16).

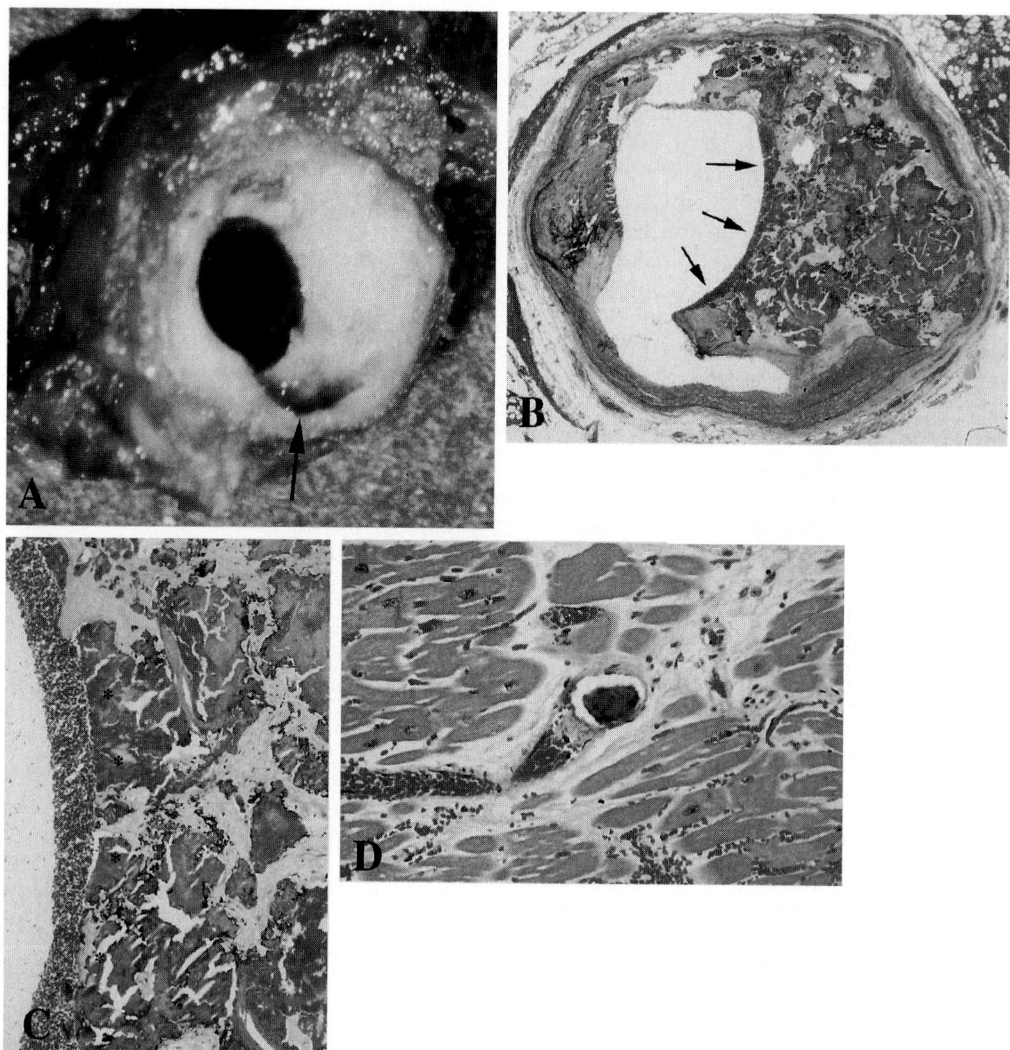

Figure 3–15. Rotational atherectomy. A 79-year-old woman underwent rotational atherectomy for severely calcified and stenotic left obtuse marginal (*LOM*) coronary artery. In *A*, the gross plaque is creamy white and markedly calcified resulting in 70% lumen area stenosis. A dissection plane (*arrow*) is present. *B* is the corresponding Movat stained section; the plaque is composed predominantly of calcified nodules with sparse collagen matrix. Rotational atherectomy produce sharp-edged smooth surface cuts with overlying red blood cells without platelet deposition (*arrows, B*). The sharp cuts (*) are seen at high power in *C*. *D* shows an intramyocardial coronary artery containing an embolized calcified nodule. Other intramyocardial arteries showed fibrin/platelet emboli (*not shown*).

Coronary restenosis atherectomy specimens demonstrate areas of smooth muscle cells and proteoglycan-rich plaque in 90% of cases; this tissue is representative of the arterial healing responses after PTCA and/or stenting. Evaluation of atherectomy specimens has provided insights into the mechanisms of the pathogenesis of acute ischemic coronary syndromes and restenosis. Mural thrombi and plaque hemorrhage are more commonly observed in atherectomy specimens from patients with unstable angina compared with stable angina.[135, 136] Increased numbers of macrophages and T-lymphocytes are more often present in plaques from patients with unstable angina versus stable angina and identify patients at increased risk of restenosis, consistent with the hypothesis that plaque inflammation plays an important role in plaque growth and clinical events.[137–139] Atherectomy specimens with smooth muscle cell-rich plaques that stain positively for acidic and basic fibroblast growth factor are more likely to be seen in patients with unstable angina versus stable angina, suggesting that rapid plaque

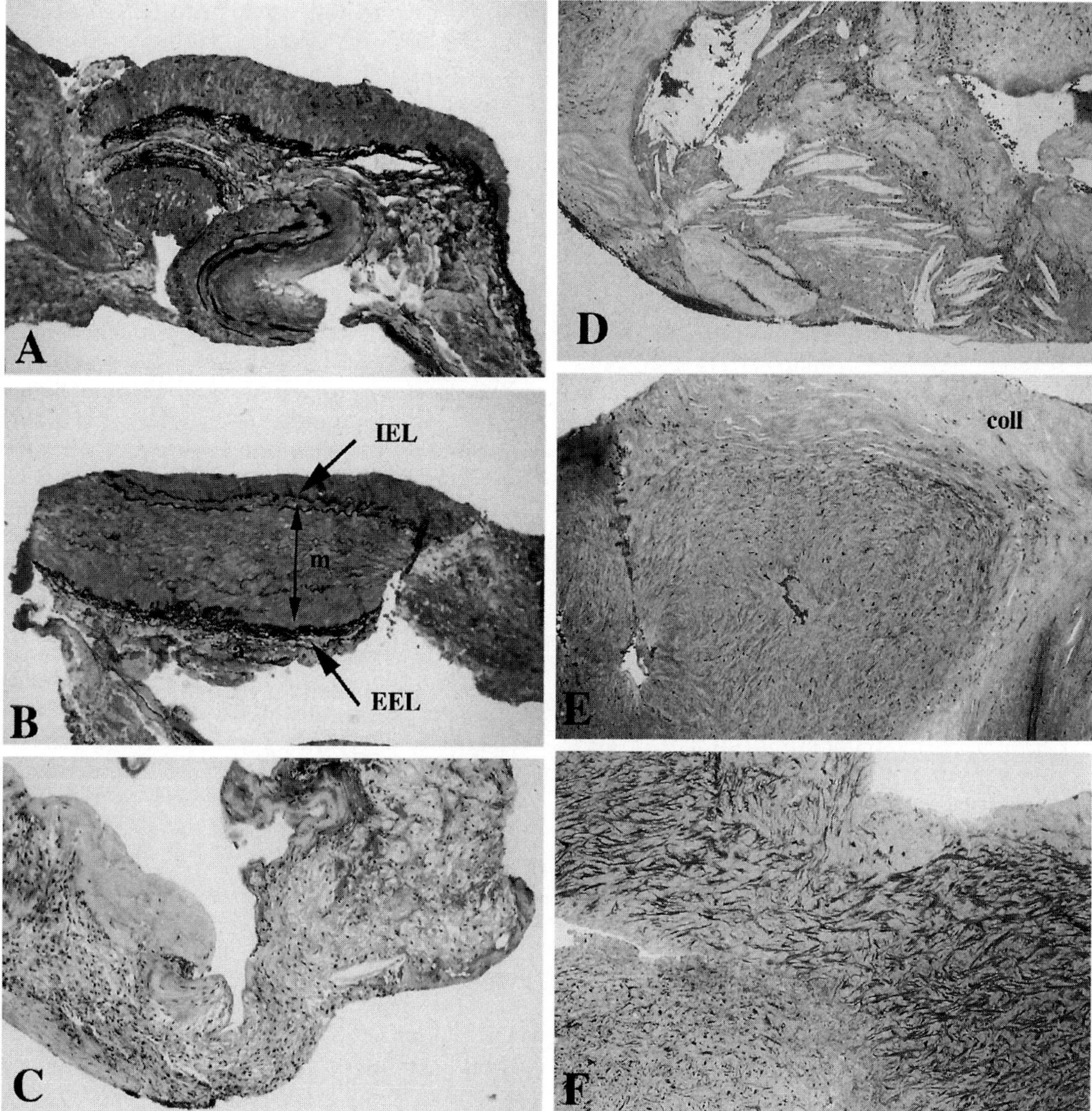

Figure 3–16. Directional coronary atherectomy. *A and B* are low- and high-power views of a portion of the media and underlying adventitia that excised along with a post-PTCA restenosis lesion. (*IEL* = internal elastic lamina. *EEL* = external elastic lamina, *m* = media, *a* = adventitia.) *C and D* show denovo atherosclerotic plaques. In *C*, numerous macrophages are present. A large, minimally calcified necrotic core containing needle-shaped cholesterol clefts and surrounding macrophages is shown in *D*. *E and F* are sections from patients who developed restenosis following PTCA. Note extensive smooth muscle cells within a proteoglycan matrix; the underlying plaque is rich in collagen (*coll, E*). *F* shows SMC arborization within a proteoglycan-rich matrix, characteristic of a coronary restenosis lesion.

growth is another mechanism of acute ischemic coronary syndromes.[135]

Lasers

Lasers (light amplification by stimulated emission of radiation) produce a narrow wavelength of photons that allow light to be focused into a precise parallel beam of high energy. The laser beam may be either continuous or pulsed in short bursts to allow the tissue to cool between laser applications to limit tissue thermal damage. The energy produced by lasers can be in ultraviolet range (short wavelengths), visible light range, or infrared range (long wavelengths). Laser energy is capable of ablating and vaporizing atherosclerotic plaque via breaking chemical bonds (ultraviolet energy), or by heating and expanding plaque (visible light and infrared energy).[140] Lasers are particularly effective in lipid-rich and fibrotic plaques; calcified plaque is much more resistant to laser energy.[140]

The lasers in use in atherosclerotic coronary arteries include: (1) the argon laser operating in the visible light spectrum; (2) solid state lasers (Nd:YAG and holmium laser) which operate in the infrared spectrum; and (3) eximer lasers, which operate in the ultraviolet spectrum.[141–143] The argon laser is not effective for heavily calcified plaque. Nd:YAG, holmium, and eximer lasers can effectively restore patency to severely stenotic coronary arteries. In general, laser-assisted balloon angioplasty is best suited for long lesions (> 2.0 cm) and chronic total occlusions.[140, 144, 145] While acute results utilizing lasers in these challenging lesions have been impressive (initial success rates approximately 65–85%), the long-term outcome has been disappointing with restenosis rates of approximately 50%.[141, 143, 146] Arterial perforation is an uncommon, but reported complication of laser-assisted angioplasty (2% of cases using the eximer laser).[140] Overall, coronary lasers are infrequently used at the present time.

Pathologically, laser energy produces a crater or hole secondary to local thermal injury to the nonvaporized edges of the lased tissue. Acutely, there is fibrin thrombus deposition along the charred, desiccated tissue edges. Over time, similar to balloon angioplasty, there is vascular smooth muscle migration and proliferation, extracellular matrix synthesis, and reendothelialization.

Coronary Artery Stenting

Dissatisfaction with the relatively high rates of restenosis following coronary balloon angioplasty (30–40%) and the less frequent, but often clinically devastating complication of abrupt arterial closure have directly led to the development of intraarterial stents. A stent is a prosthetic intraluminal scaffolding device designed to maintain lumen patency in the setting of an underlying intrinsic or extrinsic disease state. As noted earlier, negative arterial remodeling, a constrictive process that results in the overall shrinkage of the dilated artery, plays an important role in post-PTCA restenosis.[116] The semi-rigid scaffolding provided by intraarterial stents prevents both acute recoil of the dilated artery and chronic negative remodeling, both major advantages over PTCA. In the heart, emergency coronary artery stent deployment is used as a bailout procedure for abrupt or threatened artery closure due to arterial dissection following balloon angioplasty. Bailout stenting has reduced the need for urgent coronary bypass surgery.[67, 147, 148] The use of stents as primary therapy for atherosclerosis is now a standard practice based on reports of reduced restenosis rates in selected coronary lesions compared with PTCA.[149–152] Direct PTCA with placement of coronary stents is increasingly utilized as a revascularization therapy in acute myocardial infarction and is associated with high rates of arterial patency.[153, 154]

Most stents in current use in the United States come premounted and tightly wrapped ("crimped") on a balloon angioplasty catheter. The stent is delivered to its site of deployment under fluoroscopic guidance over a flexible metallic guidewire. Stents are routinely deployed and/or post-dilated at high pressure (12–16 ATM) so that the stent struts are closely apposed to the vessel wall. High pressure stent deployment and attempts to maximize lumen diameter have reduced the incidence of acute and subacute stent thrombosis; however, overexpansion is associated with increased arterial injury and neointimal growth (see following).[155]

Stent Designs

Metals that have been used in intravascular stents include surgical-grade stainless steel (316L), nickel-titanium alloy (nitinol), titanium, and gold-coated stainless steel alloys.[155] Stainless steel has excellent tensile strength and is resistant to corrosion, but is relatively thrombogenic compared with the other metals used. Titanium has high strength per unit density allowing for lighter devices, is corrosion-resistant, and has excellent biocompatibility. The shape memory property of nitinol allows for devices to be highly compressed and resume original shape upon warming. Nitinol exerts a strong radial expanding force and has good biocompatibility. Gold coating of stainless steel adds visibility via enhanced radio-opacity and inhibits corrosion and infection. The basic designs of stents previously used and in current use in the United States include the coil stent (Gianturco-Roubin II and Wiktor), mesh (Wallstent), tubular stents (Palmaz-Schatz PS-153 and Mini-Crown, MULTI-LINK Duet, Tristar, Radius), ring stents (AVE GFX and S670), and multi-design (NIR) (Fig. 3–17).[156] All of these stents are cut from 316L stainless steel except the Wallstent (cobalt alloy with a platinum

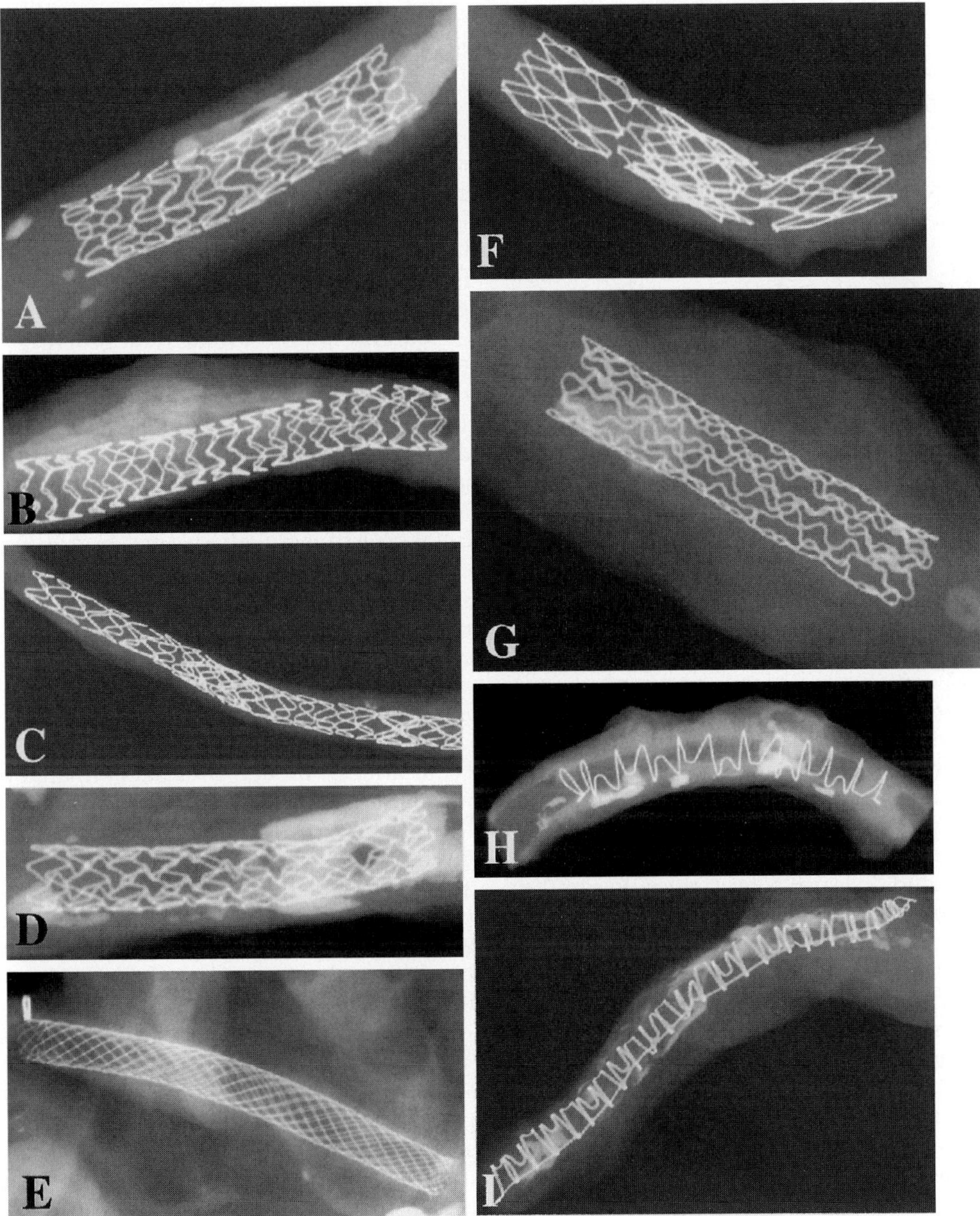

Figure 3–17. Coronary stents. Radiographs of human coronary arteries removed at surgery or autopsy showing the spectrum of the stent types that may be seen in the United States. *A* and *B* are ACS MULTI-LINK™ and ACS MULTI-LINK RX DUET™ (tubular stents), respectively. *C* is an AVE GFX (ring stent), *D* is a NIR (multi-design stent), *E* is a Magic Wallstent (mesh stent), *F* are two overlapping Palmaz-Schatz stents (articulated tubular stent), *G* is Mini-Crown Palmaz-Schatz (tubular stent), *H* is a Gianturco-Roubin (coil stent), and *I* is a Gianturco-Roubin II (coil stent).

core), Wiktor (tantalum), and nitinol (Radius). All are deployed via balloon delivery systems except the self-expanding Wallstent and Radius stents.[156]

Experimental and human studies of arterial stenting have shown a positive linear correlation between the extent of stent-induced arterial injury and neointimal growth. Limited data suggest that stent design can affect arterial injury and the inflammatory response post-deployment. At 14 days, adherent monocytes were reduced following placement of corrugated ring stents versus slotted tube stents in rabbit iliac arteries.[157] Stent strut-associated leukocyte density at 3 days was reduced by 32% with self-expanding nitinol stents compared with tubular slotted stents placed in porcine coronary arteries.[158] However, with the exception of Gianturco-Roubin coil stents which are associated with unacceptably high (> 50%) restenosis rates, the effect of different stent designs on restenosis rates has not been established in head-to-head randomized human clinical trials.

Pathologic Responses to Intracoronary Stents

Histologic findings after stenting are directly related to the duration of stent implantation. The early era of intracoronary stent deployment was plagued by a high incidence of acute stent thrombosis. Improved antiplatelet therapy (substitution of ticlopidine or clopidegel for coumadin) and especially improved deployment strategies in which stent struts are tightly apposed to the vessel wall have reduced the incidence of acute and subacute stent thrombosis to 1–2% in most published series.[159–162] Proper stent placement is shown histologically by local compression of nonruptured plaque by the stent struts.[120] Nevertheless, even with improved stent placement techniques, platelet/fibrin thrombus adherent to stent struts is almost always observed histologically within the first 3 days after stenting (Fig. 3–18).[120] In successful stent deployment, this thrombus is nonocclusive and does not compromise flow in the vast majority of cases. By 1 month post-stent placement, platelets are no longer observed around struts, and fibrin deposits eventually become incorporated into the neointima.

In human atherosclerotic arteries, penetration of stent struts through a ruptured fibrous cap into a lipid core is not uncommon and occurs in approximately 25% of arterial segments that have lipid cores (Fig. 3–19).[120] Lipid core penetration is associated with increased acute and chronic intimal inflammation and increased neointimal growth (see following). Plaques with large absolute lipid core size ($\geq 2.0\ mm^2$) and the percent of plaque occupied by the lipid core ($\geq$ 20% of total plaque area) identify lesions at increased risk for lipid core penetration by stent struts.[163]

As in PTCA, stents produce arterial injury, which provokes local inflammation. Acute inflammatory cells are commonly seen early after stent deployment and are rarely seen at > 1 month. In a study of human stents (55 stents in 35 coronary vessels from 32 patients), neutrophils associated with stent struts were present in 48/61 (79%) arterial sections examined in stents implanted ≤ 3 days, 15/18 (83%) at 4–11 days, 21/29 (72%) at 12–30 days, and 0/34 (0%) at > 30 days ($p < 0.0001$, all time points versus > 30 days).[120] In contrast, chronic inflammatory cells (macrophages and lymphocytes) may be observed at all time points after stenting, and their persistence may, in part, reflect a foreign body response. In our study of human coronary stent implants, chronic inflammatory cells (lymphocytes and macrophages) around stent struts were observed at all time points post-stent deployment [50/61 (82%) sections at ≤ 3 days), 12/18 (67%) sections at 4–11 days, 28/29 (97%) sections at 12–30 days, and 29/34 (85%) sections at > 30 days].[120] Multinucleated giant cells are commonly seen around stent struts late after stenting (> 30 days), but their contribution to neointimal growth is uncertain (Fig. 3–20).

As in balloon angioplasty, the neointima after stenting consists of a proteoglycan/collagen matrix that contains smooth muscle cells. An early neointima layer is recognized beginning approximately 2 weeks post-stenting and is always seen in routine stenting by 30 days. Intimal smooth muscle cell density within stents is similar to arteries treated with balloon angioplasty matched for the duration since treatment. Further, alcian blue staining for neointimal proteoglycans (chondroitin sulfate and hyaluronic acid) is similar after stenting and balloon angioplasty.[120] The neointimal area itself is greater with stenting compared with balloon angioplasty, but this is accounted for by a greater increase in lumen size when stents are placed.

Complete stent endothelialization in experimental animals (rabbit, dog, and pig) may be seen as early as 7 days to approximately 4 weeks post-deployment.[164–167] Data from humans regarding stent endothelialization is limited. Anderson et al. reported coronary stent endothelialization in a single stent 21 days post-implant.[168] Van Beusekom et al. demonstrated complete endothelial stent coverage by 3 months in saphenous vein bypass grafts.[169] Repair of the luminal surface via reendothelialization may be a critical process in vascular healing via prevention or limitation of luminal thrombosis. Further, inhibition of continued neointimal growth is believed to be a result of a restored endothelial surface. However, recent data demonstrate that the presence of a endothelial surface in and of itself is insufficient to inhibit the neointima; normal endothelial function and/or nonendothelium-dependent factors may be relatively more important than the presence or

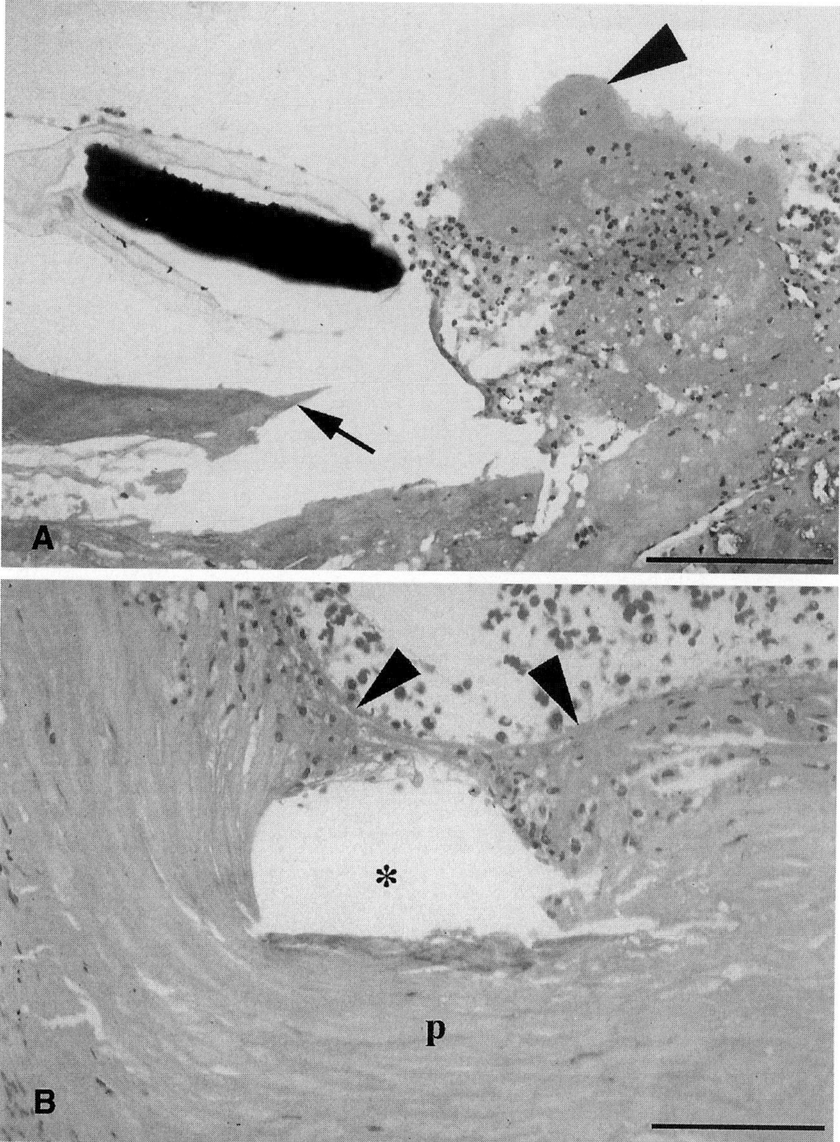

Figure 3–18. Arterial responses to stenting: thrombus deposition. A platelet-rich thrombus (*A, arrowhead*) is associated with a strut from a Gianturco-Roubin II coronary artery stent implanted 1 day antemortem. Numerous acute inflammatory cells are present within the thrombus. Focal fibrous cap disruption is seen (*arrow*). A fibrin-rich thrombus (*arrowheads*) is focally present around a stent strut (*) 1 day after placement of a Palmaz-Schatz stent (*B*). Fibrous plaque (*p*) is present below the strut. (Reproduced with permission from American Heart Association and Farb et al. Pathology of acute and chronic coronary stenting in humans. Circulation 99:44–52, 1999.)

absence of an endothelial surface in suppressing neointimal expansion.[170]

In-stent Restenosis

By providing a semi-rigid intraarterial scaffolding, stents prevent the elastic recoil and negative remodeling that contribute significantly to late lumen loss after balloon angioplasty. Therefore, with stents, the amount of subsequent smooth muscle cell and proteoglycan-rich neointimal growth alone determines whether restenosis will or will not occur (Fig. 3–21). Two angiographic definitions of restenosis have been used: (1) loss of 50% of the acute luminal gain and (2) stent lumen diameter stenosis of > 50% (defined by angiography). In assessing human pathologic stent specimens, moderate in-stent restenosis can be defined as > 50% and < 75% stent lumen narrowing by

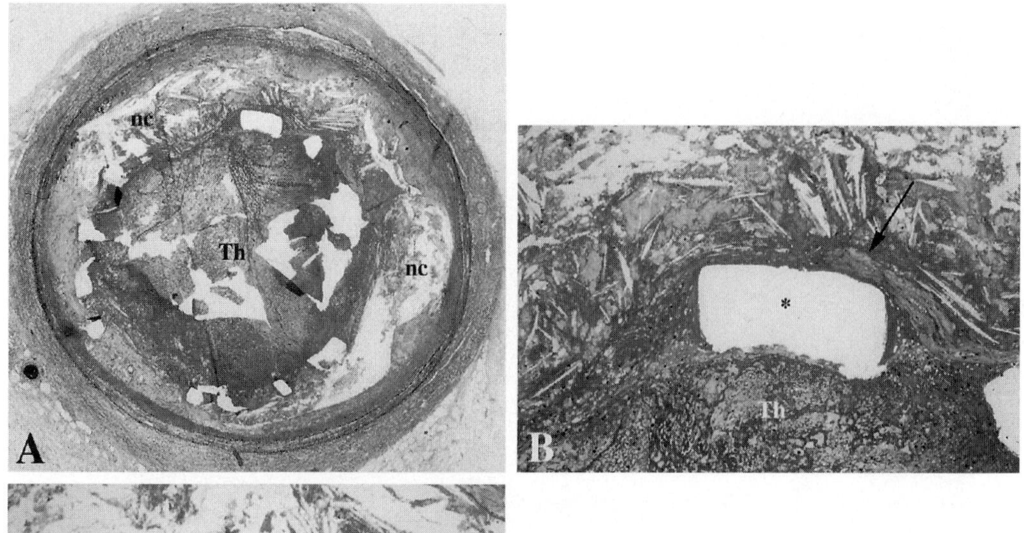

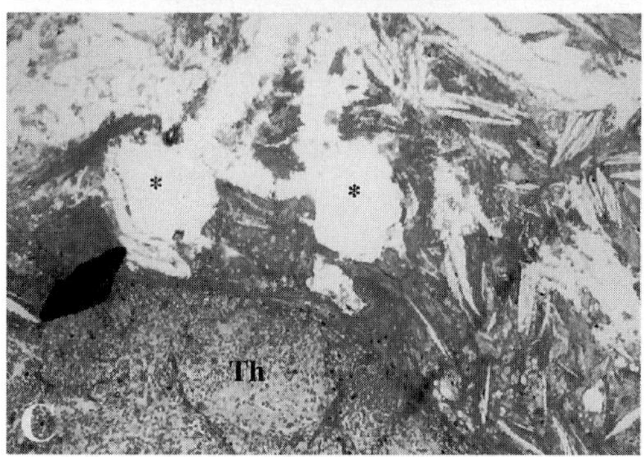

Figure 3–19. Stent strut penetration into plaque necrotic core. A 75-year-old woman with coronary atherosclerosis, hypertension, and insulin-dependent diabetes suffered a posterior wall myocardial infarction with a right coronary stent placed 2 months antemortem. In *A*, an occlusive partially organizing thrombus (*th*) is present; note the large necrotic core (*nc*). In *B*, the disrupted fibrous cap (*arrow*) overlies the necrotic core, which contains numerous cholesterol clefts. *C* shows focal prolapse of the necrotic core into the lumen. Spaces occupied by stent struts are indicated by an * in *B* and *C*.

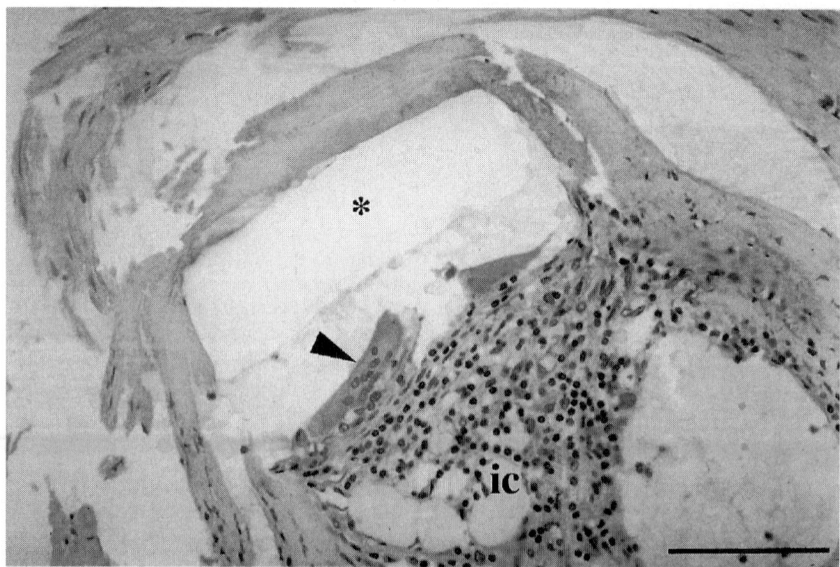

Figure 3–20. Arterial responses to stenting: chronic inflammation. Multinucleated giant cell (*arrowhead*) and numerous chronic inflammatory cells (*ic*) associated with Palmaz-Schatz stent strut (*) placed 70 days antemortem in the left anterior descending coronary artery. (Reproduced with permission from American Heart Association and Farb et al. Pathology of acute and chronic coronary stenting in humans. Circulation 99:44–52, 1999.)

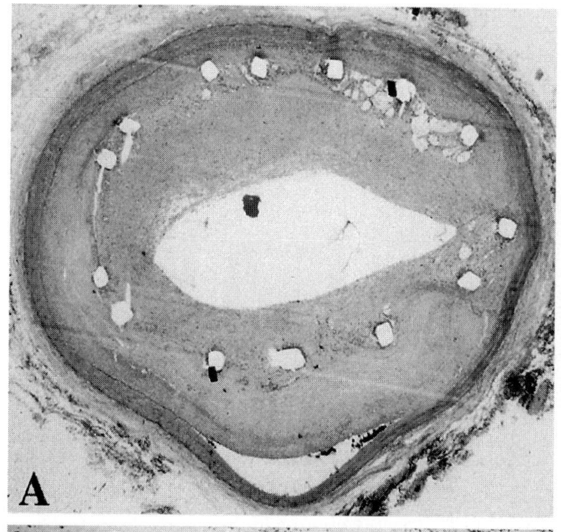

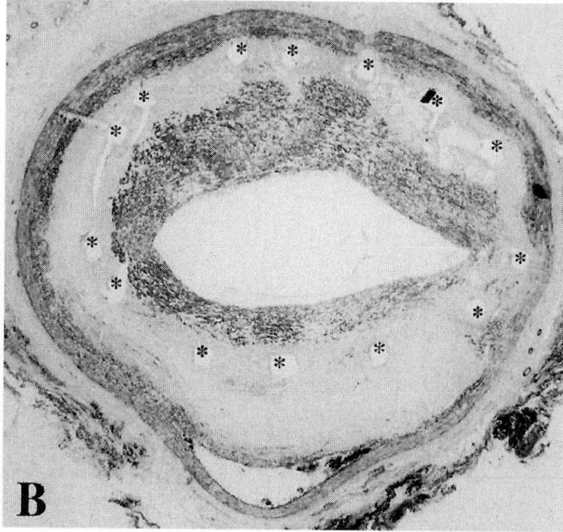

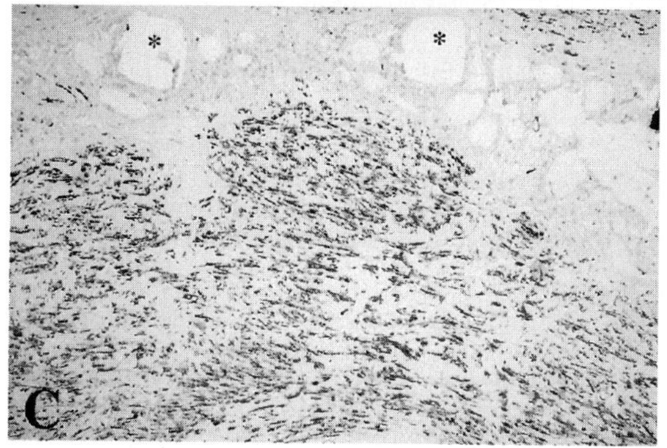

Figure 3–21. In-stent restenosis. A 69-year-old woman with coronary atherosclerosis underwent right coronary artery stenting 4 months prior to presenting with angina. Coronary angiography demonstrated in-stent restenosis, and the patient died 1 day post-CABG surgery. The right coronary artery (*A*) shows neointimal thickening within the stent (green color on Movat stain) due to the extensive deposition of proteoglycan matrix resulting in in-stent restenosis. In *B,* a section stained with antibody to α-actin, shows that the neointima contains a large number of smooth muscle cells. *C* is a high-power view of the in-stent neointima showing spindle shaped α-actin positive cells arranged parallel to the lumen. The * marks the location of stent struts.

neointima, and severe in-stent restenosis as ≥ 75% stent lumen area narrowing.

Multiple factors affect in-stent neointimal growth. Studies of arterial stenting in experimental animals suggest that increased inflammation and more severe arterial injury are associated with increased neointimal development. In stented nonatherosclerotic balloon-injured rabbit iliac arteries examined at 14 days, Rogers showed that monocyte adhesion correlated with neointimal growth ($r = 0.96$, $p < 0.008$).[157] In a subsequent study, Rogers et al. demonstrated peak RAM 11-positive monocyte adherence to the lumen surface 3 days after stenting, which correlated with intimal cellular proliferation ($r^2 = 0.916$, $p < 0.0001$).[81] Continuous heparin administration reduced neointimal monocytes by 76% at 7 days, and there was a strong correlation between adherent monocytes and intima size ($r^2 = 0.82$, $p < 0.0001$).[81] In the porcine over-sized coronary stent model, at 28 days, the severity of lymphohistiocytic cell infiltration and granuloma formation around stent struts was associated with increased intimal thickness ($r = 0.75$, $p < 0.01$) and percent lumen area stenosis ($r = 0.66$, $p < 0.01$), independent of the extent of arterial injury.[171] The effect of underlying arterial injury on subsequent neointimal growth was also addressed in a porcine double arterial injury model.[172] In areas where the arterial media was absent (damaged by balloon angioplasty 4 weeks prior to stent placement), neointimal thickness was greater than at strut sites that were adjacent to an intact internal elastic lamina and media.[172]

In human coronary arteries, the degree of stent-induced inflammation is related to the severity of vascular damage produced by stenting and adjunctive balloon angioplasty (Fig. 3–22). A more intense inflammatory response is seen when there is medial wall damage or rupture of a fibrous cap with penetration of stent struts into a lipid core; little inflammation is produced when the stent strut only compresses fibrous plaque. For example, 71% of stent struts in contact with fibrous plaque had mild (1+) inflammation, defined as ≤ 10 associated inflammatory cells, compared with 11% of struts

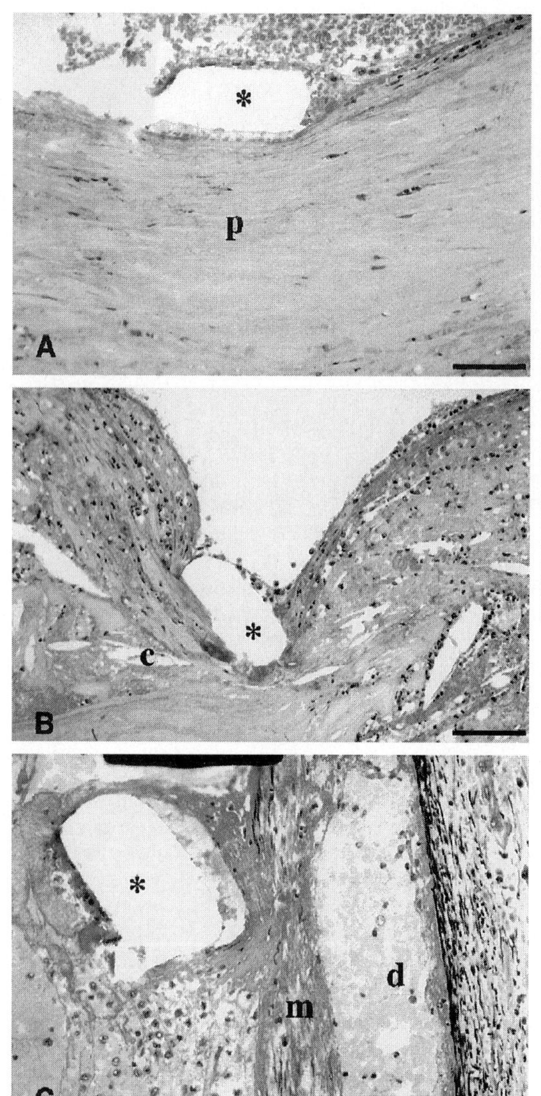

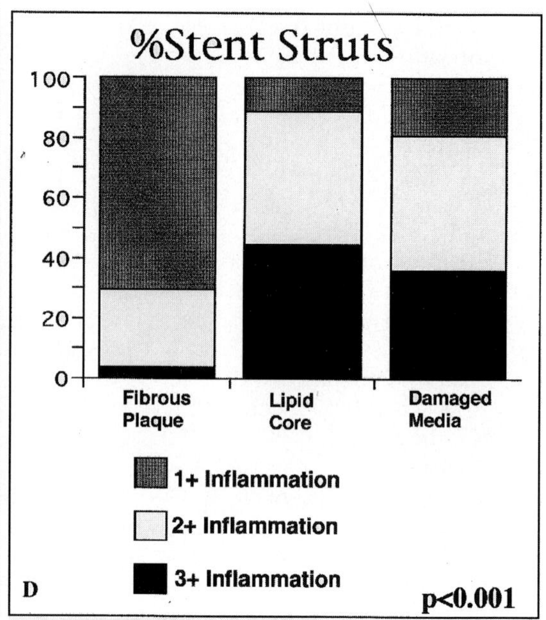

Figure 3–22. Arterial responses to stenting: inflammation. Arterial inflammation in human coronary arteries with stents placed ≤ 3 days antemortem. In *A*, few inflammatory cells are present adjacent to the stent strut (*) in contact with the fibrous plaque (*p*). Increased numbers of inflammatory cells (*B*) are associated with stent strut (*) that penetrates the necrotic core (*c*). A stent strut (*) in contact with damaged media (*m*) and dissection (*d*) and numerous associated inflammatory cells is shown in *C*. Inflammatory cell infiltrates associated with stent struts were assessed in coronary arteries containing stents of ≤ 3 days duration (*D*). There were increased numbers of inflammatory cells associated with struts in contact with lipid core and damaged media compared with fibrous plaque ($p < 0.001$). (Reproduced with permission from the American Heart Association and Farb et al. Pathology of acute and chronic coronary stenting in humans. Circulation 99:44–52, 1999.)

embedded in a lipid core and 19% of struts in contact with damaged media. In contrast, only 3% of struts in contact with fibrous plaque had severe (3+) inflammation (> 20 associated inflammatory cells) compared with 44% of struts embedded in a lipid core and 36% of struts in contact with damaged media ($p < 0.001$) (Fig. 3–22).[120]

The associations among inflammation, arterial injury, neointimal neoangiogenesis, and in-stent neointimal growth were assessed in an evaluation of 36 human coronary artery stents (mean duration of implant 263 ± 223 days).[163] Neointimal thickness was increased when there was stent strut penetration into a lipid core (0.95 ± 0.40 mm) or medial rupture (0.85 ± 0.25 mm) compared with stent struts in contact with fibrous plaque (0.65 ± 0.33 mm, $p < 0.03$). Importantly, a greater than twofold increase ($p < 0.002$) in neointimal mononuclear cell density was present with stent lipid core penetration or medial rupture versus fibrous plaque. Further, stent-induced medial injury was associated with a 3.8-fold increase and lipid core rupture a 1.9-fold increase in neointimal capillary density (neoangiogenesis) compared with stent struts in contact with fibrous plaque. There were positive correlations between neointimal inflammatory cell density and neointimal growth ($r^2 = 0.11$, $p < 0.0001$) and between neointimal neoangiogenesis and neointimal growth ($r^2 = 0.11$, $p < 0.0001$).

These data highlight the important associations among the severity of arterial injury, inflammatory cell response, and late intimal growth. Unfortunately, in current practice, the degree of arterial injury produced (plaque disruption, medial stretch, medial dissection, or medial rupture) cannot be tightly controlled. Interventional cardiologists often seek to maximize acute luminal gain when deploying stents by high-pressure balloon inflations during stent deployment. However, stent oversizing relative to the native vessel dimensions may be deleterious and lead to a greater likelihood of restenosis. There is a strong correlation ($r^2 = 0.54$, $p < 0.0001$) between increased intimal growth and stent size relative to the proximal nonstented reference artery lumen (Fig. 3–23).[120] This finding indicates the potential negative effects of the "bigger lumen is better" approach when applied to stenting. New devices and imaging techniques that limit overdilatation should reduce injury-induced inflammation.

Taken together, experimental animal studies and human autopsy data indicate that intervention-associated inflammatory responses, the underlying plaque substrate, and the severity of the stent-induced arterial injury are important contributors to late outcome. Therefore, deployment strategies that reduce medial damage and avoid stent oversizing may lower the frequency of in-stent restenosis.

Bailout Coronary Stenting

Abrupt or threatened coronary artery closure as an acute complication of PTCA is associated with a high incidence of morbidity and mortality. Emergency coronary artery stent placement (bailout stenting) for abrupt or threatened artery closure due to arterial dissection following PTCA has emerged as the treatment of choice for this complication. Clinical series have demonstrated the efficacy of bailout stents in maintaining lumen patency and reducing the need for urgent coronary bypass surgery with success rates of bailout stenting > 90% in some reports.[67, 147, 148, 173–175] While late restenosis occurs at a higher frequency in bailout stenting than stenting in nonbailout situations, the restenosis rate is similar to that reported in arteries treated with PTCA alone.[176] Bailout stenting has also been successfully employed in the setting of acute or threatened coronary closure following direct PTCA for acute myocardial infarction.[177, 178]

We recently reported pathologic findings in six cases of bailout stenting in humans.[120, 178a] There were 20 stents placed in eight coronary arteries ranging from one to five stents per artery, and all patients expired secondary to acute myocardial infarction. However, the stents themselves performed as they were intended. That is, in all six cases, the stents were well opposed to the coronary artery wall producing a relatively large lumen and compressed the balloon angioplasty-induced arterial dissection plane. However, significant residual dissection of the nonstented portion of the arteries in four of six cases was responsible for focal coronary artery luminal compression or obstruction (Fig. 3–24). These cases may be classified as being inadequately stented, reflecting the extremely long dissection (8.7 ± 1.5 cm). In bailout situa-

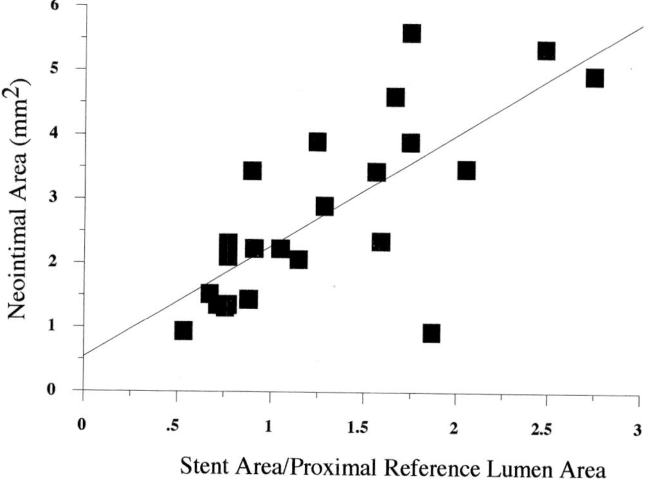

Figure 3–23. Linear regression comparing the ratio of the stent area to the lumen area of the proximal reference artery (x-axis) to the neointimal area (y-axis). Increased neointimal growth was associated with increased stent size relative to the proximal reference lumen ($R^2 = 0.54$, $p < 0.0001$). (Reproduced with permission from American Heart Association and Farb et al. Pathology of acute and chronic coronary stenting in humans. Circulation 99:44–52, 1999.)

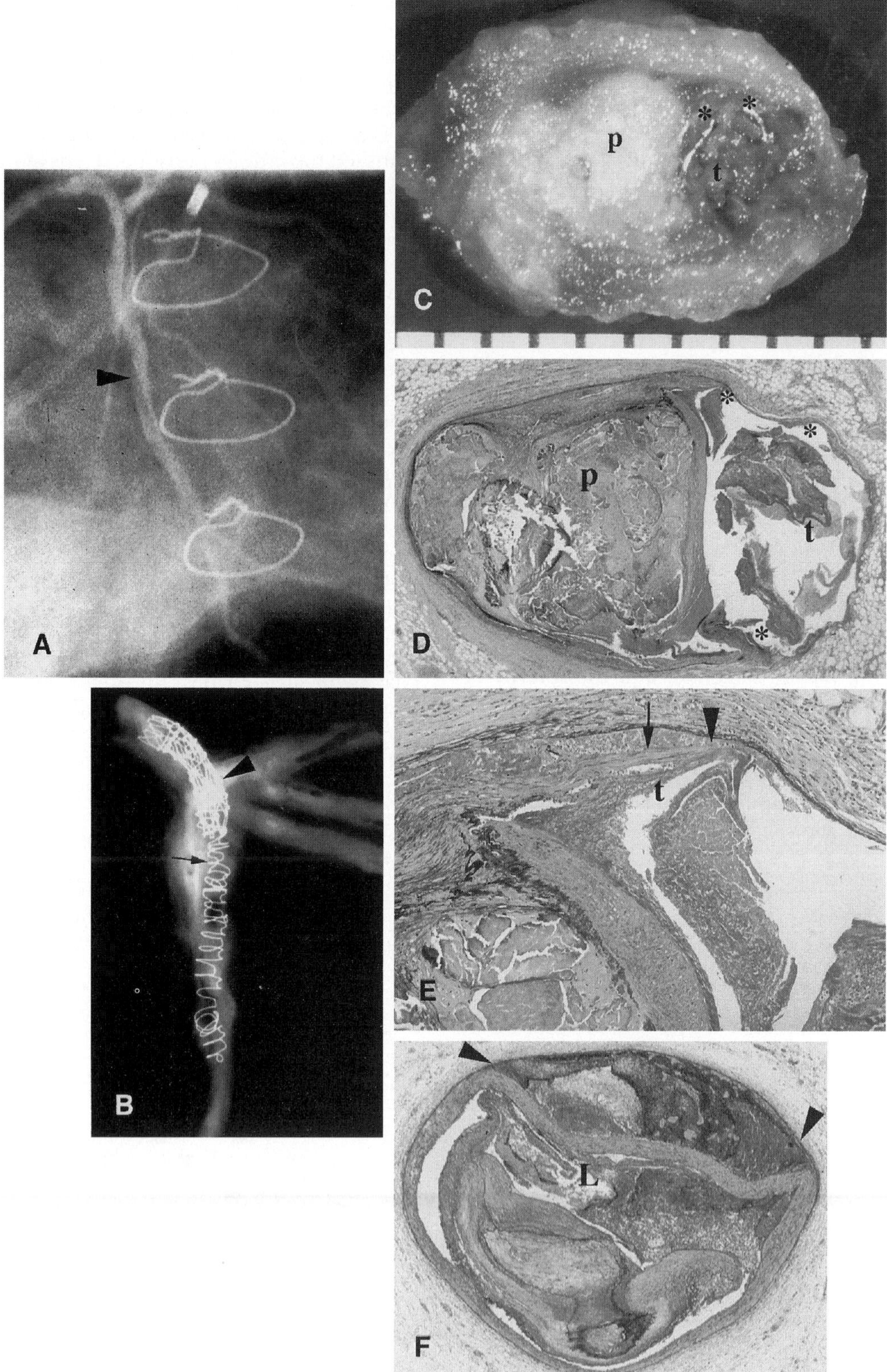

Figure 3–24. *See legend on opposite page*

tions, it should be noted that dissection-induced coronary lumen obstruction may occur proximal, distal, or between stented arteries. These findings support the need to completely cover the entire dissection with stents extending at least 0.5 to 1.0 cm into the nondissected portion of the artery.[179] In clinical studies, nonflow-limiting small residual dissections after bailout stenting have not been associated with an adverse long-term outcome.[180]

Other complications associated with bailout coronary stenting are coronary artery side-branch occlusion during deployment in the target vessel and stenting of the false lumen of the dissection plane without ultimate reentry into the true arterial lumen (Fig. 3–25).[120] These complications may also occur during coronary stenting in nonbailout situations. In problematic cases, the use of intravascular ultrasound can assure the proper placement of a coronary stent.

Handling and Processing of Coronary Stent Specimens

Initially, the heart should be radiographed to locate the artery containing the stent. The formalin-fixed stented artery is then taken off the heart and reradiographed to confirm the type of stent, measure its diameter and length, and precisely locate the stent margins. Radiographs are essential to assess the expansion of the stent and to determine whether the stent was abnormally compressed during deployment. In addition, radiographs are instrumental in confirming that the stent was placed in the proper coronary artery; failure to deliver the stent to the proper location can lead to an adverse clinical outcome (Fig. 3–26).

Histologic evaluation of intraarterial stents is a challenge for most pathology laboratories because routine cutting methods of paraffin-embedded tissues cannot be used to cut arteries containing metal devices. Attempts to remove stents whole before processing invariably results in destruction of the specimen and thus limits one's ability to accurately assess stent patency and provide clinico-pathologic correlations for clinically important events such as stent thrombosis and restenosis. The best method for evaluating stent specimens is to utilize methylmethacrylate and cut the artery with the stent *in situ*. Plastic-embedding and sectioning is the only method to properly analyze stents that have been in place for a short time ($\leq$ 1 month) in which thrombus and newly formed intimal tissue are only loosely adherent to the stent.

Following the completion of radiographic imaging, the stented portion of the vessel is placed intact into a processing vial, dehydrated with a graded series of alcohols, and embedded in methylmethacrylate plastic. Plastic sections (4–5 μm thick) are then cut with a microtome and stained with hematoxylin-eosin and Movat pentachrome. For longer-term stent implants and when methylmethacrylate is not available, it is possible to carefully remove the stent wires from a 3-mm long arterial segment as long as the stent wires are straight within the segment. The use of a dissecting microscope is a significant aide in removing stent wires. After wire removal, arterial segments can undergo routine tissue processing and paraffin embedding. Even with great care, artifacts will probably be introduced as the local morphology is disturbed by the wire-removal process. Basic

Figure 3–24. Bailout stenting. A 52-year-old man with coronary heart disease had CABG surgery 9 and 5 years antemortem. He presented with crescendo angina and underwent rotational atherectomy of the left circumflex (LCX) and left obtuse marginal arteries, which was complicated by an extensive anterograde and retrograde LCX arterial dissection. A Gianturco-Roubin stent was placed in the ostia of LCX artery with the proximal portion of the stent placed in the distal left main. The following day, he developed pulmonary edema; coronary angiography showed 70% narrowing of the LCX, and two more stents were deployed (Palmaz-Schatz in left main and another Gianturco-Roubin stent in the mid-LCX). Two days later, the patient had supraventricular arrhythmias followed by cardiac arrest. In *A*, RAO view of coronary angiogram demonstrates extensive dissection of left circumflex coronary artery (*arrowhead*). A postmortem radiograph of left coronary arteries (*B*) shows overlapping Gianturco-Roubin and Palmaz-Schatz stents in the left main and proximal left circumflex arteries (*arrowhead*) with sequential Gianturco-Roubin stents in the mid-left circumflex (*arrow*). Uneven expansion of the coils of the Gianturco-Roubin stents is present probably secondary heavy arterial calcification and arterial dissection. Gross (*C*) and corresponding histologic section (*D*) of the stented proximal left circumflex shows an eccentric, heavily calcified plaque (*p*) with a 70% cross-sectional narrowing and occlusive thrombus (*t*); stent struts are indicated (*). High-power view (in *E*) demonstrates medial rupture (*arrowhead*), resection, and dissection (*arrow*) secondary to rotational atherectomy and balloon angioplasty with adjacent thrombus (*t*). In the nonstented portion of the distal left circumflex artery (*F*), there is an extensive residual dissection (*arrowheads*) and compression of the arterial lumen (*L*). (Reproduced with permission from Farb et al. Pathology of bailout coronary stenting in humans. Am Heart J 137:621–631, 1999.)

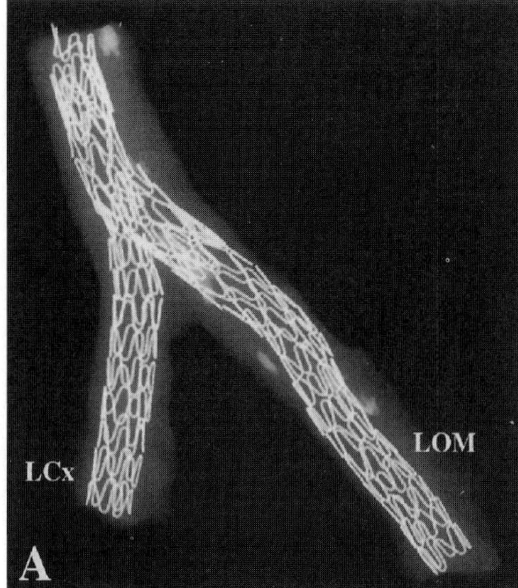

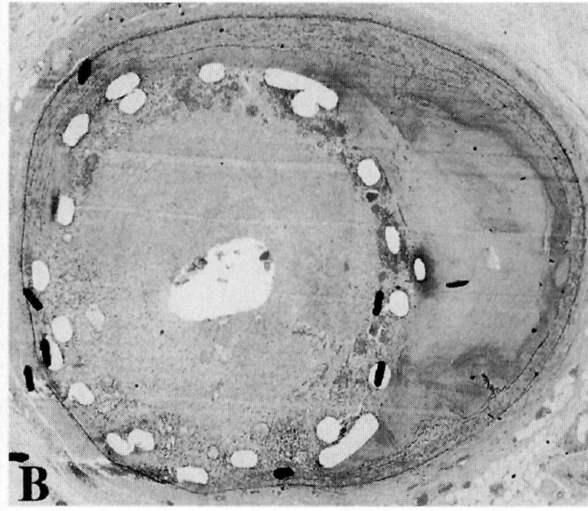

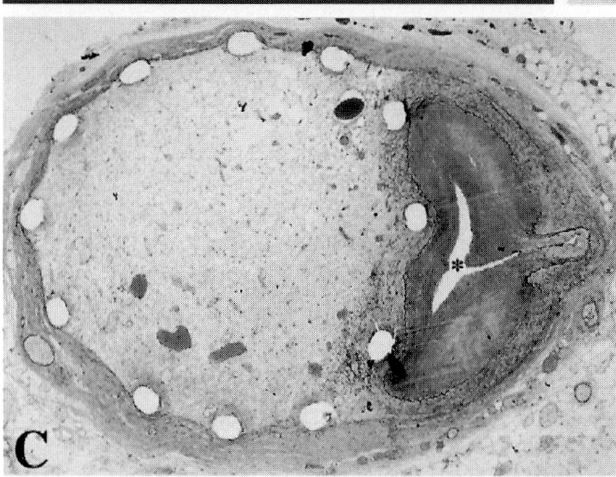

Figure 3–25. Complications of coronary stenting. A 65-year-old man with a non-Q-wave myocardial infarction underwent stenting of an occluded left circumflex (LCx) and left obtuse marginal (LOM) arteries 8 months antemortem. A nuclear stress test 1 month antemortem showed inferolateral ischemia. The patient died suddenly. In *A*, a postmortem radiograph of the LCx and LOM arteries shows multiple stents in both arteries. *B*, a section from the proximal LCx (with overlapping stents), shows severe in-stent restenosis (90% narrowing of the stent lumen) with chronic inflammation and neoangiogenesis associated with stent struts. In *C*, a section from the mid-LCx, the stent is in the false lumen of an arterial dissection. The stent lumen is occluded by an organized thrombus, and the true lumen (*) is markedly compressed.

immunohistochemical stains (actin, CD 31, KP-1) may be performed on plastic sections by established immunohistochemical methods following removal of the methylmethacrylate.

We routinely process the nonstented arterial segments just proximal and distal to the deployed stents to assess arterial injury that may cause luminal compromise. Acutely, dissections can extend proximally and distally from the stents. In long-term stent implants, post-PTCA restenosis in the nonstented arterial segments at the stent edges can compromise flow (Fig. 3–27).

At our institution, we maintain a registry of human stents and welcome contributors to submit stented arteries for plastic embedding and sectioning.

Local Arterial Treatments to Prevent Stent Thrombosis and Restenosis

The fact that restenosis and stent thrombosis are local disease processes has prompted the development of therapies that can be administered directly to the affected arterial segment. The therapeutic advantages of local drug delivery include: (1) the administration of therapy to a defined target; (2) the ability to provide agents in sufficient doses locally that could not be achieved with systemic administration; (3) the use of systemically toxic agents; (4) the need for only small total amounts of potentially expensive drugs; and (5) the ability to provide prolonged therapy. These factors have provided the rationale for "therapeutic" stents.

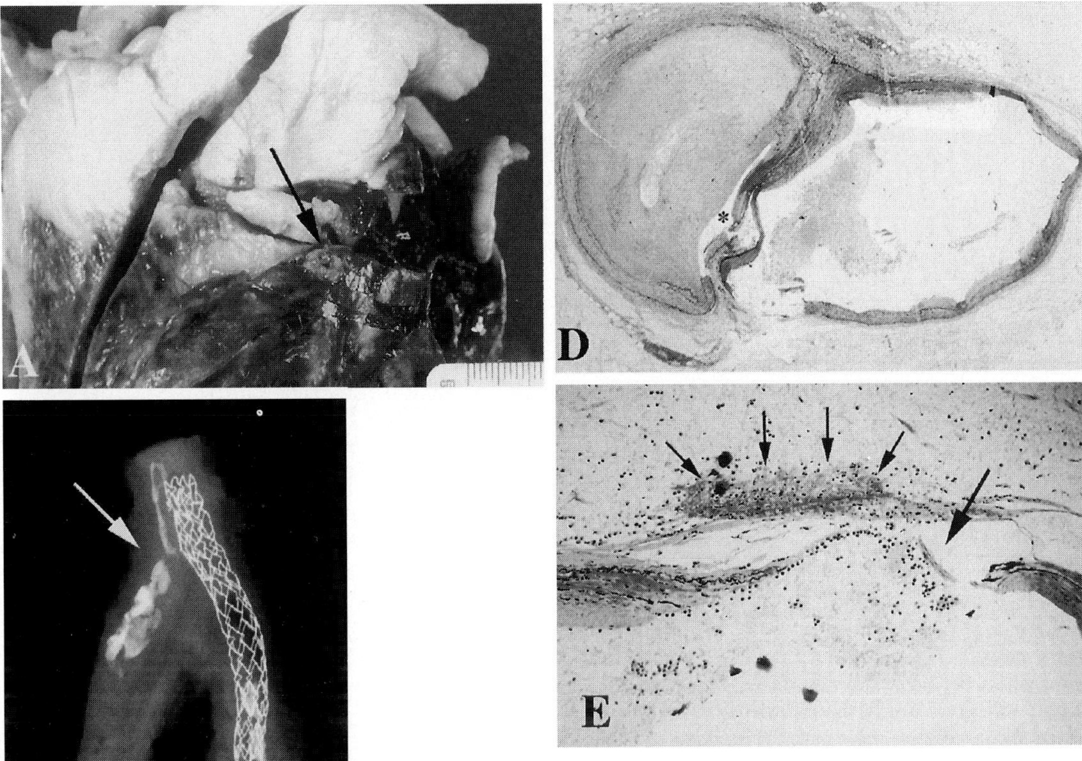

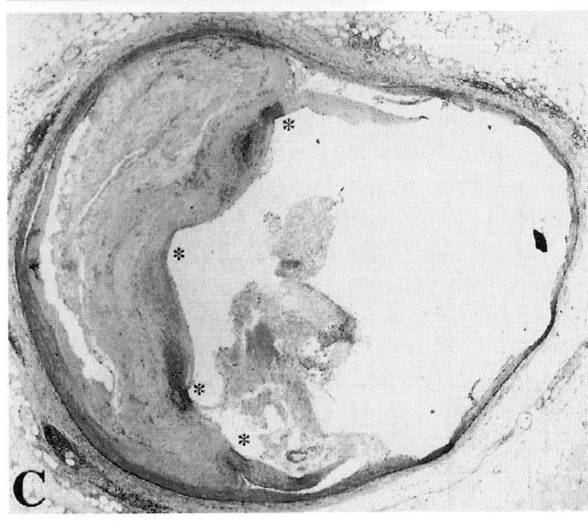

Figure 3–26. Complications of coronary stenting. A 78-year-old man with severe coronary heart disease underwent PTCA and stenting of the left anterior descending (*LAD*) coronary artery. Several hours post-catheterization, he developed hypotension, and an echocardiogram showed pericardial effusion and cardiac tamponade. The patient developed refractory hypotension and expired despite pericardiocentesis. At autopsy, hemopericardium was present, and there was an extensive hemorrhage and epicardial hematoma in the area of the stent (*A, arrow*). *B* shows the postmortem radiograph of the LAD and left diagonal (*LD*) following removal from the heart. Note that the proximal end of the stent is in the LAD, but at the bifurcation, the stent was directed into the LD, not into the LAD (where it was intended to be placed). *C* is from the proximal LAD; note compression of the plaque and tearing of the media (*on the right*). *D* is a section just distal to the LAD/LD bifurcation. The stent is in the LD (which lacks underlying atherosclerotic plaque), and there is near total compression of the lumen of the adjacent atherosclerotic LAD (* indicates the compressed LAD lumen). *E* is a high-power view of the adjoining LD showing the site of arterial rupture (*large arrow*) which led to pericardial tamponade. Note acute inflammatory cell infiltration and overlying platelet deposition (*small arrows*).

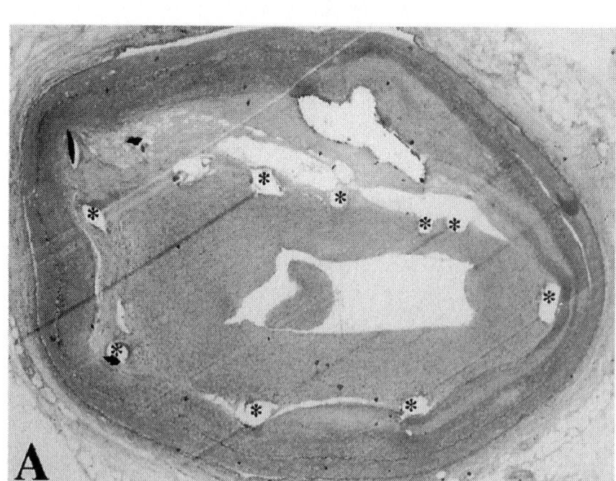

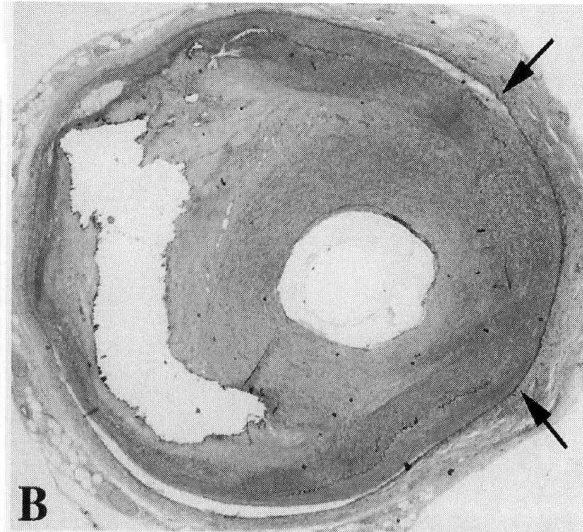

Figure 3–27. Stent edge effects. *A and B* are sections of the stented coronary artery and the native artery just proximal to the stent, respectively. In *A*, there is 60% narrowing of the stent lumen area by neointimal growth. Stent struts are indicated by *. In *B*, the nonstented arterial edge segment, there is severe stenosis (85% lumen area narrowing) as a result of post-balloon angioplasty arterial damage. Note healed balloon injury in the edge section characterized medial rupture (*arrows*) associated with marked neointimal growth. The neointima (*A and B*) is rich in proteoglycan (blue-green on Movat stain).

Stent Coatings

To date, antithrombotic drug coatings have shown promise in further reducing the incidence of stent thrombosis. Stents with an endpoint attached heparin coating had an extremely low incidence of acute stent thrombosis ($< 0.02\%$ in the BENESTENT II trial).[181] Preclinical trials with stents coated with thrombin inhibitors or platelet glycoprotein IIb/IIIa receptor antibody have also been associated with low thrombosis rates.[182–184] However, locally delivered treatments via stents or balloon catheters to inhibit neointimal growth and to treat or prevent in-stent restenosis have been less favorable. Polymeric stent coatings (biodegradable and nonbiodegradable) have been mostly disappointing secondary to excessive stent-associated inflammation.[185] Heparin coating on stents did not reduce restenosis rates in preclinical testing.[186] Stents coated with antiproliferative agents (e.g., taxol and rapamycin) are an ongoing focus of clinical testing to treat or prevent in-stent restenosis.

Brachytherapy

An alternative approach for the prevention and treatment of in-stent and post-PTCA restenosis is the local delivery of radiation therapy to create lethal DNA strand breaks in proliferating smooth muscle cells in an effort to inhibit neointimal growth. Positive studies in experimental animals have led to the initiation of human trials utilizing β-emitting (^{32}P, ^{90}Y) and γ-emitting (^{192}Ir) isotopes via catheters and stents. Initial published trials of coronary brachytherapy in patients have been encouraging with respect to a reduced restenosis rates and an overall low incidence of adverse clinical events.[187–190] However, relatively small numbers of patients have been treated with brachytherapy to date.

Effects of Local Therapy on Healing

Interventions designed to reduce neointimal growth are typically targeted against smooth muscle cell proliferation. It should be noted, however, that smooth muscle cell proliferation and extracellular matrix deposition are part of the expected healing responses following arterial injury. Therefore, restenosis-prevention therapies may delay or prevent arterial healing leading to persistent arterial inflammation. We have observed this phenomenon in two antirestenosis treatments: paclitaxel (taxol) coated stents and ^{32}P β-emitting stents. Stents coated with 20.2 or 42.0 μg paclitaxel resulted in a 36% and 49% reduction, respectively, in neointimal thickness at 28 days in rabbit iliac arteries.[191] However, there was incomplete healing characterized by intimal fibrin deposition, intraintimal hemorrhage, and increased intimal and adventitial inflammation. There was an approximate 50% reduction in rabbit iliac artery neointimal thickness by 24 and 48 μCi ^{32}P β-emitting stents at 6 months, but the intimal suppression was accompanied by persistent intimal fibrin deposition and a > twentyfold increase in intimal inflammatory cell density.[192] The presence of persistent intimal inflammation raises the question whether therapies that inhibit neointimal growth in the relative short-term will be effective in the long-term. Further, the chronically nonhealed intimal surface may increase the risk of late arterial thrombosis. For example, there was a 6.6% incidence of sudden thrombotic events 2–15 months postcoronary balloon angioplasty with or without stenting in patients treated with intracoronary β-radiation.[193]

Percutaneous Approaches to Bypass Vein Graft Disease

As noted above, the incidence of vein graft vasculopathy, particularly atherosclerosis, is increasing. These lesions are often diffuse and friable, placing them at high risk for distal embolization following catheter-based interventions. Further, restenosis rates after PTCA alone are higher than in native coronary arteries. More recently, vein graft stenting has been associated with improved clinical outcomes compared to balloon angioplasty alone. Novel aspiration and distal protection devices and stent grafts are in clinical trials in an attempt to reduce the downstream release of atheroembolic debris.[54]

The pathology of atherosclerotic bypass vein graft subjected to balloon angioplasty is similar to that seen in native coronary arteries: plaque disruption, thrombus deposition, and acute inflammation in acute angioplasty; granulation tissue and chronic inflammation in subacute cases; and neointima formation by 1 month after PTCA. Stenting of atherosclerotic saphenous vein bypass grafts can result in prolapse of the necrotic core through the stent struts (Fig. 3–28).[120] Vein graft stents in place for several months demonstrate neointimal growth (similar in composition to native coronary arteries), focal plaque compression, and chronic inflammatory cells associated with stent struts (Fig. 3–29).

Endoluminal Stent Grafts

The prevalence of abdominal aortic aneurysms is approximately 3% in patients aged 65 to 80 years (see also Chapter 13).[194,195] The traditional treatment of abdominal and thoracic aortic aneurysms is surgical with placement of a graft in the involved portion of the aorta.[196] However, abdominal aortic aneurysm surgery is associated with a mortality of 1.4 to 7.6% for nonruptured aneurysms and 10% mortality for leaking or ruptured aneurysms.[197–199] It can be expected that surgical mortality rates will remain high with the aging of the general population and the increasing incidence of coexisting morbid conditions in patients with abdominal aneurysms.[200,201] Offering the potential advantages of endovascular stents and bypass grafts, and deliverable via a percutaneous approach, stent grafts (covered stents) have been under active investigation for the treatment of aortic aneurysmal disease. The goal of this approach is to reduce the morbidity and mortality of surgery.

The graft materials used in stent grafts are typically polyester (Dacron) or expanded polytetrafluoroethylene (ePTFE). ePTFE offers the advantage that it can be dilated to the appropriate size in the target artery. In "unsupported" stent grafts, the stents are located at the ends of the graft material and act as tethering points of the stent graft to the arterial wall. "Fully-supported" stent grafts, in which the stent is present for the entire length of the graft, provide greater longitudinal support and radial strength, are less prone to kinking, and are associated with increased patency rates.[202] The stent itself may be on the inside, the outside, or completely enveloped within the graft material.

In 1969, Dotter first proposed the use of endoluminal prosthesis for the treatment of abdominal aortic aneurysms.[195] Following the first successful placement of polyurethane prostheses in dogs with an artificially induced abdominal aneurysms (in 1986), several reports of endovascular grafting in animals have been published.[196,203,204] The first human series evaluated the feasibility, safety, and effectiveness of transluminally placed self-expanding stent-grafts for the treatment of descending thoracic aortic aneurysms in 13 patients with major contraindications for surgical repair.[205] The mean diameter of the aneurysms was 6.1 cm (range 5 to 8 cm), and endovascular placement of the stent-graft prosthesis was successful in all patients. There was complete thrombosis of the thoracic aortic aneurysm surrounding the stent-graft in 12 patients, and partial thrombosis in one.[205] Two patients initially had small, residual patent proximal tracts into the aneurysm sac, but both tracts thrombosed within 2 months

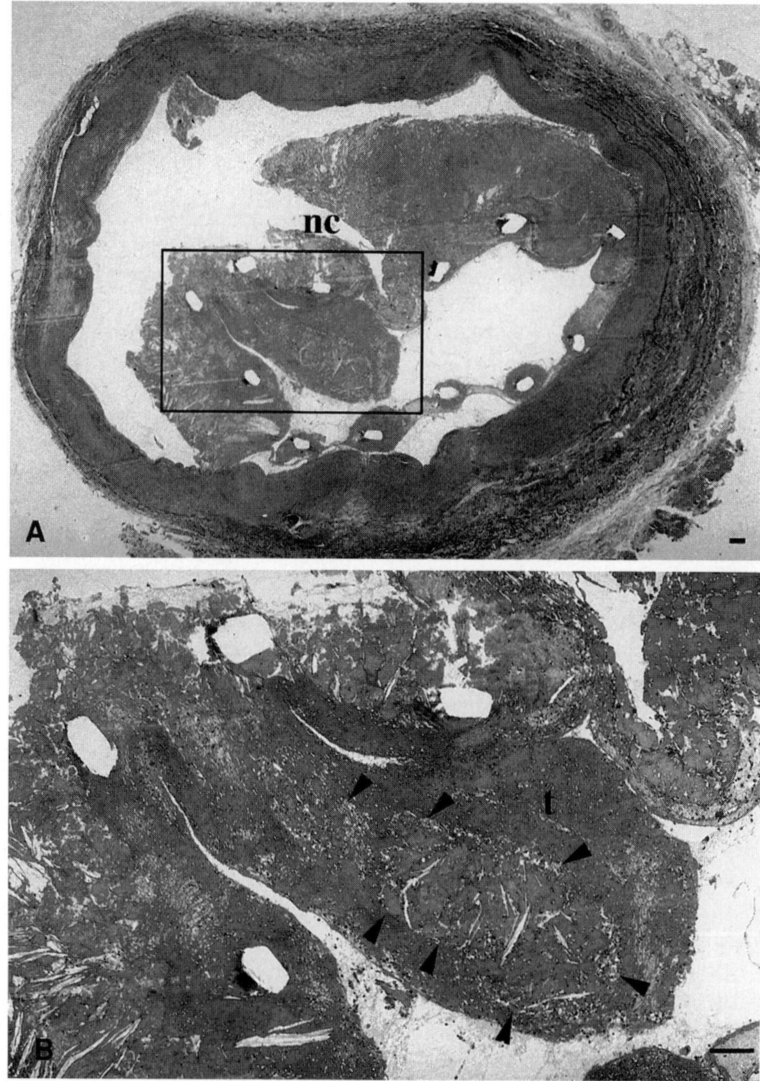

Figure 3–28. Vein graft stenting. Palmaz-Schatz stent placed 3 days antemortem in a saphenous vein graft containing a large necrotic core (*nc*, low power in *A*). In *B* (high power), there is focal extrusion of necrotic core contents (*outlined by arrowheads*) into the lumen secondary of penetration of stent struts into the lipid core. The protruding necrotic core is covered by a layer of thrombus (*t*). (Reproduced with permission from American Heart Association and Farb et al. Pathology of acute and chronic coronary stenting in humans. Circulation 99:44–52, 1999.)

after the procedure. Importantly, there were no deaths or instances of paraplegia, stroke, distal embolization, or infection during an average follow-up of 11.6 months.[205]

Major improvements in stent graft device design followed, and in 1997 Blum et al. reported their experience with endoluminal stenting for abdominal aortic aneurysms in 154 patients

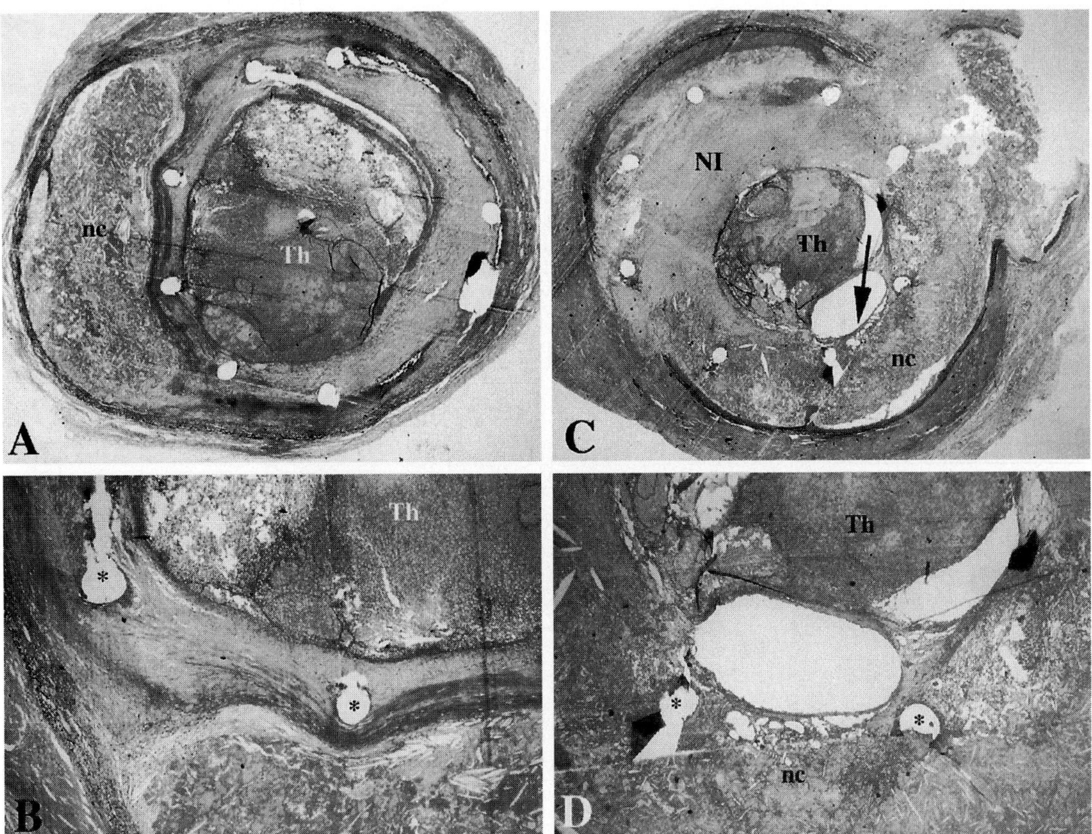

Figure 3–29. Vein graft stenting. A 73-year-old man with CABG surgery 13 years antemortem developed recurrent angina. Vein graft stenting was performed approximately 5 months antemortem. *A and B* show low- and high-power views of the vein graft with severe underlying atherosclerosis and a large necrotic core (*nc*). Note a thin neointima just above the stent struts (*, *B*) with an overlying occlusive thrombus (*Th*). *C and D* are sections from the distal portion of the stented vein graft showing the site of plaque rupture (*arrow, C*). The high-power view (*D*) shows stent struts (*) penetrating the underlying necrotic core (*nc*) and an associated luminal thrombus (*th*). On opposite wall, there is a thick neointima (*NI*) over the stent struts. Therefore, healing and plaque rupture may occur concurrently in a stented vein graft.

from three centers in Europe.[196] Of these patients, 21 without involvement of the aortic bifurcation received straight stent-grafts, and 133 with involvement of the bifurcation received bifurcating stent-grafts. The primary success rate, defined as complete exclusion of the abdominal aortic aneurysm from the circulation, was 86% in the group receiving straight grafts and 87% in the group receiving bifurcated grafts. In three patients, the procedure had to be converted to an open surgical operation. Minor (n = 13) or major (n = 3) complications associated with the procedure occurred in 10% of the patients. Major complications were rupture of the iliac artery, embolic graft occlusion, and acute hepatic failure and death. The minor complications included peripheral micro- and macroemboli, femoral-artery damage, arteriovenous fistula, groin hematoma, lymph fistula, graft occlusion, and renal failure. All patients had a postimplantation syndrome, characterized by leukocytosis and elevated serum C-reactive protein levels.[196]

With further improvements in stent graft technology, percutaneous endoluminal repair may become the standard approach for infrarenal abdominal aneurysms, especially in patients at high surgical risk. Therefore, pathologists can expect to encounter aortic stent graft specimens in their autopsy and surgical pathology labs. In the initial dissection, it is essential to remove the entire portion of the aorta that in-

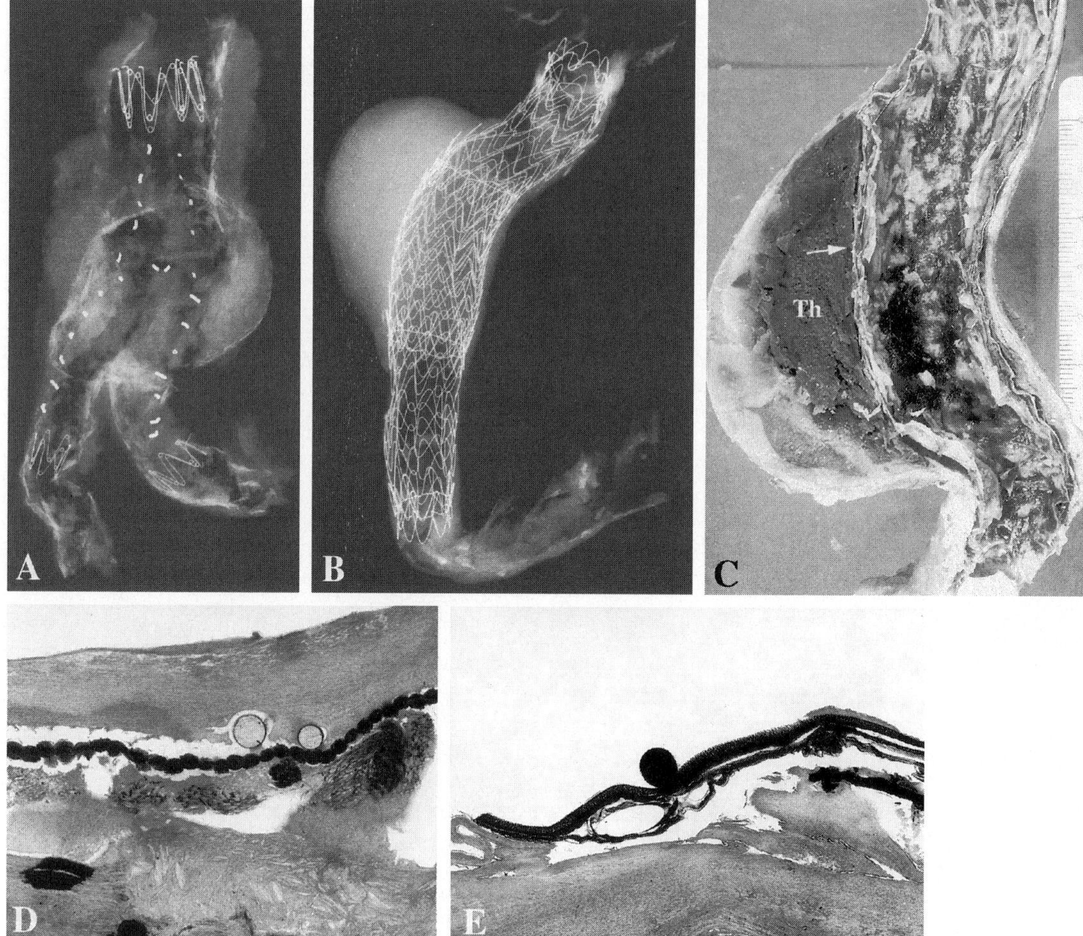

Figure 3–30. Aortic stent grafts. A 67-year-old man with hypertension, steroid dependent rheumatoid arthritis, and history of pneumonia underwent percutaneous repair of the abdominal aneurysm with stent graft. The patient did well for 6 months until he developed fever and chills, followed by septic shock and death; autopsy showed small bowel infarction. The postmortem radiograph (*A*) shows the proximal end of the Dacron stent graft in the infra-renal aorta and the distal ends in the two iliac arteries. *B* is a postmortem radiograph of a thoracic aortic aneurysm, which was treated with two percutaneously placed thoracic excluder stent grafts. The patient had carotid artery disease, and a left subclavian to left common carotid transposition procedure was performed a few days prior to stent graft placement. Following the stent graft placement, the patient suffered two strokes and died on the sixth hospital day from respiratory failure. The radiograph (*B*) shows a stent-supported ePTFE prosthesis in the thoracic aorta that fully covers the large aneurysm. *C* is the same specimen depicted in *B* cut longitudinally showing the aneurysm totally sealed off with fresh blood clot; the stent graft (*arrow*) lumen is patent. Histologic examination showed the stent graft surface to be focally covered by a thin layer of fibrin associated with a mild inflammatory infiltrate (*histologic sections not shown*). *D and E* are histologic sections of the specimen shown in *A* showing transverse and longitudinal cuts, respectively. In *D,* the dark ribbon (black) is the Dacron graft with two metal pieces towards the lumen. There is a superficial layer of fibrin thrombus and greater organization of the fibrin close to the graft. Deep to the graft is the walled-off atherosclerotic plaque. *E* (longitudinal section) shows the stent graft edge with minimal luminal thrombus. Note the absence of neointimal growth in this area of the junction with the nonstented aorta.

cludes the aneurysm and stent-graft (Fig. 3–30). Because infection is a potential complication of endoluminal aortic stenting, blood cultures and aortic cultures near the stent-graft should be performed. After overnight fixation, the specimen should be radiographed in order to locate precisely the device within the aorta.

In our laboratory, we cut the specimen transversely into 4- to 5-cm segments, keeping a portion of the adjoining nonstented aorta intact to examine the interface between stented and nonstented regions of the aorta. From these pieces we take the following sections for histologic analysis: two longitudinal sections from the proximal and distal junctions and four to five transverse sections from the stent-graft aneurysm. The longitudinal sections allow evaluation of intimal growth and thrombus formation at the junctions (Fig. 3–30). In addition, the stented and nonstented aortic interface is a location in which erosion of the graft into the aortic wall and even rupture of the aorta may occur. If possible, histologic sections that include the stent graft should be embedded in plastic and cut by the Exakt® method. This method involves sawing the plastic block into 200-μm thick segments and adhering it to a plastic slide, followed by grinding to approximately 30 to 40 μm in thickness and staining with H&E (Fig. 3–30).

Within the aneurysm sac, it is important to note the type of thrombus present; fresh thrombus indicates leakage of blood into the aneurysm sac and may be responsible for an expanded poorly sealed stent graft/aortic junction. On the stent graft luminal surface, excessive thrombus may result in distal emboli; distal vessels and organs (kidneys, spleen, and brain) should be examined for emboli. On the luminal and abluminal surfaces, the extent and type of inflammation should be noted. The presence of neutrophils or microabscesses should prompt the performance of special stains for organism identification. Aortic sections from the proximal and distal aorta close to the device are embedded in paraffin for determining the presence of medial necrosis or cystic medial change, which are commonly associated with dissections. Over time, a neointima forms over the stent graft end and may extend toward the central portion of the graft based on the porosity of the graft material used. The arterial access site (usually the femoral artery) must be examined for traumatic injuries and hemorrhage during stent-graft implantation.

An alternative to cross sections through the center of the device is a longitudinal cut through the entire stent graft (Fig. 3–30C). This type of section is less recommended, as special care is needed to maintain the relationships between the graft and native artery. The stent-graft may become detached from the aorta, unless selected instruments for cutting metal are used, especially if the stent-graft has been in the patient for only a short time.

DIRECT MYOCARDIAL REVASCULARIZATION

Despite the wide array of surgical and percutaneous interventions available to treat occlusive coronary atherosclerosis, there remains a cohort of patients with severely symptomatic, diffuse atherosclerosis who are not candidates for CABG surgery, PTCA, or stents. By noninvasive imaging utilizing scintigraphy, myocardial viability is present in these patients but is associated with chronic ischemia. These ischemic segments demonstrate impaired contractility and have been termed hibernating myocardium.[206, 207]

The clinical problem of patients with medically refractory symptoms of cardiac ischemia, evidence of myocardial viability, but no surgical or catheter-based means of improving revascularization via the epicardial coronary arteries has led to the development of techniques aimed to provide direct perfusion from blood within the left ventricular cavity. Transmyocardial laser revascularization (TMLR), a procedure performed at the time of open heart surgery, was introduced to create myocardial channels that, it was hoped, would supply oxygenated blood directly to the myocardium, and stimulate the growth of new blood vessels (angiogenesis and arteriogenesis).[208] Currently, TMLR has been approved for use in patients with refractory ischemic symptoms who are not candidates for epicardial artery revascularization. Typically, holmium:yttrium-aluminum garnet (YAG) or CO_2 lasers are used. Clinical results demonstrate that anginal symptoms are often relieved following the procedure, but no improvement in exercise tolerance, myocardial perfusion, or survival has been observed.[209–213] The mechanism of action of TMLR may thus be laser-induced myocardial denervation. Percutaneous myocardial utilizing catheter-based laser system is currently in trial.

Angiogenesis and Arteriogenesis

Angiogenesis refers to the sprouting of capillaries (endothelial-derived vascular spaces) in avascular regions from preexisting vessels and is seen in wound healing, ischemia, inflammation, in the female reproductive organs, and in tumor growth beyond a critical size.[214, 215] The ability of these vessels to provide sufficient blood to ischemic tissues is uncertain; often they end abruptly or travel in meaningless directions. Rather than supporting blood flow, capillaries formed by angiogenesis may at best be a conduit for inflammatory cells involved in the healing process. Positive regulators of angiogenesis include mitogens such as vascular endothelial growth factor (VEGF), acidic fibroblast growth factor (aFGF), basic FGF (bFGF), transforming growth factor beta (TGF-β), and tumor necrosis factor alpha (TNF-α), nitric oxide, angiopoietin (Ang-1 and -2), proteases of the plasminogen activator, matrix metalloproteinases, chymase and heparanase.[214] Of these agents, VEGF is believed to be the most important mediator of angiogenesis.

Arteriogenesis is the development of muscular collateral blood vessels *in situ* from preexisting arteriolar anastomoses supplying ischemic tissues. Initially endothelial cells and vascular smooth muscle cells proliferate accompanied by synthesis of extracellular matrix, proteoglycans, collagen, and elastin.[216] This phase is followed by remodeling, a process by which vessel diameters may increase up to twentyfold. Tissue ischemia is not required for arteriogenesis to occur; rather it is mediated by shear stress-induced upregulation of angiogenic factors and inflammatory cells such as macrophages. Experimental animal studies suggest that shear stress-induced MCP-1 (monocyte chemotactic protein) gene expression and protein secretion are upregulated in chronic ischemia.[217]

Pathology of Transmyocardial Revascularization

Histologic examination of the heart following TMLR explains the absence of improved myocardial perfusion following treatment. In experimental animal studies, laser channel closure develops 6 to 24 hours after their creation by occlusive thrombi consisting of platelets, fibrin, and red blood cells. The myocardium bordering the channel shows a band of myocyte coagulation necrosis and contraction band necrosis, which is five to seven cell layers thick. The thrombus organizes by the formation of granulation tissue, which consists of neoangiogenesis and chronic inflammatory cells with interspersed myofibroblasts, which are visible between 1 to 2 weeks following laser injury. The granulation tissue is finally replaced by collagenous scar tissue interspersed by a paucity of capillaries; these capillaries have never been conclusively shown to increase blood flow into the myocardium surrounding the region of the laser channels.[208, 218–220]

Human autopsy findings after TMLR are similar to animal experimental results. Soon after the laser channels are formed, platelets, fibrin, red blood cells, and acute inflammatory cells occlude channels (Fig. 3–31). The myocardium surrounding the channel shows a clear zone of myocyte coagulation necrosis with infiltration of neutrophils. Between the viable myocardium and the region of coagulation necrosis, there is a zone of contraction band necrosis. The surrounding vessels are congested, and occasionally the laser may disrupt muscular arteries, resulting in extravasation of red blood cells and thrombosis, if they happen to be in the laser energy field.[221, 222] On the epicardial surface, the channels are funnel shaped and are occluded by fibrinous material. The endocardial channels are also sealed by fibrinous material, which either is on the same level with the surrounding endocardium or may protrude into the ventricular cavity.[221]

At 1 to 3 weeks after TMLR, there is a pronounced healing response at the mouth of the channel created by the laser tract relative to the subjacent myocardium. This accelerated phase of healing is characterized by fibrin and collagen deposition in association with macrophages, lymphocytes, scattered red blood cells, and rare neutrophils. In contrast, intramyocardial channels show a greater accumulation of fibrin, red blood cells, macrophages, and inflammatory cells compared to the mouth of the channel. At this phase, a few cells within the laser tract react positively with antibodies to CD31 and von Willebrand Factor (vWf), providing evidence for the presence of endothelium.

Late histologic changes (> 2 months) following clinical TMLR consist of fibrous tissue scarring, sparse macrophage infiltration with an interspersed capillary network, scattered small veins, and rare arterioles (Fig. 3–31). With time, the fibrous tissue is transformed into a dense collagenous scar with fewer endothelial-lined capillaries. The capillary lining of endothelial cells are both CD31 and vWf positive. The mouth of the channel becomes completely filled with fibrous tissue, and there is no direct communication between the ventricular cavity and the capillary network within the fibrous channel.[221] Similarly, epicardial openings are completely filled with fibrous scars and may appear as depressions microscopically. No evidence of cellular proliferation has been found at early, intermediate, or late phases of healing.

Overall, the myocardial changes associated with TMLR in humans consist of limited angiogenesis within scar tissue and no arteriogenesis. A better understanding of the mediators of arteriogenesis will likely be necessary before a sig-

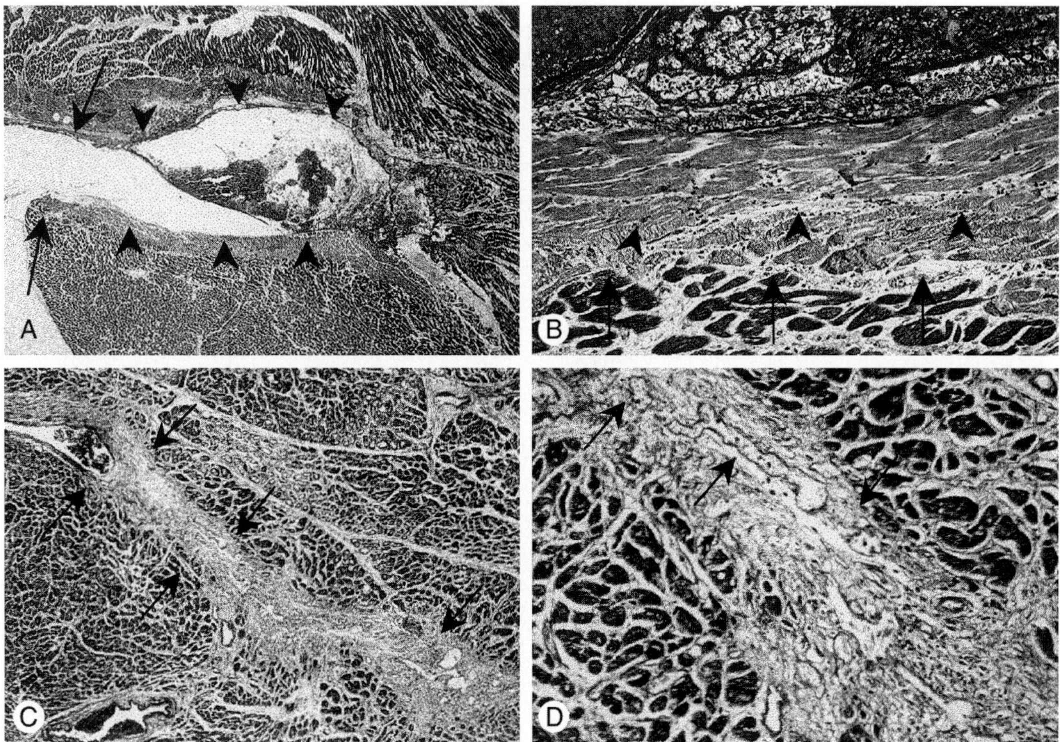

Figure 3–31. Transmyocardial revascularization (*TMLR*). A 66-year-old woman underwent TMLR 3 days antemortem. At autopsy, myocardial channels could be easily discerned grossly with focal areas of hemorrhage within the myocardium and fibrinous pericarditis. Microscopic sections (*A*) show the mouth of the channel (*arrows*) on the endocardial surface with focal fibrin clot and platelet deposition. A border zone of surrounding myocardial necrosis (*arrowheads*) is present. A high-power view of a channel in the mid-myocardium is shown in *B*. The channel is filled with thrombus (*top of the image*), and the surrounding myocardium has a zone of coagulation necrosis. The normal myocardium is separated from the zone of coagulation necrosis by a layer of contraction band necrosis (*arrows*). At the border zone between viable and necrotic myocardium, neutrophils are present. *C and D* are from a 61-year-old man who died 70 days following TMLR. The channels at this stage could not be identified by gross examination. Histologically (*C*), in the area of TMLR treatment, loosely filled fibrocollagenous tracts could be identified (*arrows*). Within the channel (*D*), multiple capillaries (*arrows*) were identified with only rare arterioles.

nificant increase in myocardial perfusion is achieved.

MECHANICAL CIRCULATORY SUPPORT

Heart failure occurs at a rate of at least 400,000 new cases per year, and is the principal cause of death in 40,000 patients per year in the United States.[223] The broad differential diagnosis of heart failure includes the most common etiologies: coronary atherosclerosis, valvular heart disease, cardiomyopathies, myocarditis, and congenital cardiac malformations.[224]

Mechanical circulatory support was first used clinically in 1953 leading to the development of surgical treatments for heart disease.[225] Subsequently, intraaortic balloon pumps to support patients with acute heart failure were developed.[226] In the 1960s, cardiopulmonary bypass, ventricular assist devices, and total artificial hearts were used as temporary supports in patients in acute heart failure (Fig. 3–32). However, it was not until the 1970s that research efforts were directed towards improvements in mechanical circulatory support devices for long-term care.

Currently, a mechanical circulatory support system is most often used as a bridge to cardiac transplantation. Clinical experience of > 15 years with mechanical assist devices as bridges-to-transplant show higher hospital discharge rates in patients with left ventricular assist devices (89%) vs. controls (60%).[227, 228] Sixty-two to 69% of patients eventually undergo transplantation, and the rate of ultimate hospital

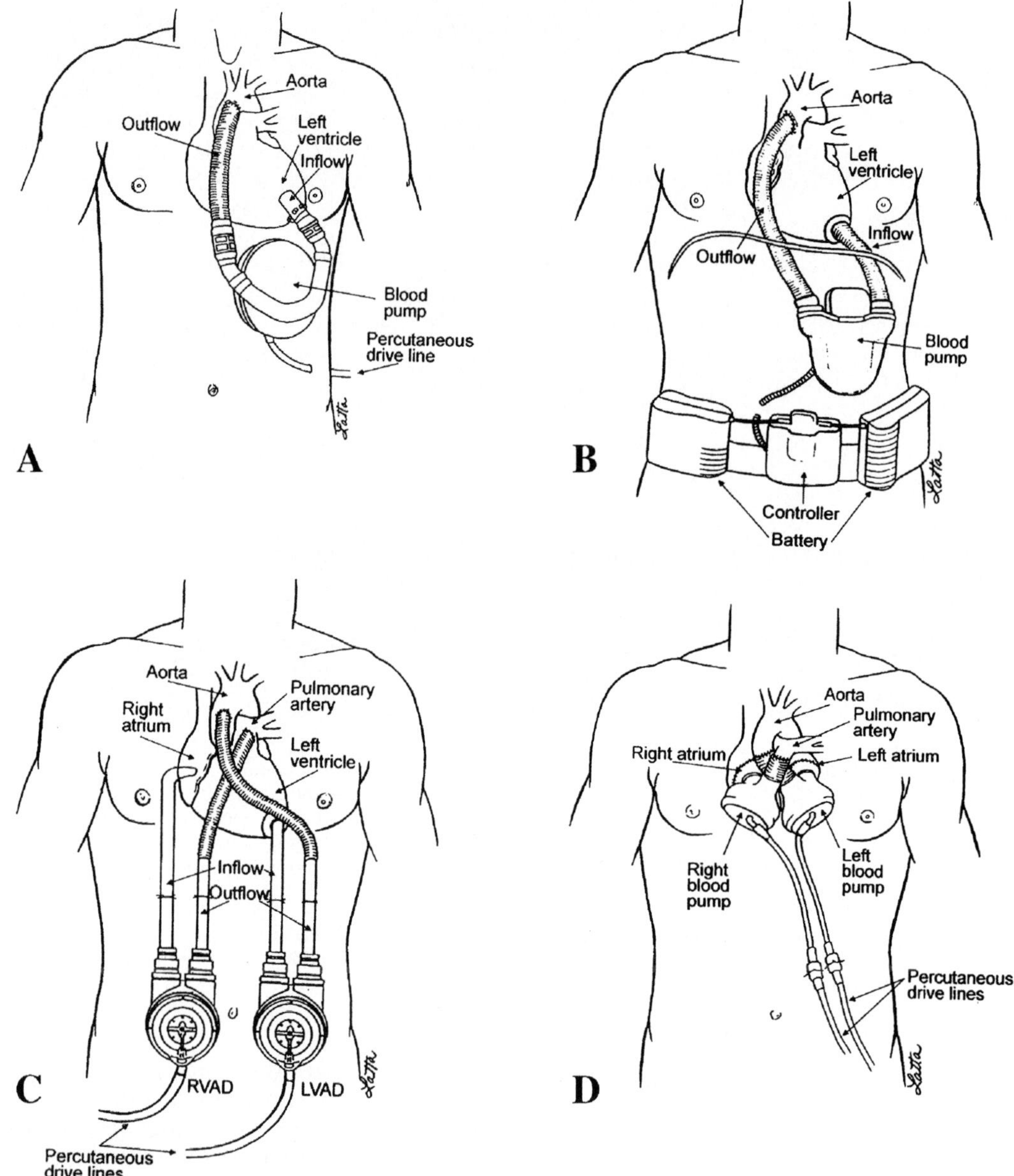

Figure 3–32. *A,* The HeartMate Implantable pneumatic left ventricular assist system. *B,* The Novacor wearable left ventricular assist system. *C,* The Thoratec ventricular assist system in the biventricular support configuration (*RVAD* = right ventricular assist device; *LVAD* = left ventricular assist device). *D,* The CardioWest total artificial heart. (Reproduced with permission from Hunt SA, Frazier OH. Mechanical circulatory support and cardiac transplantation. Circulation 97:2079–2090, 1998.)

discharge after transplant is 65 to 69%. In one controlled study of cardiac transplantation, patients receiving an implantable pneumatic left ventricular assist device had a better survival rate at 90 days (71%) than controls (36%).[229]

Assist Devices

Two available systems, the HeartMate and the Novacor, are fully implantable left ventricular assist systems, which allow mechanical bypass of the left ventricle without removal of the native heart. The HeartMate implantable device is portable, and is available in two versions: an implantable pneumatic and a vented electric version, which differ only in their method of activation. The Thoratec ventricular assist system is a paracorporeal system that can provide a right, left, or biventricular support. The CardioWest total artificial heart, also called the Jarvik or Symbion total artificial heart, is a pulsatile biventricular replacement system.

Each circulatory support device has its own characteristics and implant methods, which are relevant to pathologic evaluation (autopsy or surgical explant) for the detection of thrombus and infection at anastomotic sites (see following). In the HeartMate, the blood lining surfaces encourages the deposition of circulating cells allowing for the development of a "pseudointima."[230] The advantage of this surface is that during prolonged support, the patient can be managed with minimal or no anticoagulation.[231] The inflow and the outflow conduits contain porcine valves, and the pump is positioned below the diaphragm. The inflow tube crosses the diaphragm and is inserted in the apex of the left ventricle, whereas the outflow graft exits the pump as a 20-mm Dacron tube, crosses the diaphragm, and is inserted into the ascending aorta.[232] The HeartMate device was approved by the FDA in April 1998, and has been implanted in > 1,000 patients worldwide as a bridge to transplantation. It is reported to have a low risk of thromboembolism and mechanical failure.[224]

The Novacor is also a portable, implantable device and differs from the HeartMate design in the method of pump actuation and blood contacting surface[233] such that the patient requires heparin and warfarin as anticoagulants.[224] The Novacor pump is surgically implanted in a preperitoneal pocket just anterior to the posterior rectus sheath, between the left costal margin and the iliac crest.[233]

The Thoratec ventricular assist device is a paracorporeal, pneumatically powered system that can operate as either a univentricular or biventricular support system. The device is implanted through a median sternotomy, but cardiopulmonary bypass is not required for all patients. For left ventricular support, the inflow cannula is placed in the apex of the left ventricle or the left atrium and the pump outflow conduit is anastomosed to the ascending aorta. For right ventricular support, the inflow cannula is placed in the right atrium and the outflow cannula is sewn to the main pulmonary artery.[234] Bjork-Shiley concavo-convex tilting disc valves are in place in the inflow and the outflow conduits. Patients with the device require anticoagulation with dextran, heparin, warfarin, and dipyridamole.[235] The Thoratec system has been approved by the FDA as a bridge to heart transplantation.[224]

The CardioWest total artificial heart is a polyurethane-lined pulsatile biventricular pump. The pump has a rigid frame, with a flexible polyurethane diaphragm that separates the pump from the air chambers. Two Medtronic Hall mechanical valves provide the unidirectional blood flow. It is surgically implanted in the mediastinal space after the ventricles are excised and the atria are retained, and the pneumatic drives are exteriorized and attached to a percutaneous drive console.[224, 236, 237]

Complications of Assist Devices

The most frequent complications associated with assist devices are bleeding, infection, thromboembolism, renal failure, and neurological impairment.[227, 238–240] These complications were recently reported in 258 patients who had mechanical circulatory support (pneumatic ventricular assist device in 56%, electromechanical left ventricular assist devices in 6%, total artificial hearts in 30%, and centrifugal pumps in 8%) in the period 1986–1993. Bleeding occurred in 84 patients (33%); infections in 83 patients (32%); 21 embolic complications were reported in 16 patients (6%); renal failure in 64 cases (25%, requiring dialysis in 33 [13%]); respiratory failure in 47 (18%); and neurological impairment in 22 patients (9%).

Bleeding occurs secondary to coagulopathy as a result of hepatic dysfunction and platelet activation caused by blood-pump rheology. Bleeding is most frequent in patients requiring biventricular assist devices. Infections, often associated with morbidity and mortality, are most frequent in patients with bleeding and multiorgan failure[241–243] and are classified into four types depending on the location of the infection: (1) Class I are patient infections not of the assist device or of the blood; (2) Class II are blood-born infections; (3) Class III are percutaneous site infections; and (4) Class IV involve the intracorporeal ventricular assist device components and are the most serious infections.[243] The most frequent isolated organism is *Staphylococcus epidermidis,* which tends to persist and is refractory to antimicrobial therapies.[244] However, infectious complications do not preclude successful cardiac transplantation.[245, 246] The proposed pathogenesis of support device-associated infections are protein absorption to surfaces, bacterial adhesion to plasma and matrix proteins, metabolic state of bacteria, adhesion of leukocytes to protein-adsorbed surfaces, biofilm production by adherent bacteria, procoagulant activity of adherent bacteria and leukocytes, fibrin formation, inhibition of inflammatory response, and resistance to antomicrobials.[247]

In a recent comparison study of the HeartMate and Novacor left ventricular assist devices, neurologic complications occurred significantly more often among the Novacor group, whereas the HeartMate group had a higher incidence of infections and technical problems.[248] Survival to transplantation was 65% for the Novacor group and 60% for the HeartMate group.[248]

Autopsy Evaluation of Ventricular Assist Devices

The objectives of the autopsy in cases with ventricular assist devices are to determine the cause of death, define the underlying cardiopulmonary pathology, and document patient-prosthesis interactions. Examination of the device is preferably done in consultation with the manufacturer, who may send a representative or provide telephonic consultation regarding evaluation of the device's functions. All devices must be rinsed with heparinized solution, cultured, and then photographed. Photography

Table 3–1. Tissue Interaction with Ventricular Assist System Components

Blood-contacting surfaces
Blood pump (inner housing surface, diaphragm)
Valves (valve, valve mount, quick connectors)
Conduits (inflow cannula and graft, outflow cannula and graft)
Tissue-surface interactions
Blood pump (outer surface)
Conduits (inflow cannula and graft, outflow cannula and graft)
Compliance chamber
Secondary coil
Internal battery (electrical ventricular assist device)*
Engine-thermal battery-module (thermal electrical ventricular assist device)*
Pneumatic and vent lines*

* Components variably present, depending on device configuration

From Schoen et al. Ventricular assist devise (VAD) pathology analyses. J Appl Biomater 1:49–56, 1990, with permission.

Table 3–2. Pathologic Analysis of Pump Components and Surrounding Tissues

Inflow Cannula
Angulation
Depth of cannula in heart
External surface deposition
Internal surface deposition
Damage to endocardium/myocardium
Inflow Valve
Orifice diameter
Occluder/cuspmovement
Vegetations
Thrombus
Defects
Suture line dehiscence
Calcification
Inflow Graft
Outer apsule
Wire spring (if present)
Angulation
Twisting
Inner capsule
Inner housing
Deformity
Defect
Screw loosened
Leakage
Blood-contracting surface
Diaphragm
Deformity
Defects
Delamination
Discoloration
Thrombus
Calcification
Outflow valve (see above for inflow valve)
Outflow graft (see above for inflow graft)
Compliance Chamber
External tissue
Fluid leak
Deformity
Wall Damage
Chamber volume
Gas Analysis
Energy source and related components
External tissue
Casing integrity
Deformation

From Schoen et al. Ventricular assist device (VAD) pathology analyses. J Appl Biomater 1:49–56, 1990, with permission.

and diagrams should document the appearance of the components of the device as the device is disassembled: blood contact surfaces, valves, conduits, compliance chambers, housings, and energy source (Tables 3–1 and 3–2), with special attention on the luminal surface.[249] Valves should be carefully examined for vegetations and thrombi or any other defects that may be present (Table 3–2).[250, 251]

Evaluation of infections related to ventricular assist devices include histologic analysis of cardiac and aortic anastomotic sites and the percutaneous drive site lines.[252] Cultures are taken from biomaterial surfaces to determine the site of infection, and scrapings are obtained from adjoining tissues for histologic analysis and special stains for organisms. For microbiologic culture of tissue sites, homogenates should be prepared in consultation with the microbiology personnel, who should be notified prior to starting the autopsy. Tissues recommended for microbiological culture include the skin, subcutaneous tissue, intramuscular tissue, fibrous capsule in the region of the device, relevant vascular junctions, and components of the device, especially at sites of thrombus deposition.[249] The pathologist should carefully investigate for emboli (acute or healing) in visceral organs, particularly the brain, lungs, kidney, and spleen. A standard autopsy protocol, including microscopic examination of heart, lung, brain, liver, spleen, kidneys, adrenal glands, small and large bowels, bone marrow, and mediastinal lymph nodes is recommended. Gross abnormalities of any other organs or device components should also be further studied by histologic analysis.[249, 252]

REFERENCES

1. Yusuf S, Zucker D, Peduzzi P, et al. Effect of coronary artery bypass graft surgery on survival: Overview of 10-year results from randomised trials by the Coronary Artery Bypass Graft Surgery Trialists Collaboration. Lancet 344:563–570, 1994.
2. Eagle KA, Guyton RA, Davidoff R, et al. ACC/AHA Guidelines for Coronary Artery Bypass Graft Surgery: A Report of the American College of Cardiology/American Heart Association Task Force on Practice Guidelines (Committee to Revise the 1991 Guidelines for Coronary Artery Bypass Graft Surgery). American College of Cardiology/American Heart Association. J Am Coll Cardiol 34:1262–1347, 1999.
3. Coronary angioplasty versus coronary artery bypass surgery: The Randomized Intervention Treatment of Angina (RITA) trial. Lancet. 341:573–580, 1993.
4. King SB III, Lembo NJ, Weintraub WS, et al. A randomized trial comparing coronary angioplasty with coronary bypass surgery. Emory Angioplasty versus Surgery Trial (EAST). N Engl J Med 334:1044–1050, 1994.
5. Hamm CW, Reimers J, Ischinger T, et al. A randomized study of coronary angioplasty compared with bypass surgery in patients with symptomatic multivessel coronary disease. German Angioplasty Bypass Surgery Investigation (GABI). N Engl J Med 331:1037–1043, 1994.
6. Investigators TBARIB. Comparison of coronary bypass surgery with angioplasty in patients with multivessel disease. N Engl J Med 335:217–225, 1996.
7. Kirklin JW, Barratt-Boyes BG. Cardiac Surgery, pp 285–382. New York: Churchill Livingstone, 1993.
8. Barner HB, Swartz MT, Mudd JG, et al. Late patency of the internal mammary artery as a coronary bypass conduit. Ann Thorac Surg 34:408–412, 1982.
9. Loop FD, Lytle BW, Cosgrove DM, et al. Influence of the internal-mammary-artery graft on 10-year survival and other cardiac events. N Engl J Med 314:1–6, 1986.
10. Acinapura AJ, Rose DM, Jacobowitz IJ, et al. Internal mammary artery bypass grafting: Influence on recurrent angina and survival in 2,100 patients. Ann Thorac Surg 48:186–191, 1989.
11. Loop FD, Lytle BW, Cosgrove DM, et al. Free (aorta-coronary) internal mammary artery graft. Late results. J Thorac Cardiovasc Surg 92:827–831, 1986.
12. Motwani JG, Topol EJ. Aortocoronary saphenous vein graft disease: Pathogenesis, predisposition, and prevention. Circulation 97:916–931, 1998.
13. Shapira OM, Alkon JD, Aldea GS, et al. Clinical outcomes in patients undergoing coronary artery bypass grafting with preferred use of the radial artery. J Card Surg 12:381–388, 1997.
14. Acar C, Ramsheyi A, Pagny JY, et al. The radial artery for coronary artery bypass grafting: Clinical and angiographic results at five years. J Thorac Cardiovasc Surg 116:981–989, 1998.
15. Tatoulis J, Buxton BF, Fuller JA, et al. The radial artery as a graft for coronary revascularization: Techniques and follow-up. Adv Card Surg 11:99–128, 1999.
16. Yeh CH, Chang CH, Lin PJ, et al. Totally minimally invasive cardiac surgery for coronary artery disease. Eur J Cardiothorac Surg 14 Suppl 1:S43–47, 1998.
17. Watanabe G, Misaki T, Kotoh K, et al. Multiple minimally invasive direct coronary artery bypass grafting for the complete revascularization of the left ventricle. Ann Thorac Surg 68:131–136, 1999.
18. Subramanian VA. Clinical experience with minimally invasive reoperative coronary bypass surgery. Eur J Cardiothorac Surg 10:1058–1062; discussion 1062–1063, 1996.
19. Cremer JT, Wittwer T, Boning A, et al. Minimally invasive coronary artery revascularization on the beating heart. Ann Thorac Surg 69:1787–1791, 2000.
20. Doty JR, Fonger JD, Salazar JD, et al. Early experience with minimally invasive direct coronary artery bypass grafting with the internal thoracic artery [comment]. J Thorac Cardiovasc Surg 117:873–880, 1999.
21. Magovern JA, Benckart DH, Landreneau RJ, et al. Morbidity, cost, and six-month outcome of minimally invasive direct coronary artery bypass grafting. Ann Thorac Surg 66:1224–1229, 1998.
22. Ribakove GH, Miller JS, Anderson RV, et al. Minimally invasive port-access coronary artery bypass grafting with early angiographic follow-up: Initial clinical experience. J Thorac Cardiovasc Surg 115:1101–1110, 1998.

23. Subramanian VA, McCabe JC, Geller CM. Minimally invasive direct coronary artery bypass grafting: Two-year clinical experience. Ann Thorac Surg 64:1648–1653; discussion 1654–1655, 1997.
24. Virmani R, Atkinson JB, Forman MB. Aortocoronary bypass grafts and extracardiac conduits. In: Silver MD (ed): Cardiovascular Pathology, 1607–1648. New York: Churchill Livingstone, 1991.
25. Griffith LS, Bulkley BH, Hutchins GM, et al. Occlusive changes at the coronary artery—bypass graft anastomosis. Morphologic study of 95 grafts. J Thorac Cardiovasc Surg 73:668–679, 1977.
26. Spray TL, Roberts WC. Status of the grafts and the native coronary arteries proximal and distal to coronary anastomotic sites of aortocoronary bypass grafts. Circulation 55:741–749, 1977.
27. Shelton ME, Forman MB, Virmani R, et al. A comparison of morphologic and angiographic findings in long-term internal mammary artery and saphenous vein bypass grafts. J Am Coll Cardiol 11:297–307, 1988.
28. Berger PB, Alderman EL, Nadel A, et al. Frequency of early occlusion and stenosis in a left internal mammary artery to left anterior descending artery bypass graft after surgery through a median sternotomy on conventional bypass: Benchmark for minimally invasive direct coronary artery bypass. Circulation 100:2353–2358, 1999.
29. Kay HR, Korns ME, Flemma RJ, et al. Atherosclerosis of the internal mammary artry. Ann Thorac Surg 21:504–507, 1976.
30. Mestres CA, Rives A, Igual A, et al. Atherosclerosis of the internal mammary artery. Histopathological analysis and implications on its results in coronary artery bypass graft surgery. Thorac Cardiovasc Surg 34:356–358, 1986.
31. Bulkley BH, Hutchins GM. Accelerated atherosclerosis. A morphologic study of 97 saphenous vein coronary artery bypass grafts. Circulation 55:163–169, 1977
32. Kern WH, Dermer GB, Lindesmith GG. The intimal proliferation in aortic-coronary saphenous vein grafts. Light and electron microscopic studies. Am Heart J 84:771–777, 1972.
33. Vlodaver Z, Edwards JE. Pathologic changes in aortic-coronary arterial saphenous vein grafts. Circulation 44:719–728, 1971.
34. Barboriak JJ, Batayias GE, Pintar K, et al. Pathological changes in surgically removed aortocoronary vein grafts. Ann Thorac Surg 21:524–527, 1976.
35. Bourassa MG. Fate of venous grafts: The past, the present and the future. J Am Coll Cardiol 17:1081–1083, 1991.
36. Fitzgibbon GM, Kafka HP, Leach AJ, et al. Coronary bypass graft fate and patient outcome: Angiographic follow-up of 5,065 grafts related to survival and reoperation in 1,388 patients during 25 years [see comments]. J Am Coll Cardiol 28:616–626, 1996.
37. Campeau L, Enjalbert M, Lesperance J, et al. The relation of risk factors to the development of atherosclerosis in saphenous-vein bypass grafts and the progression of disease in the native circulation. A study 10 years after aortocoronary bypass surgery. N Engl J Med 311:1329–1332, 1984.
38. Lie JT, Lawrie GM, Morris GC, Jr. Aortocoronary bypass saphenous vein graft atherosclerosis. Anatomic study of 99 vein grafts from normal and hyperlipoproteinemic patients up to 75 months postoperatively. Am J Cardiol 40:906–914, 1977.
39. Atkinson JB, Forman MB, Vaughn WK, et al. Morphologic changes in long-term saphenous vein bypass grafts. Chest 88:341–348, 1985.
40. Neitzel GF, Barboriak JJ, Pintar K, et al. Atherosclerosis in aortocoronary bypass grafts. Morphologic study and risk factor analysis 6 to 12 years after surgery. Arteriosclerosis 6:594–600, 1986.
41. Ratliff NB, Myles JL. Rapidly progressive atherosclerosis in aortocoronary saphenous vein grafts. Possible immune-mediated disease. Arch Pathol Lab Med 113:772–776, 1989.
42. Kalan JM, Roberts WC. Morphologic findings in saphenous veins used as coronary arterial bypass conduits for longer than 1 year: Necropsy analysis of 53 patients, 123 saphenous veins, and 1865 five-millimeter segments of veins. Am Heart J 119:1164–1184, 1990.
43. Solymoss BC, Nadeau P, Millette D, et al. Late thrombosis of saphenous vein coronary bypass grafts related to risk factors. Circulation 78:I140–143, 1988.
44. Linden T, Bondjers G, Karlsson T, et al. Serum triglycerides and HDL cholesterol—major predictors of long-term survival after coronary surgery. Eur Heart J 15:747–752, 1994.
45. Daida H, Yokoi H, Miyano H, et al. Relation of saphenous vein graft obstruction to serum cholesterol levels. J Am Coll Cardiol 25:193–197, 1995.
46. The effect of aggressive lowering of low-density lipoprotein cholesterol levels and low-dose anticoagulation on obstructive changes in saphenous-vein coronary-artery bypass grafts. The Post Coronary Artery Bypass Graft Trial Investigators. N Engl J Med 336:153–162, 1997.
47. FitzGibbon GM, Leach AJ, Kafka HP. Atherosclerosis of coronary artery bypass grafts and smoking. CMAJ 136:45–47, 1987.
48. Walts AE, Fishbein MC, Matloff JM. Thrombosed, ruptured atheromatous plaques in saphenous vein coronary artery bypass grafts: Ten years' experience. Am Heart J 114:718–723, 1987.
49. Pintar K, Barboriak JJ, Johnson WD, et al. Atherosclerotic aneurysm in aortocoronary vein graft. Arch Pathol Lab Med 102:287–288, 1978.
50. Taliercio CP, Smith HC, Pluth JR, et al. Coronary artery venous bypass graft aneurysm with symptomatic coronary artery emboli. J Am Coll Cardiol 7:435–473, 1986.
51. Liang BT, Antman EM, Taus R, et al. Atherosclerotic aneurysms of aortocoronary vein grafts. Am J Cardiol 61:185–188, 1988.
52. Farb A, Weber DW, Burke AP, et al. Morphology of stenosis progression and rupture in saphenous vein bypass grafts. Circulation 100 (suppl 1):I-599, 1999.
53. Kockx MM, De Meyer GR, Bortier H, et al. Luminal foam cell accumulation is associated with smooth muscle cell death in the intimal thickening of human saphenous vein grafts. Circulation 94:1255–1262, 1996.
54. Webb JG, Carere RG, Virmani R, et al. Retrieval and analysis of particulate debris after saphenous vein graft intervention. J Am Coll Cardiol 34:468–475, 1999.
55. Chang Y, Shih CT, Lai ST. Early results of the advanced coronary endarterectomy combined with CABG in the treatment of coronary artery occlusive disease. Chung Hua I Hsueh Tsa Chih (Taipei) 54:156–159, 1994.
56. Asimakopoulos G, Taylor KM, Ratnatunga CP. Outcome of coronary endarterectomy: A case-control study. Ann Thorac Surg 67:989–993, 1999.

57. Christenson JT, Simonet F, Schmuziger M. Extensive endarterectomy of the left anterior descending coronary artery combined with coronary artery bypass grafting. Coron Artery Dis 6:731–737, 1995.
58. Shapira OM, Akopian G, Hussain A, et al. Improved clinical outcomes in patients undergoing coronary artery bypass grafting with coronary endarterectomy. Ann Thorac Surg 68:2273–2278, 1999.
59. Gruntzig AR, Senning A, Siegenthaler WE. Nonoperative dilatation of coronary-artery stenosis: Percutaneous transluminal coronary angioplasty. N Engl J Med 301:61–68, 1979.
60. Ryan TJ, Bauman WB, Kennedy JW, et al. Guidelines for percutaneous transluminal coronary angioplasty. A report of the American Heart Association/American College of Cardiology Task Force on Assessment of Diagnostic and Therapeutic Cardiovascular Procedures (Committee on Percutaneous Transluminal Coronary Angioplasty). Circulation 88:2987–3007, 1993.
61. Parisi AF, Folland ED, Hartigan P. A comparison of angioplasty with medical therapy in the treatment of single-vessel coronary artery disease. Veterans Affairs ACME Investigators. N Engl J Med 326:10–16, 1992.
62. Pitt B, Waters D, Brown WV, et al. Aggressive lipid-lowering therapy compared with angioplasty in stable coronary artery disease. Atorvastatin versus Revascularization Treatment Investigators. N Engl J Med 341:70–76, 1999.
63. Brodison A, More RS, Chauhan A. The role of coronary angioplasty and stenting in acute myocardial infarction. Postgrad Med J 75:591–598, 1999.
64. Dangas G, Stone GW. Primary mechanical reperfusion in acute myocardial infarction: The United States experience. Semin Interv Cardiol 4:21–33, 1999.
65. Lange RA, Cigarroa JE, Hillis LD. Thrombolysis versus primary percutaneous transluminal coronary angioplasty for acute myocardial infarction. Cardiol Rev 7:77–82, 1999.
66. de Feyter PJ, de Jaegere PPT, Serruys PW. Incidence, predictors, and management of acute coronary occlusion after coronary angioplasty. Am Heart J 127:643–651, 1994.
67. Lau KW, Gao W, Ding ZP, et al. Single bailout stenting for threatened coronary closure complicating balloon angioplasty: Acute and mid-term outcome. Coron Artery Dis 7:327–333, 1996.
68. Farb A, Virmani R, Atkinson JB, et al. Plaque morphology and pathologic changes in arteries from patients dying after coronary balloon angioplasty [see comments]. J Am Coll Cardiol 16:1421–1429, 1990.
69. Waller BF, Pinkerton CA, Orr CM, et al. Morphological observations late (greater than 30 days) after clinically successful coronary balloon angioplasty. Circulation 83 (Suppl 2):I28–51, 1991.
70. Nobuyoshi M, Kimura T, Ohishi H, et al. Restenosis after percutaneous transluminal coronary angioplasty: Pathologic observations in 20 patients. J Am Coll Cardiol 17:433–439, 1991.
71. Farb A, Virmani R, Atkinson JB, et al. Long-term histologic patency after percutaneous transluminal coronary angioplasty is predicted by the creation of a greater lumen area. J Am Coll Cardiol 24:1229–1235, 1994.
72. Virmani R, Farb A, Burke AP. Coronary angioplasty from the perspective of atherosclerotic plaque: Morphologic predictors of immediate success and restenosis. Am Heart J 127:163–179, 1994.
73. Ajluni SC, Glazier S, Blankenship L, et al. Perforations after percutaneous coronary interventions: Clinical, angiographic, and therapeutic observations. Cathet Cardiovasc Diagn 32:206–212, 1994.
74. Virmani R, Farb A. Rotational coronary atherectomy. J Am Coll Cardiol 18:1702–1703, 1991.
75. Kockx MM, De Meyer GRY, Jacob WA, et al. Triphasic sequence of neointimal formation in the cuffed carotid artery of the rabbit. Athero Thromb 12:1447–1457, 1992.
76. Carter AJ, Laird JR, Farb A, et al. Morphologic characteristics of lesion formation and time course of smooth muscle cell proliferation in a porcine proliferative restenosis model. J Am Coll Cardiol 24:1398–1405, 1994.
77. Edelman ER, Rogers C. Pathobiologic responses to stenting. Am J Cardiol 81:4E-6E, 1998.
78. Chung I-M, Reidy MA, Schwartz SM, et al. Enhanced extracellular matrix synthesis may be important for restenosis of arteries after stent deployment. Circulation 94 (Supplement I):I-349, 1996.
79. Kearney M, Pieczek A, Haley L, et al. Histopathology of in-stent restenosis in patients with peripheral artery disease. Circulation 95:1998–2002, 1997.
80. Tanaka H, Sukova GK, Swanson SJ, et al. Sustained activation of vascular cells and leukocytes in the rabbit aorta after balloon injury. Circulation 88 [part 1]:1788–1803, 1993.
81. Rogers C, Welt FGP, Karnovsky MJ, et al. Monocyte recruitment and neointimal hyperplasia in rabbits: Coupled inhibitory effects of heparin. Arterioscler Thromb Vasc Biol 16:1312–1318, 1996.
82. Farb A, Virmani R. Arterial restenosis: Focus on inflammatory cell infiltration and adhesion molecules. Curr Opin Anti-Inflam & Immunomod Invest Drugs 2:206–218, 2000.
83. De Servi S, Mazzone A, Ricevuti G, et al. Granulocyte activation after coronary angioplasty in humans. Circulation 82:140–146, 1990.
84. Tsutsui M, Shimokawa H, Tanaka S, et al. Granulocyte activation in restenosis after percutaneous transluminal coronary angioplasty. Jpn Circ J 60:27–34, 1996.
85. Ricevuti G, Mazzone A, Pasotti D, et al. Role of granulocytes in endothelial injury in coronary heart disease in humans. Atherosclerosis 91:1–14, 1991.
86. Peri G, Chiaffarino F, Bernasconi S, et al. Cytotoxicity of activated monocytes on endothelial cells. J Immunol 144:1444–1448, 1990.
87. Leibovich SJ, Ross R. A macrophage-dependent factor that stimulates the proliferation of fibroblasts in vitro. Am J Pathol 84:501–514, 1976.
88. Martinet Y, Bitterman PB, Mornex J-F, et al. Activated human monocytes express the c-sis proto-oncogene and release a mediator showing PDGF-like activity. Nature 319:158–160, 1986.
89. Assoian RK, Fleurdelys BE, Stevenson HC, et al. Expression and secretion of type β transforming growth factor by activated human macrophages. Natl Acad Sci USA 84:6020–6024, 1987.
90. Inoue T, Sakai Y, Morooka S, et al. Expression of polymorphonuclear leukocyte adhesion molecules and its clinical significance in patients treated with percutaneous transluminal coronary angioplasty. J Am Coll Cardiol 28:1127–1133, 1996.
91. Altieri DC, Bader R, Manucci PM, et al. Oligospecificity of the cellular adhesion receptor Mac-1 encompasses an inducible recognition specificity for fibrinogen. J Cell Biol 107:1893–1900, 1988.

92. Diacovo TG, Roth SJ, Buccola JM, et al. Neutrophil rolling, arrest, and transmigration across activated, surface-adherent platelets via sequential action of P-selectin and beta-2 integrin CD11b/CD18. Blood 88:146–157, 1996.
93. Ikeda H, Nakayama H, Oda T, et al. Neutrophil activation after percutaneous transluminal coronary angioplasty. Am Heart J 128:1091–1098, 1994.
94. Mickelson JK, Lakkis NM, Villarreal-Levy G, et al. Leukocyte activation with platelet adhesion after coronary angioplasty: A mechanism for recurrent disease? J Am Coll Cardiol 28:345–353, 1996.
95. Neumann FJ, Ott I, Gawaz M, et al. Neutrophil and platelet activation at balloon-injured coronary artery plaque in patients undergoing angioplasty. J Am Coll Cardiol 27:819–824, 1996.
96. Serrano CV, Jr., Ramires JA, Venturinelli M, et al. Coronary angioplasty results in leukocyte and platelet activation with adhesion molecule expression. Evidence of inflammatory responses in coronary angioplasty. J Am Coll Cardiol 29:1276–1283, 1997.
97. Lasky LS. Selectins: Interpreters of cell-specific carbohydrate information during inflammation. Science 258:964–969, 1992.
98. Kurz RW, Graf B, Gremmel F, et al. Increased serum concentrations of adhesion molecules after coronary angioplasty. Clin Sci (Colch) 87:627–633, 1994.
99. Ishiwata S, Tukada T, Nakanishi S, et al. Postangioplasty restenosis: Platelet activation and the coagulation-fibrinolysis system as possible factors in the pathogenesis of restenosis. Am Heart J 133:387–392, 1997.
100. Inoue T, Hoshi K, Yaguchi I, et al. Serum levels of circulating adhesion molecules after coronary angioplasty. Cardiology 91:236–242, 1999.
101. Kamijikkoku S, Murohara T, Tayama S, et al. Acute myocardial infarction and increased soluble intercellular adhesion molecule-1: A marker of vascular inflammation and a risk of early restenosis? Am Heart J 136:231–236, 1998.
102. Wang X, Feuerstein GZ, Clark RK, et al. Enhanced leucocyte adhesion to interleukin-1 beta stimulated vascular smooth muscle cells is mainly through intercellular adhesion molecule-1. Cardiovasc Res 28:1808–1814, 1994.
103. Wang X, Feuerstein GZ, Gu JL, et al. Interleukin-1 beta induces expression of adhesion molecules in human vascular smooth muscle cells and enhances adhesion of leukocytes to smooth muscle cells. Atherosclerosis 115:89–98, 1995.
104. Couffinhal T, Duplaa C, Labat L, et al. Tumor necrosis factor-α stimulates ICAM-1 expression in human vascular smooth muscle cells. Athero Thromb 13:407–414, 1993.
105. Couffinhal T, Duplaa C, Moreau C, et al. Regulation of vascular cell adhesion molecule-1 and intercellular adhesion molecule-1 in human vascular smooth muscle cells. Circ Res 74:225–234, 1994.
106. Pietersma A, Kofflard M, de Wit LEA, et al. Late lumen loss after coronary angioplasty is associated with the activation status of circulating phagocytes before treatment. Circulation 91:1320–1325, 1995.
107. Wilcox JN. Molecular biology: Insight into the causes and prevention of restenosis after arterial intervention. Am J Cardiol 72:88E–95E, 1993.
108. Davies MG, Hagen PO. Pathobiology of intimal hyperplasia. Br J Surg 81:1254–1269, 1994.
109. Schwartz SM, Reidy MA, O'Brien ER. Assessment of factors important in atherosclerotic occlusion and restenosis. Thromb Haemost 74:541–551, 1995.
110. O'Brien ER, Bennett KL, Garvin MR, et al. Beta ig-h3, a transforming growth factor-beta-inducible gene, is overexpressed in atherosclerotic and restenotic human vascular lesions. Arterioscler Thromb Vasc Biol 16:576–584, 1996.
111. Honye J, Mahon DJ, Jain A, et al. Morphological effects of coronary balloon angioplasty in vivo assessed by intravascular ultrasound imaging. Circulation 85:1012–1025, 1992.
112. Kuntz RE, Safian RD, Carrozza JP, et al. The importance of acute luminal diameter in determining restenosis after coronary atherectomy or stenting. Circulation 86:1827–1835, 1992.
113. Kuntz RE, Hinohara T, Safian RD, et al. Restenosis after directional coronary atherectomy. Effects of luminal diameter and deep wall excision. Circulation 86:1394–1399, 1992.
114. Kuntz RE, Safian RD, Levine MJ, et al. Novel approach to the analysis of restenosis after the use of three new coronary devices. J Am Coll Cardiol 19:1493–1499, 1992.
115. Glagov S, Weisenberg E, Zarins CK, et al. Compensatory enlargement of human atherosclerotic coronary arteries. N Engl J Med 316:1371–1375, 1987.
116. Mintz GS, Popma JJ, Pichard AD, et al. Arterial remodeling after coronary angioplasty: A serial intravascular ultrasound study. Circulation 94:35–43, 1996.
117. Sangiorgi G, Taylor AJ, Farb A, et al. Histopathology of postpercutaneous transluminal coronary angioplasty remodeling in human coronary arteries. Am Heart J 138:681–687, 1999.
118. Potkin BN, Keren G, Mintz GS, et al. Arterial responses to balloon coronary angioplasty: An intravascular ultrasound study. J Am Coll Cardiol 20:942–951, 1992.
119. Ueda M, Becker AE, Tsukada T, et al. Fibrocellular tissue response after percutaneous transluminal coronary angioplasty. An immunocytochemical analysis of the cellular composition. Circulation 83:1327–1332, 1991.
120. Farb A, Sangiorgi G, Carter AJ, et al. Pathology of acute and chronic coronary stenting in humans. Circulation 99:44–52, 1999.
121. Tierstein PS, Warth DC, Haq N, et al. High speed rotational coronary atherectomy for patients with diffuse coronary artery disease. J Am Coll Cardiol 18:1694–1701, 1991.
122. Stertzer SH, Rosenblum J, Shaw RE, et al. Coronary rotational atherectomy: Initial experience in 302 procedures. J Am Coll Cardiol 21:287–295, 1993.
123. Dietz U, Erbel R, Rupprecht HJ, et al. High frequency rotational ablation: An alternative in treating coronary artery stenoses and occlusions. Br Heart J 70:327–336, 1993.
124. Ellis SG, Popma JJ, Buchbinder M, et al. Relation of clinical presentation, stenosis morphology, and operator technique to the procedural results of rotational atherectomy and rotational atherectomy-facilitated angioplasty. Circulation 89:882–889, 1994.
125. Hansen DD, Auth DC, Hall M, et al. Rotational endarterectomy in normal canine coronary arteries: Preliminary report. J Am Coll Cardiol 11:1073–1077, 1988.
126. Hansen DD, Auth DC, Vracko R, et al. Rotational atherectomy in atherosclerotic rabbit arteries. Am Heart J 115:160–165, 1988.
127. Borrione M, Hall P, Almagor Y, et al. Treatment of simple and complex coronary stenosis using rotational ablation followed by low pressure balloon angioplasty. Cathet Cardiovac Diagn 30:131–137, 1993.

128. Farb A, Roberts DK, Pichard AD, et al. Coronary artery morphologic features after coronary rotational atherectomy: Insights into mechanisms of lumen enlargement and embolization. Am Heart J 129:1058–1067, 1995.
129. Freed MS, Safian RD. Directional coronary atherectomy. In: Freed MS, Grines CL (eds): Manual of Interventional Cardiology, pp 275–287. Birmingham: Physician's Press, 1992.
130. Topol EJ, Leya F, Pinkerton CA, et al. A comparison of directional atherectomy with coronary angioplasty in patients with coronary artery disease. The CAVEAT Study Group. N Engl J Med 329:221–227, 1993.
131. Elliott JM, Berdan LG, Holmes DR, et al. One-year follow-up in the Coronary Angioplasty versus Excisional Atherectomy Trial (CAVEAT I). Circulation 91:2158–2166, 1995.
132. Adelman AG, Cohen EA, Kimball BP, et al. A comparison of directional atherectomy with balloon angioplasty for lesions of the left anterior descending coronary artery. N Engl J Med 329:228–233, 1993.
133. Boehrer JD, Ellis SG, Pieper K, et al. Directional atherectomy versus balloon angioplasty for coronary ostial and nonostial left anterior descending coronary artery lesions: Results from a randomized multicenter trial. The CAVEAT-I investigators. Coronary Angioplasty versus Excisional Atherectomy Trial. J Am Coll Cardiol 25:1380–1386, 1995.
134. Garratt KN, Edwards WD, Kaufmann UP, et al. Differential histopathology of primary atherosclerotic and restenotic lesions in coronary arteries and saphenous vein bypass grafts: Analysis of tissue obtained from 73 patients by directional atherectomy. J Am Coll Cardiol 17:442–448, 1991.
135. Flugelman MY, Virmani R, Correa R, et al. Smooth muscle cell abundance and fibroblast growth factors in coronary lesions of patients with nonfatal unstable angina. A clue to the mechanism of transformation from the stable to the unstable clinical state. Circulation 88:2493–2500, 1993.
136. Mann JM, Kaski JC, Pereira WI, et al. Histological patterns of atherosclerotic plaques in unstable angina patients vary according to clinical presentation. Heart 80:19–22, 1998.
137. Moreno PR, Falk E, Palacios IF, et al. Macrophase infiltration in acute coronary syndromes. Implications for plaque rupture. Circulation 90:775–778, 1994.
138. Moreno PR, Bernardi VH, Lopez-Cuellar J, et al. Macrophage infiltration predicts restenosis after coronary intervention in patients with unstable angina. Circulation 94:3098–3102, 1996.
139. Piek JJ, van der Wal AC, Meuwissen M, et al. Plaque inflammation in restenotic coronary lesions of patients with stable or unstable angina. J Am Coll Cardiol 35:963–967, 2000.
140. Grines CL, Bakalyar DM. Laser angioplasty: Technical and clinical aspects. In: Freed MS, Grines CL (eds): Manual of Interventional Cardiology, pp 301–318. Birmingham: Physician's Press, 1992.
141. Topaz O, Rozenbaum EA, Schumacher A, et al. Solid-state mid-infrared laser facilitated coronary angioplasty: Clinical and quantitative coronary angiographic results in 112 patients. Lasers Surg Med 19:260–272, 1996.
142. Appelman YE, Piek JJ, Strikwerda S, et al. Randomised trial of excimer laser angioplasty versus balloon angioplasty for treatment of obstructive coronary artery disease [see comments]. Lancet 347:79–84, 1996.
143. de Marchena E, Larrain G, Posada JD, et al. Holmium laser-assisted coronary angioplasty in acute ischemic syndromes. Clin Cardiol 19:315–319, 1996.
144. Schofer J, Kresser J, Rau T, et al. Recanalization of chronic coronary artery occlusions using laser followed by balloon angioplasty. Am J Cardiol 78:836–838, 1996.
145. Schofer J, Rau T, Schluter M, et al. Short-term results and intermediate-term follow-up of laser wire recanalization of chronic coronary artery occlusions: A single-center experience. J Am Coll Cardiol 30:1722–1728, 1997.
146. Appelman YE, Koolen JJ, Piek JJ, et al. Excimer laser angioplasty versus balloon angioplasty in functional and total coronary occlusions. Am J Cardiol 78:757–762, 1996.
147. Goy J-J, Eeckhout E, Stauffer J-C, et al. Emergency endoluminal stenting for abrupt vessel closure following coronary angioplasty: A randomized comparison of the Wiktor and Palmaz-Schatz stents. Cath Cardiovasc Diag 34:128–132, 1995.
148. Schomig A, Kastrati A, Dietz R, et al. Emergency coronary stenting for dissection during purcutaneous transluminal coronary angioplasty: Angiographic follow-up after stenting and after repeat angioplasty of the stented segment. J Am Coll Cardiol 23:1053–1060, 1994.
149. Ellis SG, Savage M, Fischman D, et al. Restenosis after placement of Palmaz-Schatz stents in native coronary arteries: Initial results of a multicenter experience. Circulation 86:1836–1844, 1992.
150. Fischman DL, Leon MB, Baim DS, et al. A randomized comparison of coronary stent placement and balloon angioplasty in the treatment of coronary artery disease. N Engl J Med 331:496–501, 1994.
151. Serruys PW, de Jaegere P, Kiemeneij F, et al. A comparison of balloon-expandable stent implantation with balloon angioplasty in patients with coronary artery disease. N Engl J Med 331:489–495, 1994.
152. Eeckhout E, Kappenberger L, Goy JJ. Stents for intracoronary placement: Current status and future directions. J Am Coll Cardiol 27:757–765, 1996.
153. Stone GW, Brodie BR, Griffin JJ, et al. Prospective, multicenter study of the safety and feasibility of primary stenting in acute myocardial infarction: In-hospital and 30-day results of the PAMI stent pilot trial. Primary Angioplasty in Myocardial Infarction Stent Pilot Trial Investigators. J Am Coll Cardiol 31:23–30, 1998.
154. Stone GW, Brodie BR, Griffin JJ, et al. Clinical and angiographic follow-up after primary stenting in acute myocardial infarction: The Primary Angioplasty in Myocardial Infarction (PAMI) stent pilot trial. Circulation 99:1548–1554, 1999.
155. Taylor A. Metals. In: Sigwart U (ed): Endoluminal Stenting, pp 28–33. London: W.B. Saunders Co., 1996.
156. Kutryk MJB, Serruys PW. Coronary Stenting: Current Perspectives, pp 17–85. London: Martin Dunitz Ltd, 1999.
157. Rogers C, Edelman ER. Endovascular stent design dictates experimental restenosis and thrombosis. Circulation 91:2995–3001, 1995.
158. Carter AJ, Scott D, Laird JR, et al. Progressive vascular remodeling and reduced neointimal formation after placement of a thermoelastic self-expanding nitinol stent in an experimental model. Cathet Cardiovas Diagn 44:193–201, 1998.

159. Leon MB, Baim DS, Popma JJ, et al. A clinical trial comparing three antithrombotic-drug regimens after coronary-artery stenting. Stent Anticoagulation Restenosis Study Investigators. N Engl J Med 339:1665–1671, 1998.
160. Werner GS, Gastmann O, Ferrari M, et al. Risk factors for acute and subacute stent thrombosis after high-pressure stent implantation: A study by intracoronary ultrasound. Am Heart J 135:300–309, 1998.
161. De Servi S, Repetto S, Klugmann S, et al. Stent thrombosis: Incidence and related factors in the R.I.S.E. Registry (Registro Impianto Stent Endocoronarico). Catheter Cardiovasc Interv 46:13–18, 1999.
162. Berger PB, Bell MR, Rihal CS, et al. Clopidogrel versus ticlopidine after intracoronary stent placement [see comments]. J Am Coll Cardiol 34:1891–1894, 1999.
163. Farb A, Weber DK, Jones R, et al. Plaque substrate and arterial damage are predictors of restenosis after coronary stenting in humans. J Am Coll Cardiol 35(Suppl. A):4, 2000.
164. Palmaz JC, Sibbitt RR, Tio FO, et al. Expandable intraluminal vascular graft: A feasibility study. Surgery 99:199–205, 1986.
165. Schatz RA, Palmaz JC, Tio FO, et al. Balloon-expandable intracoronary stents in the adult dog. Circulation 76:450–457, 1987.
166. van der Giessen WJ, Serruys PW, van Beusekom MM, et al. Coronary stenting with a new radiopaque balloon-expandable endoprosthesis in pigs. Circulation 83:1788–1798, 1991.
167. Karas SP, Gravanis MB, Santoian EC, et al. Coronary intimal proliferation after balloon injury and stenting in swine: An animal model of restenosis. J Am Coll Cardiol 20:467–474, 1992.
168. Anderson PG, Bajaj RK, Baxley WA, et al. Vascular pathology of balloon-expandable flexible coil stents in humans. J Am Coll Cardiol 19:272–381, 1992.
169. van Beusekom HMM, van der Geissen WJ, van Suylen RJ, et al. Histology after stenting of human saphenous vein bypass grafts: Observations from surgically excised grafts 3 to 320 days after stent implantation. J Am Coll Cardiol 21:45–54, 1993.
170. van Beusekom HMM, Whelan DM, Krabbendam SC, et al. Early reendothelialization after stent implantation does not influence late intimal hyperplasia. Circulation 98:I-190, 1998.
171. Kornowski R, Hong MK, Tio FO, et al. In-stent restenosis: Contributions of inflammatory responses and arterial injury to neointimal hyperplasia. J Am Coll Cardiol 31:224–230, 1998.
172. Carter AJ, Laird JR, Kufs WM, et al. Coronary stenting with a novel stainless steel balloon-expandable stent: Determinants of neointimal formation and changes in arterial geometry after placement in an atherosclerotic model. J Am Coll Cardiol 27:1270–1277, 1996.
173. Antoniucci D, Santoro GM, Bolognese L, et al. Bailout Palmaz-Schatz coronary stenting in 39 patients with occlusive dissection complicating conventional angioplasty. Cathet Cardiovasc Diagn 35:204–209, 1995.
174. Kiemeneij F, Laarman GJ. Bailout techniques for failed coronary angioplasty using 6 French guiding catheters. Cathet Cardiovasc Diagn 32:359–366, 1994.
175. Metz D, Urban P, Camenzind E, et al. Improving results of bailout coronary stenting after failed balloon angioplasty. Cathet Cardiovasc Diagn 32:117–124, 1994.
176. Agrawal SK, Ho DSW, Liu MW, et al. Predictors of thrombotic complications after placement of the flexible coil stent. Am J Cardiol 73:1216–1219, 1994.
177. Steffenino G, Dellavalle A, Ribichini F, et al. Coronary stenting after unsuccessful emergency angioplasty in acute myocardial infarction: Results in a series of consecutive patients. Am Heart J 32:1115–1118, 1996.
178. Thomas CN, Weintraub WS, Shen Y, et al. "Bailout" coronary stenting in patients with a recent myocardial infarction. Am J Cardiol 77:653–655, 1996.
178a. Farb A, Lindsay J, Virmani R. Pathology of bailout coronary stenting in humans. Am Heart J 137:621–631, 1999.
179. Dean LS, Roubin GS. "Bail out" stenting: Case closed. Semin Intervent Cardiol 1:275–281, 1996.
180. Alfonso F, Hernandez R, Goicolea J, et al. Coronary stenting for acute coronary dissection after coronary angioplasty: Implications of residual dissection. J Am Coll Cardiol 24:989–995, 1994.
181. Serruys PW, Emanuelsson H, van der Giessen W, et al. Heparin-coated Palmaz-Schatz stents in human coronary arteries. Early outcome of the Benestent-II Pilot Study. Circulation 93:412–422, 1996.
182. Aggarwal RK, Ireland DC, Azrin MA, et al. Antithrombotic potential of polymer-coated stents eluting platelet glycoprotein IIb/IIIa receptor antibody. Circulation 94:3311–17, 1996.
183. Herrmann R, Schmidmaier G, Markl B, et al. Antithrombogenic coating of stents using a biodegradable drug delivery technology. Thromb Haemost 82:51–57, 1999.
184. Kruse KR, Crowley JJ, Tanguay JF, et al. Local drug delivery of argatroban from a polymeric-metallic composite stent reduces platelet deposition in a swine coronary model. Catheter Cardiovasc Interv 46:503–507, 1999.
185. Bertrand OF, Sipehia R, Mongrain R, et al. Biocompatibility aspects of new stent technology. J Am Coll Cardiol 32:562–571, 1998.
186. De Scheerder I, Wang K, Wilczek K, et al. Experimental study of thrombogenicity and foreign body reaction induced by heparin-coated coronary stents. Circulation 95:1549–1553, 1997.
187. King SB III, Williams DO, Chougule P, et al. Endovascular beta-radiation to reduce restenosis after coronary balloon angioplasty: Results of the beta energy restenosis trial (BERT). Circulation 97:2025–2030, 1998.
188. Teirstein PS, Massullo V, Jani S, et al. Three-year clinical and angiographic follow-up after intracoronary radiation: Results of a randomized clinical trial. Circulation 101:360–365, 2000.
189. Waksman R, Bhargava B, White L, et al. Intracoronary beta-radiation therapy inhibits recurrence of in-stent restenosis. Circulation 101:1895–1898, 2000.
190. Waksman R, White RL, Chan RC, et al. Intracoronary gamma-radiation therapy after angioplasty inhibits recurrence in patients with in-stent restenosis. Circulation 101:2165–2171, 2000.
191. Farb A, Heller P, Carter, J, et al. Paclitaxel polymer-coated stents reduce neointima. Circulation 96:I-608, 1997.
192. Farb A, Tang AL, Shroff S, et al. Neointimal responses 3 months after ^{32}P β-emitting stent placement. Int J Radioation Oncology Biol Phys 48:889–898, 2000.
193. Waksman R, Bhargava B, Leon MB. Late thrombosis following intracoronary brachytherapy. Catheter Cardiovasc Interv 49:344–347, 2000.
194. Collin J, Araujo L, Walton J, et al. Oxford screening programme for abdominal aortic aneurysm in men aged 65 to 74 years. Lancet 2:613–615, 1988.

195. Scott RA, Ashton HA, Kay DN. Abdominal aortic aneurysm in 4237 screened patients: Prevalence, development and management over 6 years. Br J Surg 78:1122–1125, 1991.
196. Blum U, Voshage G, Lammer J, et al. Endoluminal stent-grafts for infrarenal abdominal aortic aneurysms. N Engl J Med 336:13–20, 1997.
197. Roger VL, Ballard DJ, Hallett JW, Jr., et al. Influence of coronary artery disease on morbidity and mortality after abdominal aortic aneurysmectomy: A population-based study, 1971–1987. J Am Coll Cardiol 14:1245–1252, 1989.
198. Katz DJ, Stanley JC, Zelenock GB. Operative mortality rates for intact and ruptured abdominal aortic aneurysms in Michigan: An eleven-year statewide experience. J Vasc Surg 19:804–815; discussion 816–817, 1994.
199. Greenhalgh RM. Prognosis of abdominal aortic aneurysm. Bmj 301:136, 1990.
200. Brown OW, Hollier LH, Pairolero PC, et al. Abdominal aortic aneurysm and coronary artery disease. Arch Surg 116:1484–1488, 1981.
201. Crawford ES, Saleh SA, Babb JWD, et al. Infrarenal abdominal aortic aneurysm: Factors influencing survival after operation performed over a 25-year period. Ann Surg 193:699–709, 1981.
202. Cragg A, Lund G, Rysavy J, et al. Percutaneous arterial grafting. Radiology 150:45–49, 1984.
203. Balko A, Piasecki GJ, Shah DM, et al. Transfemoral placement of intraluminal polyurethane prosthesis for abdominal aortic aneurysm. J Surg Res 40:305–309, 1986.
204. Palmaz JC, Sibbitt RR, Tio FO, et al. Expandable intraluminal vascular graft: A feasibility study. Surgery 99:199–205, 1986.
205. Dake MD, Miller DC, Semba CP, et al. Transluminal placement of endovascular stent-grafts for the treatment of descending thoracic aortic aneurysms. N Engl J Med 331:1729–1734, 1994.
206. Rahimtoola SH. The hibernating myocardium. Am Heart J 117:211–221, 1989.
207. Rahimtoola SH. Concept and evaluation of hibernating myocardium. Annu Rev Med 50:75–86, 1999.
208. Mirhoseini M, Cayton MM. Revascularization of the heart by laser. J Microsurg 2:253–260, 1981.
209. Mirhoseini M, Shelgikar S, Cayton MM. New concepts in revascularization of the myocardium. Ann Thorac Surg 45:415–420, 1988.
210. Cooley DA, Frazier OH, Kadipasaoglu KA, et al. Transmyocardial laser revascularization: Clinical experience with twelve-month follow-up. J Thorac Cardiovasc Surg 111:791–797; discussion 797–799, 1996.
211. Horvath KA, Cohn LH, Cooley DA, et al. Transmyocardial laser revascularization: Results of a multicenter trial with transmyocardial laser revascularization used as sole therapy for end-stage coronary artery disease. J Thorac Cardiovasc Surg 113:645–653; discussion 653–654, 1997.
212. March RJ. Transmyocardial laser revascularization with the CO_2 laser: One year results of a randomized, controlled trial. Semin Thorac Cardiovasc Surg 11:12–18, 1999.
213. Schofield PM, Sharples LD, Caine N, et al. Transmyocardial laser revascularisation in patients with refractory angina: A randomised controlled trial. Lancet 353:519–524, 1999.
214. Pepper MS. Manipulating angiogenesis. From basic science to the bedside. Arterioscler Thromb Vasc Biol 17:605–619, 1997.
215. Cines DB, Pollak ES, Buck CA, et al. Endothelial cells in physiology and in the pathophysiology of vascular disorders. Blood 91:3527–3561, 1998.
216. Schaper W, Ito WD. Molecular mechanisms of coronary collateral vessel growth. Circ Res 79:911–919, 1996.
217. Wang DL, Wung BS, Shyy YJ, et al. Mechanical strain induces monocyte chemotactic protein-1 gene expression in endothelial cells. Effects of mechanical strain on monocyte adhesion to endothelial cells. Circ Res 77:294–302, 1995.
218. Whittaker P, Kloner RA, Przyklenk K. Laser-mediated transmural myocardial channels do not salvage acutely ischemic myocardium. J Am Coll Cardiol 22:302–309, 1993.
219. Horvath KA, Smith WJ, Laurence RG, et al. Recovery and viability of an acute myocardial infarct after transmyocardial laser revascularization. J Am Coll Cardiol 25:258–263, 1995.
220. Fisher PE, Khomoto T, DeRosa CM, et al. Histologic analysis of transmyocardial channels: Comparison of CO_2 and holmium: YAG lasers. Ann Thorac Surg 64:466–472, 1997.
221. Gassler N, Wintzer HO, Stubbe HM, et al. Transmyocardial laser revascularization. Histological features in human nonresponder myocardium. Circulation 95:371–375, 1997.
222. Sigel JE, Abramovich CM, Lytle BW, et al. Transmyocardial laser revascularization: Three sequential autopsy cases. J Thorac Cardiovasc Surg 115:1381–1385, 1998.
223. Association AH. Heart and Stroke Facts: Statistical Supplement. 1998.
224. Hunt SA, Frazier OH. Mechanical circulatory support and cardiac transplantation. Circulation 97:2079–2090, 1998.
225. Gibbon JH. Application of a heart and lung apparatus to cardiac surgery. Minn Med 37:171–180, 1954.
226. Kantrowitz A, Tjonneland S, Freed PS, et al. Initial clinical experience with intraaortic balloon pumping in cardiogenic shock. Jama 203:113–118, 1968.
227. Quaini E, Pavie A, Chieco S, et al. The Concerted Action 'Heart' European registry on clinical application of mechanical circulatory support systems: Bridge to transplant. The Registry Scientific Committee. Eur J Cardiothorac Surg 11:182–188, 1997.
228. Mehta SM, Aufiero TX, Pae WE, Jr., et al. Combined registry for the clinical use of mechanical ventricular assist pumps and the total artificial heart in conjunction with heart transplantation: Sixth official report—1994. J Heart Lung Transplant 14:585–593, 1995.
229. Frazier OH, Rose EA, McCarthy P, et al. Improved mortality and rehabilitation of transplant candidates treated with a long-term implantable left ventricular assist system. Ann Surg 222:327–336; discussion 336–338, 1995.
230. Rose EA, Levin HR, Oz MC, et al. Artificial circulatory support with textured interior surfaces. A counterintuitive approach to minimizing thromboembolism. Circulation 90:II87–91, 1994.
231. Slater JP, Rose EA, Levin HR, et al. Low thromboembolic risk without anticoagulation using advanced-design left ventricular assist devices. Ann Thorac Surg 62:1321–1327; discussion 1328, 1996.
232. Radovancevic B, Frazier OH, Duncan JM. Implantation technique for the HeartMate left ventricular assist device. J Card Surg 7:203–207, 1992.

233. Pennington DG, McBride LR, Swartz MT. Implantation technique for the Novacor left ventricular assist system. J Thorac Cardiovasc Surg 108:604–608, 1994.
234. Farrar DJ, Hill JD. Univentricular and biventricular Thoratec VAD support as a bridge to transplantation. Ann Thorac Surg 55:276–282, 1993.
235. Reedy JE, Swartz MT, Lohmann DP, et al. The importance of patient mobility with ventricular assist device support. ASAIO J 38:M151–153, 1992.
236. Arabia FA, Copeland JG, Smith RG, et al. CardioWest total artificial heart: A retrospective controlled study. Artif Organs 23:204–207, 1999.
237. Copeland JG, Pavie A, Duveau D, et al. Bridge to transplantation with the CardioWest total artificial heart: The international experience 1993 to 1995. J Heart Lung Transplant 15:94–99, 1996.
238. Mehta SM, Aufiero TX, Pae WE, Jr., et al. Mechanical ventricular assistance: An economical and effective means of treating end-stage heart disease. Ann Thorac Surg 60:284–290; discussion 290–291, 1995.
239. Livingston ER, Fisher CA, Bibidakis EJ, et al. Increased activation of the coagulation and fibrinolytic systems leads to hemorrhagic complications during left ventricular assist implantation. Circulation 94:II227–234, 1996.
240. Sun BC, Catanese KA, Spanier TB, et al. 100 long-term implantable left ventricular assist devices: The Columbia Presbyterian interim experience. Ann Thorac Surg 68:688–694, 1999.
241. Moroney DA, Vaca KJ. Infectious complications associated with ventricular assist devices. Am J Crit Care 4:204–209; quiz 210–211, 1995.
242. Holman WL, Murrah CP, Ferguson ER, et al. Infections during extended circulatory support: University of Alabama at Birmingham experience 1989 to 1994. Ann Thorac Surg 61:366–371; discussion 372–373, 1996.
243. Holman WL, Skinner JL, Waites KB, et al. Infection during circulatory support with ventricular assist devices. Ann Thorac Surg 68:711–716, 1999.
244. Wang IW, Anderson JM, Marchant RE. Staphylococcus epidermidis adhesion to hydrophobic biomedical polymer is mediated by platelets. J Infect Dis 167:329–336, 1993.
245. McBride LR, Swartz MT, Reedy JE, et al. Device related infections in patients supported with mechanical circulatory support devices for greater than 30 days. ASAIO Trans 37:M258–259, 1991.
246. Herrmann M, Weyand M, Greshake B, et al. Left ventricular assist device infection is associated with increased mortality but is not a contraindication to transplantation. Circulation 95:814–817, 1997.
247. Anderson JM. Mechanism of inflammation and infection with implanted devices. Cardiovasc Pathol 2:33S–41S, 1993.
248. El-Banayosy A, Arusoglu L, Kizner L, et al. Novacor left ventricular assist system versus HeartMate vented electric left ventricular assist system as a long-term mechanical circulatory support device in bridging patients: A prospective study. J Thorac Cardiovasc Surg 119:581–587, 2000.
249. Anderson JM. Cardiovascular device retrieval and evaluation. Cardiovasc Pathol 2:199S–208S, 1993.
250. Schoen FJ, Palmer DC, Bernhard WF, et al. Clinical temporary ventricular assist. Pathologic findings and their implications in a multi-institutional study of 41 patients. J Thorac Cardiovasc Surg 92:1071–1081, 1986.
251. Fyfe B, Schoen FJ. Pathologic analysis of 34 explanted symbionventricular assist devices and 10 explanted Jarvik-7 total artificial hearts. Cardiovasc Pathol 3:187–197, 1993.
252. Schoen FJ, Anderson JM, Didisheim P, et al. Ventricular assist device (VAD) pathology analyses: Guidelines for clinical studies. J Appl Biomater 1:49–56, 1990.

Chapter

4

NONATHEROSCLEROTIC CORONARY ARTERY DISEASE

Over 90% of myocardial infarctions occurring in the industrialized western world are the result of coronary artery atherosclerosis. However, there are many other diseases, congenital or acquired, that can give rise to myocardial ischemia. In this chapter we describe both congenital as well as acquired diseases of the epicardial and intramyocardial coronary arteries that may result in myocardial necrosis. We classify these entities into congenital coronary diseases, coronary artery vasculitis, transplant arterial disease, spontaneous coronary artery dissections, embolic coronary disease, and nonatherosclerotic coronary thrombosis. Although encountered uncommonly, it is essential to be familiar with these processes, as they are all too often overlooked or misdiagnosed by the examining pathologist.

CONGENITAL CORONARY DISEASES

Anomalous Coronary Origin

Classification

A classification of coronary artery anomalies is presented in Table 4–1. The practicing autopsy pathologist will likely encounter incidental anomalies (separate conus ostium, anomalous left circumflex), as well as those that cause sudden death (anomalous left from pulmonary trunk in children, and anomalous left and right from contralateral sinuses of Valsalva in adults).[1,2]

Left from Pulmonary Trunk

The origin of the left main coronary artery from the pulmonary trunk should always be considered in cases of infantile and pediatric sudden death, as well as in infantile and childhood cases of dilated cardiomyopathy or endocardial fibroelastosis. The incidence of this anomaly ranges from 1/50,000 to 1/300,000 per live births.[1] There is a female-to-male ratio in incidence of 2 to 1. Most cases are identified within the first year of life, but some patients accommodate the low pressures within the left coronary system, and live well into the second decade without a diagnosis. Approximately 75% of patients will die before age 1 year if the lesion is not repaired, and the remainder die or come to clinical attention between 1 and 20 years of age. Symptoms occur in the majority of patients, although sudden unexpected death in the absence of prior symptoms has been reported.[3] In adolescents surviving with the disease, sudden death may be exertional, which is typical for adults dying suddenly with anomalous origin of the left from the aorta. In infants, the clinical course in the adolescent can mimic dilated cardiomyopathy.[4]

Pathologically, the left main coronary artery arises from the pulmonary trunk, generally the left pulmonary sinus (Fig. 4–1), or rarely from the anterior pulmonary sinus. The left main coronary artery is thin walled and appears like a vein. The right coronary artery is in the normal location, but is tortuous and ectatic, with en-

The opinions or assertions contained herein are the private views of the authors and are not to be construed as official or reflecting the views of the Department of the Army, the Department of the Air Force, or the Department of Defense.

Table 4–1. Classification of Coronary Artery Anomalies

Anomalous origin of one or more coronary artery (CA) arising from the pulmonary trunk
Left main coronary arteries or left anterior descending from pulmonary trunk
Both coronary arteries from pulmonary trunk
Right coronary artery from pulmonary trunk
Anomalous origin of one or more coronary arteries from aorta
Anomalous left: left main and right coronary arteries from right aortic sinus
Anomalous right: left main and right coronary arteries from left aortic sinus
Anomalous origin of left circumflex from right aortic sinus or right coronary
Anomalous origin of coronary arteries from posterior aortic sinus
Right coronary and left anterior descending from right aortic sinus
Single coronary artery ostium from aorta
Single right coronary ostium
Single left coronary ostium
Congenital hypoplastic coronary arteries
Coronary artery fistula

larged collaterals often visible on the epicardial surface. In general, the heart is enlarged, and there is extensive scarring and thinning of the anterolateral wall of the left ventricle, with involvement of the anterolateral papillary muscle. In infants, there is typically dilatation of the left ventricle with endocardial fibroelastosis.[1]

The treatment of the anomalous left main coronary artery arising from the pulmonary trunk is surgery, and long-term survivors have been reported.[5] For this reason, clinical identification of this anomaly, by angiography or newer methods of transthoracic echocardiography, is essential.

Left from Right Sinus

The most common coronary artery anomaly that results in ischemia and sudden death in young adults is the anomalous left coronary artery. In hearts demonstrating this anomaly, both the left and right coronary arteries arise in the right sinus of Valsalva. The anomalous left artery is one of the most common causes of sudden death, especially exertional sudden death, in young men and women. The diagnosis cannot be overlooked if care is taken to examine the origin of the coronary arteries as a routine in every autopsy (see Chapter 1).

There have been over 100 cases of anomalous left coronary artery reported, and may account for sudden death from infancy to adulthood. Almost 60% of patients with this anomaly die suddenly, more than half of these during exercise; therefore, this is a highly lethal anomaly. Seventy-five percent of patients who die suddenly from an anomalous left coronary artery are less than 30 years of age and the majority of the remainder younger than 40.[6] Symptoms include syncope and chest pain, and frequently occur immediately before death. Unfortunately, screening tests—including stress electrocardiography and echocardiography—are often negative, underscoring the need for more sensitive echocardiographic studies or angiography in young patients with exertion-related

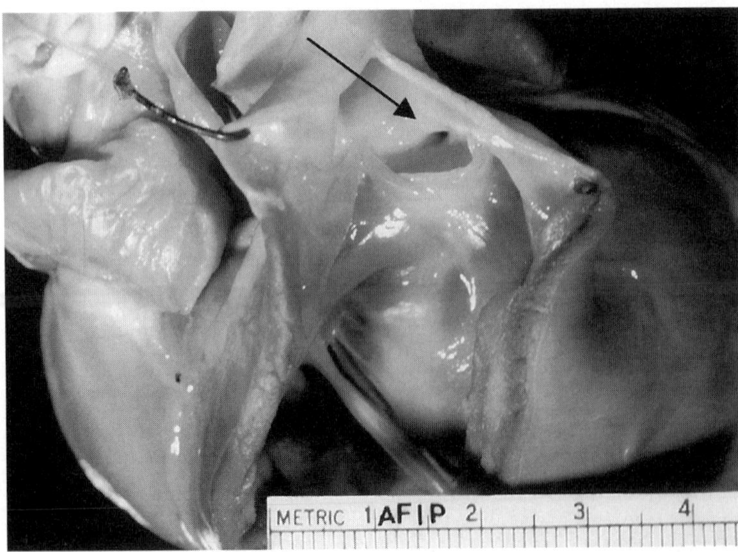

Figure 4–1. Anomalous left from pulmonary trunk. An 8-month-old boy developed heart failure and endocardial fibroelastosis. At autopsy, the heart was dilated, with left ventricular endocardial fibroelastosis. The left main coronary ostium was located in the pulmonary trunk in the left sinus (*arrow*).

cardiac symptoms.[7] It has been stated that any child or young adult who has evidence of cardiac ischemia or exercise-induced syncope should be investigated angiographically for an anomalous origin of the left coronary artery.[2] Surgical correction for the anomaly is feasible, but identifying the defects in life, and those likely to result in ischemia or sudden death, is difficult.[8] It is suspected that the mechanism of sudden death is due to compression of the origin of the artery during diastole by an ostial ridge covering the initial acute angle (Fig. 4–2). Pathologic studies to compare incidental anomalies with those resulting in sudden death have, however, been unable to prove this hypothesis.[6]

There are four possible courses of the abnormal left main coronary artery in this condition[9]; all subtypes of this anomaly have been associated with sudden death. In by far the most common pattern, the left main arises from a separate ostium, often higher than that of the right coronary and near the commissure within the right sinus of Valsalva (Figs. 4–3*A* and 4–3*B*), and passes obliquely between the aorta and pulmonary trunk. Occasionally in this pattern, the origin of the left main may be from the proximal right coronary. Less common patterns of the anomalous left main coronary artery include a course anterior to the pulmonary trunk, dividing into the circumflex and the anterior descending coronary artery in the anterior interventricular groove; a course to the right and posteriorly behind the aorta; and a course inferiorly and intramurally to the subendocardial region of the crista supraventricularis, surfacing to the anterior interventricular groove. In all subtypes, the ostium is in the right sinus of Valsalva or proximal right coronary. Approximately 25% of anomalous arteries demonstrate atherosclerosis in patients who survive into adulthood. The extent of coronary atherosclerosis may be accelerated from the turbulence in the bloodstream created by the acute angle takeoff. Left ventricular fibrosis and necrosis in the myocardium which is supplied by the anomalous left coronary artery is common. In our experience,[1] one of every three hearts from patients dying with anomalous left coronary artery have evidence of myocardial fibrosis, and approximately 60% show acute infarction.

Right from Left Sinus

This anomaly is the "mirror image" of the anomalous left, in that the origin of the right

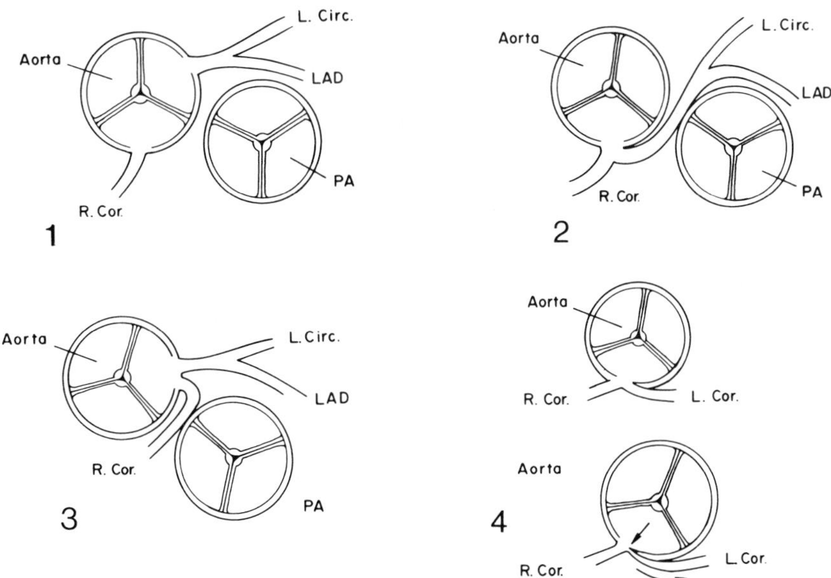

Figure 4–2. Common types of anomalous origin of coronary ostia from the aorta. (1) Normal origin of right and left coronary arteries arising form the right and left coronary sinus. (2) Origin of the left coronary artery from the right coronary sinus with course between the aorta and pulmonary trunk (*PA*) before dividing into left anterior descending (*LAD*) and left circumflex (*L. Circ.*) coronary arteries. (3) Origin of right coronary (*R. Cor.*) artery from the left coronary artery sinus. (4) The probable mechanism of obstruction, which is due to leftward or rightward passage of the coronary artery along the aortic wall causing the ostium to be slit-like. Aortic and pulmonary trunk distention may further compress the coronary artery at the onset of takeoff.

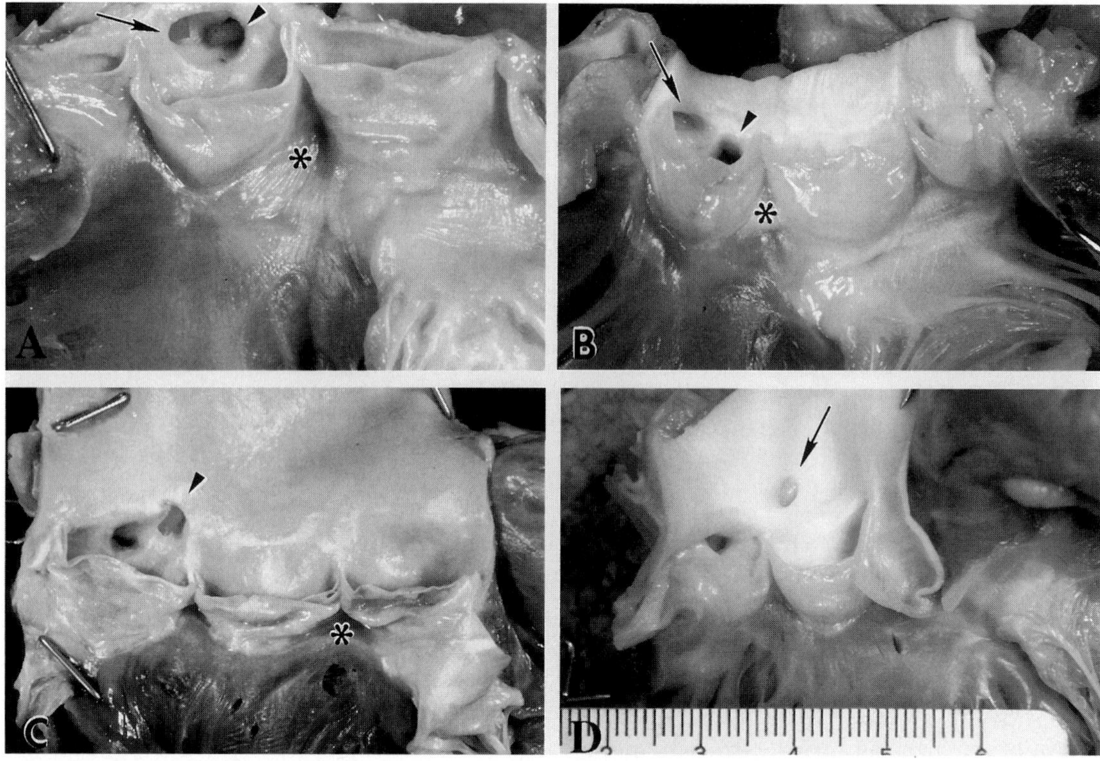

Figure 4–3. Ectopic origin of coronary ostia from aorta. *A. Anomalous left:* A 31-year-old female died suddenly after a negative stress electrocardiogram for exertional syncope. An *arrowhead* marks the position of the right ostium within the right coronary sinus, and the *arrow* the left ostium in the same sinus. A probe is present within the proximal portions of the right and left coronary ostia, which arise from a common opening. *B. Anomalous left:* A 9-year-old boy died suddenly after complaining of shortness of breath after running; there was no prior history of syncope or palpitations. An anomalous left origin is demonstrated by the *arrow* in the right sinus of Valsalva. As is typical, the origin is higher than the normal right ostium (*arrowhead*). *C. Anomalous right coronary:* A 60-year-old white male was found dead in living room due to secobarbitol intoxication. An incidental anomaly was found in which the right coronary arose in the left sinus with a slightly high takeoff near the commissure. A probe is inserted in the ostium (*arrowhead*). Although often incidental, anomalous right coronary may also be a cause of sudden death. In figures *A–C* the asterisk shows the location of the membranous septum between the right and noncoronary cusps. *D.* High takeoff, coronary ostium. The right coronary ostium is high above the sinotubular junction above the commissure between the right and left coronary cusps (*arrow*). A 5-year-old boy with a history of mental retardation and multiple syncopal episode died suddenly after a fall; other causes of death were not found at autopsy.

coronary is the left sinus of Valsalva, and both ostia arise from the left coronary sinus. In the majority of cases, the anomalous coronary passes between the aorta and pulmonary trunk. Only 25% of patients die from as a result of the anomaly. Therefore, it is much more likely to be incidental than the anomalous left (Fig. 4–3*C*), possibly because of the smaller region of the myocardium supplied by the right coronary artery, as compared with the left. However, the association between the anomalous right coronary artery and sudden death is well established.[1, 2, 10, 11] As with the anomalous left, patients with an anomalous right coronary artery who become symptomatic often develop exertion-related ischemia or sudden death. The role of surgery in correcting this anomaly is less clear than the role of surgery in correcting an anomalous left, as most patients remain asymptomatic.

High Takeoff Coronary Arteries

The coronary artery ostia are normally present within the sinus of Valsalva beneath the aortic ridge (sinotubular junction). When situated higher, there is an increased risk for ostial ridges and acute angles that may precipitate ischemia and sudden death (Fig. 4–3*D*), especially during exertion.[12] There are no complete data regarding the incidence of high coronary takeoffs, but in our experience they occur in approximately 1% of autopsies. High takeoffs are considered a form of ostial anomaly that may be a causative factor for sudden death.[7, 13, 14] Although there is no specific distance from the sinotubular junction above which an abnormally high takeoff may result in ischemia, we considered at least 3 to 5 mm significant (depending on the age of the patient), or if there are other abnormalities, such as acute angles or ridges. High takeoffs have been associated with other coronary anomalies,[15] and the position of the ostia in anomalous left and right coronary arteries arising from the aorta is often at or slightly above the aortic ridge.

Incidental Anomalies

The practicing pathologist should be aware of normal variations in ostial location. In approximately 30% of patients, as demonstrated angiographically, there is a separate ostium in the right sinus of Valsalva for the conus branch of the right coronary artery. The frequency is somewhat less at autopsy. In this variation, two separate ostia will be clearly seen in the right sinus of Valsalva.

The other relatively common incidental anomaly is the ectopic origin of the left circumflex from the right coronary artery (Fig. 4–4). In this anomaly, which has no hemodynamic consequences, the left circumflex arises either from a separate ostium in the right sinus of Valsalva or as a first branch of the right coronary artery. The subsequent course of the left circumflex is posterior to the aortic root, between the ascending aorta and left atrial appendage, and then within the atrioventricular sulcus, the final normal location of the left circumflex. This anomaly should be suspected if no circumflex is seen taking off from the left main coronary artery.

Miscellaneous Anomalies of Variable Clinical Significance

There are a number of variations on the anomalous origin of one or more coronary artery from the pulmonary trunk. If only the left circumflex or right coronary artery arises from the pulmonary trunk, the condition is far less lethal than if the left main arises from the pulmonary artery. Ectopic origin of the right coronary artery from the pulmonary trunk occurs in 0.003% of patients undergoing coronary arteriography; most patients are free of cardiac symptoms. The left anterior descending arising from the pulmonary artery, with origin of the circumflex and right coronary arteries from the aorta, is extremely rare. Most patients with this condition are asymptomatic, the anomaly being discovered incidentally at autopsy or angiography. Typically, the right and left circumflex are dilated and tortuous, and the left anterior descending fills from collateral circulation. A likewise rare anomaly is the condition in which both arteries arise from the sinuses of the pulmonary valve, with two ostia supplying the left main and right coronary. Most patients with both arteries arising from the pulmonary artery have other major congenital anomalies of heart, and most are symptomatic before 3 days of life. This condition is incompatible with normal life and development.

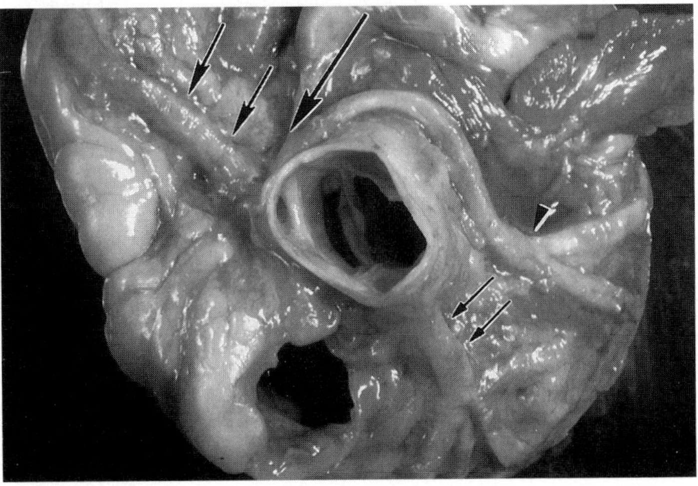

Figure 4–4. Anomalous circumflex coronary artery. A 36-year-old man was the driver of a vehicle that left the road and landed upside down in shallow water; he was pronounced dead without evidence of drowning or trauma. The presumed cause of death was left ventricular hypertrophy (540 gram heart); no other cause of death was identified at autopsy. The anomalous origin of the left circumflex artery within the right sinus of Valsalva is identified by the *large arrow.* The proximal course of the circumflex is between the left atrial appendage and aortic root; the takeoff of the marginal branch is identified by the *arrowhead.* The left anterior descending is shown by the *two small arrows;* and the right coronary, the *two middle-sized arrows.*

Single coronary ostium is a condition similar to the anomalous left or right coronary artery arising from the aorta, in that both arteries arise from a single sinus of Valsalva. In the single coronary ostium, however, one ostium supplies a common artery which, after a course of variable length, gives rise to the three epicardial arteries (Fig. 4–5). Possibly because of an absence of an acute angle or ostial ridge, which are frequently associated with anomalous left or right coronary arteries, the single coronary ostium is infrequently observed with sudden death. However, sudden death related to single coronary ostium, similar to other coronary artery anomalies, is often exertional.[1]

A variety of rare anomalies, in addition to those discussed, are generally of no clinical significance and are presented for completeness in Table 4–1.

Tunnel Coronary Artery

Tunneling primarily occurs in the left anterior descending artery, and refers to the presence of a myocardial bridge overlying a segment of the vessel, typically in the middle portion of the vessel.[16–19] The tunnel left anterior descending coronary artery is usually an incidental finding, occurring in 30% of autopsy heart specimens. However, when deep, a tunnel can result in myocardial ischemia, caused by compression of the artery by the overlying myocardial bridge. What constitutes

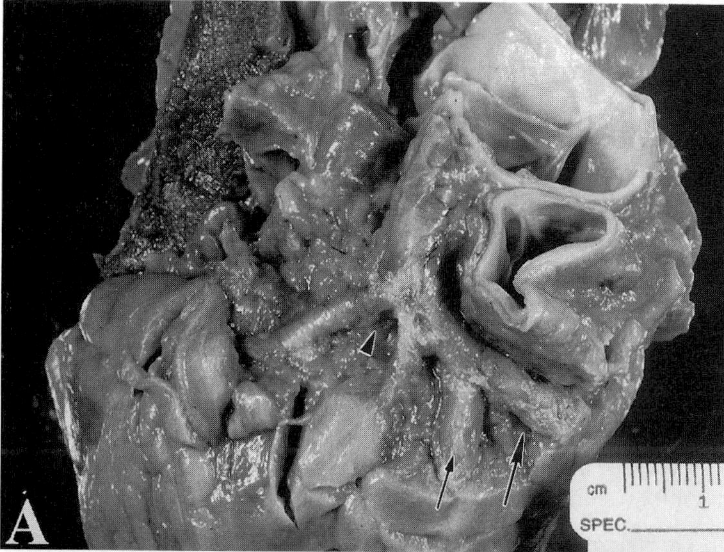

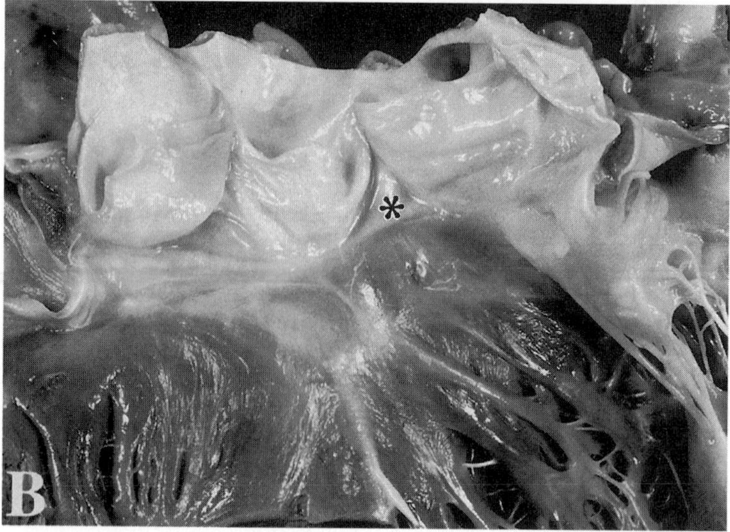

Figure 4–5. Single coronary ostium, situs inversus. *A.* The anterior aspect of the heart demonstrates a large single coronary artery branching into the left circumflex and ramus intermedius (*arrowhead*), left anterior descending (*small arrow*); the right coronary continues around the left portion of the heart under the pulmonary trunk (*large arrow*). The configuration of the heart is mirror-image (situs inversus). *B.* The left ventricular outflow shows a single coronary ostium. The asterisk marks the position of the membranous septum; the right-sided (anatomically left) ostium is to the right, and the anatomically right cusp to the left of the membranous septum; the noncoronary cusp has been cut through. The association between single coronary ostium and situs inversus is rare. (Reproduced with permission, Turchin A, Radentz SS, Burke A. Situs inversus totalis and single coronary ostium. A coincidence or a pattern? Cardiovasc Pathol 9:127–129, 2000.)

"deep" is not well established; however, we considered an arterial segment that is greater than 3 mm within the myocardial a potential cause for ischemia or sudden death. Most deaths due to coronary artery anomalies are exertional; for this reason, the finding of a deep tunnel in an exercise-related death is more likely significant than in a death that occurred at rest. The mechanism of sudden death in myocardial bridges may involve more than compression. Other myocardial findings that have been associated with myocardial bridges of the left anterior descending and that may contribute to sudden death include scarring in the myocardium overlying the tunneled artery (Fig. 4–6), a small posterior descending coronary artery, and tunneling of other epicardial arteries.[19] As with all cases of anomalous origin of coronary arteries, the finding of ischemia lesions (subendocardial necrosis or fibrosis) within the distribution of the abnormal vessel is evidence that the anomaly was hemodynamically significant.

Hypoplastic Coronary Arteries

At this time, the term hypoplastic coronary arteries[15, 20, 21] is not a specific diagnosis, as criteria for this entity have not been standardized, nor has a specific clinicopathologic syndrome been defined. Before considering a diagnosis of hypoplastic coronary arteries, we require that a large portion of the myocardium, usually the posterior wall, be devoid of a major blood supply. In these cases, which are extremely rare,[22] there is no posterior descending coronary artery. In addition, there is no extension of the left anterior descending coronary artery around the apex providing

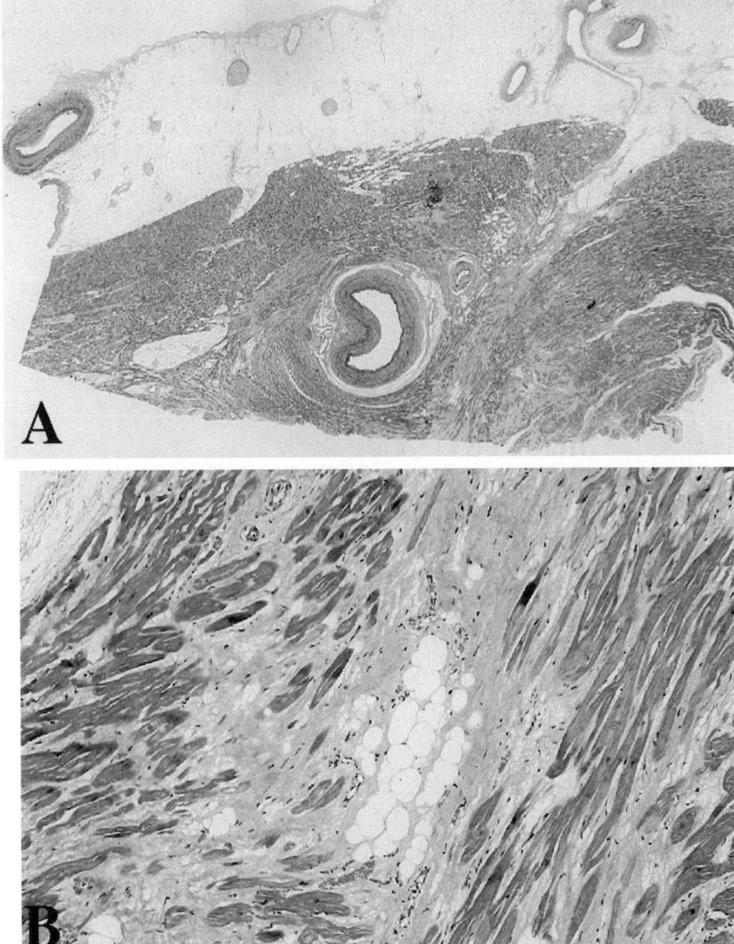

Figure 4–6. Tunnel coronary artery. A 36-year-old man died during a soccer match; no other cause of death was identified other than a tunnel left anterior descending artery, 4 mm deep, 2 cm in length. *A.* A histologic section demonstrates the anterior portion of the myocardium, with the left ventricle on the left side, and a diagonal branch in the upper left. The left anterior descending is buried within the myocardium. *B.* There is scarring and focal fat replacement in the area of myocardial bridging (Masson trichrome).

blood supply to the posterior wall, nor is there a branch of the obtuse marginal extending rightwards and branching to provide vascularization to the posterior ventricular septum. Verification of a hemodynamic compromise in such cases is important in establishing a diagnosis, and we carefully examine the posterior left ventricle for evidence of ischemia. An alternate definition of hypoplastic coronary arteries is that of diffusely narrowed arteries, with normal length.[20, 21] We would be very hesitant to ascribe sudden death only on the basis of arteries of relatively small caliber, in the absence of histologic evidence of ischemia.

Coronary Ostial Stenosis, Congenital

Congenital coronary occlusion isolated to the ostium is usually a component of congenital heart disease, especially supravalvar aortic stenosis, in which a flap or membrane exists occluding the orifice. Other forms of congenital heart disease, such as pulmonary atresia with intact ventricular septum, are associated with absence of a coronary ostium. Rarely, congenital ostial stenosis is isolated (Fig. 4–7), and may result in sudden death or ischemic symptoms in infants and adults.[13, 23–25] In adults, especially women, Takayasu's disease should be carefully excluded, as ostial stenosis is common in Takayasu's aortitis and should be the primary differential diagnostic consideration. The histologic features of congenital ostial stenosis have not been carefully described, but, unlike Takayasu's disease, there is no evidence of an inflammatory process.

Congenital Coronary Artery Aneurysms

Coronary artery aneurysms are generally categorized as either acquired or congenital. The incidence of coronary aneurysms at autopsy is in the range of 1–2%[26] and varies with the definition of aneurysm. Generally, an ectasia is considered an aneurysm if the area of dilatation exceeds the normal adjacent segments or the diameter of the patient's largest coronary vessel by 1.5 times. Acquired aneurysms are usually atherosclerotic or a sequela of vasculitis, particularly Kawasaki disease.[27] Those coronary aneurysms that have no specific features of an acquired process are usually considered congenital, partly by process of elimination, as there are no specific histologic features in most cases that identify a congenital aneurysm (Fig. 4–8).

Congenital coronary aneurysms are rare. Most cases are found at autopsy, although detection during life has been reported[28] as has successful surgical excision.[29] Rupture and thrombosis are the most common causes of death, and distal embolization may result in myocardial infarction.[30] Secondary causes of aneurysms—such as Kawasaki disease, Takayasu's disease, and syphilitic aortitis—must be excluded before the diagnosis of congenital aneurysm is accepted. Some cases of congenital coronary aneurysms are found in patients with inherited connective tissue disorders, especially

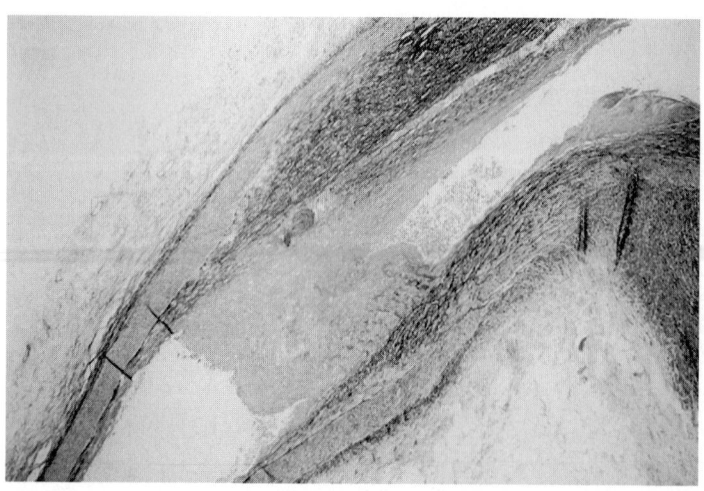

Figure 4–7. Congenital ostial stenosis. A 5-year-old girl died suddenly with no prior history of heart problems or syncope. At autopsy, the left main coronary ostium could not be grossly identified, although the left main and anterior descending arteries had a normal course. Histologically, there was fibrointimal proliferation occluding the left main ostium (Movat pentachrome).

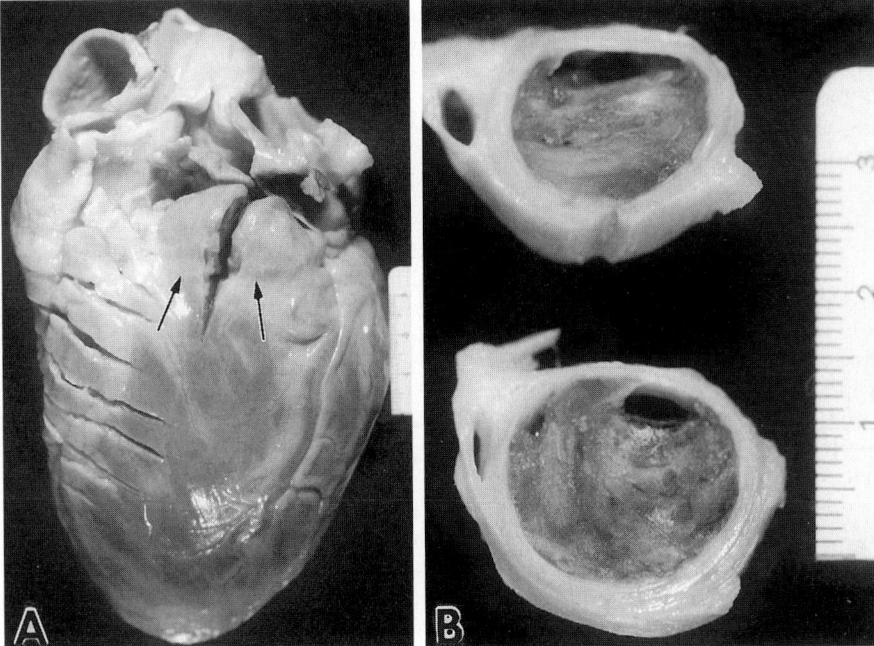

Figure 4–8. Congenital aneurysm. A 50-year-old man was found dead; he had a history of hypertension and recent "viral infection" treated with an antibiotic; an aortic dissecting aneurysm of the descending thoracic aorta was the presumed cause of death. *A*. A large aneurysm of the left circumflex artery is seen under the left atrial appendage, already cut. *B*. Cross sections of the aneurysm demonstrate organized thrombus. The etiology of the aneurysm was unclear, and may have been exacerbated by hypertension. However, the lack of atherosclerosis, association with rare dissection of the distal aorta, and focal nature of the aneurysm (other arteries were normal) suggest a significant congenital component to the etiology.

Marfan syndrome. In these cases, and in some sporadic coronary aneurysms, cystic medial necrosis is seen histologically (Fig. 4–9). Congenital aneurysms are generally single; if an adult is diagnosed to have multiple aneurysms, they are often considered to represent sequelae of occult Kawasaki's disease.[31]

Congenital coronary aneurysms are most common in the RCA and are usually asymptomatic. Histologic studies on congenital coronary aneurysms are extremely few. The basis of the medial weakness is in most cases unclear, as histologic studies show nonspecific fibrosis in the wall of the artery, or less typically, medial

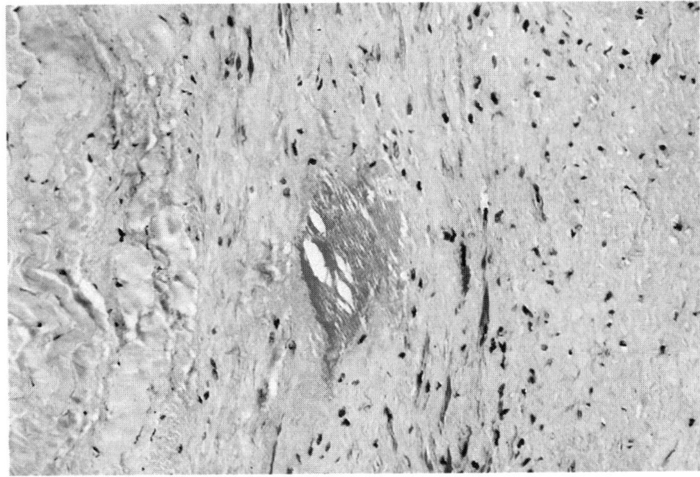

Figure 4–9. Cystic medial necrosis, congenital coronary aneurysm. A 35-year-old man developed palpitations, with mass on chest X-ray. Coronary catheterization demonstrated a giant aneurysm of the left main coronary artery; at surgery, a left circumflex aneurysm measuring 7 cm and a smaller one involving the left anterior descending coronary artery were removed, with ligation of the left main coronary artery and multiple bypass grafts. The surgically removed specimen demonstrates fragments of arterial wall with marked proteoglycan deposition of the medial wall; the adventitia is seen on the left. The patient died postoperatively.

degeneration. The lumen typically contains thrombus, organization, and calcification with minimal atherosclerosis. The major differential considerations are inflammatory aneurysms, especially Kawasaki's disease, and atherosclerotic aneurysms.

Coronary Artery Fistulae

Coronary artery fistulae in the absence of complex congenital heart disease are rare. The sites of communication are numerous, and include the right coronary artery to right atrium or to right ventricle, from the left coronary artery to right atrium or coronary sinus, from left coronary artery to right ventricle, or from right and left coronary artery to right ventricle.[32, 33] In fewer than 20% of cases they terminate in the pulmonary trunk or in the left side of the heart. The usual symptom is congestive heart failure, although coronary fistulae may also result in myocardial infarction due to coronary steal syndrome,[34] sudden death due to ischemia and myocardial hypertrophy,[35] and endocarditis. Coronary artery fistulae may be associated with ostia atresia, coronary aneurysms, and anomalous origin of one or more coronary arteries.[36] When associated with complex heart defects, they are especially common in pulmonary atresia with intact ventricular septum, and other forms of atrioventricular valve atresia.

Pathologically, the fistulae may be difficult to identify, especially the exact site of communication with the ventricle. The artery proximal to the fistula is tortuous, with dilated communications between the artery and the cardiac cavity or pulmonary trunk.

CORONARY ARTERY VASCULITIS

Classification

The precise classification of vasculitis is not always possible, especially when localized to a specific organ. In most cases of vasculitis that is localized primarily in the heart and adjacent great arteries, the diagnosis is Kawasaki disease, especially in children, or Takayasu's disease, especially in adults. However, coronary vasculitis may be a manifestation of patients with systemic vasculitis of virtually all types, and is classified in part by clinical and extracardiac findings. In some cases of isolated coronary vasculitis, the histologic features are not diagnostic of a specific pathologic entity; in such cases, a descriptive diagnosis is rendered.[37–40]

Kawasaki Disease

Epidemiology and Etiology

Kawasaki disease, or mucocutaneous lymph node syndrome,[41] is a pediatric inflammatory illness of unknown etiology with an incidence of 20–100/100,000 in Japan in children less than 5 years and from 4–15/100,000 in the United States.[42] In the United States, the incidence is highest in Asians, followed by Blacks, Caucasians, and Native Americans.[42, 43] There is a slight male predisposition, with a male-to-female ratio of 1.5 to 1. The etiology is unknown, but there have been links to viruses, bacterial infection, autoimmunity triggered by superantigens of staphylococci and streptococci, toxins found in rug cleaners, dust mites, and other factors.[44–46] Features of Kawasaki disease, such as infiltration of T cells into vascular lesions, elevation of soluble interleukin-2 receptors in serum, an imbalance of T-cell subsets, and transient depletion of T cells with CD11/CD18, suggest that the activation of T cells is pathogenetically involved, suggesting T-cell activation by as-of-yet unproven superantigen.[47]

Clinical Course and Treatment

The clinical diagnosis is based on the findings of a high fever of abrupt onset, persisting 5 days or more, unresponsive to antibiotics; redness of palms and soles, with indurative edema that evolves to desquamation; bilateral conjunctival congestion; redness of lips, strawberry tongue, and diffuse infection of oral pharyngeal mucosa; acute nonpurulent cervical lymphadenopathy; and the presence of coronary aneurysms demonstrated by echocardiography.[44] Infants < 6 months may present atypically with an unusually aggressive form of the disease. These small children develop coronary aneurysms without any other signs and symptoms of Kawasaki's disease and may have nodular thickening without aneurysms.[48] The aggressive treatment of Kawasaki disease with the inclusion of intravenous gamma globulin reduces the risk for the development of coronary aneurysms, especially giant lesions. Two gm/kg gamma globulin combined with 30 to 50 mg/kg per day of aspirin is the current recommended treatment,[49] although the possible role of corticosteroids is still debated.[50]

Aneurysms: Pathology

Cardiac complications of Kawasaki disease occur in approximately 25% of patients who receive no treatment.[51, 52] The initial phase of cardiac involvement is a pancarditis with the subsequent formation of epicardial coronary aneurysms. Detailed pathologic studies of Japanese patients with Kawasaki disease have stressed the findings of coronary artery aneurysms that occur in all but the earliest stages of disease. Kawasaki disease begins as a pancarditis with vasculitis of small vessels (stage 1), progressing to panvasculitis of the epicardial coronary arteries with proximal aneurysms (stage II), granulation of the aneurysms with disappearance of microvascular inflammation (stage III), and scarring of the coronary arteries with stenoses (stage IV).[53–57] Stage I typically lasts from 0 to 9 days after symptoms, and is characterized by perivasculitis and vasculitis of the microvessels (arterioles, capillaries, and venules) and small arteries, and acute perivasculitis and endarteritis of the epicardial coronary arteries. Pericarditis, myocarditis, inflammation of the AV node, and endocarditis with valvulitis may also be present at this stage. Stage II (12–25 days) is characterized by panvasculitis of the coronary arteries and the formation of aneurysms with thrombus at the base of the aneurysms (Fig. 4–10). Myocarditis, coagulation necrosis, lesions of the conduction system, pericarditis and endocarditis with valvulitis are also present in stage II. In stage III (28–31 days), organization of the coronary thrombi and disappearance of the inflammation in the mi-

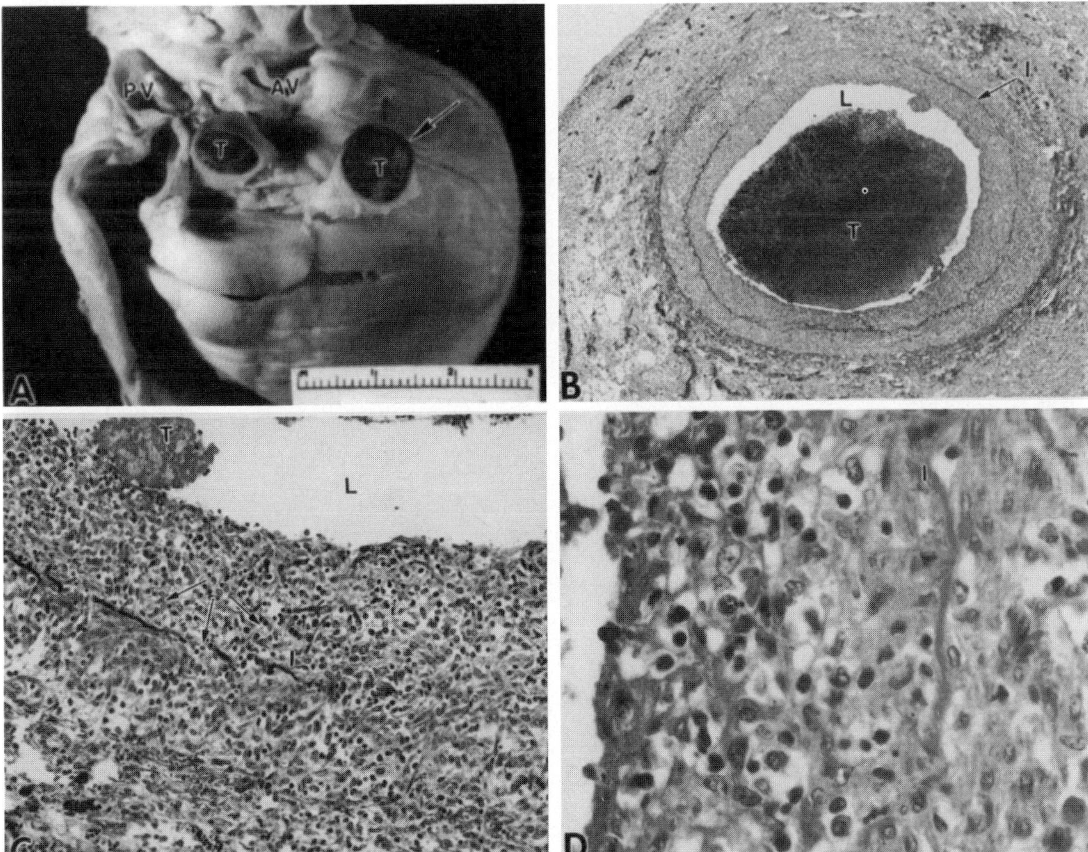

Figure 4–10. Kawasaki disease. *A.* Multiple cross sections of thrombosed left anterior descending coronary artery aneurysm in a 4½-year-old child with stage II Kawasaki disease (21 days' duration). The external diameter of the aneurysm of the left anterior descending coronary artery measured 9 mm (*arrow*). *B* and *C.* Note inflammatory infiltrate and interrupted internal elastic lamina (*arrows*) within the wall of the artery without fibrinoid necrosis. The lumen of the aneurysm is filled with thrombus. *D.* Higher power view of the inflammatory infiltrate consisting predominantly of lymphocytes (*AV,* aortic-valve; *I,* internal elastic lamina; *L,* lumen; *PV,* pulmonary valve; *T,* thrombus). (From Robinowitz M, Forman MB, Virmani R. Nonatherosclerotic coronary aneurysms. In: Virmani R, Forman MB (eds): Nonatherosclerotic Ischemic Heart Disease, pp 291, 292. New York, Raven Press, 1989, with permission).

crovessels are noted. Patients in stage IV (40 days to 4 years) (Fig. 4–11) demonstrate scarring with severe stenosis in the coronary arteries. Fibrosis of the myocardium, coagulation necrosis, lesions of the conduction system, and endocardial fibroelastosis are present to a variable degree.[53]

We recently described a form of Kawasaki disease characterized by a severe vasculitis with intimal thickening, stenosis, and absence of coronary aneurysms[58] (Fig. 4–12). This unusual form of the acute disease may be more common in children with especially severe clinical symptoms or atypical symptoms.

Fate of Coronary Lesions

Coronary aneurysms, which occur in approximately 25% of children, may result in thrombosis and long-term ischemic damage to the myocardium. For this reason, the fate of coronary aneurysms in patients with Kawasaki disease is of paramount concern. Angiographically, only the lumen of the aneurysm is identified, whereas echocardiography demonstrates the outer border of the lesion. The aneurysms are characterized clinically by the presence of calcification and their size, which is classified as small (<1.5 × normal), moderate (1.5–4 × normal) and "giant" (>4 × normal or larger than 8 mm). The persistence rate of aneurysms is 72% at 1 year and 41% at 5 years of follow-up[59]; overall, 55% show regression with a mean follow-up of 14 years.[51] In multivariate analysis, the regression of an aneurysm is inversely related to severity of the initial aneurysm (small, moderate, or giant) and male gender, and positively related to treatment.[59] Over 80% of small or moderate-sized aneurysms regress within 5 years, whereas giant aneurysms show a much slower rate of regression. The long-term rate of acute myocardial infarction is 1.9%, with a mortality rate of 0.8%; most of these children had giant aneurysms that had progressed to stenosis.[51]

Older children and young adults who present with coronary aneurysms secondary to Kawasaki disease, with or without a documented prior

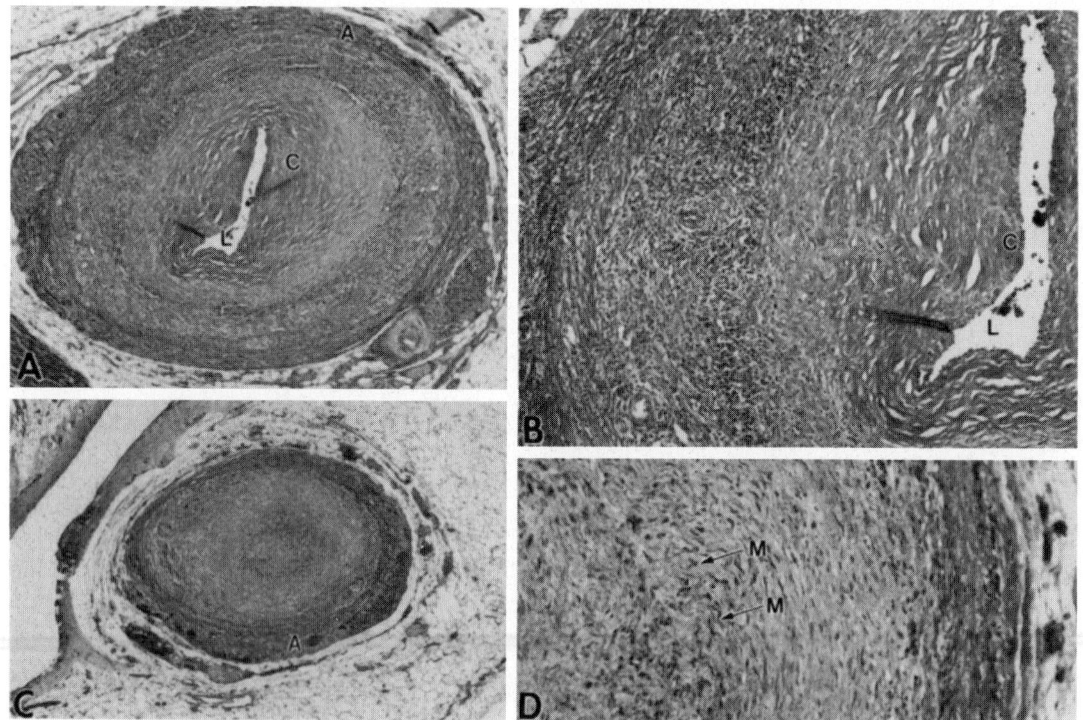

Figure 4–11. Kawasaki disease. Healed stage of Kawasaki disease (greater than 31 days' duration). *A* and *B.* Coronary artery showing severe fibrointimal proliferation and collagen deposition in a patient with healed aneurysms secondary to Kawasaki disease (stage IV). *C* and *D.* Total occlusion of the coronary lumen by fibrointimal proliferation and collagen deposition (*A,* adventitia; *C,* collagen fibers; *L,* lumen; *M,* smooth muscle cells). (From Robinowitz M, Forman MB, Virmani R. Nonatherosclerotic coronary aneurysms. In: Virmani R, Forman MB (eds): Nonatherosclerotic Ischemic Heart Disease, pp 293, 294. New York, Raven Press, 1989, with permission).

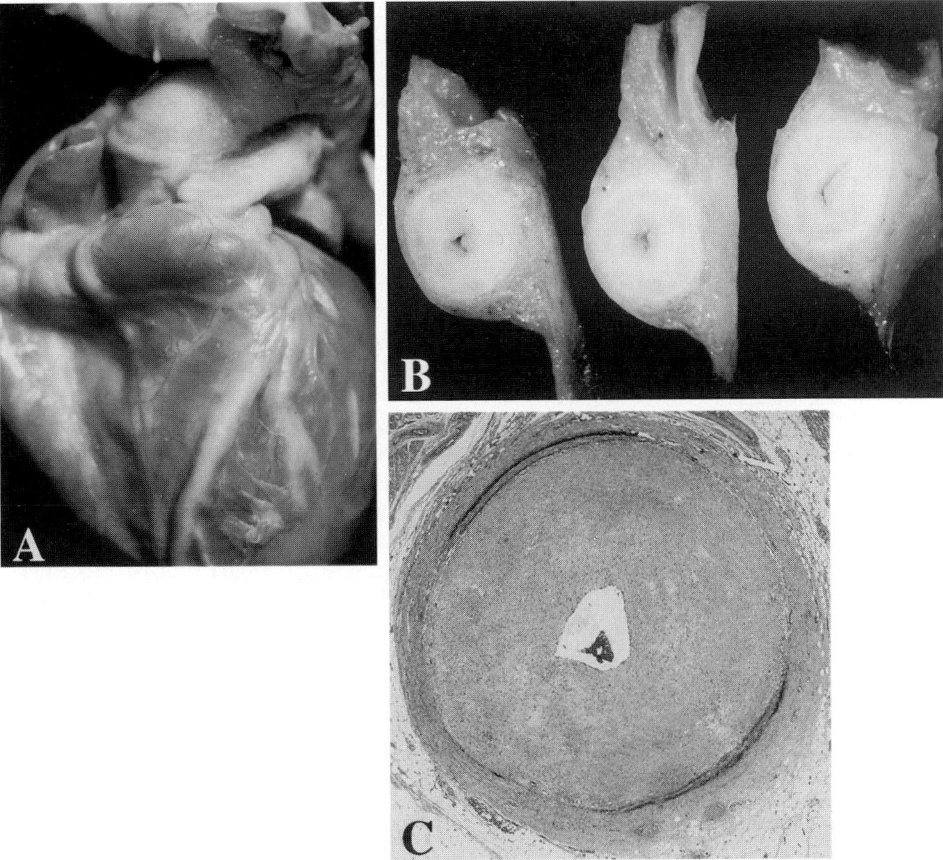

Figure 4–12. Kawasaki disease diffuse intimal type. A 20-month-old boy died suddenly 1 year after a severe case of Kawasaki disease treated with aspirin and immunoglobulin. Follow-up revealed no evidence of aneurysms. At autopsy, the major coronary-arteries were thickening, diffusely ectatic, and cord-like (*A*). On cross section, they showed diffuse intimal thickening (*B*). Histologically (*C*), there was cellular fibrointimal proliferation with focal destruction of the elastica (Movat pentachrome stain).

history, are 25 years on the average, with a range of 12–29 years.[60] The patients generally present with acute myocardial infarct, arrhythmia, or sudden death. Pathologically, the aneurysms are multiple, and histologically there is organized mural thrombus, medial thinning with focal destruction of the elastic laminae, frequent calcification, and variable numbers of residual chronic inflammatory cells in the adventitia. The calcification in these arteries is often appreciated only microscopically, as only one third demonstrate calcification on chest X-ray. Three of every four patients dying of long-term ischemic sequelae of Kawasaki disease demonstrate total occlusion of one or more epicardial arteries at autopsy, with coronary aneurysms present in every case. These findings demonstrate that the acute vasculitis of Kawasaki disease can result in coronary artery damage predisposing to thrombus and progressive atherosclerotic changes that may remain clinically silent for many years.

Other Features of Kawasaki Disease

Vessels other than the coronary arteries may be involved with vasculitis and aneurysm formation. Patients with extracoronary aneurysms almost invariably have giant coronary aneurysms.[51] Virtually any artery may be involved, including (in approximate order of incidence) the axillary artery, common iliac artery, renal artery, subclavian artery, internal iliac artery, superior mesenteric artery, internal thoracic artery, and femoral artery.[51] Other than coronary aneurysms, patients with Kawasaki disease may develop a myocarditis contributing to heart failure[61–63] and microvascular disease on the basis of abnormal perfusion scanning or intravascular ultrasound, in the absence of coronary aneurysm.[64]

Takayasu's Disease

The most common form of vasculitic syndrome with symptomatic coronary involvement in adults is Takayasu's disease, or nonspecific aortoarteritis. Unlike Kawasaki disease, the coronary arteries are only occasionally involved in Takayasu's aortitis, and when coronary involvement occurs, it is usually restricted to the proximal portions of the epicardial vessels, generally the ostia. As is the case with other vasculitic syndromes, the diagnostic criteria are often based on clinicopathologic findings, as the etiology of Takayasu's disease is unknown. It is sometimes a matter of subjective preference whether to use the term Takayasu's arteritis, or a more generic term such as nonspecific or granulomatous arteritis in adults with noninfectious coronary arteritis and aortitis without a specific clinical syndrome.[65] In fact, some reported cases of granulomatous coronary arteries secondary to Takayasu's disease may in fact represent other entities, such as giant cell arteritis, especially in elderly patients without a clinical diagnosis of Takayasu's.[66, 67]

Epidemiology and Etiology

The incidence of Takayasu's arteritis is estimated at 2.6/1,000,000 in a U.S. population of predominantly Northern European derivation.[68] The incidence is higher in Asia, including Japan, Korea, and India, and in Africa. Approximately 80% of patients are women. The etiology of Takayasu's disease is unknown; associations such as autoimmune hepatitis, chronic thyroiditis, and Sjogren syndrome strongly suggest that Takayasu's aortitis may be an autoimmune disease.[69] There is an association with HLA-B5, Bw 52, and Dw 12 antigens.

Clinical Findings

The typical patient with Takayasu's aortoarteritis generally becomes symptomatic between the ages of 20 and 40 years, although reported ages run the gamut of infancy to the elderly. Diagnosis is often delayed because the symptoms are nonspecific, the diagnosis is often not considered clinically, and there is no diagnostic laboratory test.[68] Clinical criteria for diagnosis include onset at age less than or equal to 40 years; claudication of an extremity; decreased brachial artery pulse; greater than 10 mm Hg difference in systolic blood pressure between arms; a bruit over the subclavian arteries or the aorta; and arteriographic evidence of narrowing or occlusion of the entire aorta, its primary branches, or large arteries in the proximal upper or lower extremities.[70]

Ancillary laboratory studies include elevations of acute phase reactants and sedimentation rate, low-grade leukocytosis, and mild normocytic normochromic anemia. The early phase is characterized by malaise, weakness, fever, night sweats, arthralgias, arthritis, myalgias, weight loss, pleuritic pain, and anorexia; weeks or months later, symptoms related to aorta and arch vessels intervene. These late symptoms include absent pulses (96%), bruits (94%), hypertension (74%), heart failure (28%), retinopathy (25%), and symptoms associated with carotid-artery involvement. Involvement of the aortic root and aortic valve occurs in 10–20% of patients and leads to aortic insufficiency. Angiographically, Takayasu's disease has been categorized as type I (aortic arch and arch vessels), type II (descending thoracic aorta and abdominal aorta), type III (combination of types I and II), and type IV (involvement of pulmonary arteries).

Coronary Arterial Involvement

Coronary ostial stenosis occurs in about 10–20% of patients with Takayasu's disease and can occasional predate clinically evident lesions in the aorta and systemic signs of inflammation.[71] In a series of patients seen at the Mayo clinic, 2 of 32 patients with Takayasu's disease had symptomatic coronary disease treated with angioplasty.[68] Cardiac symptoms in patients with Takayasu's disease is not necessarily caused by ischemia; in only 3 of 75 young women with heart symptoms in a series from India was there angiographically documented coronary stenoses. Other causes of heart disease in patients with Takayasu's disease include myocarditis and cardiomyopathy secondary to hypertension and aortic insufficiency.[72] Concomitant myocarditis appears to be more prominent in a series of Asian patients with Takayasu's disease compared with those in the United States.[73]

Ischemic complications of Takayasu's disease occur primarily in women. The initial clinical manifestation is angina pectoris in almost three of four patients. Angiographically, coronary ostia are involved exclusively in 73%, followed by nonostial proximal lesions, 20%; segmental and diffuse disease account for the remainder of the cases. Aortic regurgitation is seen concomitantly in nearly 50% of patients.[74]

Pathologic Findings

The gross coronary lesions in Takayasu's disease have been classified into three groups: coronary ostial lesions, diffuse coronary disease with or without skip lesions, and coronary artery aneurysms.[75] The most common manifestation is coronary ostial stenosis as an extension of aortic disease (Fig. 4–13). Diffuse disease without skip lesions, and coronary aneurysms are distinctly rare.[76] In some cases of giant coronary aneurysm, the weakness of the media may result in ectasia secondary to systemic hypertension in elderly patients with long-standing disease.[69] Aneurysms of the left main coronary artery in patients with Takayasu's disease may occur concomitantly with aortic aneurysms.[77]

The histopathologic features of Takayasu's arteritis have not been well defined, resulting in a great confusion regarding use of the term Takayasu's disease in cases of coronary arteritis in patients without a typical history of the syndrome. It has been stated that the pathologic changes are indistinguishable from those of giant-cell or temporal arteritis, suggesting that Takayasu arteritis and giant-cell arteritis are distinguished solely on clinical grounds.[68] While the distinction between the two entities may be more difficult in a muscular artery as compared with the aorta, there are histologic features enabling distinction between Takayasu's from giant-cell arteritis in a majority of cases.

If there is aortic involvement, adventitial scarring and large areas of necrosis favor Takayasu's disease over giant-cell arteritis, which is primarily a disease of the media. Giant cells are not a

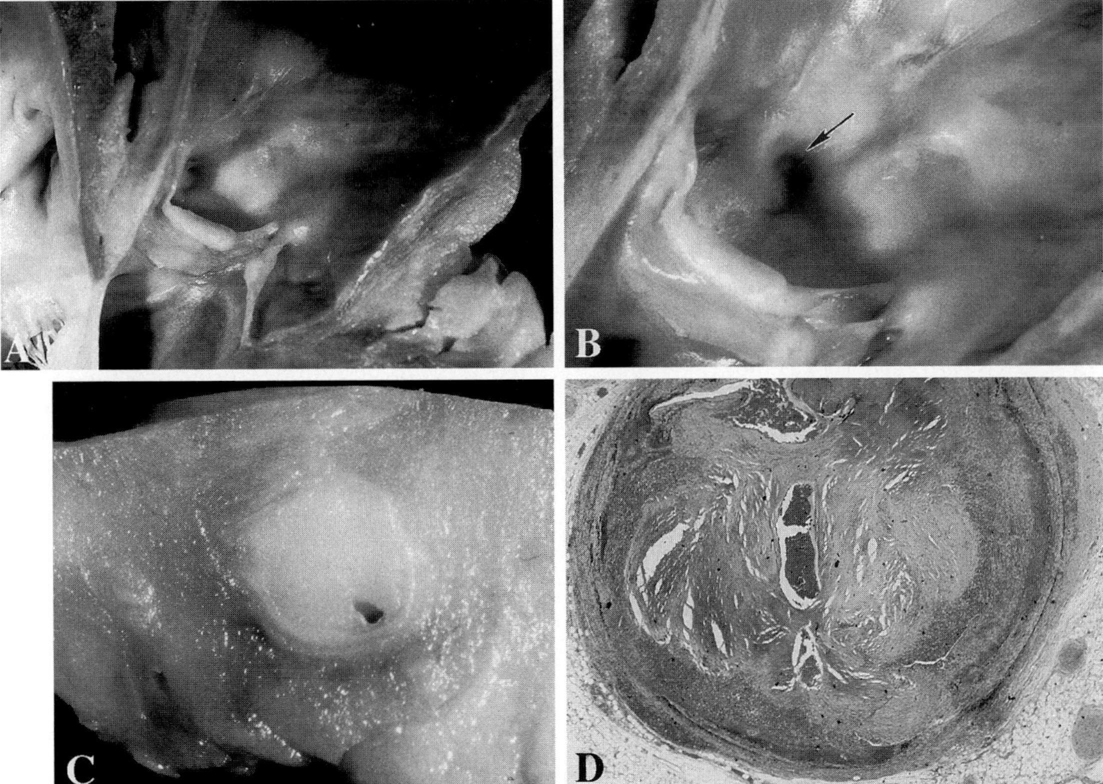

Figure 4–13. Takayasu's disease with coronary ostial involvement. A 24-year-old female developed shortness of breath and dyspnea on exertion and died suddenly. At autopsy, there was dilatation of the proximal aorta with aortic valve insufficiency (*A*). A high magnification of the valve (*B*) demonstrates rolling and thickening of the free edges indicative of insufficiency; the right ostium was pinpoint (*arrow*), as was the left ostium (not shown). A cross section of the left coronary demonstrated more than 95% luminal narrowing (C). Histologically, there was total occlusion with recanalization of the right coronary artery (*C*), with focal destruction of the elastic laminae (Movat pentachrome). The histologic features of the aorta were typical of Takayasu's aortitis (not shown).

helpful distinctive feature, as they may be prominent in either condition. In the muscular coronary arteries, giant-cell arteritis is characterized by inflammation centered on the elastic laminae, and in cases with relatively sparse inflammation, only the media will be affected. In Takayasu's arteritis, however, there is a panarteritis characterized by panarterial fibrosis and patchy chronic inflammation involving all layers of the artery, with more irregular areas of necrosis. Clearly, clinical features, especially the age of the patient are helpful in separating the two entities. Nevertheless, there are certain cases of coronary arteritis that defy classification, and in which, because of the lack of corroborating clinical history, a specific diagnosis cannot be made.

Treatment

The treatment of coronary arteritis in Takayasu's disease consists of anti-inflammatory treatment with steroids, percutaneous angioplasty,[78, 79] and coronary artery bypass graft surgery. In some patients, aortic valve replacement, aortic root reconstruction, and coronary implantation into a tube graft is necessary (Bentall procedure). Use of an internal mammary artery may be contraindicated due to development of arteritis in this vessel.[80] Other surgical issues involve the difficulty of suturing the inflamed aortic wall, necessitating use of special surgery techniques including Teflon-reinforced strips at the anastomotic sites.[80] Endarterectomy of coronary ostial lesions has also been performed in patients with valve replacement.[81]

Lupus Arteritis

Clinical Findings

The cardiac manifestations of lupus erythematosus include pericarditis, endocarditis, and myocarditis.[82] As is the case with patients with rheumatoid arthritis, coronary arteritis may occur, but is less common than atherosclerosis, especially in older patients. In young patients with ischemic cardiac symptoms, the clinical differential between coronary arteritis and premature atherosclerosis may be difficult. It has been appreciated that patients with lupus have a fivefold increased risk for developing premature atherosclerosis; it is unclear how much of this risk is related to autoimmune inflammatory effects of lupus and traditional risk factors for coronary atherosclerosis.[83] In areas with low rates of coronary atherosclerosis, death due to coronary disease in patients with lupus is extremely low,[84] suggesting that the majority of coronary disease in lupus patients is atherosclerotic. Risk factors for atherosclerosis in lupus patients include steroid therapy, hyperlipidemia, hypertension, and elevated homocysteine.[85] There is some evidence that antiphospholipid antibodies may be associated with increased coronary disease in patients with lupus.[86] Angiographic studies have demonstrated an increase in coronary aneurysms, some giant, in patients with lupus coronary disease.[87–89] Coronary aneurysms are generally considered a feature of arteritis, as opposed to atherosclerosis.

The clinical distinction between arteritis and atherosclerosis is important in the young patient, as steroids could exacerbate the atherosclerosis, but help to resolve arteritis. Clinical parameters of activity of the autoimmune disorder are helpful in this distinction, as patients with lupus vasculitis often are systemically ill with marked elevations of disease activity index. Angiographic features that suggest arteritis, in addition to aneurysm, are rapidly changing lesions.

Pathologic Studies

Autopsy studies characterizing the coronary lesions of patients dying with lupus erythematosus are few.[82] The distinction between coronary arteritis and atherosclerosis is often blurred in clinical and pathologic reports of the disease. In a series of 58 autopsies reviewed at the Armed Forces Institute of Pathology (unpublished data), 19 men (mean age 52) and 38 women (mean age 42) had a history of lupus erythematosus. Coronary artery disease was present in 23 (40%), with a mean age of 55 years, and coronary arteritis in 5 (9%), with a mean age of 45 years. In some cases, the distinction between atherosclerosis and arteritis was difficult, as there were features of both processes. Morphologic features characteristic of atherosclerosis were eccentric, lipid-rich lesions with calcification. In contrast, arteritic lesions demonstrated more diffuse, concentric disease, with less calcification and lipid, and often began as an acute arteritis phase, and healed in a fibrotic phase (Figs. 4–14 and 4–15). Approximately two thirds of patients with coronary disease had evidence of acute or healed myocardial infarction, and there was no difference in the arteritis groups versus the atherosclerotic group.

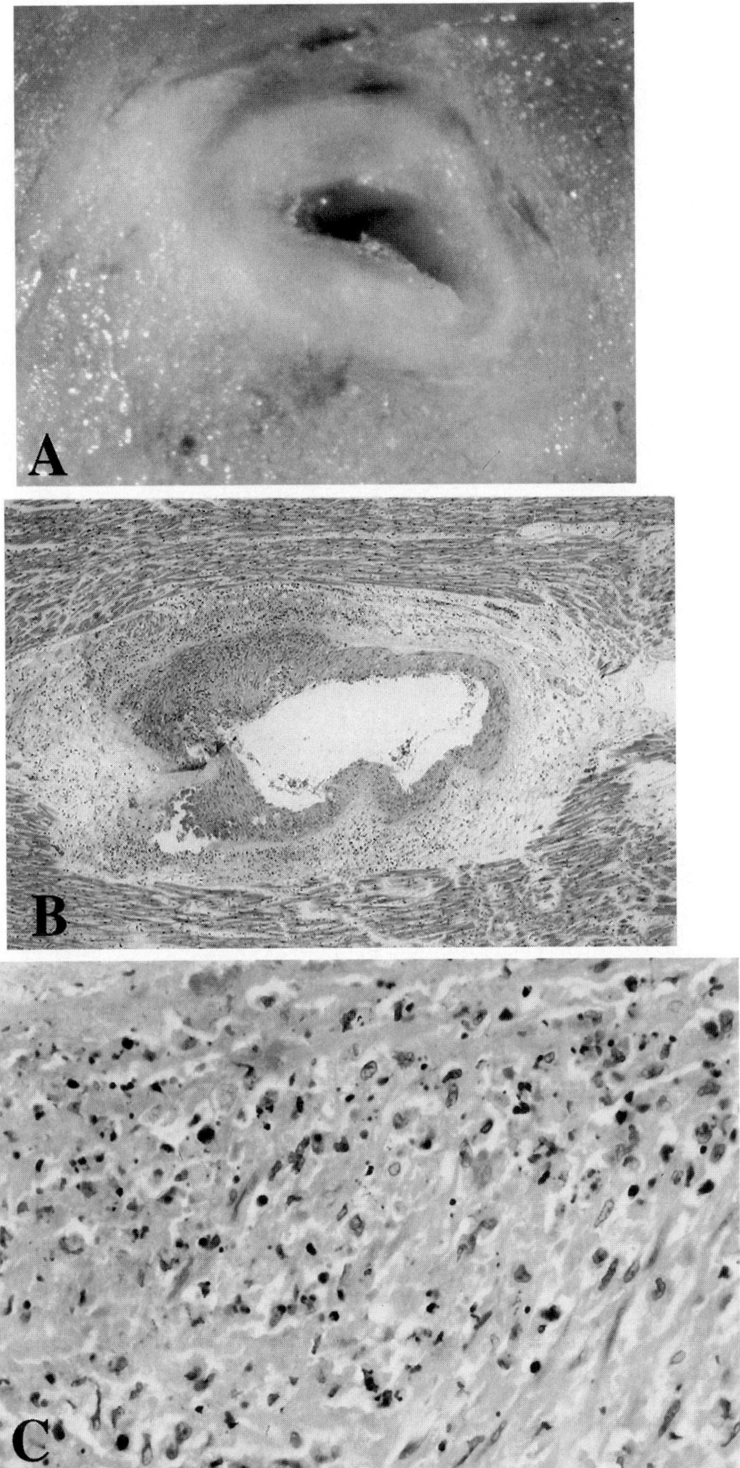

Figure 4–14. Lupus arteritis, acute. A 35-year-old woman with a long history of lupus erythematosus treated with prednisone, depression, and schizophrenia, was found dead. At autopsy there was severe three-vessel disease with total occlusion of the left anterior descending. (*A*) demonstrates a section of right coronary artery with moderate luminal narrowing; in this segment, there was an ongoing acute arteritis (*B*). A higher magnification of the arterial wall (*C*) demonstrates acute inflammation of the media with degenerating neutrophils.

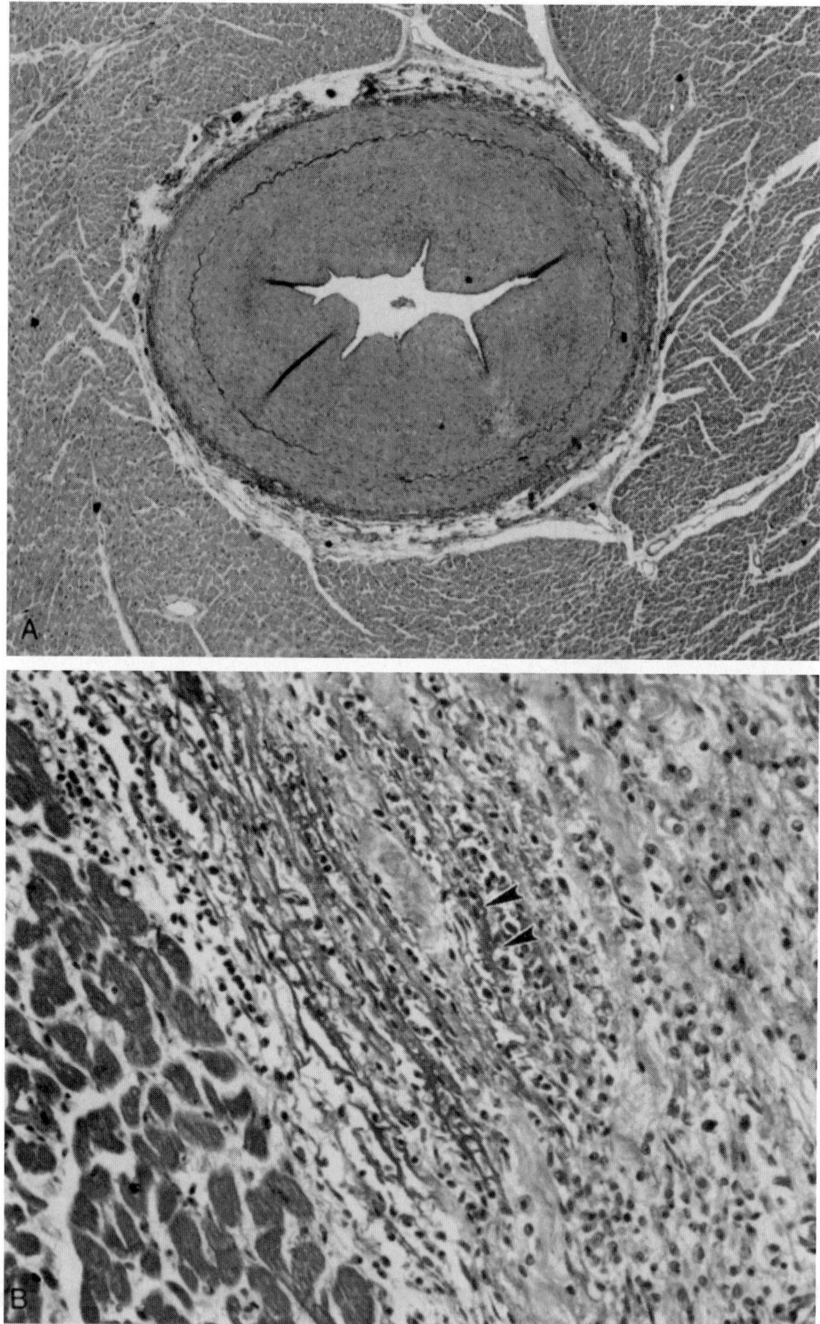

Figure 4–15. Lupus arteritis, healed. Systemic lupus erythematosus. *A.* Marked concentric fibrointimal proliferation in an intramyocardial muscular artery in a patient with lupus who presented with angina. *B.* Fibrinoid change involving the interstitium and a small vessel (*arrowheads*) in the active stage of the disease. (From Darcy TP, Virmani R. Coronary vasculitis. In: Virmani R, Forman MB (eds): Nonatherosclerotic Ischemic Heart Disease, p 267. New York, Raven Press, 1989, with permission.)

Rheumatoid Arteritis

Rheumatoid arthritis is the most likely of the autoimmune disorders to result in arteritis of the muscular arteries. The incidence of clinically diagnosed rheumatoid vasculitis is estimated at 12.5/1,000,000 population annually,[90] a rate higher than that for polyarteritis nodosa or Wegener's granulomatosis. However, coronary arteritis in patients with rheumatoid arthritis is uncommon and tends to occur in patients with long-standing disease and high titers of rheumatoid factor.[91–93] In an autopsy study of 188 patients with severe rheumatoid arthritis, evidence of systemic arteritis was present in seven, four of whom had coronary involvement with associated ischemic lesions.[94] In a smaller study from the Armed Forces Institute of Pathology,[95] five of 48 patients with rheumatoid arthritis had epicardial arteritis (Fig. 4–16). Small-vessel disease has also been described in rheumatoid arthritis,[96] and rheumatoid nodules may be present within the media and adventitia of the arteries and within the myocardium itself. The histologic features of rheumatoid arteritis are nonspecific, and include chronic inflammation, disruption of the elastic lamina, and, in some cases, necrobiosis typical of rheumatoid nodules. The presence of necrosis in areas that do not show rheumatoid nodules is variable, but large areas of necrosis similar to that seen in polyarteritis is rare.

The major differential diagnosis in rheumatoid arteritis is coronary atherosclerosis. There is far less evidence of accelerated atherosclerosis in patients with rheumatoid arthritis, as com-

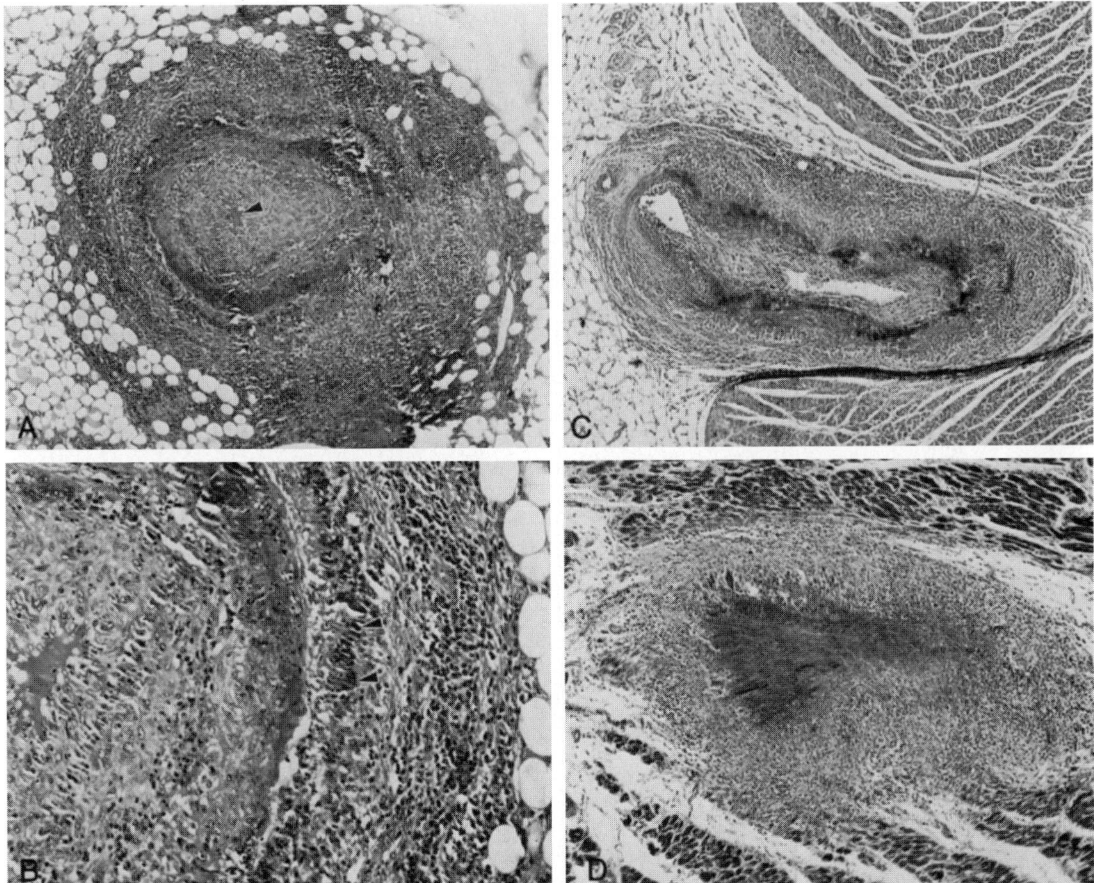

Figure 4–16. Rheumatoid arteritis. *A.* Epicardial coronary artery involved by rheumatoid arteritis. Inflammation involves all layers of the vessel wall, and the lumen is markedly narrowed by fibrointimal proliferation (*arrowhead*). *B.* High-power view of the artery wall with fibrinoid necrosis and palisading histiocytes (*arrowhead*). *C.* Penetrating muscular artery involved by rheumatoid granulomas. *D.* Myocardial rheumatoid nodule. (From Darcy TP, Virmani R. Coronary vasculitis. In: Virmani R, Forman MB, (eds): Nonatherosclerotic Ischemic Heart Disease, pp 244, 245. New York, Raven Press, 1989, with permission.)

pared with patients with lupus erythematosus. However, patients with rheumatoid arthritis may have elevated cholesterol and lower high-density lipoprotein cholesterol, independent of steroid treatment, that may predispose to coronary artery disease.[90] A population-based study has suggested that women with rheumatoid arthritis are more likely to die as a result of coronary artery disease (presumably atherosclerotic) than women without arthritis.[97]

The histologic features of atherosclerosis may include abundant inflammatory infiltrates, making the distinction difficult in some cases. However, the presence of necrotic core and calcification are features of atherosclerosis, whereas the absence of these findings in the presence of inflammation, scarring, and destruction of the elastic laminae, especially if there is fibrinoid necrosis, are features of vasculitis. In some cases, both processes may coexist. In patients with rheumatoid arthritis and coronary lesions, atherosclerosis should be expected as the most likely diagnosis in men over the age of 40 and women over the of 50 years, whereas arteritis is equally likely in younger patients.

Giant-Cell Arteritis

Aortic involvement occurs in approximately 10–15% of patients with giant-cell arteritis. Coronary involvement is, however, quite rare and published information regarding giant-cell coronary arteritis is restricted to case reports.[98–102] Because of the uncertainty in the diagnosis of some cases of granulomatous coronary arteritis in the elderly, it is possible the condition is underdiagnosed.[65, 66] Giant-cell arteritis, when involving the coronary arteries, may cause ischemic heart disease and sudden death.[98, 99] The diagnosis should be considered in elderly patients with ischemic heart disease and coronary lesions who do not demonstrate typical histologic features of atherosclerosis, in whom there is aortitis with aortic root dilatation.

The histologic features of giant-cell arteritis of the coronary arteries are identical to those of the muscular arteries in the temporal region (Fig. 4–17). The inflammatory process begins at the level of the internal elastic lamina. Giant cells are not necessarily present, but granulomatous inflammation rich in macrophages is pres-

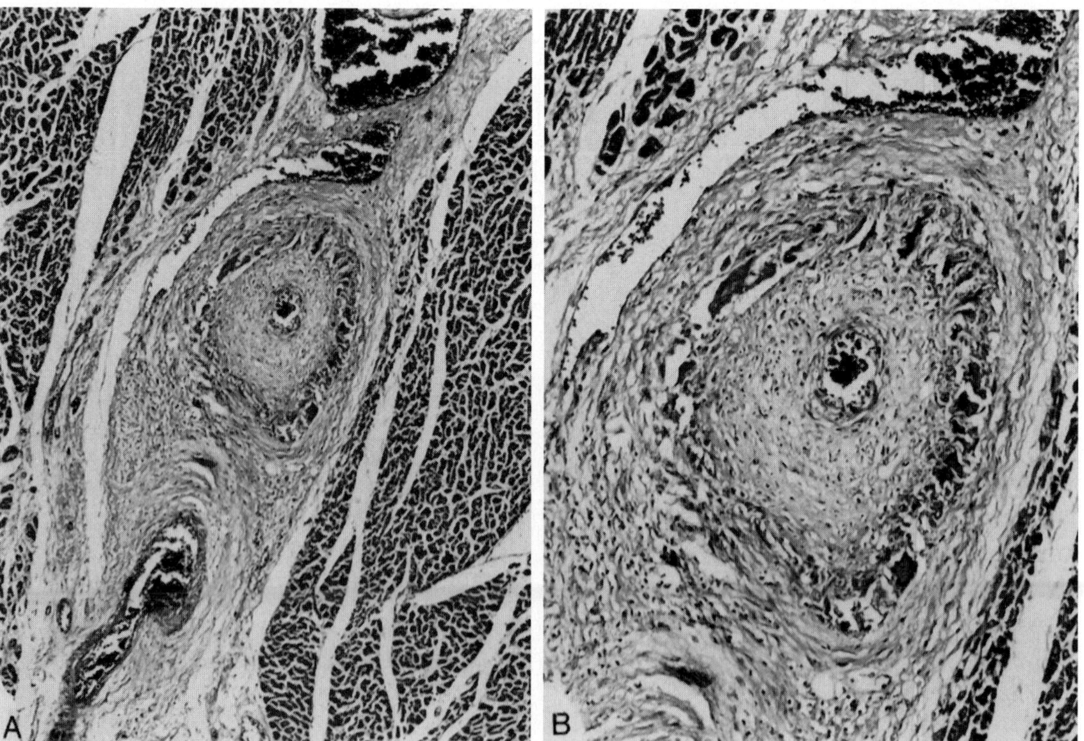

Figure 4–17. Giant-cell arteritis. *A.* Giant-cell arteritis involving a small muscular artery in the left ventricular myocardium. *B.* Intimal thickening with marked luminal narrowing, fragmentation of internal elastic lamina, and profuse giant cell reaction. (From Darcy TP, Virmani R. Coronary vasculitis. In: Virmani R, Forman MB (eds): Nonatherosclerotic Ischemic Heart Disease, p 241. New York, Raven Press, 1989, with permission.)

ent in areas of destruction of the elastic lamellae. In contrast to Takayasu's disease, adventitial scarring is not a feature of giant-cell arteritis. Necrosis may be prominent in either giant-cell or Takayasu disease, or may be absent altogether.

Polyarteritis Nodosa

Coronary artery involvement in polyarteritis nodosa rarely gives rise to ischemic symptoms and sudden death.[37, 103] Histologic features include fibrinoid necrosis and transmural inflammation, often with aneurysms (Fig. 4–18). There are no reliable histologic features to distinguish polyarteritis nodosa from necrotizing arteritis of autoimmune diseases, especially lupus erythematosus or Wegener's granulomatosis. Idiopathic arteritis with fibrinoid necrosis, when discovered in patients without a known vasculitic syndrome, is often classified as polyarteritis nodosa, even if systemic vasculitis or coronary aneurysms are identified (Figs. 4–19 and 4–20).[104] The rate of coronary involvement in patients with known polyarteritis nodosa is unknown, because coronary symptoms rarely become evident during life. The single large autopsy series of patients dying with fulminant polyarteritis nodosa[105] demonstrated that 62% of patients had coronary vasculitis, and the majority was associated with myocardial infarction. The vasculitis in this study was found to affect both epicardial as well as intramural arterial branches, in contrast to atherosclerosis. A substantial minority of cases demonstrated only intramural coronary artery involvement. The histopathologic features of polyarteritis include fibrinoid necrosis as a required finding, often segmental and involving the entire thickness of the media. Giant cells and adventitial scarring are not generally present, which help differentiate polyarteritis from giant-cell arteritis and Takayasu's disease. However, there are no reliable histologic features to distinguish polyarteritis from necrotizing arteritis associated with lupus or Wegener's granulomatosis.

Wegener's Granulomatosis

Wegener's granulomatosis is a necrotizing and granulomatous vasculitis that usually affects the upper and lower respiratory tracts and the kidneys, and is associated with antibodies to cytoplasmic components of neutrophils (ANCA), including proteinase-3 and myeloperoxidase. Cardiac involvement is unusual, although pericarditis, coronary arteritis, myocarditis, valvulitis, and arrhythmias have been described. Approximately 12% of patients with Wegener's granulomatosis demonstrate cardiac involvement, largely manifested by pericarditis and coronary arteritis.[106–110] Acute myocardial infarction with clinical expression is rare.[108] The histologic features of arteritis in Wegener's granulomatosis is indistinguishable from necrotizing arteritis of polyarteritis nodosa (Fig. 4–21).[111] The characteristic geographic necrosis that is typical of lung lesions of polyarteritis have not been reported in the myocardium.

Churg–Strauss Angiitis and Eosinophilic Periarteritis

Inflammation of the coronary arteries with marked infiltrates of eosinophils is associated with three conditions: coronary artery dissection, which in some cases is purported to be precipitated by an eosinophilic vasculitis; Churg–Strauss angiitis (allergic angiitis with granulomatosis); and a recently described entity, eosinophilic periarteritis. Coronary dissection is a distinct entity, clinically and pathologically, although a variant of arteritis with features of both Churg–Strauss angiitis and dissection has been reported.[112]

Churg–Strauss angiitis is a clinical syndrome characterized by peripheral eosinophilia, pulmonary infiltrates, and asthma. The histologic features of Churg–Strauss angiitis include necrotizing arteritis, often involving both arteries and veins, a mixed inflammatory infiltrate including eosinophils, and necrotizing granulomas in the surrounding periadventitial soft tissue. Coronary involvement in the systemic forms of Churg–Strauss angiitis has been described, as well as localized Churg–Strauss syndrome isolated to the coronary arteries.[113] In the original autopsy series reported by Churg and Strauss, the heart was the most common site of inflammation, with 11 of 13 patients having some form of cardiac lesion, with pericarditis and fibrosis secondary to coronary vasculitis. In a more recent clinical series of patients with Churg–Strauss angiitis,[114] 50% of patients had abnormal electrocardiograms; 75%, hypertension; 12%, pericarditis; and 25%, heart failure. Forty-eight percent of deaths were due to con-

Text continued on page 133.

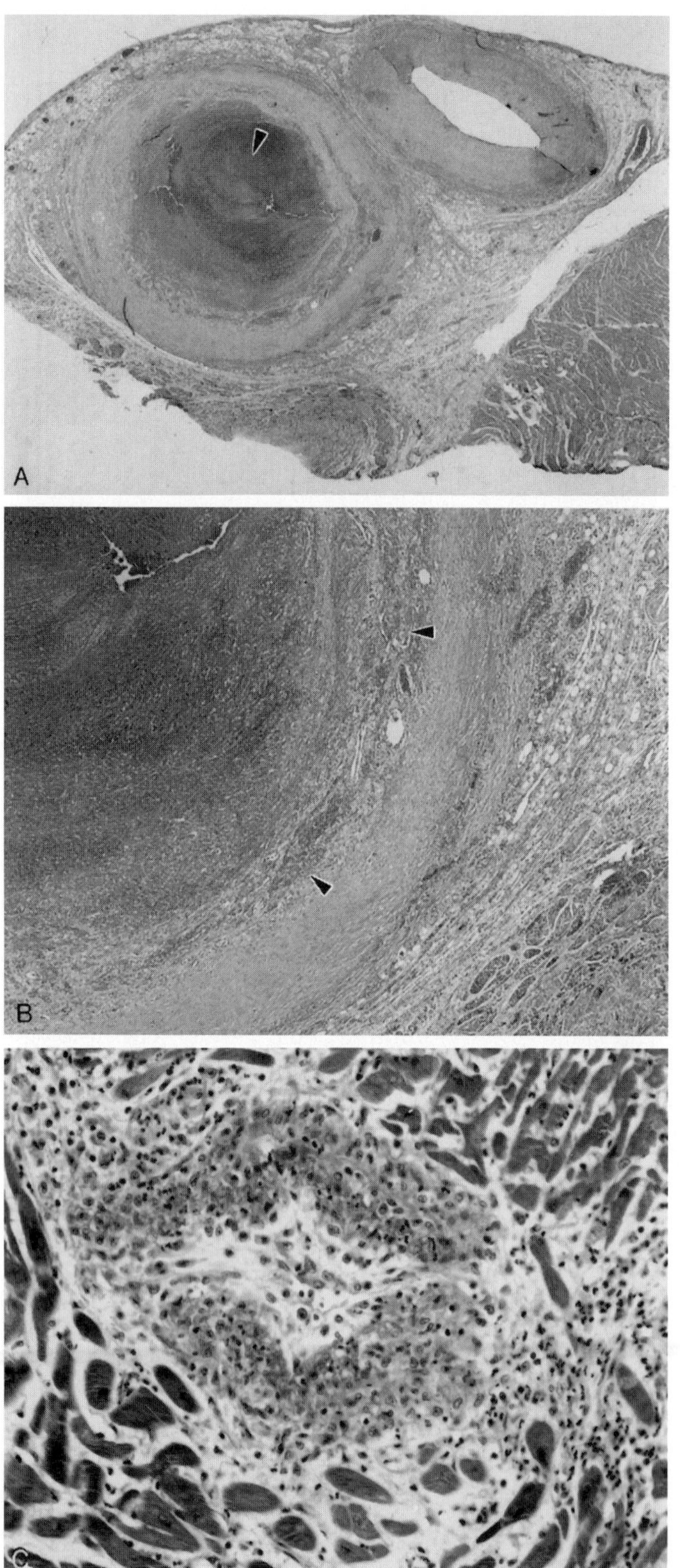

Figure 4–18. Polyarteritis nodosa. *A.* Polyarteritis nodosa involving an epicardial coronary artery near a branch point. Note aneurysmal dilation of the vessel and occlusive luminal thrombus (*arrowhead*). *B.* Higher power view of the artery wall demonstrating fibrinoid necrosis (*arrowheads*). *C.* Intramyocardial small artery with fibrinoid necrosis and acute inflammation. (From Darcy TP, Virmani R. Coronary vasculitis. In: Virmani R, Forman MB (eds): Nonatherosclerotic Ischemic Heart Disease, pp 255, 256. New York, Raven Press, 1989, with permission.)

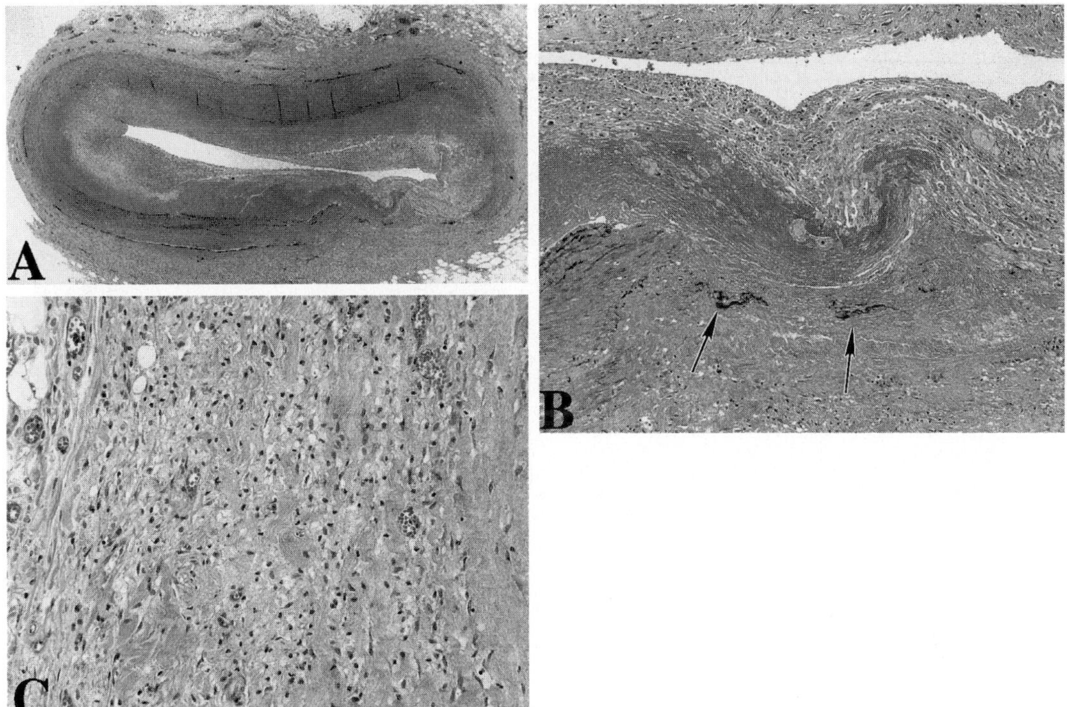

Figure 4–19. Isolated polyarteritis nodosa, acute. A 35-year-old man died suddenly during a karate class; there was no history of autoimmune disease. Autopsy findings were limited to the coronary arteries, where there was a necrotizing arteritis. *A*. The left anterior descending coronary artery demonstrates ectasia. *B*. A high magnification demonstrates destruction of the elastic laminae (*arrows*) with overlying area of fibrinoid necrosis. (*A* and *B*. Movat pentachrome.) *C*. A high magnification of the media demonstrates a chronic inflammatory infiltrate composed primarily of macrophages (Hematolyxin-eosin).

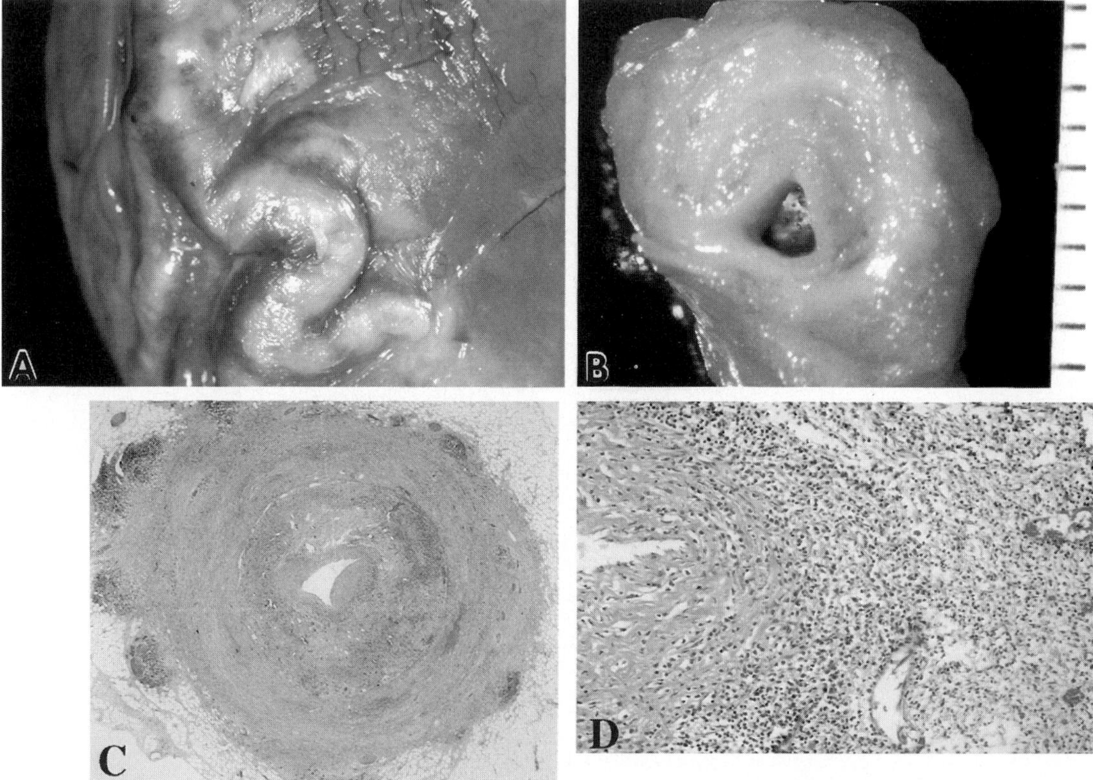

Figure 4–20. Isolated polyarteritis, healed. A 52-year-old man was found dead after exercising; there was no prior history of syncope or history of autoimmune disease. At autopsy, significant findings were limited to the coronary arteries. There was a segmental arteritis affecting the left obtuse marginal artery, manifest by focal aneurysm/ectasia (*A*). A cross section demonstrated marked luminal compromise by intimal thickening (*B*). Histologically, there was a concentric intimal thickening with inflammation in the adventitial seen on low magnification (*C*). On higher magnification, there were areas of inflammation in the intima as well as in the adventitia with total destruction of the media (*D*). Acute fibrinoid necrosis was not identified, but the features were consistent with a healed arteritis.

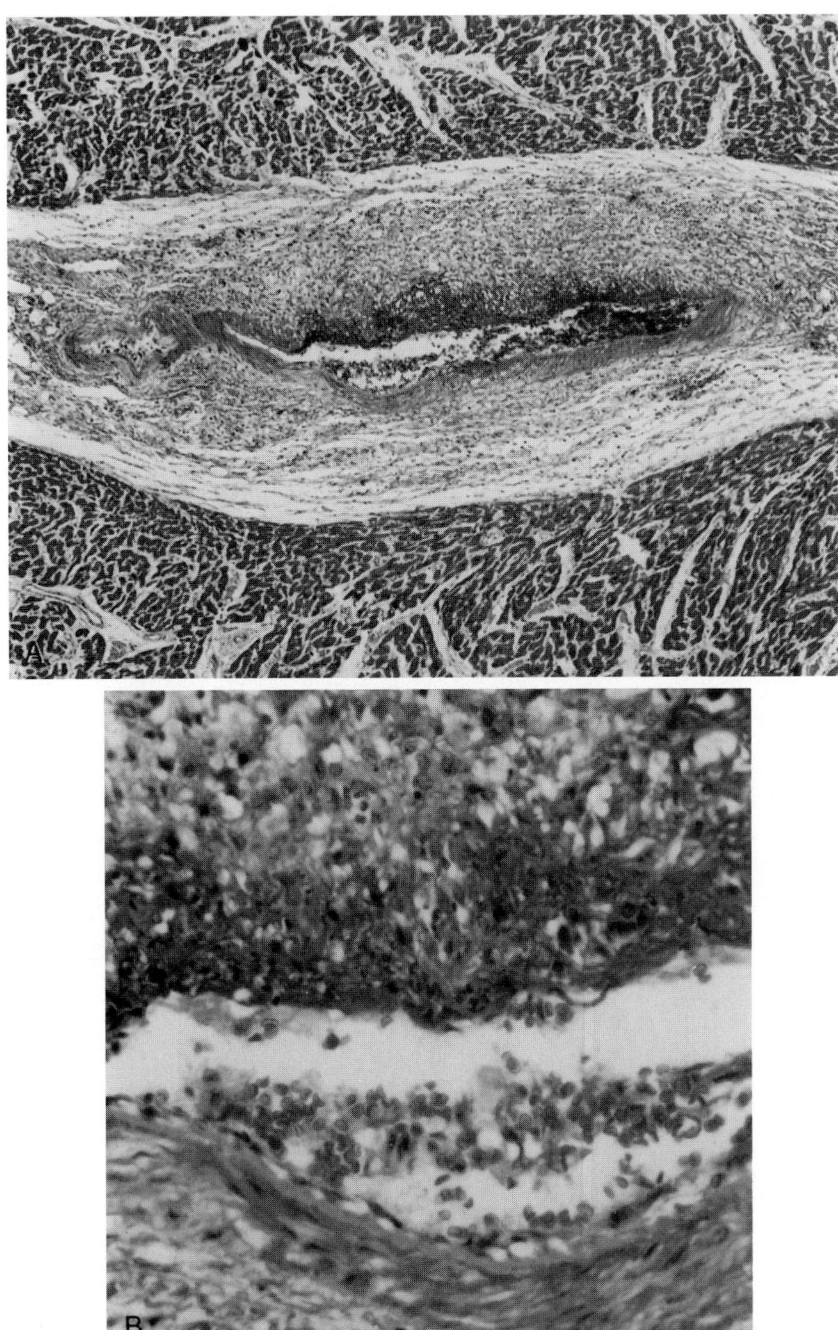

Figure 4–21. *A.* Wegener's granulomatosis involving an intramyocardial muscular artery. Note intense segmental inflammation involving the full thickness of the vessel wall. *B.* High-power view of the arterial wall with fibrinoid necrosis and inflammation (*top*). Below the media is intact. (From Darcy TP, Virmani R. Coronary vasculitis. In: Virmani R, Forman MB (eds): Nonatherosclerotic Ischemic Heart Disease, p 258. New York, Raven Press, 1989, with permission.)

gestive heart failure and/or myocardial infarction.

Eosinophilic periarteritis is distinct from Churg–Strauss angiitis in that necrosis and soft-tissue granulomas are absent. The process is entirely adventitial, and the media of the surrounding artery is intact with a patent lumen. The process may cause ischemia and sudden death, presumably from coronary vasospasm, but the etiology and associations are poorly understood due to its rarity. Only one case has been reported,[115] and we have seen a similar process in a woman who died suddenly with no other finding at autopsy (Fig. 4–22).

Ankylosing Spondylitis

One of the seronegative spondyloarthropathies, ankylosing spondylitis is a systemic disease associated with HLA B27 haplotype, skeletal disease, uveitis, and heart disease.[116] Cardiac manifestations include aortic insufficiency and heart block, which occur in 3–10% of patients with long-standing disease.[117, 118] Occasionally, aortic disease can involve the coronary ostia.[119]

Pathologically, ankylosing spondylitis primarily results in dilatation of the aortic valve ring and fibrosis of the aortic valve, which prolapses into the left ventricular cavity. The aortic wall of the sinus of Valsalva is involved along with a few centimeters of the tubular portion of the ascending aorta. In the active phase of the disease, there is endarteritis obliterans and perivascular infiltration by lymphocytes and plasma cells. The media is also involved with destruction of the elastic fibers and muscle cells. The inflammation extends to the anterior mitral leaflet, causing its thickening and eventually fibrosis.[120] A subaortic ridge or bump eventually forms on the septal surface of the anterior mitral leaflet, which is characteristic of the disease. Coronary artery involvement in ankylosing spondylitis results from the extension of the aortic inflammation and fibrosis into the coronary ostia (Fig. 4–23).

Infectious Coronary Vasculitis

Syphilis

With the adequate treatment of syphilis in Western countries, syphilitic coronary arteritis has become something of a historic curiosity.[121]

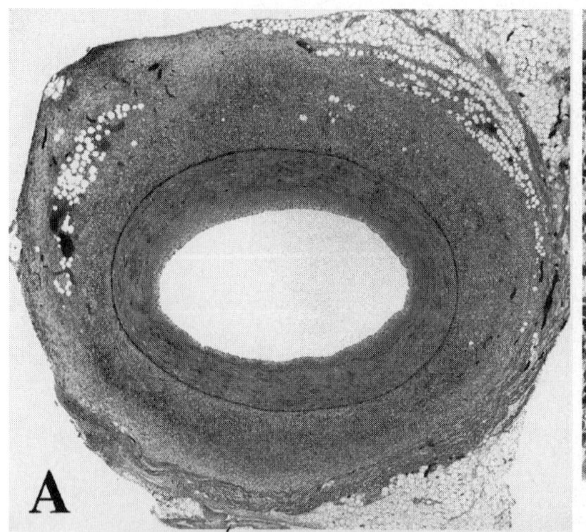

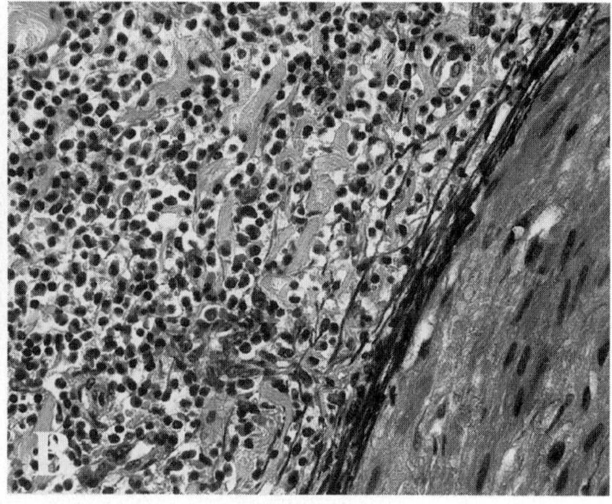

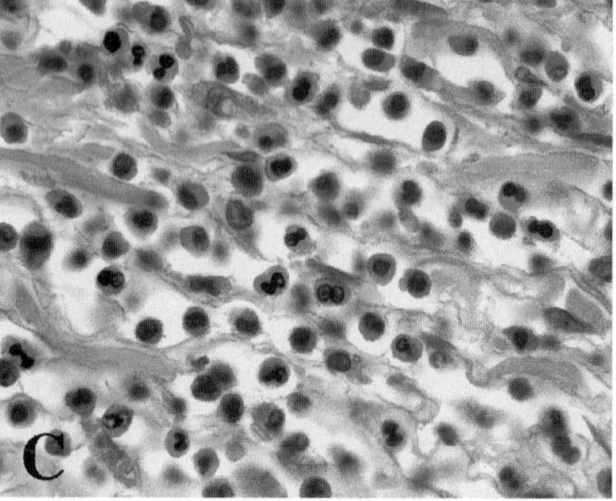

Figure 4–22. Eosinophilic periarteritis. A young woman died suddenly and unexpectedly without significant prior medical history. At autopsy, the left circumflex coronary artery was diffusely thickened and firm. The other epicardial arteries were grossly and histologically normal. Histologically, there was an intense adventitial infiltrate without luminal involvement of the circumflex (*A*). On high magnification, the external elastic lamina was intact (*B*). The predominant inflammatory cells were eosinophils and macrophages (*C*).

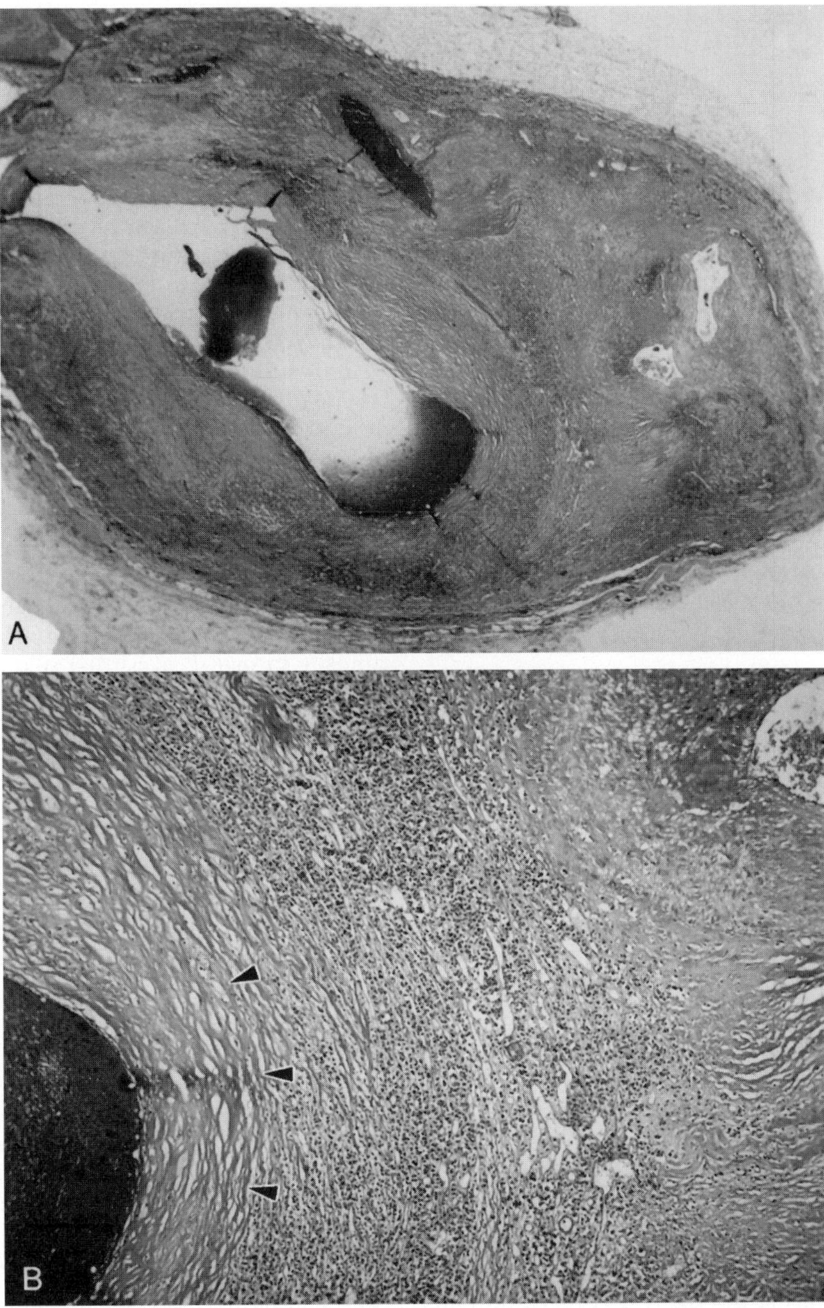

Figure 4–23. A 58-year-old man had ankylosing spondylitis and a past history of myocardial infarctions, congestive heart failure, and mitral and aortic regurgitation. *A.* Left anterior descending coronary artery with marked fibrous thickening and inflammatory infiltrates (*arrowheads*) in the vessel wall. *B.* Predominantly plasma cell infiltrate. (From Darcy TP, Virmani R. Coronary vasculitis. In: Virmani R, Forman MB (eds): Nonatherosclerotic Ischemic Heart Disease, p 248. New York, Raven Press, 1989, with permission).

In patients studied in the 1950s and 1960s with syphilitic aortitis, ostial involvement was described in 20–30% of patients.[95] Occasionally, there can be sparing of the ostium with proximal coronary artery involvement.[121] Pathologically, there is marked thickening of the vessel wall by plasma cells, lymphocytes, and macrophages. The vasa vasorum characteristically show endarteritis obliterans, and microgummas—zones of necrosis surrounded by mononuclear inflammatory cells and plasma cells—may be present in the wall of the vessel. In advanced lesions, the lumen of the vessel may be obliterated by a fibrointimal proliferation with or without superimposed atherosclerosis. Spirochetes are difficult to locate in the lesions.

Syphilis is often in the differential diagnosis of aortitis with or without coronary ostial involvement. Serologic tests for syphilis should identify past infection with the spirochete in most patients. Pathologically, the distribution and gross appearance of lesions in the aorta is important, as syphilitic aortitis is characterized by marked aneurysmal dilatation, whereas Takayasu's disease is more typically associated with narrowing or relatively mild ectasia, with skip lesions and involvement of the arch vessels. Histologically it may be difficult to differentiate the two conditions, as endarteritis obliterans may be present in Takayasu's disease as well as syphilis, and both are characterized by adventitial scarring.

Septic Vasculitis

Infectious coronary arteritis is usually the result of infection of an atherosclerotic plaque in a patient with bacteremia, often with concomitant renal failure.[122] Other sources of infection include adjacent ring abscess and embolization of infected material (see following). Most common organisms implicated in septic coronary arteritis include staphylococci and streptococci.

TRANSPLANT ARTERIAL DISEASE

Acute cardiac rejection is the result of T-cell mediated myocyte damage that is routinely suppressed by cyclosporine and other drugs (see Chapter 9). More recently, immunologically mediated vascular disease, affecting the epicardial and intramural coronary arteries, has been described in heart transplant recipients. There are various terms for this process, including cardiac allograft vasculopathy, graft vascular disease, transplant arteriopathy, transplant arteriosclerosis, and others. Because typical atherosclerotic lesions also occur in transplant hearts, the term "graft atherosclerosis" probably should not be used synonymously with graft vasculopathy.

The sequelae of graft vasculopathy are manifest later than those of acute rejection. For this reason, graft arterial disease has historically been called "chronic rejection." Hammond and others maintain that a significant proportion of acute rejection involves deposition of complement and immunoglobulin in small vessels in the absence of a significant cellular response (acute vascular rejection, or humoral rejection).[123, 124] The association between acute vascular rejection and graft vasculopathy in mural and epicardial arteries remains to be elucidated fully. It is unclear if eventually this form of acute rejection will be classified under the umbrella of graft vasculopathy, thus rendering the distinction between "acute" and "chronic" rejection obsolete.

Graft vascular disease is the major cause of late death in cardiac transplant recipients, and differs from atherosclerosis in that it is concentric, diffuse, progresses rapidly, and rarely calcifies.[125] Although no definitive cause for cardiac allograft vasculopathy has been established, a combination of immunologic and nonimmunologic damage to endothelial cells results in myointimal proliferation. Intravascular ultrasound and coronary angioscopy are more sensitive diagnostic measures of cardiac allograft vasculopathy than coronary angiography. Although retransplantation currently seems to be the only definitive therapy for cardiac allograft vasculopathy, it has shown only fair results.[126]

Clinical

Symptomatic graft vascular disease occurs in 15–20% of transplant recipients, and is the most common cause of death after the first year of heart transplantation. Clinical detection of graft vascular disease is difficult because it is diffuse and concentric, and coronary angiography underestimates the degree of disease. Clinical symptoms are nonspecific, as typical angina does not occur in allograft hearts. Intracoronary ultrasound is more sensitive in diagnosis than angiography, and thallium-201 scintigraphy is a useful diagnostic adjunct. By clinical detection methods, graft vasculopathy occurs in approximately 25% of patients in the first eight years of transplant. Sudden death is a relatively common complication of graft vascular disease. Aggressive monitoring and treatment of early episodes of graft vascular disease has been shown to cause regression of coronary disease,[127] but the effect of immunosuppression on graft vasculopathy is unclear (see following).

Pathogenesis and Etiology

Various etiologies for transplant arteriopathy have been proposed, including cytomegalovirus infection and immune-mediated vasculitis. Risk factors for the development of graft arteriopathy include nonimmunologic (lipids, hypertension, donor age, cytomegalovirus infection, diabetes mellitus, time after transplantation, and cold ischemic time), immunologic factors (histocompatibility, episodes of treated rejection, and average first-year biopsy rejection score), and immunosuppressive regimens. By multivariate analysis, high prednisone dosage, low cyclosporine dosage, increased cellular rejection, and increased donor age were significantly associated with the development of ischemic events in transplant recipients.[128] The effect of cyclosporine on the development of graft arteriopathy is controversial, as experimental models have shown a cyclosporine-induced vasculitis and arteriopathy, although lowering cyclosporine does not reduce the risk for graft vascular disease in humans.[129] A relationship between cytomegalovirus infection and endothelialitis of small vessels in transplant biopsies has been demonstrated, but the relationship between endothelialitis and graft arteriopathy is unclear. In experimental rabbits, hypercholesterolemia may augment allograft atherosclerosis, T-cell accumulation, and intimal neovascularization,[130] and may be associated with fatty-rich lesions of graft vascular disease.[131]

Experimental models of transplant arteriopathy have shown that it is mediated by histocompatibility antigens and that it is antibody-dependent.[132, 133] The intimal thickening typical of the disease has been shown to be the result of injury associated with inflammation occurring after transplant, not as a result of injury incurred as a result of transplant, that is, procurement, preservation, and reperfusion injury.[134] The initial recruitment of inflammatory cells involves interferon gamma, a pro-inflammatory cytokine, as interferon gamma deficient animals do not develop graft vasculopathy and have reduced expression of murine histocompatibility class II antigens and leukocyte adhesion molecules.[135, 136] Ongoing histocompatibility class II expression in donor vascular cells, as well as in recipient macrophages, may contribute to sustained activation of host T cells with consequent release of cytokines that ultimately promote the development of graft arteriosclerosis.[137]

Studies from Peter Libby's laboratory have suggested that graft arteriosclerosis resembles delayed-type hypersensitivity localized in the graft's arteries, a manifestation of cellular immunity mediated in large part by a regionally acting cytokine network. The chronic immunologic process involves inappropriate expression of histocompatibility antigens, the participation of cytokines derived from vascular cells and infiltrating leukocytes. The involvement of helper T cells interacting with class II HLA may distinguish transplantation-associated arteriosclerosis from typical acute rejection, which may involve primarily cytolytic T cells interacting with class I HLA.[138, 139]

Although the precise mechanisms are unclear, the bulk of animal studies indicated that the intimal thickening of graft coronary arteries begins as an inflammatory cell-mediated activation of vascular endothelial cells, resulting in up-regulation of endothelial-derived mesenchymal growth factors capable of stimulating smooth muscle cell proliferation and migration.[140]

Pathologic Findings

Autopsy Studies

Descriptions of graft vasculopathy are almost entirely derived from autopsy studies and explanted hearts retrieved during retransplantation, as it is a disease primarily of epicardial and larger intramural coronary arteries. Sequential evaluation of vascular changes is limited in human biopsy material by their general absence in endomyocardial specimens. Changes in arterioles and capillaries, constituting so-called vascular rejection, have been described primarily in biopsy specimens early in the course of transplant, and have an unclear relationship with graft arteriopathy.

Autopsy studies have shown three types of epicardial coronary disease in patients dying with heart allografts: diffuse proliferative arteriopathy that extends into the intramural and smaller branches (Fig. 4–24); acute vasculitis, with or without necrosis (Fig. 4–25); and typical atherosclerotic disease in the epicardial arteries. The last type, atherosclerosis, may in part be due to preexisting disease in the donor. Tissue immunofluorescence analysis has demonstrated vascular deposition of immunoglobulin and complement in acute vasculitis, similar to findings in acute vascular rejection in arterioles.[141] Studies in short- and long-term survivors performed by Johnson et al. have classified graft vascular disease on the basis of proximal versus diffuse epicardial disease. Proximal graft disease is primarily fibrointimal and begins to demonstrate typical fibroatheroma after 1 year of transplantation, whereas diffuse coronary lesions show more inflammation and necrosis.

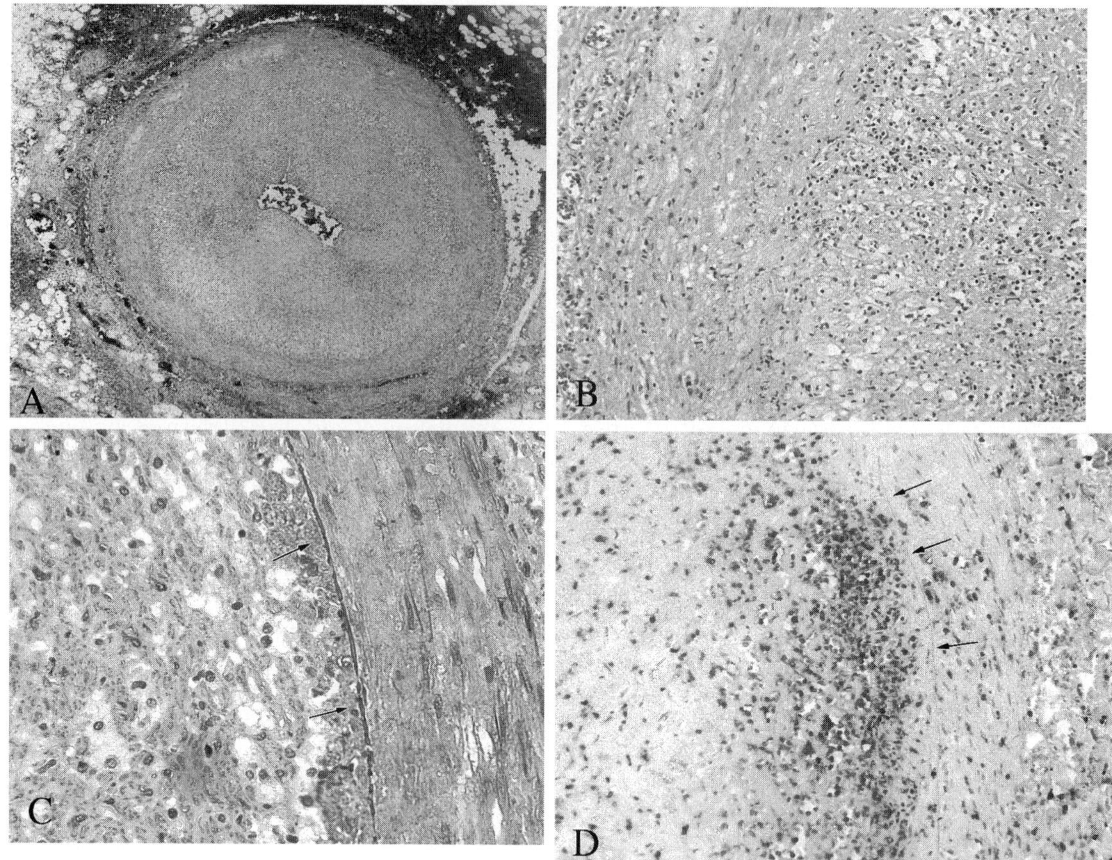

Figure 4–24. Epicardial arterial graft vasculopathy. A 65-year-old man underwent orthotopic transplant for dilated cardiomyopathy, and died suddenly 16 months after transplant. *A.* The epicardial arteries demonstrated diffuse intimal thickening with mild chronic inflammation of all arterial layers. *B.* A higher magnification of the media and outer intima demonstrate a chronic inflammatory infiltrate. *C.* The intimal elastic lamina is intact (*arrows*). *D.* The inflammation is present in the outer intima; the cells are stained for UCHL, T-cell marker. The arrows outline the internal elastic lamina. (Courtesy of Dr. Thomas Aretz.)

Early diffuse necrotizing vasculitis was invariably associated with acute myocardial rejection; this type of diffuse disease progressed to fibrous or fibrofatty intimal lesions of the large and small epicardial and intramyocardial arteries.[142] In this study, the pattern of lesions most strongly associated with ischemic death was diffuse disease, followed by proximal atherosclerotic plaques, and proximal fibrointimal lesions without significant lipid.

The relationship between small-vessel disease and epicardial fibrointimal proliferation in allograft hearts is unclear. Medial lymphocytic vasculitis in intramural myocardial arteries was associated with vasculitis in the vasa vasorum of the epicardial coronary arteries, independent of the occurrence of myocardial fiber rejection, in a study of autopsy hearts.[143] There are fewer data corroborating an association between disease of arterioles and capillaries and epicardial coronary disease, possibly because of the different time course between small-vessel disease, which presumably occurs before epicardial fibrointimal proliferation.

The arteriopathy of epicardial coronary arteries is diffuse and concentric, involving proximal, distal, and small branch segments. Smooth muscle cells in a lipid- and glycosaminoglycan-rich matrix are the predominant components of this expanded intima, with various amounts of collagen. Early changes in vessels (before 14 months) have shown that the medial inflammation of epicardial and medium-sized coronary arteries begins primarily in the outer two thirds of the media and adventitia, suggesting that the early vascular manifestations may reflect tissue rejection similar to that seen in the myocardium.[144] The pattern of inflammation in the intima is different, in that there is a superficial and, to a lesser degree, deep, band-like infiltrate of T cells and macrophages, suggesting a progression of endothelialitis (see next section). The mononuclear infiltrate is more prominent in early lesions as compared with more severely narrowed arteries from longer-term, susceptible grafts.[125]

Virtually all of the coronary features are seen in the medium to large arteries of liver, pancreas, and kidney allografts. A finding perhaps unique to epicardial coronary arteries of heart allografts is the presence of eccentric lesions more typical of native atherosclerosis, which may represent preexistent, undetected donor disease.[125]

Endothelialitis

Endothelialitis refers to a subendothelial collection of lymphocytes and other mononuclear cells in graft arteries (Figs. 4–25*A* and 4–25*B*) and arterioles. It is believed to represent an early form of vascular injury, and has been described primarily in renal and hepatic allografts. More recently, a similar phenomenon has been described in heart transplants.[132, 145–147] Endothelialitis is believed to be a precursor lesion to intimal hyperplasia in animal models.[134]

Accelerated transplant arteriosclerosis accounts for approximately 20% of deaths due to graft failure within 1 year. In the first cases of "endothelialitis" noted in human autopsy transplants, a very prominent inflammation with T cells was noted in the subendothelial space in addition to intimal proliferation in the first-order and second-order intramuscular branches of the major coronary arteries.[147] In these hearts there was only a minimal inflammatory reaction in the vascular adventitia and media.[147] This study suggests that endothelialitis may be a precursor lesion to graft intimal proliferation, as hypothesized by animal models.

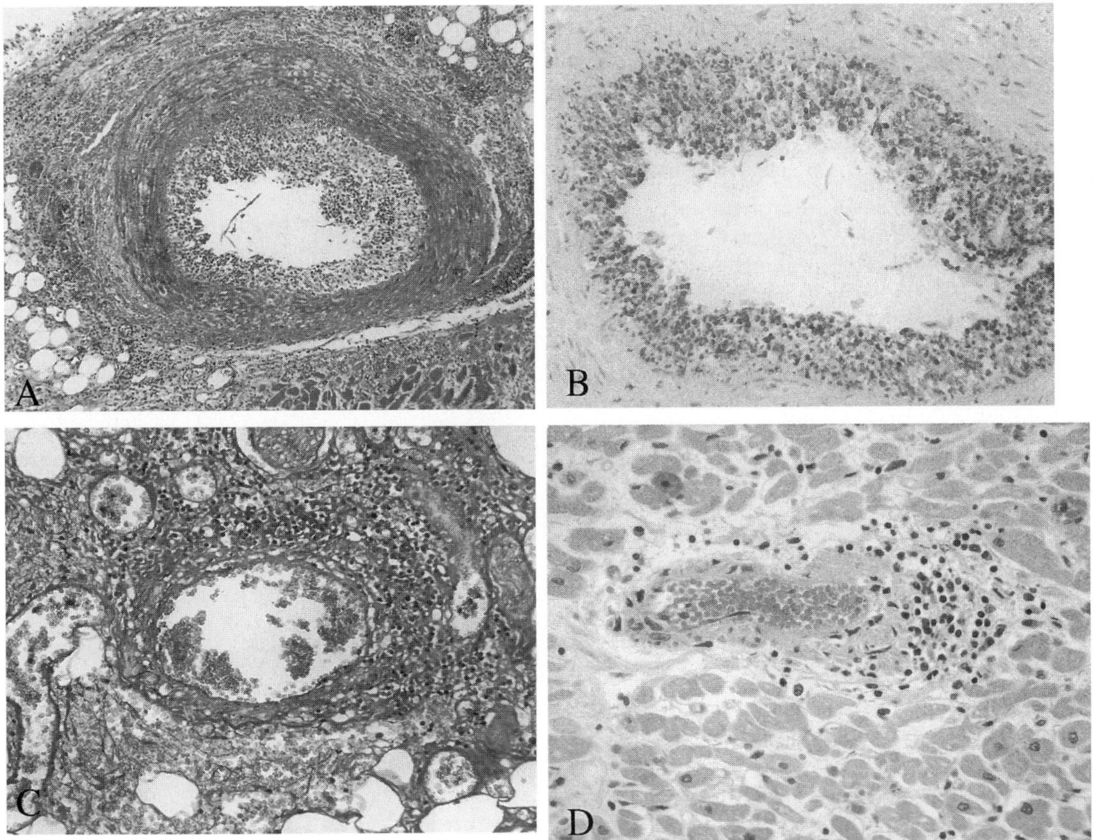

Figure 4–25. Transplant vasculitis. A middle-aged man died suddenly 1 year after transplant. *A.* An epicardial artery with relatively normal media, and inflammation within the intima. *B.* Many of the cells in the intima stain for UCHL, T-cell marker. Smaller vessels in the heart also demonstrated inflammation. *C.* An elastic stains shows inflammation with destruction of the elastica in a large arteriole/small muscular artery. *D.* Inflammation in an arteriole. (Courtesy of Dr. Thomas Aretz.)

Subsequent autopsy studies have shown that endothelialitis was highly associated with transplant-related arteriosclerosis ($P < 0.005$), that macrophages were an additional component of the inflammatory response, and that the lymphocytes were cytotoxic T cells (CD8+, CD2+).[145] Endomyocardial biopsy studies of endothelialitis in transplant recipients have shown a strong correlation with cytomegalovirus infection.[146]

Endomyocardial Biopsy

Because graft arteriopathy is primarily a disease of large- and medium-sized arteries, endomyocardial biopsies cannot be used for the diagnosis. Secondary ischemic changes may be present in the subendocardial myocytes in cases of graft arterial disease, and are important changes to note in reports of transplant biopsies.[148] As mentioned earlier, acute vascular rejection (humoral) is not currently considered a form of graft vasculopathy, as it is unclear whether it is associated with epicardial disease. Experience from the University of Utah suggests that over 20% of allografts demonstrate acute vascular rejection, characterized by the absence of inflammation, endothelial swelling, and vascular deposition of immunoglobulin and complement by immunofluorescence on frozen sections. Furthermore, the group from Utah has reported that vascular rejection is associated with decreased graft survival[123] and graft coronary disease.[124] However, the incidence of vascular rejection is not so high as 20% in other centers, and the significance of vascular rejection remains controversial.

Endothelialitis has not been extensively reported in biopsy specimens from heart allografts. In a report from Finland, 3% of endomyocardial biopsies show T-cell endothelialitis of small intramyocardial arterioles, almost exclusively in patients with evidence of cytomegalovirus infection.[146]

Effect of Treatment and Acute Rejection on Graft Vasculopathy

Despite the toxic affect that cyclosporine exhibits on small vessels in renal arteries,[149] a similar effect has not been demonstrated in cardiac allografts. In fact, lowering the dose of cyclosporine does not decrease the incidence of graft vasculopathy,[129] and, paradoxically, there is evidence that the incidence of epicardial disease is inversely related to cyclosporine dose.[128] Because of the difficulty in assessing the presence of graft vasculopathy and its various definitions, a clear-cut relationship with acute rejection has not been demonstrated. However, the presumed earliest phase of the disease, acute vasculitis of medium sized arteries, has been found to be associated with acute rejection in an autopsy study.[142] Furthermore, a study evaluating the occurrence of ischemic graft disease by various clinical and autopsy modalities demonstrated an association between graft vasculopathy and acute rejection, in addition to donor age, lower overall cyclosporine dose, and increased steroid dose.[128] Treatment of angiographic or scintigraphic evidence of coronary vasculopathy with 3-day methylprednisolone pulse and antithymocyte globulin has been shown to result in regression of coronary lesions,[127] and, in animals, treatment with anti CD8 antibody has shown to be effective for graft arteriosclerosis.[150]

SPONTANEOUS CORONARY ARTERY DISSECTION

Incidence and Prevalence

The incidence of spontaneous coronary artery dissection is unknown. Based on population data from the state of Maryland, we estimate the incidence of sudden death due to idiopathic coronary artery dissection to be 2/1,000,000 young and middle-aged women annually. At angiography, the rate of nonfatal coronary dissection has been reported to be as high as 1.1% of patients presenting with angina pectoris.[151] However, the dissections in this study were primary atherosclerotic and relatively limited; the incidence of nonatherosclerotic nonfatal spontaneous dissection was 0.18%.[151]

Etiology

There are several etiologic classifications of spontaneous coronary artery dissections.[152] In the surgical literature, they have been classified into peripartum dissections, idiopathic dissections (presumed vasospastic), and atherosclerotic dissections.[153] Cocaine has been reported to result in vasospasm-induced spontaneous coronary artery dissection.[154]

It is unclear if vasculitis is a cause of spontaneous coronary artery dissection. Pathologically, the majority of dissections are encountered in cases of sudden unexpected death in young women without coronary disease. The histologic findings in the majority of these dissections demonstrate a normal media, with abundant adventitial eosinophils. It is debated if the eosinophils in these dissections are secondary to the hemorrhage or causative.[155–157] A report of coronary artery dissection with true vasculitis consisting of medial inflammation and features of Churg–Strauss syndrome has been reported, but true vasculitis in spontaneous dissection is exceptional.[112]

Cystic medial necrosis is only infrequently seen in the media of spontaneous dissections,[158] and most patients do not have evidence of Marfan syndrome. Spontaneous coronary dissections occurring in patients with Marfan syndrome are almost always extensions of aortic dissections.[152] Rare spontaneous coronary dissections demonstrate angiomatosis of the adventitia; to our knowledge, medial dysplasia as a cause of spontaneous coronary artery dissection has not been reported.

Although the association between puerperium and spontaneous coronary artery dissections is often emphasized, the majority of women dying with coronary artery dissection are not peripartum,[158, 159] and few women with angiographically documented dissection are pregnant or have recently been pregnant.[151, 160] However, there are reports of spontaneous coronary dissections in women taking oral contraceptives, and we have seen several hearts from women taking birth-control pills with spontaneous dissections.[159] Systemic hypertension may also predispose to coronary artery dissection in a minority of patients.

It has been suggested that heavy physical exertion may result in a form of traumatic, noniatrogenic dissection.[151] These patients, however, were not studied pathologically, and it is likely that the exertion merely precipitated dissection in patients otherwise susceptible.[151]

Spontaneous coronary artery dissection may also occur as an extension of aortic dissection (see Chapter 13). Nonspontaneous iatrogenic dissections are discussed in Chapter 3. Nonspontaneous noniatrogenic dissections are typically the result of blunt trauma to the chest, which may result in aortic dissections and tears, ruptured vessels, hemorrhage into an atherosclerotic plaque, and coronary spasm. Spontaneous coronary dissection occurs in approximately 10% of patients with blunt trauma and cardiac injury.[152]

Clinical Findings

The major clinical presentation of coronary artery dissection is sudden death and acute myocardial ischemia. In autopsy series, over 80% of patients are women aged 20–50.[152] In 80%, the left anterior descending coronary artery is involved, and the majority of the remainder involve the right coronary artery. Occasionally, a branch of the left anterior descending or the left main coronary artery is the site of the dissection.[152] About one third of patients have premonitory chest pain, and a similar percent will have a history of hypertension. In the largest autopsy series, which was composed entirely of women, only one in 16 patients was peripartum.[152]

Clinical findings in a series of patients diagnosed during angiography differ significantly from those of a autopsy series. The female preponderance in clinical series varies from 18–80%,[151, 160] but the male predominance is due solely to inclusion of large numbers of dissections induced by atherosclerosis.[151] Dissection is most frequently located in the left anterior descending coronary artery (approximately 50%), followed by the right coronary artery (30%) and the left circumflex coronary artery (20%).[151] Only 10–25% of spontaneous dissections diagnosed angiographically occur in peripartum women.[151, 160] Most patients present with acute myocardial infarction[160–162] or unstable angina.[151]

Pathology

Pathologic studies of spontaneous coronary dissection are derived from autopsy series (Figs. 4–26*A–D*). In a literature review, 42% of cases demonstrated adventitial eosinophils (Fig. 4–26*D*); 35%, cystic medial degeneration. However, in the largest series from a single institution, eosinophils were present in over 85%, and significant medial degeneration was not encountered in the affected coronary arteries.[152] In rare cases, the dissection may be precipitated by a Churg–Strauss syndrome, polyarteritis nodosa, or angiomatosis of the adventitia.[112, 158, 163] In three of four cases, the dissection occurs in the outer third of the media (Fig. 4–26), and, in the remainder, the middle third. An entry tear can usually not be demonstrated in acute dissections. Acute myocardial

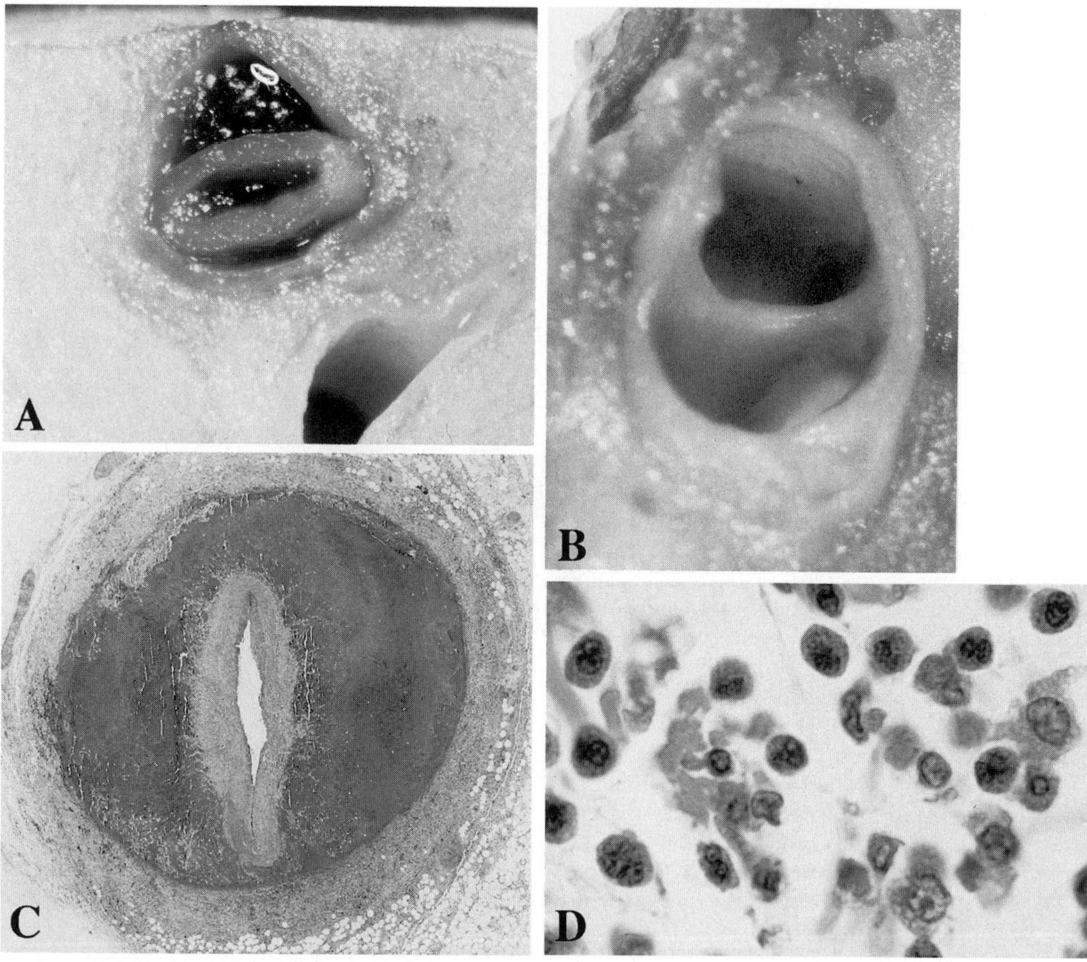

Figure 4–26. *A*. Acute coronary dissection in the left anterior descending coronary artery. The vein is seen below within the epicardial fat. A 38-year-old woman died suddenly after complaining of chest pain; there was no prior history of syncope or recent pregnancy. *B*. Chronic coronary dissection. A 70-year-old man had focally severe coronary disease and aortic stenosis that were treated with bypass surgery and valve replacement. A chronic dissection was noted at angiography; prior instrumentation had not been performed. The patient died of surgical complications. At autopsy, there was a chronic dissection involving much of the left anterior descending artery. The point of intimal connection to the false lumen did not demonstrate atherosclerotic plaque. *C*. Histologic findings, acute dissection. The dissection is typically in the outer media with an intramural hematoma. The media often appears unremarkable. *D*. Often, there are numerous eosinophils within the adventitial inflammation.

infarction is found in 50% of patients, and healed infarction in 10%. Chronic dissections are characterized by a double-lumen chamber, one of which is lined by elastica, and the other by organizing fibrointimal cells (Fig. 4–27).

Treatment and Prognosis

In early clinical studies of spontaneous coronary artery dissection, the condition was nearly uniformly fatal.[152] However, with better recognition of the entity and improved angiographic techniques, the mortality rate has decreased dramatically, reported less than 5%.[151, 159–162] Treatment includes coronary artery bypass grafting, which may be technically difficult due to friability of the arteries,[160] balloon angioplasty with or without coronary stents,[151] and medical treatment alone, including nitrates and beta blockade.[159, 161] The use of thrombolytic therapy during acute coronary dissection may result in exacerbation of clinical symptoms. Inappropriate treatment of spontaneous dissection with thrombolytic treatment may occur if there is no angiographic diagnosis in patients admitted for acute myocardial infarction.[164]

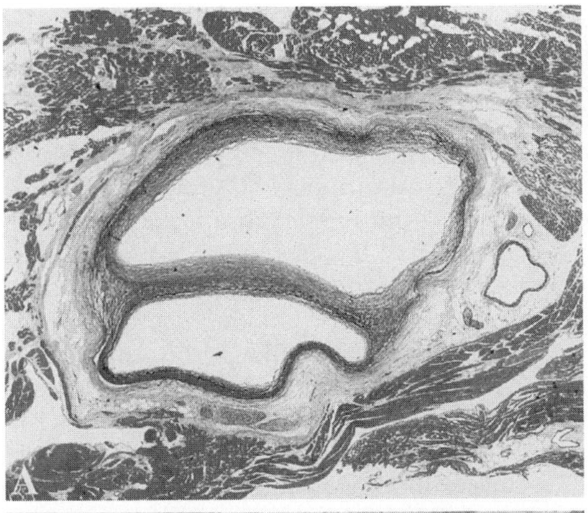

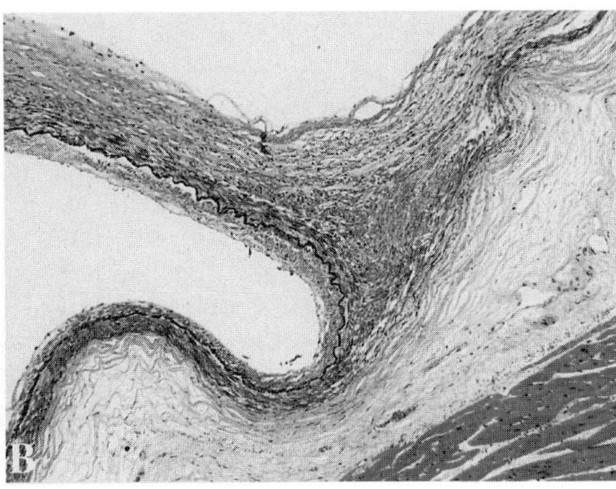

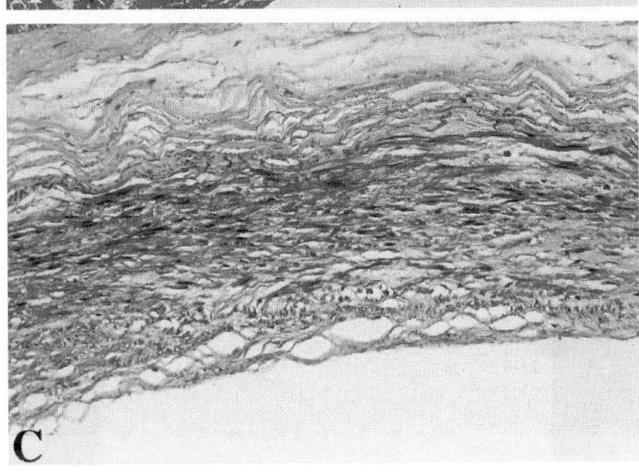

Figure 4–27. Coronary dissection, healed, histologic findings. The dissection illustrated in Figure 4–24*B* is shown histologically. *A*. The intramural portion of the left anterior descending coronary artery demonstrates a double-barrel chamber. *B*. Higher magnification demonstrates the true lumen (*below*) showing an intact internal elastic lamina, with the false lumen (*above* and *left*) lined by fibrointimal tissue. *C*. A higher magnification of the false lumen with an absence of elastica. (Movat pentachrome.)

EMBOLIC CORONARY ARTERY DISEASE

Etiology and Incidence

The etiology of noniatrogenic coronary embolism includes thrombotic, infectious, and neoplastic conditions (see Table 4–2). Iatrogenic causes, which are covered in Chapter 3, are becoming more common. These include cardiac catheterization, cardiac surgery, cardioversion, and external cardiac massage. Coronary artery obstruction associated with prosthetic valve replacement most often is due to coronary embolism, and noninfective valvular heart disease has now replaced infective endocarditis as the most frequent source of coronary emboli.[165]

Table 4–2. Causes of Coronary Embolism

Natural
Endocarditis—nonbacterial and infective
Mural thrombi—atrial fibrillation, MI, cardiomyopathy
Tumor—myxoma, bronchogenic, etc.
Myocardial infarction with rupture (myocardial embolus)

Trauma
Fat embolus

Iatrogenic
Cardiac catheterization
Cardiac surgery (platelet–fibrin emboli, calcium, talc, suture, cholesterol, myocardium, silicon, cloth, etc.)
Prosthetic valve replacement
Debridement of calcified valve
Percutaneous balloon angioplasty (necrotic debris from native CA or saphenous vein bypass grafts)
External cardiac massage

In a review of 32 cases of coronary embolism from the files at the Armed Forces Institute of Pathology, it was found that the most frequent underlying condition was infective endocarditis (10 patients), followed by valve replacement (5 patients), nonbacterial thrombotic endocarditis (4 patients), myxoma (2 patients), mural thrombus in the heart (3 patients), abdominal surgery (2 patients), and one patient each had renal cell carcinoma, coronary artery bypass surgery, scuba-diving accident, and atherosclerosis with atheroembolism.[165] The composition of the embolus in these cases was fibrin and platelets (50%), infected clot (16%), atheroembolism (6%), myxoma (2%), air (6%) (patient with splenorenal shunt placement and scuba accident), calcium (6%), foreign body (3%), healed thrombus (3%), and bone marrow (3%, case of renal cell carcinoma).[165]

Before the 1960s, coronary embolism was considered a rare event, most often resulting from active infective endocarditis, with the remainder due to mural thrombus in the left atrium associated with mitral stenosis, or left ventricular mural thrombus associated with myocardial infarction or dilated cardiomyopathy.[165] As more invasive methods of treating cardiac disease have evolved—such as valve replacement and cardiac catheterization and percutaneous coronary interventions—coronary embolism is more commonly being recognized. Prior to the 1960s, the incidence of coronary embolism had been reported in the range of .06–0.8%, and up to 5% in cases of acute myocardial infarction.[165]

General Clinicopathologic Features of Coronary Embolization

Coronary embolism may be diagnosed clinically, and should be suspected when acute myocardial infarction occurs in association with an underlying condition that predisposes to embolism.[166] The most common predisposing conditions are valvular heart disease, a prosthetic heart valve, infective endocarditis, and cardiomyopathy or chronic arrhythmia with mural thrombus. The diagnosis is supported clinically by the demonstration of angiographically normal coronary arteries. Coronary emboli have a predilection for the left coronary arterial system, possibly because there are fewer angles in the proximal course of the left coronary, as compared with the right and circumflex, and also because of its relatively large size. Myocardial infarction occurs in 75% of cases of coronary embolism probably because of poor collateral coronary circulation in patients who have little underlying ischemic heart disease. The appearance of an embolus will vary, depending on its course and composition, and whether or not it directly caused the patient's death or was an incidental finding. Small, distal asymptomatic thromboemboli of no clinical consequence may appear as fibrotic, recanalized occlusions, whereas larger, more recent emboli may comprise a recent platelet-fibrin clot. If a proximal embolus organizes without causing death, large channels consisting of muscular arterial walls with well-developed elastic lamellae may form, and the arterial lumen on angiography may appear normal because such channels are capable of carrying large amounts of blood.

Coronary embolism may present as an acute cardiac event with angina, myocardial infarction, or pulmonary edema. For an embolus to become clinically apparent, however, it usually must become lodged in a large epicardial coronary artery. If myocardial ischemia due to embolic vegetations is treated as coronary thrombosis with streptokinase and aspirin, hemorrhagic infarction may result, underscoring the need to consider embolization as a possible cause of myocardial infarction in patients prone to the development of endocarditis.[167] If infectious embolic coronary stenoses are inadvertantly treated by balloon angioplasty, mycotic aneurysm or cerebral hemorrhage may result.[168] In the absence of treatment, aneurysm formation secondary to coronary embolism may occur if there is no collateral supply.[165]

Treatment of known coronary embolism is possible when diagnosed during life. For thromboembolism in patients with cardiomyopathy, treatment with long-term anticoagulants may prevent further emboli. Additional antiplatelet drugs are also necessary in patients with prosthetic heart valves. Immediate treatment depends on the composition of the embolism. In cases of endocarditis with embolism and myocardial infarction, coronary stenting has been used to regain patency of the artery.[169]

Atheroembolism

Embolism caused by atherosclerotic coronary lesions are generally composed of fibrin platelet clot (see Chapter 2). In some cases, especially after intervention, the embolic material may be primarily cholesterol clefts and calcified deposits (see Chapter 3). As this chapter exclusively deals with nonatherosclerotic disease, the reader is referred to Chapters 2 and 3 for further discussion of this entity.

Calcium Embolism

Embolism of calcified fragments may occur in patients with calcified aortic or mitral stenosis[170] (Fig. 4–28) and after procedures such as valvuloplasty and coronary interventions. More commonly, valve disease results in embolization of infected or sterile vegetations.

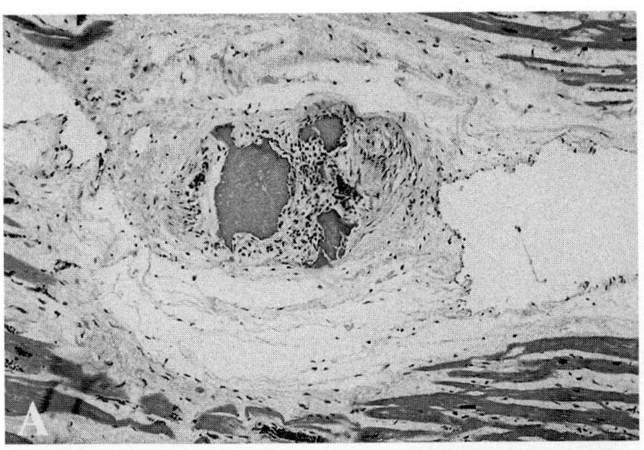

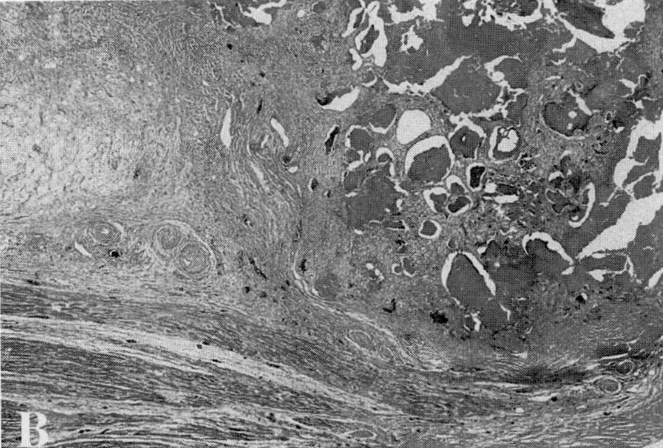

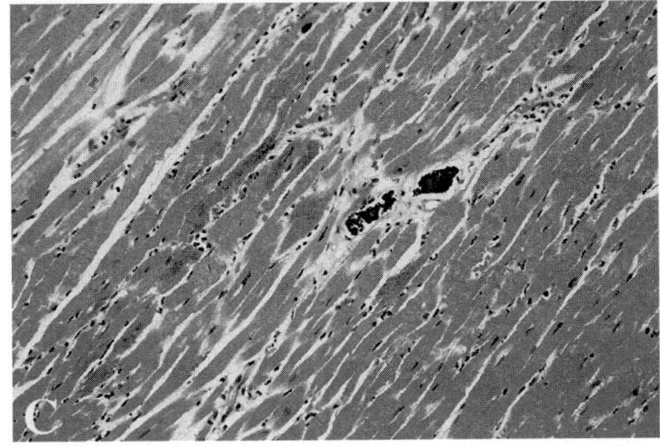

Figure 4–28. Calcium embolism. A 26-year-old man developed refectory arrhythmias and died. At autopsy, there was a congenitally bicuspid aortic valve with severe stenosis and calcification. There were multiple mural calcific emboli (*A*). A 32-year-old male had renal failure, tertiary hyperparathyroidism, and severely calcified mitral valve, with moderate regurgitation, and moderate calcified aortic valve. He died suddenly during dialysis. At autopsy, the heart weighed 820 grams. The mitral annulus was severely calcified (*B*). Many intramural arteries demonstrated calcified emboli (*black areas*) (*C*).

Thromboembolism

Thromboembolism occurs primarily in patients with nonbacterial thrombotic endocarditis,[169] or patients with mural thrombi due to ischemic heart disease or cardiomyopathy.[171, 172] Some patients with cardiomyopathy may die from an acute myocardial infarction, in the absence of coronary atherosclerosis. In such patients, coronary embolism dislodged from the ventricular wall must be suspected, even if not documented at autopsy.[173]

Septic Embolism

Myocardial infarction secondary to infectious endocarditis is one of the more common causes of symptomatic coronary embolization,[174] and occurs in adults, children, and infants.[167–169, 175] In a series from the Armed Forces Institute of Pathology, the most common organisms responsible for fatal septic embolism in the coronary arteries were *S. aureus,* phycomycytes, and candida.[95]

Tumor Embolism

The majority of tumor emboli originate from left atrial myxoma (Fig. 4–29) or aortic papillary fibroelastoma[176, 177] (see Chapter 12). In the case of papillary fibroelastoma, the embolic fragments are typically composed of fibrin that has dislodged from the surface of the tumor. In symptomatic or fatal cases of embolic myxoma, however, the embolic fragments are typically composed of myxoid tumor fragments (Fig. 4–29). Other tumors that have been reported to embolize into coronary arteries include malignant teratoma, colon carcinoma, lung carcinoma, retroperitoneal fibrosarcoma, Hodgkin's disease, myelogenous leukemia, breast carcinoma, liposarcoma, cardiac sarcoma, and malignant fibrous histiocytoma.[165]

Miscellaneous Embolism

Myocardial embolism is extremely rare, and generally the sequela of ruptured myocardial infarction.[165] Iatrogenic myocardial embolism may result from septal myectomy in patients with hypertrophic cardiomyopathy.[178] Bone marrow embolism is rare in the systemic circulation, but may occur paradoxically in patients with patient foramen valve who have been resuscitated, or with extensive bone marrow replacement by tumor.

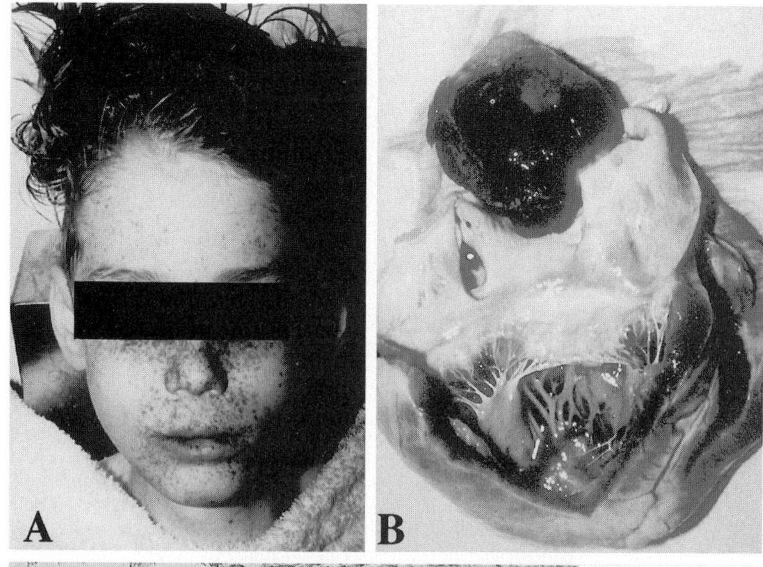

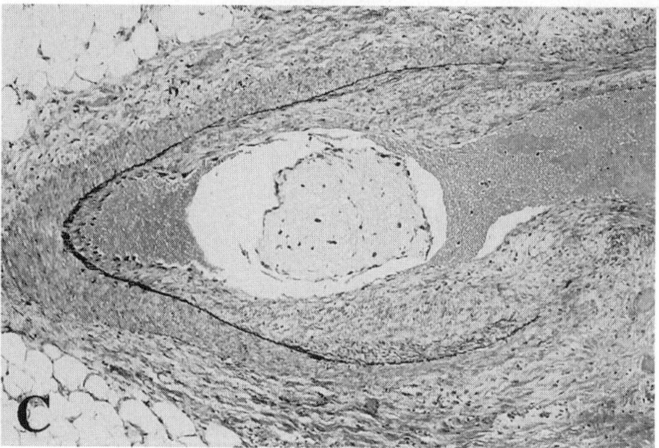

Figure 4–29. Myxoma embolism. A young child died suddenly while taking a walk with his father, who had had surgical removal of a cardiac myxoma 15 years prior. At autopsy, there were multiple ephelides of the face and lips characteristic of the myxoma syndrome (*A*). The left atrium showed a hemorrhagic mass (*B*). There were microscopic embolic tumor fragments in the epicardial coronary arteries (*C*).

NONATHEROSCLEROTIC CORONARY THROMBOSIS

Coagulopathy-related Thrombosis

Congenital Defects in Specific Coagulation Factors

Several reports suggest that congenital defects of coagulation factors may precipitate coronary thrombosis in the absence of atherosclerosis. Protein C deficiency may result in venous and arterial thrombosis, as well as coronary thrombosis in the absence of significant atherosclerosis.[179] Similarly, protein S deficiency as well as the lupus anticoagulant (antiphospholipid syndrome) have been associated with premature coronary thrombosis[180] and clotting of saphenous vein bypass grafts.[181, 182] There is anecdotal evidence that deficiencies of factor XII (Hageman factor) may result in decreased fibrinolysis and coronary thrombosis in the absence of coronary atherosclerosis.[183] It appears that congenital variations in coagulant factors may be important in nonatherosclerotic coronary thrombosis, but that the occurrence of thrombi in normal coronary arteries is rare—other arterial and venous vessels being more often affected.[184]

There has been intense interest in the association between congenital defects in the levels of blood-coagulation factors and the risk for acute coronary atherothrombosis. Polymorphisms of platelet glycoproteins have been associated with atherothrombosis, especially in patients who are smokers (see Chapter 2).[185–187] Elevations of fibrinogen may increase the risk of myocardial infarction; overall, up to 50% of variations in plasma fibrinogen are genetically based.[188] Although the factor V Leiden polymorphism is associated with venous thrombosis, current evidence does not support an increased risk for myocardial infarction,[189, 190] unless there is a concomitant mutation in prothrombin.[191] There is some evidence that increased levels of activated factor VIIa and genetic polymorphisms resulting in increased factor VII levels are associated with coronary thrombosis[192–194]; this association may be enhanced by smoking.[195] Elevations of factor VIII, in association with activated protein C resistance, may be related to premature coronary thrombosis.[196]

Heparin-induced thrombocytopenia (HIT) may result in arterial and venous thrombi, but these complications typically occur in the extremities, and rarely in the coronary arteries.[197] Coronary thrombosis, including clotting of saphenous vein bypass grafts, has been reported in patients who have undergone coronary artery bypass surgery (Fig. 4–30).[198] A series of 1,500 open heart surgeries with cardiopulmonary bypass revealed that 11 patients developed HIT with serious thromboembolic complications, including two cases with graft closure.[199] Pathologically, the clots caused by heparin-induced thrombocytopenia are grossly white, and histologically are rich in platelets.

Polycythemia Vera and Essential Thrombosis

Patients with polycythemia and essential thrombocytosis with platelet counts of over 400,000/mm^3 may develop myocardial ischemia, in up to 19% of patients.[165] However, pathological documentation of the coronary thrombosis in the absence of atherosclerosis has been only rarely achieved.[200] As expected, the coronary thrombi in these patients are rich in platelets, with relatively little fibrin.

Miscellaneous Procoagulant Conditions

Coronary thrombosis in the absence of significant preexisting coronary occlusion has been reported to occur after strenuous exercise[201] and may in part be due to altered coagulation. Although coronary spasm may play a role in such circumstances, long-distance running causes an increase in the number of circulating platelets and alters platelet aggregability. It is well known that cigarette smoking results in alterations in the clotting cascade and platelet

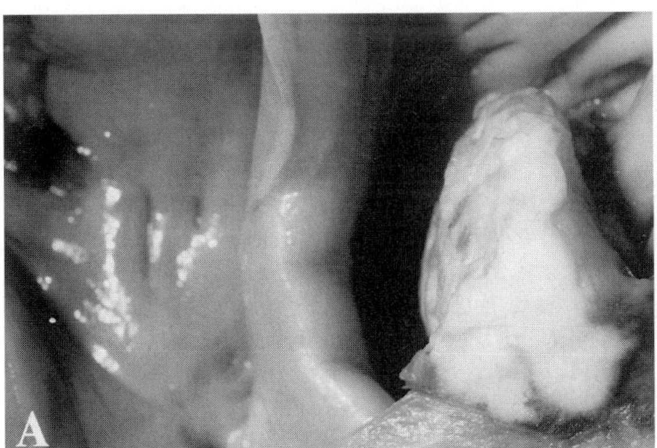

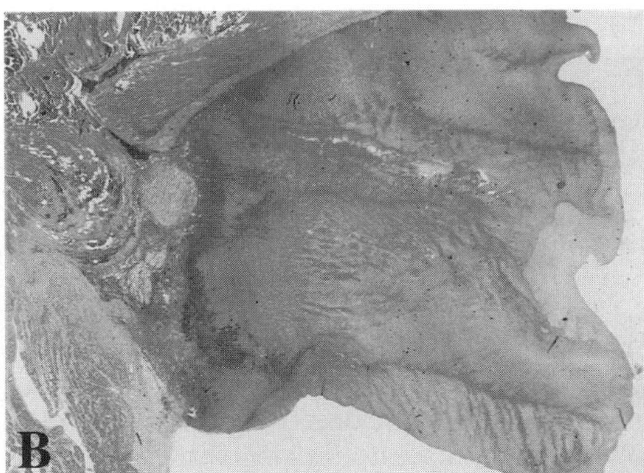

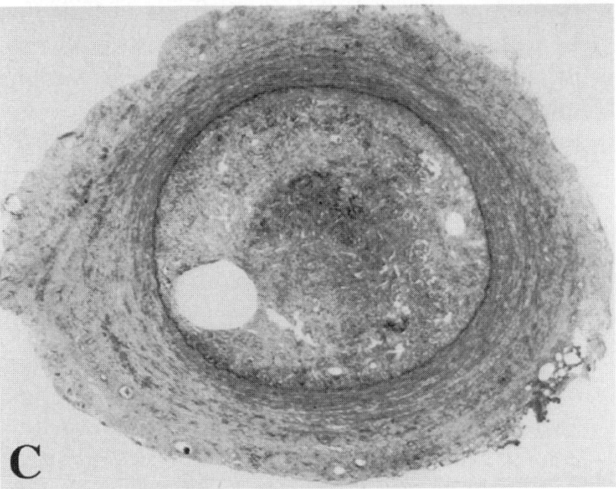

Figure 4–30. Heparin induced thrombocytopenia. A 54-year-old woman developed heparin-induced thrombocytopenia after bypass graft surgery. At autopsy, there were mural thrombi in the right atrium (*A*). Histologic sections of the thrombus demonstrated an arborizing, platelet-rich thrombus (*B*). There were diffuse thrombi within the saphenous vein grafts (*C*), but the native coronary arteries were free of thrombosis. (From Burke AP, Farb A, Mezzetti T, Zech ER, Virmani R. Multiple coronary artery graft occlusion in a fatal case of heparin-induced thrombocytopenia, Chest 144:1494, 1998, with permission.)

aggregability. However, coronary thrombosis in the absence of coronary lesions has not been proven to occur solely on the basis of smoking. As discussed in Chapter 2, cigarette smoking appears to predispose to thrombosis overlying plaque erosion and ruptured atherosclerotic plaques. The effects of smoking are increased in patients with congenital defects in clotting factors (see earlier) and those taking oral contraceptives (see following).

Drug-related Thrombosis

Oral Contraceptive Use

There have been several reports of coronary thrombosis occurring in young women without apparent coronary atherosclerosis.[202–206] Unfortunately, it is unknown if there were concomitant coagulation defects in these patients that may have unmasked an estrogen-induced propensity for thrombosis. In general, it is considered that there is no increased risk for premature myocardial infarction in women taking contraceptives, unless there is concomitant smoking and the age is older than 35 years.[203] A putative association between estrogens and birth-control pills and plaque erosion, a common form of coronary thrombosis in premenopausal women (see Chapter 2), has not yet been documented.

Cocaine

Cocaine abuse is known to predispose to premature coronary thrombosis, as well as arterial spasm.[165] In the few autopsy reports of cocaine-induced coronary thrombosis, approximately 2 of 3 patients had underlying atherosclerosis, and the remainder did not. It appears likely that many patients in the latter category may have developed thrombi overlying eroded coronary plaques, which differ from more typical fibroatheroma (see Chapter 2). There are several potential mechanisms of cocaine-induced myocardial ischemia in addition to vasospasm. Cocaine-induced enhancement of sympathetic activity may increase oxygen demand and decrease myocardial reserve by producing coronary constriction. Acute coronary occlusion by platelet thrombi through alpha-adrenergic mediated increase in platelet aggregability may lead to thrombosis. An autopsy study has demonstrated that there are increased mast cells in the adventitia of cocaine abusers, indicating a possible mechanism of cocaine-induced spasm.[207–211]

Thrombotic Thrombocytopenic Purpura

Clinical Findings and Pathogenesis

Thrombotic microangiopathy (thrombotic thrombocytopenic purpura/hemolytic uremic syndrome) is characterized by hemolytic anemia, red-cell schistocytes on peripheral smear, and thrombocytopenia in the absence of activation of the clotting cascade. Platelet microthrombi occur in various organs, but have a predilection for the heart.[116] In the hemolytic uremic syndrome, renal symptoms dominate, whereas the central nervous system and to a lesser degree the heart are involved in thrombotic thrombocytopenic purpura. Thrombotic thrombocytopenic purpura is primarily seen in females with a peak incidence in the fourth decade. The pathogenetic basis of thrombotic thrombocytopenic purpura is unknown, but probably results from toxic endothelial damage following infections by verotoxin producing *E. coli,* viral infections including HIV, or autoimmune damage by circulating immune complexes. There is evidence that decreased levels of protease results in multimers of von Willebrand factor that contribute to the pathogenesis of thrombotic thrombocytopenic purpura. In sporadic cases, the decreased levels are likely caused by an acquired inhibitor, which is an immunoglubin G,[212, 213] representing a form of autoimmunity. There is an inherited lack of protease in familial cases. Conditions that may trigger thrombotic thrombocytopenic purpura include pregnancy, systemic disease, malignant hypertension, HIV infection, cancer, systemic lupus erythematosus, sickle cell disease, and treatment with anticancer drugs. Clinically, heart failure may occur, and is occasionally rapidly progressive resulting in death. Treatment includes plasma infusion and exchange, sometimes accompanied by antiplatelet drugs, prostacyclin analogs, or steroids. If instituted early in the disease course, treatment results in remission in the majority of patients.[116]

Pathologic Findings

Thrombi are found at autopsy (in decreasing order of frequency) in the brain, heart, lungs, kidneys, adrenals, spleen, and liver. Characteristic cardiac findings include subepicardial hemorrhages, usually grossly evident, with microscopic platelet thrombus present within intramyocardial arterioles (see Fig. 10–6 in Chapter 10). These microthrombi may be difficult to discern on hematoxylin eosin-stained slides, unless there is an index of suspicion. Immunohistochemical stains for platelet glycoprotein receptor and fibrin are helpful in highlighting the thrombi if they are difficult to discern on routine sections.

REFERENCES

1. Virmani R, Rogan K, Cheitlin M. Congenital coronary artery anomalies: Pathologic aspects. In: Virmani R, Forman MD (eds): Nonatherosclerotic ischemic heart disease, pp 153–183. New York: Raven Press, 1989.
2. Virmani R, Burke AP, Farb A, Kark J. Causes of sudden death in young and middle-aged competitive athletes. Cardiol Clin 15:439–466, 1999.
3. Frescura C, Basso C, Thiene G, et al. Anomalous origin of coronary arteries and risk of sudden death: A study based on an autopsy population of congenital heart disease. Hum Pathol 29:689–695, 1998.
4. Daniels C, Bacon J, Fontana ME, Eaton G, Cohen D, Leier CV. Anomalous origin of the left main coronary artery from the pulmonary trunk masquerading as peripartum cardiomyopathy. Am J Cardiol 79:1307–1308, 1997.
5. Nakano A, Konishi T. Long term follow-up in a case of anomalous origin of the left coronary artery from the pulmonary artery. Int J Cardiol 65:301–303, 1998.
6. Taylor AJ, Byers JP, Cheitlin MD, Virmani R. Anomalous right or left coronary artery from the contralateral coronary sinus: "High-risk" abnormalities in the initial coronary artery course and heterogeneous clinical outcomes. Am Heart J 133:428–435, 1997.
7. Basso C, Maron BJ, Corrado D, Thiene G. Clinical profile of congenital coronary artery anomalies with origin from the wrong aortic sinus leading to sudden death in young competitive athletes. J Am Coll Cardiol 35:1493–1501, 2000.
8. Thomas D, Salloum J, Montalescot G, Drobinski G, Artigou JY, Grosgogeat Y. Anomalous coronary arteries coursing between the aorta and pulmonary trunk: Clinical indications for coronary artery bypass. Eur Heart J 12:832–834, 1991.
9. Roberts WC, Shirani J. The four subtypes of anomalous origin of the left main coronary artery from the right aortic sinus (or from the right coronary artery). Am J Cardiol 70:119–121, 1992.
10. Roberts WC, Siegel RJ, Zipes DP. Origin of the right coronary artery from the left sinus of Valsalva and its functional consequences: Analysis of 10 necropsy patients. Am J Cardiol 49:863–868, 1982.
11. Taylor A, Rogan KM, Virmani R. Sudden cardiac death associated with isolated congenital coronary artery anomalies. J Am Coll Cardiol 20:640–647, 1992.
12. Virmani R, Chun P, Goldstein R, Robinowitz M, McAllister H. Acute takeoffs of the coronary arteries along the aortic wall and congenital coronary ostial valve-like ridges: Association with sudden death. J Am Coll Cardiol 3:766–771, 1984.
13. Basso C, Frescura C, Corrado D, et al. Congenital heart disease and sudden death in the young. Hum Pathol 26:1065–1072, 1995.
14. Basso C, Corrado D, Thiene G. Cardiovascular causes of sudden death in young individuals including athletes. Cardiol Rev 7:127–135, 1999.
15. Menke D, Waller B, Pless J. Hypoplastic coronary arteries and high takeoff position of the right coronary ostium. A fatal combination of congenital coronary artery anomalies in an amateur athlete. Chest 88:299, 1985.
16. Shotar A, Busuttil A. Myocardial bars and bridges and sudden death. Forensic Sci Int 68:143–147, 1994.
17. Raizner A, Ishimori T, Verani M. Surgical relief of myocardial ischemia due to myocardial bridges. Am J Cardiol 45:417, 1980.
18. Pittaluga J, de Marchena E, Posada JD, Romanelli R, Morales A. Left anterior descending coronary artery bridge. A cause of early death after cardiac transplantation. Chest 111:511–513, 1997.
19. Morales AR, Romanelli R, Tate LG, Boucek RJ, de Marchena E. Intramural left anterior descending coronary artery: Significance of the depth of the muscular tunnel. Hum Pathol 24:693–701, 1993.
20. Buchika S, Morrow PL, Adams SP. Hypoplastic coronary artery disease within the spectrum of sudden unexpected death in young and middle age adults. Am J Forensic Med Pathol 17:86, 1996.
21. Zugibe FT, Zugibe FT, Jr., Costello JT, Breithaupt MK. Hypoplastic coronary artery disease within the spectrum of sudden unexpected death in young and middle age adults. Am J Forensic Med Pathol 14:276–283, 1993.
22. Taylor AJ, Farb A, Ferguson M, Virmani R. Myocardial infarction associated with physical exertion in a young man. Circulation 96:3201–3204, 1997.
23. Lobo FV, Cairns JA, Stolberg HO, Heggtveit HA. Death following coronary angiography in a young woman with isolated left coronary ostial stenosis. Can J Cardiol 5:149–154, 1989.
24. Knobel B, Rosman P, Kriwisky M, Tamari I. Sudden death and cerebral anoxia in a young woman with congenital ostial stenosis of the left main coronary artery. Catheter Cardiovasc Interv 48:67–70, 1999.
25. Lea JWT, Page DL, Hammon JW, Jr. Congenital ostial stenosis of the right coronary artery repaired by vein patch angioplasty. J Thorac Cardiovasc Surg 92:796–798, 1986.
26. Syed M, Lesch M. Coronary artery aneurysm: A review. Prog Cardiovasc Dis 40:77–84, 1997.
27. Virmani R, Robinowitz M, Atkinson JB, Forman MB, Silver MD, McAllister HA. Acquired coronary arterial aneurysms: An autopsy study of 52 patients. Hum Pathol 17:575–583, 1986.
28. Wong CK, Cheng CH, Lau CP, Leung WH. Asymptomatic congenital coronary artery aneurysm in adulthood. Eur Heart J 10:947–949, 1989.
29. Wei J, Wang DJ. A giant congenital aneurysm of the right coronary artery. Ann Thorac Surg 41:322–324, 1986.
30. Cohle SD. Sudden unexpected death due to atherosclerotic coronary artery aneurysm. Am J Forensic Med Pathol 6:153–157, 1985.
31. Letac B, Cazor JL, Cribier A, Sibille C, Toussaint C. Large multiple coronary artery aneurysm in adult patients: A report on three patients and a review of the literature. Am Heart J 99:694–700, 1980.
32. Schumacher G, Roithmaier A, Lorenz HP, et al. Congenital coronary artery fistula in infancy and childhood: Diagnostic and therapeutic aspects. Thorac Cardiovasc Surg 45:287–294, 1997.

33. Sunder KR, Balakrishnan KG, Tharakan JA, et al. Coronary artery fistula in children and adults: A review of 25 cases with long-term observations. Int J Cardiol 58:47–53, 1997.
34. Kiuchi K, Nejima J, Kikuchi A, Takayama M, Takano T, Hayakawa H. Left coronary artery–left ventricular fistula with acute myocardial infarction, representing the coronary steal phenomenon: A case report. J Cardiol 34:279–284, 1999.
35. Lau G. Sudden death arising from a congenital coronary artery fistula. Forensic Sci Int 73:125–130, 1995.
36. Topcuoglu MS, Salih OK, San M, Kayhan C, Ulus T. Aorto-left atrial fistula with bicuspid aortic valve and coronary artery origin anomaly. Ann Thorac Surg 63:854–856, 1997.
37. Swalwell CI, Reddy SK, Rao VJ. Sudden death due to unsuspected coronary vasculitis. Am J Forensic Med Pathol 12:306–312, 1991.
38. Pereira MC, Filho AA, Lastoria S, Franco M. Inflammatory aneurysm of the abdominal aorta with coronary arteritis. Arch Pathol Lab Med 105:678–679, 1981.
39. Cohle SD, Lie JT. Inflammatory aneurysm of the aorta, aortitis, and coronary arteritis. Arch Pathol Lab Med 112:1121–1125, 1988.
40. Dettmeyer R, Amberg R, Varchmin-Schultheiss K, Madea B. Sudden cardiac death due to atypical isolated coronary arteritis? Forensic Sci Int 95:193–200, 1998.
41. Laupland KB, Dele Davies H. Epidemiology, etiology, and management of Kawasaki disease: State of the art. Pediatr Cardiol 20:177–183, 1999.
42. Holman RC, Belay ED, Clarke MJ, Kaufman SF, Schonberger LB. Kawasaki syndrome among American Indian and Alaska Native children, 1980 through 1995. Pediatr Infect Dis J 18:451–455, 1999.
43. Davis RL, Waller PL, Mueller BA, Dykewicz CA, Schonberger LB. Kawasaki syndrome in Washington State. Race-specific incidence rates and residential proximity to water. Arch Pediatr Adolesc Med 149:66–69, 1995.
44. Rowley AH, Shulman ST. Kawasaki syndrome. Pediatr Clin North Am 46:313–329, 1999.
45. Rauch AM, Glode MP, Wiggins JW, Jr., et al. Outbreak of Kawasaki syndrome in Denver, Colorado: Association with rug and carpet cleaning. Pediatrics 87:663–669, 1991.
46. Leung DY. Kawasaki syndrome: Immunomodulatory benefit and potential toxin neutralization by intravenous immune globulin. Clin Exp Immunol 104 Suppl 1:49–54, 1996.
47. Uchiyama T, Kato H. The pathogenesis of Kawasaki disease and superantigens. Jpn J Infect Dis 52:141–145, 1999.
48. Burns JC, Wiggins JW, Jr., Toews WH, et al. Clinical spectrum of Kawasaki disease in infants younger than 6 months of age. J Pediatr 109:759–763, 1986.
49. Terai M, Shulman ST. Prevalence of coronary artery abnormalities in Kawasaki disease is highly dependent on gamma globulin dose but independent of salicylate dose. J Pediatr 131:888–893, 1997.
50. Shinohara M, Sone K, Tomomasa T, Morikawa A. Corticosteroids in the treatment of the acute phase of Kawasaki disease. J Pediatr 135:465–469, 1999.
51. Kato H, Sugimura T, Akagi T, et al. Long-term consequences of Kawasaki disease. A 10- to 21-year follow-up study of 594 patients. Circulation 94:1379–1385, 1996.
52. Landing BH, Larson EJ. Pathological features of Kawasaki disease (mucocutaneous lymph node syndrome). Am J Cardiovasc Pathol 1:218–229, 1987.
53. Fujiwara H, Hamashima Y. Pathology of the heart in Kawasaki disease. Pediatrics 61:100–107, 1978.
54. Fujiwara H, Fujiwara T, Kao T-C, Ohshio G, Hamashima Y. Pathology of Kawasaki disease in the healed stage. Acta Pathol Jpn 36:857–867, 1986.
55. Fujiwara T, Fujiwara H, Nakano H. Pathological features of coronary arteries in children with Kawasaki disease in which coronary arterial aneurysm was absent at autopsy. Quantitative analysis. Circulation 78:345–350, 1988.
56. Kawasaki T, Kosaki F, Okawa S, Shigematsu I, Yanagawa H. A new infantile acute febrile mucocutaneous lymph node syndrome (MLNS) prevailing in Japan. Pediatrics 54:271–276, 1974.
57. Hirose K, Nakaumura Y, Yanagawa H. Cardiac sequelae of Kawasaki disease in Japan over 10 years. Acta Paediatr Jpn 37:667–671, 1995.
58. Bruke AP, Virmani R, Perry LW, Li L, King TM, Smialek J. Fatal Kawasaki disease with coronary arteritis and no coronary aneurysms. Pediatrics 101:108, 1998.
59. Akagi T, Rose V, Benson LN, Newman A, Freedom RM. Outcome of coronary artery aneurysms after Kawasaki disease. J Pediatr 121:689–694, 1992.
60. Burns JC, Shike H, Gordon JB, Malhotra A, Schoenwetter M, Kawasaki T. Sequelae of Kawasaki disease in adolescents and young adults. J Am Coll Cardiol 28:253–257, 1996.
61. Ino T, Akimoto K, Nishimoto K, et al. Myocarditis in Kawasaki disease. Am Heart J 17:1400–1401, 1989.
62. Takahashi M. Myocarditis in Kawasaki syndrome. A minor villain? Circulation 79:1398–1400, 1989.
63. Matsuura H, Ishikita T, Yamamoto S, et al. Gallium-67 myocardial imaging for the detection of myocarditis in the acute phase of Kawasaki disease (mucocutaneous lymph node syndrome): The usefulness of single photon emission computed tomography. Br Heart J 58:385–392, 1987.
64. Muzik O, Paridon SM, Singh TP, Morrow WR, Dayanikli F, Di Carli MF. Quantification of myocardial blood flow and flow reserve in children with a history of Kawasaki disease and normal coronary arteries using positron emission tomography. J Am Coll Cardiol 28:757–762, 1996.
65. Aufderheide AC, Henke BW, Parker EH. Granulomatous coronary arteritis (Takayasu's disease). Arch Pathol Lab Med 105:647–649, 1981.
66. Payan HM, Gilbert EF. Granulomatous coronary arteritis. Arch Pathol Lab Med 108:136–137, 1984.
67. Tanaka A, Fukayama M, Funata N, Koike M, Saito K. Coronary arteritis and aortoarteritis in the elderly males. A report of two autopsy cases with review of the literature. Virchows Arch A Pathol Anat Histopathol 414:9–14, 1988.
68. Hall S, Barr W, Lie JT, Stanson AW, Kazmier FJ, Hunder GG. Takayasu arteritis. A study of 32 North American patients. Medicine (Baltimore) 64:89–99, 1985.
69. Suzuki H, Daida H, Tanaka M, et al. Giant aneurysm of the left main coronary artery in Takayasu aortitis. Heart 81:214–217, 1999.
70. Arend WP, Michel BA, Bloch DA, et al. The American College of Rheumatology 1990 criteria for the classification of Takayasu arteritis. Arthritis Rheum 33:1129–1134, 1990.

71. Noma M, Sugihara M, Kikuchi Y. Isolated ostial stenosis in Takayasu's arteritis: Case report and review of the literature. Angiology 44:839–844, 1993.
72. Panja M, Kar AK, Dutta AL, Chhetri M, Kumar S, Panja S. Cardiac involvement in non-specific aortoarteritis. Int J Cardiol 34:289–295, 1992.
73. Talwar KK, Kumar K, Chopra P, et al. Cardiac involvement in nonspecific aortoarteritis (Takayasu's arteritis). Am Heart J 122:1666–1670, 1991.
74. Amano J, Suzuki A. Coronary artery involvement in Takayasu's arteritis. Collective review and guideline for surgical treatment. J Thorac Cardiovasc Surg 102:554–560, 1991.
75. Matsubara O, Kuwata T, Nemoto T, Kasuga T, Numano F. Coronary artery lesions in Takayasu arteritis: Pathological considerations. Heart Vessels Suppl 7:26–31, 1992.
76. Noma M, Kikuchi Y, Yoshimura H, Yamamoto H, Tajimi T. Coronary ectasia in Takayasu's arteritis. Am Heart J 126:459–461, 1993.
77. Kumar S, Subramanyan R, Mandalam KR, et al. Aneurysmal form of aortoarteritis (Takayasu's disease): Analysis of thirty cases. Clin Radiol 42:342–347, 1990.
78. Dev V, Shrivastava S, Rajani M. Percutaneous transluminal balloon angioplasty in Takayasu's aortitis: Persistent benefit over two years. Am Heart J 120:222–224, 1990.
79. Essop MR, Rothlisberger C, Skoularigis J, Sareli P. Angioplasty for treatment of Takayasu's arteriopathy: Case reports. Angiology 44:833–837, 1993.
80. Amano J, Suzuki A. Surgical treatment of cardiac involvement in Takayasu arteritis. Heart Vessels Suppl 7:168–178, 1992.
81. Fujiwara T, Masaki H, Yamane H, Yoshida H, Katsumura T. Coronary ostial endarterectomy in Takayasu's aortitis—confirmation of patency nine years postsurgically. Jpn Circ J 56:556–559, 1992.
82. Doherty NE, Siegel RJ. Cardiovascular manifestations of systemic lupus erythematosus. Am Heart J 110:1257–1265, 1985.
83. Bruce IN, Gladman DD, Urowitz MB. Premature atherosclerosis in systemic lupus erythematosus. Rheum Dis Clin North Am 26:257–278, 2000.
84. Kim WU, Min JK, Lee SH, Park SH, Cho CS, Kim HY. Causes of death in Korean patients with systemic lupus erythematosus: A single center retrospective study. Clin Exp Rheumatol 17:539–545, 1999.
85. Petri M. Detection of coronary artery disease and the role of traditional risk factors in the Hopkins Lupus Cohort. Lupus 9:170–175, 2000.
86. Moder KG, Miller TD, Tazelaar HD. Cardiac involvement in systemic lupus erythematosus. Mayo Clin Proc 74:275–284, 1999.
87. Chu PH, Ko YS, Hsu TS, Luo SF, Chiang CW. Unusual coronary artery ectasia and stenosis in a patient with systemic lupus erythematosus and acute myocardial infarction. J Rheumatol 25:807–809, 1998.
88. Nobrega TP, Klodas E, Breen JF, Liggett SP, Higano ST, Reeder GS. Giant coronary artery aneurysms and myocardial infarction in a patient with systemic lupus erythematosus. Cathet Cardiovasc Diagn 39:75–79, 1996.
89. Wilson VE, Eck SL, Bates ER. Evaluation and treatment of acute mycoardial infarction complicating systemic lupus erythematosus. Chest 101:420, 1992.
90. Lakatos J, Harsagyi A. Serum total, HDL, LDL cholesterol, and triglyceride levels in patients with rheumatoid arthritis. Clin Biochem 21:93–96, 1998.
91. Morris PB, Imber MJ, Heinsimer JA, Hlatky MA, Reimer KA. Rheumatoid arthritis and coronary arteritis. Am J Cardiol 57:689–690, 1986.
92. Rudge SR, Jones JK, Macfarlane A. Coronary and peripheral vascular occlusion due to rheumatoid arthritis. Postgrad Med J 57:196–198, 1981.
93. van Albada-Kuipers GA, Bruijn JA, Westedt ML, Breedveld FC, Eulderink F. Coronary arteritis complicating rheumatoid arteritis. Ann Rheum Dis 45:963–965, 1986.
94. Gravallese EM, Corson JM, Coblyn JS, Pinkus GS, Weinblatt ME. Rheumatoid aortitis: A rarely recognized but clinically significant entity. Medicine (Baltimore) 68:95–106, 1989.
95. Darcy TP, Virmani R. Coronary vasculitis. In: Virmani R, Forman MB (eds): Nonatherosclerotic ischemic heart disease, pp 237–275. New York: Raven Press, 1989.
96. Bely M, Apathy A, Beke-Martos E. Cardiac changes in rheumatoid arthritis. Acta Morphol Hung 40:149–186, 1992.
97. Kvalvik AG, Jones MA, Symmons DP. Mortality in a cohort of Norwegian patients with rheumatoid arthritis followed from 1977 to 1992. Scand J Rheumatol 29:29–37, 2000.
98. Lie JT, Failoni DD, Davis DC, Jr. Temporal arteritis with giant cell aortitis, coronary arteritis, and myocardial infarction. Arch Pathol Lab Med 110:857–860, 1986.
99. Freddo T, Price M, Kase C, Goldstein MP. Myocardial infarction and coronary artery involvement in giant cell arteritis. Optom Vis Sci 76:14–18, 1999.
100. Martin JF, Kittas C, Triger DR. Giant cell arteritis of coronary arteries causing myocardial infarction. Br Heart J 43:487–489, 1980.
101. Saito S, Arai H, Kim K, Aoki N. Acute myocardial infarction in a young adult due to solitary giant cell arteritis of the coronary artery diagnosed antemortemly by primary directional coronary atherectomy. Cathet Cardiovasc Diagn 33:245–249, 1994.
102. Bloch T, Waller BF, Vakili ST. Giant cell arteritis of the coronary arteries. Indiana Med 80:262–264, 1987.
103. Paul RA, Helle MJ, Tarssanen LT. Sudden death as sole symptom of coronary arteritis. Ann Med 22:161–162, 1990.
104. Cassling RS, Lortz JB, Olson DR, Hubbard TF, McManus BM. Fatal vasculitis (periarteritis nodosa) of the coronary arteries: Angiographic ambiguities and absence of aneurysms at autopsy. J Am Coll Cardiol 6:707–714, 1985.
105. Holsinger DR, Osmundson PJ, Edwards JE. The heart in periarteritis nodosa. Circulation 25:610–618, 1962.
106. Gatenby PA, Lytton DG, Bulteau VG, O'Reilly B, Basten A: Myocardial infarction in Wegener's granulomatosis. Aust N Z J Med 6:336–340, 1976.
107. Parry SD, Clark DM, Campbell J. Coronary arteritis in Wegener's granulomatosis causing fatal myocardial infarction. Hosp Med 61:284–285, 2000.
108. Fuertes Beneitez J, Garcia-Iglesias F, Gallego Garcia de Vinuesa P, et al. Acute myocardial infarction secondary to Wegener's granulomatosis. Rev Esp Cardiol 51:336-339, 1998.
109. Schiavone WA, Ahmad M, Ockner SA. Unusual cardiac complications of Wegener's granulomatosis. Chest 88:745–748, 1985.
110. Allen DC, Doherty CC, O'Reilly DP. Pathology of the heart and the cardiac conduction system in Wegener's granulomatosis. Br Heart J 52:674–678, 1984.

111. Morbini P, Dal Bello B, Arbustini E. Coronary artery inflammation and thrombosis in Wegener's granulomatosis–polyarteritis nodosa overlap syndrome. G Ital Cardiol 28:377–382, 1998.
112. Hunsaker JCD, O'Connor WN, Lie JT. Spontaneous coronary arterial dissection and isolated eosinophilic coronary arteritis: Sudden cardiac death in a patient with a limited variant of Churg–Strauss syndrome. Mayo Clin Proc 67:761–766, 1992.
113. Lie JT, Bayardo RJ. Isolated eosinophilic coronary arteritis and eosinophilic myocarditis. A limited form of Churg–Strauss syndrome. Arch Pathol Lab Med 113:199–201, 1989.
114. Lanham JG, Elkon KB, Pusey CD, Hughes GR. Systemic vasculitis with asthma and eosinophilia: A clinical approach to the Churg–Strauss syndrome. Medicine (Baltimore) 63:65–81, 1984.
115. Kajihara H, Kato Y, Takanashi A, et al. Periarteritis of coronary arteries with severe eosinophilic infiltration. A new pathologic entity (eosinophilic periarteritis)? Pathol Res Pract 184:46–52, 1988.
116. Ruggenenti P, Lutz J, Remuzzi G. Pathogenesis and treatment of thrombotic microangiopathy. Kidney Int Suppl 58:S97–101, 1997.
117. Townend JN, Emery P, Davies MK, Littler WA. Acute aortitis and aortic incompetence due to systemic rheumatological disorders. Int J Cardiol 33:253–258, 1991.
118. de Almeida FA, Albanesi Filho FM, de Albuquerque EM, Magalhaes EC, de Menezes ME. Echocardiography in the evaluation of cardiac involvement in seronegative spondylo-arthropathies. Medicina (B Aires) 55:231–236, 1995.
119. Hoogland YT, Alexander EP, Patterson RH, Nashel DJ. Coronary artery stenosis in Reiter's syndrome: A complication of aortitis. J Rheumatol 21:757–759, 1994.
120. Bulkley BH, Roberts WC. Ankylosing spondylitis and aortic regurgitation: Description of the characteristic cardiovascular lesion from study of eight necro patients. Circulation 48:1014–1018, 1973.
121. Herskowitz A, Cho S, Factor SM. Syphilitic arteritis involving proximal coronary arteries. N Y State J Med 80:971–974, 1980.
122. Dishop MK, Yoneda K. Staphylococcal coronary arteritis as a complication of septicemia. Arch Pathol Lab Med 123:332–334, 1999.
123. Hammond EH, Yowell RL, Nunoda S, et al. Vascular (humoral) rejection in heart transplantation: Pathologic observations and clinical implications. J Heart Transplant 8:430–443, 1989.
124. Hammond EH, Yowell RL, Price GD, et al. Vascular rejection and its relationship to allograft coronary artery disease. J Heart Lung Transplant 11:S111–119, 1992.
125. Radio S, Wood S, Wilson J, Lin H, Winters G, McManus B. Allograft vascular disease: Comparison of heart and other grafted organs. Transplant Proc 28:496–499, 1996.
126. Ventura HO, Mehra MR, Smart FW, Stapleton DD. Cardiac allograft vasculopathy: Current concepts. Am Heart J 129:791–799, 1995.
127. Lamich R, Ballester M, Marti V, et al. Efficacy of augmented immunosuppressive therapy for early vasculopathy in heart transplantation. J Am Coll Cardiol 32:413–419, 1998.
128. Mehra MR, Ventura HO, Chambers RB, Ramireddy K, Smart FW, Stapleton DD. The prognostic impact of immunosuppression and cellular rejection on cardiac allograft vasculopathy: Time for a reappraisal. J Heart Lung Transplant 16:743–751, 1997.
129. Vassalli G, Kaski JC, Tousoulis D, et al. Low-dose cyclosporine treatment fails to prevent coronary luminal narrowing after heart transplantation. J Heart Lung Transplant 15:612–619, 1996.
130. Tanaka H, Sukhova GK, Libby P. Interaction of the allogeneic state and hypercholesterolemia in arterial lesion formation in experimental cardiac allografts. Arterioscler Thromb 14:734–745, 1994.
131. Esper E, Glagov S, Karp RB, et al. Role of hypercholesterolemia in accelerated transplant coronary vasculopathy: Results of surgical therapy with partial ileal bypass in rabbits undergoing heterotopic heart transplantation. J Heart Lung Transplant 16:420–435, 1997.
132. Russell PS, Chase CM, Colvin RB. Alloantibody- and T cell-mediated immunity in the pathogenesis of transplant arteriosclerosis: Lack of progression to sclerotic lesions in B cell-deficient mice. Transplantation 64:1531–1536, 1997.
133. Madsen JC, Yamada K, Allan JS, et al. Transplantation tolerance prevents cardiac allograft vasculopathy in major histocompatibility complex class I-disparate miniature swine. Transplantation 65:304–313, 1998.
134. Aziz S, McDonald TO, Gohra H. Transplant arterial vasculopathy: Evidence for a dual pattern of endothelial injury and the source of smooth muscle cells in lesions of intimal hyperplasia. J Heart Lung Transplant 14:S123–136, 1995.
135. Furukawa Y, Becker G, Stinn JL, Shimizu K, Libby P, Mitchell RN. Interleukin-10 (IL-10) augments allograft arterial disease: Paradoxical effects of IL-10 in vivo. Am J Pathol 155:1929–1939, 1999.
136. Nagano H, Mitchell RN, Taylor MK, Hasegawa S, Tilney NL, Libby P. Interferon-gamma deficiency prevents coronary arteriosclerosis but not myocardial rejection in transplanted mouse hearts. J Clin Invest 100:550–557, 1997.
137. Hasegawa S, Becker G, Nagano H, Libby P, Mitchell RN. Pattern of graft- and host-specific MHC class II expression in long-term murine cardiac allografts: Origin of inflammatory and vascular wall cells. Am J Pathol 153:69–79, 1998.
138. Libby P, Salomon RN, Payne DD, Schoen FJ, Pober JS. Functions of vascular wall cells related to development of transplantation-associated coronary arteriosclerosis. Transplant Proc 21:3677–3684, 1989.
139. Libby P, Tanaka H. The pathogenesis of coronary arteriosclerosis ("chronic rejection") in transplanted hearts. Clin Transplant 8:313–318, 1994.
140. Hosenpud JD, Morris TE, Shipley GD, Mauck KA, Wagner CR. Cardiac allograft vasculopathy. Preferential regulation of endothelial cell-derived mesenchymal growth factors in response to a donor-specific cell-mediated allogeneic response. Transplantation 61:939–948, 1996.
141. Foerster A. Vascular rejection in cardiac transplantation. A morphological study of 25 human cardiac allografts. APMIS 100:367–376, 1992.
142. Johnson DE, Gao SZ, Schroeder JS, DeCampli WM, Billingham ME. The spectrum of coronary artery pathologic findings in human cardiac allografts. J Heart Transplant 8:349–359, 1989.
143. Higuchi ML, Benvenuti LA, Demarchi LM, Libby P. Histological evidence of concomitant intramyocardial and epicardial vasculitis in necropsied heart allografts:

A possible relationship with graft coronary arteriosclerosis. Transplantation 67:1569–1576, 1999.
144. Gravanis MB. Allograft heart accelerated atherosclerosis: Evidence for cell-mediated immunity in pathogenesis. Mod Pathol 2:405–505, 1989.
145. Hruban RH, Beschorner WE, Baumgartner WA, et al. Accelerated arteriosclerosis in heart transplant recipients in associated with a T-lymphocyte-mediated endothelialitis. Am J Pathol 137:871–882, 1990.
146. Koskinen P, Lemstrom K, Bruggeman C, Lautenschlager I, Hayry P. Acute cytomegalovirus infection induces a subendothelial inflammation (endothelialitis) in the allograft vascular wall. A possible linkage with enhanced allograft arteriosclerosis. Am J Pathol 144:41–50, 1994.
147. Paavonen T, Mennander A, Lautenschlager I, Mattila S, Hayry P. Endothelialitis and accelerated arteriosclerosis in human heart transplant coronaries. J Heart Lung Transplant 12:117–122, 1993.
148. Winters GL, Schoen FJ. Graft arteriosclerosis-induced myocardial pathology in heart transplant recipients: Predictive value of endomyocardial biopsy. J Heart Lung Transplant 16:985–993, 1997.
149. Antonovych TT, Sabnis SG, Austin HA, et al. Cyclosporine-A induced arteriolopathy. Transplant Proc 20, Supplement 3:951–958, 1988.
150. Allan JS, Choo JK, Vesga L, et al. Cardiac allograft vasculopathy is abrogated by anti-CD8 monoclonal antibody therapy. Ann Thorac Surg 64:1019–1025, 1997.
151. Hering D, Piper C, Hohmann C, Schultheiss HP, Horstkotte D. Prospective study of the incidence, pathogenesis and therapy of spontaneous, by coronary angiography diagnosed coronary artery dissection. Z Kardiol 87:961–970, 1998.
152. Virmani R, Forman MB. Coronary Artery Dissections. In: Virmani R, Forman MB (eds): Nonatherosclerotic Ischemic Heart Disease, pp 325–354. New York: Raven Press, 1989.
153. Yoshida K, Mori S, Tomari S, et al. Coronary artery bypass grafting for spontaneous coronary artery dissection: A case report and a review of the literature. Ann Thorac Cardiovasc Surg 6:57–60, 2000.
154. Jaffe BD, Broderick TM, Leier CV. Cocaine-induced coronary–artery dissection. N Engl J Med 330:510–511, 1994.
155. Virmani R, Forman MB, Robinowitz M, McAllister HA, Jr. Coronary artery dissections. Cardiol Clin 2:633–646, 1984.
156. Borczuk AC, van Hoeven KH, Factor SM. Review and hypothesis: The eosinophil and peripartum heart disease (myocarditis and coronary artery dissection)—coincidence or pathogenetic significance? Cardiovasc Res 33:527–532, 1997.
157. Robinowitz M, Virmani R, McAllister HA, Jr. Spontaneous coronary artery dissection and eosinophilic inflammation: A cause and effect relationship? Am J Med 72:923–928, 1982.
158. Basso C, Morgagni GL, Thiene G. Spontaneous coronary artery dissection: A neglected cause of acute myocardial ischaemia and sudden death. Heart 75:451–454, 1996.
159. Zampieri P, Aggio S, Roncon L, et al. Follow up after spontaneous coronary artery dissection: A report of five cases. Heart 75:206–209, 1996.
160. Jorgensen MB, Aharonian V, Mansukhani P, Mahrer PR. Spontaneous coronary dissection: A cluster of cases with this rare finding. Am Heart J 127:1382–1387, 1994.
161. Lee TM, Liau CS. Spontaneous coronary artery dissection in an elderly woman with acute inferior myocardial infarction. A case report. Angiology 46:847–851, 1995.
162. Kouvaras G, Tsamis G, Polydorou A. Spontaneous left anterior descending coronary artery dissection. Case report presentation and review of the relevant literature. Jpn Heart J 34:639–642, 1993.
163. Chu KH, Menapace FJ, Blankenship JC, Hausch R, Harrington T. Polyarteritis nodosa presenting as acute myocardial infarction with coronary dissection. Cathet Cardiovasc Diagn 44:320–324, 1998.
164. Elming H, Kober L. Spontaneous coronary artery dissection. Case report and literature review. Scand Cardiovasc J 33:175–179, 1999.
165. Atkinson JB, Forman MB, Virmani R. Emboli and thrombi in coronary arteries. In: Virmani R, Forman M (eds): Nonatherosclerotic Ischemic Heart Disease, pp 355–385. New York: Raven Press, 1989.
166. Charles RG, Epstein EJ. Diagnosis of coronary embolism: A review. J R Soc Med 76:863–869, 1983.
167. Connolly DL, Dardas PS, Crowley JJ, Kenny A, Petch MC. Acute coronary embolism complicating aortic valve endocarditis treated with streptokinase and aspirin. A case report. J Heart Valve Dis 3:245—246, 1994.
168. Herzog CA, Henry TD, Zimmer SD. Bacterial endocarditis presenting as acute myocardial infarction: A cautionary note for the era of reperfusion. Am J Med 90:392–397, 1991.
169. Glazier JJ, McGinnity JG, Spears JR. Coronary embolism complicating aortic valve endocarditis: Treatment with placement of an intracoronary stent. Clin Cardiol 20:885–888, 1997.
170. Charles RG, Epstein EJ, Holt S, Coulshed N. Coronary embolism in valvular heart disease. Q J Med 51:147–161, 1982.
171. Aiello VD, Mansur AJ, Favaratto D. Rupture of posteromedial papillary muscle as a mechanism of death in dilated cardiomyopathy. Int J Cardiol 54:73–75, 1996.
172. Maddoux GL, Goss JE, Ramo BW, et al. Left main coronary artery embolism: A case report. Cathet Cardiovasc Diagn 13:394–397, 1987.
173. Simoes MV, Felix PR, Marin-Neto JA. Acute myocardial infarction complicating the clinical course of dilated cardiomyopathy in childhood. Chest 101:271–272, 1992.
174. Perera R, Noack S, Dong W. Acute myocardial infarction due to septic coronary embolism. N Engl J Med 342:977–978, 2000.
175. Ueda M, Becker AE, Fujimoto T, Tamai H. Bacterial endocarditis of the aortic valve with septic coronary embolism and myocardial infarction in a 4-month old baby. Eur Heart J 7:449–451, 1986.
176. Abascal VM, Kasznica J, Aldea G, Davidoff R. Left atrial myxoma and acute myocardial infarction. A dangerous duo in the thrombolytic agent era. Chest 109:1106–1108, 1996.
177. Eckstein FS, Schafers HJ, Grote J, Mugge A, Borst HG. Papillary fibroelastoma of the aortic valve presenting with myocardial infarction. Ann Thorac Surg 60:206–208, 1995.
178. Chan S, Silver MD. Fatal myocardial embolus after myectomy. Can J Cardiol 16:207–211, 2000.
179. Bux-Gewehr I, Nacke A, Feurle GE. Recurring myocardial infarction in a 35-year-old woman. Heart 81:316–317, 1999.
180. Mills TJ, Safford RE, Kazmier FJ. Myocardial infarction, persistent coronary artery thrombosis and lupus anticoagulant. Int J Cardiol 21:190–194, 1988.

181. De Paulis R, Bognolo G, Tomai F, Bassano C, Tracey M, Chiariello L. Early coronary artery bypass graft thrombosis in a patient with protein S deficiency. Eur J Cardiothorac Surg 10:470–472, 1996.
182. Beattie S, Norton M, Doll D. Coronary thrombosis associated with inherited protein S deficiency: A case report. Heart Lung 26:76–79, 1997.
183. Penny WJ, Colvin BT, Brooks N. Myocardial infarction with normal coronary arteries and factor XII deficiency. Br Heart J 53:230–234, 1985.
184. Lande G, Dantec V, Trossaert M, Godin JF, Le Marec H. Do inherited prothrombotic factors have a role in myocardial infarction with normal coronary arteriogram? J Intern Med 244:543–544, 1998.
185. Moshfegh K, Wuillemin WA, Redondo M, et al. Association of two silent polymorphisms of platelet glycoprotein Ia/IIa receptor with risk of myocardial infarction: A case-control study. Lancet 353:351–354, 1999.
186. Ridker PM, Hennekens CH, Schmitz C, Stampfer MJ, Lindpaintner K. PIA1/A2 polymorphism of platelet glycoprotein IIIa and risks of myocardial infarction, stroke, and venous thrombosis. Lancet 349:385–388, 1997.
187. Sperr WR, Huber K, Roden M, et al. Inherited platelet glycoprotein polymorphisms and a risk for coronary heart disease in young central Europeans. Thromb Res 90:117–123, 1998.
188. Kannel WB, Wolf PA, Vastelli WP, D'Agostino RB. Fibrinogen and the risk of cardiovascular disease: The Framingham study. JAMA 258:1183–1186, 1987.
189. Gowda MS, Zucker ML, Vacek JL, et al. Incidence of factor V Leiden in patients with acute myocardial infarction. J Thromb Thrombolysis 9:43–45, 2000.
190. Mangoni ED, Davies GJ, Tuddenham EG, Ruggiero G. Factor V Leiden in patients with acute coronary syndromes. Ann Ital Med Int 14:15–19, 1999.
191. Doggen CJ, Cats VM, Bertina RM, Rosendaal FR. Interaction of coagulation defects and cardiovascular risk factors: Increased risk of myocardial infarction associated with factor V Leiden or prothrombin 20210A. Circulation 97:1037–1041, 1998.
192. Iacoviello L, Di Castelnuovo A, De Knijff P, et al. Polymorphisms in the coagulation factor VII gene and the risk of myocardial infarction. N Engl J Med 338:79–85, 1998.
193. Heinrich J, Balleisen L, Schulte H, Assmann G, van de Loo J. Fibrinogen and factor VII in the prediction of coronary risk. Results from the PROCAM study in healthy men. Arterioscler Thromb 14:54–59, 1994.
194. Carvalho de Sousa J, Azevedo J, Soria C, et al. Factor VII hyperactivity in acute myocardial thrombosis. A relation to the coagulation activation. Thromb Res 51:165–173, 1988.
195. Junker R, Heinrich J, Schulte H, van de Loo J, Assmann G. Coagulation factor VII and the risk of coronary heart disease in healthy men. Arterioscler Thromb Vasc Biol 17:1539–1544, 1997.
196. Gorog DA, Rakhit R, Parums D, Laffan M, Davies GJ. Raised factor VIII is associated with coronary thrombotic events. Heart 80:415–417, 1998.
197. Warkentin TE, Chong BH, Greinacher A. Heparin-induced thrombocytopenia: Towards consensus. Thromb Haemost 79:1–7, 1998.
198. Burke AP, Farb A, Mezzetti T, Zech ER, Virmani R. Multiple coronary artery graft occlusion in a fatal case of heparin-induced thrombocytopenia. Chest 114:1492–1495, 1998.
199. Singer RL, Mannion JD, Bauer TL, Armenti FR, Edie RN. Complications from heparin-induced thrombocytopenia in patients undergoing cardiopulmonary bypass. Chest 104:1436–1440, 1993.
200. Virmani R, Poposky MA, Roberts WC. Thrombocytosis, coronary thrombosis and acute myocardial infarction. Am Med J 67:498–506, 1979.
201. Chan KL. Coronary thrombosis and subsequent lysis after a marathon. J Am Col Cardiol 4:1322–1325, 1984.
202. Nakagawa T, Yasuno M, Tanahashi H, et al. A case of acute myocardial infarction. Intracoronary thrombosis in two major coronary arteries due to hormone therapy. Angiology 45:333–338, 1994.
203. Thorneycroft IH. Oral contraceptives and myocardial infarction. Am J Obstet Gynecol 163:1393–1397, 1990
204. Engel HJ, Hundeshagen H, Lichtlen P. Transmural myocardial infarction in young women taking oral contraceptives. Evidence of reduced regional coronary flow in spite of normal coronary arteries. Br Heart J 39:477–484, 1977.
205. Motte G, Vogel M, Coatantiec G, Mariette P, Welti JJ. Acute coronary thrombosis in a 28-year-old woman. Arch Mal Coeur Vaiss 68:91–96, 1975.
206. Maleki M, Lange RL. Coronary thrombosis in young women on oral contraceptives: Report of two cases and review of the literature. Am Heart J 85:749–754, 1973.
207. Kolodgie FD, Farb A, Virmani R. Pathobiological determinants of cocaine-associated cardiovascular syndromes. Hum Pathol 26:583–586, 1995.
208. Kuhn FE, Gillis RA, Virmani R, Visner MS, Schaer GL. Cocaine produces coronary artery vasoconstriction independent of an intact endothelium. Chest 102:581–585, 1992.
209. Kolodgie FD, Virmani R, Cornhill JF, Herderick EE, Smialek J. Increase in atherosclerosis and adventitial mast cells in cocaine abusers: An alternative mechanism of cocaine-associated coronary vasospasm and thrombosis. J Am Coll Cardiol 17:1553–1560, 1991.
210. Virmani R. Cocaine-associated cardiovascular disease: Clinical and pathological aspects. NIDA Res Monogr 108:220–229, 1991.
211. Virmani R, Robinowitz M, Smialek JE, Smyth DF. Cardiovascular effects of cocaine: An autopsy study of 40 patients. Am Heart J 115:1068–1076, 1988.
212. Tsai HM, Lian EC. Antibodies to von Willebrand factor-cleaving protease in acute thrombotic thrombocytopenic purpura. N Engl J Med 339:1585–1594, 1998.
213. Furlan M, Robles R, Galbusera M, et al. von Willebrand factor-cleaving protease in thrombotic thrombocytopenic purpura and the hemolytic-uremic syndrome. N Engl J Med 339:1578–1584, 1998.

Chapter

5

PATHOLOGY OF MYOCARDIAL INFARCTION

More than 1.5 million Americans suffer from an acute myocardial infarct (MI) annually. Acute myocardial infarction is the major cause of morbidity and mortality in the United States and accounts for 500,000 deaths each year.[1] In-hospital admissions for acute myocardial infarction are more than 1 million annually and of these only in 30% to 50% is the diagnosis of MI confirmed. Myocardial infarction is most frequent under the age of 70 years.[2] Hospital mortality rates from myocardial infarction have declined from 22% to 17% since the establishment of coronary care units.[2] Mortality is highest in patients > 65 years of age.[3] Males have a fivefold higher risk of MI than females between the age of 45 to 54 years and it decreases to twofold difference in the eighth decade. Women have a higher mortality than men after an MI and older (65–74 years) patients have a higher mortality than younger (< 65 years) independent of infarct size.[4,5] The major cause of acute myocardial infarction is coronary atherosclerosis with superimposed luminal thrombus, accounting for > 80% of all infarcts and less frequently infarction may occur from nonatherosclerotic diseases of the coronary arteries (see Chapter 4).

CLINICAL EVALUATION OF PATIENT WITH ACUTE MYOCARDIAL INFARCTION

For the clinical diagnosis of acute myocardial infarction, the World Health Organization requires that at least two of the following three criteria be present: (1) a history of chest pain or discomfort; (2) a rise and subsequent fall in serum cardiac enzymes; and (3) the development of electrocardiogram (ECG) abnormalities (new Q-waves or ST segment or T-wave changes) on serially obtained ECGs.[6] Because the ECG lacks sufficient sensitivity and specificity to detect myocardial necrosis, the presence of myocardial injury is often dependent upon the release of cardiac-specific serum markers such as troponin T, troponin I, and CK-MB.[7–10] It has been shown that infarct size generally correlates with the peak rise in serum CK-MB level.[11]

Most patients who present with chest pain and ST-segment elevation on ECG are likely to develop Q-waves.[12, 13] Conversely, the majority of patients who present without ST-segment elevation do not evolve Q-waves and have either unstable angina or non-Q wave MI, based on the presence of elevated serum cardiac enzymes.[13–16] The extent of infarction is classified as transmural (extending from endocardium to epicardium) or subendocardial (involving only the subendocardial region to the middle myocardium), terms originally correlated with Q-wave and non-Q wave infarction, respectively.[16–19] However, autopsy studies have shown that the ECG lacks specificity and sensitivity to distinguish transmural from subendocardial MI based on presence and absence of Q-waves; Q-wave infarcts can be as frequently subendocardial as non-Q wave infarcts can be transmural.[20] Nevertheless, short-term clinical studies show that Q-wave infarcts are associated with greater myocardial necrosis and have a higher short-term mortality than non-Q wave infarcts, but

The opinions or assertions contained herein are the private views of the authors and are not to be construed as official or reflecting the views of the Department of the Army, the Department of the Air Force, or the Department of Defense.

the long-term mortality is similar in both (31% versus 26%).[15]

MYOCARDIAL ISCHEMIA

Myocardial ischemia occurs when there is an imbalance between oxygen supply and demand. Myocardial infarction or necrosis occurs when ischemia is severe and prolonged. Two zones of myocardial damage occur: a central zone with no flow or very low flow, and a zone of collateral vessels in a surrounding marginal zone. The survival of the marginal zone is dependent on the level and the duration of ischemia. The infarct size is of critical importance as it is a predictor of survival. In 1971, Page et al. showed that infarcts ≥ 40% of left ventricle are predictors of cardiogenic shock and death.[21]

DEVELOPMENT OF COLLATERAL VESSELS AND RELATIONSHIP TO EXTENT OF CORONARY DISEASE

The underlying coronary disease appears to play a large role in the extent of myocardial necrosis. It has been observed that patients with transmural myocardial infarction usually have total occlusion of the coronary artery supplying the bed with the infarct and usually have poorly developed collateral vessels.[22] In contrast, patients with subendocardial or nonconfluent infarcts often have noncritical underlying stenosis with a superimposed nonocclusive thrombus.[22–24] The degree and rate of development of coronary stenosis is related to the development of collateral circulation. Graded ischemia developing with the gradual narrowing of the coronary artery lumen allows for the development of collateral vessels supplying the bed with critical stenosis.[22, 25]

THE WAVE FRONT PHENOMENON

The extent of myocardial necrosis is also dependent on the duration of coronary occlusion, the so-called "wave front phenomenon." Reimer and Jennings, in a landmark paper in 1979, showed in the dog that if the coronary artery was occluded for 15 or 40 minutes, 3 hours, or permanently for 4 days myocardial necrosis progressed as a "wave front phenomenon" (Fig. 5–1*A*).[26] After only 15 minutes of occlusion, no infarct occurred. At 40 minutes, the infarct was subendocardial, involving only the papillary muscle, resulting in 28% of the myocardium at risk. At 3 hours following coronary artery occlusion and reperfusion, the infarct was significantly smaller compared with nonreperfused permanently occluded infarct (62% of area at risk). The infarct size was the greatest in permanent occlusion (4 days until sacrifice), becoming transmural involving 75% of the area at risk[27] (Fig. 5–1*B*). In the dog model 100% of area at risk is never infarcted because the dog has inherently good collateral blood supply.

CONSEQUENCES OF REDUCTION IN ARTERIAL BLOOD FLOW

The main consequence of reduced blood flow is the depletion of high energy phosphate (~P) within the involved myocardium and the accumulation of metabolic products.[27–29] When the oxygen supply becomes limited, the aerobic or mitochondrial respiration ceases, and the myocardium begins to depend upon the ~P reserves. Because these reserves are small, consisting entirely of creatine phosphate, which is utilized rapidly following the cessation of aerobic metabolism, anaerobic glycolysis begins almost immediately in order to counter the decline of ATP supplies. At first, anaerobic glycolysis supplies 80% of the ~P, but within 60–90 seconds this decreases because acidosis develops secondary to lactate accumulation. The net ATP decreases very quickly during the first 10 minutes of low flow, decreasing to 10% of the ~P released by glucose metabolism[27] (Fig. 5–2). Myocardial changes of ischemia are fully reversible only up to 15 minutes of ischemia in the dog.[30, 31] There is virtually no ATP at 40 minutes, at which point lactate ranges from 200 to 250 μmol/g dry weight and irreversible injury sets in.[32] Upon depletion of ATP, anaerobic glycolysis ceases and the tissue undergoes contracture-rigor, resulting in myofibrillar shortening and extrusion of erythrocytes out of the area of ischemia with acquisition of a pale color.[26, 27] Once the changes of contracture-rigor set in, myocardial injury is irreversible even if the blood flow is restored.[27]

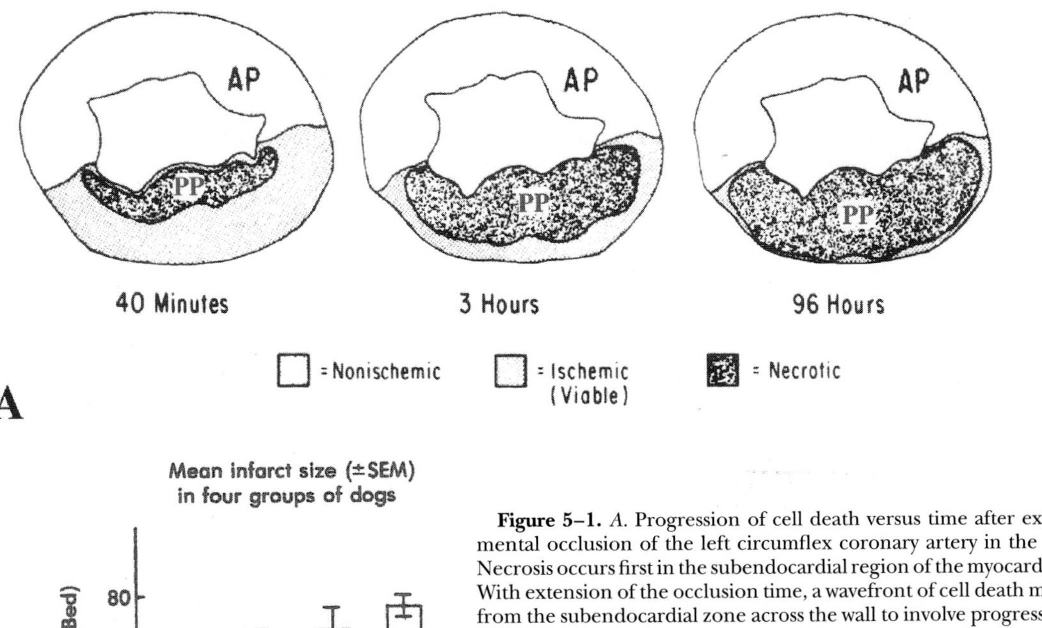

Figure 5–1. *A.* Progression of cell death versus time after experimental occlusion of the left circumflex coronary artery in the dog. Necrosis occurs first in the subendocardial region of the myocardium. With extension of the occlusion time, a wavefront of cell death moves from the subendocardial zone across the wall to involve progressively more of the transmural thickness of the ischemic zone (*AP* = anterior; *PP* = posterior). *B.* Infarct size variation with increasing duration of coronary occlusion. Infarct size dramatically increases from 40 minutes to 3 hours; however, there is very little increase between 3 and 6 hours and between 6 and 96 hours of coronary artery occlusion (*LCC* = left circumflex coronary bed). (From Reimer KA, Jennings RB. The "wavefront phenomenon" of myocardial ischemic cell death. II. Transmural progression of necrosis with the framework of ischemic bed size (myocardium at risk) and collateral flow. Lab Invest 40:633–644, 1979, with permission.)

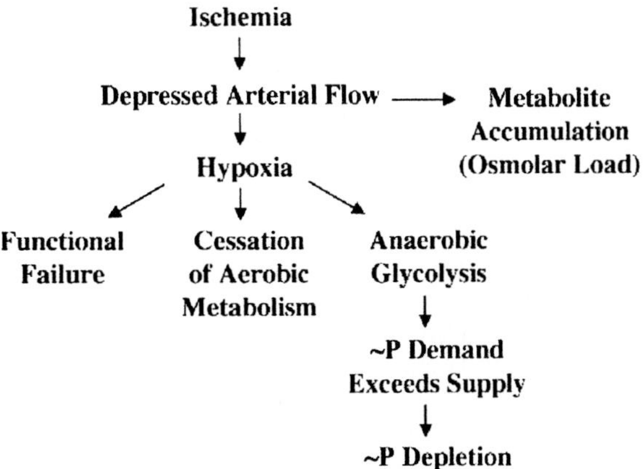

Figure 5–2. Principal consequences of ischemia are shown in this diagram. Metabolites are produced intracellularly by hypoxic metabolism where they accumulate and equilibrate to a variable extent with extracellular fluid. Because tissue demand for high-energy phosphate (~P) exceeds supply, the net level of adenosine triphosphate decreases until it is virtually zero in zones of low-flow ischemia. (From Jennings RB, Reimer KA, Steenbergen C, Jr, Murray CE. Energy metabolism in myocardial ischemia. In: Dhalla NS, Innes IR, Beamish RE (eds): Myocardial Ischemia. Boston: Martinus Nijhoff, pp. 185–198, 1987, with permission.)

ELECTRON MICROSCOPIC CHANGES OF REVERSIBLE AND IRREVERSIBLE INJURY

Electron microscopic criteria for reversible versus irreversible myocardial ischemic injury are well established.[33, 34] Reversible injury is defined as injury that can be reversed to normal functioning state without any structural damage, if the offending agent is removed.[35] An irreversible injury is said to set in if the cell can no longer perform its normal metabolic functions, even when the offending agent is removed.

Reversibly injured myocytes are edematous and swollen from the osmotic overload. The cell size is increased with a decrease in the glycogen content.[27, 36] The myocyte fibrils are relaxed and thinned; I-bands are prominent secondary to noncontracting ischemic myocytes.[27] The nuclei show mild condensation of chromatin at the nucleoplasm. The cell membrane (sarcolemma) is intact and no breaks can be identified. The mitochondria are swollen, with loss of normal dense mitochondrial granules and incomplete clearing of the mitochondrial matrix, but without amorphous or granular flocculent densities (Fig. 5–3*A* and *B*).

Irreversibly injured myocytes contain shrunken nuclei with marked chromatin margination. The two hallmarks of irreversible injury are cell membrane breaks and mitochondrial presence of small osmiophilic amorphous densities.[27, 33] The densities are composed of lipid, denatured proteins, and calcium.[33, 37, 38] The cell membrane breaks are small and are associated with subsarcolemmal blebs of edema fluid[27] (Figure 5–3*B*).

GROSS PATHOLOGY OF ACUTE MYOCARDIAL INFARCTION

In hearts with acute myocardial infarction, it is essential to state the region of involvement (such as anteroseptal); the level of involvement, that is, basal, midventricle, or apical; and whether the infarct is subendocardial or transmural (Fig. 5–4). An estimation of the percent of the infarcted left ventricular myocardium should be made.

The most frequent site of coronary thrombosis of an atherosclerotic plaque is the left anterior descending coronary artery, constituting 40 to 50% of the total. In cases of thrombus in the left anterior descending, the area of infarction is in the anterior wall of the left ventricle and the anterior two thirds of the ventricular septum. The next most frequently thrombosed artery causing acute myocardial infarction is the right coronary, representing 30–40% of the total. In cases of right coronary thrombosis, the resulting infarct occurs in the posterior wall of the left ventricle ± right-ventricle posterior wall. The least frequent major epicardial artery resulting in acute myocardial infarction is the left circumflex (15–20% of acute infarcts). With occlusion of the left circumflex, the infarct is located on the lateral wall of the left ventricle. No coronary thrombosis is found in fewer than 5% of acute myocardial infarcts.

The earliest gross change can be discerned at 12 hours after infarction, and consists of pallor of the myocardium. The gross detection of infarction can be enhanced and made possible within 2 to 3 hours after infarct by immersion of the fresh heart slices in a solution of triphenyltetrazolium chloride or nitro-blue tetrazolium. Tetrazolium salts are dyes that are sensitive to the presence of tissue dehydrogenase enzyme activity, which is depleted in the infarcted region. Red color (triphenyl-tetrazolium chloride) or blue color (nitro-blue tetrazolium) will only form in the normal noninfarcted myocardium, thus revealing the pale nonstained infarcted region (Fig. 5–4).

Around 24 hours the pallor is enhanced (Fig. 5–5). However, in this era of thrombolytic therapy, most in-hospital patients will have received tissue plasminogen activator, streptokinase, or IIb/IIIa inhibitors, which lyse the thrombus and restore blood flow into the area of infarction. Therefore, in a reperfused infarct the infarcted region will appear red from trapping of the red cells and hemorrhage from the rupture of the necrotic capillaries (Fig. 5–6). However, if there has been no reperfusion, the area of the infarct is better defined at 2 to 3 days with a central area of yellow discoloration that is surrounded by a thin rim of highly vascularized hyperemia (Fig. 5–5). At 5 to 7 days the regions are much more distinct, with a central soft area and a depressed hyperemic border.[39–41] At 1 to 2 weeks the infarct begins to heal with infiltration by macrophages as well as early fibroblasts at the margins. At the same time the infarct begins to be more depressed, especially at the margins where organization takes place, and there is a white hue border (Table 5–1) (Fig. 5–5). Healing may be complete as early as 4 to 6 weeks in small infarcts, or may take as long as 2 to 3 months when the area of infarction is

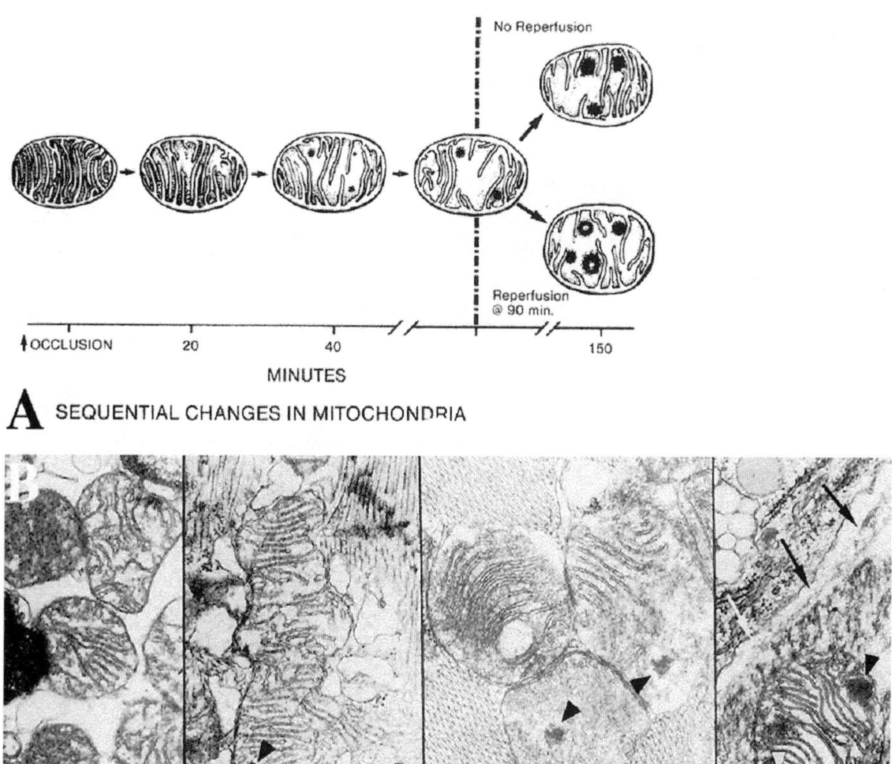

Figure 5–3. *A.* Sequential changes within mitochondria with varying time intervals of myocardial ischemia. At 20 minutes of ischemia, there is mild mitochondrial swelling. Matrix space between cristae show disorganization. At 40 minutes of ischemia, there is greater mitochondrial swelling, and prominent amorphous matrix densities are present, which indicate irreversible injury. With longer duration of coronary occlusion, mitochondria show larger amorphous matrix densities, and they also become more numerous. On reperfusion, both amorphous and granular densities are seen. Granular densities, however, seem larger and more fully developed. (Adapted with permission of American Heart Association. Jennings RB, Ganote CE. Structural changes in myocardium during acute ischemia. Circ Res 35(suppl III):III156–III172, 1974) *B.* Electron micrographs showing progressive changes in mitochondria as a result of ischemia in the canine model. *Panel a.* Mitochondria showing reversible changes of ischemia after 10 minutes of coronary occlusion and reperfusion: Mitochondria are swollen, there is clearing of mitochondrial matrix, and some cristae show disorganization. *Panel b.* Similar changes as in *panel a* with only one of the mitochondria showing amorphous matrix densities (*arrowhead*) after 90 minutes of ischemia. *Panel c.* Note the presence of large amorphous matrix densities (*arrowheads*) in two of the three mitochondria, in a dog with 120 minutes of coronary occlusion. *Panel d.* Ischemic myocyte with mitochondria containing multiple large amorphous matrix densities (*arrowheads*) after 3 days of permanent coronary occlusion. Note the break in the plasma lemma (*arrow*). (From the American Heart Association. Virmani R, Forman MB, Kolodgie FD. Circulation 81(suppl IV):IV57–IV68, 1990, with permission.)

large. Healed infarcts are white from the scarring and the ventricular wall may or may not be thinned (aneurysmal). In general, infarcts that are transmural and confluent are likely to result in thinning, whereas subendocardial and nonconfluent infarcts are not.

LIGHT MICROSCOPIC FINDINGS IN NONREPERFUSED INFARCTION

The earliest change, 1 to 3 hours after onset of ischemia, is described as the appearance of wavy fibers[42] (Fig. 5–7). It is hypothesized that the wavy fibers result from the stretching of the ischemic noncontractile fibers by the adjoining viable contracting myocytes.[42] We have observed this change quite commonly in the right ventricle even in the absence of ischemia. For this reason, this morphologic change is not a specific marker for the detection of the early ischemic change, and is not useful within 6 hours after occlusion of the vessel.

The earliest morphologic characteristic of myocardial infarction that can be discerned, between 12 to 24 hours after onset of chest

(Text continued on page 162.)

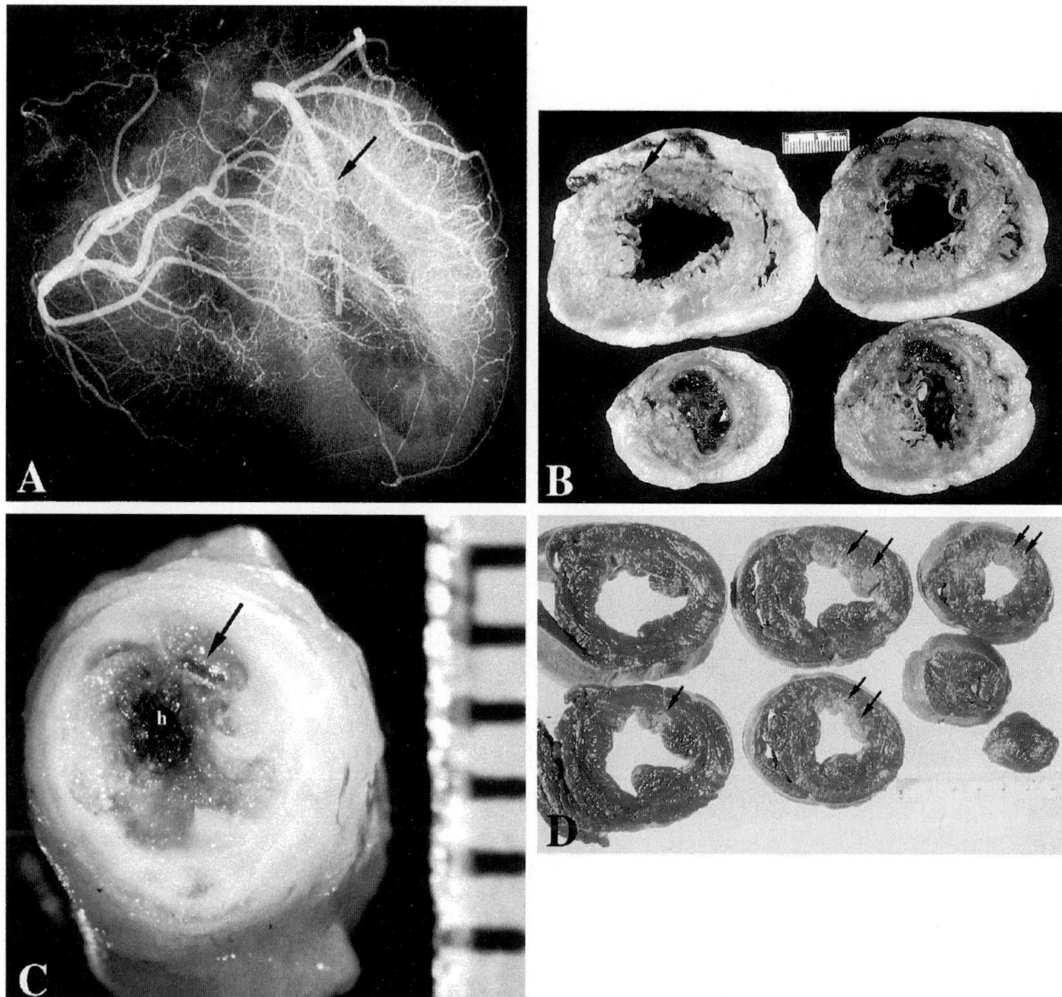

Figure 5–4. Regional distribution of vascular supply to the ventricles with right coronary artery dominance. *A.* Postmortem angiogram of the heart in a patient with acute myocardial infarction with total occlusion (*arrow*) of the proximal left anterior descending coronary artery in a 65-year-old female who presented with persistent chest pain of 6 hours' duration. *B.* At autopsy she had a hemopericardium with rupture site (*arrow*) identified on the anterior wall of the left ventricle. Note extensive hemorrhagic transmural infarction involving the anterior wall of the left ventricle near the base of the heart (*upper slices*) and extending into the septum in the mid and apical slices (*lower slices*). *C.* A gross photograph of the left anterior descending coronary artery showing hemorrhage into the necrotic core and a > 90% luminal narrowing; barium is seen within the lumen (*arrow*). *D.* Canine heart slices following 15 minutes incubation in 2% triphenyltetrazolium chloride (*TTC*) at 37°C. The animal had under gone 60 minutes of left anterior descending (LAD) coronary artery occlusion distal to the first diagonal branch followed by reperfusion and sacrifice at 24 hours. Injecting monastral dye, following reocclusion of the LAD just prior to sacrifice, identified the myocardium at risk of infarction. The heart was sliced and then immersed in TTC. The viable myocardium at risk stains red and area not at risk is blue-red, whereas the infarcted region is creamy white (*arrows*).

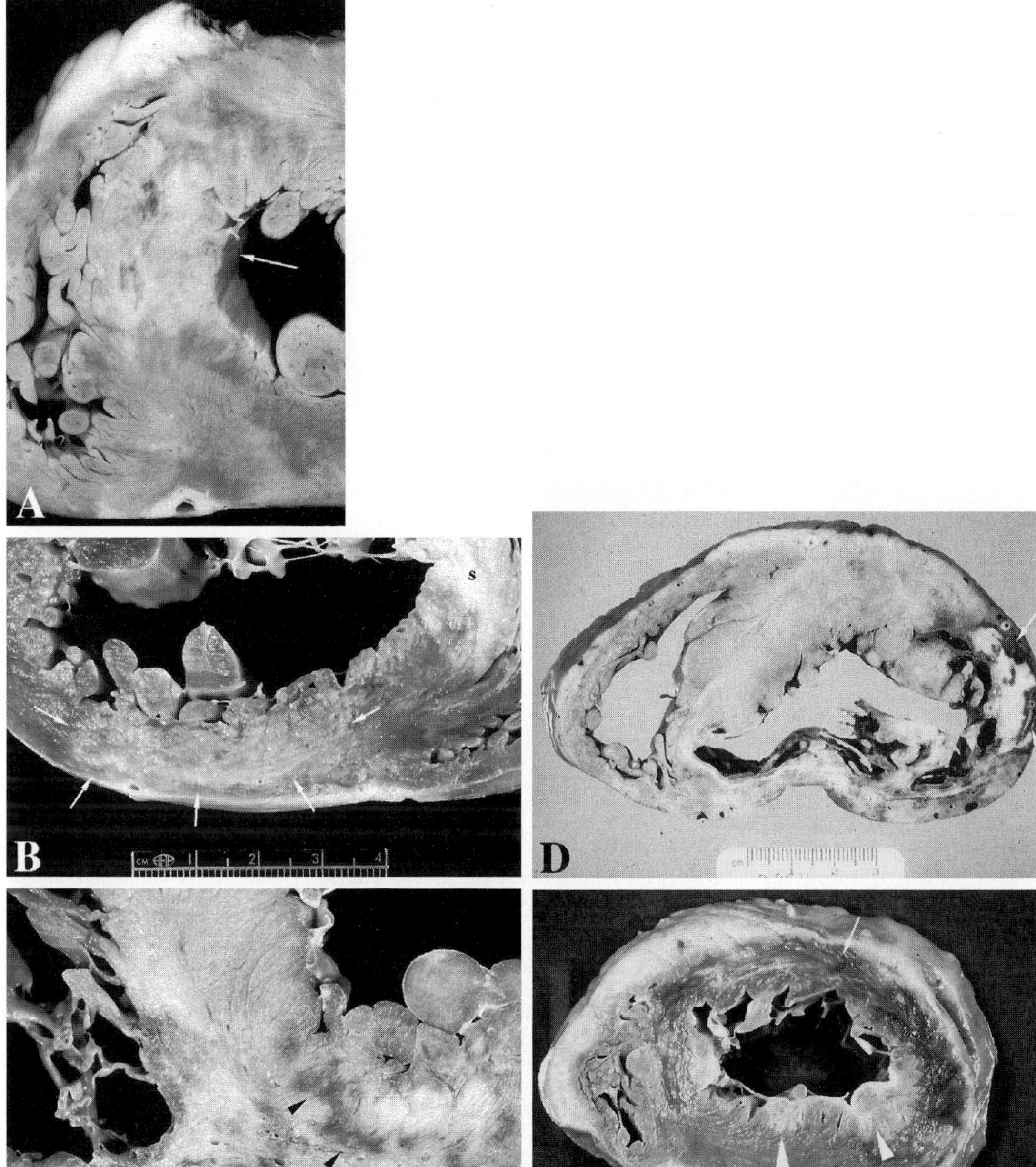

Figure 5–5. Gross photographs of hearts with varying ages of acute myocardial infarction. *A.* A 50-year-old hyperlipidemic and hypertensive male presented with unstable angina, underwent emergency PTCA of the LAD, died 20 hours following onset of chest pain. At autopsy, heart had a pale ill defined, slightly raised region in the anterior ventricular septum suggestive of an acute transmural infarct (*arrow*) which was confirmed by the presence of hypereosinophilic myocytes localized to the septum with sparing of the subendocardial myocytes. The *LAD* at the PTCA site was totally occluded by a luminal thrombus and an underlying 60% atherosclerotic lesion. *B.* Another high power of a different acute transmural myocardial infarct involving the posterior wall of the heart; well-defined pale, creamy tan, slightly raised infarct; note absence of hyperemia in the border region—the infarct is 24 to 36 hours old. An older infarct can be seen in the septum(*s*).*C.* An older infarct dated 36 to 72 hours showing hyperemic areas (*arrowheads*) surrounding the subendocardial infarct (age 3 days), with paler area in the outer half of the posterior wall of the left ventricle (infarct extension). The more recent infarct involves the posterior portion of the ventricular septum and the posterior wall of the right ventricle (36 to 48 hours). *D.* Gross photograph of a heart slice. Close to the base of the heart shows 1-week-old acute transmural myocardial infarct involving the posterolateral wall of the heart; note the marked pale region in the inner two thirds of the infarct with surrounding prominent hyperemic zone (*arrows*). Also present is a healed transmural myocardial infarct involving the posterior wall and posteroseptal region of the heart. The patient died in severe congestive heart failure. *E.* Gross photograph of a transmural healing myocardial infarct involving the septum, anterior, and the lateral wall of the left ventricle in an apical slice of the heart. Note the depressed, gelatinous appearance (*arrow*) of the infarct, which is 3 weeks old. Focal areas of scarring can be seen (*arrowheads*).

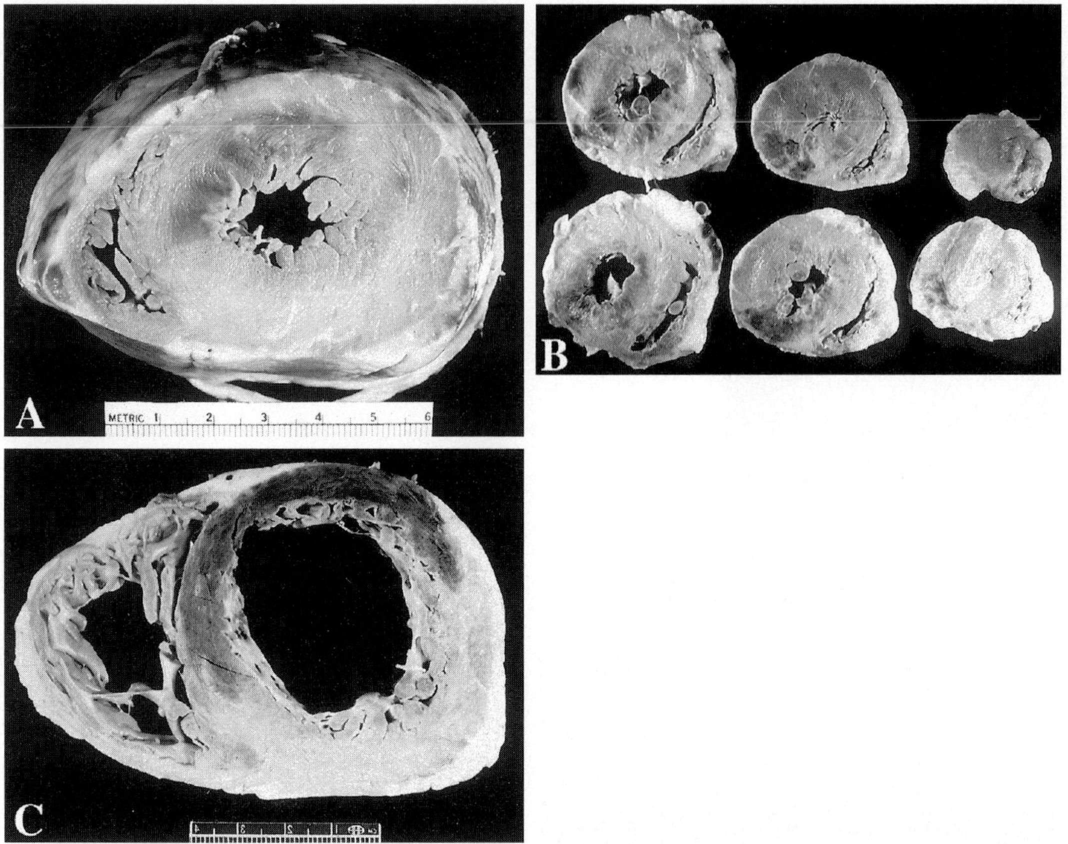

Figure 5–6. *A.* A 47-year-old black male presented with unstable angina, evolved into a Q wave infarct. On catheterization had a total occlusion of the left anterior descending coronary artery and had severe stenosis of the right and left circumflex coronary arteries; underwent emergency bypass graft to all three vessels. Died secondary to refractory arrhythmias on the third hospital day. Note subendocardial hyperemic region in the anteroseptal wall of the left ventricle. *B.* Patient presented with acute myocardial infarction of 6 hours' duration, received streptokinase in the emergency room with successful reperfusion, died 2 days later of a cerebral bleed. Note a hemorrhagic transmural infarct involves the posteroseptal wall of the left ventricle, extending from the base to the apex of the heart with approximately 20–25% of the myocardium infarcted. *C.* A 60-year-old male admitted with onset of chest pain while mowing the lawn did not seek medical treatment until 8 hours after onset of chest pain. Received streptokinase, developed arrhythmias, was treated with lidocaine, went into cardiogenic shock, died 3 days following infarction. Note transmural confluent hemorrhagic infarct of the anteroseptal wall of the left ventricle involving at least 40% of the left ventricle.

pain, is the hypereosinophilic myocyte (Fig. 5–7). Despite the hypereosinophilia of the cytoplasm, which is seen best on routine hematoxylin-eosin staining, the myocyte striations appear normal and some chromatin condensation may be seen in the nucleus. The area of infarction may show interstitial edema; however, this change is difficult to appreciate in human autopsy hearts and better appreciated in animal experiments. Neutrophil infiltration is present by 24 hours at the border areas. As the infarct progresses between 24 to 48 hours, coagulation necrosis is established with various degrees of nuclear pyknosis, early karyorrhexis, and karyolysis. The myocyte striations are preserved and the sarcomeres elongate. The border areas show prominent neutrophil infiltration by 48 hours (Fig. 5–7).

At 3 to 5 days the central portion of the infarct shows loss of myocyte nuclei and striations; in smaller infarcts, neutrophils invade within the infarct and fragment, resulting in more severe karyorrhexis (nuclear dust). Loss of myocyte striations is best appreciated by Mallory's trichrome stain. Macrophages and fibroblasts begin to appear in the border areas. By one week, neutrophils decline and granulation tissue is established with neocapillary invasion, macrophages, lymphocytic, and plasma cell infiltration. Although lymphocytes may be seen as early

Table 5–1. Gross and Microscopic Evolution of Reperfused and Nonreperfused Acute Myocardial Infarct

Time of Occlusion	Permanent occlusion/no reperfusion		Reperfusion following occlusion	
	Gross	**Histologic**	**Gross**	**Histologic**
12 hours	No change/pallor	Wavy fibers	Mottled, prominent hemorrhage	CBN
24–48 hours	Pallor—yellow, soft	Hypereosinophilic fibers, PMNs at borders	Prominent hemorrhage	Hypereosinophilic fibers + CBN + PMNs + hemorrhage throughout
3–5 days	Yellow center, hyperemic borders	Large number of PMNs at border, coagulation necrosis, loss of nuclei	Prominent hemorrhage	Aggressive phagocytosis, profuse fibroblast infiltration + early collagen
6–10 days	Yellow, depressed central infarct, tan-red margins	Mummified fibers in center, macrophage phagocytosis + granulation tissue at borders	Depressed red-brown infarct with gray-white intermingled	Aggressive healing with greater collagen + macrophages
10–14 days	Grey-red borders, infiltrating central ten–yellow infarct if large	Marked granulation tissue, collagen deposition, subendocardial myocyte sparing	Gray-white intermingled with brown	Aggressive healing with greater collagen
2–8 weeks	Gelatinous to grey-white scar, greater healing at border zone	Collagen deposition with prominent large capillaries	White intermingled with areas of red myocardium	Collagen intermingled with groups of myocytes

PMN = polymorphonuclear neutrophil leukocytes
CBN = contraction band necrosis

as 2 to 3 days, they are not prominent in any stage of infarct evolution. Eosinophils may be seen within the inflammatory infiltrate but are only present in 24% of infarcts.[43] There is phagocytic removal of the necrotic myocytes by macrophages, and pigment is seen within macrophages.

By the second week, fibroblasts are prominent but their appearance may be seen as early as day 4 at the periphery of the infarct. There is continued removal of the necrotic myocytes as the fibroblasts are actively producing collagen and angiogenesis occurs in the area of healing. The healing continues and, depending on the extent of necrosis, the healing may be complete as early as 4 weeks, or require 8 weeks or longer to complete (Fig. 5–7). The central area of infarction may remain unhealed showing mummified myocytes for extended periods, despite the fact that the infarct borders are completely healed. For this reason, it is important to evaluate the age of the infarct by examining the border with noninfarcted muscle.

The magnitude of repair and healing is dependent not only on infarct size, but also upon local and systemic factors. If there is good collateral blood flow locally, healing will be relatively rapid, especially at the lateral borders where viable myocardium interdigitates with necrotic myocardium. There may be various levels of healing within an infarct, because of differences in blood flow in adjoining vascular beds caused by variable extent of coronary narrowing. The border areas may show hemorrhage and contraction band necrosis, depending upon regional variations in blood flow. Systemic factors that influence repair of myocardium are the systemic blood pressure and cardiac output, which are severely decreased in hearts of patients with multisystem failure.

LIGHT MICROSCOPIC APPEARANCE OF REPERFUSED ACUTE MYOCARDIAL INFARCTION

Data from animal experiments in the dog have demonstrated that myocardium can be salvaged if the artery supplying the area of infarction is opened following varying periods of total

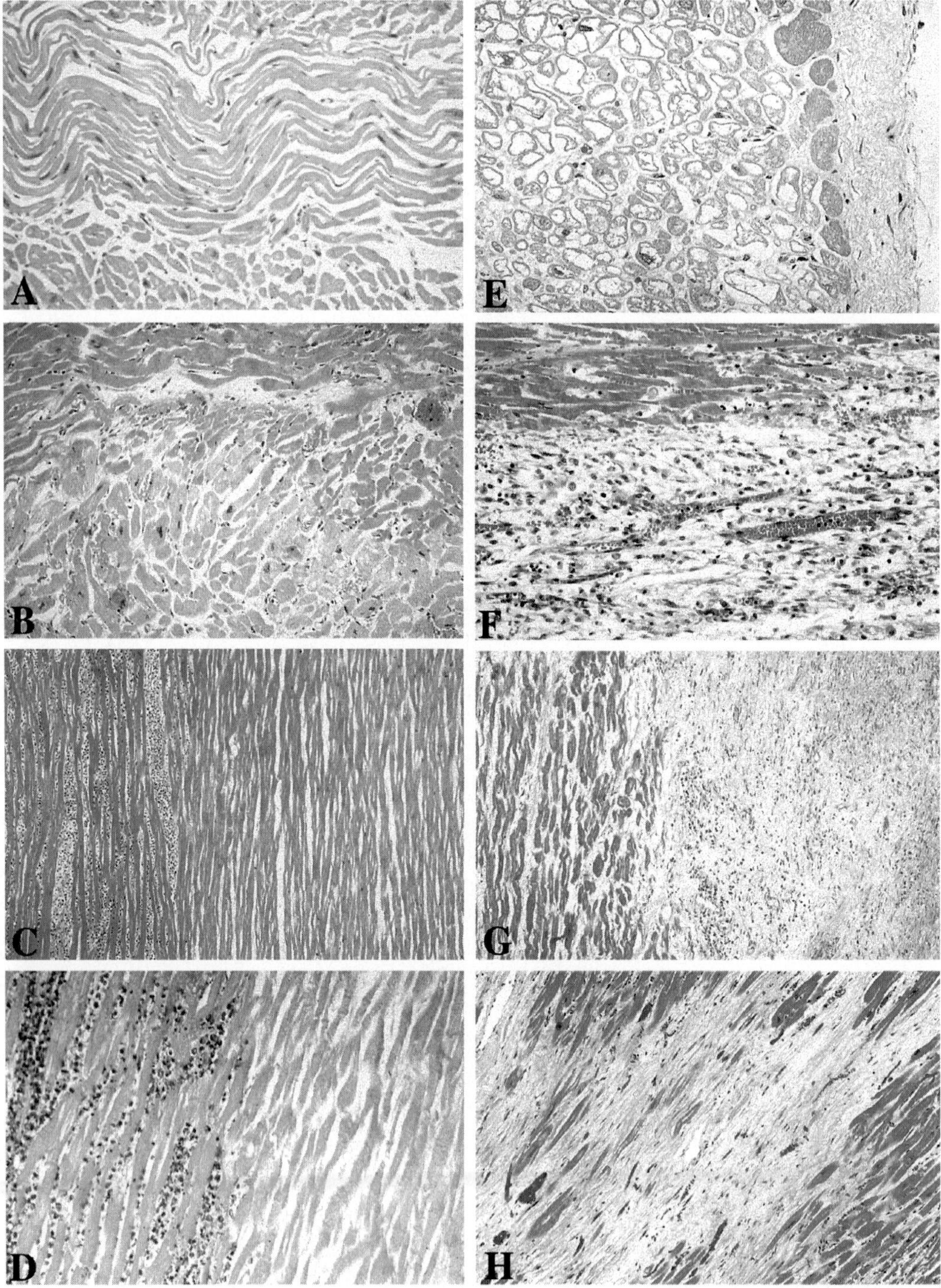

Figure 5–7 *See legend on opposite page*

occlusion. The maximal salvage is possible, both in dogs and humans, if the artery is opened within 6 hours of occlusion. The myocardium in the dog following 90 minutes of occlusion followed by reperfusion and sacrifice at 24 hours shows a hemorrhagic infarct limited to the area of infarction, which is subendocardial in extent. Hemorrhage occurs when the myocardial blood flow during the occlusion period is less than one fifth of normal. The myocytes are thin, hypereosinophilic, devoid of nuclei or showing karyorrhexis, with ill-defined borders and interspersed areas of interstitial hemorrhage. There is a diffuse but mild neutrophil infiltration. Within 2 to 3 days, macrophage infiltration is obvious and there is phagocytosis of necrotic myocytes and early stages of granulation tissue. The infarct healing in the dog is more rapid than that in humans, most likely due to nondiseased adjoining coronary arteries and a healthy myocardium. There is often chronic ischemia secondary to extensive atherosclerotic disease in humans with acute myocardial infarction.

If reperfusion occurs in a human within 4 to 6 hours following onset of chest pain or ECG changes, there is myocardial salvage and the infarct is likely to be subendocardial without transmural extension. There will be a nearly confluent area of hemorrhage within the infarcted myocardium, with extensive contraction band necrosis. The extent of hemorrhage is dependent upon the extent of reperfusion of the infarct as well as the extent of capillary necrosis. The larger the infarct, and the longer the duration of the infarct, the more the hemorrhage. The degree of hemorrhage may be variable and nonuniform, as blood flow is dependent upon the residual area of coronary narrowing and the amount of thrombolysis. Within a few hours of reperfusion, neutrophils are evident within the area of necrosis, but they are usually sparse (Fig. 5–8). In contrast to nonreperfused infarcts, neutrophils do not show concentration at the margins. However, reperfused infarcts often demonstrate areas of necrosis at the periphery with interdigitation with noninfarcted myocardium. Macrophages begin to appear by day 2 or 3 and stromal cells show enlarged nuclei and nucleoli by days 3 and 4 (Fig. 5–8). Neutrophil debris, which may be concentrated at the border areas in cases of incomplete reperfusion, is seen by 3 to 5 days. By days 3 to 5 fibroblasts appear, with an accelerated rate of healing as compared with nonreperfused infarcts. By one week there is collagen deposition with disappearance of neutrophils and prominence of macrophages containing pigment derived from ingested myocytes (Fig. 5–8). Angiogenesis is prominent and lymphocytes are often seen. Infarcts at 5 to 10 days are more cellular and there is prominent myocytolysis (loss of myofibrils). As early as 2 to 3 weeks subendocardial infarcts may be fully healed (Fig. 5–8). Five to ten layers of subendocardial myocytes are spared without necrosis. However, myofibrillar loss, which is a result of ischemia not severe enough to cause cell death, is prominent in this subendocardial zone. Larger infarcts, and those reperfused after 6 hours, take longer to heal. Infarcts reperfused after 6 hours show larger areas of hemorrhage as compared with occlusions with more immediate reperfusion (Fig. 5–6). However, myocytes maintain their striations, become stretched and elongated, and—as they do not respond to calcium influx—do not show significant contraction band necrosis. Despite the fact that reperfusion should occur within 6 hours of occlusion for maximal myocyte salvage, there appears to be

Figure 5–7. Histologic characteristics of myocardial infarction following total occlusion of a coronary artery. *A.* The earliest change seen is within 12 hours after the onset of chest pain and has been described as wavy fibers with elongation of myocytes, and narrowing of the myocyte diameter. *B.* Hypereosinophilic myocyte fibers representing early features of coagulation necrosis can be seen between 12 to 24 hours after onset of chest pain, the nucleus is intact, and the cross-striation are well seen. *C.* By 48 to 72 hours the neutrophils are now concentrated at the border of the infarcted and viable myocardium, the extent of neutrophil infiltration depends upon the collateral flow as well as the extent of coronary perfusion of the adjacent bed. The central zone of infarction now shows all the features of coagulation necrosis with karyolysis and loss of cross striations. *D.* Photomicrograph showing high-power view of the border zone of a 5-day-old infarct with marked neutrophil infiltration that has undergone karyopyknosis and karyorrhexis. The adjoining infarcted myocardium shows coagulation necrosis with loss of nuclei and cross-striations. *E.* A high-power view of the subendocardial region that is usually ischemic but viable showing myocyte vacuolization and loss of myofibrils. *F.* Almost complete removal of the necrotic myocardium; note presence of neovascular channels and surrounding macrophages and few lymphocytes (granulation tissue) at 7 to 10 days following acute myocardial infarction. *G.* The infarct is heavily infiltrated with fibroblasts with early collagen deposition and interspersed neocapillaries and few lymphocytes; infarct age 3 to 4 weeks. *H.* A fully healed infarct with dense collagen and few interspersed myocytes at the border region of the healed infarct. Infarct age may be 6 weeks and greater.

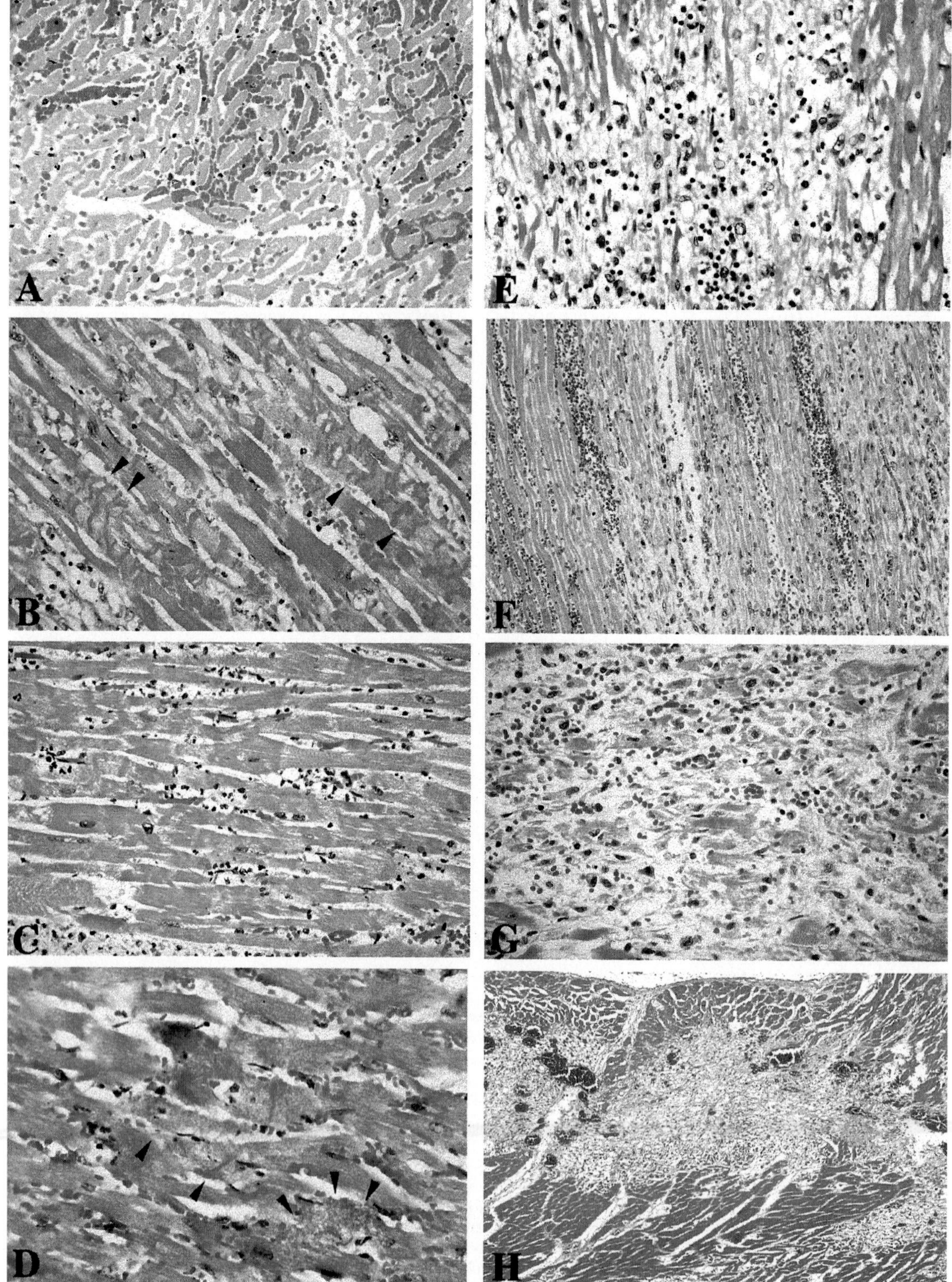

Figure 5–8 *See legend on opposite page*

some benefit in opening an artery regardless of the duration of coronary occlusion.

COMPLICATIONS OF ACUTE MYOCARDIAL INFARCTION

The complications of myocardial infarction may be immediate or remote, and are dependent upon the extent of infarction. The acute complications consist of sudden death, arrhythmias, cardiogenic shock, infarct extension, fibrinous pericarditis, cardiac rupture including papillary muscle rupture, and embolization.

Sudden Death and Arrhythmias

Sudden death occurs in 25% of patients after myocardial infarction, often before reaching the hospital. The proportion of deaths from ischemic heart disease that are sudden is almost 60%; therefore, it is crucial to understand the cause and mechanism of sudden death. Arrhythmias are common after acute myocardial infarction, occurring soon after the onset of symptoms.[17, 44] Most arrhythmias that are the result of increased autonomic activity are bradycardia, and some are associated with atrioventricular block and hypotension.[17] However, most arrhythmias responsible for out-of-hospital sudden coronary deaths are ventricular tachycardia and fibrillation, which may be monomorphic or polymorphic. In all patients, ventricular tachyarrhythmias are seen in 67% of cases within the first 12 hours of acute myocardial infarction.[45] Nonsustained ventricular tachycardia is not associated with increased mortality, whereas sustained ventricular tachycardia seen during the first 48 hours following acute myocardial infarction is associated with 20% hospital mortality.[46] Arrhythmias most likely arise from the adjoining ischemic but noninfarcted myocardium. In this acidotic arrhythmogenic zone, there is the release of metabolites such as potassium, calcium, and catecholamines, with low levels ATP and oxygen.[47, 48] Arrhythmias may occur later in the course of myocardial infarction as a result of scar tissue surrounding viable myocytes.[49] The conduction system is relatively protected against ischemic injury because conduction fibers are relatively inactive metabolically, as their function is not to provide contractility but the propagation of the impulse.[50, 51]

Cardiogenic Shock

Cardiogenic shock after myocardial infarction usually occurs if there is loss of at least 40% of the left ventricular mass, either acutely or in combination with scarred myocardium from old healed infarcts.[21, 52, 53] In about 10% of patients who develop cardiogenic shock, shock occurs before hospitalization immediately upon presentation. Much more commonly, shock develops while the patient is in the hospital, presumably from infarct extension (Fig. 5–9*A*).[54, 55] As a proportion of short-term deaths after myocardial infarction, cardiogenic shock accounts for 44%. The remainder of deaths are the result of cardiac rupture (26%) and arrhythmias (16%).[49] Patients with extension of infarction (reinfarction) into subendocardial zones remote from the larger infarct may develop cardiogenic shock (Fig. 5–9*B*). In turn, cardiogenic shock renders the remaining viable myocardium prone to ischemic necrosis because of poor perfusion.[56]

Two related but distinct complications of myocardial infarction are infarct extension and

Figure 5–8. Histologic characteristics of a reperfused infarct following occlusion and reperfusion either with thrombolysis (t-PA, streptokinase, or IIb/IIIa) or balloon angioplasty with or without stenting or surgical revascularization. *A.* Shows a cross section of myocytes showing necrosis with interstitial hemorrhage. Note pale myocyte nuclei and very early neutrophil infiltration. *B.* Myocytes cut longitudinally in a patient who was admitted with chest pain of 2 hours' duration followed by infusion of streptokinase. The patient died within 6 hours. Note the extensive contraction band necrosis (dark bands alternating with lighter bands, *arrowheads*), a hallmark of reperfusion injury. There are interstitial red cells and a few neutrophils that were scattered throughout the infarct. *C.* Note the number of neutrophils is greater than the previous example. There is mild red cell extravasation and contraction band necrosis. The duration of chest pain was 3 hours prior to reperfusion and the patient died 24 hours later. *D.* It is not uncommon to see single or a few necrotic myocytes with calcification (*arrowheads*) in patients with reperfused infarcts. *E.* Note presence of macrophages and lymphocytes with early dissolution of the necrotic myocytes. These areas of necrosis are interdigitating with viable noninfarcted myocardium (4–5 days old reperfused infarct). *F.* Note infiltrating macrophages and interstitial hemorrhage in the lower one fifth and the right one third of photomicrograph. *G.* High-power view of another infarct showing dissolution of the infarct and replacement with macrophages and early angiogenesis. Hemorrhage is still present; but no neutrophils are seen (5–7 day infarct). *H.* Low-power view of a healing infarct at 7–10 days; note angiogenesis and early replacement fibrosis.

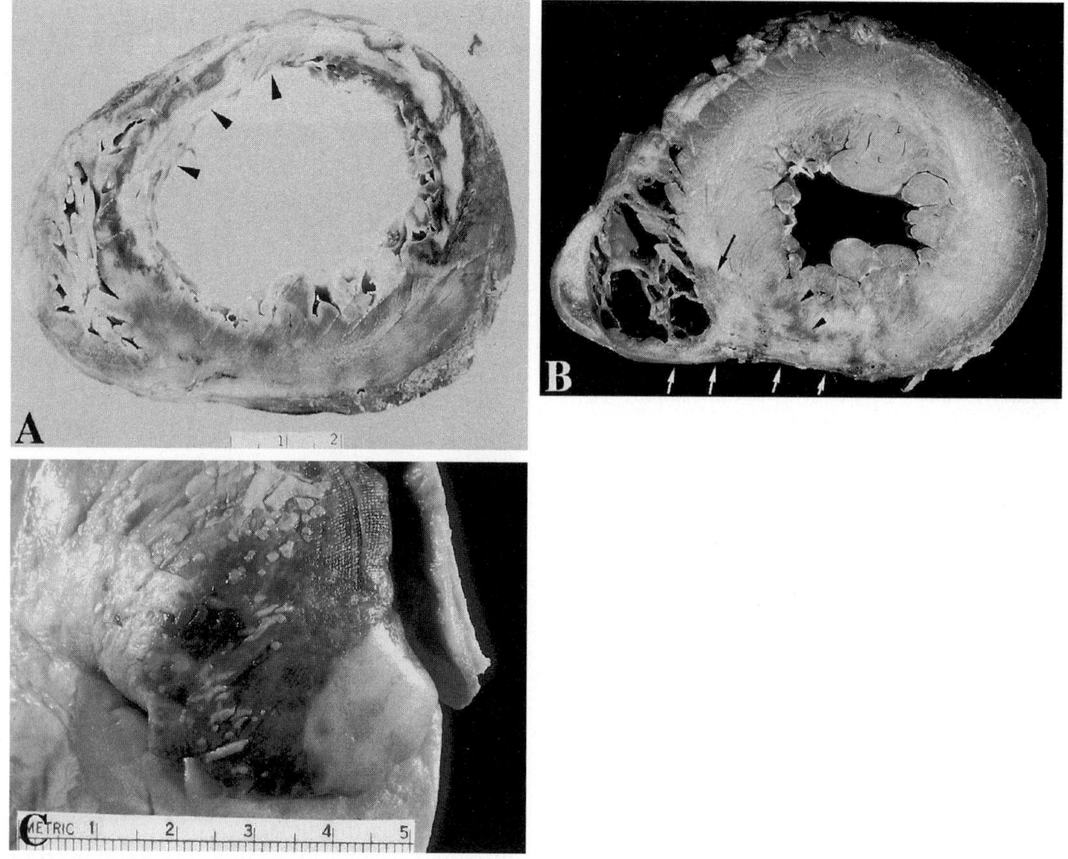

Figure 5–9. A 54-year-old male with history of acute myocardial infarction had an anteroseptal transmural myocardial infarction; on day 3 patient went into severe congestive heart failure and died on day 10. Note markedly thinned transmural anteroseptal infarct (*arrowheads*) involving 60% of the basal slice of the heart. The anteroseptal region shows infarct expansion. *B.* A 47-year-old man presented with chest pain, elevated CK and CK-MB; on ECG had a non Q-wave myocardial infarction involving the posterior wall of the left ventricle. Patient had an uneventful hospital course with cardiac enzymes (CK-MB) falling close to base line. On third hospital day he developed another episode of chest pain with rise in cardiac enzymes and new ECG changes of ST segment elevation in precordial leads and the patient was diagnosed with infarct extension and right ventricular infarction. The ventricular slice shows an older subendocardial infarct with hyperemic border (*arrowheads*) and a more recent infarction involving full thickness of the posterior wall and portion of the ventricle septum with extension into the posterior wall of the right ventricle (*arrows*). *C.* A 51-year-old male presented with chest pain of > 24 hours' duration and a diagnosis of acute myocardial infarction was made involving the inferior wall of the left ventricle and a right atrial infarction. Note the hemorrhagic right atrial border and the tip is pale and dusky, the surface shows fibrin deposits on the pericardial surface.

infarct expansion. Infarct extension results from an incremental increase in absolute necrotic myocardium, and may be the result of infarction remote from the original infarct in either the right or left ventricle (Fig. 5–9). It has been suggested that the more general term "recurrent infarction" be used for infarct extension.[57] Infarct extension usually occurs between 2 to 10 days following infarction, at a time when ECG changes are evolving and the troponin I or T is still high. However, the rapidly falling serum creatine kinase (CK-MB) after the first 24 hours may be useful for the detection of infarct extension along with new Q wave on ECG.[58] The risk factors associated with infarct expansion are cardiogenic shock, subendocardial infarct, female gender, and previous infarcts.[59]

Infarct expansion is the thinning of the area of the infarcted region and is not an increase in myocardial necrosis. In contrast, infarct expansion is caused by stretching of myocyte bundles reducing the density of myocytes in the area of the infarcted wall, and resulting in loss of tissue within the necrotic myocardium.[60] Infarct expansion typically results in dilatation and thinning of the infarct, and is associated with heart failure, ventricular aneurysm, and high mortality.[61] Risk factors for infarct expansion are anterior transmural infarcts and life-threatening arrhythmias.[61] Another term often applied to infarct expansion is ventricular remodeling, and involves remodeling of both the infarcted and the noninfarcted myocardium. As so defined, infarct expansion is a combination of changes of left ventricular dilation and hypertrophy of noninfarcted myocardium.[62, 63]

Rupture of the Myocardial Free Wall

At autopsy, cardiac rupture is the cause of death in 8 to 15% of patients dying of acute transmural myocardial infarction.[64–67] Following rupture of the free wall of the left ventricle, death occurs rapidly from hemopericardium and cardiac tamponade (Fig. 5–10). Risk factors for cardiac rupture after myocardial infarction include multivessel atherosclerotic disease, female gender and age older than 60 years, hypertension, absence of hypertrophy and previous infarction, poor collateral flow, the presence of a transmural infarct involving at least 20% of the wall, and location of the infarct in the mid anterior or lateral wall of the left ventricle.[65, 68–72] Cardiac rupture usually occurs in the first few days (1 to 4 days) following the infarct when coagulation necrosis and neutrophilic infiltration are at their peak and have weakened the left ventricular wall.[16, 17] Left ventricular wall rupture is seven times more common than the right ventricle rupture.[17] We have observed that infarcts with rupture contain more extensive inflammation and are more likely to demonstrate eosinophils (30% eosinophilic infiltration, as compared with 12% eosinophils in nonruptured infarcts[66]). However, at least 13 to 28% of ruptures occur within 24 hours of onset of infarction when inflammation and necrosis are not prominent.[64] Rupture most frequently occurs at the border of the infarcted region with the viable myocardium.[16, 17] Ruptures usually are not seen beyond 10 days after healing occurs. However, ruptures in infarcts with healing generally occur in the center of the infarct, unlike earlier ruptures (Fig. 5–10).[17] Nearly half the deaths from cardiac rupture occur as out-of-hospital sudden deaths and therefore are never seen by the clinician.[64] Clinical signs of cardiac rupture in patients who survive to the hospital include new murmur, a palpable thrill, and an echocardiographic finding of pericardial effusion.[73]

Rupture of the free wall occurs in 10% of acute transmural infarcts, and rupture of the ventricular septum in only 2%.[67] The two common locations of septal rupture are the anteroapical portion of the septum and inferobasal portion of the posterior septum extending into the right ventricular free wall. The posteroseptal rupture is associated with a worse prognosis and is rarely accompanied by rupture into the pericardium through the right ventricle (Fig. 5–10).[74] Septal ruptures are seen in the first week after transmural infarct with the development of a right-to-left shunt, murmur, and severe acute heart failure. Mortality is high, but emergency surgical intervention with placement of an umbrella-shaped device via catheter may successfully close the acquired defect and prolong survival.[17, 75, 76]

Rupture of a papillary muscle is less common than septal or free wall ruptures, and may occur as a complication of small subendocardial or larger transmural myocardial infarctions.[67, 77] More than 80% of infarcts underlying papillary muscle rupture involve the posteromedial muscle, which has a single blood supply from the right coronary artery (Fig. 5–10). Because the anterolateral papillary muscle has a dual blood supply from the left anterior descending and the left circumflex coronary artery, it rarely undergoes isolated ischemic rupture.[16, 77, 78] The patient with papillary muscle rupture presents with sudden mitral regurgitation with variable severity. Complete transection of a left ventricular papillary muscle is incompatible with life because of massive sudden mitral regurgitation.[17]

Right-Sided Infarction

Right ventricular infarction is a common complication of inferior transmural myocardial infarction (Fig. 5–9*B*). In a series reported by Isner et al., as many as 30% of patients with transmural posteroseptal left ventricular infarction had posterior right ventricular infarction. Extension into the anterior wall is uncommon in cases of right ventricular infarction.[79, 80] We reported that 78% of right ventricular infarctions occurring in patients with inferior left ventricular infarcts had concomitant right ventricular hypertrophy.[81] Isolated right ventricular infarction may infrequently occur in the absence of coronary disease in patients with chronic lung disease and right ventricular hypertrophy.[82] Atrial infarction occurs in 10% of

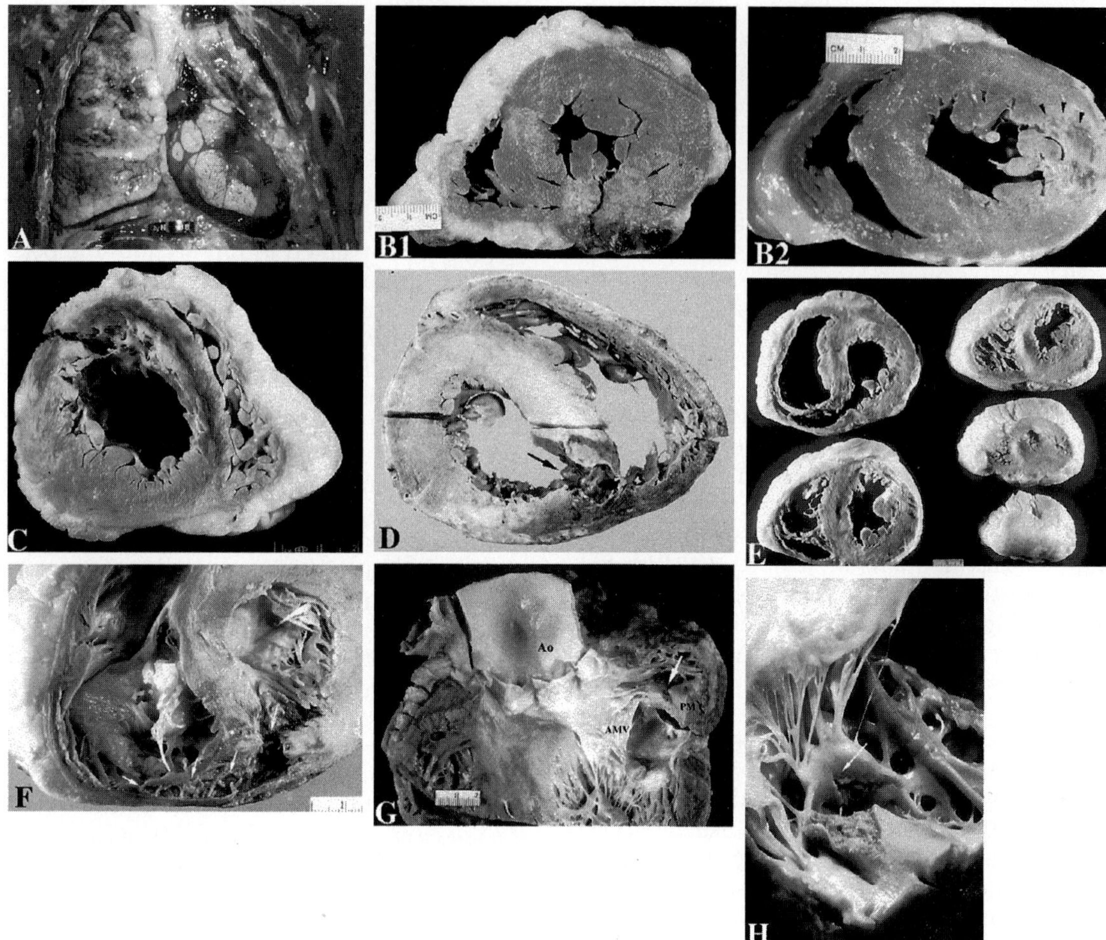

Figure 5–10. Ruptured acute myocardial infarction. *A.* Hemopericardium in a 70-year-old male with history of chest pain and diagnosis of acute transmural infarction died suddenly while walking to the bathroom 24 hours following admission. *B1.* The pericardium contained 300 ml of blood and a rupture site was identified on the posterior wall of the left ventricle. Note an early transmural infarct (pale area on the posterior wall [*arrows*] with rupture site close to the viable myocardium but within the infarct zone. *B2.* Shows a lateral wall rupture; note the rupture site is close to the viable and the infarcted myocardium (*arrowheads*). *C.* A 50-year-old man presented with 7-hour duration of chest pain. He received streptokinase and underwent balloon angioplasty of the proximal left anterior descending coronary artery. At autopsy, the patient had hemopericardium and a transmural hemorrhagic reperfused infarct involving the anteroseptal wall of the left ventricle. The rupture occurred close to the viable myocardium on the anterior wall. *D.* Rupture of the posterior ventricular septum (*arrow*) 2 weeks following an acute myocardial infarction. The patient died with severe congestive heart failure, and the diagnosis of ventricular septal rupture was clinically missed. (A four-chamber cut had been made prior to breadloaf). *E.* Ventricular septal rupture involving the inferobasal portion of the heart, which extends through the posterior septum and into the right ventricle causing a dissection of the posterior wall of the right ventricle. *F.* A high-power view of the inferobasal portion of the heart showing the rupture through the septum extending into the right ventricle and piercing the right ventricular wall (*arrow* along the rupture tract). *G.* A patient with transmural myocardial infarction of the posterior wall of the left ventricle with rupture of one of the two heads of posteromedial (*PM*) papillary muscle (*arrow*). The base of the heart has been opened along the left ventricular outflow tract (*Ao* = aorta, *AMV* = anterior mitral leaflet). *H.* High-power view showing total severance of one of the papillary heads (*arrow*) of the posteromedial papillary muscle.

all left ventricular inferior wall infarcts, and typically involves the right atrium.[83]

Pericardial Effusion and Pericarditis

Pericardial effusion is reported in 25% of patients with acute myocardial infarcts and is more common in patients with anterior myocardial infarction, large infarcts, and congestive heart failure.[84, 85] Pericardial effusion secondary to acute myocardial infarction may occur as a transudative effusion, or as an exudate, in association with acute pericarditis.

Pericarditis occurs less often than pericardial effusion, and is seen only in transmural acute myocardial infarction (see Chapter 11). Pericarditis, in contrast to postinfarction effusions, may be localized to the area of necrosis, and is accompanied by chest pain. Pericarditis consists of fibrin deposition in addition to inflammation, and may be present from day 1 postinfarction to as late as 6 weeks. Risk factors for the development of postinfarction pericarditis include heparinization and thrombolytic therapy.[86] Dressler syndrome, also called postmyocardial infarction syndrome, is a form of postinfarction pericarditis, which was said to occur in 3 to 4% of all myocardial infarctions in 1957.[17] At autopsy, there is localized fibrinous pericarditis along with neutrophil infiltration. The cause of Dressler syndrome is unknown, but antibodies to cardiac tissue have been reported, suggesting an immunologic process.[87]

Chronic Congestive Heart Failure

Patients with large acute myocardial infarction and persistent ischemia are the most likely to develop heart failure. Patients with chronic congestive heart failure have a poor prognosis.[88] Congestive heart failure occurs usually in the presence of two- or three-vessel disease and may develop even in the presence of well-developed collaterals.[89] Grossly, the atria and the ventricles are dilated and the ventricle shows either a large healed infarct (Fig. 5–11) or multiple smaller infarcts with or without a transmural scar.[90] Scarring of the inferior wall of the left ventricle often involves the posteromedial papillary muscle that gives rise to mitral regurgitation contributing to congestive heart failure (Fig. 5–11).[89] Microscopically the subendocardial regions of ischemia will show myocytes with myofibrillar loss and rich in glycogen suggesting a state of "hibernation" (see following).[91] Sometimes it is difficult to differentiate ischemic cardiomyopathy from idiopathic dilated cardiomyopathy when infarcts are few and small and only one vessel disease is present; in such situations we tend to call these idiopathic dilated cardiomyopathy with coronary artery disease.[92]

True and False Aneurysms

A large acute transmural myocardial infarct that has undergone expansion is the most likely infarct that will result in a true aneurysm.[93, 94] The pulsatile force from the blood in the cavity stretches and thins the necrotic muscle, which heals forming the wall of a true aneurysm.[95] An aneurysm is defined clinically as a discrete thinned segment of the left ventricle that protrudes during both systole and diastole and has a broad neck (Fig. 5–12). Morphologically the wall of a true aneurysm consists of fibrous tissue with interspersed myocytes. In contrast, a false aneurysm has a small neck (from a prior rupture of the infarct) and a wall formed by pericardium, thrombus, and fibrous tissue (Figure 5–12).

The incidence of true aneurysm following a myocardial infarction is 5 to 10% and is more frequent in transmural infarction than subendocardial infarction.[17] Aneurysms are usually associated with two- or more vessel coronary disease with poorly developed collaterals.[96] Most aneurysms involve the anteroapical wall of the left ventricle (80%)[16] and are four times more frequent in this wall than the inferior or posterior wall.[17] The pericardium is usually adherent to the aneurysm and may calcify. True aneurysms rarely rupture, whereas rupture is more common of a false aneurysm (Fig. 5–12).[97] The cavity of the aneurysm usually contains an organizing thrombus and the patient may present with embolic complications (see following). The mortality is six times higher in patients with aneurysm than without.[98]

False aneurysms occur when a rupture is sealed off by the pericardium (Fig. 5–12). Pericardial adhesions that have formed either prior to the infarct or prior to rupture (if late after an infarction) contain the hematoma. The cavity of the false aneurysm is usually filled with large blood clot, both old and new. The wall of a pseudoaneurysm lacks cardiac muscle.[99–101] Once recognized clinically, generally by echocardiography, treatment is operative repair.[72]

Mural Thrombus and Embolization

Mural thrombus forming on the endocardial surface over the area of the acute infarction occurs in 20% of all patients. However, the incidence is 40% for anterior infarcts and 60% for apical infarcts.[102–105] Patients with left ventricular thrombi have poorer global left ventricular function and poorer prognosis as compared with those without thrombi.[102] The poor prognosis is secondary to complications of a large infarct and not from emboli.[103] It has been reported that those who form thrombi have endocardial inflammation during the phase of acute infarction. The thrombi tend to organize, but the superficial portions may embolize in about

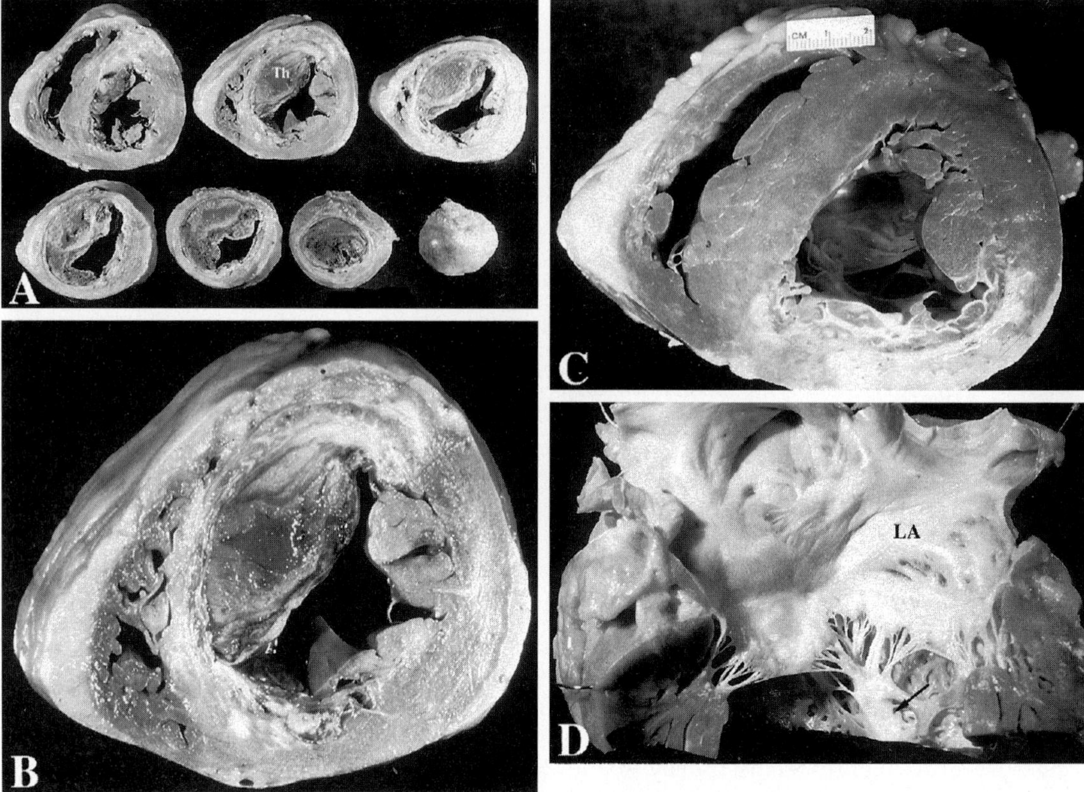

Figure 5–11. Thrombus left ventricle with healed myocardial infarct. *A*. Ventricular slices of a heart with healed myocardial infarction involving the anteroseptal wall of the left ventricle with extension from the base to the apex; note dilatation of the left ventricular cavity and presence of an organizing thrombus (*Th*). *B*. Close up of the basal ventricular slice (middle slice from top row in *A*); note large transmural healed infarct with overlying organizing infarct. Patient at autopsy had multiple infarcts in the kidneys and one in the spleen. *C*. A 60-year-old man with congestive heart failure and mitral regurgitation had a healed myocardial infarction of the posterolateral wall of the left ventricle at autopsy. *D*. Note scarred and thinned posteromedial papillary muscle (*arrow*) whereas the anterolateral papillary muscle is hypertrophied. Note dilated left atrium (*LA*).

10% of cases (Fig. 5–13).[102] The usual sites of symptomatic embolization are the brain, eyes, kidney, spleen, bowel, legs, and coronary arteries. Symptomatic emboli are usually due to larger fragments, whereas small particles of thrombus that embolize generally do not cause symptoms.[104] The risk of embolization is greatest in the first few weeks of acute myocardial infarction.[106] Anticoagulation has been shown to reduce the incidence of left ventricular thrombus formation.[17]

MYOCARDIAL STUNNING

Myocardial stunning is a term that expresses mechanical myocardial dysfunction that persists following coronary occlusion of variable duration and reperfusion, in the absence of irreversible damage to the myocardium.[91] The term is applied solely to a physiologic derangement of cardiac contractility, as the involved myocardium is histologically normal. The first description of the entity is credited to Heyndrickx et al. in 1975[107] and the majority of animal studies have been performed in the dog model or isolated heart preparations. Stunning may occur following a single coronary occlusion lasting less than 20 minutes followed by reperfusion[107, 108] following multiple repeated occlusions and reperfusion lasting 5 to 10 minutes[109]; following partially reversible and partially irreversible ischemia lasting from 20 minutes to 3 hours, causing no or some necrosis, respectively[91]; following global ischemia *in vitro* (isolated heart preparation)[91]; following global ischemia *in vivo* (cardioplegic arrest)[110]; and following exercise-induced ischemia.[111] The pathogenesis of myocardial stunning is poorly understood and is thought to be multifactorial. The

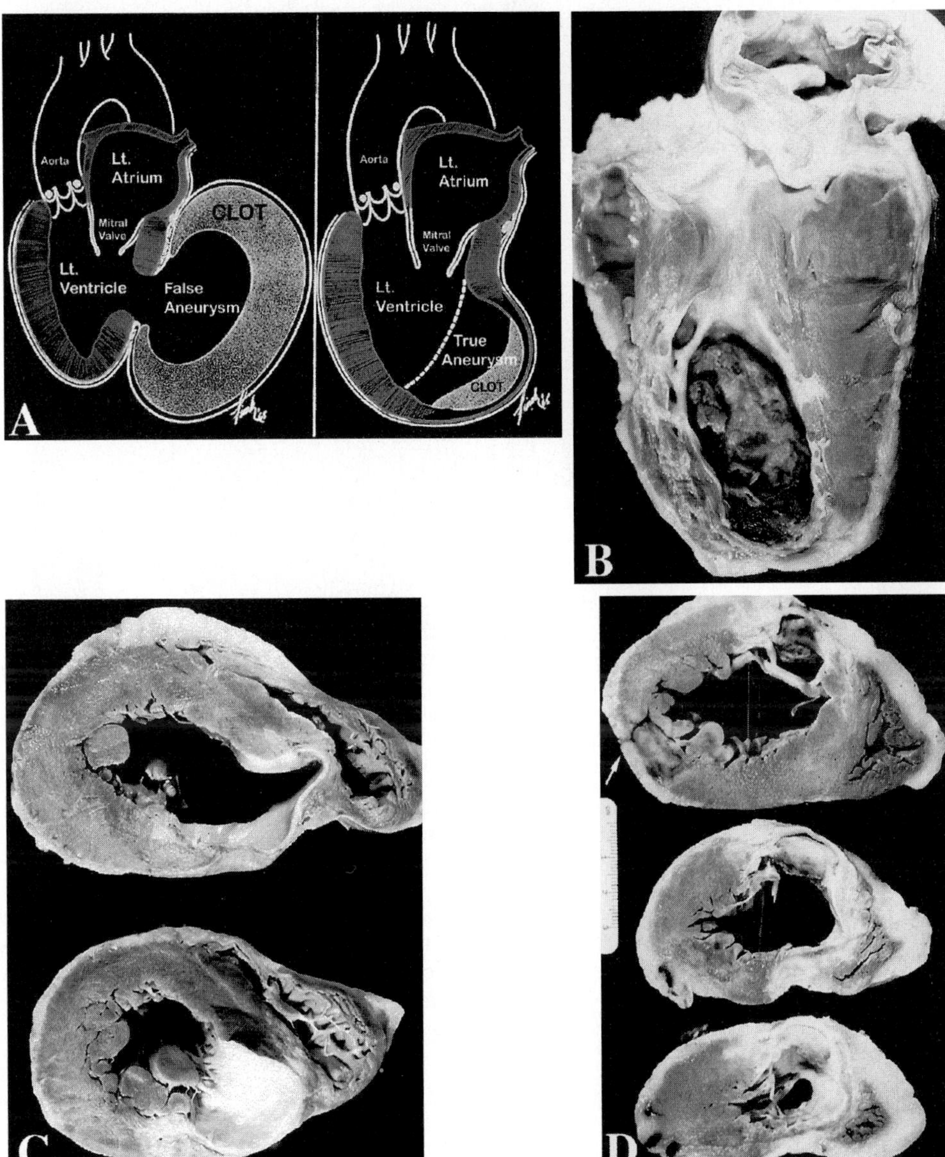

Figure 5–12. Diagram of a false (*left*) and a true (*right*) aneurysm. Note a rupture of the left ventricular wall with the blood contained by the pericardial wall. The left ventricle does not form the wall of the aneurysm and the neck of the aneurysm is narrow. The wall of the true aneurysm is formed by the wall of the infarcted myocardium and the neck of the aneurysm is wide (Courtesy of Dr. William C. Roberts). *B.* A true aneurysm is seen at the apex of the heart involving the anteroseptal apical two thirds of the left ventricle. The aneurysm is filled with a thrombus and there is endocardial thickening around the edges of the infarct. *C.* Healed transmural infarction of the posteroseptal wall of the left ventricle; note the thinned and bulging aneurysm of the posterior and septal wall with marked endocardial thickening. No thrombus was identified within the cavity of the aneurysm. *D.* A 54-year-old man died suddenly without any significant medical history. At autopsy there was cardiac tamponade with ventricular rupture of the posterolateral wall (*arrow*) secondary to a transmural acute infarction. Ventricular slices of the heart showing presence of a localized small anterior aneurysm from a healed myocardial infarction involving the anterior and septal wall of the left ventricle. Note organizing thrombus in the aneurysmal cavity.

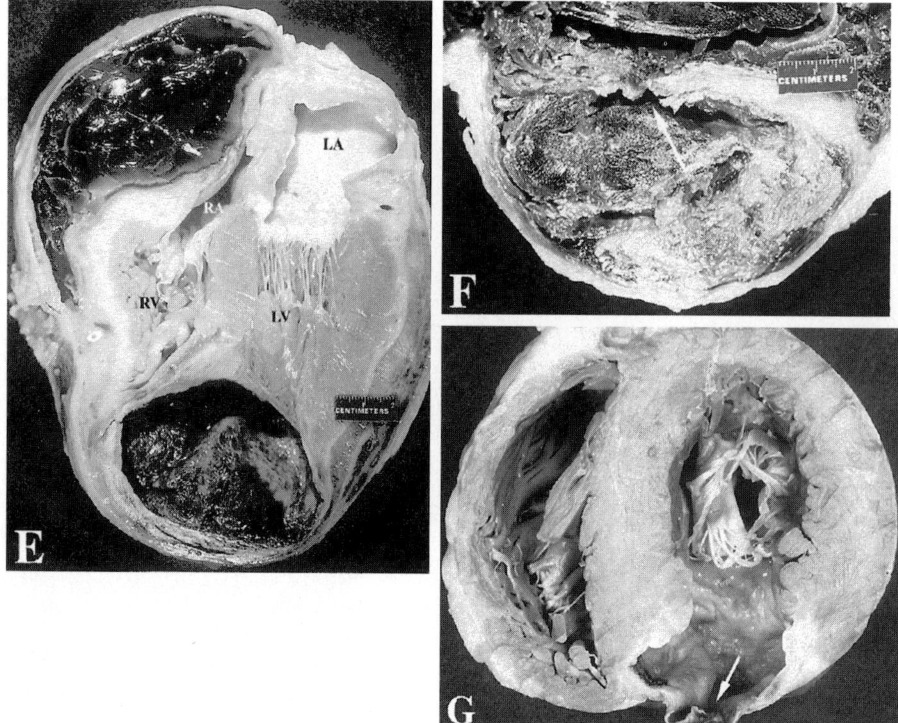

Figure 5–12 *Continued. E.* False aneurysm. A 47-year-old male presented with sudden onset shortness of breath and died in the emergency room. At autopsy there was a loculated hemopericardium and a left ventricular anteroapical aneurysm secondary to a healed myocardial infarction with overlying thrombus. Four-chamber cut of the heart showed extensive adhesions between the visceral and the parietal pericardium and loculated fresh blood was present in the pericardial space above the right atrium (*RA*) and right ventricle (*RV*) as well as organizing hemorrhage around the heart (*LA* = left atrium, *LV* = left ventricle). *F.* A deeper posterior cut revealed the rupture site in the aneurysmal wall (*arrow*). Note the narrow, communicating neck of the true aneurysm with the false aneurysm. A diagnosis of rupture of a true aneurysm with a secondary false aneurysm was made. *G.* Rupture of a healed inferior wall aneurysm (*arrow*) in a 56-year-old male who developed chest pain and died while undergoing a stress test. At autopsy, there was hemopericardium (500 mL).

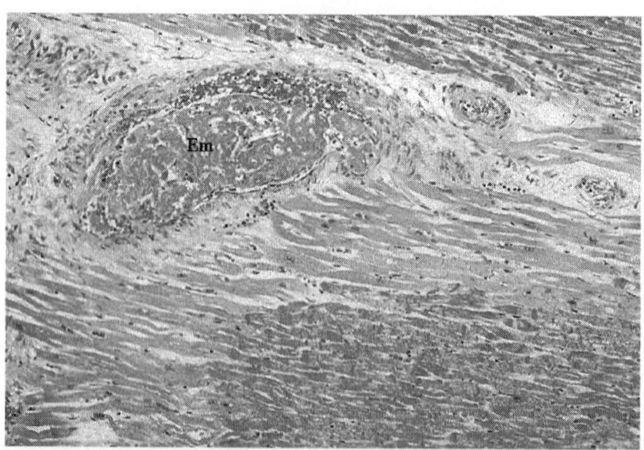

Figure 5–13. Intramyocardial thrombus with surrounding acute myocardial infarction in a patient with history of myocardial infarction 6 months prior to current presentation with chest pain. On echocardiography he had a thrombus in the left ventricular cavity overlying the healed infarct. No acute thrombus was seen in any of the epicardial coronary arteries at autopsy. However, the anterolateral wall of the left ventricle showed intramyocardial coronary emboli (*Em*) and surrounding infarction of less than 24 hours' duration.

most accepted mechanisms of myocardial stunning involve damage by oxygen-free radicals and altered calcium homeostasis resulting in cellular calcium overload during the early phase of reperfusion.[91]

HIBERNATING MYOCARDIUM

In the early 1980s Rahimtoola found significant improvement in left ventricular function after coronary revascularization in a subset of patients with depressed ventricular performance.[112] He postulated that the mechanism of poor myocardial contractility was chronic ischemia, which could be improved by revascularization. The premise behind this rationale was dependent on the surviving myocardium being in a functional albeit depressed "hibernating" state,[113, 114] suggesting that the myocardium may adapt to chronic ischemia by decreasing its contractility but preserving viability.

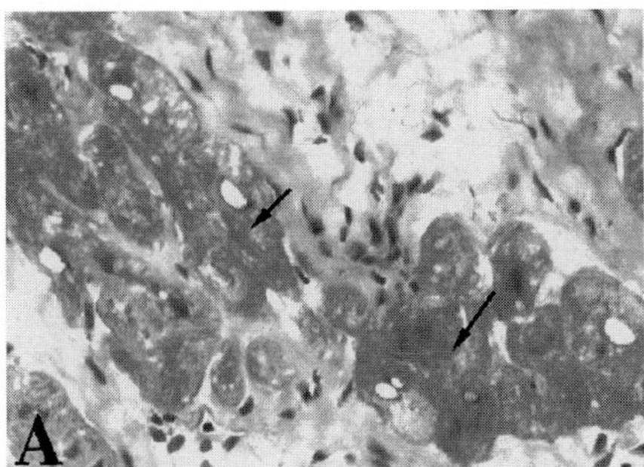

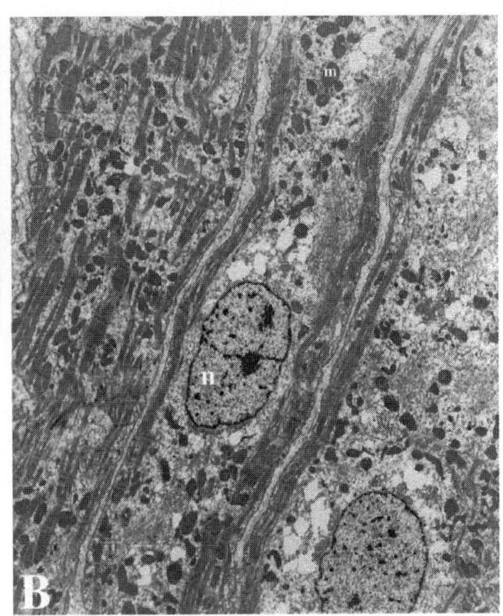

Figure 5–14. Hibernating myocardium in a dog heart. *A*. Note subendocardial myocytes showing perinuclear intracellular glycogen (*arrow*) (PAS stain). *B*. Corresponding electron micrograph showing small mitochondria (*m*) of varying sizes and shapes surrounded by empty spaces representative of glycogen. Note loss of myofibrils and nuclei (*n*) showing loss of heterochromatin.

Morphologically hibernating myocytes show loss of contractile elements, especially in the perinuclear region, and occasionally throughout the cytoplasm. The space left by the dissolution of the myofibrils is occupied by glycogen, as evidenced by the strong PAS positivity (Fig. 5–14). Ultrastructurally, there is depletion of sarcomeres, most pronounced in the perinuclear region, with increased glycogen. The nuclei are enlarged, with a tortuous nuclear membrane and evenly distributed heterochromatin. The mitochondria are elongated, shrunken, and osmiophilic (Fig. 5–14).[115]

REFERENCES

1. Tavazzi L. Clinical epidemiology of acute myocardial infarction. Am Heart J 138:48–54, 1999.
2. Norris RM. The natural history of acute myocardial infarction. Heart 83:726–730, 2000.
3. Pashos CL, Newhouse JP, McNeil BJ. Temporal changes in the care and outcomes of elderly patients with acute myocardial infarction, 1987 through 1990. JAMA 270:1832–1836, 1993.
4. Miller TD, Christian TF, Hodge DO, Hopfenspirger MR, Gersh BJ, Gibbons RJ. Comparison of acute myocardial infarct size to two-year mortality in patients < 65 to those > or = 65 years of age. Am J Cardiol 84:1170–1175, 1999.
5. Rosamond WD, Chambless LE, Folsom AR. Survival trends, coronary event rates, and the MONICA project. Monitoring trends and determinants in cardiovascular disease [letter; comment]. Lancet 354:864–865, 1999.
6. Tunstall-Pedoe H, Kuulasmaa K, Amouyel P, Arveiler D, Rajakangas AM, Pajak A. Myocardial infarction and coronary deaths in the World Health Organization MONICA Project. Registration procedures, event rates, and case-fatality rates in 38 populations from 21 countries in four continents. Circulation 90:583–612, 1994.
7. Hedges JR, Young GP, Henkel GF, Gibler WB, Green TR, Swanson JR. Serial ECGs are less accurate than serial CK-MB results for emergency department diagnosis of myocardial infarction. Ann Emerg Med 21:1445–1450, 1992.
8. Young GP, Gibler WB, Hedges JR, et al. Serial creatine kinase-MB results are a sensitive indicator of acute myocardial infarction in chest pain patients with nondiagnostic electrocardiograms: The second Emergency Medicine Cardiac Research Group Study. Acad Emerg Med 4:869–877, 1997.
9. Morrow DA, Rifai N, Tanasijevic MJ, Wybenga DR, de Lemos JA, Antman EM. Clinical efficacy of three assays for cardiac troponin I for risk stratification in acute coronary syndromes: A Thrombolysis In Myocardial Infarction (TIMI) 11B Substudy. Clin Chem 46:453–460, 2000.
10. Antman EM, Grudzien C, Sacks DB. Evaluation of a rapid bedside assay for detection of serum cardiac troponin T. JAMA 273:1279–1282, 1995.
11. Hackel DB, Reimer KA, Ideker RE, et al. Comparison of enzymatic and anatomic estimates of myocardial infarct size in man. Circulation 70:824–835, 1984.
12. Cannon CP. Defining acute myocardial infarction by ST segment deviation [editorial; comment]. Eur Heart J 21:266–267, 2000.
13. Cannon CP, Rutherford JD. The clinical spectrum of ischemic heart disease. In: Antman EM, Rutherford JD (eds): Coronary Care Medicine: A Practical Approach. Boston: Marinus Nijhoff, 1996.
14. Buja LM, Willerson JT. The role of coronary artery lesions in ischemic heart disease: Insights from recent clinicopathologic, coronary arteriographic, and experimental studies. Hum Pathol 18:451–461, 1987.
15. Gibson RS. Non-Q-wave myocardial infarction: Diagnosis, prognosis, and management. Curr Probl Cardiol 13:9–72, 1988

16. Edwards WD. Pathology of myocardial infarction and reperfusion. In: Gersh BJ, Rahimatoola SH (eds): Acute Myocardial Infarction, pp 14–48. New York: Elsevier, 1991.
17. Antman EM, Braunwald E. Acute myocardial infarction. In: Braunwald E (ed): Heart Disease. A Text Book of Cardiovascular Disease. Vol. 2, pp 1184–1288. Philadelphia: WB Saunders, 1997.
18. van der Laarse A, van Leeuwen FT, Krul R, Tuinstra CL, Lie KI. The size of infarction as judged enzymatically in 1974 patients with acute myocardial infarction. Relation with symptomatology, infarct localization and type of infarction. Int J Cardiol 19:191–207, 1988.
19. Freifeld AG, Schuster EH, Bulkley BH. Nontransmural versus transmural myocardial infarction. A morphologic study. Am J Med 75:423–432, 1983.
20. Braunwald E, Cannon CP. Non-Q wave and ST segment depression myocardial infarction: Is there a role for thrombolytic therapy? J Am Coll Cardiol 27:1333–1334, 1996.
21. Page DL, Caulfield JB, Kastor JA, DeSanctis RW, Sanders CA. Myocardial changes associated with cardiogenic shock. N Engl J Med 285:133–137, 1971.
22. Piek JJ, Becker AE. Collateral blood supply to the myocardium at risk in human myocardial infarction: A quantitative postmortem assessment. J Am Coll Cardiol 11:1290–1296, 1988.
23. Falk E. Unstable angina with fatal outcome: Dynamic coronary thrombosis leading to infarction and/or sudden death. Autopsy evidence of recurrent mural thrombosis with peripheral embolization culminating in total vascular occlusion. Circulation 71:699–708, 1985.
24. Andersen HR, Falk E, Nielsen D. Clinical first myocardial infarction: Coronary artery disease and old infarcts in 53 consecutive fatal cases from a coronary care unit. Am J Cardiovasc Pathol 2:315–319, 1989.
25. Baroldi G, Manion WC. Microcirculatory disturbances and human myocardial infarction. Am Heart J 74:173–178, 1967.
26. Reimer KA, Jennings RB. The "wavefront phenomenon" of myocardial ischemic cell death. II. Transmural progression of necrosis within the framework of ischemic bed size (myocardium at risk) and collateral flow. Lab Invest 40:633–644, 1979.
27. Jennings RB, Steenbergen C, Jr., Reimer KA. Myocardial ischemia and reperfusion. Monogr Pathol 37:47–80, 1995.
28. Reimer KA, Jennings RB, Hill ML. Total ischemia in dog hearts, in vitro. 2. High energy phosphate depletion and associated defects in energy metabolism, cell volume regulation, and sarcolemmal integrity. Circ Res 49:901–911, 1981.
29. Jennings RB, Reimer KA, Hill ML, Mayer SE. Total ischemia in dog hearts, in vitro. 1. Comparison of high energy phosphate production, utilization, and depletion, and of adenine nucleotide catabolism in total ischemia in vitro vs. severe ischemia in vivo. Circ Res 49:892–900, 1981.
30. Jennings RB, Reimer KA. Lethal myocardial ischemic injury. Am J Pathol 102:241–255, 1981.
31. Jennings RB, Schaper J, Hill ML, Steenbergen C, Jr., Reimer KA. Effect of reperfusion late in the phase of reversible ischemic injury. Changes in cell volume, electrolytes, metabolites, and ultrastructure. Circ Res 56:262–278, 1985.
32. Reimer KA, Jennings RB. Energy metabolism in the reversible and irreversible phases of severe myocardial ischemia. Acta Med Scand Suppl 651:19–27, 1981.
33. Jennings RB, Ganote CE. Structural changes in myocardium during acute ischemia. Circ Res 35 Suppl 3:156–172, 1974.
34. Jennings RB, Ganote CE, Reimer KA. Ischemic tissue injury. Am J Pathol 81:179–198, 1975.
35. Virmani R, Forman MB, Kolodgie FD. Myocardial reperfusion injury. Histopathological effects of perfluorochemical. Circulation 81:IV57–68, 1990.
36. Jennings RB. Acute myocardial ischemic injury. Ultrastructural and biochemical studies of the early phase of lethal injury. Arch Inst Cardiol Mex 50:365–371, 1980.
37. Buja LM, Hagler HK, Willerson JT. Altered calcium homeostasis in the pathogenesis of myocardial ischemic and hypoxic injury. Cell Calcium 9:205–217, 1988.
38. Buja LM, Fattor RA, Miller JC, Chien KR, Willerson JT. Effects of calcium loading and impaired energy production on metabolic and ultrastructural features of cell injury in cultured neonatal rat cardiac myocytes. Lab Invest 63:320–331, 1990.
39. Schoen FJ. The heart In: Cotran RS, Kumar V, Collins T (eds): Robbins Pathologic Basis of Disease, pp 554–564. Philadelphia: WB Saunders Company, 1999.
40. Mallory GK, White PD, Salcedo-Salgar J. The speed of healing of myocardial infarction: A study of the pathologic anatomy in seventy-two cases. Am Heart J 18:647–671, 1939.
41. Lodge-Patch I. The aging of cardiac infarcts, and its influence on cardiac rupture. Br Heart J 13:37–42, 1951.
42. Bouchardy B, Majno G. Histopathology of early myocardial infarcts. A new approach. Am J Pathol 74:301–330, 1974.
43. Cowan MJ, Reichenbach D, Turner P, Thostenson C. Cellular response of the evolving myocardial infarction after therapeutic coronary artery reperfusion. Hum Pathol 22:154–163, 1991.
44. Pantridge JF, Adgey AA. Pre-hospital coronary care. The mobile coronary care unit. Am J Cardiol 24:666–673, 1969.
45. Campbell RW, Murray A, Julian DG. Ventricular arrhythmias in first 12 hours of acute myocardial infarction. Natural history study. Br Heart J 46:351–357, 1981.
46. Eldar M, Sievner Z, Goldbourt U, Reicher-Reiss H, Kaplinsky E, Behar S. Primary ventricular tachycardia in acute myocardial infarction: Clinical characteristics and mortality. The SPRINT Study Group. Ann Intern Med 117:31–36, 1992.
47. Corr PB, Gillis RA. Autonomic neural influences on the dysrhythmias resulting from myocardial infarction. Circ Res 43:1–9, 1978.
48. Corr PB, Sobel BE. Mechanisms contributing to dysrhythmias induced by ischemia and their therapeutic implications. Adv Cardiol 110–129, 1978.
49. Stevenson WG, Linssen GC, Havenith MG, Brugada P, Wellens HJ. The spectrum of death after myocardial infarction: A necropsy study. Am Heart J 118:1182–1188, 1989.
50. Bloor CM, Ehsani A, White FC, Sobel BE. Ventricular fibrillation threshold in acute myocardial infarction and its relation to myocardial infarct size. Cardiovasc Res 9:468–472, 1975.
51. Bloor CM, White FC. Coronary artery reperfusion: Effects of occlusion duration on reactive hyperemia responses. Basic Res Cardiol 70:148–158, 1975.

52. Mark DB, Naylor CD, Hlatky MA, et al. Use of medical resources and quality of life after acute myocardial infarction in Canada and the United States. N Engl J Med 331:1130–1135, 1994.
53. Califf RM, Bengtson JR. Cardiogenic shock. N Engl J Med 330:1724–1730, 1994.
54. Holmes DR, Jr., Bates ER, Kleiman NS, et al. Contemporary reperfusion therapy for cardiogenic shock: The GUSTO-I trial experience. The GUSTO-I Investigators. Global Utilization of Streptokinase and Tissue Plasminogen Activator for Occluded Coronary Arteries. J Am Coll Cardiol 26:668–674, 1995.
55. Holmes DR, Jr., Califf RM, Topol EJ. Lessons we have learned from the GUSTO trial. Global Utilization of Streptokinase and Tissue Plasminogen Activator for Occluded Arteries. J Am Coll Cardiol 25:10S–17S, 1995.
56. Gutovitz AL, Sobel BE, Roberts R. Progressive nature of myocardial injury in selected patients with cardiogenic shock. Am J Cardiol 41:469–475, 1978.
57. Califf RM. Myocardial reperfusion: Is it ever too late? J Am Coll Cardiol 13:1130–1132, 1989.
58. The TIMI Study Group. Comparison of invasive and conservative strategies after treatment with intravenous tissue plasminogen activator in acute myocardial infarction. Results of the thrombolysis in myocardial infarction (TIMI) phase II trial. N Engl J Med 320:618–627, 1989.
59. Ellis SG, Topol EJ, George BS, et al. Recurrent ischemia without warning. Analysis of risk factors for in-hospital ischemic events following successful thrombolysis with intravenous tissue plasminogen activator. Circulation 80:1159–1165, 1989.
60. Weisman HF, Bush DE, Mannisi JA, Weisfeldt ML, Healy B. Cellular mechanisms of myocardial infarct expansion. Circulation 78:186–201, 1988.
61. Weisman HF, Healy B. Myocardial infarct expansion, infarct extension, and reinfarction: Pathophysiologic concepts. Prog Cardiovasc Dis 30:73–110, 1987.
62. Gaudron P, Eilles C, Ertl G, Kochsiek K. Adaptation to cardiac dysfunction after myocardial infarction. Circulation 87:IV83–89, 1993.
63. Gaudron P, Eilles C, Kugler I, Ertl G. Progressive left ventricular dysfunction and remodeling after myocardial infarction. Potential mechanisms and early predictors [see comments]. Circulation 87:755–763, 1993.
64. Batts KP, Ackermann DM, Edwards WD. Postinfarction rupture of the left ventricular free wall: Clinicopathologic correlates in 100 consecutive autopsy cases. Hum Pathol 21:530–535, 1990.
65. Mann JM, Roberts WC, Rupture of the left ventricular free wall during acute myocardial infarction: Analysis of 138 necropsy patients and comparison with 50 necropsy patients with acute myocardial infarction without rupture. Am J Cardiol 62:847–859, 1988.
66. Atkinson JB, Robinowitz M, McAllister HA, Virmani R. Association of eosinophils with cardiac rupture. Hum Pathol 16:562–568, 1985.
67. Reeder GS. Acute myocardial infarction: Enhancing the results of reperfusion therapy. Mayo Clin Proc 70:1185–1190, 1995.
68. Reeder GS. Identification and treatment of complications of myocardial infarction. Mayo Clin Proc 70:880–884, 1995.
69. Pohjola-Sintonen S, Muller JE, Stone PH, et al. Ventricular septal and free wall rupture complicating acute myocardial infarction: Experience in the Multicenter Investigation of Limitation of Infarct Size. Am Heart J 117:809–818, 1989.
70. Reddy SG, Roberts WC. Frequency of rupture of the left ventricular free wall or ventricular septum among necropsy cases of fatal acute myocardial infarction since introduction of coronary care units. Am J Cardiol 63:906–911, 1989.
71. Shapira I, Isakov A, Burke M, Almog C. Cardiac rupture in patients with acute myocardial infarction. Chest 92:219–223, 1987.
72. Oliva PB, Hammill SC, Edwards WD. Cardiac rupture, a clinically predictable complication of acute myocardial infarction: Report of 70 cases with clinicopathologic correlations. J Am Coll Cardiol 22:720–726, 1993.
73. Reardon MJ, Carr CL, Diamond A, et al. Ischemic left ventricular free wall rupture: Prediction, diagnosis, and treatment. Ann Thorac Surg 64:1509–1513, 1997.
74. Cummings RG, Reimer KA, Califf R, Hackel D, Boswick J, Lowe JE. Quantitative analysis of right and left ventricular infarction in the presence of postinfarction ventricular septal defect. Circulation 77:33–42, 1988.
75. Pett SB, Jr., Follis F, Allen K, Temes T, Wernly JA. Posterior ventricular septal rupture: An anatomical reconstruction. J Card Surg 13:445–450; discussion 451–452, 1998.
76. Pretre R, Ye Q, Grunenfelder J, Lachat M, Vogt PR, Turina MI. Operative results of "repair" of ventricular septal rupture after acute myocardial infraction. Am J Cardiol 84:785–788, 1999.
77. Barbour DJ, Roberts WC. Rupture of a left ventricular papillary muscle during acute myocardial infarction: Analysis of 22 necropsy patients. J Am Coll Cardiol 8:558–565, 1986.
78. Wei JY, Hutchins GM. The pathogenesis of papillary muscle rupture complicating myocardial infarction: Hemorrhage accompanying contraction band necrosis. Lab Invest 39:204–209, 1978.
79. Isner JM, Roberts WC. Right ventricular infarction complicating left ventricular infarction secondary to coronary heart disease. Frequency, location, associated findings and significance from analysis of 236 necropsy patients with acute or healed myocardial infarction. Am J Cardiol 42:885–894, 1978.
80. Isner JM. Right ventricular myocardial infarction. JAMA 259:712–718, 1988.
81. Forman MB, Wilson BH, Sheller JR, et al. Right ventricular hypertrophy is an important determinant of right ventricular infarction complicating acute inferior left ventricular infarction. J Am Coll Cardiol 10:1180–1187, 1987.
82. Kopelman HA, Forman MB, Wilson BH, et al. Right ventricular myocardial infarction in patients with chronic lung disease: Possible role of right ventricular hypertrophy. J Am Coll Cardiol 5:1302–1307, 1985.
83. Lazar EJ, Goldberger J, Peled H, Sherman M, Frishman WH. Atrial infarction: Diagnosis and management. Am Heart J 116:1058–1063, 1988.
84. Galve E, Garcia-Del-Castillo H, Evangelista A, Batlle J, Permanyer-Miralda G, Soler-Soler J. Pericardial effusion in the course of myocardial infarction: Incidence, natural history, and clinical relevance. Circulation 73:294–299, 1986.
85. Sugiura T, Iwasaka T, Takayama Y, et al. Factors associated with pericardial effusion in acute Q wave myocardial infarction. Circulation 81:477–481, 1990.

86. Erhardt LR. Clinical and pathological observations in different types of acute myocardial infarction. Acta Med Scand Suppl 560:1–78, 1974.
87. Uuskiula MM, Lamp KM, Martin SI. [Relation between the clinical course of acute myocardial infarction and specific sensitization of lymphocytes and lymphotoxin production]. Kardiologiia 27:57–60, 1987.
88. Pantely GA, Bristow JD. Ischemic cardiomyopathy. Prog Cardiovasc Dis 27:95–114, 1984.
89. Schuster EH, Bulkley BH. Ischemic cardiomyopathy: A clinicopathologic study of fourteen patients. Am Heart J 100:506–512, 1980.
90. Virmani R, Roberts WC. Quantification of coronary arterial narrowing and of left ventricular myocardial scarring in healed myocardial infarction with chronic, eventually fatal, congestive cardiac failure. Am J Med 68:831–838, 1980.
91. Kloner RA, Bolli R, Marban E, Reinlib L, Braunwald E. Medical and cellular implications of stunning, hibernation, and preconditioning: An NHLBI workshop. Circulation 97:1848–1867, 1998.
92. Atkinson JB, Virmani R. Congestive heart failure due to coronary artery disease without myocardial infarction: Clinicopathologic description of an unusual cardiomyopathy. Hum Pathol 20:1155–1162, 1989.
93. Erlebacher JA, Richter RC, Alonso DR, Devereux RB, Gay WA, Jr. Early infarct expansion: Structural or functional? J Am Coll Cardiol 6:839–844, 1985.
94. Erlebacher JA, Weiss JL, Weisfeldt ML, Bulkley BH. Early dilation of the infarcted segment in acute transmural myocardial infarction: Role of infarct expansion in acute left ventricular enlargement. J Am Coll Cardiol 4:201–208, 1984.
95. Hamer DH, Lindsay J, Jr. Redefining true ventricular aneurysm. Am J Cardiol 64:1192–1194, 1989.
96. Forman MB, Collins HW, Kopelman HA, et al. Determinants of left ventricular aneurysm formation after anterior myocardial infarction: A clinical and angiographic study. J Am Coll Cardiol 8:1256–1262, 1986.
97. Vlodaver Z, Coe JI, Edwards JE. True and false left ventricular aneurysms. Propensity for the latter to rupture. Circulation 51:567–572, 1975.
98. Meizlish JL, Berger HJ, Plankey M, Errico D, Levy W, Zaret BL. Functional left ventricular aneurysm formation after acute anterior transmural myocardial infarction. Incidence, natural history, and prognostic implications. N Engl J Med 311:1001–1006, 1984.
99. Edwards WD. Aneurysms and mural thrombi of the left ventricle [editorial]. Mayo Clin Proc 56:129–131, 1981.
100. Cabin HS, Roberts WC. True left ventricular aneurysm and healed myocardial infarction. Clinical and necropsy observations including quantification of degrees of coronary arterial narrowing. Am J Cardiol 46:754–763, 1980.
101. Cabin HS, Roberts WC. Left ventricular aneurysm, intraaneurysmal thrombus and systemic embolus in coronary heart disease. Chest 77:586–590, 1980.
102. Keeley EC, Hillis LD. Left ventricular mural thrombus after acute myocardial infarction. Clin Cardiol 19:83–86, 1996.
103. Fuster V, Halperin JL. Left ventricular thrombi and cerebral embolism [editorial]. N Engl J Med 320:392–394, 1989.
104. Meltzer RS, Visser CA, Fuster V. Intracardiac thrombi and systemic embolization. Ann Intern Med 104:689–698, 1986.
105. Visser CA, Kan G, Meltzer RS, Koolen JJ, Dunning AJ. Incidence, timing and prognostic value of left ventricular aneurysm formation after myocardial infarction: A prospective, serial echocardiographic study of 158 patients. Am J Cardiol 57:729–732, 1986.
106. Kupper AJ, Verheugt FW, Peels CH, Galema TW, Roos JP. Left ventricular thrombus incidence and behavior studied by serial two-dimensional echocardiography in acute anterior myocardial infarction: Left ventricular wall motion, systemic embolism and oral anticoagulation. J Am Coll Cardiol 13:1514–1520, 1989.
107. Heyndrickx GR, Millard RW, McRitchie RJ, Maroko PR, Vatner SF. Regional myocardial functional and electrophysiological alterations after brief coronary artery occlusion in conscious dogs. J Clin Invest 56:978–985, 1975.
108. Bolli R, Zhu WX, Thornby JI, O'Neill PG, Roberts R. Time course and determinants of recovery of function after reversible ischemia in conscious dogs. Am J Physiol 254:H102–114, 1988.
109. Bolli R, Zughaib M, Li XY, et al. Recurrent ischemia in the canine heart causes recurrent bursts of free radical production that have a cumulative effect on contractile function. A pathophysiological basis for chronic myocardial "stunning." J Clin Invest 96:1066–1084, 1995.
110. Gardner TJ. Oxygen radicals in cardiac surgery. Free Radic Biol Med 4:45–50, 1988.
111. Homans DC, Sublett E, Dai XZ, Bache RJ. Persistence of regional left ventricular dysfunction after exercise-induced myocardial ischemia. J Clin Invest 77:66–73, 1986.
112. Rahimtoola SH, Grunkemeier GL, Teply JF, et al. Changes in coronary bypass surgery leading to improved survival. JAMA 246:1912–1916, 1981.
113. Rahimtoola SH. The hibernating myocardium. Am Heart J 117:211–221, 1989.
114. Rahimtoola SH. Concept and evaluation of hibernating myocardium. Annu Rev Med 50:75–86, 1999.
115. Vanoverschelde JL, Wijns W, Depre C, et al. Mechanisms of chronic regional postischemic dysfunction in humans. New insights from the study of noninfarcted collateral-dependent myocardium. Circulation 87:1513–1523, 1993.

Chapter

6

CARDIOMYOPATHY

DEFINITION AND CLASSIFICATION

The cardiomyopathies are a diverse group of myocardial diseases that are characterized by chronic ventricular dysfunction. The clinical classification of cardiomyopathy is based on hemodynamic and echocardiographic abnormalities, and consists of dilated cardiomyopathy, hypertrophic cardiomyopathy, and restrictive cardiomyopathy. Recently, arrhythmogenic right ventricular dysplasia has been added to this classification[1] (Table 6–1). Hypertrophic and right ventricular cardiomyopathies have fairly distinctive morphological manifestations. Dilated and restrictive cardiomyopathies, on the other hand, are a more heterogeneous group of disorders without uniform histologic features. For this reason, the modifier "idiopathic" often precedes restrictive and dilated cardiomyopathy to emphasize that a variety of specific cardiac and systemic illnesses that may mimic these conditions has been ruled out. Secondary cardiomyopathies are termed "specific cardiomyopathies" in the recent World Health Organization classification,[1] and are primary diseases of the valves or coronary arteries, or are systemic illnesses with cardiac manifestations.

Pathologists have historically used the term "cardiomyopathy" only for primary cardiac disorders, although clinicians often use the term (generally with modifiers) for secondary conditions (e.g., "ischemic cardiomyopathy").[2] Only after clinical and pathologic exclusion of secondary causes of myocardial dysfunction (such as pericardial, hypertensive, congenital, valvular, and ischemic disease) is the term "cardiomyopathy" strictly appropriate. However, the distinction between primary and secondary cardiomyopathy is sometimes arbitrary; for example, restrictive cardiomyopathy with endocardial fibrosis has been alternately classified as secondary or primary.[1, 2]

The opinions or assertions contained herein are the private views of the authors and are not to be construed as official or reflecting the views of the Department of the Army, the Department of the Air Force, or the Department of Defense.

DILATED CARDIOMYOPATHY

Definitions and Terms

Dilated cardiomyopathy is an idiopathic disease of heart muscle that is characterized by impaired systolic function of both ventricles.[3] Clinically, approximately 50% of patients with congestive heart failure of unknown etiology will have no specific underlying cause demonstrated after complete evaluation, including endomyocardial biopsy.[4] In the other 50%, clinical investigation will reveal myocarditis and occult coronary artery disease in the majority; a host of other inciting agents (e.g., toxic insults secondary to anthracyclines or catecholamines) and systemic diseases (e.g., renal disease, hemochromatosis, or amyloidosis) may also result in congestive heart failure. Pathologically, dilated cardiomyopathy is a term that should be restricted to cases of idiopathic global cardiac dilatation in the absence of significant coronary, valvular, and hypertensive disease, and other causes of cardiac dilatation such as cor pulmonale and congenital heart disease. In patients with conditions that are associated with dilated cardiomyopathy, such as chronic alcoholism, diabetes mellitus, and the peripartum state, the term is still often employed.

Table 6–1. Classification of Cardiomyopathies[1]

Dilated Cardiomyopathy

Hypertrophic Cardiomyopathy

Arrhythmogenic right ventricular dysplasia

Restrictive Cardiomyopathy
- Idiopathic
- Secondary
  - Amyloidosis[2]
  - Loeffler's eosinophilic endocardial fibrosis[2]
  - Tropical endocardial fibrosis (Davies' disease)

Unclassified cardiomyopathies
- Mitochondrial cardiomyopathy
- Fibroelastosis
- Noncompacted myocardium
- Systolic dysfunction with minimal dilatation[3]

Specific (secondary) cardiomyopathies
- Ischemic cardiomyopathy
- Valvular cardiomyopathy
- Hypertensive cardiomyopathy
- Inflammatory cardiomyopathy
  - Myocarditis
  - Chagas cardiomyopathy
  - HIV cardiomyopathy
- Metabolic cardiomyopathy
- General system disease
  - Connective tissue disease
  - Sarcoidosis
  - Leukemic infiltrates
- Muscular dystrophies
- Neuromuscular disorders
- Sensitivity and toxic reactions
  - Alcoholic cardiomyopathy[4]
  - Anthracycline cardiomyopathy
  - Catecholamine cardiomyopathy
  - Peripartal cardiomyopathy[4]

[1] Adapted from Richardson et al. Report of the 1995 World Health Organization/International Society and Federation of Cardiology Task Force on the definition and classification of cardiomyopathies. Circulation 93:841–842, 1996, with permission.

[2] These conditions may also result in dilated ventricles, but are classically considered restrictive cardiomyopathies.

[3] Related to minimally dilated cardiomyopathy, see text.

[4] Occasionally considered in the spectrum of idiopathic dilated cardiomyopathy (see text).

The use of "dilated cardiomyopathy" persists in the cardiology literature even for cases of cardiac dilatation secondary to coronary artery disease and other conditions.[4,5] To avoid confusion, the modifier "idiopathic" is often applied by clinicians to emphasize the absence of underlying diseases. In this chapter, however, "dilated cardiomyopathy" is synonymous with "idiopathic dilated cardiomyopathy."

Epidemiologic Features

The prevalence of dilated cardiomyopathy in the United States is about 37/100,000 individuals with a yearly incidence rate of 6/100,000.[6,7] The mean age at presentation is in the fifth decade, typically between 20 and 60 years. Men are two to three times more likely than females to develop the disease.[7,8] There is also a predilection for blacks.[9]

Clinical Features

The main criteria for diagnosis are ejection fraction of < 45–55% and ventricular dilatation (left ventricular internal diastolic dimensions > 2.7 cm/m^2 of body surface area).[10] In most patients, the ejection fraction is less than 40% and may be as low as 10% in the final stages of disease.[11] There is global hypokinesia on echocardiography. Cardiac dilatation may precede left ventricular dysfunction, or may in some cases be minimal or absent (mildly dilated cardiomyopathy).[12] Other causes of cardiac failure—especially coronary artery disease, valvular disease, infiltrative diseases, and hypertensive disease—must be ruled out clinically before entertaining the diagnosis of dilated cardiomyopathy.

The most common symptoms are dyspnea and fatigue related to heart failure. Most patients develop symptoms gradually, with a mean interval of approximately 50 months between onset and death.[8] However, the duration of disease may be quite short, and the *presenting* symptom is sudden death due to arrhythmia in approximately 3% of patients.[8] Chest pain occurs in one quarter to one half of patients and may be due to coronary microvascular disease,[13] may be related to decreased coronary dilatory capacity,[14] or may be secondary to pulmonary embolism. Systemic and pulmonary embolism is common in the course of the disease and occurs in the majority of patients.[8] Conduction disturbances and arrhythmias are common. Ambulatory Holter monitoring will demonstrate nonsustained ventricular tachycardia in about one half of patients,[15] complete bundle branch block in 50% of patients,[8] and atrial fibrillation in 25%.[8]

The prognosis varies greatly in different series, but there is at least a 35% 5-year and 15% 10-year survival rate. The most important risk factors for death are progressive ventricular dysfunction, significant arrhythmias,[11] and right ventricular dysfunction.[16] One fifth of patients with known dilated cardiomyopathy die suddenly secondary to arrhythmias, and in the majority of the remainder the cause of death is intractable heart failure.[8] The rate of sudden death or cardiac arrest due to ventricular tachyarrhythmias is about 2% per year, and is greater in patients with decreased heart rate variability.[17]

Pathologic Features

Gross Pathologic Features

Cardiomegaly is morphologically considered a requisite for the diagnosis of dilated cardiomyopathy.[18] In some patients with dilated cardiomyopathy there is very little cardiac enlargement, however, and the diagnosis must be made largely on clinical grounds.[19] The mean heart weight in a large series of dilated cardiomyopathy was 615 grams (range 360–940 grams).[8] Hearts weighing more than 700 grams are unusual, representing less than 3% of all cases in three compiled autopsy studies.[20]

Typically, there is four-chamber dilatation (Table 6–2) (Fig. 6–1), which is greater in the ventricles than the atria. In patients with a history of atrial fibrillation, atrial dilatation may be prominent. At autopsy, left ventricular dilatation is best assessed by measuring the chamber cavity at the level of the papillary muscles in a transverse cut; any measurement > 4 cm (excluding the papillary muscles) is indicative of left ventricular dilatation. Concomitant right ventricular dilatation results in the typical globular appearance of the heart.

Table 6–2. Autopsy Pathologic Features, Dilated Cardiomyopathy

Feature	Frequency[1]
Gross	
Cardiomegaly	95%
Ventricular dilatation	95–100%
Mural thrombi	50%
Mural plaques	10%
Subendocardial scars	10%
Transmural scars	2%
Histologic	
Myofiber hypertrophy	95%
Lymphocytic infiltrates	50%[2]
Subendocardial fibrosis	45%
Interstitial fibrosis, diffuse	15%
Myocarditis (Dallas criteria)	< 5%

[1] These are approximate and may vary by definitions used.
[2] >5 foci in several histologic sections.

The increase in heart weight in patients with dilated cardiomyopathy is by necessity secondary to cardiac hypertrophy. However, left ventricular wall thickness may be normal because of the ventricular dilatation.[21]

The mitral valve annulus has been described as relatively normal in circumference. Mitral insufficiency may result from papillary muscle dysfunction secondary to ventricular dilatation and changes in ventricular wall shape.[8] In contrast, tricuspid regurgitation results from annular dilatation.[8]

Right-sided mural thrombi are present in approximately one third of hearts, and left-sided thrombi in nearly one half.[8] Endocardial fibrous plaques in the ventricles are less common, occurring in about 10% of cases.[8] Endocardial plaques are believed to be the result of organized thrombi. Mild diffuse or patchy endocardial fibrosis, especially toward the ventricular outflow tracts, is frequent and is likely a result of cardiac dilatation.

The myocardium in dilated cardiomyopathy is generally grossly unremarkable. However, gross scars (excluding fibrosis of the papillary muscles), usually subendocardial, may be present in up to 23% of hearts.[8, 20–22] Transmural scars have also been reported.[23]

The coronary arteries in dilated cardiomyopathy by definition should be less than 75% narrowed in cross-sectional area (severe coronary disease).[8, 20] However, it is not rare in autopsy practice to encounter hearts with the gross features of cardiac dilatation with severe coronary disease involving one vessel, in the absence of myocardial infarcts, hypertensive or valvular disease.[24] In such cases, it is difficult to explain cardiac failure on the basis of coronary occlusion. Because of the high prevalence of severe one-vessel disease in Western populations, one would expect the coexistence of dilated cardiomyopathy and coronary artery disease. Patients with cardiac failure and limited (e.g., one vessel) severe atherosclerosis may, however be diagnosed with ischemic cardiomyopathy.[1]

Microscopic Features

The histologic features of dilated cardiomyopathy are nonspecific (Table 6–2)[1] and may be seen in failing hearts of any cause. The classic histologic triad consists of myocyte hypertrophy, myocyte atrophy, and interstitial fibrosis.[8, 18, 20, 21, 25] However, the degree of fibrosis is quite variable.[21, 26] Although myocyte hypertrophy is present in the vast majority of cases, the

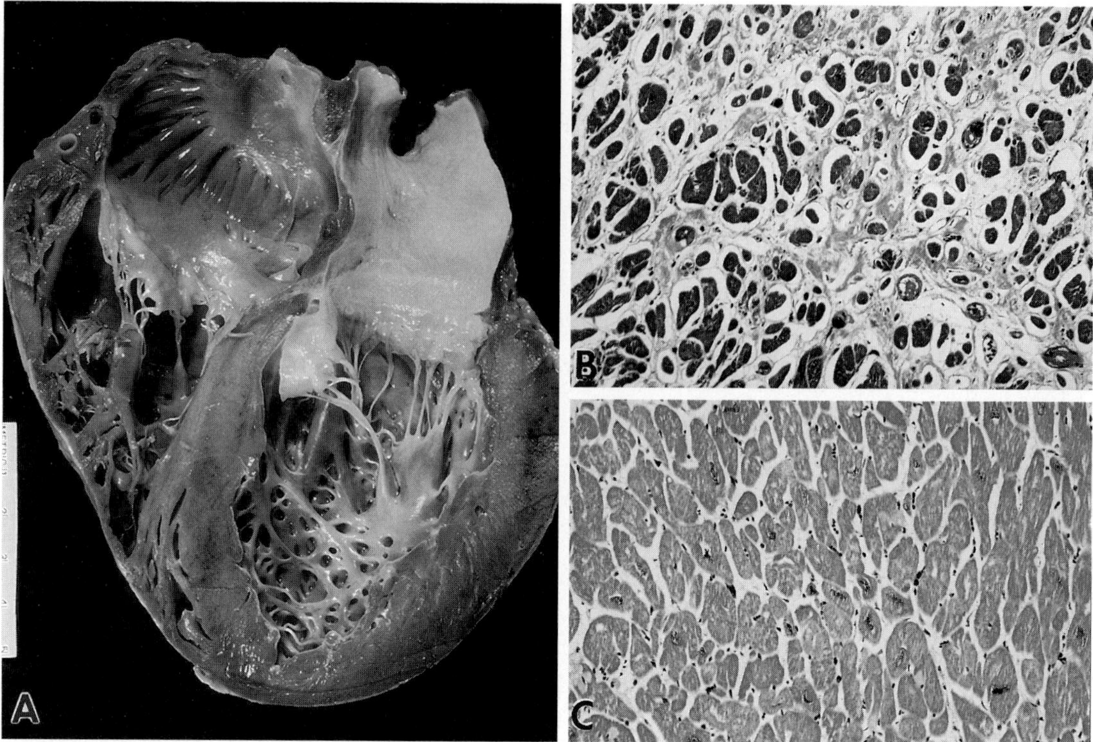

Figure 6–1. Dilated cardiomyopathy. *A.* A four-chamber cut through this heart demonstrates ventricular dilatation exceeding atrial dilatation. The diameter of the left ventricle at the level of the papillary muscles is greater than 4 cm. There is mild endocardial fibrosis in the left ventricle. The patient was a 42-year-old male with a remote history of drug abuse who died suddenly; the epicardial coronary arteries and cardiac valves were normal, and there was no clinical history of hypertension or histologic evidence of renal arteriolopathy. *B.* The characteristic histologic features of dilated cardiomyopathy are interstitial fibrosis and variation in myocyte size, seen here on cross section. The degree of interstitial fibrosis varies considerably. In this example, there is marked interstitial fibrosis. The specimen was a cardiac explant from a patient with end-stage cardiomyopathy. Interstitial fibrosis in dilated cardiomyopathy is often accentuated in subendocardial regions because of ischemic changes. *C.* In many cases of dilated cardiomyopathy, histologic findings are minimal, and there is only nonspecific myocyte hypertrophy.

histologic appearance in some cases is essentially normal,[21] supporting the concept that the primary defect is at a subcellular metabolic level.

Myocyte Changes

The myocyte hypertrophy characteristic of dilated cardiomyopathy is accompanied by increased nuclear DNA content and normal or reduced myocyte width due to myocyte attenuation.[26] The mean myocardial cell diameter in patients with dilated cardiomyopathy has been calculated at 22 microns, compared with 17 microns in control subjects.[27] It is typical to see a marked variation in myofiber size, especially when viewed on cross section (Fig. 6–2). The myofibrillar loss results in the loss of contractile filaments and vacuolization of myocytes which may be related to decrease in ventricular contractility.[26] Several investigators have noted an association between percentage area occupied by myofibers (as determined morphometrically on endomyocardial biopsy) and cardiac ejection fraction. This association suggests that the degree of myofiber loss may have prognostic significance.[28–30]

Inflammation

The degree of lymphocytic infiltrate has been a matter of debate. In autopsy hearts, Rose and Beck demonstrated no increase in lymphocytes compared with a control population,[20] and clusters of lymphocytes are found in over 40% of trauma control hearts,[31] as well as hearts with dilated cardiomyopathy.[21] Tazelaar and Billingham found no infiltrates in 13%, 1–5 foci of at least 5 inflammatory cells in 33%, 6–30 foci in 47%, and 30 or more foci in 8% in generously

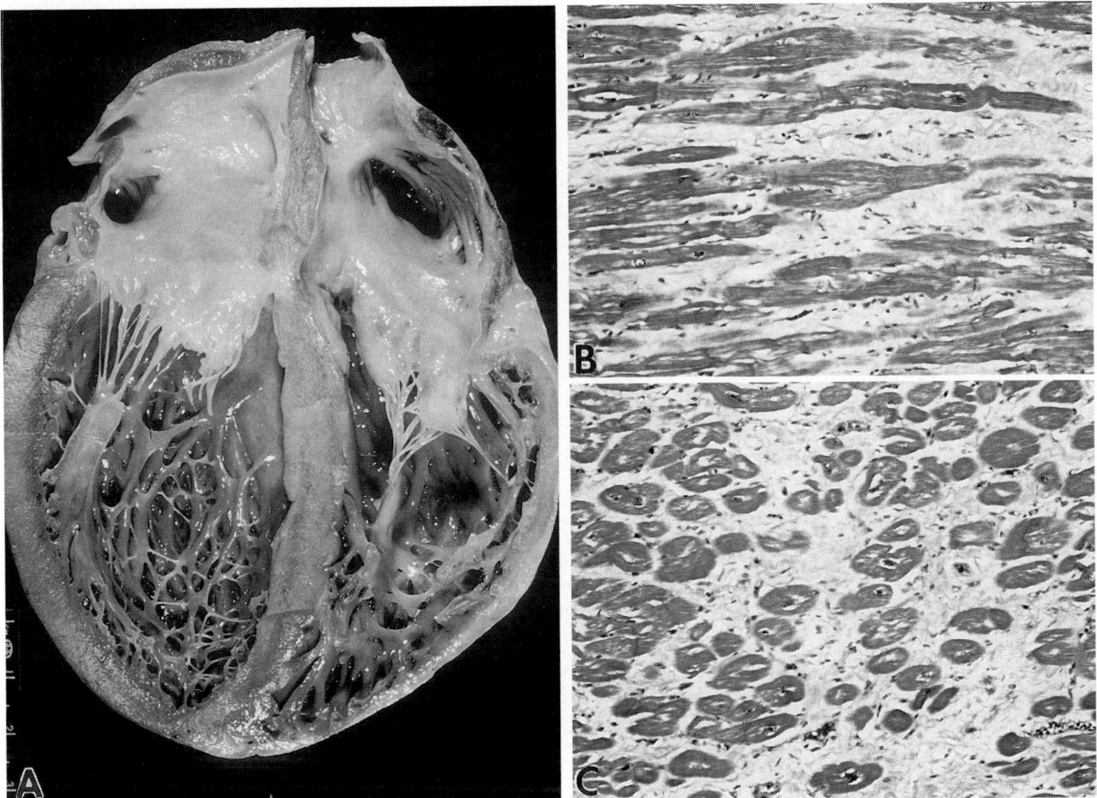

Figure 6–2. Dilated cardiomyopathy. *A*. This heart was from a 23-year-old man with recent onset dilated cardiomyopathy. Note marked dilatation of the ventricles; the ventricular walls appear relatively thinned. *B*. When cut longitudinally, the myofibers may appear attenuated due to cardiac dilatation. There is moderate interstitial fibrosis. *C*. A more transverse section demonstrates variation in myofiber size, interstitial fibrosis, and myocyte hypertrophy. The histologic features of dilated cardiomyopathy are nonspecific. The diagnosis may be made only with knowledge of clinical and gross pathologic data.

sampled hearts from patients dying with dilated cardiomyopathy.[32] Areas of true myocarditis with adjacent myocyte necrosis are seen in fewer than 5% of cases.[8] In endomyocardial biopsies from patients with recently diagnosed dilated cardiomyopathy, 13% demonstrate myocarditis by the Dallas criteria.[33] The degree of lymphocytic infiltrate varies greatly by stage of disease, methods of sampling, and methods of lymphocyte quantitation.

Fibrosis

The type of fibrosis present in dilated cardiomyopathy is typically described as interstitial,[21] although both interstitial and replacement fibrosis (with dropout of myocytes) have been described. The frequency of patchy interstitial and focal replacement fibrosis is approximately 15% and 45%, respectively.[8, 20] The types and extent of fibrosis found in cases of dilated cardiomyopathy were found to be similar to that found in hearts from patients dying of other cardiovascular and neoplastic diseases.[20] The degree of fibrosis (as determined morphometrically) increases from the epicardium to the endocardium, and is greater on the left side of the ventricular septum than the right.[27] The endocardial predilection is secondary to subendocardial ischemic damage that is frequently seen in failing hearts.

The fibrosis of dilated cardiomyopathy is associated with a selective increase in collagen type I, which imparts stiffness and may accentuate diastolic dysfunction, and which may be mediated through upregulation of transforming growth factor (TGF) beta.[34]

Small Vessel and Atrial Disease

The precapillary arterioles have been described as thickened in endomyocardial biopsies from patients with dilated cardiomyopathy.[35] By computed morphometric analysis, the degree of atrial fibrosis is increased in patients with dilated cardiomyopathy compared to other forms of congestive heart failure, suggesting an intrinsic atrial defect[36] that reflects the left atrial dysfunction that may be detected hemodynamically.[37]

Ultrastructural Features

Ultrastructural changes of dilated cardiomyopathy consist primarily of interstitial fibrosis (increased numbers of mature and developing collagen fibrils in interstitial spaces), cellular hypertrophy (increased transverse diameters of muscle cells, increased size of nuclei and Golgi complex, and increase in mitochondria, glycogen, and ribosomes), and degenerative changes (cellular edema, increased lipid droplets, lysosomes and lipofuschin, and T-tubular dilatation).[18, 25] The most striking change is rarefaction or even complete loss of contractile elements.[38, 39] Morphometrically, there is a mean increase in nuclear area, irregularity of the nuclear outline, and a decrease in mitochondrial area compared with controls.[40]

The degree of myofibrillar loss appears to be increased in patients with marked cardiac dilatation, compared with those with minimal cardiac dilatation (mildly congestive cardiomyopathy).[41]

Pathogenesis and Risk Factors

The major associations and risk factors for dilated cardiomyopathy are viral myocarditis, diabetes mellitus, pregnancy, heredity, alcoholism, and autoimmunity. In addition, black race has been identified as a risk factor in an epidemiologic study.[9] Blacks are 2 to 3 times as likely to develop the disease as compared with whites. Cigarette smoking has been associated with dilated cardiomyopathy in some studies[42] but not others.[9] The wide range of associations corroborate the hypothesis that dilated cardiomyopathy is a heterogeneous group of diseases with a common end point.[21]

Myocarditis

The proportion of cases of dilated cardiomyopathy secondary to a previous viral infection is difficult to ascertain, as is the rate of progression of myocarditis to cardiomyopathy. In series of endomyocardial biopsies in patients presenting with unexplained heart failure, inflammation is found in 0–67%,[11] but is generally around 13%.[33, 43] Most retrospective serological studies demonstrate a higher rate of enteroviral antibodies in patients with dilated cardiomyopathy compared with controls,[44] but the rate is generally less than 50%. Persistent IgM enteroviral antibodies in a small proportion of patients[45] suggests the possibility of persistent, perhaps defective replication within the heart.[44] Blot hybridization for the detection of enteroviral RNA has demonstrated a 13–50% positivity rate,[46, 47] and there have been rare reports of enteroviral RNA detection by *in situ* hybridization[48] in cardiac tissues from patients with dilated cardiomyopathy. There have been several studies that have attempted to identify enteroviral RNA sequences by the polymerase chain reaction, but these have been hampered by lack of both specificity and sensitivity of the probes selected for use.[44] A recent study of 53 patients with dilated cardiomyopathy has shown only a 7% positivity rate using a probe designed to detect a wide range of enteroviral types.[49] Other investigators find a 40% rate of enteroviral RNA in heart biopsies of patients with dilated cardiomyopathy, compared with 7% of controls.[50]

In a small prospective study of patients with clinically diagnosed myocarditis, dilated cardiomyopathy developed in approximately 15% of cases.[44] The sequential morphologic changes (inflammation to interstitial fibrosis) have rarely been studied by serial biopsy.[44] In prospective studies of patients with biopsy-proven myocarditis, the subsequent development of dilated cardiomyopathy is between 40 and 50%.[51] It is generally believed that these data overestimate the overall rate of development of cardiomyopathy because of selection of highly ill patients.

The viral-induced cell injury in dilated cardiomyopathy is likely a complex and multifactorial process. Recently, evidence has been presented that coxsackieviruses induce a superantigen-driven immune response.[52]

Autoimmune Other Inflammatory Factors and Apoptosis

Persistent viral infection and autoimmunity are two major mechanisms that may, separately or together, contribute to the pathogenesis of dilated cardiomyopathy.[53] Dilated cardiomyopathy has been reported in patients with systemic lupus erythematosus, serum sickness, polyarteritis nodosa, acquired immunodeficiency syndrome, and other immunologic disorders.[54] Recently, an association between asthma and dilated cardiomyopathy has been found.[54]

Serologic evidence supports the hypothesis that autoimmune factors may be important in the pathogenesis of dilated cardiomyopathy.[55,56] Acute myocarditis is associated with a host of circulating autoantibodies.[53] Serum antibodies that have been described in patients with dilated cardiomyopathy include anti-muscle specific and heart reactive antibodies, anti-laminin, antimitochondrial antibodies, anti-myosin heavy and light chain antibodies, and anti-β adrenoceptor antibodies.[53, 57, 58] The role of these antibodies in pathogenesis of the disease and the role of viral infection in their elaboration is under investigation.

A variety of inflammatory cytokines, especially interleukin-1, has been demonstrated in tissues of patients with dilated cardiomyopathy. Interleukin-1 beta mRNA has been found in increased levels in macrophages, endothelial cells, and myocytes of tissues from patients with dilated cardiomyopathy compared with patients with ischemic heart disease.[59] Increased expression of cell adhesion molecules has been demonstrated in endomyocardial biopsies of patients with dilated cardiomyopathy, indicating inflammatory endothelial activation.[60]

Increased numbers of apoptotic myocytes have been observed in hearts from patients dying with dilated cardiomyopathy as compared with patients with ischemic cardiomyopathy.[61] These data suggest that programmed cell death may be partly causative in the pathogenesis of dilated cardiomyopathy. More recently, the double-stranded DNA damage seen in myocytes from patients with dilated cardiomyopathy has been attributed to DNA repair as opposed to apoptosis.[62]

Alcohol

There is some debate whether alcoholic cardiomyopathy should be considered as an entity separate from dilated cardiomyopathy. Most series of dilated cardiomyopathy include alcoholics.[8] However, other investigators consider chronic alcoholics (ingesting more than 8 oz of ethanol daily for at least 6 months) with cardiomyopathy as suffering from alcoholic (toxic) cardiomyopathy.[9]

Pathologically, there are no gross or histologic features that distinguish dilated cardiomyopathy in alcoholics and nonalcoholics.[21, 63] The mechanism of cardiotoxicity is generally considered to be a direct toxic effect on the myocytes. Toxicity may involve calcium binding and transport, mitochondrial respiration, myocardial lipid metabolism, myocardial protein synthesis, myofibrillar ATPase, or a combination of these cellular functions.[64] In some patients, concomitant nutritional factors may play a role in pathogenesis.[11]

The relative risk for developing dilated cardiomyopathy is no greater in individuals who consume up to 40 fluid ounces of ethanol weekly compared with controls.[9] Beyond this amount the relative risk increases to 2.5 times that of the general population.[9] In case-controlled studies, patients with nonfamilial dilated cardiomyopathy consume on the average 3 to 4 times that of controls.[65]

At autopsy, alcoholics who succumb to cardiomyopathy have enlarged hearts, usually from 500–700 grams, but weights of up to 900 grams have been reported.[66] The ultrastructural features of alcoholic cardiomyopathy include swelling of the endoplasmic reticulum, degenerative changes of myofilaments, increased lipofuschin and lysosome-like bodies, increased lipid, mitochondrial swelling, alterations in mitochondrial cristae, and the formation of dense intramitochondrial inclusions. The majority of the ultrastructural findings are nonspecific, and may partly be due to terminal ischemic events.[67]

Diabetes

Diabetes mellitus is found in approximately 7% of patients with dilated cardiomyopathy.[8] The relative risk of dilated cardiomyopathy among diabetics was estimated at 1.6 that of the general population, but the elevated odds ratio was not statistically significant.[9] The role of coronary microangiopathy in the causation of diabetic dilated cardiomyopathy has been debated.[11]

Familial Aspects

The incidence of a positive family history in patients with dilated cardiomyopathy was 7%[68] and 20%[69] in two carefully planned studies. There is a range of 2–56% of a familial frequency with different methods of evaluation of relatives.[70, 71] Nearly 30% of relatives of patients with idiopathic dilated cardiomyopathy demonstrate echocardiographic abnormalities, and approximately one third of these affected relatives develop cardiomyopathy.[72] Histologic abnormalities have also been demonstrated in endomyocardial biopsies of family members of patients with dilated cardiomyopathy, and include increased cellularity and apoptosis in inflammatory cells.[71] The pattern of transmission is autosomal dominant with incomplete penetrance in over 90% of families.[69] However, there is likely significant genetic heterogeneity, and in some families autosomal recessive, X-linked, polygenic inheritance, and mitochondrial inheritance have been proposed.[70, 73, 74] There have been few specific gene mutations identified in familial autosomal dominant dilated cardiomyopathy, such as mutations in the lamin A/C gene.[75]

With the exception of X-linked cardiomyopathy (see following) and rare families with mutations in cardiac actin gene, specific mutations have not yet been demonstrated and there does not appear to be an association with HLA type.[70] In two families with dilated cardiomyopathy, missense mutations in the cardiac actin gene have been demonstrated in regions of the gene coding for areas of the protein near attachments sites to A bands and intercalated discs.[76] A familial dilated cardiomyopathy has been mapped to chromosome 2q31, in the region of the titan cytoskeletal protein gene.[77]

There are no pathological or clinical features that distinguish familial dilated cardiomyopathy from sporadic cases. However, it has been suggested that dilated cardiomyopathy with minimal cardiac dilatation (mildly dilated congestive cardiomyopathy) is more likely familial than typical dilated cardiomyopathy.[41]

X-Linked Dilated Cardiomyopathy

A heterogeneous group of cardiomyopathies is transmitted as an X-linked trait. The two most common forms currently recognized are X-linked dilated cardiomyopathy (a disease of teenagers and adults) and Barth syndrome (a disease of infants and children, see following).

In less than 10% of familial dilated cardiomyopathy, the mode of inheritance is X-linked.[68] X-linked dilated cardiomyopathy affects teenage boys and is secondary to a mutation in the 5′ region of the dystrophin gene on locus Xp21.[78–81] Female carriers may develop cardiomyopathy later in life.[82] Cardiac-specific regulatory sequences of the dystrophin gene may be affected,[83] there are few skeletal symptoms, and dystrophin immunofluorescent staining of skeletal muscle biopsies is relatively normal. In contrast, X-linked muscular dystrophy (Duchenne's muscular dystrophy), a related disease also characterized by a defect in dystrophin gene, is a disorder primarily of skeletal muscle. However, 50% of patients have a mild or overt form of dilated cardiomyopathy.[84]

The gross and histologic features of X-linked cardiomyopathy are not specific and do not allow distinction from nonhereditary forms of dilated cardiomyopathy.[85]

Mitochondrial Disease

It has been reported that approximately 10% of patients with idiopathic dilated cardiomyopathy who undergo preoperative evaluation for heart transplantation demonstrate mitochondrial abnormalities in endomyocardial biopsy specimens.[86] These ultrastructural abnormalities include giant organelles; angulated, tubular, and concentric cristae; and crystalloid or osmiophilic inclusion bodies. In these patients, nearly one fourth demonstrate heteroplasmic mitochondrial DNA mutations that are associated with decreased levels of cytochrome c oxidase activity. It has been suggested that elevations of trace elements, especially mercury and antimony, may be the cause of mitochondrial abnormalities in some patients with dilated cardiomyopathy.[87] The significance of mitochondrial gene mutations in infantile and adult dilated cardiomyopathy is unclear.[88]

Pregnancy

In approximately 25% of peripartum patients with heart failure, the etiology is idiopathic leading to the diagnosis of peripartal (dilated) cardiomyopathy.[89, 90] Peripartum cardiomyopathy is defined as left ventricular dilation and failure, first developing during the third trimester of pregnancy or in the first 6 months postpartum. The pathologic features are similar to dilated cardiomyopathy in patients who do not meet these criteria (Fig. 6–3). The incidence is approximately 10 in 100,000 births[91, 92] and the mortality is between 25 and 60%.[11] Risk factors for peripartum cardiomyopathy include advanced maternal age, multiparity, African descent, twinning, and long-term tocolysis.[93] The disease is occasionally familial.[94]

In general, the incidence of myocarditis in peripartal cardiomyopathy is very low, similar to that of nonperipartal dilated cardiomyopathy.[95] However, two studies have shown a high proportion (29–79%) of myocarditis at endomyocardial biopsy of patients with peripartal congestive

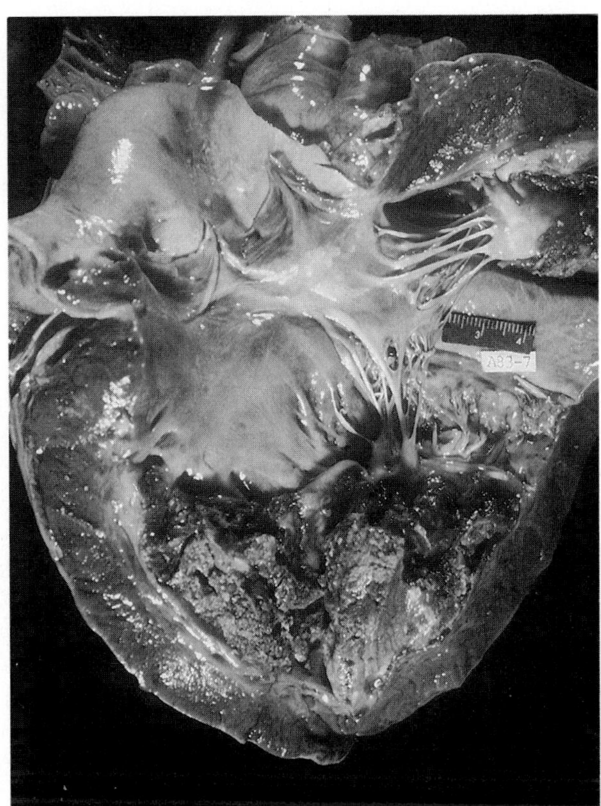

Figure 6–3. Dilated cardiomyopathy. There is a large apical thrombus, a complication of left ventricular systolic dysfunction. The patient was a young woman who had recently given birth to a healthy child; there was a family history of peripartum cardiomyopathy.

heart failure.[91, 96] The varied frequency of inflammatory infiltrates may be partly due to terminology; peripartum myocarditis is occasionally classified separately from peripartum cardiomyopathy.[67]

Although the clinical features of peripartum cardiomyopathy do not differ from those of dilated cardiomyopathy (other than earlier age at onset and shorter duration of symptoms,[91] it is often considered as an entity separate from dilated cardiomyopathy. The precise classification of this entity has not been resolved.[1]

Differential Diagnosis

A number of conditions that may result in cardiac failure must be distinguished from dilated cardiomyopathy.[11] Ischemic heart disease, especially in diabetic patients with healed silent myocardial infarction, may result in congestive heart failure in the absence of a clinical history of angina. In general, the presence of > 75% cross-sectional luminal narrowing of an epicardial coronary artery is considered an adequate cause for ischemic cardiac dilatation.

Myocarditis typically results in congestive heart failure. Because enteroviral myocarditis may progress to dilated cardiomyopathy, the distinction between it and dilated cardiomyopathy may be arbitrary. However, if there are widespread infiltrates with myocyte necrosis, and the clinical course was rapid, the diagnosis of myocarditis is preferable. Other types of myocarditis, such as hypersensitivity myocarditis and giant-cell myocarditis, may result in cardiac dilatation. These entities have distinctive histologic patterns that distinguish them from lymphocytic myocarditis or dilated cardiomyopathy.

Toxic insults, such as anthracycline toxicity, may result in a secondary form of dilated cardiomyopathy[97, 98] (Fig. 6–4), as well as restrictive hemodynamic parameters.[99] A clinical history and ultrastructural examination are required for the correct diagnosis.

Myocardial involvement by hemochromatosis is generally manifest by dilated ventricles and cardiac failure, although a restrictive

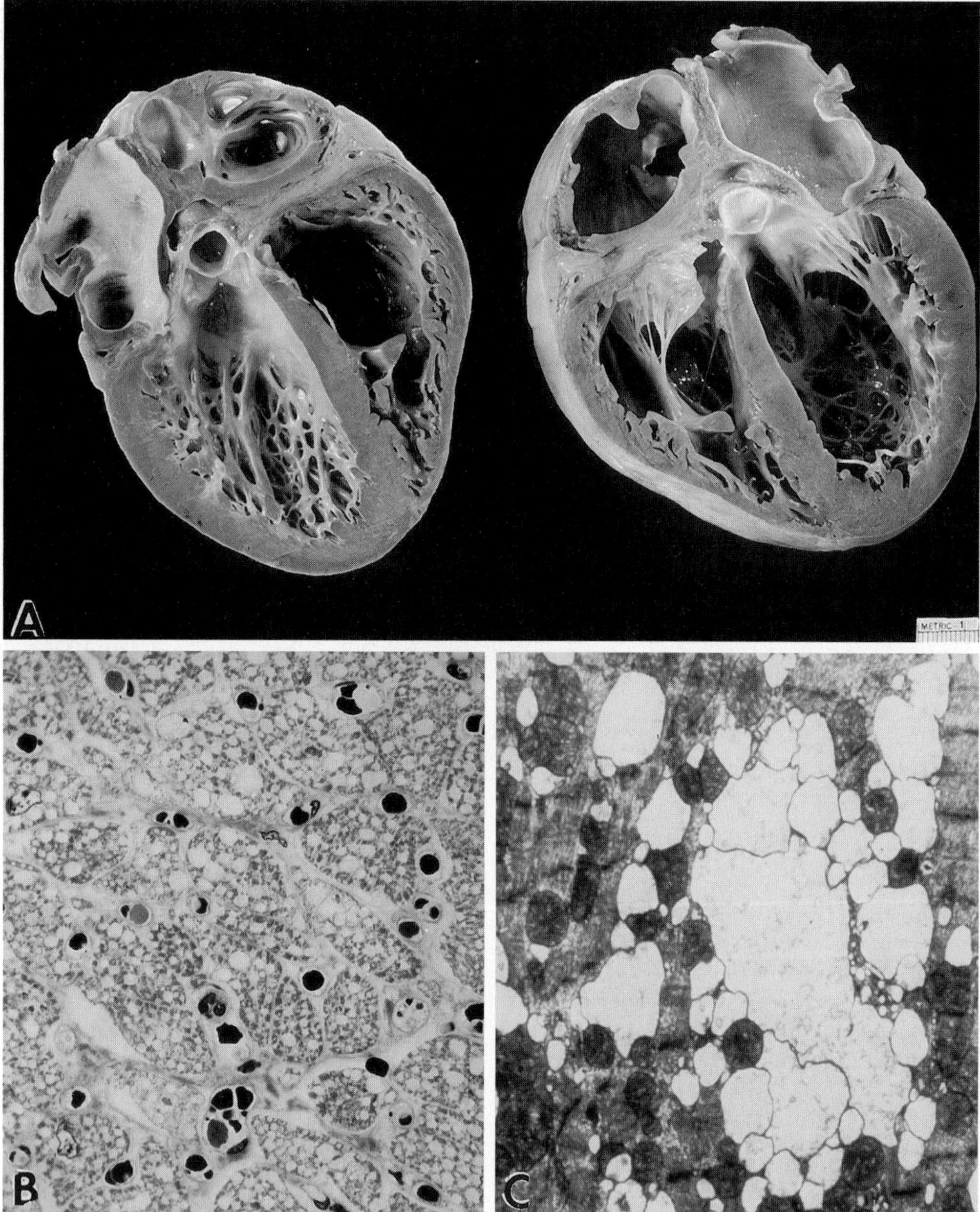

Figure 6–4. Anthracycline cardiomyopathy. A variety of conditions may result in cardiac dilatation. This patient received doxorubicin for lymphoma and died from congestive heart failure. *A.* The gross features are indistinguishable from dilated cardiomyopathy, and consist of ventricular dilatation and endocardial fibrosis, most prominent on the left side. *B.* Histologically, there were clusters of vacuolated cells, as seen on this toluidine blue-stained plastic section. *C.* Ultrastructurally, there is sarcotubular dilatation characteristic of anthracycline toxicity; myofibrillar loss, also characteristic, is not evident in this photomicrograph.

pattern may also occur. The diagnosis is made histologically by the identification of Prussian-blue positive pigment within myocytes. Because the pigment is predominantly subepicardial, endomyocardial biopsy may be falsely negative in early stages of disease.

Amyloidosis and eosinophilic endocardial disease generally result in restrictive cardiomyopathy. However, they may result in congestive heart failure. Histologic evaluation is necessary in all cases of presumed dilated cardiomyopathy in order to exclude secondary causes.

HYPERTROPHIC CARDIOMYOPATHY

Definition and Terms

Hypertrophic cardiomyopathy is idiopathic ventricular hypertrophy in the absence of ventricular dilatation. It is a diastolic disorder that is characterized by restriction of ventricular filling.[21] The clinical diagnosis rests on echocardiographic criteria, which include a nondilated hypertrophied left ventricle, with normal or increased ejection fraction.[100] The area of hypertrophy is often greatest at the base of the ventricular septum, resulting in asymmetric hypertrophy in a large proportion of patients. Left ventricular outflow obstruction occurs in a subset of patients, in whom the diagnosis of idiopathic hypertrophic subaortic stenosis or hypertrophic obstructive cardiomyopathy is occasionally rendered. Currently, the term hypertrophic cardiomyopathy is preferred for all morphologic variants of the disease, however.

Clinical and Epidemiologic Features

Epidemiologic Features

The prevalence and yearly incidence of hypertrophic cardiomyopathy in Olmsted County, Minnesota, have been estimated at about 20/100,000 and 2.5/100,000, respectively.[6] Echocardiographic abnormalities suggestive of the disease are found in a much higher proportion of the population, with a prevalence of 170–500/100,000 in the United States.[101, 102] The disease may occur at any age, although most patients are in their 30s or 40s at the time of diagnosis. In a recent clinical series of 600 patients, the mean age was 45 (range 7–79 years), and 66% of patients were men.[103] Males were affected one and one-half times as frequently as females in one multicenter study.[104] Currently, with implementation of screening regimens for relatives of patients with known disease, hypertrophic cardiomyopathy is being diagnosed frequently in adolescents and children.

Clinical Features

Symptoms

One of four patients is asymptomatic at the time of diagnosis. The most frequent presenting symptoms are chest pain and dyspnea. Chest pain is usually anginal, and is multifactorial, related to an imbalance between oxygen supply and demand, myocardial infarction, and small-vessel disease. Dyspnea is generally a consequence of elevated left ventricular diastolic pressure, which results from impaired ventricular filling. Syncope or near syncope occurs in about 25% of patients[6] and may result from inadequate cardiac output with exertion (especially if there is subaortic stenosis) or cardiac arrhythmias. In 16% the diagnosis is first made at autopsy (sudden death).[6] Sudden unexpected death occurs most frequently in young persons.

Echocardiography

The cardinal echocardiographic finding is left ventricular hypertrophy with a small ventricular cavity. The hypertrophy is asymmetric (with variability from region to region in the myocardium) in 80–98% of cases[100] and is usually greatest in the ventricular septum and anterior free wall of the left ventricle. In a recent series of 600 patients from the U.S., the anterior portion of the ventricular septum was thickened in 96%, and was also the predominant site of hypertrophy in 83% of patients. Concentric hypertrophy or hypertrophy confined to the apex were present in only 1% each.[103]

When there is subaortic obstruction, echocardiography will reveal systolic anterior motion of the anterior leaflet of the mitral valve, which is associated with elongation of the mitral leaflets with abnormalities of the coaptation sites.[105] The abnormal motion of the mitral valve is likely a result of Venturi forces related to left ventricular outflow tract obstruction. Other echocardiographic findings include a ground glass appearance of the hypertrophied myocardium, reduced septal motion during systole, and mitral valve prolapse. In a series of 528 patients, the mitral valve prolapse was found in 3% of patients, a frequency that is comparable to the general population.[106]

Hemodynamics

Hemodynamic alterations typical of hypertrophic cardiomyopathy are diminished diastolic left ventricular compliance and in about 50% of patients, a subaortic gradient. Systolic pressure gradients of up to 170 mm Hg at rest have been reported.[18] A characteristic of the gradient is its lability and variability, which result from temporal changes in ventricular volume.

Apical Hypertrophic Cardiomyopathy

In fewer than 5% of patients in the United States, but in 25% of Japanese patients, the area of hypertrophy is located in the ventricular apex. The apical form of hypertrophic cardiomyopathy is associated with giant negative T waves on electrocardiogram. The diagnosis is facilitated by a spade-like configuration on the end-diastolic left ventriculogram or apical hypertrophy as demonstrated by nuclear magnetic resonance short axis imaging.[107, 108]

Prognosis

The clinical course of hypertrophic cardiomyopathy is variable, and many patients remain stable and symptoms may even improve spontaneously. The annual attrition is 3% per year in adults and 6% per year in children.[109, 110] Symptoms increase with advancing age but do not correlate with the presence or severity of an outflow gradient.[111] The onset of atrial fibrillation usually leads to an increase in symptoms and warrants pharmacological or electrical cardioversion. In upwards of 10% of patients, heart failure with cardiac dilatation occurs. The progression to congestive cardiomyopathy appears to be related to wall thinning and scar formation as a consequence of myocardial ischemia caused by small vessel coronary artery disease.[112]

Sudden death is the most feared complication. Those features that most reliably identify high-risk patients include age younger than 30 years, and a family history of hypertrophic cardiomyopathy with sudden death, genetic abnormalities associated with increased prevalence of sudden death (see following), sustained ventricular or supraventricular tachyarrhythmias, recurrent syncope in the young, nonsustained ventricular tachycardias, and bradyarrhythmias.[109] Sudden death often occurs during exercise, and patients are often counseled against undertaking sports. Patients may die suddenly before the onset of left ventricular hypertrophy and identifiable echocardiographic evidence of the disease.[113, 114]

Differential Diagnosis

The clinical differential diagnosis of hypertrophic cardiomyopathy includes conditions that mimic the echocardiographic and hemodynamic alterations of the disease. The most common of these conditions are systemic hypertension (see following) and aortic stenosis, which may result in asymmetric hypertrophy requiring myomectomy at the time of valve replacement in approximately 5–10% of patients.[115, 116] A variety of miscellaneous diseases may result in asymmetric hypertrophy that may mimic hypertrophic cardiomyopathy echocardiographically. These include amyloidosis,[117] storage diseases (especially Fabry's disease),[118, 119] cardiac tumors (such as lymphoma),[120] and eosinophilic heart disease.[119] These conditions are readily distinguished from hypertrophic cardiomyopathy upon histologic evaluation. The outflow tract gradient of hypertrophic cardiomyopathy may be mimicked by hypercontractile states, pheochromocytoma, hyperthroidism, and hyperparathroidism.[121–125]

Pathologic Features

Gross Pathologic Features (Table 6–3)

Heart Weight

The heart is typically enlarged to approximately twice normal weight. The mean heart weight in a series of 40 autopsied cases was 634 grams[18] and weights of over 1,000 grams may be encountered.[18, 126] However, the heart weight may be minimally enlarged or even normal, especially in cases of apical hypertrophic cardiomyopathy. In sudden death, the heart may appear grossly normal and the diagnosis made only on the basis of histologic criteria.[113, 114] Recently, cardiac hypertrophy has been shown to be a predictor of sudden death in patients with hypertrophic cardiomyopathy.

Table 6–3. Autopsy Pathologic Features, Hypertrophic Cardiomyopathy

Feature	Frequency[1]
Gross	
Cardiomegaly	95%
Asymmetric hypertrophy	90%
Subendocardial scars	80%
Left ventricular outflow tract plaque	60%
Mitral valve prolapse	3%
Transmural scars	2%
Apical septal hypertrophy	1%[2]
Histologic	
Myofiber disarray > 5% of ventricular septum	85%
Intramural coronary artery thickening	83%
Interstitial fibrosis	95%

[1] These are approximate and may vary by definitions used and phase of illness.
[2] Up to 25% in the Japanese.

Site of Hypertrophy

The cardiac hypertrophy is secondary to ventricular thickening, usually asymmetrical, that may occur almost anywhere in the ventricular mass, but most often in the ventricular septum[127,128] (Fig. 6–5). Maron et al. have classified hypertrophic cardiomyopathy into four morphologic groups. Type I signifies asymmetric hypertrophy involving only the anterior segment of the ventricular septum (usually at the base). Type II is defined by diffuse thickening of the septum without free wall involvement (Fig. 6–5). Type III denotes thickening of the ventricular septum and the anterior free wall. Finally, type IV involves thickening involving any parts of the ventricle other than the anterior basal septum, including the posterior septum (Fig. 6–6), the anterolateral free wall, or the apical portion of the left ventricle. Asymmetric hypertrophy (the maximal septal thickness significantly thicker than the ventricular free wall) is present in up to 90% of cases. The minimum ratio of septal thickness to free wall thickness that signifies asymmetry is subjective and arbitrary, but is generally at least 1.3:1 pathologically and 1.5:1 by echocardiography. Portions of the right ventricle may be involved both grossly and histologically. The most common site of involvement in the right ventricle is the posterior wall, often towards the apex.

The gross features of apical hypertrophic cardiomyopathy differ from other types. The heart weight may be only mildly increased, and the apex of the ventricular septum demonstrates scarring and myofiber disarray that may be grossly visible and involve the right ventricle and left ventricular septum.

Evolution of Gross Features

In early stages of disease, the left ventricular cavity is small, and there is usually left atrial dilatation resulting from decreased left ventricular compliance. There may be relatively rapid accumulation of myocardial mass, in children, with 250% increases in ventricular thickness occurring over 3–6 years.[129] In later stages of disease, there may be gradual dilatation of the left ventricle, and areas of hypertrophy may be partly replaced by grossly discernible fibrous tissue (Figs. 6–7 and 6–8). The replacement of hypertrophied areas by scarring may transform previously hypertrophied areas of ventricular wall to normal or even thin ones,[112] and transmural scars may be present in the absence of epicardial coronary occlusions.[130] Occasionally, there may be diffuse gross myocardial scarring in late stages of disease.[11] The evolution of morphologic features must be considered if autopsy findings are compared to cardiac imaging performed years prior to death.

Endocardial and Valvular Pathology

A left ventricular outflow tract plaque is present in up to 73% of hearts[18] (Fig. 6–9). In contrast to congenital subaortic stenosis, the area of endocardial fibrosis is limited to that opposite the anterior leaflet of the mitral valve. The frequency of a left ventricular outflow tract plaque is 95% in patients with documented subaortic stenosis by catheterization, and less than 50% in patients without subaortic stenosis.[18] The area of stenosis may be surgically removed to relieve outflow tract obstruction (Figs. 6–10 and 6–11). Currently, percutaneous ethanol injection into the ventricular septum is performed in lieu of surgical correction.

The anterior leaflet of the mitral valve is typically thickened in cases of outflow tract obstruction, and there is often a mismatch in the lengths of the anterior and posterior leaflets, resulting in systolic anterior motion of the anterior leaflet.[131] In a study of 94 valves from patients with mostly the obstructive form of hypertrophic cardiomyopathy, the mean anterior leaflet length was greater than that of a control group of mitral valves, and increased mitral leaflet area was found in 58%.[132] In addition, nine patients had a congenital malformation of the mitral apparatus in which one or both papillary muscles inserted directly into anterior mitral leaflet.[132] The abnormal insertion of the papillary muscle onto the left ventricular outflow tract is an important variant to recognize before surgical myomectomy is attempted.[133] The abnormalities of the mitral valve may predispose to infectious endocarditis.[134] Endocarditis occurs in approximately 4/1,000 patients, with higher rates in patients with left atrial dilatation and left ventricular outflow tract obstruction.[135]

Microscopic Pathologic Features (Table 6–3)

Myofiber Disarray

The most characteristic microscopic feature of hypertrophic cardiomyopathy is myofiber disarray (also called myocyte disarray,[11] myocardial disarray,[136] and myocyte disorganization[137]). Unlike hypertrophy secondary to increased volume or pressure load, hypertrophic cardiomy-

Text continued on page 196.

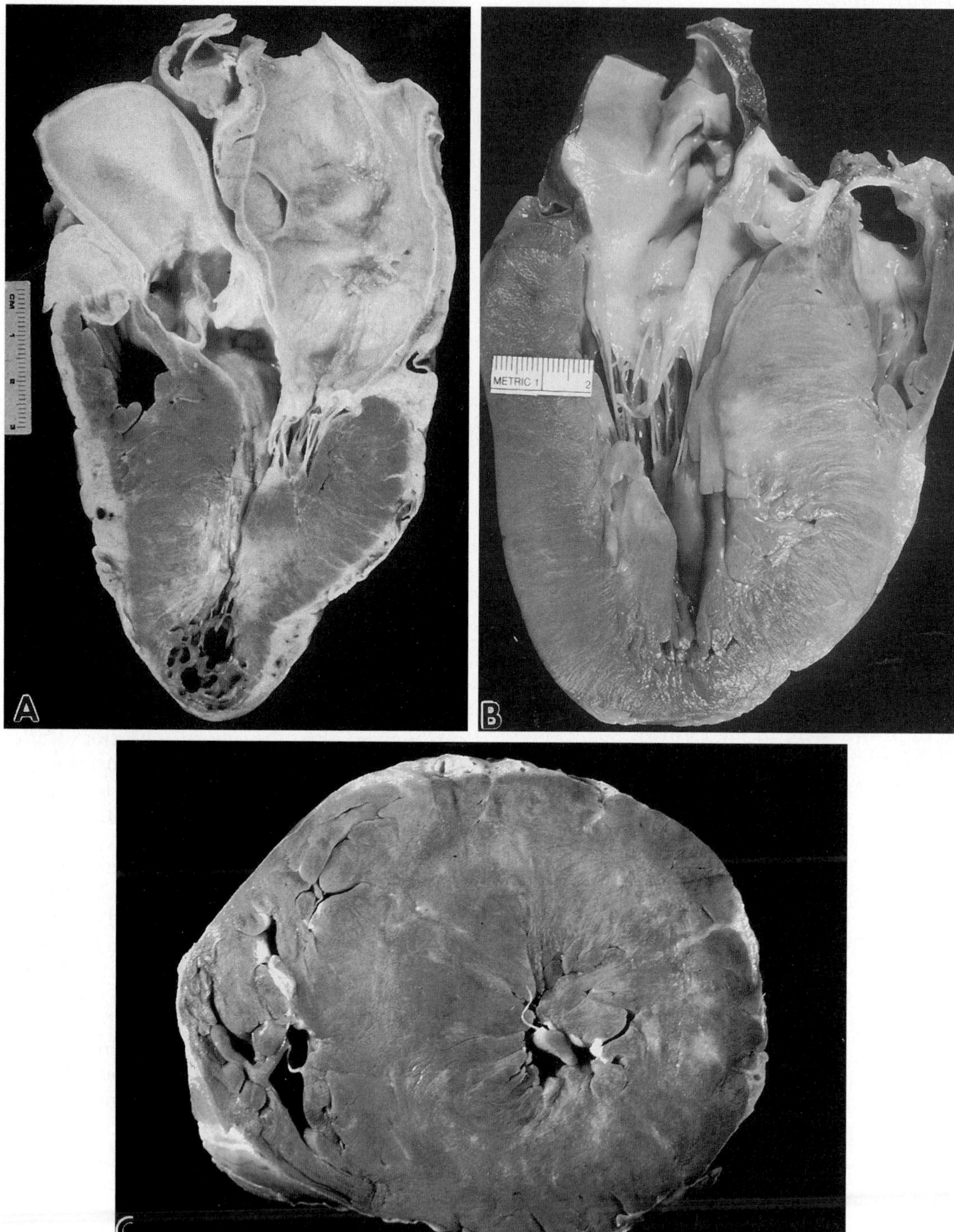

Figure 6–5. Hypertrophic cardiomyopathy. *A.* This is a long-axis echocardiographic view of the right and posterior half of the heart from a patient with hypertrophic cardiomyopathy. Note there is marked left atrial dilatation; the patient had long-standing atrial fibrillation. The thinning of the apical left ventricle was secondary to healed infarction secondary to coronary artery disease. *B.* This long-axis echocardiographic view of the left and anterior half of the heart demonstrates asymmetric hypertrophy, the ventricular septum measuring 2.6 cm, and the ventricular free wall 1.6 cm in thickness. The interstitial scarring in the septum is grossly visible near the left ventricular endocardium. *C.* A short axis view of the ventricular myocardium demonstrates diffuse thickening of the ventricular septum; often only the anterior portion is involved.

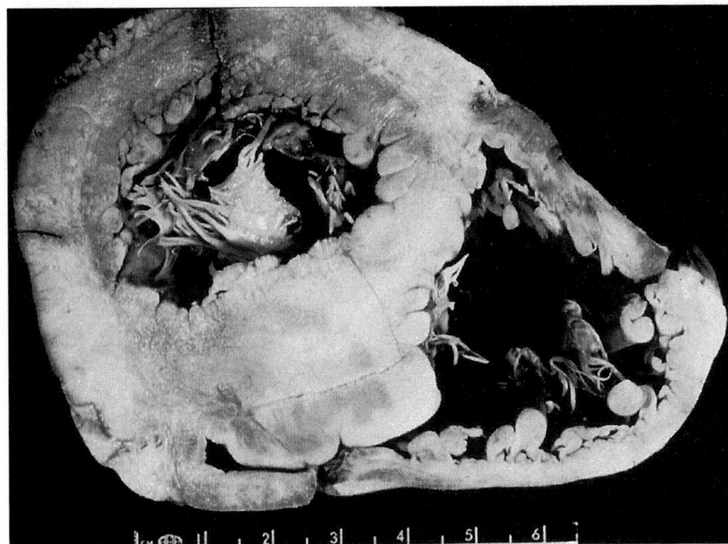

Figure 6–6. Hypertrophic cardiomyopathy, asymmetric hypertrophy. In this example, the anterior portion of the septum is thickened, which is the most common area in the septum to demonstrate hypertrophy.

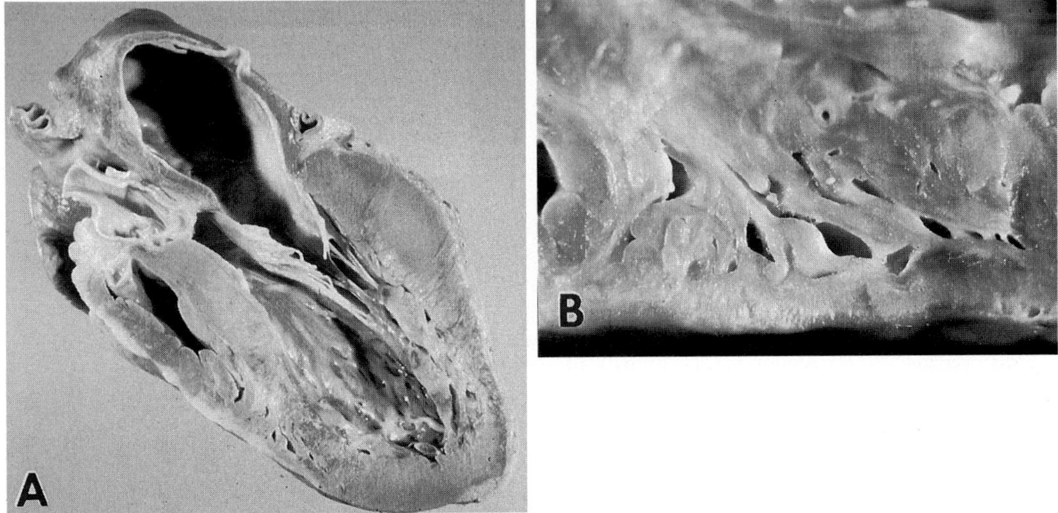

Figure 6–7. Hypertrophic cardiomyopathy, ventricular scarring. *A.* In later stages of disease, the thickened portion of septum may be replaced by scarring and hypertrophy is no longer evident. *B.* A higher magnification demonstrates grossly visible myocardial scars.

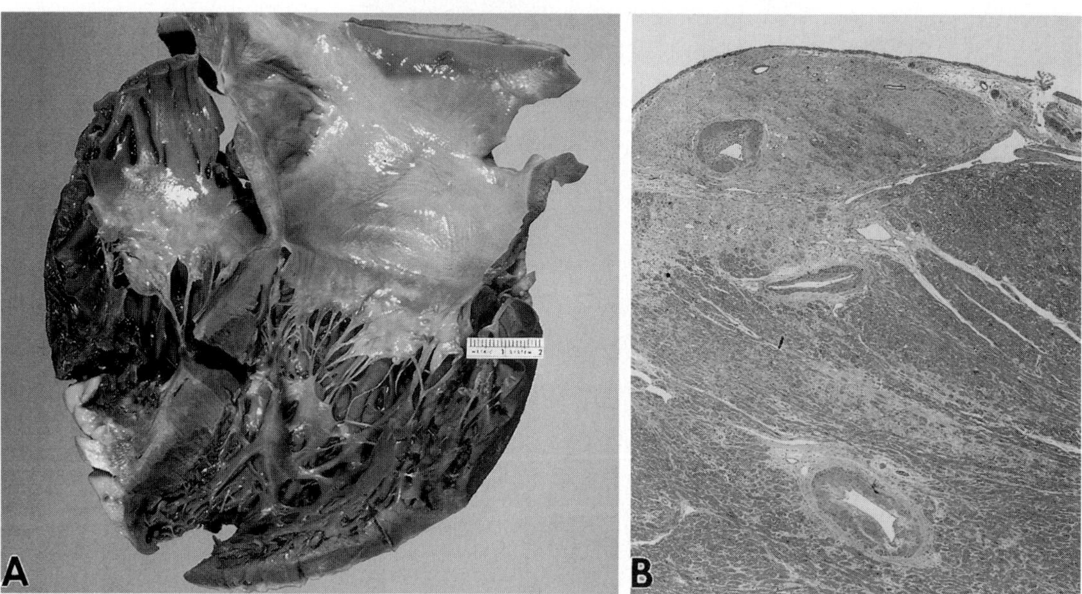

Figure 6–8. Hypertrophic cardiomyopathy, ventricular scarring. *A*. In this case of an elderly woman with hypertrophic cardiomyopathy, the septum was thinned, with diffuse scarring and marked vascular thickening. *B*. Histologically, there was diffuse scarring with marked intramural coronary artery thickening.

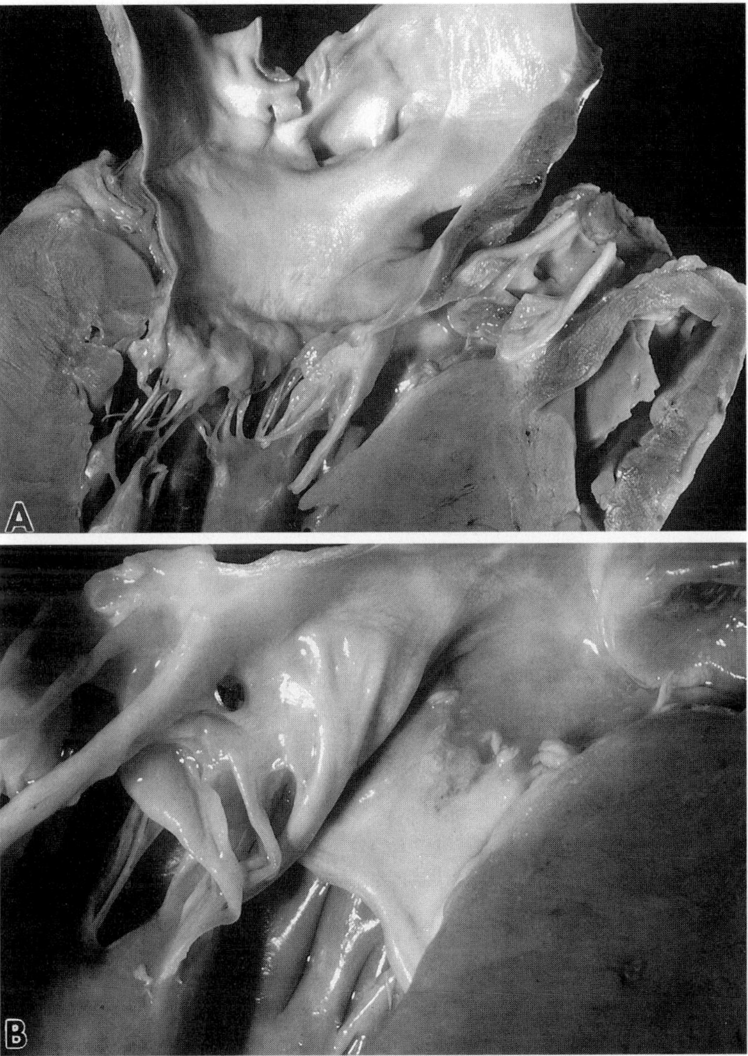

Figure 6–9. Hypertrophic cardiomyopathy, left ventricular outflow tract plaque. *A.* The left atrium, left ventricular inflow, and portion of the left ventricular outflow tract are demonstrated for orientation. *B.* A higher magnification of the outflow tract, with the anterior leaflet of the mitral valve lifted back, shows a discrete outflow tract plaque. In contrast to congenital subaortic stenosis, the thickening is not circumferential, the aortic valve leaflets are normal (not shown), and there is myofiber disarray histologically (not shown). Left ventricular outflow tract plaques are seen in about one half to three quarters of hearts with hypertrophic cardiomyopathy.

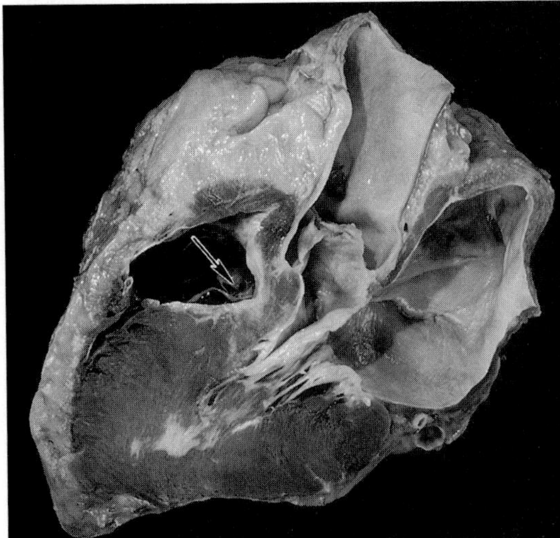

Figure 6–10. Hypertrophic cardiomyopathy, surgical relief of subaortic stenosis. In the early days of surgical treatment of hypertrophic cardiomyopathy, a right ventricular approach was sometimes used; note indentation representing myomectomy in the right ventricular outflow (*arrow*).

opathy results in a very uneven increase in myocyte size reflected by myocyte disorganization at a subcellular level. The histologic manifestations of myocyte disarray include oblique alignment of myocytes, producing a whorled, tangled, or pinwheel configuration[138, 139] (Fig. 6–12). In addition, the shape of myocytes is abnormal, with branching fibers common, and lateral attachments are increased. The degree of myofiber disarray is variable, but averages 30% of the septal myocardium and is usually greater than 5%.[137, 140]

The proper histologic evaluation of myofiber disarray is dependent on taking cross sections of the ventricular septum, to avoid artifacts of tangential or longitudinal sections.

The sensitivity and specificity of the histologic diagnosis of myofiber disarray (compared with hearts from normal controls and hearts with other cardiac diseases resulting in cardiac hypertrophy) is approximately 86% and 90%, respectively. These high sensitivity and specificity figures result when a cut-off point of 5% of septal cross-sectional areas is used for the designation of myofiber disarray.[137, 140] For pathologic practice, we section 5 to 6 areas of ventricular septum in cases of suspected hypertrophic cardiomyopathy: 3 from the basal septum (anterior, mid-septum, and posterior), and 2 to 3 from the apical septum. Because sections of ventricular septum are typically large, it is occasionally necessary to divide the section of septum into two pieces. However, the need for cross sections cannot be overemphasized in the proper evaluation of myofiber disarray. In many cases of hypertrophic cardiomyopathy, myofiber disarray is also present in the ventricular free wall, corresponding to the gross subtypes described by Maron et al.[100]

Conditions that may result in myofiber disarray other than hypertrophic cardiomyopathy include other causes of ventricular hypertrophy,

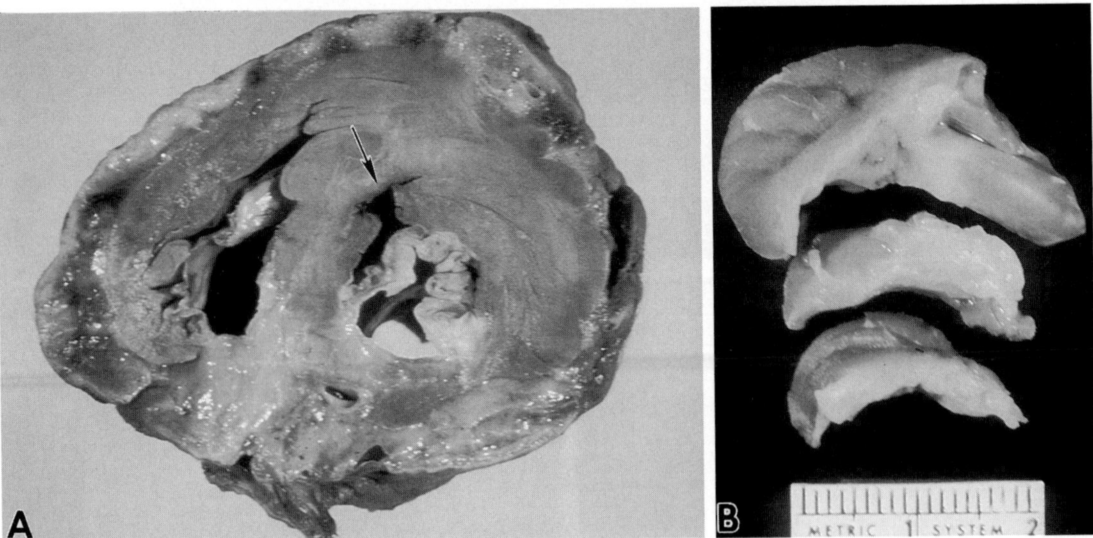

Figure 6–11. Hypertrophic cardiomyopathy, myomectomy. *A.* Currently, a left ventricular approach is used; note the indentation in the left ventricle where the myomectomy was performed (*arrow*). *B.* The surgical specimen demonstrates endocardial fibrosis of the left ventricular outflow tract plaque.

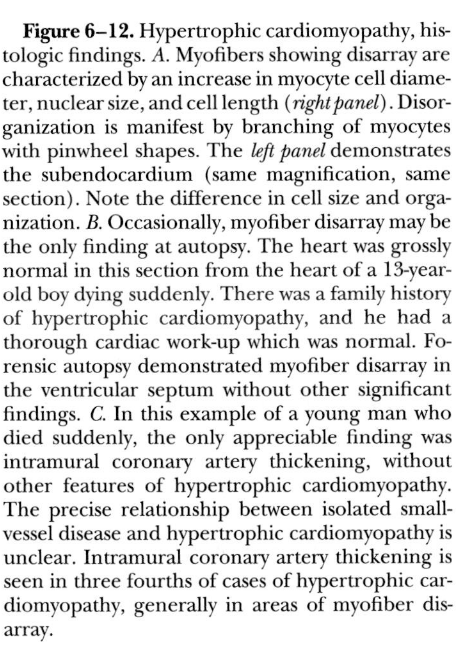

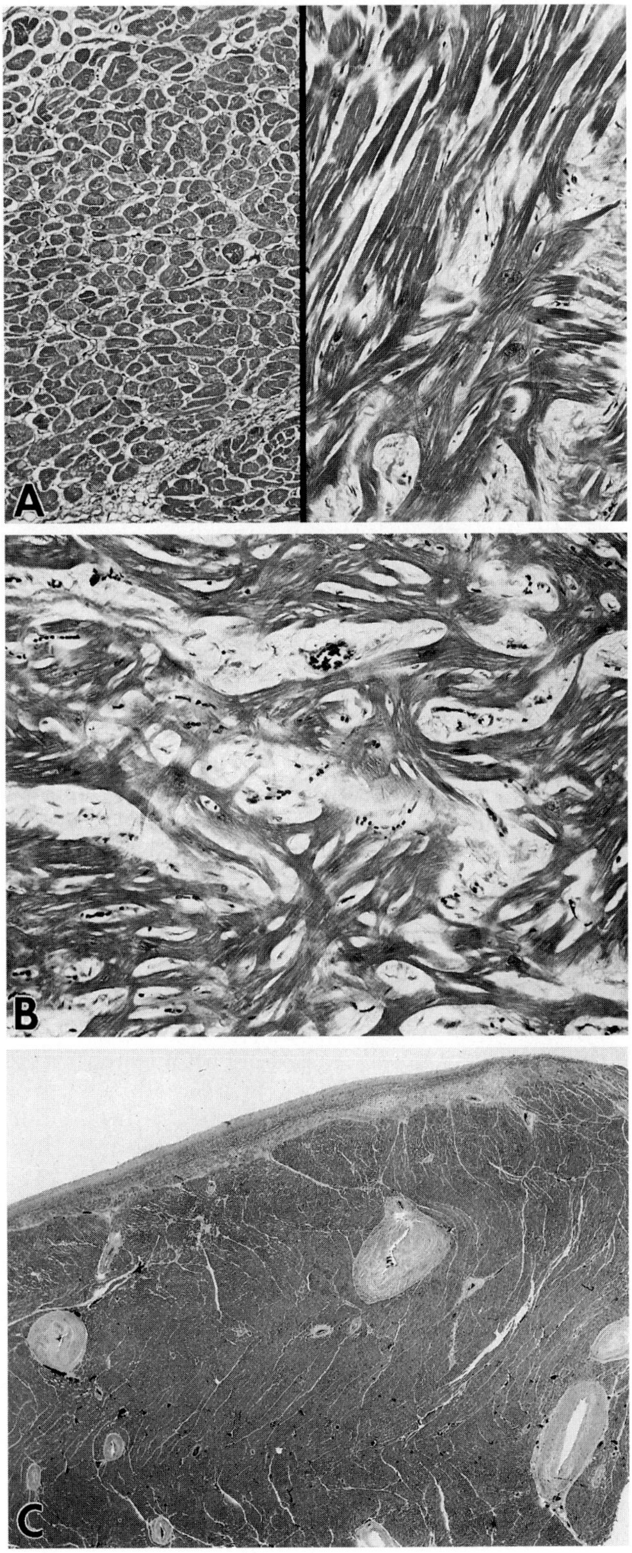

Figure 6–12. Hypertrophic cardiomyopathy, histologic findings. *A.* Myofibers showing disarray are characterized by an increase in myocyte cell diameter, nuclear size, and cell length (*right panel*). Disorganization is manifest by branching of myocytes with pinwheel shapes. The *left panel* demonstrates the subendocardium (same magnification, same section). Note the difference in cell size and organization. *B.* Occasionally, myofiber disarray may be the only finding at autopsy. The heart was grossly normal in this section from the heart of a 13-year-old boy dying suddenly. There was a family history of hypertrophic cardiomyopathy, and he had a thorough cardiac work-up which was normal. Forensic autopsy demonstrated myofiber disarray in the ventricular septum without other significant findings. *C.* In this example of a young man who died suddenly, the only appreciable finding was intramural coronary artery thickening, without other features of hypertrophic cardiomyopathy. The precise relationship between isolated small-vessel disease and hypertrophic cardiomyopathy is unclear. Intramural coronary artery thickening is seen in three fourths of cases of hypertrophic cardiomyopathy, generally in areas of myofiber disarray.

including aortic stenosis and chronic hypertension.[11, 141] However, the degree of myofiber disarray in these conditions is generally minimal, and less than 5%. Normal hearts may demonstrate myofiber disarray at the junction of the free walls and septum. The myocyte disarray of hypertrophic cardiomyopathy is characterized by a greater enlargement of myocyte size in the affected region (usually in the middle third of the ventricular septum) than in the subendocardial areas in the same section of myocardium. Myofiber disarray is usually accompanied by increase in fibroblasts and collagen, the former predominating in early stages, and the latter in later stages of disease.[142–144]

Abnormal patterns of desmin immunoreactivity have been described in areas of myofiber disarray. These include decrease or loss of labeling of intercalated discs and Z bands; longitudinal arrangement of desmin intermediate filaments; focal intense, granular staining of myocytes.[145] Ultrastructually, malalignment of sarcomeric myosin filaments has been described in patients with hypertrophic cardiomyopathy with known genetic mutations.[146]

Fibrosis

In addition to an increase in fibrosis in areas of myofiber disarray, there may be patchy interstitial fibrosis to extensive and grossly visible scars that may even be transmural.[18, 130]

Coronary Artery Abnormalities

Abnormal intramural coronary arteries, characterized by thickening of the vessel wall with a decrease in lumen size, are found within the ventricular septum in 83% of hearts, with a mean of 3 per tissue section[147] (Fig. 6–12). Intramural coronary artery thickening is more common in hearts with fibrosis than those without significant fibrosis.[147] The vessels are dysplastic without a well-developed internal elastic lamina and smooth muscle cells are in disarray.

Epicardial coronary arteries are usually normal in hypertrophic cardiomyopathy. However, the presence of a myocardial bridge over a portion of the left anterior descending artery (tunnel) has been associated with an increased risk of sudden death, especially in children.[148]

Histologic Findings of Myomectomy Specimens

Patients with > 50mm Hg subaortic gradient are often treated surgically with myomectomy and/or myotomy for the relief of outflow tract obstruction. In a study of 89 myomectomy specimens from patients with hypertrophic cardiomyopathy, myofiber disarray was present in 58%, generally in the deepest portion of the specimen. In contrast, myofiber disarray is present in a smaller proportion of endomyocardial biopsies, secondary to sampling error.[149] Other histologic features of hypertrophic cardiomyopathy that may be seen in myomectomy specimens include intramural artery thickening and endocardial fibrous plaque.[149]

Familial Hypertrophic Cardiomyopathy

Inheritance

The autosomal dominant inheritance of hypertrophic cardiomyopathy was established 13 years after its initial description in 1958.[150, 151] An echocardiographic study of 70 families of index cases demonstrated that in 55% of families, at least one member had echocardiographic evidence of hypertrophic cardiomyopathy.[152]

Genetic Basis

The genetic basis for familial hypertrophic cardiomyopathy is heterogeneous. In most cases of familial hypertrophic cardiomyopathy, and in less than half of all cases, there is a mutation of the gene coding for β cardiac myosin heavy chain (a component of the thick filament of striated muscle in cardiac and slow skeletal muscle) (Fig. 6–13), located on chromosome 14q1. A variety of mutations of this gene have been identified, most of which are single-point missense mutations occurring in exons 7, 9, 13, 14, 16, 19, 20, or 23.[153, 154] Certain of these mutations, especially those in exons 13 and 14, are associated with an especially poor prognosis.[155–157] The amino acid position 403 on exon 13, an apparent "hot spot" for the disease, may affect the myosin-actin dissociation in the contractile cycle.[158] Mutant messenger RNA has been identified in both cardiac and skeletal muscle[159] although symptoms related to skeletal involvement are rare.

Other sarcomeric proteins that may show mutations include cardiac troponin T, cardiac troponin I, alpha-tropomyosin, ventricular myosin essential light chain, ventricular myosin regulatory light chain, and cardiac myosin binding protein C.[153, 159, 160] Mutations in cardiac troponin T are associated with an especially poor prognosis with relatively mild hypertrophy,[161] although more benign mutations of this gene

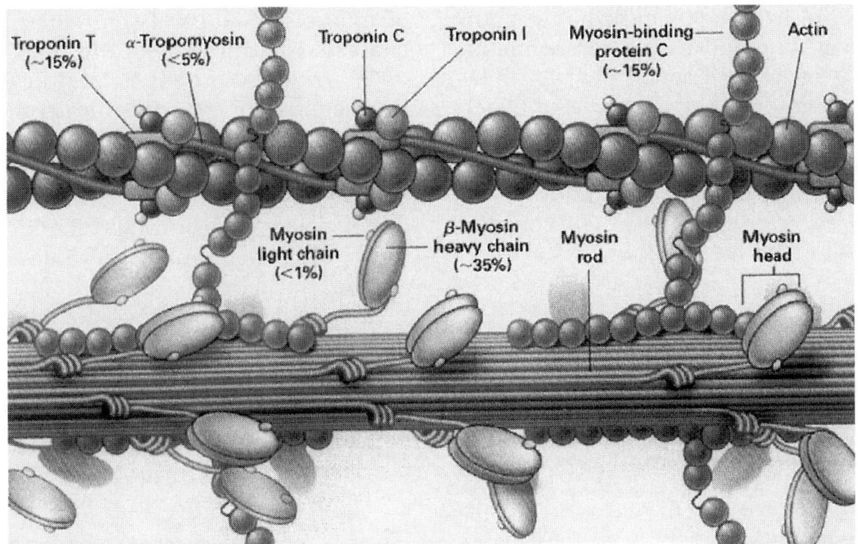

Figure 6–13. Hypertrophic cardiomyopathy, sites of genetic defects. The defects of hypertrophic cardiomyopathy involve sarcomeric proteins, most commonly β cardiac myosin heavy chain. Less commonly, there may be mutations in cardiac myosin binding protein C and troponin T. Unusual sites are ventricular myosin, α-tropomyosin essential light chain 1, the ventricular myosin regulatory light chain 2, cardiac troponin I, and α-tropomyosin. Contraction involves bindings and releasing of actin by the myosin heavy-chain region, as mediated by Ca^{++} concentration. (Used with permission, Spirito P et al. The management of hypertrophic cardiomyopathy. N Engl J Med 336:775–785, 1997.)

have also been described.[162] Mutations in tropomyosin are relatively more common in Finland than mutations in myosin heavy chain among patients with hypertrophic cardiomyopathy.[163] The clinical expression of mutations in the gene for cardiac myosin-binding protein C is often delayed until middle age or old age.[164, 165] There is evidence that coexisting mitochondrial mutations may effect the course of the disease, resulting in a higher incidence of congestive heart failure.[166, 167]

Disease in the Elderly and in Hypertensives

Hypertrophic cardiomyopathy is frequently diagnosed in the elderly,[168, 169] in whom it is often associated with subaortic obstruction resulting from distortion of the left ventricular outflow tract rather than true septal hypertrophy.[170] In many elderly patients with hypertrophic cardiomyopathy, the systolic anterior motion of the mitral valve results from a combination of anterior motion of the mitral valve and posterior excursion (bowing) of the ventricular septum.[170] Mitral annular calcification is frequently found, which may contribute to left ventricular outflow obstruction.[168] The left ventricular contour has been described echocardiographically as more ovoid than that of younger patients with the disease, and the reversed curvature of the ventricular septum, typically seen in younger patients, is absent.[171]

Age-associated bowing of the ventricular septum has been termed the sigmoid septum or angled interventricular septum.[172–174] The angle between the aortic outflow and ventricular septum is 90 to 110 degrees in elderly patients with subaortic stenosis, as compared with 140–145 degrees in younger patients with hypertrophic obstructive cardiomyopathy or control hearts. The sigmoid or angled septum may result in subaortic endocardial plaques, but symptoms related to subaortic obstruction are infrequent.[174]

Mild systolic hypertension is frequent in elderly patients with hypertrophic cardiomyopathy, and is present in up to one third of patients in autopsy series.[18] Large clinical series often exclude some patients with hypertension because of overlap between the echocardiographic findings of systemic hypertension and hypertrophic cardiomyopathy.[103] Patients with so-called hypertensive hypertrophic cardiomyopathy are often female[175] and often present in heart failure. The echocardiographic findings are indistinguishable from hypertrophic cardiomyopathy in normotensives, although the left ventricular wall is thicker.[176, 177]

It is likely that hypertrophic cardiomyopathy in the elderly is a heterogeneous entity, including true cases of hypertrophic cardiomyopathy as well as cases of hemodynamic derangements secondary to age-related septal bowing or hypertension. At autopsy, the diagnosis of hypertrophic cardiomyopathy in the elderly should be made only if there are unequivocal histologic features of myofiber disarray or a family history of hypertrophic cardiomyopathy, in conjunction with true septal hypertrophy or scarring.

Differential Diagnosis

At autopsy, the most difficult differential diagnosis involves asymmetric hypertrophy secondary to chronic hypertension. The evaluation of multiple sections of ventricular septum for characteristic findings of myofiber disarray in $> 5\%$ of septal area is helpful in establishing the diagnosis of hypertrophic cardiomyopathy. As discussed earlier age-related angulation of the ventricular septum may also suggest the diagnosis of hypertrophic cardiomyopathy, but true septal hypertrophy and the histologic features of hypertrophic cardiomyopathy are absent.

In concentric and apical forms of hypertrophic cardiomyopathy, the diagnosis may not be considered until histologic sections are evaluated for myofiber disarray and intramural coronary artery thickening. Because these forms comprise less than 10% of cases in the U.S.,

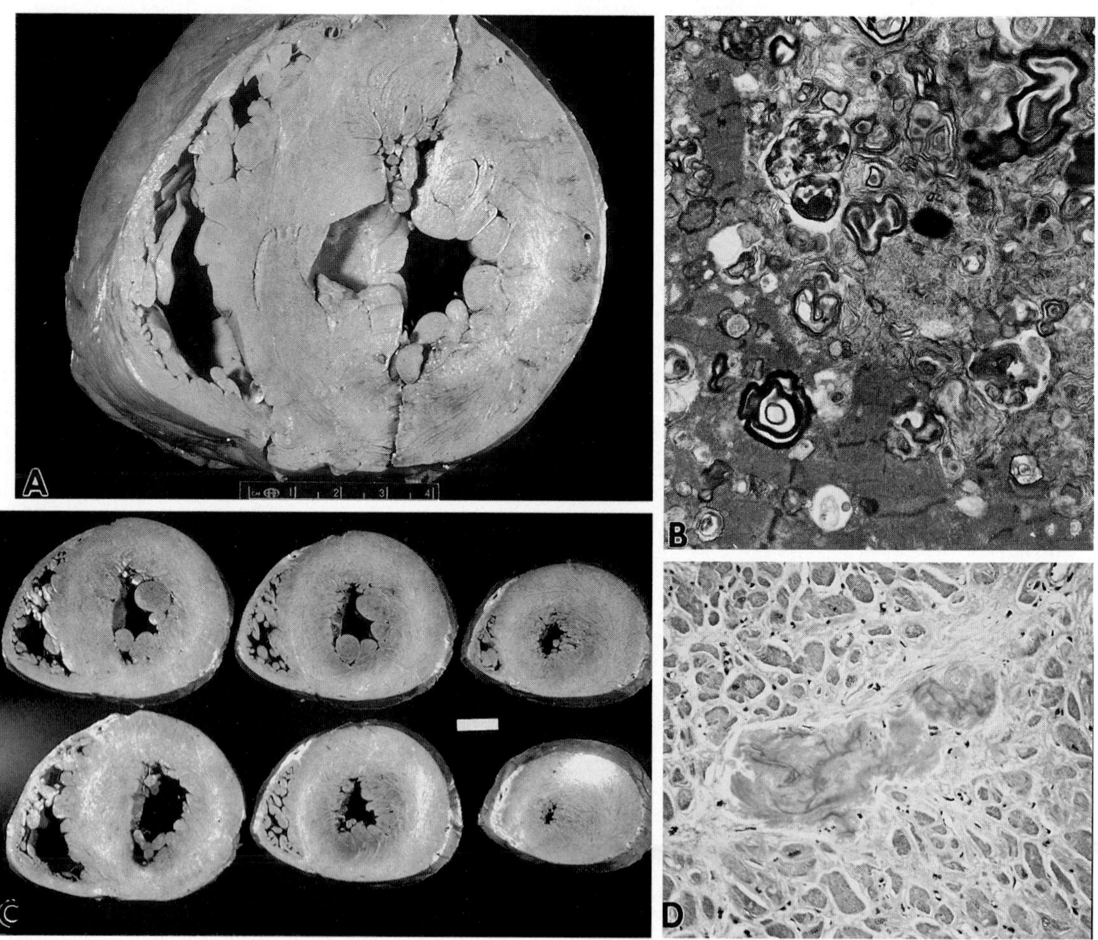

Figure 6–14. Mimickers of hypertrophic cardiomyopathy. A variety of conditions may result in asymmetric hypertrophy and grossly mimic hypertrophic cardiomyopathy, emphasizing that all cases must be confirmed histologically. *A.* Fabry's disease. There is asymmetric left ventricular hypertrophy with a normal chamber cavity, typical of hypertrophic cardiomyopathy. However, the patient had a history of cutaneous angiokeratomas. Histologically, there was diffuse myocyte vacuolization, which ultrastructurally demonstrated typical lamellated bodies of Fabry's disease (*B*). *C.* Amyloidosis may occasionally result in asymmetric hypertrophy, best appreciated in this example in the lower left panel. *D.* Histologically, amyloid forms amorphous deposits in the cardiac interstitium and intramyocardial vessel walls.

these types of hypertrophic cardiomyopathy are not frequently encountered.

Myofiber disarray is absent in asymmetric hypertrophy secondary to aortic stenosis. However, the aortic stenosis and hypertrophic cardiomyopathy may coexist in the same patient.[115]

Several conditions that may result in asymmetric hypertrophy—such as amyloidosis, Fabry's disease, lymphoma, and eosinophilic endomyocardial disease—are readily distinguished from hypertrophic cardiomyopathy by histologic evaluation (Fig. 6–14).

The various differential features separating hypertrophic from dilated cardiomyopathy are presented in Table 6–4.

ARRHYTHMOGENIC RIGHT VENTRICULAR DYSPLASIA

Definition

Right ventricular cardiomyopathy has many synonyms and related terms, including right ventricular dysplasia, arrhythmogenic right ventricular dysplasia, arrhythmogenic right ventricular dysplasia-cardiomyopathy, parchment heart, partial absence of the right ventricle, and Uhl's anomaly. The current preferred term is arrhythmogenic right ventricular dysplasia-cardiomyopathy.[1, 178]

The definition of arrhythmogenic right ventricular dysplasia is based on pathologic criteria of "transmural fibrofatty replacement of the right ventricular myocardium."[179] As will be pointed out, the pathologic criteria are not yet uniformly accepted, as is the case for most types of cardiomyopathy.

There is ongoing debate about the nature of arrhythmogenic right ventricular dysplasia.[180] Originally considered a genetically determined congenital malformation, it may represent a healed form of myocarditis.[181–183]

Clinical Features

The major clinical manifestations of arrhythmogenic right ventricular dysplasia arise from structural and functional abnormalities of the right ventricle, electrocardiographic depolarization/repolarization changes, and arrhythmias of right ventricular origin.[179] Imaging studies (especially echocardiography) typically demonstrate segmental dilatation of the right ventricle, localized right ventricular aneurysms, or global dilatation of the right ventricle without left ventricular involvement. Depolarization and conduction abnormalities typical of arrhythmogenic right ventricular dysplasia are epsilon waves or localized prolongation (> 110 ms) of the QRS complex in right precordial leads. Arrhythmias that are commonly diagnosed are left bundle branch block-type ventricular tachycardia, sustained and nonsustained, and frequent ventricular extrasystoles.[179] Diagnosis rests on demonstration of fibrofatty replacement of full-thickness right ventricular

Table 6–4. Differential Features, Hypertrophic versus Dilated Cardiomyopathy

	Dilated Cardiomyopathy	Hypertrophic Cardiomyopathy
Incidence (yearly)	6/100,000	2.5/100,000
Mean age at diagnosis	45	30s
Familial	7–20%	50–60%
Genetic basis	Unknown; rarely dystrophin gene abnormality	Beta myosin heavy chain and others
Viral etiology	10–20%	None implicated
Functional defect	Systolic	Diastolic
LV chamber size	Increased	Decreased or normal
LV mass	Increased	Greatly increased
Sudden death	20%	40%
At presentation	3%	20%
Congestive heart failure	> 95%	10%
Arrhythmias	Common	Common
10-year survival	15%	60%

myocardium generally at autopsy; clinical diagnosis rests on the presence of two major criteria, one major and two minor criteria, or four minor criteria (Table 6–5).

The incidence of arrhythmogenic right ventricular dysplasia is unknown, although it has been estimated to afflict one in 5,000 persons.[184] It accounts for 1–20% of cases of sudden cardiac death depending on the geographic location.

Most patients are young adults at the time of diagnosis. The mean age for patients dying suddenly is usually in the third decade,[185, 186] and the average age of patients diagnosed with the disease is 30 years.[187] Patients may be as young as 3 years old, and the disease is also diagnosed in the elderly. Syncope, ventricular tachyarrhythmias, and sudden death are more common in adolescent than adult patients.[188] There is no sex predilection.[185–187]

In a series of 20 patients from the Mayo Clinic, the initial clinical presentation was right ventricular arrhythmia (45%), congestive heart failure (25%), heart murmur (10%), asymptomatic (10%), complete heart block (5%), and sudden death (5%).[187]

Table 6–5. Clinical Criteria for the Diagnosis of Right Ventricular Dysplasia

I Functional and structural abnormalities
MAJOR
Severe dilatation and reduction of RV ejection fraction with no or mild LV impairment
Localized RV aneurysms
Severe segmental dilatation of RV
MINOR
Mild global RV dilatation and/or ejection fraction reduction with normal LV
Mild segmental dilatation of the RV
Regional RV hypokinesia
II Tissue characterization of walls
MAJOR
Fibrofatty replacement of myocardium on endomyocardial biopsy
III Repolarization abnormalities
MINOR
Inverted T waves in right precordial leads (> 12 years of age, in the absence of right bundle branch block)
IV Depolarization/conduction abnormalities
MAJOR
Epsilon waves or localized prolongation (> 110 ms) of the QRS complex in right precordial leads
MINOR
Late potentials (signal averaged ECG)
V Arrhythmias
MINOR
Left bundle branch block type ventricular tachycardia
Frequent ventricular extrasystoles (> 1000/24 hrs)
VI Family history
MAJOR Familial disease confirmed at autopsy or surgery
MINOR
Familial history of premature sudden death (< 35 years) due to suspected RV dysplasia
Familial history based on current clinical criteria

Adapted from McKenna et al. Diagnosis of arrhythmogenic right ventricular dysplasia/cardiomyopathy. Task Force of the Working Group Myocardial and Pericardial Disease of the European Society of Cardiology and of the Scientific Council on Cardiomyopathies of the International Society and Federation of Cardiology. Br Heart J 71:215–218, 1994, with permission.

Associations

A familial occurrence of arrhythmogenic right ventricular dysplasia was first reported in 1982.[189] First-order relatives are affected in approximately 30% of patients.[185] The mode of inheritance is autosomal dominant. Although the genetic basis is unknown, linkage studies have suggested a heterogeneous group of genetic defects. The most common locus linked to arrhythmogenic right ventricular dysplasia is 14q23-q24, followed by 1q42-q43, 14q12-q22, 3p23, and probably others.[183, 184, 190, 191]

Arrhythmogenic right ventricular dysplasia has been described in patients with hypertrophic cardiomyopathy,[192] in identical and nonidentical twins,[193–195] and in a patient with dermatomyositis.[196] There is a possibility that it may represent, in some patients, a form of healed myocarditis.[181, 182, 197, 198]

Pathologic Features

Gross Findings

The heart is generally normal in size or slightly enlarged.[180, 186, 199] The right ventricle is dilated often only focally, and there is usually an area of myocardial thinning to 2 mm or less (Figs. 6–15 and 6–16). Aneurysmal thinning may occur anywhere in the right ventricle, especially the right ventricular outflow tract (infundibulum), apex, and posterobasal segment. The epicardial fat may be thickened over the affected areas. The left ventricle is normal in two thirds of cases, although subepicardial scars may be present, most frequently in the posterior wall.[200] The presence of gross left ventricular enlargement identifies a subset of patients who tend to be older and develop heart failure more frequently than patients with grossly normal left ventricles.[201]

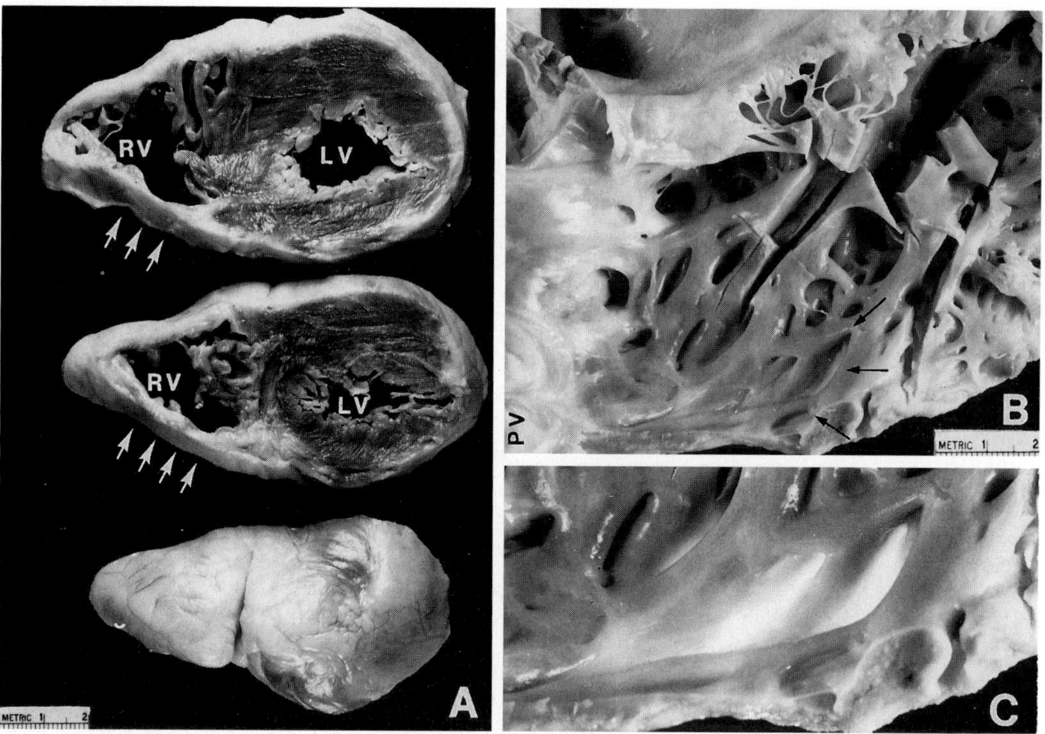

Figure 6–15. Arrhythmogenic right ventricular dysplasia. *A.* Grossly, there is marked thinning of the posterior wall of the right ventricle (*RV*) (*arrows*). *B.* The right ventricular outflow tract shows marked thinning (*arrows*) subjacent to the pulmonary valve (*PV*). *C.* Transillumination demonstrates the paper-thin quality of the ventricle in this area. (Reproduced with permission, Virmani R, et al. Sudden death and partial absence of the right ventricular myocardium. A report of three cases and a review of the literature. Arch Pathol Lab Med 106:165, 1982.

Histologic Findings

The histologic features of arrhythmogenic right ventricular dysplasia include fibrosis, fat, and inflammation (Figs. 6–15 and 6–16). Fat infiltration of the right ventricular myocardium is usually considered a *sine qua non* for the diagnosis of arrhythmogenic right ventricular dysplasia. Fibrosis, on the other hand, is only sometimes considered a required feature.[179] The disease has been pathologically subclassified based on the proportion of fat and fibrous tissue present. Italian investigators recognize a lipomatous and fibrolipomatous pattern[183, 186] and Lobo et al. add a third type, in which there is an absence of myocardium with apposition of endocardium and epicardial tissue.[180]

The autopsy diagnosis of arrhythmogenic right ventricular dysplasia should not be made entirely based on the presence of fat. Fat infiltration of the anterior wall of over 50% of myocardial area is not unusual in hearts from trauma victims, especially in the anterior wall near the apex[202, 203] Thin myocardial fascicles dispersed within epicardial fat (in the absence of fibrosis) is also a normal finding and not pathognomonic for cardiomyopathy. The hallmark of arrhythmogenic right ventricular dysplasia is transmural fat infiltration accompanied by fibrosis and thinning of the ventricular wall. The myocytes in the affected regions typically possess a characteristic bubbly or foamy cytoplasm[203] which, on ultrastructural analysis, represents marked mitochondrosis.

Massive fat infiltration of the myocardium, with a thickened ventricular wall (> 4 mm) instead of a thin one, has been associated with sudden death.[204] Massive fat infiltration of the myocardium should probably be considered separately from arrhythmogenic right ventricular dysplasia, because the right ventricle is generally thicker than normal and cardiac dilatation is not a prominent feature.

Lymphocytic infiltrates are frequently found in affected areas of myocardium, and have been described in up to 70% of cases of arrhythmogenic right ventricular dysplasia.[198, 205, 206]

With histologic evaluation of autopsy cases, it has become evident that arrhythmogenic right

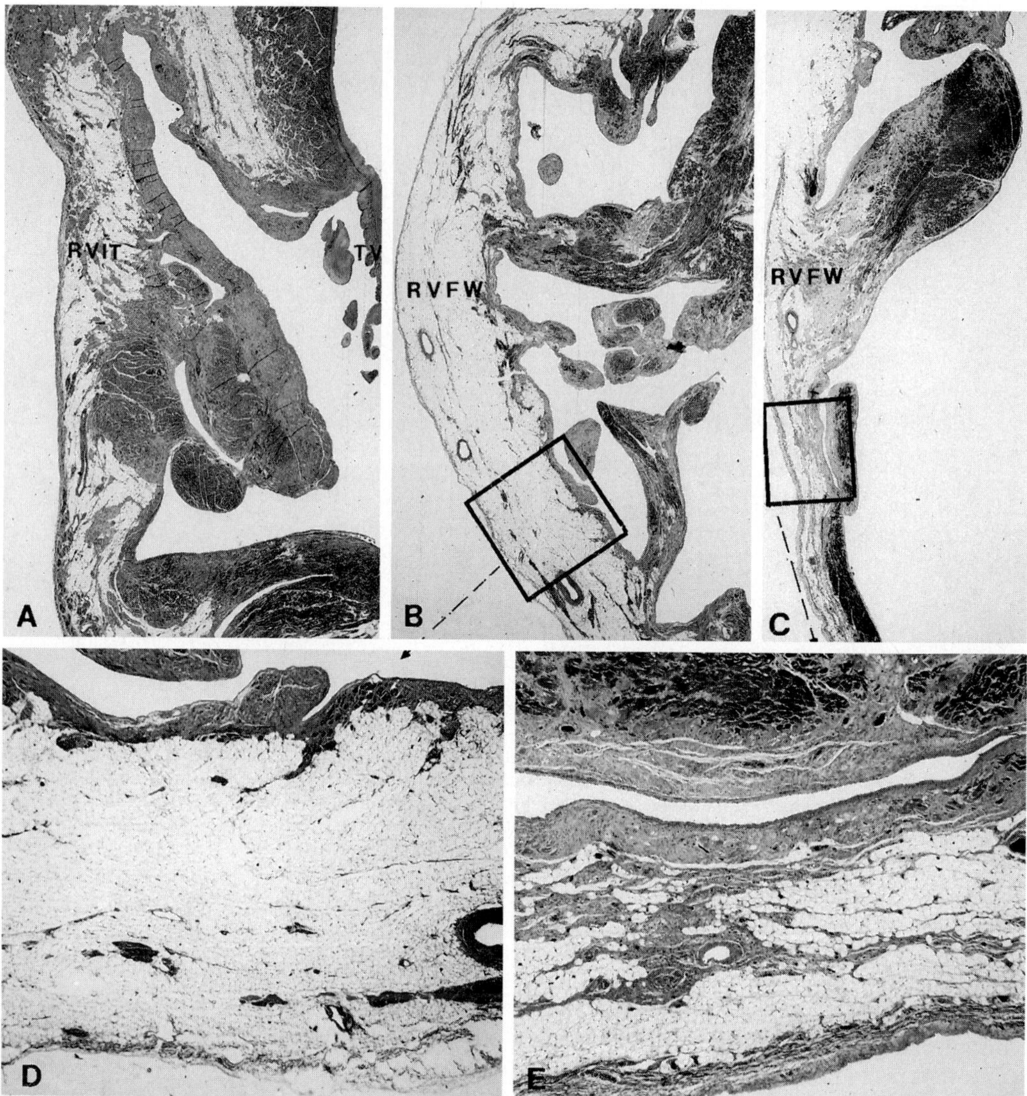

Figure 6–16. Arrhythmogenic right ventricular dysplasia. *A.* A low magnification demonstrates thinned right ventricular inflow tract (*RVIT*) adjacent to the tricuspid valve (*TV*). *B.* The free wall (*RVFW*) is largely replaced by fat and scar tissue in the subendocardial area. *C.* A low magnification of the right ventricular free wall (*RVFW*) in a different area of the same case demonstrates fibrofatty infiltration. *D,E.* Higher magnifications of *B* and *C* highlight the fat and fibrous tissue infiltrates that characterize arrhythmogenic right ventricular dysplasia. (Reproduced with permission, Virmani R, et al. Sudden death and partial absence of the right ventricular myocardium. A report of three cases and a review of the literature. Arch Pathol Lab Med 106:166, 1982.

ventricular dysplasia is a biventricular disease.[207] Subepicardial scars, fatty infiltrates, or inflammatory foci are present in approximately 75% of left ventricles, usually in the lateral wall.[205, 206, 208] Patients with gross or microscopic evidence of left ventricular involvement are more likely to have ventricular arrhythmias and enlarged hearts as compared with those patients with isolated right ventricular involvement.[201]

The endomyocardial biopsy diagnosis of arrhythmogenic right ventricular dysplasia is hampered by sampling error, and a negative biopsy does not exclude the diagnosis. If excess fat and fibrous tissue is present in an endomyocardial biopsy, the diagnosis may be suggested in the appropriate clinical setting.[187, 188, 209–211] By morphometric study, the degree of fat in endomyocardial biopsies is greater in patients with arrhythmogenic right ventricular dysplasia than control patients and those with dilated cardiomyopathy. Interstitial fibrosis is also increased, but similar to that seen in dilated cardiomyopathy.[210]

Differential Diagnosis

In typical cases of right ventricular dysplasia, the combined features of aneurysmal right ventricular dilatation, marked myocardial thinning, and fibrofatty replacement of the affected right ventricular myocardium allow for a straightforward diagnosis. However, when some of these features are absent, the diagnosis may be quite difficult, especially in the absence of a clinical or family history.

In the absence of significant fibrosis, fat infiltration of the right ventricle may be a normal variant. Unless there is greater than 50% fat infiltration of the posterior wall or basal region of the right ventricle, the diagnosis of arrhythmogenic right ventricular dysplasia should not be made. The anterior wall of the mid and apical right ventricle is frequently a site of intramural fat.

If there is extensive biventricular scarring with inflammatory infiltrates, the diagnosis of healing myocarditis should be considered. There is likely an overlap between healing myocarditis, dilated cardiomyopathy, and arrhythmogenic right ventricular dysplasia, and the precise distinction among these three entities is not always possible.

RESTRICTIVE CARDIOMYOPATHY

Definition and Causes

The hemodynamic parameters of restrictive cardiomyopathy reflect diastolic dysfunction due to stiff (noncompliant) ventricles.[212] Poor filling of the ventricles results in increased end-diastolic left atrial pressure, pulmonary and hepatic venous congestion, and biatrial enlargement. Cardiac hypertrophy or ventricular dilatation are absent, in contrast to the other major forms of cardiomyopathy. The underlying pathologic causes include infiltrative diseases, myocardial diseases, endocardial fibrosis, and idiopathic ventricular fibrosis. Clinically, it may be difficult to distinguish restrictive cardiomyopathy from constrictive pericarditis without endomyocardial biopsy.[213]

The most common causes of restrictive cardiomyopathy worldwide are amyloidosis, endocardial fibrosis (Davies disease), and endocardial disease with eosinophilia (Loeffler's disease). In addition to constrictive pericarditis, a variety of other myocardial conditions may result in restrictive parameters (Table 6–6), including storage diseases, carcinoid heart disease, methysergide therapy, pseudoxanthoma elasticum, radiation therapy, sarcoidosis, lupus erythematosus, and scleroderma.[11, 214]

Idiopathic Restrictive Cardiomyopathy

Clinical Features

In a group of patients with the clinical diagnosis of restrictive cardiomyopathy based on hemodynamic assessment, no secondary causes (including endocardial disease) are found even after endomyocardial biopsy. In some series of patients with restrictive cardiomyopathy, especially those of children, most cases are idiopathic.[215–217] An idiopathic enzymatic or metabolic disturbance has been postulated in some patients.[99] The clinical features include severe pulmonary congestion, arrhythmias, heart block, and cardiac failure. There is usually a rapidly fatal course in children.[215, 217] whereas survival is generally longer than 5 years in adults.[218] Families with idiopathic restrictive car-

Table 6–6. Secondary Causes of Restrictive Cardiomyopathy

Disease related to toxic eosinophil products
Idiopathic hypereosinophilic syndrome
Eosinophilia myalgia syndrome
Parasitic infections
Malignancy-associated eosinophilia
Eosinophilic leukemia
Infiltrative and fibrotic diseases
Amyloidosis
Carcinoid heart disease
Metastatic disease
Methysergide therapy
Radiation therapy
Sarcoidosis
Scleroderma
Myocardial diseases
Hemochromatosis
Fabry's disease
Glycogen storage disease
Hypertrophic cardiomyopathy
Pseudoxanthoma elasticum

Adapted from Edwards WD. Cardiomyopathies. In Virmani R, Atkinson JB, Fenoglio JJ (eds): Cardiovascular Pathology. Philadelphia: WB Saunders, 1991, with permission.

diomyopathy have been reported, but the familial incidence is lower than for hypertrophic or dilated cardiomyopathy.[219, 220]

Pathologic Findings

The gross pathologic features of restrictive cardiomyopathy are biatrial dilatation, a normal or small ventricular cavity, and ventricular walls of normal thickness (Fig. 6–17). Histologic studies in cases of idiopathic restrictive cardiomyopathy are few. In general, the light microscopic features are nonspecific and are similar to those of dilated cardiomyopathy.[41] Marked interstitial fibrosis has been described in some cases, some with associated myofiber disarray.[215, 218, 220–222] Ultrastructurally, myofibrillar loss is not seen, in contrast to dilated cardiomyopathy.[41] In autopsy studies, some patients with the clinical diagnosis of restrictive cardiomyopathy were found to have a form of hypertrophic cardiomyopathy with diffuse scarring.[216, 221] It is likely that what is now considered to be idiopathic restrictive cardiomyopathy will prove to be a heterogeneous group of disorders. Recently, it has been reported that in nearly 50% of patients with idiopathic restrictive cardiomyopathy, endomyocardial biopsy will demonstrate intracellular granulofilamentous dense deposits that by immunogold labeling, consist of desmin.[223] Desmin cardiomyopathy is also associated with atrioventricular block and overt or subclinical myopathy, and may be familial.[223]

Endomyocardial Disease with Hypereosinophilia

Pathogenesis

Eosinophilic endomyocardial disease (also known as eosinophilic endomyocarditis or Loeffler's eosinophilic endomyocarditis) is a result of the toxic effects of hypereosinophilia, generally defined as an increase in circulating eosinophils of greater than 1500/mm^3 for 6 months or

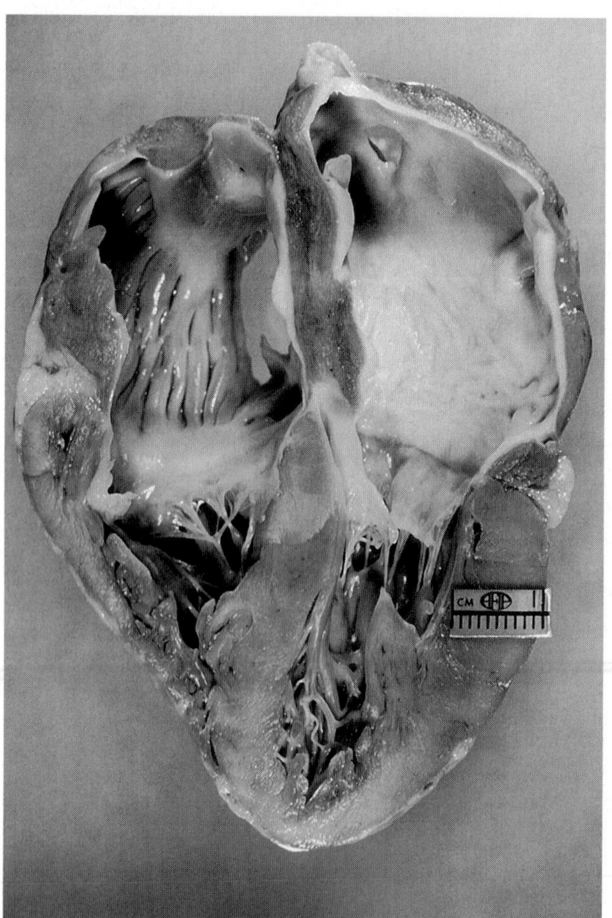

Figure 6–17. Idiopathic restrictive cardiomyopathy. There is marked biatrial dilatation secondary to decreased compliance of the ventricles. The ventricular walls are of normal thickness and the ventricular cavities of normal size. The patient was a child with dyspnea and pulmonary congestion; histologic features were nonspecific and there were no infiltrative or endocardial diseases diagnosed.

more. The mechanism of endocardial damage secondary to toxic products within eosinophil granules is poorly understood but may involve tissue damage by major basic and cationic proteins.[224–228] Because some patients with hypereosinophilia do not develop cardiac tissue damage, there are likely unknown factors other than hypereosinophilia that are responsible for the toxic endomyocardial damage.

In addition to increased numbers of eosinophils, patients have intrinsic abnormalities in circulating eosinophils. These include cytoplasmic vacuolization, abnormal cytoplasmic granules, increased tendency for degranulation, phagocytosis of red blood cells, a prolonged half-life, an increase in receptors for C3 and IgG, and abnormal cellular kinetics.[229]

A variety of conditions that lead to peripheral eosinophilia are associated with endocardial disease, but in Western countries, idiopathic hypereosinophilic syndrome is by far the most common cause.[230] Other causes of eosinophilic endomyocardial disease include the Churg–Strauss syndrome, eosinophilic leukemia, malignancy-associated hypereosinophilia, and parasitic-related eosinophilia.[11] Recently, eosinophilic endomyocardial disease has been described as a complication of the eosinophilia myalgia syndrome.[231]

Epidemiologic and Clinical Considerations

Endomyocardial disease is the least frequent type of cardiomyopathy in Western countries, but is endemic in the tropics. For unknown reasons, endocardial disease in the tropics is less frequently associated with hypereosinophilia than endomyocardial disease in the West. In a series of restrictive cardiomyopathy from tropical countries, the proportion of patients with eosinophilia ranges from 0 to less than 25%,[232–234] whereas in Western countries hypereosinophilia is a constant finding. A male predominance has been described,[230] and all patients were male in one autopsy series of eight patients.[18] Davies et al. have postulated that in patients with the tropical form of disease, there is a high load of parasites and persistent low level of eosinophilia that required years to develop cardiac toxicity. In contrast, Western cases are characterized by the sudden onset of eosinophilia, usually caused by the hypereosinophilic syndrome, and a relatively rapid onset of disease within 6 months.[230]

The mean age at onset of eosinophilic endomyocardial disease is approximately 40 years. In about one half of patients, the initial symptom is cardiac failure,[235] and in the other half, other manifestations of the hypereosinophilic syndrome predate the cardiac symptoms. In a series of 50 patients with hypereosinophilic syndrome, the heart and central nervous system were the most frequently involved organs.[226] Cardiac symptoms occur in almost three fourths of patients,[236, 237] and the most frequent cardiac symptom is biventricular congestive heart failure.[18] Occasionally, there may be septal hypertrophy mimicking hypertrophic cardiomyopathy.[119] The cardiac manifestations initially are related to cardiac dilatation with thrombosis and mitral insufficiency; at later stages, a restrictive cardiomyopathy often develops.[226, 236] Arrhythmias and conduction system disturbances, including AV block, right bundle branch block, and atrial fibrillation, may occur.[238] Mitral valve replacement may be required for severe mitral insufficiency.[239–241] Surgical removal of ventricular thrombi in both ventricles or the left ventricle with mitral or tricuspid valve replacement has shown to slightly prolong survival.[241] Treatment with prednisone is often effective in ameliorating the effects of cardiac failure and atrioventricular valve regurgitation.[235]

Pathologic Features

In clinical and autopsy series, biventricular disease is found in most patients,[18, 230] although univentricular involvement, usually of the left ventricle, has been said to occur in up to 50% of cases.[99] The pathologic features of eosinophilic endomyocardial disease may be divided into three stages.[11]

1. The necrotic stage is an eosinophilic myocarditis characterized by tissue necrosis, eosinophilic granulomas, eosinophil breakdown products, and intramural coronary artery thrombi.[242–244] This phase is not typically characterized as a cardiomyopathy. Patients dying in this phase of illness have generally been ill for a short time, and the clinical course resembles fulminant myocarditis.

2. The thrombotic stage is associated with a mural thrombus that begins apically and extends toward the base of the heart, entrapping papillary muscle, chordae tendineae, and atrioventricular valve leaflets[99, 226, 235] (Fig. 6–18). The cause of death is often related to thromboembolism or cardiac failure, and the course of illness is months to years. At this stage of disease, mitral valve replacement may be required. The ex-

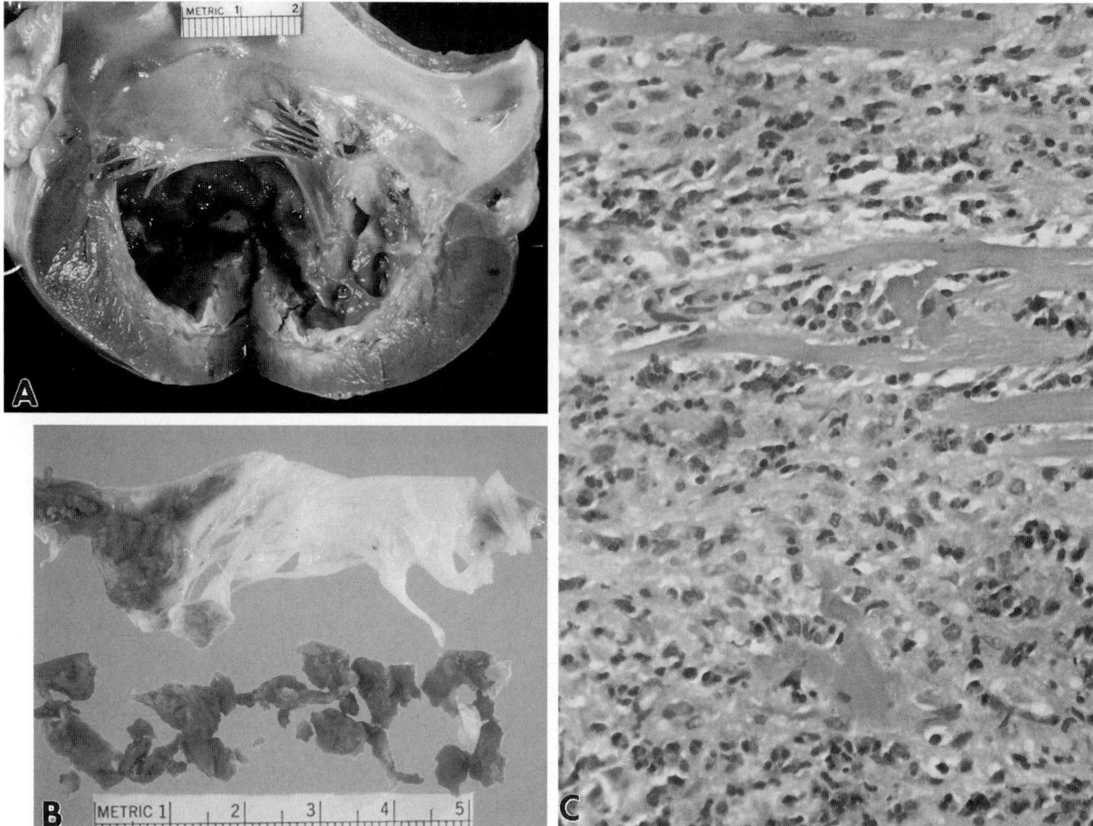

Figure 6–18. Eosinophilic endomyocardial disease. *A.* There is an organized thrombus that fills the left ventricular apex and extends to the mitral valve. *B.* Occasionally, mitral insufficiency is severe, caused by thrombus on the ventricular surface of the valve leaflets adhering the valve to the endocardium. Valve replacement may be necessary, as shown in this excised mitral valve with attached thrombus. *C.* Histologically, eosinophilic endomyocardial disease is characterized by eosinophilic infiltrates, eosinophil breakdown products.

cised valve demonstrates thrombus adherent to the posterior leaflet, only on the ventricular surface. Histologically, there is acute and organizing thrombus with sheets of eosinophils, eosinophil breakdown products, and Charcot–Leyden crystals.

3. The fibrotic stage resembles endocardial fibrosis as seen in the tropics and that which is generally described at autopsy.[18] There is ventricular apical thrombus with thick endocardial fibrous plaques that often have distinct borders with rolled edges.[99, 245] The atrioventricular valves show thickening with adherence to the underlying ventricular surface, resulting in valvular insufficiency. The ventricles are generally mildly dilated with thickened walls.[18] Histologically, the predominant finding is fibrosis. Eosinophils and eosinophil breakdown products may be detectable in some hearts, but are dependent on the stage of disease.[18] Intramural coronary thrombi with adjacent necrosis are present in a minority of hearts.[18]

Endomyocardial Disease Without Hypereosinophilia (Endocardial Fibrosis)

Definition

Also known as Davies' disease, endomyocardial fibrosis is an idiopathic condition that is found exclusively in tropical zones, and is not associated with overt hypereosinophilia. However, it is believed that endocardial fibrosis may represent an end stage of eosinophilic disease or the result of chronic low levels of hypereosinophilia related to chronic parasitic infection.[11, 230] Endomyocardial disease with and without eosinophilia are often considered as a single entity with differing morphologic and clinical expressions (Table 6–7).[11]

Clinical Findings

The mean age at presentation is approximately 30 years and there is no sex predilec-

Table 6–7. Differentiating Characteristics, Endocardial Fibrosis with and Without Hypereosinophilia

Feature	With Hypereosinophilia	Without Hypereosinophilia
Sex predilection	Males	None
Underlying cause	Toxic eosinophil damage	Unknown
Geographic distribution	Worldwide	Tropics
Eosinophilic myocarditis	Present in initial stages	Absent
Mural thrombi	Usually present	Usually absent
Univentricular involvement	Uncommon	Common

tion.[18, 232, 233, 246] The clinical features differ from those of endomyocardial disease with hypereosinophilia in that patients are younger, there is no male predominance, and isolated left ventricular disease is common.[230] The mean duration of clinical symptoms before death is about 7 months.[18] The most common symptoms are those of heart failure,[232, 247] although embolic symptoms may occur in up to one third of patients.[232] Ventricular involvement is influenced by the geographic location. The majority of patients in Venezuela have left-sided involvement,[232] whereas in Egypt—where there is a high rate of infection with schistosomiasis—right ventricular involvement is the rule.[234]

Pathologic Findings

At autopsy, the heart weight is mildly increased, and endocardial fibrous plaques are present in one or both ventricles.[18] (Figs. 6–19 and 6–20). The involved ventricles are typically normal in size or constricted, and the atria are dilated. With left ventricular involvement, there is generally a shrunken left ventricular cavity and biatrial dilatation generating the appearance of a heart with mitral stenosis.[18] Endomyocardial biopsy will demonstrate nonspecific findings of endocardial fibrosis without eosinophils.[233, 234]

Cardiac Amyloidosis

Definition

Cardiac amyloidosis is characterized by the extracellular deposition of fibrillary proteins, often resulting in diastolic and systolic dysfunction. Amyloid proteins are diverse, but share

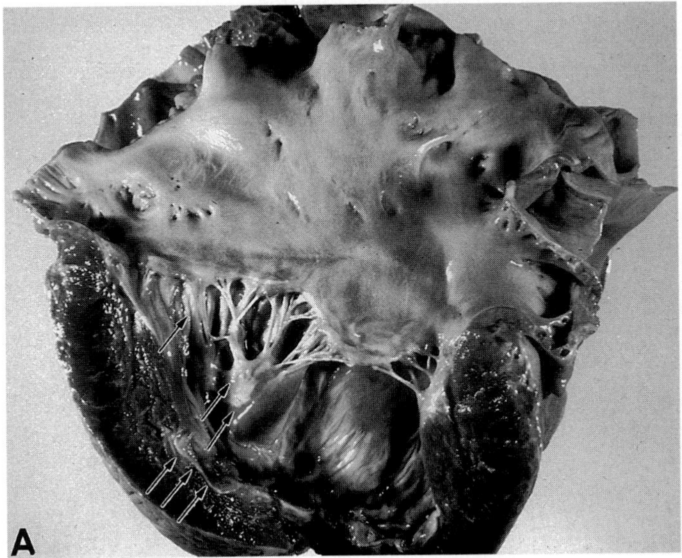

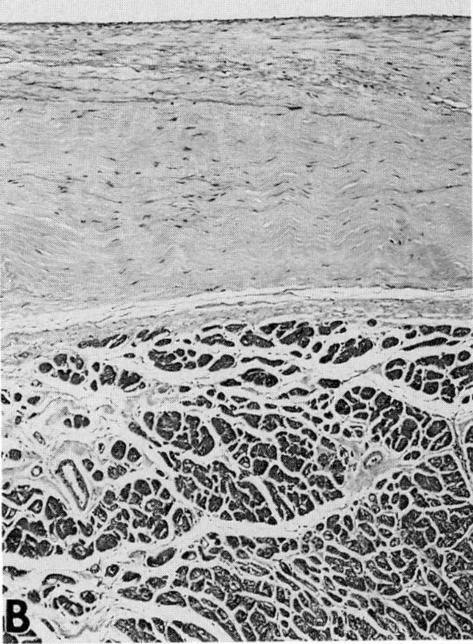

Figure 6–19. Idiopathic endocardial fibrosis (Davies' disease). *A.* In this case from Africa, there are endocardial plaques (*arrows*) involving the chordae of the posterior leaflet of the mitral valve and in the left ventricular apex (*arrows*). *B.* Histologically, these areas demonstrated dense endocardial fibrous thickening.

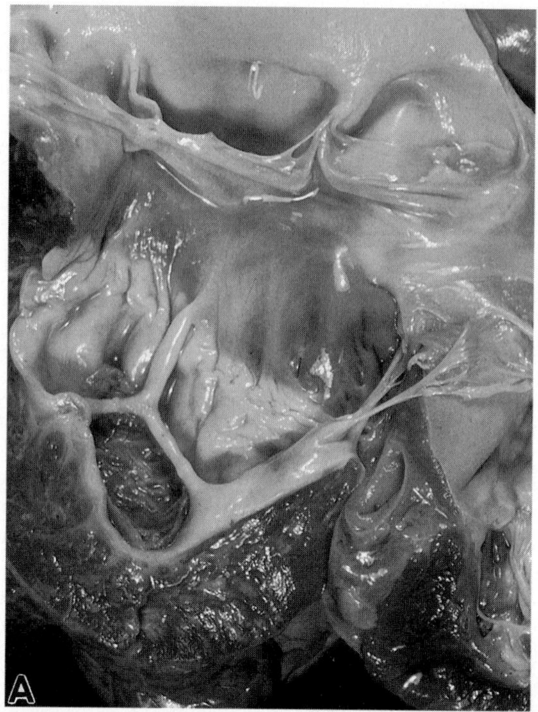

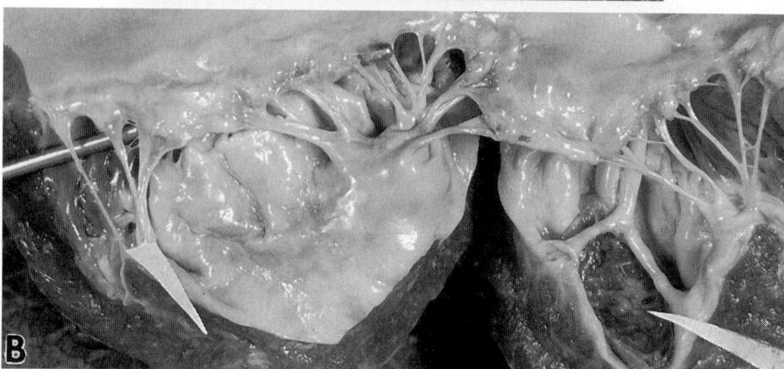

Figure 6–20. Idiopathic endocardial fibrosis (Davies' disease). *A.* There are dense endocardial plaques in the left ventricular outflow area along with an organizing thrombus (*right arrow in B*). *B.* The plaques result in plastering of the posterior leaflet of the mitral valve against the endocardial surface. Note subendocardial fibrosis in the wall of the left ventricle (*left arrow*). (Figure courtesy of Dr. Prem Chopra, All Indian Institute of the Medical Sciences, New Delhi.)

several characteristics. By light microscopy, amyloid is amorphous and eosinophilic, demonstrating apple-green birefringence with polarized light after Congo-red staining. Ultrastructurally, amyloid fibrils measure 7–10 nm in diameter and do not branch. The protein demonstrates a crossed β-pleated sheet structure by infrared and X-ray diffraction techniques.[248]

Classification and Protein Composition

Cardiac amyloid is classified according to the protein responsible for the fibril structure (Table 6–8). The precursor proteins responsible for amyloid cardiomyopathy are transthyretin (prealbumin), immunoglobulin light chains, and (rarely) amyloid A protein. Each of these three types of amyloid is virtually always accompanied by extracardiac amyloid deposition. The common names that correspond to these three types of cardiac amyloid are senile systemic amyloid, primary amyloid, and secondary amyloid, respectively.

A fourth form of cardiac amyloidosis, hereditary cardiac amyloidosis, may also result in cardiomyopathy. It is caused by an accumulation of transthyretin modified by a mutation in the

Table 6–8. Major Types of Cardiac Amyloidosis

Type	Age (mean)	Protein Precursor	% of Affected Patients with Heart Infiltrates	% of Patients with Symptomatic Heart Disease	Frequency in Patients Diagnosed with Cardiac Amyloid by Biopsy
Senile	70+	Transthyretin (ASc) (ATTR)	100%	low	20%
Familial	60	Transthyretin (ATTR)	Probably > 50%	20–50%	< 5%
Primary	60	Light chains (AL)	High	20–30%	75%
Secondary	50	SAA	Unknown	0–5%	0–5%
Isolated atrial	80+	AANF	100%	0	0
Hemodialysis	—	β-2 macro globulin	60–70%	0	0

ASc = amyloid senile (cardiac); ATTR = amyloid transthyretin; AL = amyloid light chains; SAA = serum amyloid A protein; AANF = amyloid atrial natriuretic factor

gene coding for the protein, and is transmitted as an autosomal dominant condition. Over 28 separate mutations have been described.[249, 250] Families with this condition were first reported in Portugal, Japan, and Sweden.[251]

It is a matter of debate whether there is an underlying mutation in transthyretin in cases of senile systemic amyloid. The transthyretin precursor for senile amyloid is generally believed to be normal,[248, 252] although transthyretin variant isoleucine-122 has been described in a patient with senile cardiac amyloid.[253] Senile cardiac amyloidosis in African Americans is associated with the isoleucine-122 variant, which is present in approximately 3% of Blacks but is rare in Caucasians. An autopsy study demonstrated that nearly 20% of Blacks, compared with 0% of Caucasians with senile cardiac amyloidosis possess the isoleucine-122 variant of transthyretin, and that the majority of Blacks possessing this variant harbor microscopic quantities of amyloid in their cardiac ventricles.[254]

There are other forms of hereditary amyloidosis that may involve the heart but usually do not result in cardiomyopathy. The precursor protein in Finnish hereditary amyloidosis is gelsolin, an actin-binding protein.[255, 256] Other forms of hereditary amyloid arising from deposits of cystatin C and apolipoprotein A1 do not have a predilection for the myocardium.[251]

The type of cardiac amyloid that is considered the most frequent[257, 258] is an entity currently designated "isolated atrial amyloid." This form of cardiac amyloid has not been clearly linked to cardiac dysfunction or cardiomyopathy, however.[248] Before the protein composition of amyloid was known, isolated atrial amyloid and senile systemic amyloid were considered as the same entity (senile amyloidosis). Unlike senile systemic amyloidosis, the precursor protein for isolated atrial amyloid is related to atrial natriuretic factor[259] and ventricular involvement is uncommon. Isolated atrial amyloidosis is seen as an incidental autopsy finding in about 80% of patients over 80 years of age.[257]

Amyloidosis is an uncommon complication of chronic long-term hemodialysis. The principal component of hemodialysis-associated amyloid is β-2 microglobulin. Clinical symptoms result from the carpal tunnel syndrome, bone cysts, and spondyloarthropathy. The heart is the most common viscus involved at autopsy, with effacement of small blood vessels.[260] However, symptomatic cardiac disease does not occur.

In addition to the protein that is responsible for the fibril structure that is the basis for classification, other proteins and glycoproteins are consistently found in the amyloid deposits. Serum amyloid P is a 25 kilodalton protein that forms doughnut-shaped pentamers that are stacked at right angles to the fibril. It is useful in the immunohistochemical detection of amyloid (regardless of the type) in tissues[261] as well as scintigraphic localization of amyloid within patients.[262] Heparan sulfate, perlecan, laminin, collagen IV, fibronectin, and entactin are also deposited in many or all forms of amyloid[248]

Clinical Findings

The average age of patients presenting with cardiac amyloidosis is approximately 60 years, and there is a male:female predominance of 2:1[263] to 4:1.[261] The major clinical expressions of cardiac amyloidosis are restrictive cardiomyopathy (diastolic dysfunction), systolic dysfunction, orthostatic hypotension, and arrhythmias.[64, 264] The diastolic dysfunction of restrictive cardiomyopathy results from increased stiffness of the ventricles. Systolic dysfunction may be precipitated by atrial deposits that result in the loss of atrial transport function and congestive heart failure; patients with predominantly systolic dysfunction have a relentless course that may be complicated by anginal chest pain in the absence of epicardial coronary artery disease.[265] Angina pectoris is usually a result of concomitant atherosclerosis, however. Right-sided findings, such as peripheral edema, are usually prominent. Orthostatic hypotension may be a result of amyloid infiltration of the autonomic nervous system, and conduction system disturbance may result from amyloid infiltrates of the conduction system. Syncope is often a manifestation of late stages of disease, and may herald impending sudden death.[266]

Typical echocardiographic features include normal left ventricular cavity dimension, increased ventricular wall thickness, a granular sparkling texture of the myocardium, and decreased systolic function. In 10–20% of patients, the echocardiographic features are suggestive of dilated cardiomyopathy or hypertrophic cardiomyopathy, and in the remainder a restrictive pattern is seen.[267] More recently developed imaging techniques, such as magnetic resonance imaging, may differentiate amyloid deposits from idiopathic cardiomyopathy by high-resolution evaluation of the myocardial wall.[268]

Senile Systemic Amyloidosis (Amyloid AS)

Before the distinction between primary atrial and senile systemic amyloidosis was made, senile amyloidosis was often considered a benign condition.[267] In recent series of biopsy-diagnosed cases of symptomatic cardiac amyloidosis, in which the type of amyloidosis is carefully established by immunohistochemical stains and serum tests for light chains, approximately 20% of cases represent senile amyloidosis.[261, 267] Similar to other types of cardiac amyloidosis, the presenting symptom is usually dyspnea; palpitations and syncope related to left ventricular outflow tract obstruction may also occur.[267] The prognosis of senile systemic cardiac amyloidosis is far better than that of primary cardiac amyloidosis, and most patients are alive after 2 years.[267] The mean age of patients with senile amyloidosis is over 70 years, and even higher in autopsy series[257, 261]

Familial Amyloidosis

Rukavina et al. described the first series of patients with familial amyloidosis.[269] In contrast to senile amyloidosis, the dominant symptoms in patients with familial amyloidosis are usually polyneuropathy and autonomic dysfunction.[270–272] In a series of 52 North American patients with familial amyloidosis, the median age was 64 years, 83% had peripheral neuropathy and 27% had cardiomyopathy.[273] In this study, the median survival was 5.8 years, and the cause of death in 55% was cardiac. In some families with hereditary amyloidosis, however, the cardiac symptoms predominate.[274, 275] In the majority of families with hereditary amyloidosis, mutations to transthyretin have been identified.[276, 277] Familial amyloidosis presents similar echocardiographic features as primary amyloidosis, although low-voltage patterns are less frequent by electrocardiogram. Compared to primary amyloidosis, however, survival is far better in patients with hereditary amyloid.[278]

Primary (AL) Amyloidosis

Primary amyloidosis is generally synonymous with light-chain amyloidosis or amyloid AL disease. Amyloidosis associated with overt multiple myeloma is sometimes classified separately from primary amyloidosis,[264, 279] but the two entities form a spectrum.[280] Approximately 25% of patients with AL amyloidosis have multiple myeloma.[264, 281] The remainder of patients suffer from premalignant plasma cell dyscrasia, manifest by plasmacytosis of the bone marrow and free monoclonal light chain in the serum or urine. The mean age of patients presenting with primary amyloidosis is approximately 60 years, and 60% of patients are men.[282]

Over 20% of patients with primary amyloidosis present with cardiac symptoms, most often congestive heart failure.[264, 280] Similar to all patients with primary amyloidosis, the mean age of patients with cardiac involvement is 60 years, and about three of four patients are men.[261] Survival among patients with symptomatic cardiac involvement averages only 6 months,[283] although occasional patients respond to alkylating agents and live for years.[280, 284] A significant negative prognostic finding in patients with cardiac amyloidosis is right ventricular dilatation.[285]

Because of its high rate of symptoms, primary cardiac amyloidosis is more common than senile systemic amyloidosis in clinical series. Three of four patients with biopsy-proven cardiac amyloidosis have primary amyloidosis,[261] and a similar fraction has been reported at autopsy.[279, 286] The most common cause of death in primary amyloidosis is cardiac failure, accounting for 30% of fatalities.[264]

Secondary Amyloidosis (Amyloid AA)

The incidence of symptomatic heart involvement in secondary amyloidosis is low. In an autopsy study of 54 patients with cardiac amyloidosis causing cardiac dysfunction, no patient had secondary amyloid.[279] Of 64 patients seen at the Mayo Clinic with AA amyloid documented by rectal or abdominal fat biopsy, none had symptomatic cardiac involvement.[287] Cardiac symptoms in 18 patients with secondary amyloidosis reported by Wright and Calkins[288] were all attributed to causes other than amyloid, with the possible exception of two patients. In a review of several studies of type AA amyloid secondary to familial Mediterranean fever, Meyerhoff et al. did not find significant evidence of cardiac involvement.[289] In a clinical study of localization of amyloidosis by ^{123}I-labeled serum amyloid P component, none of 25 patients with secondary amyloidosis had positive uptake in the myocardium, compared with a majority of 25 patients with primary amyloidosis.

A recent echocardiographic study has demonstrated evidence of cardiac involvement in 3/30 patients with secondary amyloidosis and in 13/24 patients with primary amyloidosis.[290] The patients in this study were not severely symptomatic. Of 108 autopsies of patients with cardiac amyloidosis at the Johns Hopkins Hospital, five patients had secondary amyloidosis.[286]

Gross Pathologic Findings

The mean heart weight in an autopsy series of 54 cases of symptomatic cardiac amyloidosis was 554 grams, with a range of 300–900 grams.[279] The gross consistency of the myocardium is often described as firm, rubbery or waxy, a feature that allows the gross diagnosis in a large proportion of cases[279] (Fig. 6–21). Atrial dilatation is a constant feature, and ventricular dilatation is infrequent and reported in about 20% of cases.[279]

Focal, tan, waxy endocardial deposits are generally observed in the mural endocardium of one or both atria and frequently on the valve leaflets. The most frequently involved valves are the tricuspid and mitral, demonstrating amyloid deposits in 80–85% of cases, followed by the semilunar valves, one half of which contain amyloid.[279] Although amyloid commonly involves the valves histologically, it does not cause symptomatic valvular disease.

Transmural myocardial scarring or acute infarction occurs in approximately 13% of autopsy cases of fatal cardiac amyloidosis,[291] and may occur in the absence of significant epicar-

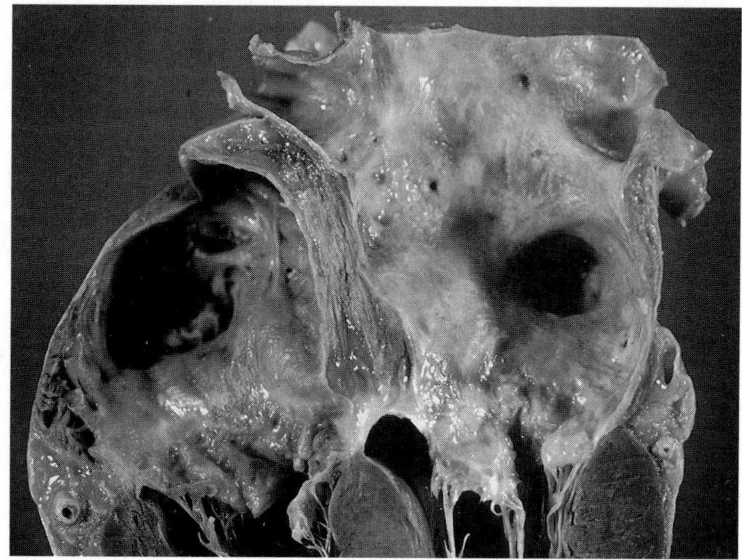

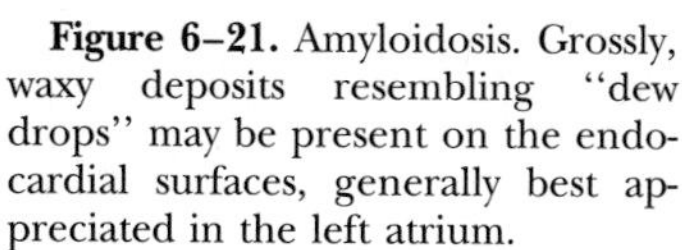

Figure 6–21. Amyloidosis. Grossly, waxy deposits resembling "dew drops" may be present on the endocardial surfaces, generally best appreciated in the left atrium.

dial coronary disease. Myocardial infarction in cardiac amyloid has been ascribed to narrowing of intramyocardial arteries by amyloid deposits.[286]

Microscopic Pathologic Findings

The histologic appearance of cardiac amyloid is identical to that of amyloidosis of other organs. There are a battery of stains that identify the amorphous eosinophilic infiltrates as amyloid. These include the sulfated alcian blue stain,[292] metachromatic stains, Congo-red stains, thioflavin T, crystal violet, and Sirius red.[248]

There are four major patterns of amyloid deposition within the myocardium: pericellular, vascular, nodular, and endocardial (Fig. 6–22). There have been few studies correlating histologic findings with the type of amyloid. In a series of 47 hearts from 21 patients with primary amyloidosis and 26 patients with senile amyloidosis, Smith et al. found that primary amyloid was associated with extensive infiltrates and a high frequency of interstitial and vascular amyloid. In contrast, senile amyloid was associated with less extensive infiltrates, which correlate with overall fewer cardiac symptoms, and a high incidence of nodular deposits.[293] Similar findings have been reported in endomyocardial biopsies from patients with cardiac amyloidosis,[261] although in the latter the interstitial pattern was seen in equal frequency in both groups. The presence of nodular deposits, thick perimyocytic layers of amyloid, and small myocyte diameters have been associated with shorter survival.[294]

The role of endomyocardial biopsy in the diagnosis of cardiac amyloidosis includes establishing the diagnosis, characterizing of the immunohistochemical protein, and assessing myocyte damage.[294] Periumbilical fat biopsy may also be helpful in establishing a diagnosis of

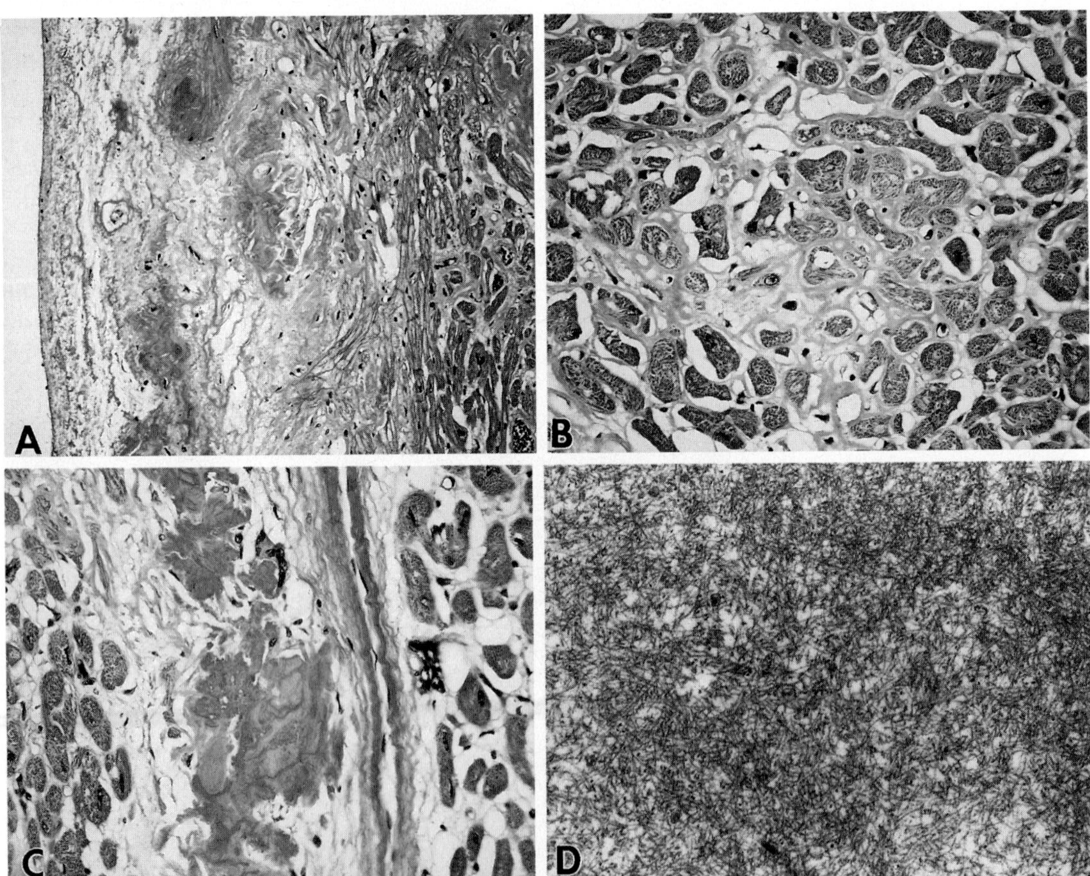

Figure 6–22. Amyloidosis. Histologic patterns of cardiac amyloidosis include subendocardial (*A*), perimyocytic (*B*), nodular (*C*), and vascular (not shown). There may be a macrophage reaction to the amyloid (*C*). Ultrastructurally, there are nonbranching 10-nm filaments within the interstitium (*D*).

amyloid without the need for a more invasive procedure.

Immunohistochemical techniques are helpful in the diagnosis of amyloid and in differentiating between the subtypes of amyloid.[294] Antibodies against serum amyloid P will react with all forms of amyloid, and antibodies against amyloid AA protein, kappa and lambda light chains, and transthyretin have been applied to frozen and paraffin-embedded tissues.[261, 267] Frozen tissues or immunogold labeling of electron microscopic samples are preferred for diagnosis, because paraffin-embedded tissues often result in nonspecific or absent staining.

In senile systemic amyloidosis, there is typically small arterial involvement in the lungs, liver, and kidneys.[295] Primary amyloidosis virtually always affects viscera, and there is a high frequency of splenic involvement in secondary amyloidosis. The distribution of amyloidosis in familial amyloidosis is similar to primary amyloidosis, with subcutaneous fat and rectal biopsy positivity in 75% of cases.[273]

MISCELLANEOUS INFANTILE AND HEREDITARY CARDIOMYOPATHIES

Overview of Genetic Cardiomyopathies in Infants and Children

Clinical Approach

The diagnosis of cardiomyopathy in infants and children is a multifaceted task involving genetics, biochemical testing, and neuromuscular evaluation. Genetic conditions associated with cardiomyopathy can be classified into overlapping categories: inborn errors of metabolism, neuromuscular disorders, and isolated genetic cardiomyopathies.[296] Only isolated cardiomyopathies will be discussed in any detail in this chapter.

Inborn Errors of Metabolism

Storage diseases result from disorders of glycogen metabolism, mucopolysaccharide degradation, glycosphingolipid degradation (Fabry's disease), glucosylceramide degradation (Gaucher's disease), oxalic acid metabolism (oxalosis), or ganglioside degradation. Cardiac involvement may occur in all of these conditions,[296] and is generally considered secondary.

Disorders of energy metabolism that may result in cardiomyopathy include defects of pyruvate metabolism and disorders of oxidative phosphorylation. In the latter group, Barth syndrome and mitochondrial cardiomyopathies are specific entities that may result in morphologic alterations of the mitochondria. Histiocytoid cardiomyopathy is occasionally considered an inborn error of metabolism[296] because of an association with a deficiency of complex III in the mitochondrial electron transport chain.[297] Cardiac phosphorylase kinase deficiency is a rare metabolic defect that results in isolated cardiomyopathy with an autosomal recessive inheritance.[298, 299]

Barth Syndrome

Barth syndrome is an X-linked skeletal and cardiac myopathy in infants and children that is related to a genetic defect in locus Xq28 resulting in mitochondrial respiratory chain dysfunction. Type II X-linked 3-methylglutaconic aciduria is a related condition[300] that is sometimes considered synonymous with Barth syndrome.[296]

In addition to myopathy, affected boys have short stature, neutropenia, and ultrastructural mitochondrial abnormalities.[301, 302] In some families the primary disease is a lethal dilated cardiomyopathy affecting male infants who do not have skeletal myopathy or neutropenia.[78] Carnitine levels in Barth syndrome may be low, but the metabolic abnormalities are believed to be epiphenomena, the primary defect lying in mitochondrial electron transport.[302]

The pathologic features of Barth syndrome include dilated cardiomyopathy, left ventricular hypertrophy, and endocardial fibroelastosis. Ultrastructural abnormalities of mitochondria are found, including abnormal mitochondrial crystal condensations and paracrystalline inclusions.[303–305]

Cardiomyopathies with Mitochondrial Inheritance

Mutations of the mitochondrial genome may cause defective mitochondrial respiration and cardiac dysfunction.[306] The mitochondrial electron transport chain is composed of five complexes: complex I, NADH-ubiquinone oxidoreductase; complex II, succinate-ubiquinone oxidoreductase; complex III, ubiquinone-cytochrome c oxidoreductase; complex IV, cytochrome oxidase; and complex V, ATPase. Mitochondrial DNA codes for a subset of proteins forming complexes I, III, IV, and V, and the remainder of the proteins are encoded in nuclear DNA. Mitochondrial genes that have been associated with cardiomyopathy include those that code for transport chain complexes as well as those that code for mitochondrial ribosomal RNAs, organelle-specific transfer RNAs, and genes regulating transcription and replication.

Mutations in mitochondrial DNA occur at a rate many times higher than that of nuclear DNA. In many patients with mitochondrial cardiomyopathy, the mutations are acquired, resulting in sporadic disease, and in the remainder of patients the disease is inherited maternally. Multiple mutations, often combined deficiencies of complex I and IV, are typically found in these patients.

Isolated Mitochondrial Cardiomyopathy

In adults, mitochondrial cardiomyopathy may resemble hypertrophic cardiomyopathy, dilated cardiomyopathy, or the failing heart may be normal in size.[306] The mean age at presentation is in the third decade, and there appears to be a male predominance.[306] Families with isolated mitochondrial cardiomyopathy have been reported worldwide.[306] There is very little information regarding the pathology of adult mitochondrial cardiomyopathy, although expanded mitochondria with inclusions and glycogen granules have been described.[306]

Infantile forms of mitochondrial cardiomyopathy without clinical muscle disease have been reported. The infants have dilated ventricles with diastolic dysfunction[307] but pathologic data is lacking. Infants with "hypertrophic cardiomyopathy" have been shown to have abnormal cytochrome oxidase levels in frozen samples of endomyocardial biopsies, suggesting a mitochondrial disorder.[308]

A 3-year-old boy with cardiac failure and massive left ventricular hypertrophy and lipid deposits within the myocardium has been described.[309] Ultrastructurally, lipid was associated with mitochondria. The authors speculate that the disease in this child may represent a form of mitochondrial cardiomyopathy.

MELAS (mitochondrial myopathy, encephalopathy, lactic acidosis, and stroke-like episodes) and Other Multiorgan Mitochondrial Diseases

Mitochondrial cardiomyopathy is more often part of a multisystem disease than an isolated condition. Patients with MELAS suffer from muscle weakness, recurrent episodic vomiting, headache, and stroke-like episodes; the mitochondrial mutation is characteristically at position 3243 in the tRNA Leu gene.[310] Cardiomyopathy, which may be clinically classified as hypertrophic cardiomyopathy or dilated cardiomyopathy,[311] is frequently observed with onset in the second and third decades, but may occur in infancy.[312] Cardiac evaluation demonstrates early cardiac failure with hypoperfusion in dipyridamole stress scintigraphy suggestive of small vessel angiopathy.[313]

Histologic studies of myocardium demonstrate interstitial fibrosis and myocardial cell vacuolization. Ragged red fibers, which are perinuclear deposits that stain red-purple on Masson trichrome, are occasionally identified in cardiac myocytes, and appear similar to those seen in skeletal muscle.[313] Ultrastructural examination of myocytes mirror those of skeletal muscle, and reveal increased numbers and size of mitochondria, concentric configuration of cristae, decreased myofibrils, and swollen endothelial cells[313] (Fig. 6–23). In general, the ultrastructural findings in mitochondrial disorders include large aggregates of abnormal mitochondria, usually under the sarcolemma, with parallel or concentric lamellae with crystalline inclusions or globular bodies.[314]

Other mitochondrial respiratory chain disorders, such as myoclonic epilepsy with ragged red fibers (MERRF)[315] and Kearns–Sayre syndrome may occasionally present with cardiomyopathy. There are reports of infants and adults with mitochondrial cardiomyopathies and skeletal muscle disease who do not fit neatly into one of the mitochondrial syndromes.[314, 316–318] In general, the infantile forms are not associated with endocardial fibrosis.[318] On occasion, ventricular tachycardia is the presenting symptom in such patients.[319]

Neuromuscular Disorders

Neuromuscular disorders associated with cardiomyopathy include the muscular dystrophies, centronuclear myopathy, nemaline rod myopathy, Friedreich's ataxia, and Refsum disease.[296] There is an overlap among X-linked dilated cardiomyopathy, dystrophin abnormalities, and muscular dystrophy (see earlier).[82, 320]

Isolated Inherited Cardiomyopathies

The major types of inherited cardiomyopathy that are not usually accompanied by extracar-

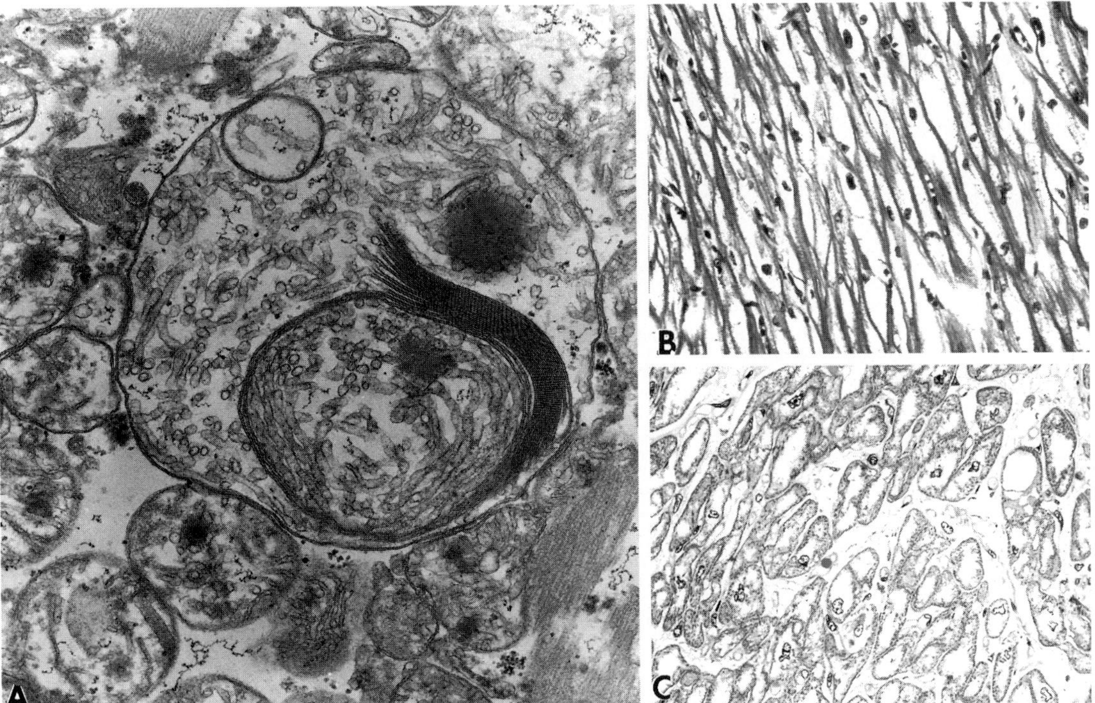

Figure 6–23. Mitochondrial disease. *A.* Morphologic ultrastructural abnormalities of mitochondrial disease include abnormal whorls of cristae and intramyocardial inclusions. *B.* The light microscopic features are nonspecific and there is vacuolization secondary to increased mitochondria. *C.* A plastic section (Toluidine blue) demonstrates vacuolization.

diac involvement are hypertrophic cardiomyopathy, dilated cardiomyopathy, restrictive cardiomyopathy, arrhythmogenic right ventricular dysplasia, and mitochondrial cardiomyopathy. The incidence of familial involvement and genetic bases for hereditary forms of these diseases have been discussed earlier. A list of inherited cardiomyopathies is provided in Table 6–9.

Perimortem Evaluation

Because of the numerous entities and syndromes that may manifest as cardiomyopathy in infants, it is recommended that a variety of specimens be collected and tests performed at autopsy or perimortem evaluation in a patient without a specific premortem diagnosis.[296] Blood should be studied for electrolytes, glucose, renal function tests, lactate and pyruvate, ammonia, creatinine kinase, cholesterol and triglyceride, transaminases, acylcarnitines, carnitine, quantitative amino acids, and chromosome analysis (if the patient is dysmorphic). Urine or vitreous should be sampled for ketones, organic acids (including 3-methylglutaconic acids for males), quantitative amino acids, acylglycines, mucopolysaccharides, and oligosaccharides. A skeletal X-ray survey and gross photographs should be taken, as well as frozen tissue from heart, skeletal muscle, liver, kidney, brain, and skin. Tissue should be preserved for ultrastructural examination in addition to routine histology.

Endocardial Fibroelastosis (Infantile Dilated Cardiomyopathy)

Idiopathic endocardial fibroelastosis is a descriptive term embracing a heterogeneous group of disorders resulting in infantile dilated cardiomyopathy. Ventricular dilatation in the very young results in a greater degree of endocardial fibrosis than that which is seen in adults with dilated cardiomyopathy.

The underlying causes for endocardial fibroelastosis, which is an end-stage condition, include viral infection and Barth syndrome.[303] Most cases are idiopathic. It has been argued that it should not be considered a specific entity.[321]

The clinical definition of endocardial fibroelastosis requires the onset of congestive heart failure before age 2, voltage criteria for left ven-

Table 6–9. Inherited Forms of Isolated Cardiomyopathy

Morphologic Type	Inheritance	Gene Product	Chromosome
Hypertrophic	Autosomal dominant	Cardiac myosin β heavy chain Troponin T α tropomyosin	14q11-q12 1q3 15q2
	Autosomal recessive (rare)	Unknown	
Dilated	Autosomal dominant	Unknown	
	X-linked	Dystrophin Mitochondrial transport chain (?)[1]	Xp21 Xq28
	Autosomal recessive	Unknown	
Right ventricular	Autosomal dominant	Unknown	14q23-q24, 1q42-q43 14q12-q22
Mixed[2]	Maternal	Mitochondrial tRNA	Mitochondrial
Ventricular noncompaction	Probable autosomal dominant	Unknown	Unknown

[1] Barth syndrome; almost always associated with skeletal disease and neutropenia.
[2] Usually associated with skeletal disease and encephalopathy.

tricular hypertrophy, dilated and poorly contractile left ventricle by echocardiography or angiography, and the exclusion of structural abnormalities.[322] The mean age at onset is 7 months, and there may be female predisposition.[322]

At autopsy, the heart is globular and enlarged, and the endocardium of the left ventricle is opaque, resembling porcelain (Fig. 6–24). The trabeculae are flattened and the papillary muscles are often incorporated into the fibrotic process.

Histologically, the endocardium is thickened by collagen deposition and duplication of elastic fibers. The myocardium is generally unremarkable, although there may be foci of inflammation suggesting a remote myocarditis.[323]

In a follow-up study of infants with endocardial fibrosis, 77% of patients were alive at 4 years,[322] although a more recent study suggests a mortality closer to 50%.[324] Poor prognostic indicators are low ejection fraction and cardiac index at the time of diagnosis, marked endocardial fibroelastosis, need for anticoagulation reflective of severe left ventricular function, and right ventricular dysfunction.

The major differential diagnosis at autopsy is an anomalous left main coronary artery arising from the pulmonary trunk. In this condition, the heart is typically globoid and dilated, and

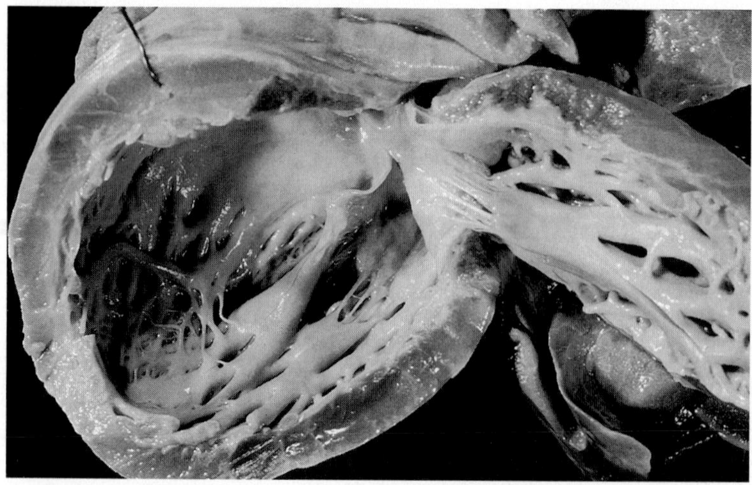

Figure 6–24. Endocardial fibroelastosis. A 6-month-old infant had a short history of poor feeding and lethargy. One morning before seeking medical attention for the child, the mother found her dead. At autopsy, there was ventricular dilatation, primarily of the left ventricle, with a "porcelain" appearance to the thickened left ventricular endocardium.

endocardial fibrosis is often striking. Other structural anomalies such as congenital mitral valve defects should also be excluded before making the diagnosis of endocardial fibroelastosis at autopsy.

Infantile Hypertrophic Cardiomyopathy

Like endocardial fibroelastosis, infantile cardiac hypertrophy is a heterogeneous disorder that includes mitochondrial cardiomyopathy,[308] Barth syndrome,[303] Noonan syndrome,[325, 326] and infants of diabetic mothers.[327, 328] It has recently been emphasized that the molecular abnormalities of infantile hypertrophic cardiomyopathy differ widely from those seen in adults with hypertrophic cardiomyopathy.[329] In almost all cases of diabetes-associated hypertrophic cardiomyopathy, cardiac enlargement regresses within the first month of life, regardless of therapy, and cardiac function returns to normal.[11]

In some infants with hypertrophic cardiomyopathy, the disease is likely a form of the adult disease, with asymmetric hypertrophy documented echocardiographically in first-degree family members.[330] Specific mutations of the beta myosin heavy chain gene are associated with expression of the disease early in childhood.[331] In contrast to the adult form, right ventricular outflow tract obstruction is common, and occasionally as great as that on the left side. Asymmetric hypertrophy with outflow tract obstruction may occur before 6 months of age, suggesting a congenital malformation. The initial presentation is often a systolic murmur, bradycardia, cyanosis, or heart failure. Earlier studies have emphasized that prognosis is poor, especially if there is congestive heart failure.[330] Prognosis has improved significantly with the use of beta blockade[332]; poor prognostic variables include increasing posterior left ventricular thickness and an underlying metabolic defect or Noonan's syndrome.[326] Grossly, the heart is enlarged, with a mean septal thickness of 16 mm.[325] Histologically, myofiber disarray occurs in $> 5\%$ of the ventricular septum. A septum-free wall ratio of ≥ 1.3 is common in neonates and not specific for the diagnosis, and histologic confirmation is mandatory.

Desmin Cardiomyopathy

Desmin is an intermediate filament that is integral to the structure of striated muscle cells. It is normally localized at the Z lines, in the interfibrillar space between adjacent Z bands, and close to the intercalated disc.[38] An increase in disordered desmin has been described in hypertrophied hearts[333] and in those with dilated[38] and hypertrophic cardiomyopathy.[145]

A rare cardiomyopathy with excessive accumulation and disorganization of desmin microfilaments has been described in families.[334, 335] The disease has since been termed desmin cardiomyopathy or desminopathy.[336–338] It is characterized by progressive congestive heart failure, occurring usually in the second and third decades of life; males and females may be affected. At initial presentation, the clinical diagnosis is often that of idiopathic restricitve cardiomyopathy, often with atrioventricular block.[223] Light microscopic features are nonspecific, but ultrastructurally there are degenerative alterations characterized by the accumulation of granular-disordered filaments that stain positive for desmin by immunolabeling. Skeletal myopathy often accompanies the cardiomyopathy,[337, 338] and PAS-positive intracytoplasmic inclusions containing phosphorylated desmin may be seen in skeletal muscle.[337] Abnormal collections of intermediate filaments have also been described in intestinal smooth muscle cells and the spinal cord in desmin myopathy.[336] An association with mental retardation has been reported.[339]

Noncompaction of the Myocardium

Definition

Noncompaction of the myocardium[340] denotes the persistence of the trabecular network of sponge-like muscle characteristic of early fetal life, when myocardial blood is supplied by diffusion from the intertrabecular spaces that communicate with the heart chambers. Coronary vessels develop only during the second embryonal month. Their growth is associated with the disappearance of "sinusoids" and the transformation of the spongy myocardium into compact musculature. Other terms for persistent noncompacted myocardium include "spongy myocardium"[341] and "persistence of myocardial sinusoids."[342] The latter designation has been criticized because the intramyocardial vessels communicate with the cardiac chambers and, as such, are invaginations rather than sinusoids.[340]

Associations

Persistence of noncompacted myocardium may be associated with structural heart defects or be isolated. Associated conditions include coronary artery anomalies (anomalous origin of the left main coronary artery from the pulmonary trunk and coronary ventricular fistulae) and conotruncal anomalies (absent pulmonary valve, pulmonary atresia, tricuspid atresia, and transposition of the great arteries).[340, 341, 343] Syndromes associated with noncompaction of the ventricles include Barth syndrome, which may be genetically related,[344] and Melnick–Needles syndrome.[345]

Clinical Features

Isolated persistence of noncompacted myocardium is rare.[340, 346] The age range at presentation is 1 week to 23 years (mean 9 years). As the echocardiographic features of the disease have been better described, more adult patients with isolated noncompaction of the ventricles have been described.[347, 348] Clinical presentations include systolic ventricular dysfunction, restrictive cardiomyopathy, ventricular arrhythmias, and systemic embolism; the disease may also be detected incidentally. The echocardiographic findings consist of a prominent apical trabecular meshwork with deep intertrabecular recesses in the left ventricle. The syndrome is familial in 44% of patients,[346] in whom facial dysmorphism may be prominent. Many patients die suddenly from presumed tachyarrhythmias or cerebral emboli.[340, 341] Ventricular pacing, calcium channel blockers, and quinidine may suppress arrhythmias. Patients with ventricular noncompaction have been successfully treated with heart transplantation.[348]

Pathologic Features

The gross pathologic findings consist of numerous, prominent trabeculations and deep intertrabecular recesses of the left ventricular apex.[340, 341] The involved myocardium is mottled and spongy, and there may be sparing of the base of the heart, which is compact. Histologically, there are interanastomosing channels within the myocardium that are lined by endothelial cells. The channels communicate with the ventricular cavity and trabecular arteries may communicate with the sinusoidal channels.[341] The intervening myocardium has prominent elastic tissue,[341] lacks the normal cardiac structure, and has been likened to the organization of hepatocytes forming single layers surrounding sinuses.[340, 341]

REFERENCES

1. Richardson P, McKenna W, Bristow M, Maisch B, Mautner B, O'Connell J, Olsen E, Thiene G, Goodwin J, Gyarfas I, Martin K, Nordet P. Report of the 1995 World Health Organization/International Society and Federation of Cardiology Task Force on the definition and classification of cardiomyopathies. Circulation 93:841–842, 1996.
2. Waller BF. Pathology of the cardiomyopathies. J Am Soc Echocardiogr 1:4–19, 1988.
3. Dec G, Fuster V. Idiopathic dilated cardiomyopathy. N Engl J Med 331:1564–1575, 1994.
4. Felker GM, Hu W, Hare JM, Hruban RH, Baughman KL, Kasper EK. The spectrum of dilated cardiomyopathy. The Johns Hopkins experience with 1,278 patients. Medicine (Baltimore) 78:270–283, 1999.
5. Kasper EK, Agema WR, Hutchins GM, Deckers JW, Hare JM, Baughman KL. The causes of dilated cardiomyopathy: A clinicopathologic review of 673 consecutive patients. J Am Coll Cardiol 23:586–590, 1994.
6. Codd MB, Sugrue DD, Gersh BJ, Melton LJD. Epidemiology of idiopathic dilated and hypertrophic cardiomyopathy. A population-based study in Olmsted County, Minnesota, 1975–1984. Circulation 80:564–572, 1989.
7. Gillum RF. Idiopathic cardiomyopathy in the United States. 1970–1982. Am Heart J 111, 1986.
8. Roberts WC, Siegel RJ, McManus BM. Idiopathic dilated cardiomyopathy: Analysis of 152 necropsy patients. Am J Cardiol 60:1340–1355, 1987.
9. Coughlin SS, Szklo M, Baughman K, Pearson TA. The epidemiology of idiopathic dilated cardiomyopathy in a biracial community. Am J Epidemiol 131:48–56, 1990.
10. Manolio TA, Baughman KL, Rodeheffer R, Pearson TA, Bristow JD, Michels VV, Abelmann WH, Harlan WR. Prevalence and etiology of idiopathic dilated cardiomyopathy. Am J Cardiol 69:1458–1466, 1992.
11. Edwards WD. Cardiomyopathies. In: Virmani R, Atkinson JB, Fenoglio JJ (eds): Cardiovascular Pathology. Philadelphia: WB Saunders, 1991.
12. Gavazzi A, DeMaria R, Renosto G. The spectrum of left ventricular size in dilated cardiomyopathy: Clinical correlates and prognostic implications. Am Heart J 125:410–422, 1993.
13. Treasure CB, Vita JA, Cox DA, Fish RD, Gordon JB, Mudge GH, Coluci WS, Sutton MG, Selwyn AP, Alexander RW. Endothelium-dependent dilation of the coronary microvasculature is impaired in dilated cardiomyopathy. Circulation 81:772–779, 1990.
14. Opherk D, Schwarz F, Mall G, Manthey J, Baller D, Kubler W. Coronary dilatory capacity in idiopathic dilated cardiomyopathy: Analysis of 16 patients. Am J Cardiol 51:1657–1662, 1983.
15. Milechman G, Scheinman MM. Ventricular dysrhythmias and sudden death in dilated cardiomyopathy. In Zipes DP, Rowlands DJ (eds): Progress in Cardiology, pp 85–94. Philadelphia: Lea and Febiger, 1989.
16. La Vecchia L, Paccanaro M, Bonanno C, Varotto L, Ometto R, Vincenzi M. Left ventricular versus biventricular dysfunction in idiopathic dilated cardiomyopathy. Am J Cardiol 83:120–122, 1999.
17. Fauchier L, Babuty D, Cosnay P, Fauchier JP. Prognostic value of heart rate variability for sudden death and major arrhythmic events in patients with idiopathic

dilated cardiomyopathy. J Am Coll Cardiol 33:1203–1207, 1999.
18. Roberts WC, Ferrans VJ. Pathologic anatomy of the cardiomyopathies. Idiopathic dilated and hypertrophic types, infiltrative types, and endomyocardial disease with and without eosinophilia. Hum Pathol 6:287–342, 1975.
19. Keren A, Billingham ME, Weintraub D, Sintson EB, Popp RL. Mildly dilated congestive cardiomyopathy. Circulation 72:302–309, 1985.
20. Rose AG, Beck W. Dilated (congestive) cardiomyopathy: A syndrome of severe cardiac dysfunction with remarkably few morphological features of myocardial damage. Histopathology 9:367–379, 1985.
21. Edwards WD. Cardiomyopathies. Hum Pathol 18:625–637, 1987.
22. Waller TA, Hiser WL, Capehart JE, Roberts WC. Comparison of clinical and morphologic cardiac findings in patients having cardiac transplantation for ischemic cardiomyopathy, idiopathic dilated cardiomyopathy, and dilated hypertrophic cardiomyopathy. Am J Cardiol 81:884–894, 1998.
23. Isner JM, Virmani R, Itscoitz SB, Roberts WC. Clinical pathologic conference. Left and right ventricular myocardial infarction in idiopathic dilated cardiomyopathy. Am Heart J 99:235–242, 1980.
24. Atkinson JB, Virmani R. Congestive heart failure due to coronary artery disease without myocardial infarction: Clinicopathologic description of an unusual cardiomyopathy. Hum Pathol 20:1155–1162, 1989.
25. Ferrans VJ. Pathologic anatomy of the dilated cardiomyopathies. Am J Cardiol 64:9C–11C, 1989.
26. Davies MJ, McKenna WJ. Dilated cardiomyopathy: An introduction to pathology and pathogenesis. Br Heart J 72:S24, 1994.
27. Unverferth DV, Baker PB, Swift SE, Chaffee R, Fetters JK, Uretsky BF, Thompson ME, Leier CV. Extent of myocardial fibrosis and cellular hypertrophy in dilated cardiomyopathy. Am J Cardiol 57:816–820, 1986.
28. Pelliccia F, d'Amati G, Cianfrocca C, Bernucci P, Nigri A, Marino B, Gallo P. Histomorphometric features predict 1-year outcome of patients with idiopathic dilated cardiomyopathy considered to be at low priority for cardiac transplantation. Am Heart J 128:316–325, 1994.
29. Chopra P, Misra A, Talwar KK. Prognostic significance of pathological parameters of endomyocardial biopsy in clinical outcome of patients with dilated cardiomyopathy—I. Quantitative morphometric analysis. Indian Heart J 43:415–420, 1991.
30. Schwarz F, Mall G, Zebe H, Blickle J, Derks H, Manthey J, Kubler W. Quantitative morphologic findings of the myocardium in idiopathic dilated cardiomyopathy. Am J Cardiol 51:501–506, 1983.
31. Anderson DW, Virmani R, Reilly JM, O'Leary T, Cunnion RE, Robinowitz M, Macher AM, Punja U, Villaflor ST, Parrillo JE, Roberts C. Prevalent myocarditis at necropsy in the acquired immunodeficiency syndrome. J Am Coll Cardiol 11:792–799, 1988.
32. Tazelaar HD, Billingham ME. Leukocytic-infiltrates in idiopathic dilated cardiomyopathy. Am J Surg Pathol 10:405–412, 1986.
33. Latham RD, Mulrow JP, Virmani R, Robinowitz M, Moody JM. Recently diagnosed idiopathic dilated cardiomyopathy: Incidence of myocarditis and efficacy of prednisone therapy. Am Heart J 117:876–882, 1989.
34. Pauschinger M, Knopf D, Petschauer S, Doerner A, Poller W, Schwimmbeck PL, Kuhl U, Schulthesis HP. Dilated cardiomyopathy is associated with significant changes in collagen type I/III ratio. Circulation 99:2750–2756, 1999.
35. Tanganelli P, Pierli C, Bravi A, Del Sordo M, Salvi A, Bussani R, Silvestri F, Camerini F. Small vessel disease (SVD) in patients with unexplained ventricular arrhythmia and dilated congestive cardiomyopathy. Am J Cardiovasc Pathol 3:13–19, 1990.
36. Ohtani K, Yutani C, Nagata S, Koretsune Y, Hori M, Kamada T. High prevalence of atrial fibrosis in patients with dilated cardiomyopathy. J Am Coll Cardiol 25:1162–1169, 1995.
37. Triposkiadis F, Pitsavos C, Boudoulas H, Trikas A, Toutouzas P. Left atrial myopathy in idiopathic dilated cardiomyopathy. Am Heart J 128:308–315, 1994.
38. Schaper J, Froede R, Hein S, Buck A, Hashizume H, Speiser B, Friedl A, Bleese N. Impairment of the myocardial ultrastructure and changes of the cytoskeleton in dilated cardiomyopathy. Circulation 83:504–514, 1991.
39. Unverferth BJ, Leier CV, Magorien RD, Unverferth DV. Differentiating characteristics of myocardial nuclei in cardiomyopathy. Hum Pathol 14:974–983, 1983.
40. Rowan RA, Masek MA, Billingham ME. Ultrastructural morphometric analysis of endomyocardial biopsies. Idiopathic dilated cardiomyopathy, anthracycline cardiotoxicity, and normal myocardium. Am J Cardiovasc Pathol 2:137–144, 1988.
41. Keren A, Billingham ME, Popp RL. Features of mildly dilated congestive cardiomyopathy compared with idiopathic restrictive cardiomyopathy and typical dilated cardiomyopathy. J Am Soc Echocardiogr 1:78–87, 1988.
42. Hartz AJ, Anderson AJ, Brooks HJ. The association of smoking and cardiomyopathy. N Engl J Med 311:1201, 1984.
43. Virmani R, Atkinson JB. Endomyocardial biopsy in the diagnosis of heart diseases. In: Virmani R, Atkinson JB, Fenoglio JJ, Jr. (eds): Cardiovascular Pathology. Vol. 23, pp 220–245. Philadelphia: WB Saunders, 1991.
44. Keeling PJ, Tracy S. Link between enteroviruses and dilated cardiomyopathy: Serological and molecular data. Br Heart J 72:S25–S29, 1994.
45. Muir P, Nicholson F, Tilzey AJ, Signy M, English TA, Banatvala JE. Chronic relapsing pericarditis and dilated cardiomyopathy: Serological evidence of persistent enterovirus infection. Lancet i:804–807, 1989.
46. Wiegand V, Tracy S, Chapman N, Wucherpfennig C. Enteroviral infection in end stage dilated cardiomyopathy. Klin Wochenschr 68:914–920, 1990.
47. Archard LC, Bowles NE, Cunningham L. Molecular probes for detection of persisting enterovirus infection of human heart and their prognostic value. Eur Heart J 12:56–59, 1991.
48. Easton AJ, Eglin RP. The detection of Coxsackievirus RNA in cardiac tissue by *in situ* hybridization. J Gen Virol 69:285–291, 1988.
49. Giacca M, Severini GM, Mestroni L, Salvi A, Lardieri G, Falaschi A, Camerini F. Low frequency of detection by nested polymerase chain reaction of enterovirus ribonucleic acid in endomyocardial tissue of patients with idiopathic dilated cardiomyopathy. J Am Coll Cardiol 24:1033–1140, 1994.
50. Archard LC, Khan MA, Soteriou BA, Zhang H, Why HJ, Robinson NM, Richardson PJ. Characterization of Coxsackie B virus RNA in myocardium from patients

with dilated cardiomyopathy by nucleotide sequencing of reverse transcription-nested polymerase chain reaction products. Hum Pathol 29:578–584, 1998.

51. Quigley PJ, Richardson PJ, Meany DT. Long term follow-up in biopsy proven myocarditis: Progression to dilated cardiomyopathy. Circulation 74(Suppl II): 142, 1986.
52. Luppi P, Rudert WA, Zanone MM, Stassi G, Trucco G, Finegold D, Boyle GJ, Del Nido P, McGowan FX Jr., Trucco M. Idiopathic dilated cardiomyopathy: A superantigen-driven autoimmune disease. Circulation 98:777–785, 1998.
53. Caforio AL. Role of autoimmunity in dilated cardiomyopathy. Br Heart J 72:S30–S34, 1994.
54. Coughlin SS, Szklo M, Baughman K, Pearson TA. Idiopathic dilated cardiomyopathy and atopic disease: Epidemiologic evidence for an association with asthma. Am Heart J 118:768–774, 1989.
55. Caforio AL, Bonifacio E, Stewart JT, Neglia D, Parodi O, Bottazzo GF, McKenna WJ. Novel organ-specific circulating cardiac autoantibodies in dilated cardiomyopathy. J Am Coll Cardiol 15:1527–1534, 1990.
56. Caforio AL, Keeling PJ, Zachara E, Mestroni L, Camerini F, Mann JM, Bottazzo GF, McKenna WJ. Evidence from family studies for autoimmunity in dilated cardiomyopathy. Lancet 344:773–777, 1994.
57. Limas CJ, Goldenberg IF, Limas C. Autoantibodies against beta-adrenoceptors in human idiopathic dilated cardiomyopathy. Circ Res 64:97–103, 1989.
58. Ansari AA, Wang YC, Danner DJ, Gravanis MB, Mayne A, Neckelmann N, Sell KW, Herskowitz A. Abnormal expression of histocompatibility and mitochondrial antigens by cardiac tissue from patients with myocarditis and dilated cardiomyopathy. Am J Pathol 139:337–354, 1991.
59. Francis SE, Holden H, Holt CM, Duff GW. Interleukin-1 in myocardium and coronary arteries of patients with dilated cardiomyopathy. J Mol Cell Cardiol 30:215–223, 1998.
60. Noutsias M, Seeberg B, Schultheiss HP, Kuhl U. Expression of cell adhesion molecules in dilated cardiomyopathy: Evidence for endothelial activation in inflammatory cardiomyopathy. Circulation 99:2124–2131, 1999.
61. Narula J, Haider N, Virmani R, DiSalvo TG, Kolodgie FD, Hajjar RJ, Schmidt U, Semigran MJ, Dec GW, Khaw BA. Apoptosis in myocytes in end-stage heart failure. N Engl J Med 335:1182–1189, 1996.
62. Kanoh M, Takemura G, Misao J, Hayakawa Y, Aoyama T, Nishigki K, Noda T, Fujiwara T, Fukuda K, Minatoguchi S, Fujiwara H. Significance of myocytes with positive DNA in situ nick end-labeling (TUNEL) in hearts with dilated cardiomyopathy: Not apoptosis but DNA repair. Circulation 99:2757–2764, 1999.
63. Urbano-Marquez A, Estruch R, Navarro-Lopez F, Grau JM, Mont L, Rubin E. The effects of alcoholism on skeletal and cardiac muscle. N Engl J Med 320:409–415, 1989.
64. Wynne J, Braunwald E. The cardiomyopathies and myocarditides: Toxic, chemical, and physical damage to the heart. In: Braunwald E (ed): Heart Disease. Philadelphia: WB Saunders, 1992.
65. McKenna CJ, Codd MB, McCann HA, Sugrue DD. Alcohol consumption and idiopathic dilated cardiomyopathy: A case control study. Am Heart J 135:833–837, 1998.
66. Rubin E, Urbano-Marquez A. Alcoholic cardiomyopathy. Alcohol Clin Exp Res 18:111–114, 1994.
67. Hibbs RG, Ferrans VJ, Black WC, Weilbaecher DG, Walsh JJ, Burch GE. Alcoholic cardiomyopathy. An electron microscopic study. Am Heart J 69:766–779, 1963.
68. Mestroni L, Miani D, Di Lenarda A, Silvestri F, Bussani R, Filippi G, Camerini F. Clinical and pathologic study of familial dilated cardiomyopathy. Am J Cardiol 65:1449–1453, 1990.
69. Michels VV, Moll PP, Miller FA, Tajik AJ, Chu JS, Driscoll DJ, Burnett JC, Rodeheffer RJ, Chesebro JK, Tazelaar HD. The frequency of familial dilated cardiomyopathy in a series of patients with idiopathic dilated cardiomyopathy. N Engl J Med 326:77–82, 1992.
70. Mestroni L, Krajinovic M, Severini GM, Pinamonti B, DiLenarda A, Giacca M, Falaschi A, Camerini F. Familial dilated cardiomyopathy. Br Heart J 72:S35–S41, 1994.
71. McKenna CJ, Sugrue DD, Kwon HM, Sangiorgi G, Carlson PJ, Mahon N, McCann HA, Edwards WD, Holmes DR, Jr., Schwartz RS. Histopathologic changes in asymptomatic relatives of patients with idiopathic dilated cardiomyopathy. Am J Cardiol 83:281–283, A6, 1999.
72. Baig MK, Goldman JH, Caforio AL, Coonar AS, Keeling PJ, McKenna WJ. Familial dilated cardiomyopathy: Cardiac abnormalities are common in asymptomatic relatives and may represent early disease. J Am Coll Cardiol 31:195–201, 1998.
73. Keeling PJ, McKenna WJ. Clinical genetics of dilated cardiomyopathy. Herz 19:91–96, 1994.
74. Mestroni L, Rocco C, Gregori D, Sinagra G, Di Lenarda A, Miocic S, Vatta M, Pinamonti B, Muntoni F, Caforio AL, McKenna WJ, Falaschi A, Giacca M, Camerini. Familial dilated cardiomyopathy: Evidence for genetic and phenotypic heterogeneity. Heart Muscle Disease Study Group. J Am Coll Cardiol 34:181–190, 1999.
75. Brodsky GL, Muntoni F, Miocic S, Sinagra G, Sewry C, Mestroni L. Lamin A/C gene mutation associated with dilated cardiomyopathy with variable skeletal muscle involvement. Circulation 101:473–476, 2000.
76. Olson TM, Michels W, Thibodeau SN, Tai YS, Keating MT. Actin mutations in dilated cardiomyopathy, a heritable form of heart failure. Science 280:750–752, 1998.
77. Siu BL, Niimura H, Osborne JA, Fatkin D, MacRae C, Solomon S, Benson DW, Seidman JG, Seidman CE. Familial dilated cardiomyopathy locus maps to chromosome 2q3l. Circulation 99:1022–1026, 1999.
78. Gedeon AK, Wilson MJ, Colley AC, Sillence DO, Mulley JC. X linked fatal infantile cardiomyopathy maps to Xq28 and is possibly allelic to Barth syndrome. J Med Genet 32:383–338, 1995.
79. Franz WM, Cremer M, Herrmann R, Grunig E, Fogel W, Scheffold T, Goebel HH, Kircheisen R, Kubler W, Voit T, et al. X-inked dilated cardiomyopathy. Novel mutation of the dystrophin gene. Ann N Y Acad Sci 752:470–491, 1995.
80. Oldfors A, Eriksson BO, Kyllerman M, Martinsson T, Wahlstrom J. Dilated cardiomyopathy and dystrophin gene: An illustrated review. Br Heart J 72:344–348, 1994.
81. Mestroni L, Krajinovic M, Severini GM, Falaschi A, Giacca M, Camerini F. Molecular genetics of dilated cardiomyopathy. Herz 19:97–104, 1994.
82. Towbin JA, Hejtmancik JF, Brink P, Gelb B, Zhu XM, Chamberlain JS, McCabe ER, Swift M. X-linked dilated cardiomyopathy. Molecular genetic evidence of link-

age to the Duchenne muscular dystrophy (dystrophin) gene at the Xp21 locus. Circulation 87:1854–1865, 1993.

83. Muntoni F, Wilson L, Marrosu G, Marrosu MG, Cianchetti C, Mestroni L, Ganau A, Dubowitz V, Sewry C. A mutation in the dystrophin gene selectively affecting dystrophin expression in the heart. J Clin Invest 96:693–699, 1995.
84. Angelini C, Fanin M, Pegoraro E, Freda MP, Cadaldini M, Martinello F. Clinical-molecular correlation in 104 mild X-linked muscular dystrophy patients: Characterization of sub-clinical phenotypes. Neuromuscul Disord 4:349–358, 1994.
85. Berko BA, Swift M. X-linked dilated cardiomyopathy. N Engl J Med 316:1186–1191, 1987.
86. Arbustini E, Diegoli M, Fasani R, Grasso M, Morbini P, Banchieri N, Bellini O, Dal Bello B, Pilotto A, Magrini G, Campana C, Fortina P, Gavazzi A, Narula J, Vigano M. Mitochondrial DNA mutations and mitochondrial abnormalities in dilated cardiomyopathy. Am J Pathol 153:1501–1510, 1998.
87. Frustaci A, Magnavita N, Chimenti C, Caldarulo K, Sabbioni E, Pietra R, Cellini C, Possati GF, Maseri A. Marked elevation of myocardial trace elements in idiopathic dilated cardiomyopathy compared with secondary cardiac dysfunction. J Am Coll Cardiol 33:1578–1583, 1999.
88. Wallace DC. Mitochondrial defects in cardiomyopathy and neuromuscular disease. Am Heart J 139:S70–S85, 2000.
89. Pearson GD, Veille JC, Rahimtoola S, Hsia J, Oakley CM, Hosenpud JD, Ansari A, Baughman KL. Peripartum cardiomyopathy: National Heart, Lung, and Blood Institute and Office of Rare Diseases (National Institutes of Health) workshop recommendations and review. JAMA 283:1183–1188, 2000.
90. Cunningham FG, Pritchard JA, Hankins GD, Anderson PL, Lucas MJ, Armstrong KF. Peripartum heart failure: Idiopathic cardiomyopathy or compounding cardiovascular events? Obstet Gynecol 67:157–168, 1986.
91. O'Connell JB, Costanzo-Nordin MR, Subramanian R, Robinson JA, Wallis DE, Scanlon PJ, Gunnar RM. Peripartum cardiomyopathy: Clinical, hemodynamic, histologic and prognostic characteristics. J Am Coll Cardiol 8:52–56, 1986.
92. Homans DC, Peripartum cardiomyopathy. N Engl J Med 312:1432–1437, 1985.
93. Lampert MB, Lang RM. Peripartum cardiomyopathy. Am Heart J 130:860–870, 1995.
94. Pearl W. Familial occurrence of peripartum cardiomyopathy. Am Heart J 129:421–422, 1995.
95. Rizeq MN, Rickenbacher PR, Fowler MB, Billingham ME. Incidence of myocarditis in peripartum cardiomyopathy. Am J Cardiol 74:474–477, 1994.
96. Midei MG, DeMent SH, Feldman AM, Hutchins GK Baughman KL. Peripartum myocarditis and cardiomyopathy. Circulation 81:922–928, 1990.
97. Bristow MR, Thompson PD, Martin RP, Mason JW, Billingham ME, Harrison DC. Early anthracycline cardiotoxicity. Am J Med 65:823–832, 1978.
98. Bristow MR, Mason JW, Billingham ME, Daniels JR. Doxorubicin cardiomyopathy: Evaluation by phonocardiography, endomyocardial biopsy, and cardiac catheterization. Ann Intern Med 88:168–178, 1978.
99. Child JS, Perloff JK. The restrictive cardiomyopathies. Cardiol Clin 6:289–316, 1988.
100. Maron BJ, Bonow RO, Cannon RO, Leon MB, Epstein SE. Hypertrophic cardiomyopathy, N Engl J Med 316:780–789, 1987.
101. Maron BJ, Gardin JM, Flack JM, Gidding SS, Kurosaki TT, Bild DE. Prevalence of hypertrophic cardiomyopathy in a general population of young adults. Echocardiographic analysis of 4111 subjects in the CARDIA study. Circulation 92:785–789, 1995.
102. Savage DD, Castelli WP, Abbott RD, Garrison RJ, Anderson SJ, Kannell WB, Feinleib M. Hypertrophic cardiomyopathy and its markers in the general population: The great masquerader revisited: The Framingham Study. J Cardiovascul Ultrason 2:41–47, 1983.
103. Klues HG, Schiffers A, Maron BJ. Phenotypic spectrum and patterns of left ventricular hypertrophy in hypertrophic cardiomyopathy: Morphologic observations and significance as assessed by two-dimensional echocardiography in 600 patients. J Am Coll Cardiol 26:1699–1708, 1995.
104. Shah PM, Adelman AG, Wigle ED, Gobel FL, Burchell BB, Hardarson T, Curiel R, De La Calzada C, Oakley CM, Goodwin JF. The natural (and unnatural) history of hypertrophic obstructive cardiomyopathy. Circ Res 35:suppl II:179–195, 1974.
105. Grigg LE, Wigle ED, Williams WG, Daniel LB, Rakowski H. Transesophageal Doppler echocardiography in obstructive hypertrophic cardiomyopathy: Clarification of pathophysiology and importance in intraoperative decision making. J Am Coll Cardiol 20:42–52, 1992.
106. Petrone RK, Klues HG, Panza JA, Peterson EE, Maron BJ. Coexistence of mitral valve prolapse in a consecutive group of 528 patients with hypertrophic cardiomyopathy assessed with echocardiography. J Am Coll Cardiol 20:55–61, 1992.
107. Suzuki J, Watanabe F, Takenaka K, Amano K, Amano W, Igarashi T, Aoki T, Serizawa T, Sakamoto T, Sugimoto T, et al. New subtype of apical hypertrophic cardiomyopathy identified with nuclear magnetic resonance imaging as an underlying cause of markedly inverted T waves. J Am Coll Cardiol 22:1175–1181, 1993.
108. Casolo GC, Trotta F, Rostagno C, Poggesi L, Galanti G, Masotti G, Bartolozzi C, Dabizzi RP. Detection of apical hypertrophic cardiomyopathy by magnetic resonance imaging. Am Heart J 117:468–472, 1989.
109. McKenna WJ. The natural history of hypertrophic cardiomyopathy. Cardiovasc Clin 19:135–156, 1988.
110. Spirito P, Bellone P. Natural history of hypertrophic cardiomyopathy. Br Heart J 72:S10–S12, 1994.
111. Frank S, Braunwald E. Idiopathic hypertrophic subaortic stenosis. Clinical analysis of 126 patients with emphasis on the natural history. Circulation 37:759–766, 1968.
112. Spirito P, Maron BJ, Bonow RO, Epstein SE. Occurrence and significance of progressive left ventricular wall thinning and relative cavity dilatation in hypertrophic cardiomyopathy. Am J Cardiol 60:123–129, 1987.
113. Maron BJ, Kragel AH, Roberts WC. Sudden death in hypertrophic cardiomyopathy with normal left ventricular mass. Br Heart J 63:308–310, 1990.
114. McKenna WJ, Stewart JT, Nihoyannopoulos P, McGinty F, Davies MJ. Hypertrophic cardiomyopathy without hypertrophy: Two families with myocardial disarray in the absence of increased myocardial mass. Br Heart J 63:287–290, 1990.
115. Dare AJ, Veinot JP, Edwards WD, Tazelaar HD, Schaff HV. New observations on the etiology of aortic valve

disease: A surgical pathologic study of 236 cases from 1990. Hum Pathol 24:1330–1338, 1993.
116. Panza JA, Maron BJ. Valvular aortic stenosis and asymmetric septal hypertrophy: Diagnostic considerations and clinical and therapeutic implications. Eur Heart J 9 Suppl E:71–76, 1988.
117. Presti CF, Waller BF, Armstrong WF. Cardiac amyloidosis mimicking the echocardiogrpahic appearance of obstructive hypertrophic myopathy. Chest 93:881–883, 1988.
118. Colucci WS, Lorell BH, Schoen FJ, Warhol MJ, Grossman W. Hypertrophic obstructive cardiomyopathy due to Fabry's disease. N Engl J Med 307:926–928, 1982.
119. Miller W, Walsh R, McCall D. Eosinophilic heart disease presenting with features suggesting hypertrophic obstructive cardiomyopathy. Cathet Cardiovasc Diagn 13:185–188, 1987.
120. Cabin HS, Costello RM, Vasudevan G, Maron BJ, Roberts WC. Cardiac lymphoma mimicking hypertrophic cardiomyopathy. Am Heart J 102:466–468, 1981.
121. Come PC, Burkley BH, Goodman ZD, Hutchins GM, Pitt B, Fortuin NJ. Hypercontractile cardiac states simulating hypertrophic cardiomyopathy. Circulation 55:901–908, 1977.
122. Shub C, Williamson MD, Tajik AJ, Eubanks DR. Dynamic left ventricular outflow tract obstruction associated with pheochromocytoma. Am Heart J 102:286–290, 1981.
123. Wilson R, Gibson TC, Terrien CM, Jr., Levy AM. Hyperthyroidism and familial hypertrophic cardiomyopathy. Arch Intern Med 143:379–380, 1983.
124. Symons C; Richardson PJ, Feizi O. Hypertrophic cardiomyopathy and hyperthyroidism: A report of three cases. Thorax 29:713–719, 1974.
125. Symons C, Fortune F, Greenbaum RA, Dandona P. Cardiac hypertrophy, hypertrophic cardiomyopathy, and hyperparathyroidism—an association. Br Heart J 54:539–542, 1985.
126. Roberts CS, Roberts WC. Hypertrophic cardiomyopathy as a cause of massive cardiomegaly (greater than 1,000 g). Am J Cardiol 64:1209–1210, 1989.
127. Maron BJ, Gottdiener JS, Bonow RO, Epstein SE. Hypertrophic cardiomyopathy with unusual locations of left ventricular hypertrophy undetectable by M-mode echocardiography. Circulation 63:409–417, 1981.
128. Wigle ED, Sasson Z, Henderson MA, Ruddy TD, Fulop J, Rakowski H, Williams WG. Hypertrophic cardiomyopathy. The importance of the site and the extent of hypertrophy. A review. Prog Cardiovasc Dis 28:1–83, 1985.
129. Maron BJ, Spirito P, Wesley Y, Arce J. Development or progression of left ventricular hypertrophy in children with hypertrophic cardiomyopathy: Identification by two-dimensional echocardiography. N Engl J Med 315:610–614.
130. St. John Sutton MG, Lie JT, Anderson KR, O'Brien PC, Frye RL. Histopathological specificity of hypertrophic obstructive cardiomyopathy: Myocardial fiber disarray and myocardial fibrosis. Br Heart J 44:433–443, 1980.
131. Schwammenthal E, Nakatani S, He S, Hopmeyer J, Sagie A, Weyman AE, Lever HM, Yoganathan AP, Thomas JD, Levine RA. Mechanism of mitral regurgitation in hypertrophic cardiomyopathy: Mismatch of posterior to anterior leaflet length and mobility. Circulation 98:856–865, 1998.
132. Klues HG, Maron BJ, Dollar AL, Roberts WC. Diversity of structural mitral valve alterations in hypertrophic cardiomyopathy. Circulation 85:1651–1660, 1992.
133. Maron BJ, Nishimura RA, Danielson GK. Pitfalls in clinical recognition and a novel operative approach for hypertrophic cardiomyopathy with severe outflow obstruction due to anomalous papillary muscle. Circulation 98:2505–2508, 1998.
134. Chagnac A, Rudniki C, Loebel H, Zahavi I. Infectious endocarditis in idiopathic hypertrophic subaortic stenosis: Report of three cases and review of the literature. Chest 81:346–349, 1982.
135. Spirito P, Rapezzi C, Bellone P, Betocchi S, Autore C, Conte MR, Bezante GP, Bruzzi P. Infective endocarditis in hypertrophic cardiomyopathy: Prevalence, incidence, and indications for antibiotic prophylaxis. Circulation 99:2132–2137, 1999.
136. Davies MJ, McKenna WJ: Hypertrophic cardiomyopathy: An introduction to pathology and pathogenesis. Br Heart J 72:S2–S3, 1994.
137. Maron BJ, Roberts WC. Quantitative analysis of cardiac muscle disorganization in the ventricular septum of patients with hypertrophic cardiomyopathy. Circulation 4:689–706, 1979.
138. Davies MJ. The current status of myocardial disarray in hypertrophic cardiomyopathy. Br Heart J 51:361–363, 1984.
139. Davies MJ. Hypertrophic cardiomyopathy: One disease or several? Br Heart J 63:263–264, 1990.
140. Maron BJ, Anan TJ, Roberts WC. Quantitative analysis of the distribution of cardiac muscle cell disorganization in the left ventricular wall of patients with hypertrophic cardiomyopathy. Circulation 63:882–894, 1981.
141. van der Bel-Kahn J. Muscle fiber disarray in common heart diseases. Am J Cardiol 40:355–364, 1977.
142. Fujiwara H, Hoshino T, Yamana K, Fujiwara T, Furuta M, Hamashima Y, Kawai C. Number and size of myocytes and amount of interstitial space in the ventricular septum and in the left ventricular free wall in hypertrophic cardiomyopathy. Am J Cardiol 52:818–823, 1983.
143. Unverferth DV, Baker PB, Pearce LI, Lautman J, Roberts WC. Regional myocyte hypertrophy and increased interstitial myocardial fibrosis in hypertrophic cardiomyopathy. Am J Cardiol 59:932–936, 1987.
144. Frenzel H, Schwartzkopff B, Reinecke P, Kamoni K, Losse B. Evidence of muscle fiber hyperplasia in the septum of patients with hypertrophic obstructive cardiomyopathy. Quantitative examination of endocardial biopsies and myectomy specimens. Z Kardiol 76:S14–S19, 1987.
145. Francalanci P, Gallo P, Bernucci P, Silver NM, d'Amati G. The pattern of desmin filaments in myocardial disarray. Hum Pathol 26:262–266, 1995.
146. Muraishi A, Kai H, Adachi K, Nishi H, Imaizumi T. Malalignment of the sarcomeric filaments in hypertrophic cardiomyopathy with cardiac myosin heavy chain gene mutation. Heart 82:625–629, 1999.
147. Maron BJ, Wolfson JK, Epstein SE, Roberts WC. Intramural (small vessel) coronary artery disease in hypertrophic cardiomyopathy. J Am Coll Cardiol 8:545–557, 1986.
148. Yetman AT, Hamilton RM, Benson LN, McCrindle BW. Long-term outcome and prognostic determinants in children with hypertrophic cardiomyopathy. J Am Coll Cardiol 32:1943–1950, 1998.
149. Tazelaar HD, Billingham, ME. The surgical pathology of hypertrophic cardiomyopathy. Arch Pathol Lab Med 111:257–260, 1987.
150. Teare D. Asymmetrical hypertrophy of the heart in young adults. Br Heart J 20:1–8, 1958.

151. Emanuel R, Withers R, O'Brien K. Dominant and recessive modes of inheritance in idiopathic cardiomyopathy. Lancet ii:1065–1067, 1971.
152. Maron BJ, Nichols PFI, Pickles LW, Wesley YE, Mulvihill JJ, Patterns of inheritance in hypertrophic cardiomyopathy: Assessment by M-mode and two-dimensional echocardiography. Am J Cardiol 53:1087–1094, 1984.
153. Watkins H. Multiple disease genes cause hypertrophic cardiomyopathy. Br Heart J 72:S4–S9, 1994.
154. Bundgaard H, Havndrup O, Andersen PS, Larsen LA, Brandt NJ, Vuust J, Kjeldsen K, Christiansen M. Familial hypertrophic cardiomyopathy associated with a novel missense mutation affecting the ATP-binding region of the cardiac beta-myosin heavy chain. J Mol Cell Cardiol 31:745–750, 1999.
155. Geisterfer-Lowrance AA, Kass S, Tanigawa G, Vosberg HP, McKenna W, Seidman JG. A molecular basis for familial hypertrophic cardiomyopathy: A beta cardiac myosin heavy chain gene missense mutation. Cell 62:999–1006, 1990.
156. Epstein MD, Cohn GM, Cyran F, Fananapazir L. Differences in clinical expression of hypertrophic cardiomyopathy associated with two distinct mutations in the beta-myosin heavy chain gene. A 908Leu-> Val mutation and a 403Arg-> Gln mutation. Circulation 1992:345–352, 1992.
157. Watkins H, Rosenzweig A, Hwang DS, Levi T, McKenna W, Seidman CE, Siedman JG. Characteristics and prognostic implications of myosin missense mutations in familial hypertrophic cardiomyopathy. N Engl J Med 326:1108–1114, 1992.
158. Vosberg HP. Myosin mutations in hypertrophic cardiomyopathy and functional implications. Herz 19:75–83, 1994.
159. Hengstenberg C, Carrier L, Schwartz K, Maisch B. Clinical and genetical heterogeneity of familial hypertrophic cardiomyopathy. Herz 19:84–90, 1994.
160. Bonne G, Carrier L, Richard P, Hainque B, Schwartz K. Familial hypertrophic cardiomyopathy: From mutations to functional defects. Circ Res 83:580–593, 1998.
161. Forissier JF, Carrier L, Farza K, Bonne G, Bercovici J, Richard P, Hainque B, Townsend PJ, Yacoub MH, Faure S, Dubourg O, Millaire A, Hagege AA, Desnos M, Komajda M, Schwartz K. Codon 102 of the cardiac troponin T gene is a putative hot spot for mutations in familial hypertrophic cardiomyopathy. Circulation 94:3069–3073, 1996.
162. Anan R, Shono H, Kisanuki A, Arima S, Nakao S, Tanaka H. Patients with familial hypertrophic cardiomyopathy caused by a Phe110Ile missense mutation in the cardiac troponin T gene have variable cardiac morphologies and a favorable prognosis. Circulation 98:391–397, 1998.
163. Jaaskelainen P, Soranta M, Miettinen R, Saarinen L, Pihlajamaki J, Silvennoinen K, Tikanoja T, Laakso M, Kuusisto J. The cardiac beta-myosin heavy chain gene is not the predominant gene for hypertrophic cardiomyopathy in the Finnish population. J Am Coll Cardiol 32:1709–1716, 1998.
164. Niimura H, Bachinski LL, Sangwatanaroj S, Watkins H, Chudley AE, McKenna W, Kristinsson A, Roberts R, Sole M, Maron BJ, Seidman JG, Seidman CE. Mutations in the gene for cardiac myosin-binding protein C and late-onset familial hypertrophic cardiomyopathy. N Engl J Med 338:1248–1257, 1998.
165. Carrier L, Bonne G, Bahrend E, et al. Organization and sequence of human cardiac myosin binding protein C gene (MYBPC3) and identification of mutations predicted to produce truncated proteins in familial hypertrophic cardiomyopathy. Circ Res 80:427–434, 1997.
166. Arbustini E, Fasani R, Morbini P, Diegoli M, Grasso M, Dal Bello B, Marangoni E, Banfi P, Banchieri N, Bellini O, Comi G, Narula J, Campana C, Gavazzi A, Danesino C, Vigano M. Coexistence of mitochondrial DNA and beta myosin heavy chain mutations in hypertrophic cardiomyopathy with late congestive heart failure. Heart 80:548–585, 1998.
167. Odawara K, Yamashita K. Mitochondrial DNA abnormalities in hypertrophic cardiomyopathy. Lancet 353:150, 1999.
168. Aronow WS, Kronzon I. Prevalence of hypertrophic cardiomyopathy and its association with mitral anular calcium in elderly patients. Chest 94:1295–1296, 1988.
169. Shenoy MM, Khanna A, Nejat M, Greif E, Friedman SA. Hypertrophic cardiomyopathy in the elderly. A frequently misdiagnosed disease. Arch Intern Med 146:658–661, 1986.
170. Lewis JF, Maron BJ. Elderly patients with hypertrophic cardiomyopathy: A subset with distinctive left ventricular morphology and progressive clinical course late in life. J Am Coll Cardiol 13:36–45, 1989.
171. Lever HM, Karam RF, Currie PJ, Healy BP. Hypertrophic cardiomyopathy in the elderly. Distinctions from the young based on cardiac shape. Circulation 79:580–589, 1989.
172. Goor D, Lillehei CW, Edwards JE. The sigmoid septum. Variation in the contour of the left ventricular outlet. Am J Roentgenol Radium Ther Nucl Med 107:366–376, 1969.
173. Fowles RE, Martin RP, Popp RL. Apparent asymmetric septal hypertrophy due to angled interventricular septum. Am J Cardiol 46:386–392, 1980.
174. Dalldorf FG, Willis PW. Angled aorta (sigmoid septum) as a cause of hypertrophic subaortic stenosis. Hum Pathol 16:457–462, 1985.
175. Topol EJ, Traill TA, Fortuin N. Hypertensive hypertrophic cardiomyopathy in the elderly. N Engl J Med 312:277–283, 1985.
176. Pearson AC, Gudipati CV, Labovitz AJ. Systolic and diastolic flow abnormilities in elderly patients with hypertensive hypertrophic cardiomyopathy. J Am Coll Cardiol 12:989–995, 1988.
177. Karam R, Lever HM, Healy BP. Hypertensive hypertrophic cardiomyopathy or hypertrophic cardiomyopathy with hypertension? A study of 78 patients. J Am Coll Cardiol 13:580–584, 1989.
178. Corrado D, Fontaine G, Marcus FI, McKenna WJ, Nava A, Thiene G, Wichter T. Arrhythmogenic right ventricular dysplasia/cardiomyopathy: Need for an international registry. Study Group on Arrhythmogenic Right Ventricular Dysplasia/Cardiomyopathy of the Working Groups on Myocardial and Pericardial Disease and Arrhythmias of the European Society of Cardiology and of the Scientific Council on Cardiomyopathies of the World Heart Federation. Circulation 101:E101–E106, 2000.
179. McKenna WJ, Thiene G, Nava A, Fontaliran F, Blomstrom-Lundqvist C, Fontaine G, Camerini F. Diagnosis of arrhythmogenic right ventricular dysplasia/cardiomyopathy. Task Force of the Working Group Myocardial and Pericardial Disease of the European Society of Cardiology and of the Scientific Council on Cardiomyopathies of the International Society and

Federation of Cardiology. Br Heart J 71:215–218, 1994.

180. Lobo FV, Heggtveit HA, Butany J, Silver MD, Edwards JE. Right ventricular dysplasia: Morphological findings in 13 cases. Can J Cardiol 8:261–268, 1992.

181. Hofmann R, Trappe HJ, Klein H, Kemnitz J. Chronic (or healed) myocarditis mimicking arrhythmogenic right ventricular dysplasia. Eur Heart J 14:717–720, 1993.

182. Sabel KG, Blomstrom-Lundqvist C, Olsson SB, Enestrom S. Arrhythmogenic right ventricular dysplasia in brother and sister: Is it related to myocarditis? Pediatr Cardiol 11:113–116, 1990.

183. Basso C, Thiene G, Corrado D, Angelini A, Nava A, Valente M. Arrhythmogenic right ventricular cardiomyopathy. Dysplasia, dystrophy, or myocarditis? Circulation 94:983–991, 1996.

184. Ahmad F, Li D, Karibe A, Gonzalez O, Tapscott T, Hill R, Weilbaecher D, Blackie P, Furey M, Gardner M, Bachinski LL, Roberts R. Localization of a gene responsible for arrhythmogenic right ventricular dysplasia to chromosome 3p23. Circulation 98:2791–2795, 1998.

185. Nava A, Thiene G, Canciani B, Scognamiglio R, Daliento L, Buja G, Martini B, Stritoni P, Fasoli G. Familial occurrence of right ventricular dysplasia: A study involving nine families. J Am Coll Cardiol 12:1222–1228, 1988.

186. Thiene G, Nava A, Corrado D, Rossi L, Pennelli N. Right ventricular cardiomyopathy and sudden death in young people. N Engl J Med 318:129–133, 1988.

187. Kullo IJ, Edwards WD, Seward JB. Right ventricular dysplasia: The Mayo Clinic experience. Mayo Clin Proc 70:541–548, 1995.

188. Daliento L, Turrini P, Nava A, Rizzoli G, Angelini A, Buja G, Scognamiglio R, Thiene G. Arrhythmogenic right ventricular cardiomyopathy in young versus adult patients: Similarities and differences. J Am Coll Cardiol 25:655–664, 1995.

189. Marcus FI, Fontaine GH, Guiraudon G, Frank R, Laurenceau JL, Malergue C, Grosgogeat Y. Right ventricular dysplasia: A report of 24 adult cases. Circulation 65:384–398, 1982.

190. Rampazzo A, Nava A, Danieli GA, Buja G, Daliento L, Fasoli G, Scognamiglio R, Corrado D, Thiene G. The gene for arrhythmogenic right ventricular cardiomyopathy maps to chromosome l4q23-q24. Hum Mol Genet 3:959–962, 1994.

191. Rampazzo A, Nava A, Erne P, Eberhard K, Vian E, Slomp P, Tiso N, Thiene G, Danieli GA. A new locus for arrhythmogenic right ventricular cardiomyopathy (ARVD2) maps to chromosome Iq42-q43. Hum Mol Genet 4:2151–2154, 1995.

192. Anguera Ferrando N, Pujadas Capmany R, Abardia Oliva X, Casasus Ramon A. Familial association of arrhythmogenic dysplasia of the right ventricle and obstructive hypertrophic myocardiopathy. Med Clin (Barc) 101:798, 1993.

193. Buja G, Nava A, Daliento L, Scognamiglio R, Morelli M, Canciani B, Alampi G, Thiene G. Right ventricular cardiomyopathy in identical and nonidentical young twins. Am Heart J 126:1187–1193, 1993.

194. Hiraoka E, Koide M, Sakamoto S, Miki T, Ohga N, Suzuki S, Mizutani K Kintaka T, Matsuo T. Identical twins with arrhythmogenic right ventricular dysplasia. Am J Cardiol 76:1099–1100, 1995.

195. Solenthaler M, Ritter M, Candinas R, Jenni R, Amann FW. Arrhythmogenic right ventricular dysplasia in identical twins. Am J Cardiol 74:303–304, 1994.

196. Imakita M, Yutani C, Ishibashi-Ueda H, Miyatake K. A case of overlap syndrome of systemic sclerosis and dermatomyositis with right ventricular dysplasia. Hum Pathol 22:504–506, 1991.

197. McFalls EO, van Suylen RJ. Myocarditis as a cause of primary right ventricular failure. Chest 103:1607–1608, 1993.

198. Burke AP, Farb A, Virmani R. Arrhythmogenic right ventricular dysplasia-cardiomyopathy: A form of healing myocarditis? J Am Coll Cardiol 27:399A, 1996.

199. Goodin JC, Farb A, Smialek JE, Field F, Virmani R. Right ventricular dysplasia associated with sudden death in young adults. Mod Pathol 4:702–706, 1991.

200. Gallo P, d'Amati G, Pelliccia F. Pathologic evidence of extensive left ventricular involvement in arrhythmogenic right ventricular cardiomyopathy. Hum Pathol 23:948–952, 1992.

201. Corrado D, Basso C, Thiene G, McKenna WJ, Davies MJ, Fontaliran F, Nava A, Silvestri F, Blomstrom-Lundqvist C, Wlodarska EK, Fontaine G, Camerini F. Spectrum of clinicopathologic manifestations of arrhythmogenic right ventricular cardiomyopathy/dysplasia: A multicenter study. J Am Coll Cardiol 30:1512–1520, 1997.

202. Fontaliran F, Fontaine G, Fillette F, Aouate P, Chomette G, Grosgogeat Y. Nosologic frontiers of arrhythmogenic dysplasia. Quantitative variations of normal adipose tissue of the right heart ventricle. Arch Mal Coeur Vaiss 84:33–38, 1991.

203. Burke AP, Farb A, Tashko G, Virmani R. Arrhythmogenic right ventricular cardiomyopathy and fatty replacement of the right ventricular myocardium. Are they different diseases? Circulation 97:1571–1580, 1998.

204. Voigt J, Agdal N. Lipomatous infiltration of the heart: An uncommon cause of sudden, unexpected death in a young man. Arch Pathol Lab Med 106:497–498, 1982.

205. Fontaliran F, Fontaine G, Brestescher C, Labrousse J, Vilde F. Significance of lymphoplasmocytic infiltration in arrhythmogenic right ventricular dysplasia. Apropos of 3 own cases and review of the literature. Arch Mal Coeur Vaiss 88:1021–1028, 1995.

206. Fontaine G. Arrhythmogenic right ventricular dysplasia. Curr Opin Cardiol 10:16–20, 1995.

207. Pinamonti B, Pagnan L, Bussani R, Ricci C, Silvestri F, Camerini F. Right ventricular dysplasia with biventricular involvement. Circulation 98:1943–1945, 1998.

208. Burke AP, Farb A, Virmani R. Inflammation, fibrosis, and fat in right ventricular dysplasia. Mod Pathol 9:28A, 1996.

209. Iesaka Y, Hiroe M, Aonuma K, Nitta J, Nogami A, Tokunaga T, Amemiya H, Fujiwara H, Sekiguchi M. Usefulness of electrophysiologic study and endomyocardial biopsy in differentiating arrhythmogenic right ventricular dysplasia from idiopathic right ventricular tachycardia. Heart Vessels Suppl 5:65–69, 1990.

210. Angelini A, Thiene G, Boffa G, Calliari I, Daliento L, Valente M, Chioin R, Nava A, Volta S, Calliari I. Endomyocardial biopsy in right ventricular cardiomyopathy. Int J Cardiol 40:273–282, 1993.

211. Sotozono K, Imahara S, Masuda H, Akashi K, Kamegai M, Miyake F, Murayama M, Sugai J. Detection of fatty tissue in the myocardium by using computerized tomography in a patient with arrhythmogenic right ventricular dysplasia. Heart Vessels Suppl 5:59–61, 1990.

212. Kushwaha SS, Fallon JT, Fuster V. Restrictive cardiomyopathy. N Engl J Med 336:267–276, 1997.

213. Schoenfeld MH, Supple EW, Dec GW, Jr., Fallon JT, Palacios IF. Restrictive cardiomyopathy versus constrictive pericarditis: Role of endomyocardial biopsy in avoiding unnecessary thoracotomy. Circulation 75:1012–1017, 1987.
214. Durand I, Blaysat G, Chauvaud S, Tron P, Tron F, Mallet E, Lebranchu Y, Kachaner J. Extensive fibrous endocarditis as first manifestation of systemic lupus erythematosus. Arch Fr Pediatr 50:685–688, 1993.
215. Ortolani P, Rapezzi C, Binetti G, Baroni M, Mirri A, Alampi G, Benati A, Branzi A, Magnani B. Idiopathic restrictive cardiomyopathy: Clinical, hemodynamic, histologic and prognostic profile. Cardiologia 34:759–768, 1989.
216. Hirota Y, Shimizu G, Kita Y, Nakayama Y, Suwa M, Kawamura K, Nagata S, Sawayama T, Izumi T, Nakano T, et al. Spectrum of restrictive cardiomyopathy: Report of the national survey in Japan. Am Heart J 120:188–194, 1990.
217. Cetta F, O'Leary PW, Seward JB, Driscoll DJ. Idiopathic restrictive cardiomyopathy in childhood: Diagnostic features and clinical course. Mayo Clin Proc 70:634–640, 1995.
218. Siegel RJ, Shah PK, Fishbein MC. Idiopathic restrictive cardiomyopathy. Circulation 70:165–169, 1984.
219. Aroney C, Bett N, Radford D. Familial restrictive cardiomyopathy. Aust N Z J Med 18:877–878, 1988.
220. Fitzpatrick AP, Shapiro LM, Rickards AF, Poole-Wilson PA. Familial restrictive cardiomyopathy with atrioventricular block and skeletal myopathy. Br Heart J 63:114–118, 1990.
221. Nishikawa T, Tanaka Y, Sasaki Y, Kawataki M, Miyazawa Y, Yasui S, Takarada M, Kasajima T. A case of pediatric cardiomyopathy with severely restrictive physiology. Heart Vessels 7:206–210, 1992.
222. Miyazaki A, Ichida F, Suzuki Y, Okada T. Long-term follow-up of a child with idiopathic restrictive cardiomyopathy. Heart Vessels Suppl 5:74–76, 1990.
223. Arbustini E, Morbini P, Grasso M, Fasani R, Verga L, Bellini O, Dal Bello B, Campana C, Piccolo G, Febo O, Opasich C, Gavazzi A, Ferrans VJ. Restrictive cardiomyopathy, atrioventricular block and mild to subclinical myopathy in patients with desmin-immunoreactive material deposits. J Am Coll Cardiol 31:645–653, 1998.
224. Tai PC, Ackerman SJ, Spry CJ, Dunnette S, Olsen EG, Gleich GJ. Deposits of eosinophil granule proteins in cardiac tissues of patients with eosinophilic endomyocardial disease. Lancet 1:643–647, 1987.
225. Kudenchuk PJ, Hosenpud JD, Fletcher S. Eosinophilic endomyocardiopathy. Clin Cardiol 9:344–348, 1986.
226. Fauci AS, Harley JB, Roberts WC, Ferrans VJ, Gralnick HR, Bjornson BH. NIH conference. The idiopathic hypereosinophilic syndrome. Clinical, pathophysiologic, and therapeutic considerations. Ann Intern Med 97:78–92, 1982.
227. Sasano H, Virmani R, Patterson RH, Robinowitz M, Guccion JG. Eosinophilic products lead to myocardial damage. Hum Pathol 20:850–857, 1989.
228. deMello DE, Liapis H, Jureidini S, Nouri S, Kephart GM, Gleich GJ. Cardiac localization of eosinophil-granule major basic protein in acute necrotizing myocarditis. N Engl J Med 323:1542–1545, 1990.
229. Spry CJ. Eosinophils in eosinophilic endomyocardial disease. Postgrad Med J 62:609–613, 1986.
230. Davies J, Spry CJ, Vijayaraghavan G, De Souza JA. A comparison of the clinical and cardiological features of endomyocardial disease in temperate and tropical regions. Postgrad Med J 59:179–185, 1983.
231. Berger PB, Duffy J, Reeder GS, Karon BL, Edwards WD. Restrictive cardiomyopathy associated with the eosinophilia-myalgia syndrome. Mayo Clin Proc 69:162–165, 1994.
232. Puigbo JJ, Combellas I, Acquatella H, Marsiglia I, Tortoledo F, Casal H, Suarez JA. Endomyocardial disease in South America—report on 23 cases in Venezuela. Postgrad Med J 59:162–169, 1983.
233. Fawzy ME, Ziady G, Halim M, Guindy R, Mercer EN, Feteih N. Endomyocardial fibrosis: Report of eight cases. J Am Coll Cardiol 5:983–988, 1985.
234. Rashwan MA, Ayman M, Ashour S, Hassanin MM, Zeina AA. Endomyocardial fibrosis in Egypt: An illustrated review. Br Heart J 73:284–289, 1995.
235. Davies J, Spry CJ, Sapsford R, Olsen EG, de Perez G, Oakley CM, Goodwin JF. Cardiovascular features of 11 patients with eosinophilic endomyocardial disease. Q J Med 52:23–39, 1983.
236. Parrillo JE, Borer JS, Henry WL, Wolff SM, Fauci AS. The cardiovascular manifestations of the hypereosinophilic syndrome. Prospective study of 26 patients, with review of the literature. Am J Med 67:572–582, 1979.
237. Parrillo JE. Heart disease and the eosinophil. N Engl J Med 323:1560–1566, 1990.
238. Arnold M, McGuire L, Lee JC. Leoffler's fibroplastic endocarditis. Pathology 20:79–82, 1988.
239. Blake DP, Palmer TE, Olinger GN. Mitral valve replacement in idiopathic hypereosinophilic syndrome. J Thorac Cardiovasc Surg 89:630–632, 1985.
240. Boustany CW, Jr., Murphy GW, Hicks GL, Jr. Mitral valve replacement in idiopathic hypereosinophilic syndrome. Ann Thorac Surg 51:1007–1009, 1991.
241. Schneider U, Jenni R, Turina J, Turina M, Hess OM. Long-term follow up of patients with endomyocardial fibrosis: Effects of surgery. Heart 79:362–367, 1998.
242. Herzog CA, Snover DC, Staley NA. Acute necrotising eosinophilic myocarditis. Br Heart J 52:343–348, 1984.
243. Tanino M, Kitamura K, Ohta G, Yamamoto Y, Sugioka G. Hypereosinophilic syndrome with extensive myocardial involvement and mitral valve thrombus instead of mural thrombi. Acta Pathol Jpn 33:1233–1242, 1983.
244. Lie JT, Bayardo RJ. Isolated eosinophilic coronary arteritis and eosinophilic myocarditis. A limited form of Churg–Strauss syndrome. Arch Pathol Lab Med 113:199–201, 1989.
245. Olsen EG. Restrictive cardiomyopathy. Postgrad Med J 62:607–608, 1986.
246. Hutt MS. Epidemiology aspects of endomyocardial fibrosis. Postgrad Med J 59:142–146, 1983.
247. Falase AO. Endomyocardial fibrosis in Africa. Postgrad Med J 59:170–178, 1983.
248. Walley VM, Kisilevsky R, Young ID. Amyloid and the cardiovascular system: A review of pathogenesis and pathology with clinical correlations. Cardiovasc Pathol 4:79–102, 1995.
249. Benson MD. "Primary systemic amyloidosis": The seeds of our present research. Medicine (Baltimore) 72:63–65, 1993.
250. Hesse A, Altland K, Linke RP, Almeida MR, Saraiva MJ, Steinmetz A, Maisch B. Cardiac amyloidosis: A review and report of a new transthyretin (prealbumin) variant. Br Heart J 70:111–115, 1993.
251. Skinner M. Familial amyloidotic cardiomyopathy. J Lab Clin Med 117:171–172, 1991.
252. Westermark P, Sletten K, Johansson B, Cornwell GG. Fibril in senile systemic amyloidosis is derived from

normal transthyrtein. Proc Natl Acad Sci (USA) 1990:2843–2845, 1990.

253. Nichols WC, Liepnieks JJ, Snyder EL, Benson MD. Senile cardiac amyloidosis associated with homozygosity for a transthyretin variant (ILE-122). J Lab Clin Med 117:175–180, 1991.
254. Jacobson DR, Pastore RD, Yaghoubian R, Kane I, Gallo G, Buck FS, Buxbaum JN. Variant-sequence transthyretin (isoleucine 122) in late-onset cardiac amyloidosis in black Americans. N Engl J Med 336:466–473, 1997.
255. Loeffler KU, Edward DP, Tso MO. An immunohistochemical study of gelsolin immunoreactivity in corneal amyloidosis. Am J Ophthalmol 113:546–554, 1992.
256. Maury CP. Gelsolin-related amyloidosis. Identification of the amyloid protein in Finnish hereditary amyloidosis as a fragment of variant gelsolin. J Clin Invest 87:1195–1199, 1991.
257. Cornwell GG, Murdoch WL, Kyle RA, Westermark P, Pitkanen P. Frequency and distribution of senile cardiovascular amyloid: A clinicopathologic correlation. Am J Med 75:618–623, 1983.
258. Storkel S, Bohl J, Schneider H-M. Senile amyloidosis: Principles of localization in a heterogeneous form of amyloidosis. Virchows Arch [A] 44:145–161, 1983.
259. Johansson B, Westermark P. The relation of atrial natriuretic factor to isolated atrial amyloid. Exp Mol Pathol 52:266–278, 1990.
260. Gal R, Korzets A, Schwartz A, Rath-Wolfson L, Gafter U. Systemic distribution of beta 2-microglobulin-derived amyloidosis in patients who undergo long-term hemodialysis. Report of seven cases and review of the literature. Arch Pathol Lab Med 118:718–721, 1994.
261. Crotty TB, Li C-Y, Edwards WD, Suman VJ. Amyloidosis and endomyocardial biopsy: Correlation of extent and pattern of deposition with amyloid immunophenotype in 100 cases. Cardiovasc Pathol 4:39–42, 1995.
262. Hawkins PN, Lavender JP, Pepys MB. Evaluation of systemic amyloidosis by scintigraphy with 123I-labeled serum amyloid P component. N Engl J Med 323:508–513, 1990.
263. Klein AL, Hatle LK, Taliercio CP, Oh JK, Kyle RA, Gertz MA, Bailey KR, Seward JB, Tajik AJ. Prognostic significance of Doppler measures of diastolic function in cardiac amyloidosis. A Doppler echocardiography study. Circulation 83:808–816, 1991.
264. Kyle RA, Bayrd ED. Amyloidosis: Review of 236 cases. Medicine (Baltimore) 54:271–299, 1975.
265. Benson MD. Hereditary amyloidosis and cardiomyopathy. Am J Med 93:1–14, 1992.
266. Chamarthi B, Dubrey SW, Cha K, Skinner M, Falk RH. Features and prognosis of exertional syncope in light-chain associated AL cardiac amyloidosis. Am J Cardiol 80:1242–1245, 1997.
267. Olson LJ, Gertz MA, Edwards WD, Li CY, Pellikka PA, Holmes DR, Jr., Tajik AJ, Kyle RA. Senile cardiac amyloidosis with myocardial dysfunction. Diagnosis by endomyocardial biopsy and immunohistochemistry. N Engl J Med 317:738–742, 1987.
268. Celletti F, Fattori R, Napoli G, Leone O, Rocchi G, Reggiani LB, Gavelli G. Assessment of restrictive cardiomyopathy of amyloid or idiopathic etiology by magnetic resonance imaging. Am J Cardiol 83:798–801, A10, 1999.
269. Rukavina JG, Block WD, Jackson CE, Falls HF, Carey JH, Curtis AC. Primary systemic amyloidosis: A review and an experimental, genetic, and clinical study of 29 cases with particular emphasis on the familial form. Medicine (Baltimore) 35:239–334, 1956.
270. Dwulet FE, Benson MD. Characterization of a transthyretin (prealbumin) variant associated with familial amyloidotic polyneuropathy type II (Indiana/Swiss). J Clin Invest 78:880–886, 1986.
271. Ikeda S, Hanyu N, Hongo M, Yoshioka J, Oguchi H, Yanagisawa N, Kobayashi T, Tsukagoshi H, Ito N, Yokota T. Hereditary generalized amyloidosis with polyneuropathy. Clinicopathological study of 65 Japanese patients. Brain 110:315–337, 1987.
272. Staunton H, Dervan P, Kale R, Linke RP, Kelly P. Hereditary amyloid polyneuropathy in north west Ireland. Brain 110:1231–1245, 1987.
273. Gertz MA, Kyle RA, Thibodeau SN. Familial amyloidosis: A study of 52 North American-born patients examined during a 30-year period. Mayo Clin Proc 67:428–440, 1992.
274. Ranlov I, Alves IL, Ranlov PJ, Husby G, Costa PP, Saraiva MJM. A Danish kindred with familial amyloid cardiomyopathy revisited: Identification of a mutant transthyretin-methionine111 variant in serum from patients and carriers. Am J Med 93:3–8, 1992.
275. Benson MD, Wallace MR, Tejada E, Baumann H, Page B. Hereditary amyloidosis: Description of a new American kindred with late onset cardiomyopathy. Appalachian amyloid. Arthritis Rheum 30:195–200, 1987.
276. Staunton H, Davis MB, Guiloff RJ, Nakazato M, Miyazato N, Harding AE. Irish (Donegal) amyloidosis is associated with the transthyretin ALA60 (Appalachian) variant. Brain 114:2675–2679, 1991.
277. Ueno S, Fujimura H, Yorifuji S, Nakamura Y, Takahashi M, Tarui S, Yanagihara T. Familial amyloid polyneuropathy associated with the transthyretin Cys114 gene in a Japanese kindred. Brain 115:1275–1289, 1992.
278. Dubrey SW, Cha K, Skinner M, LaValley M, Falk RH. Familial and primary (AL) cardiac amyloidosis: Echocardiographically similar diseases with distinctly different clinical outcomes. Heart 78:74–82, 1997.
279. Roberts WC, Waller BF. Cardiac amyloidosis causing cardiac dysfunction: Analysis of 54 necropsy patients. Am J Cardiol 52:138–146, 1983.
280. Gertz MA, Kyle RA, Greipp PR. Response rates and survival in primary systemic amyloidosis. Blood 77:257–262, 1991.
281. Gertz MA, Kyle RA, O'Fallon WM. Dialysis support of patients with primary systemic amyloidosis. A study of 211 patients. Arch Intern Med 152:2245–2250, 1992.
282. Gertz MA, Kyle RA, Greipp PR, Katzmann JA, O'Fallon WM. Beta 2-microglobulin predicts survival in primary systemic amyloidosis. Am J Med 89:609–614, 1990.
283. Kyle RA, Greipp PR, O'Falon WM. Primary systemic amyloidosis: Multivariate analysis for prognostic factors in 168 cases. Blood 68:220–226, 1986.
284. Kyle RA, Gertz MA, Greipp PR, Witzig TE, Lust JA, Lacy MQ, Therneau TM. A trial of three regimens for primary amyloidosis: Colchicine alone, melphalan and prednisone, and melphalan, prednisone, and colchicine. N Engl J Med 336:1202–1207, 1997.
285. Patel AR, Dubrey SW, Mendes LA, Skinner M, Cupples A, Falk RH, Davidoff R. Right ventricular dilation in primary amyloidosis: An independent predictor of survival. Am J Cardiol 80:486–492, 1997.
286. Smith RRL, Hutchins GM. Ischemic heart disease secondary to amyloidosis of intramyocardial arteries. Am J Cardiol 52:137–146, 1979.

287. Gertz MA, Kyle RA. Secondary systemic amyloidosis: Response and survival in 64 patients. Medicine (Baltimore) 70:246–256, 1991.
288. Wright JR, Calkins E. Clinical-pathologic differentiation of common amyloid syndromes. Medicine (Baltimore) 60:429–448, 1981.
289. Meyerhoff J. Familial Mediterranean fever: Report of a large family, review of the literature, and discussion of the frequency of amyloidosis. Medicine (Baltimore) 59:66–77, 1980.
290. Hamer JP, Janssen S, van Rijswijk MH, Lie KI. Amyloid cardiomyopathy in systemic nonhereditary amyloidosis. Clinical, echocardiographic and electrocardiographic findings in 30 patients with AA and 24 patients with AL amyloidosis. Eur Heart J 13:623–627, 1992.
291. Barbour DJ, Roberts WC. Frequency of acute and healed myocardial infarcts in fatal cardiac amyloidosis. Am J Cardiol 62:1134–1135, 1988.
292. Pomerance A, Slavin G, McWatt J. Experience with the sodium sulphate-Alcian Blue stain for amyloid in cardiac pathology. J Clin Pathol 29:22–28, 1976.
293. Smith TJ, Kyle RA, Lie JT. Clinical significance of histopathologic patterns of cardiac amyloidosis. Mayo Clin Proc 59:547–555, 1984.
294. Arbustini E, Merlini G, Gavazzi A, Grasso M, Diegoli M, Fasani R, Bellotti V, Marinone G, Morbini P, Dal Bello B, et al. Cardiac immunocyte-derived (AL) amyloidosis: An endomyocardial biopsy study in 11 patients. Am Heart J 130:528–536, 1995.
295. Pitkanen P, Westermark P, Cornwell GGI. Senile systemic amyloidosis. Am J Pathol 117:391–399, 1984.
296. Schwartz ML, Cox GF, Lin AE, Korson MS, Perez-Atayde A, Lacro RV, Lipshultz SE. Clinical approach to genetic cardiomyopathy in children. Circulation 94:2021–2038, 1996.
297. Papadimitriou A, Neustein HB, DiMauro S, Stanton R, Bresolin N. Histiocytoid cardiomyopathy of infancy: Deficiency of reducible cytochrome b in heart mitochondria. Pediatr Res 18:1023–1028, 1984.
298. Eishi Y, Takemura T, Sone R, Yamamura H, Narisawa K, Ichinohasama R, Tanaka M, Hatakeyama S. Glycogen storage disease confined to the heart with deficient activity of cardiac phosphorylase kinase: A new type of glycogen storage disease. Hum Pathol 16:193–197, 1985.
299. Servidei S, Metlay LA, Chodosh J, DiMauro S. Fatal infantile cardiopathy caused by phosphorylase b kinase deficiency. J Pediatr 113:82–85, 1988.
300. Ostman-Smith I, Brown G, Johnson A, Land JM. Dilated cardiomyopathy due to type II X-linked 3-methylglutaconic aciduria: Successful treatment with pantothenic acid. Br Heart J 72:349–353, 1994.
301. Ades LC, Gedeon AK, Wilson MJ, Latham M, Partington MW, Mulley JC, Nelson J, Lui K, Sillence DO. Barth syndrome: Clinical features and confirmation of gene localisation to distal Xq28. Am J Med Genet 45:327–334, 1993.
302. Christodoulou J, McInnes RR, Jay V, Wilson G, Becker LE, Lehotay DC, Platt BA, Bridge PJ, Robinson BH, Clarke JT. Barth syndrome: Clinical observations and genetic linkage studies. Am J Med Genet 50:255–264, 1994.
303. Orstavik KH, Skjorten F, Hellebostad M, Haga P, Langslet A. Possible X linked congenital mitochondrial cardiomyopathy in three families. J Med Genet 30:269–272, 1993.
304. Neustein HB, Lurie PR, Dahms B, Takahashi M. An X-linked recessive cardiomyopathy with abnormal mitochondria. Pediatrics 64:24–29, 1979.
305. Barth PG, Scholte HR, Berden JA, Van der Klei-Van Moorsel JM, Luyt-Houwen IE, Van't Veer-Korthof ET, Van der Harten JJ, Sobotka-Plojhar MA. An X-linked mitochondrial disease affecting cardiac muscle, skeletal muscle and neutrophil leucocytes. J Neurol Sci 62:327–355, 1983.
306. Ozawa T. Mitochondrial cardiomyopathy. Herz 19:105–118, 1994.
307. Romero NB, Marsac C, Paturneau-Jouas M, Magnier S, Fardeau M. Infantile familial cardiomyopathy due to mitochondrial complex I and IV associated deficiency. Neuromusc Disord 3:31–42, 1993.
308. Rustin P, Lebidois J, Chretien D, Bourgeron T, Piechaud JF, A. R, Munnich A, Sidi D. Endomyocardial biopsies for early detection of mitochondrial disorders in hypertrophic cardiomyopathies. J Pediatr 124:224–228, 1994.
309. Zimmerman A, Wyss P, Stocker F. Primary lipid cardiomyopathy. Virchows Archiv [A] 416:453–459, 1990.
310. Goto YI, Nonaka K, Horai S. A mutation in the tRNA (Leu[UUR]) gene associated with the MELAS subgroup of mitochondrial encephalomyopathies. Nature 348:651–653, 1990.
311. Taniike M, Fukushima H, Yanagihara I, Tsukamoto H, Tanaka J, Fujimura H, Nagai T, Sano T, Yamaoka K, Inui K, et al. Mitochondrial tRNA(Ile) mutation in fatal cardiomyopathy. Biochem Biophys Res Commun 186:47–53, 1992.
312. Silvestri G, Santorelli FM, Shanske S, Whitley CB, Schimmenti LA, Smith SA, DiMauro S. A new mtDNA mutation in the tRNA (Leu[UUR]) gene associated with maternally inherited cardiomyopathy. Hum Mutat 3:37–43, 1994.
313. Sato W, Tanaka M, Sugiyama S, Nemoto T, Harada K, Miura Y, Kobayashi Y, Goto A, Takada G, Ozawa T. Cardiomyopathy and angiopathy in patients with mitochondrial myopathy, encephalopathy, lactic acidosis and strokelike episodes. Am Heart J 128:733–741, 1994.
314. Lindal S, Torbergsern T, Aasly J, Mellgren SI, Borud O, Monstad P. Mitochondrial diseases and myopathies: A series of muscle biopsy specimens with ultrastructural changes in the mitochondria. Ultrastruct Pathol 16:263–274, 1992.
315. Lombes A, Mendell JR, Nakase H, Barohn RJ, Bonilla E, Zeviani M, Yates AJ, Omerza J, Gales TL, Nakahara K, Rizzuto R, Engle WK, DiMauro S. Myoclonic epilepsy and rugged-red fibers with cytochrome oxidase deficiency: Neuropathology, biochemistry, and molecular genetics. Ann Neurol 26:20–33, 1989.
316. Van Hove JLK, Shanske S, Ciacci F, Ballinger S, Shoffner JS, Wallace DC, Hanioka T, Folkers K, Bossen EH, Kussin PS, Kpoita JM, Kahler SG. Mitochondrial myopathy with anemia, cardiomyopathy, and lactic acidosis: A distinct late onset mitochondrial disorder. Am J Med Genetics 51:114–120, 1994.
317. Nishizawa Y, Tanaka K, Shinozawa K, Kuwabara T, Atsumi T, Myatake T, Ohama E. A mitochondrial encephalomyopathy with cardiomyopathy. A case revealing a defect of complex I in the respiratory chain. J Neurol Sci 78:189–201, 1987.
318. Muller-Hocker J, Ibel H, Paetzke I, Deufel T, Endres W, Kadenbach B, Gokel JM, Hubner G. Fatal infantile mitochondrial cardiomyopathy and myopathy with heterogeneous tissue expression of combined respiratory chain deficiencies. Virchows Archiv [A] 419:355–362, 1991.

319. Schwartzkopff B, Zierz S, Frenzel H, Block M, Neuen-Jacob E, Reiners K, Stratuer BE. Ultrastructual abnormalities of mitochondria and deficiency of myocardial cytochrome c oxidase in a patient with ventricular tachycardia. Virchows Archiv [A] 419:63–68, 1992.
320. Cziner DG, Levin RI. The cardiomyopathy of Duchenne's muscular dystrophy and the function of dystrophin. Med Hypotheses 40:169–173, 1993.
321. Lurie PR. Endocardial fibroelastosis is not a disease. Am J Cardiol 62:468, 1988.
322. Ino T, Benson LN, Freedom RM, Rowe RD. Natural history and prognostic risk factors in endocardial fibroelastosis. Am J Cardiol 62:431–434, 1988.
323. Hutchins GM, Vie SA. The progression of interstitial myocarditis in idiopathic endocardial fibroelastosis. Am J Pathol 66:483–491, 1972.
324. Arola A, Tuominen J, Ruuskanen O, Jokinen E. Idiopathic dilated cardiomyopathy in children: Prognostic indicators and outcome. Pediatrics 101:369–376, 1998.
325. Ehlers KH, Engle MA, Levin AR, Deely WJ. Eccentric ventricular hypertrophy in familial and sporadic instances of 46 XX, XY Turner phenotype. Circulation 45:639–645, 1972.
326. Suda K, Kohl T, Kovalchin JP, Silverman NH. Echocardiographic predictors of poor outcome in infants with hypertrophic cardiomyopathy. Am J Cardiol 80:595–600, 1997.
327. Way GL, Wolfe RR, Eshaghpour E. The natural history of hypertrophic cardiomyopathy in infants of diabetic mothers. J Pediatr 95:1920–1927, 1979.
328. Gutgesell HP, Speer ME, Rosenberg HS. Characterization of the cardiomyopathy in infants of diabetic mothers. Circulation 61:441–447, 1980.
329. Towbin JA, Lipshultz SE. Genetics of neonatal cardiomyopathy. Curr Opin Cardiol 14:250–262, 1999.
330. Maron BJ, Tajik AJ, Ruttenberg HD, Graham TP, Atwood GF, Victorica BE, Lie JT, Roberts WC. Hypertrophic cardiomyopathy in infants: Clinical features and natural history. Circulation 65:7–17, 1982.
331. Hwang TH, Lee WH, Kimura A, Satoh M, Nakamura T, Kim MK, Choi SK, Park JE. Early expression of a malignant phenotype of familial hypertrophic cardiomyopathy associated with a Gly716Arg myosin heavy chain mutation in a Korean family. Am J Cardiol 82:1509–1513, 1998.
332. Skinner JR, Manzoor A, Hayes AM, Joffe HS, Martin RP. A regional study of presentation and outcome of hypertrophic cardiomyopathy in infants. Heart 77:229–233, 1997.
333. Thornell LE, Johanson B, Erikson A, Lehto VP, Virtanen I. Intermediate filament and associated proteins in the human heart: An immunofluorescence study of normal and pathologic hearts. Eur Heart J 5:231–241, 1984.
334. Stoeckel ME, Osborn M, Porte A, Sacrez A, Batzenschlager A, Weber K. An unusual familial cardiomyopathy characterized by aberrant accumulation of desmin-type intermediate filaments. Virchows Archiv [A] 393:53–60, 1981.
335. Porte A, Stoeckel ME, Sacrez A, Batzenschlager A, Weber K. Unusual familial cardiomyopathy with storage of intermediate filaments in the cardiac muscular cells. Virchows Arch [A] 1980:43–58, 1980.
336. Ariza A, Coll J, Fernandez-Figueras MT, Lopez MD, Mate JL, Garcia O, Fernandez-Vasalo A, Navas-Palacios JJ. Desmin myopathy: A multisystem disorder involving skeletal, cardiac, and smooth muscle. Hum Pathol 26:1032–1037, 1995.
337. Cameron CH, Mirakhur M, Allen IV. Desmin myopathy with cardiomyopathy. Acta Neuropathol (Berl) 89:560–566, 1995.
338. Vajsar J, Becker LE, Freedom RM, Murphy EG. Familial desminopathy: Myopathy with accumulation of desmin-type intermediate filaments. J Neurol Neurosurg Psychiatry 56:644–648, 1993.
339. Muntoni F, Catani G, Mateddu A, Rimoldi M, Congiu T, Faa G, Marrosu MG, Cianchetti C, Porcu M. Familial cardiomyopathy, mental retardation and myopathy associated with desmin-type intermediate filaments. Neuromuscul Disord 4:233–241, 1994.
340. Chin TK, Perloff JK, Williams RG, Jue K, Mohrmann R. Isolated noncompaction of left ventricular myocardium. A study of eight cases. Circulation 82:507–513, 1990.
341. Steiner I, Hrubecky J, Pleskot J, Kokstejn Z. Persistence of spongy myocardium with embryonic blood supply in an adult. Cardiovasc Pathol 5:47–53, 1996.
342. Jenni R, Goebel N, Tartini R, Schneider J, Arbenz U, Oswald O. Persisting myocardial sinusoids of both ventricles as an isolated anomaly. Echocardiographic, angiographic, and pathological anatomical findings. Cardiovasc Intervent Radiol 9:127–131, 1986.
343. Rose AG. Multiple coronary arterioventricular fistulae. Circulation 58:178–180, 1978.
344. Bleyl SB, Mumford BR, Thompson V, Carey JC, Pysher TJ, Chin TK, Ward K. Neonatal, lethal noncompaction of the left ventricular myocardium is allelic with Barth syndrome. Am J Hum Genet 61:868–872, 1997.
345. Wong JA, Bofinger MK. Noncompaction of the ventricular myocardium in Melnick–Needles syndrome. Am J Med Genet 71:72–75, 1997.
346. Ichida F, Hamamichi Y, Miyawaki T, et al. Clinical features of isolated noncompaction of the ventricular myocardium: Long-term clinical course, hemodynamic properties, and genetic background. J Am Coll Cardiol 34:233–240, 1999.
347. Shah CP, Nagi KS, Thakur RK, Boughner DR, Xie B. Spongy left ventricular myocardium in an adult. Tex Heart Inst J 25:150–151, 1998.
348. Ritter M, Oechslin E, Sutsch G, Attenhofer C, Schneider J, Jenni R. Isolated noncompaction of the myocardium in adults. Mayo Clin Proc 72:26–31, 1997.

Chapter

7

PATHOLOGY OF CARDIAC VALVES

The last four decades have witnessed significant changes in the epidemiology of valvular heart disease. Post-rheumatic valve scarring is no longer the dominant lesion. There has been an increased recognition of myxomatous degeneration, and with the general increasing age of the population, the prevalence of fibrocalcific valve disease affecting previously normal and congenitally abnormal valves has increased. Large numbers of patients now survive in chronic immunosuppressed states, which has established a population of individuals who are at increased risk of infective endocarditis.

With dramatic improvements in clinical imaging techniques readily available to clinical cardiologists, many morphologic aspects of valvular heart disease can now be appreciated during life. However, clinical impressions of valve lesions are often imperfect, and the anatomic pathologist still plays a central role in establishing a definitive diagnosis and providing important pathologic correlations for the functional abnormalities (stenosis and regurgitation) defined by imaging tools (particularly echocardiography).

Role of the Pathologist

In establishing a diagnosis, the anatomic pathologist should describe lesions (fibrosis, calcification, perforation, vegetations, thrombi) affecting the various parts of the valve (cusps, leaflets, commissures, chordae, papillary muscles) in detail. For clinico-pathologic correlation, pathologists should also report the functional consequences of valve pathology and assess whether the valve was likely to have produced stenosis, regurgitation, both stenosis and regurgitation, or neither stenosis nor regurgitation. In autopsy cases, other cardiac findings associated with underlying valve disease should be sought (e.g., left atrial dilatation associated with mitral stenosis and left ventricular hypertrophy secondary to aortic stenosis). For most valve diseases, especially those associated with degenerative calcification, histologic examination is not necessary, and a gross diagnosis is often sufficient; exceptions include valve vegetations and valve abnormalities associated with systemic diseases and drug exposures. However, photography of the gross specimen is recommended for a permanent record of the case.

Classification of Valvular Heart Disease

The major cardiac valvular diseases may be classified according to the underlying etiology: congenital, degenerative, postinflammatory, or infectious (Table 7–1). It should be recognized, however, that overlap in the various etiologies often contribute to clinically significant valve disorders; for example, aortic stenosis occurs in congenitally bicuspid valves following degenerative calcification of valve cusps. This chapter will focus on cardiac valve disease in adults. Normal valve anatomy is illustrated. The pathology of the mitral and aortic valves is discussed based on underlying etiology. Diseases of the tricuspid and pulmonary valves are presented individually, and endocarditis is treated as a separate section. Valve pathology associated with systemic diseases is presented, and a final

Table 7–1. Classification of Valvular Heart Disease

Mitral Valve

Congenital Disorders: Parachute Mitral Valve, Cleft Mitral Valve

Myxomatous Degeneration (Mitral Valve Prolapse)

Acute Rheumatic Fever and Post-Rheumatic Scarring

Mitral Annular Calcification

Papillary Muscle Ischemia and Infarction

Mitral Annular Dilatation (Dilated Cardiomyopathy)

Hypertrophic Cardiomyopathy

Tricuspid Valve

Post-Rheumatic Scarring

Tricuspid Insufficiency Secondary to Annular Dilatation (Pulmonary Hypertension)

Ebstein's Anomaly

Myxomatous degeneration (Tricuspid Valve Prolapse)

Aortic Valve

Aortic Stenosis
- Congenial: Unicuspid and Bicuspid Valves
- Degenerative Tricuspid Aortic Stenosis
- Post-Rheumatic Scarring

Aortic Insufficiency
- Diseases of Valve
  - Congenital Bicuspid Valve
  - Post-Rheumatic Scarring
  - Myxomatous Degeneration (Aortic Valve Prolapse)
- Diseases of the Aortic Root
  - Hypertension
  - Marfan Syndrome
  - Ehlers–Danlos Syndrome
  - Pseudoxanthoma Elasticum
  - Idiopathic Aortic Dilatation (Annuloaortic Ectasia)
  - Aortic Dissection
  - Trauma

Pulmonary Valve

Congenital Bicuspid Valve
- Isolated Pulmonic Stenosis
- Tetralogy of Fallot

Pulmonic Insufficiency Secondary to Annular Dilatation (Pulmonary Hypertension)

Post-Rheumatic Scarring

Valvular Abnormalities in Systemic Disease

Carcinoid Heart Disease

Valve Lesions Associated with Drugs
- Appetite suppressants
- Ergotamine

Systemic Lupus Erythematosus

Rheumatoid Arthritis

Seronegative Spondyloarthropathy (HLA-B27 Disease)

Whipple's Disease

Hypereosinophilic Syndrome

Endocarditis: Infective and Noninfective

Prosthetic Valves

Bioprosthetic Valves
- Heterografts (Porcine, Bovine)
- Homografts

Mechanical Valves
- Ball-Cage
- Tilting Disc

Modified with permission from Farb A, Virmani R, Burke AP. Pathogenesis and pathology of valvular heart disease. In: Alpert JS, Dalen JE, Rahimtoola SH (eds): Valvular Heart Disease, p 2. Philadelphia: Lippincott Williams & Wilkins, 2000.

section deals with prosthetic valves. For the clinically important etiologies of valvular heart disease, basic demographics, pathophysiology, clinical findings, and descriptive pathology are discussed.

ATRIOVENTRICULAR VALVES

Mitral Valve

Anatomy of the Mitral Valve

The normal mitral valve is comprised of an anterior leaflet connected by the commissures to a posterior leaflet (Fig. 7–1*A*). The anterior leaflet length (typically 1.5–2.5 cm [mean 2.0 cm]) is greater than the posterior leaflet (0.8–1.4 cm [mean 1.1 cm]). The mean anterior leaflet width is 3.3±0.5 cm, and the mean posterior leaflet width is 4.8±0.9 cm. The chordae from each leaflet insert into the anterolateral and the posteromedial papillary muscles. The "strut" chordae tendineae of the anterior leaflet arise at 45-degree angles from leaflet edge and insert on its ventricular surface. The commissural chordae branch and fan out from the papillary muscle, while the leaflet chordae are usually single and branch and fan out near their leaflet insertion sites. Normal chordae are

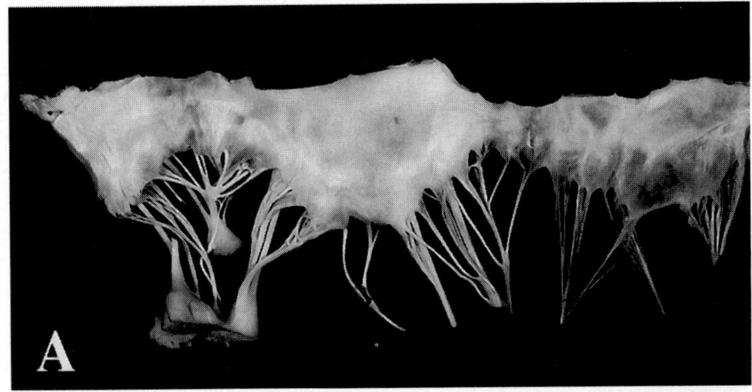

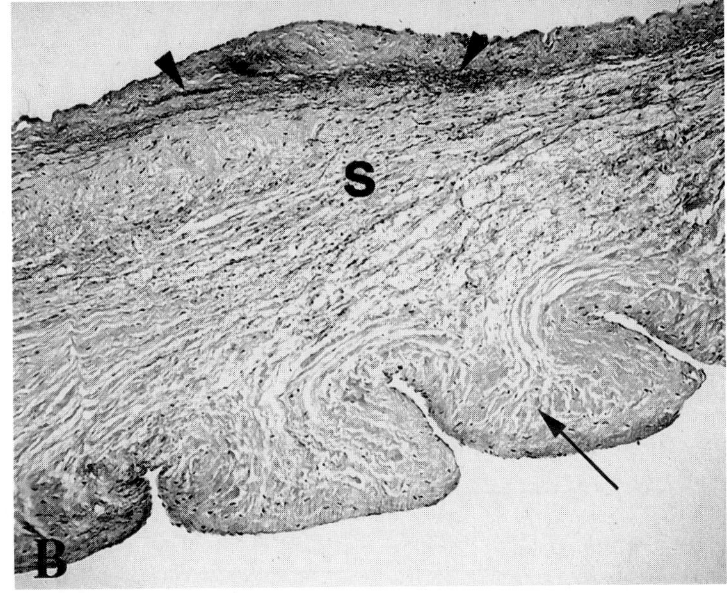

Figure 7–1. Normal mitral valve. Gross photograph of the mitral valve (*A*) showing anterior and posterior leaflets. The anterior leaflet is larger and the chordae arise from the ventricular surface at 45-degree angle. The anterior leaflet is separated from the posterior leaflet by the commissures and by fan-shaped branching commissural chordae. The posterior leaflet has three, often poorly defined, scallops, each with chordal attachments. A photomicrograph of a mitral valve leaflet (*B*, Movat pentachrome stain) demonstrates the atrial surface which is rich in elastic fibers (*arrowheads*), proteoglycan-rich spongiosa (*s*) in the mid-portion, and dense collagenous tissue (*arrow*) which extends toward the ventricular surface of the leaflet. (From Farb A, Virmani R, Burke AP. Pathogenesis and pathology of valvular heart disease. In: Alpert JS, Dalen JE, Rahimtoola SH (eds): Valvular Heart Disease, p 3. Philadelphia: Lippincott Williams & Wilkins, 2000, with permission.)

thin and delicate, and their length varies from 1/6 to 1/7 the length of the left ventricle. The normal annular circumference is < 10 cm, and the normal mitral valve orifice area is 4 to 6 cm^2. The anterior mitral leaflet is in direct continuity (without intervening myocardium) with the posterior (noncoronary) cusp of the aortic valve. There is considerable variability in the sizes of the three scallops of the posterior leaflet. Similarly, variability exists in the number of papillary muscle heads and the extension of the muscle bundles into the chordae tendineae. The mitral valve consists of three histologic layers (Fig. 7–1*B*): (1) the atrialis (a fibroelastic layer on the atrial aspect of the leaflet); (2) the spongiosa (loose fibro-myxomatous tissue rich in proteoglycans in the mid-portion of the valve); and (3) the fibrosa (a dense collagenous layer that extends toward the ventricular surface and provides basic structural support) which is covered by thin fibroelastic tissue (ventricularis). The mitral annulus, a "C"-shaped structure with the gap located at the anterior mitral leaflet, does not form a complete ring around the mitral valve.

Etiology and Epidemiology of Mitral Valve Disease (Tables 7–2 to 7–4)

Mitral valve disease can be classified as congenital or acquired.[1] Congenital conditions that may be corrected surgically include myxomatous degeneration, cleft mitral leaflet (almost always associated with primum atrial septal defect), parachute mitral valve (part of the Shone syndrome), and deformed valves in which there are direct leaflet attachments to the papillary muscles without intervening chordae tendineae. Acquired mitral valve diseases include acute rheumatic fever, post-rheumatic scarring, infective endocarditis, mitral annular calcification, connective tissue diseases, radiation heart

Table 7–2. Classification of Mitral Valve Disease by Functional Abnormality, Etiology, and Mean Age at Presentation

Functional Abnormality	Diagnosis	Total (%)	Mean Age (years)
Mitral stenosis ± regurgitation	Postinflammatory disease (post-rheumatic scarring)	25–40*	55
	Ergotamine-induced valve disease	< 1	Adult
	Fenfluramine-phentermine	Unknown, Probably < 1	Adult
	Mucopolysaccharidosis	< 1	Childhood
	Congenital valve disease	< 1	First decade of life
Mitral regurgitation	Mitral valve prolapse	15–30*	65
	Postinflammatory disease (post-rheumatic scarring)	10	55
	Ischemic heart disease	4–8	70
	Endocarditis	2–5	50
	Carcinoid	< 1	Adult
	Hypertrophic cardiomyopathy	< 1	Adult
	Post-radiation therapy	< 1	Young adult
	Congenital valve disease	< 1	Childhood
	Idiopathic chordal rupture	< 1	Adult

* The relative proportion of valve replacement for mitral valve prolapse has risen in recent years, with a concomitant drop in the proportion of valves removed for postinflammatory valve disease.

From Virmani R, Burke AP, Farb A. Atlas of Cardiovascular Pathology, p 39. Philadelphia: W.B. Saunders Co., 1996, with permission.

Table 7–3. Pathology of Mitral Regurgitation Treated Surgically as a Function of Patient Age

	Incidence (%)	
Diagnosis	*Age > 60 Years*	*Age > 60 Years*
Postinflammatory disease	40	20
Mitral valve prolapse	33	45
Ischemic heart disease	5	18
Endocarditis	7	5
Other	15	12

Adapted from Olson LJ, Subramanian R, Ackermann DM, Orszulak TA, Edwards WD. Surgical pathology of the mitral valve: A study of 712 cases spanning 21 years. Mayo Clin Proc 62:22–34, 1987, with permission.

Table 7–4. Pathology of Surgically Excised Mitral Valves from 1965 to 1996

Etiology	Olson (1965)	Olson (1985)	Dare (1990)	AFIP (1992–1996)
Post-rheumatic	124 (89%)	43 (51%)	47 (49%)	47 (35%)
Myxomatous mitral valve	5 (4%)	21 (25%)	27 (29%)	57 (43%)
Papillary muscle ischemia	0	8 (10%)	7 (7%)	5 (4%)
Endocarditis	1	2 (2%)	5 (5%)	10 (8%)
Miscellaneous	10 (7%)	10 (12%)	9 (9%)	14 (11%)
Age (years) and range	47 (12–61)	61 (15–82)	61 (8–85)	56 (12–87)
Total	140	84	95	133

From Farb A, Virmani R, Burke AP. Pathogenesis and pathology of valvular heart disease. In: Alpert JS, Dalen JE, Rahimtoola SH (eds): Valvular Heart Disease, p 5. Philadelphia: Lippincott Williams & Wilkins, 2000, with permission.

disease, ergotamine-induced valvular disease,[2] and the recently described valvular pathology associated with the use of the weight-reducing agents fenfluramine–phentermine.[3] Other diseases that secondarily lead to mitral valve dysfunction include coronary artery disease with papillary muscle dysfunction and cardiomyopathies (hypertrophic, dilated, and restrictive).

Rheumatic mitral stenosis was the predominant etiology leading to mitral valve surgery prior to the 1960s. Since then, the incidence of untreated streptococcal infections and subsequent acute rheumatic fever has declined in the United States and in other industrialized nations.[1, 4, 5] Currently, the most frequent cause of mitral valve disease leading to surgical intervention is myxomatous degeneration of the mitral valve (mitral valve prolapse).[6] In 1987, Olson et al. reported the frequency of the various causes of mitral valve disease in 712 patients who had undergone mitral valve replacement at various time points from 1965 to 1985.[6] Mitral stenosis was present in 452 valves, 99% secondary to postinflammatory (presumably post-rheumatic) disease, and 1% secondary to congenital mitral stenosis. There were 262 cases of pure mitral incompetence with myxomatous degeneration accounting for 38%, postinflammatory disease 31%, ischemic mitral regurgitation 11%, and idiopathic chordal rupture 4%. Notably, the frequency of post-rheumatic valvular scarring declined from 89% in 1965 to 51% in 1985. In 1993, Dare et al. reported a similar frequency of post-rheumatic valves (49%, Table 7–4).[7] The incidence of post-rheumatic disease among surgically excised mitral valves seen at our Institute from 1992 to 1996 was even lower (35%), highlighting the continued decline in acute rheumatic fever and subsequent rheumatic heart disease in the United States.

Mitral Valve Pathology

Myxomatous Degeneration of the Mitral Valve

Myxomatous degeneration of the mitral valve includes mitral valve prolapse, systolic click-murmur syndrome, Barlow syndrome, billowing mitral cusp syndrome, floppy mitral valve syndrome, and redundant mitral valve. The most common form of valvular heart disease in the United States, myxomatous degeneration of the mitral valve is present in 3–5% in the population, is twice as frequent in women than in men, and is reported in all age groups.[8] Familial clusters of myxomatous degeneration of the mitral valve are inherited as autosomal dominant traits, but no consistent chromosomal abnormalities associated with this valve lesion have been identified.[9] Most patients with Marfan syndrome, Ehlers–Danlos syndrome, osteogenesis imperfecta, and pseudoxanthoma elasticum have myxomatous degeneration of the mitral valve; all are disorders of connective tissue with autosomal dominate inheritance.

Most patients with myxomatous degeneration of the mitral valve are asymptomatic and suffer no long-term consequences with a diagnosis made by physical examination (mid-systolic click) or echocardiography.[10] Common symptoms in patients with mitral prolapse with no or mild valvular regurgitation include palpitations and atypical chest pain. Supraventricular and ventricular arrhythmias may be seen in individuals with mild to severe prolapse. Advanced mitral regurgitation occurs in 10–15% of patients and is more common in men > 50 years old.[11] In these individuals, signs and symptoms of left-sided heart failure may be present, often associated with atrial fibrillation. Chronic severe mitral regurgitation can ultimately lead to pulmonary hypertension and resultant right-sided heart failure.

The clinical cardiac complications of myxomatous degeneration of the mitral valve (mitral regurgitation, need for valve surgery, endocarditis, and sudden death) are associated with increased severity of myxomatous change (i.e., increased leaflet thickness and length).[12] Although the incidence of sudden death in myxomatous degeneration in the absence of significant mitral regurgitation is extremely low, it is not zero (estimated annual rate of 1.9–40/10,000 patients with mitral prolapse).[12–16] The mechanism of sudden death in these cases is uncertain. In one study, mitral valve prolapse was present in 25% of patients with otherwise normal hearts referred for evaluation of idiopathic ventricular tachycardia.[17] Sudden-death cases evaluated at autopsy demonstrated that mitral annulus circumference, anterior leaflet length, posterior leaflet length, and posterior leaflet thickness were significantly larger (20%, 15%, 22%, and 33%, respectively) than these structures measured in hearts in which mitral prolapse was an incidental finding.[16] Additionally, subvalvular friction lesions caused by contact of elongated chordae tendineae and the posterior leaflet with the adjacent ventricular endocardium of the posterobasal wall are more frequently observed in sudden-death cases than incidental mild myxomatous degeneration. Further, in sudden death associated with myxomatous degeneration of the mitral valve, dysplasia of the atrioventricular nodal artery is common (75% of cases in our series), resulting in lumen narrowing and associated with myocardial fibrosis in the base of the interventricular septum.[18]

Currently, myxomatous degeneration of the mitral valve is the most common pathology seen in patients undergoing mitral valve surgery.[8] Valve surgery is indicated in symptomatic patients with chronic severe mitral regurgitation and in asymptomatic patients with severe regurgitation associated with left ventricular dilatation (left ventricular end systolic cavity diameter > 45 mm) or dysfunction (left ventricular ejection fraction < 60%).[19] Less commonly, surgery is performed secondary to acute severe mitral regurgitation as a result of chordal rupture producing a flail leaflet. Previously, the entire mitral valve, including chordae and papillary muscles, was removed. More recently, the important role played by the subleaflet valve apparatus in preserving left ventricular function and preventing left ventricular dilatation is appreciated.[20] Currently, valve repair without valve replacement is performed by segmental valve resection (mitral valvuloplasty), often accompanied by placement of an annuloplasty ring.[21] In valve repair, a portion of the posterior leaflet (which has maximal myxomatous degeneration) is typically excised. Chordal shortening may also be performed. When valve repair is not possible, the anterior leaflet is resected, the posterior leaflet and chordal attachments to the papillary muscles and mitral annulus are often spared, and a prosthetic valve is placed.[6]

The pathologic spectrum of myxomatous degeneration of the mitral valve ranges from mild to severe valvular changes (Fig. 7–2).[16] In mild cases, the posterior mitral leaflet (especially the middle [or intermediate] scallop) demonstrates myxoid thickening, increased length, and mild prolapse toward the left atrium. This mild form of the condition is typically an incidental finding diagnosed by the presence of a mid-systolic click on physical examination and is not associated with significant mitral regurgitation. In the more severe form of myxomatous valvular degeneration, all scallops of posterior leaflet are involved (with or without involvement of the anterior leaflet), and the degree of myxomatous change, valve thickening, and elongation is substantially more pronounced than incidental mitral prolapse.[22, 23] Chordal elongation is typically present (Fig. 7–2*B*) resulting in extensive leaflet prolapse into the left atrium. Further, the normal pattern of chordal insertion on the ventricular leaflet surface is often effaced; chordae insert chaotically producing poor leaflet structural support (Fig. 7–2*D*).[24] The frequency of chordal rupture (Fig. 7–2*E*) varies between 20 to 74% in surgically excised mitral valves. Functional prolapse is most marked when there are multiple ruptured chords resulting in a flail leaflet(s). Annular calcification may be present and is frequent in patients with significant chronic mitral regurgitation.

A gross diagnosis is usually sufficient in routine autopsy or surgical cases of myxomatous degeneration of the mitral valve; histologic sectioning of the valve is not necessary unless infective endocarditis is suspected. If performed, histology shows an expanded leaflet spongiosa layer, and there is multi-focal disruption of the fibrosa by the proteoglycan-rich spongiosa (Fig. 7–2*F*). These pathologic changes are best appreciated when the valve is appropriately embedded in saggital section and stained for proteoglycans by Movat pentachrome or alcian blue stain.

In autopsy cases of myxomatous degeneration of the mitral valve, the presence (or absence) of cardiac findings consistent with mitral regurgitation deserves comment. Significant mitral regurgitation is associated with cardiomegaly and a volume-overloaded heart characterized by left atrial and left ventricular dilatation. Myocardial histology demonstrates myocyte hypertrophy and increased interstitial fibrous tissue. The mitral valve annulus circumference is increased. In patients with pulmonary hypertension secondary to chronic severe mitral regurgitation, right-sided cavity dilatation is present. Biatrial dilatation is further augmented by chronic atrial fibrillation.

Acute and Chronic Rheumatic Mitral Valve Disease

Acute rheumatic fever, a noninfectious immune-mediated complication of pharyngitis secondary to Group A β-hemolytic streptococcus, remains highly prevalent today in the third world with the highest rates in the Middle East and sub-Saharan Africa.[25] Rheumatic fever and subsequent post-rheumatic heart disease are the leading cause of worldwide cardiovascular morbidity and mortality.[25] However, the incidence of acute rheumatic fever remains in

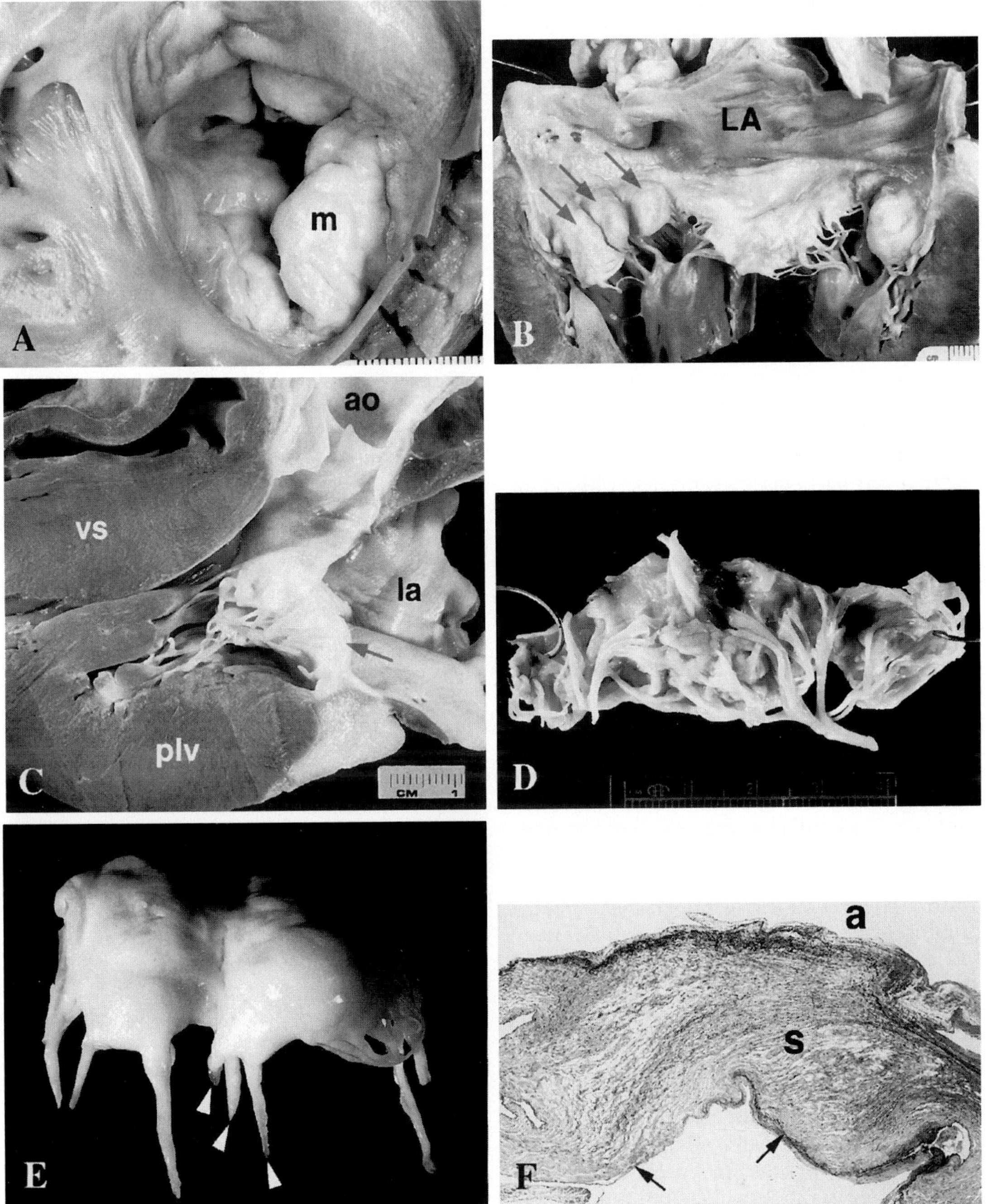

Figure 7–2. Myxomatous degeneration of the mitral valve. An atrial view of the mitral valve (*A*) shows marked posterior leaflet hooding and prolapse toward the left atrium. The middle scallop (*m*) of the posterior leaflet is maximally affected. *B.* Opened left atrium and ventricle from a patient with severe mitral regurgitation and heart failure secondary to myxomatous mitral valve degeneration. Note elongated chordae and increased posterior mitral leaflet length (*arrows*) with prominent scallops. The left atrium and ventricle are dilated. A parasternal long axis echocardiogram view is demonstrated in *C.* The thickened, redundant posterior mitral leaflet (*arrow*) prolapses into the left atrium (*la*); the aorta (*ao*), ventricular septum (*vs*), and posterior left ventricular wall (*plv*) are indicated in this "clinical" orientation. Multiple haphazardly inserted chordae are present on a surgically excised posterior leaflet (*D*) viewed from the ventricular surface. One scallop excised in mitral valve repair (*E*) shows hooding and myxomatous degeneration with chordal rupture (*arrowheads*). Histologically (*F*), the atrial surface (*a*) of a prolapsed mitral valve shows elastic fibers; the spongiosa (*s*) is expanded and disrupts the collagenous fibrosa and ventricularis layers (*arrows*). (*D* and *F* from Farb A, Virmani R, Burke AP. Pathogenesis and pathology of valvular heart disease. In: Alpert JS, Dalen JE, Rahimtoola SH (eds): Valvular Heart Disease, p 6. Philadelphia: Lippincott Williams & Wilkins, 2000, with permission.) (*E* from Virmani R, Burke AP, Farb A. Pathology of valvular heart disease. In: Valvular Heart Disease, p 1.11. Rahimtoola SH (volume ed.). Volume XI of Atlas of Heart Diseases. Braunwald E (series ed). St. Louis: Mosby, 1997, with permission.)

sharp decline in the industrialized world over the last three to four decades. The reasons for this epidemiological change are multifactorial and are secondary to a combination of improved socioeconomic conditions, a lower incidence of untreated streptococcal infections, and the widespread use of antibiotics. In the 1980s, there were sporadic outbreaks of acute rheumatic fever in several geographic locations in the United States. The two most important factors responsible for these cases were: (1) the significant increase in the number of immigrants entering the United States from parts of the world where acute rheumatic fever is still endemic, and (2) the appearance of virulent strains of streptococci (such as M types 5 and 18) that are particularly associated with acute rheumatic fever and carditis. The largest number of recent nonimmigrant cases of acute rheumatic fever were seen in Utah in 1985, and over 80% of the cases occurred in middle class families.[3, 4] Because up to one third of streptococcal throat infections are asymptomatic, cases of acute rheumatic fever will continue to be seen.[25]

The pathophysiology of acute rheumatic carditis involves an altered immune response to Group A β-hemolytic streptococcus infection. Multiple streptococcal antigens cross-react with antibodies to cardiac structures. For example, an N-acetyl glucosamine moiety of the Group A polysaccharide cross-reacts with heart valve tissue.[26] There is an increased synthesis of antistreptococcal, antistreptolysin, anti-DNAase, and antihyaluronidase antibodies that characterize the immune response. Glycoproteins, myocardial and smooth muscle cell sarcolemma (which cross-react with streptococcal membrane antigens), and myocyte myosin (which shares antigens with streptococcal M protein) are the immunologic targets within the heart. The stimulation of T-cells cytotoxic for cardiac muscle by Group A streptococcal membrane antigens suggests that cellular immunity is involved in the pathogenesis of acute rheumatic fever. Host factors likely play an important role in rheumatic fever, as attacks have been linked to histocompatibility antigens DR4 in the United States and Saudi Arabia, and DR3 and DQw2 in India.[25]

Clinical signs and symptoms of rheumatic fever occur 2 to 6 weeks after the initial streptococcal pharyngitis with an overall attack rate of $< 5\%$.[27] A diagnosis of acute rheumatic fever is made by serologic evidence of a preceding streptococcal infection plus either (1) two of the major Jones criteria (carditis, polyarthritis, chorea, erythema marginatum, subcutaneous nodules) or (2) one major and two minor Jones criteria (fever, arthralgias, previous rheumatic fever or rheumatic heart disease, elevated erythrocyte sedimentation rate, positive C-reactive protein, or prolonged P-R interval on electrocardiogram).[27–29] Currently, echocardiography has become a useful diagnostic tool. The frequency of cardiac involvement in patients with acute rheumatic fever is highly variable, ranging from nearly one third to over 50% of cases.[30, 31] The incidence of clinical carditis was 72% in the most recent outbreak of acute rheumatic fever in the United States in Utah.[31] Nearly 80% of patients with carditis develop this complication within the first 2 weeks of the onset of acute rheumatic fever.[25]

Clinically, valvular involvement is suggested by the appearance of a new regurgitation murmur (mitral and/or aortic insufficiency). The mechanism of mitral regurgitation involves a combination of inflammatory valvulitis, functional prolapse, and annular dilatation. Most cases of mild to moderate mitral regurgitation resolve; however, marked mitral involvement can result in severe mitral regurgitation and resultant heart failure. Medical treatment consists of antibiotics and salicylates with a short course of corticosteroids. Mitral regurgitation resulting in severe congestive heart failure can be treated successfully with mitral valve repair or replacement.

Pathologically, a pancarditis may be present in which there is inflammation present in all three layers of the heart: endocarditis, myocarditis, and pericarditis. The histologic hallmark of acute rheumatic carditis is the Aschoff nodule, which can be found in the myocardium (atria and papillary muscles in surgically removed tissue or ventricular myocardium in endomyocardial biopsy specimens) and on valve leaflets.[32, 33] The Aschoff nodule contains lymphocytes, macrophages, and plasma cells with focal fibrinoid necrosis. Two types of macrophages may be seen in an Aschoff nodule: (1) an Anitschkow's cell (also known as an Aschoff's cell, caterpillar cell, and owl-eyed cell) and (2) a multinucleated Anitschkow's cell (Aschoff's giant cell). The Anitschkow's cells have round to oval nuclei and condensation of the chromatin toward the nuclear periphery. In the center of the nucleus, chromatin strands connect the periphery of the nucleus to the center with an intervening clear space. The most frequent location of Aschoff nodules is the endocardium of the atria and in the perivascular spaces of the ventricular myocardium.

In acute rheumatic valvulitis, the mitral valve is affected in 70–75% of cases with simultaneous mitral and aortic valve involvement in an additional 20%. Isolated aortic valve disease occurs in 5–8% of patients.[25] Tricuspid valve involvement is not uncommon (up to 30% of cases in some series) with recurrent attacks of acute rheumatic carditis,[34] and pulmonary valve lesions are exceedingly rare. Pathologically, valves appear dull and thickened. Small verrucous vegetations (Fig. 7–3*A*) are located along the lines of valve closure (atrial surface of the mitral valve and ventricular surface of the aortic valve). Histologically (Fig. 7–3*B*), vegetations are composed of fibrin with associated palisading mononuclear cells within the valve tissue. Aschoff nodules may be present (Fig. 7–3*C*). Healing lesions demonstrate granulation tissue. Because myocardial and pericardial lesions typically heal without clinical sequelae, it is the valvular lesions of acute rheumatic fever that are associated with long-term complications.

In post-rheumatic mitral valve disease, a history of previous acute rheumatic fever is present in only up to 50% of patients with mitral stenosis.[6] Therefore, chronic rheumatic heart disease will continue to be encountered in adults who may have had subclinical acute rheumatic carditis. Postinflammatory valvular scarring is presumed to be post-rheumatic, unless there is a history of some other nonrheumatic inflammatory disease. The latency period between the

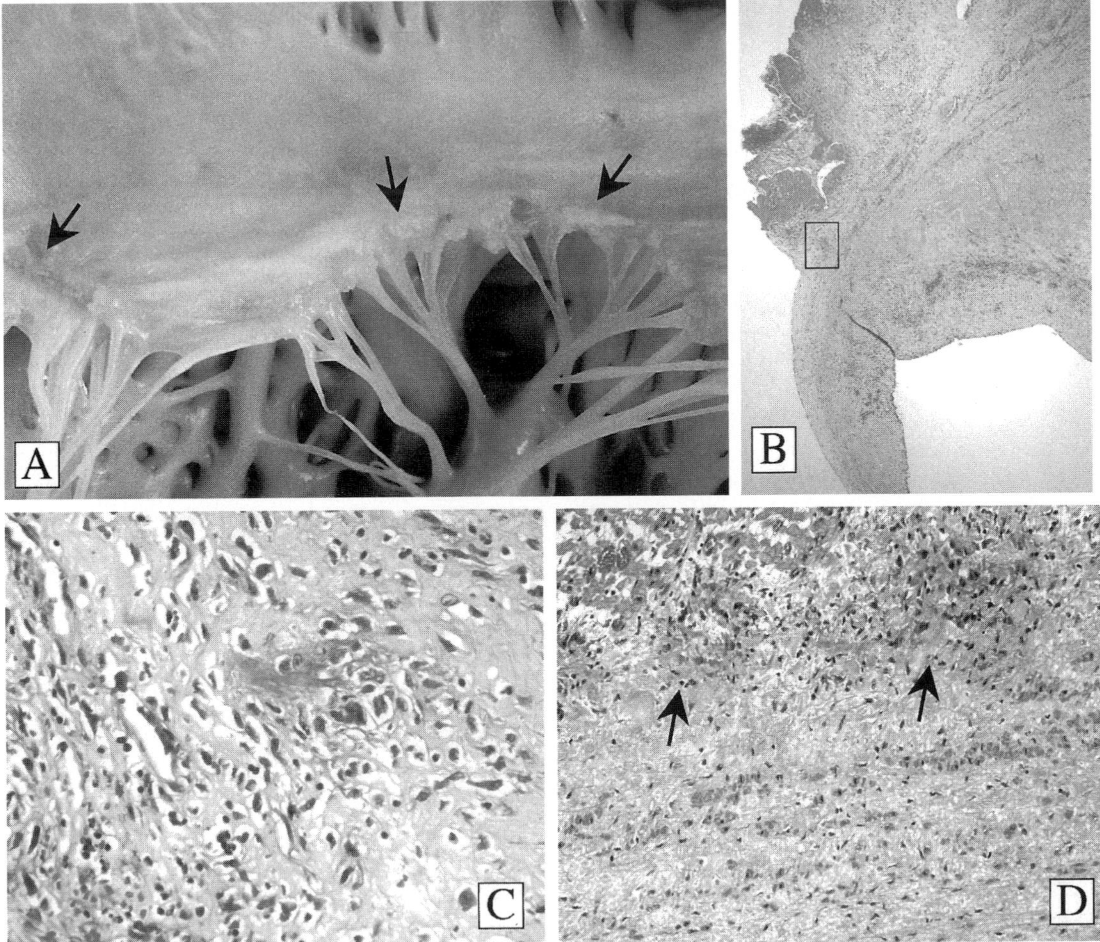

Figure 7–3. Acute rheumatic carditis and mitral valvulitis in a 14-year-old boy who died suddenly. Multiple small firm vegetations are present along the line of valve closure (*A, arrows*) of both the anterior and posterior leaflets. Histologically (*B*), there is fibrin deposition on the surface of the vegetation with inflammation and organization towards its base. The rectangular selected area is shown at high magnification (*C*), demonstrating an Aschoff nodule with central fibrinoid change. Multiple small Aschoff nodules are shown in the endocardium (*D, arrows*).

development of acute rheumatic fever and chronic rheumatic valve disease can be as long as 10 to 20 years, but an interval as short as 2 years has also been reported.[29] The pathogenesis of the long latency period is believed to be due to ongoing valve damage as a result of abnormal blood flow patterns caused by the initial valvulitis.[35] Like most immune-mediated diseases, post-rheumatic valvular scarring is more common in women with a male:female ratio of approximately 0.4:1. In the industrialized world, signs and symptoms of chronic valvular scarring typically appear in the third and fourth decades, and valve surgery is usually performed in patients in their fifth decade. In underdeveloped countries, however, severe post-rheumatic valve disease may occur in adolescents. The risk of developing chronic valvular deformities is highest in patients who had a history of rheumatic carditis associated with congestive heart failure as part of the spectrum of their acute rheumatic fever.

Rheumatic mitral stenosis is by far the most frequent pathologic manifestation of chronic rheumatic heart disease; mixed mitral stenosis and regurgitation is not uncommon and pure mitral regurgitation is rare. Roberts and Virmani reviewed surgically excised valves from patients treated at the NIH from 1964–1975.[32] Aschoff nodules were present in the atrial appendages almost exclusively in patients with mitral stenosis with or without regurgitation and with or without other valve involvement; only one patient with pure mitral regurgitation had Aschoff nodules.

The valve area in mild mitral stenosis is < 2 to 4 cm^2, moderate mitral stenosis 1 to 2 cm^2, and severe stenosis < 1 cm^2. Signs and symptoms of mitral stenosis are due to progressive pulmonary venous hypertension. Patients initially experience dyspnea on exertion followed by orthopnea, paroxysmal nocturnal dyspnea, and signs of left-sided heart failure as the severity of mitral stenosis increases. Acute pulmonary edema can be precipitated by rapid atrial fibrillation (via a reduced duration of left atrial emptying), conditions that increase cardiac output (hyperthyroidism, infection, fever), and pregnancy (increased heart rate and intravascular volume). In some patients, chronic severe pulmonary venous hypertension ultimately leads to pulmonary artery vasoconstriction, right ventricular pressure overload, and eventual right-sided heart failure. Clinically significant symptoms typically correlate with a mitral valve orifice area of < 1 cm^2, and mechanical intervention is indicated in symptomatic patients with severe stenosis and/or regurgitation.[36] Patients with post-rheumatic valve scarring are at increased risk for infective endocarditis, and individuals with atrial fibrillation associated with mitral stenosis are at particularly high risk for systemic thromboembolic events.

Mechanical treatment (surgery or percutaneous valvuloplasty) is indicated in mitral stenosis patients with symptoms of pulmonary venous congestion.[35] Over the past 50 years, mitral stenosis treatment has evolved from closed commissurotomy to open commissurotomy to the current era of mitral valve replacement, repair, and balloon dilatation. Percutaneous mitral valvuloplasty, which utilizes balloon dilatation of the mitral orifice, is an effective treatment for many patients with mitral stenosis with no or minimal mitral regurgitation, pliable noncalcified leaflets, and mild subvalvular chordal fusion.[37,38] Surgery is recommended for patients with advanced subvalvular chordal disease or leaflet calcification and those with mixed stenosis and regurgitation. At valve replacement surgery, the anterior leaflet is removed, and an attempt is made to retain the posterior leaflet and its chordal attachment to the papillary muscles. Preservation of chordal structures is associated with improved cardiac function and reduced risk of postoperative left ventricular rupture or dilatation. However, severe chordal thickening may preclude their complete preservation in order to assure an adequate valve orifice. When technically feasible, mitral repair rather than replacement may be attempted. Valve repair is more likely to be performed in younger patients, and is associated with a superior long-term survival than valve replacement; however, the need for subsequent reoperation is greater in valve repair than replacement.[39]

Post-rheumatic scarring results in fusion of parts of the mitral valve apparatus—commissures, leaflets, and/or chordae—leading to stenosis (Fig. 7–4). Commissural fusion alone is seen in 30%, fusion of leaflets alone in 15%, and fusion of the chordae alone in 10%; in the remainder, more than one portion of the mitral valve structure is involved. Valve leaflets become fibrotically thickened, and calcification may be focally observed at the fused commissures and ulcerate the leaflet surface. Chordal thickening, fusion, and shortening result in the formation of a fibrous tunnel below the leaflets and provides the classic "fish mouth" appearance of severe mitral stenosis when the valve is viewed from the left ventricular aspect (Fig.

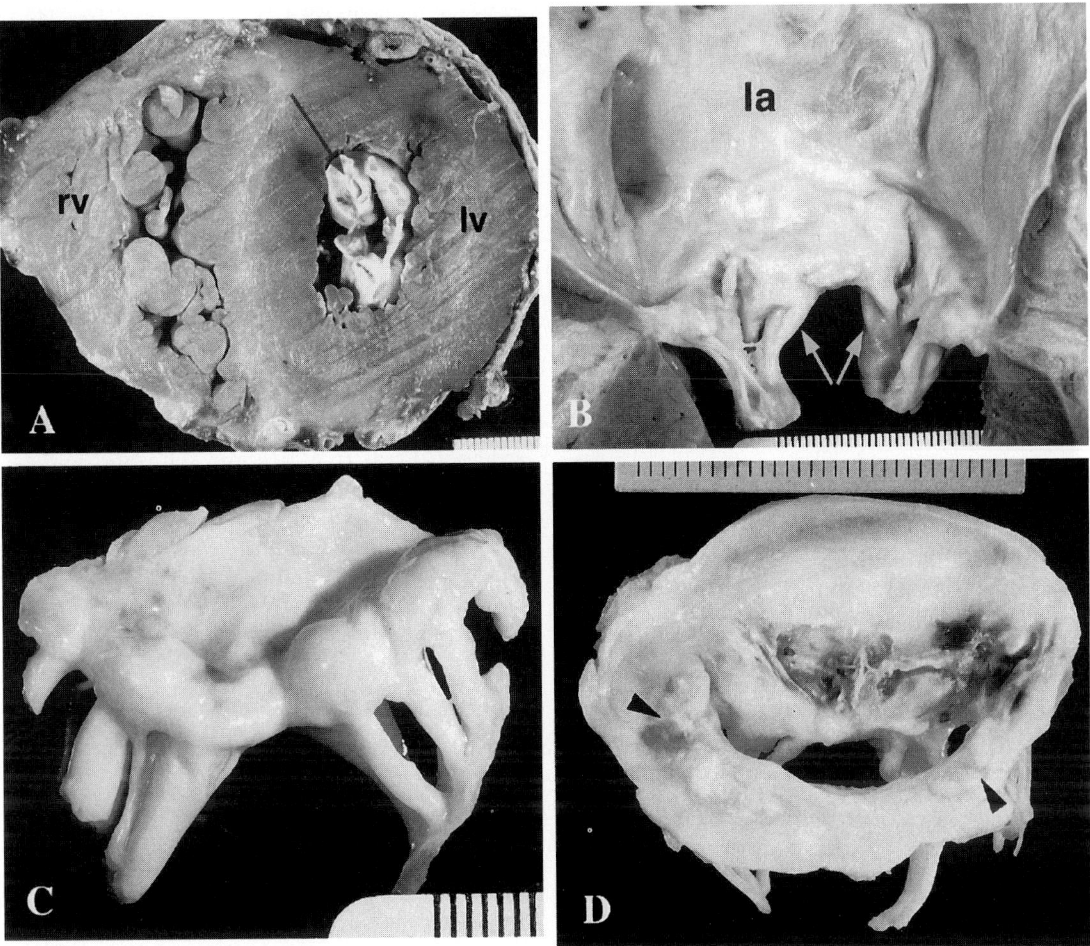

Figure 7–4. Rheumatic mitral stenosis. The mitral valve as viewed from the ventricular surface (*A*) shows a markedly stenotic orifice with chordal fusion and fibrosis (*arrow*). Marked hypertrophy of the right ventricle (*rv*) is present secondary to pulmonary hypertension. The left ventricular (*lv*) cavity has a "D"-shaped configuration as a result of right ventricular pressure overload. Marked dilatation of the left atrium (*la*) is shown (*B*) secondary to post-rheumatic mitral stenosis. Note leaflet fibrosis, commissural fusion, and severe chordal fusion and shortening (*arrows*). A fibrotic anterior mitral leaflet with chordal fusion and shortening was resected during mitral valve replacement (*C*). Viewed from the atrial surface, an entire surgically excised mitral valve (*D*) shows commissural fusion, leaflet thickening, and focal calcification (*arrowheads*). (*D* from Farb A, Virmani R, Burke AP. Pathogenesis and pathology of valvular heart disease. In: Alpert JS, Dalen JE, Rahimtoola SH (eds): Valvular Heart Disease, p 9. Philadelphia: Lippincott Williams & Wilkins, 2000, with permission.)

7–4*A*). Histologically, the normal connective tissue layers of the valve are replaced by collagen with interspersed fibroblasts and focal neoangiogenesis. Focal chronic inflammatory cell infiltrates, consisting of lymphocytes, plasma cells and macrophages, are not uncommon. Aschoff nodules are rarely seen in surgical valve specimens, but are more frequently present in patients from areas that have a high prevalence of rheumatic heart disease. In patients undergoing surgery for chronic post-rheumatic mitral scarring in the United States, the frequency of Aschoff nodules in excised atrial appendages and papillary muscles is 11% and 1%, respectively.[32] Gross inspection of post-rheumatic mitral valve disease is sufficient for diagnostic purposes, but histology should be performed if endocarditis is suspected.

At autopsy, severe mitral stenosis is associated with marked left atrial dilatation (Fig. 7–4*B*) with or without right ventricular hypertrophy and right atrial dilatation (secondary to pulmonary hypertension). The left ventricular cavity size is small with normal wall thickness because the left ventricle is "protected" from increased pressure by the stenotic mitral valve. Severe right ventricular pressure overload results in flattening of the interventricular septum so that the left ventricular cavity has a "D"-shaped configuration (Fig. 7–4*A*). In patients with significant mitral regurgitation, the left ventricular and left atrial cavities are dilated, the extent of which is dependent upon the severity of mitral incompetence.[40] A focal area of left atrial endocardial thickening (MaCallum's patch) represents a regurgitant jet lesion. If there is concurrent aortic stenosis, left ventricular hypertrophy is present. For the surgical pathologist, the submitted specimen consists of either the anterior leaflet (with or without portion of the posterior leaflet) or the entire mitral valve (Fig. 7–4*D*).

Aging Changes and Mitral Annular Calcification

At birth, the mitral leaflets are translucent, gelatinous and transmit light, but become opaque after the age of 20. The anterior leaflet is opaque and fibrotic and heavily infiltrated with lipids by age 50. By the age of 70, the lines of closure along both mitral leaflets are thickened and nodular, and annular calcification is often present. Mitral annular calcification is frequently seen in earlier ages in patients with Marfan syndrome, myxomatous degeneration of the mitral valve, end-stage renal disease with secondary hyperparathyroidism, and the Hurler syndrome. Risk factors for coronary atherosclerosis—hypertension, hyperlipidemia, and diabetes mellitus—are also associated with mitral annular calcification.[41]

Mitral annular calcification is found at autopsy in 10% of individuals dying after the age of 50 years. In most cases, annular calcification is an incidental finding; however, when severe, it may be responsible for significant mitral regurgitation. Calcification remains localized to the mitral annulus in 77% of cases[42] and is more common in women.[41] Annular calcification is especially common in patients with end-stage renal disease;[43] in these individuals, calcification may be severe, extend into the body of the valve leaflets and/or left atrium and ventricle, and cause mitral stenosis. Over 50% of patients with severe mitral annular calcification have involvement of the aortic valve, but rarely does it lead to aortic stenosis. In the elderly, echocardiographic evidence of mitral annular calcification is associated with a twofold increase in the incidence of stroke.[44]

Pathologically, annular calcification develops between the mitral valve cusp and the ventricular wall (Figs. 7–5*A* and 7–5*B*). The severity of calcification ranges from mild, with focal small calcific deposits, to severe with large calcific nodules involving the entire annulus projecting into the left ventricular cavity or as spurs which project into the left ventricular posterolateral basal wall. Calcification involves more than one third of the annulus in 88% of patients, the posterior annulus alone in 10.5%, and the whole annulus in 1.5%.[42] The calcification extends into the myocardium in 12% of patients and into the papillary muscles in 4.5%.[42] When severe annular calcification causes significant mitral stenosis (Figs. 7–5*C* and 7–5*D*), valve replacement is indicated. Occasionally large calcified areas may become semisolid and necrotic and may mimic an annular abscess cavity when seen by echocardiography. Gross examination alone is sufficient to establish a diagnosis of mitral annular calcification. Left atrial dilatation is present in cases of significant mitral regurgitation (or stenosis).

Ischemic Mitral Regurgitation

Mitral regurgitation is present in 30% of patients with coronary artery atherosclerosis who are being considered for coronary bypass surgery.[45,46] The regurgitation is mild in most cases; however, chronic severe regurgitation secondary to coronary atherosclerosis is associated with a poor prognosis. Ischemic mitral regurgitation is more common in men, secondary to the higher prevalence of ischemic heart disease in males. Chronic ischemic mitral regurgitation occurs as a result of papillary muscle dysfunction, mitral annular dilatation, or both. In contrast, the mechanism of acute severe mitral regurgitation is infarction and rupture of a papillary muscle, a mechanical complication of acute myocardial infarction. Either the entire papillary muscle may rupture or only one of the muscle heads. Acute papillary muscle rupture occurs in 0.9–5% of patients dying after acute myocardial infarction and typically occurs between days 2 to 5 following acute myocardial infarction. This serious complication is often fatal with 50% of patients dying within 24 hours and 80% within 14 days.[47]

The posteromedial papillary muscle has a single blood supply from the posterior descending coronary artery and is more susceptible to ischemic injury than the anterolateral papillary muscle, which has a dual blood supply from diagonal branches (from the left anterior descending coronary artery) and marginal

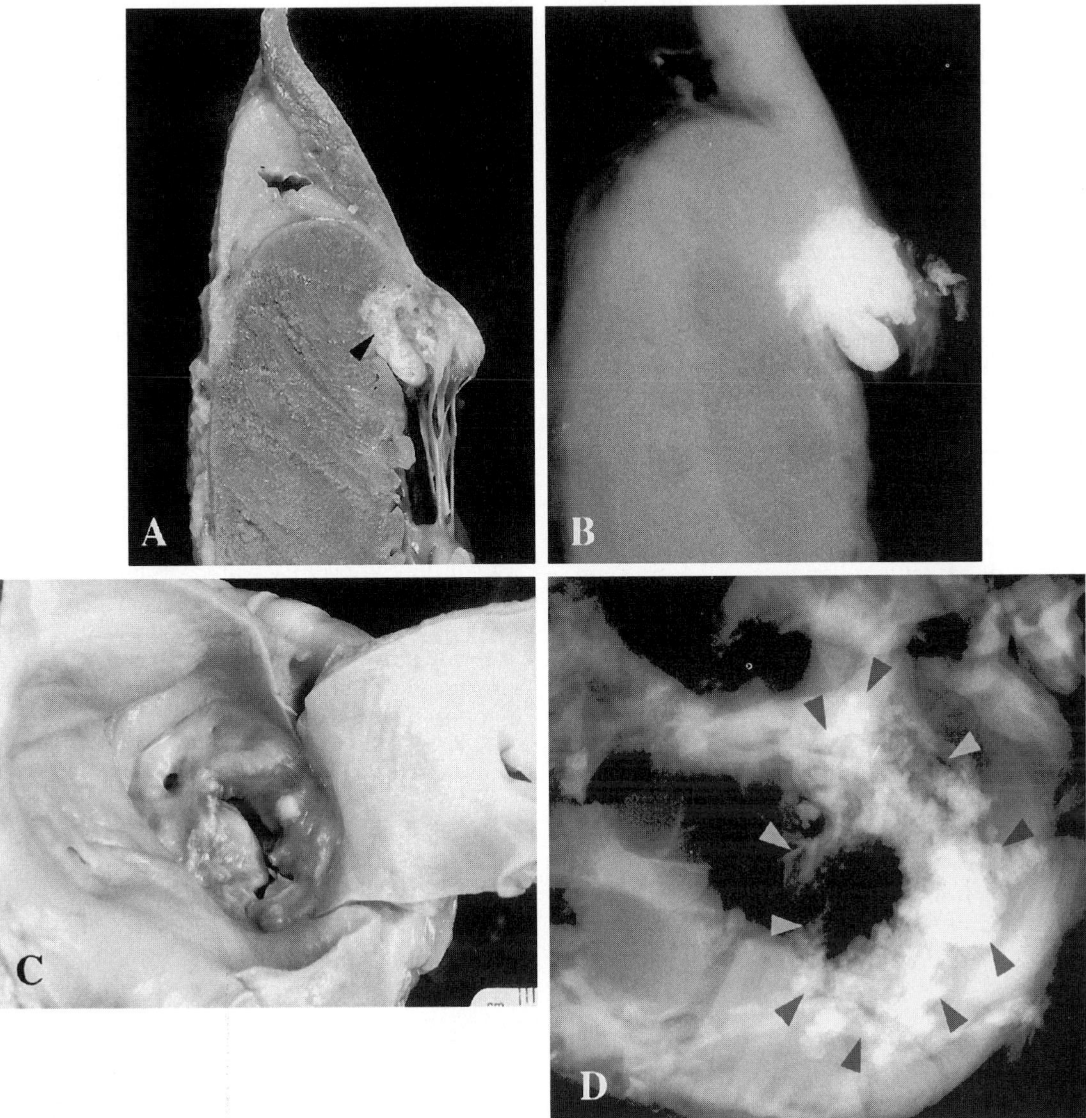

Figure 7–5. Mitral annular calcification. Heavy calcification of the mitral annulus is present at the insertion of the posterior mitral leaflet (*arrowhead:* gross photo, *A;* corresponding radiograph, *B*). Heart from a 51-year-old woman with diabetes mellitus, end-stage renal disease, and hypertension with severe mitral stenosis secondary to annular calcification (*C* and *D*). Note calcific nodules focally erupting through the atrial endocardium around the stenotic mitral orifice (*C*). A small perforation in the anterior mitral leaflet is present. A postmortem radiograph (*D*) of the heart in *C* shows marked mitral annular calcification (*arrowheads*) that extends almost circumferentially around the annulus. (*A* and *B* from Farb A, Virmani R, Burke AP. Pathogenesis and pathology of valvular heart disease. In: Alpert JS, Dalen JE, Rahimtoola SH (eds): Valvular Heart Disease, p 11. Philadelphia: Lippincott Williams & Wilkins, 2000, with permission.)

branches (from the left circumflex coronary artery). While papillary muscle dysfunction is most frequently seen in the setting of ischemic heart disease, it can also result from shock, severe anemia, coronary arteritis, anomalous coronary arteries, abscess formation, congenital malposition of the papillary muscles, and infiltration of the papillary muscles by sarcoidosis, neoplasms, and amyloid deposits. Mitral annular dilatation, secondary to myocardial infarction or dilated cardiomyopathy, results in the alteration of the anatomic relationship among the papillary muscles and the chordae tendineae resulting in progressive mitral regurgitation.

Because the pathologic findings are in the papillary muscles, the valve leaflets and the chordae tendineae are usually unremarkable except for age-related changes. In surgical pathology specimens from patients with chronic regurgitation that contain the papillary muscle, the muscle is atrophic and scarred in patients with chronic regurgitation. In papillary muscle rupture from acute ischemic injury, myocyte coagulation necrosis is present, and platelets and fibrin line the ruptured papillary muscle surface. Histologic examination is recommended to confirm myocardial scarring in chronic regurgitation and acute infarction in papillary muscle rupture. In autopsy cases, one sees healed infarction of one or both papillary muscles in chronic regurgitation cases (Fig. 7–6). There is associated transmural healed myocardial infarction with left atrial and left ventricular dilatation secondary to mitral regurgitation. In acute papillary muscle rupture involving the posteromedial papillary muscle (Fig. 7–6), an acute subendocardial or transmural posterior myocardial infarction is present. The infarction need not be extensive and can be localized to the region of the papillary muscle. Neither the left atrium nor the left ventricle is dilated as the mitral regurgitation is acute.

Surgical treatment of ischemic mitral regurgitation typically consists of resection of the entire valve or just the anterior mitral leaflet.[45, 46] Papillary muscle reimplantation, annuloplasty, chordal shortening, and leaflet resection have also been utilized to treat acute and chronic ischemic mitral regurgitation.[48–50]

Tricuspid Valve

Anatomy of the Tricuspid Valve

Tricuspid valve structure is the most variable of the four cardiac valves. The tricuspid valve normally measures 10 to 12.5 cm in circumference and consists of three leaflets—an anterior, septal, and posterior leaflets—each separated from one another by commissures. However, the size of the septal leaflet is highly variable, and the septal leaflet is often rudimentary or absent without any clinical consequences.[51] The septal leaflet forms a useful landmark, because just above its insertion in the right atrium lies the atrioventricular node, and the membranous septum lies on its most anterior insertion. The anterior leaflet is the largest of the three tricuspid leaflets; it is suspended across the anterior wall of the right ventricular cavity and separates the inflow portion of the right ventricle from the outflow. The chordae tendineae from the anterior and the posterior leaflets attach to a large single anterior papillary muscle that arises from the anterior free wall of the right ventricle and fuses with the moderator band. Several small posterior papillary muscles are attached to the posterior wall into which insert the chordae tendineae from the posterior and the septal leaflets. Chordae from the septal and anterior leaflet insert either into the small septal papillary muscles or directly into the ventricular

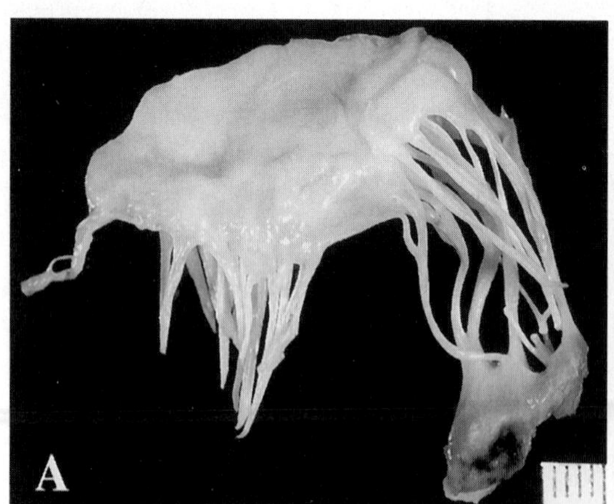

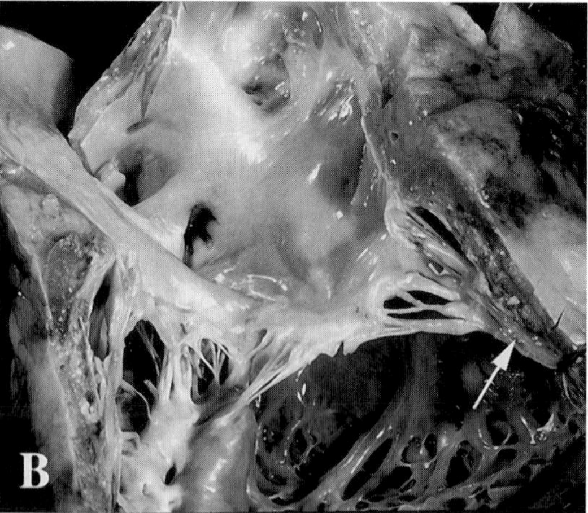

Figure 7–6. Ischemic mitral valve disease. A 65-year-old man presented with an acute inferior myocardial infarction with acute mitral regurgitation secondary to the rupture of the posteromedial papillary muscle. The anterior mitral leaflet (*A*) with its ruptured and infarcted papillary muscle was excised. Chronic mitral regurgitation and congestive heart failure secondary to healed posterior wall myocardial infarction was present in this 60-year-old man (*B*). Note scarred and thinned posterior papillary muscle (*arrow*) and left atrial dilatation. (From Farb A, Virmani R, Burke AP. Pathogenesis and pathology of valvular heart disease. In: Alpert JS, Dalen JE, Rahimtoola SH (eds): Valvular Heart Disease, p11. Philadelphia: Lippincott Williams & Wilkins, 2000, with permission.)

septum. The histologic valve layers are similar to the mitral valve.

Post-Rheumatic Tricuspid Valve Disease

Post-rheumatic tricuspid valve disease is uncommon. Of the 543 autopsy cases of rheumatic heart disease reported by Roberts and Virmani, significant tricuspid valve stenosis occurred in eight cases (2%) and was only seen in the presence of mitral and aortic valve stenosis. Overall, some degree of tricuspid valve involvement was seen in 64 cases (12%).[32] While post-rheumatic scarring is the most frequent cause of pure tricuspid valve stenosis, post-rheumatic tricuspid scarring most often results in valvular regurgitation. Of 363 surgically excised tricuspid valves studied by Hauck et. al., post-rheumatic disease was observed in 194 (53%); of these, pure tricuspid valve stenosis was seen in 3% of cases, tricuspid stenosis and regurgitation in 41%, and tricuspid regurgitation in 56%.[52] All 194 cases with post-rheumatic tricuspid valve disease had concurrent mitral valve disease, with 68% having combined mitral stenosis and incompetence, 26% with pure mitral stenosis, and 12% with pure mitral incompetence.

Pathologically, post-rheumatic tricuspid valve disease consists of leaflet thickening and fusion of one or more commissures (Fig. 7–7). Chordal thickening and fusion are usually less pronounced than in the mitral valve. The severity of leaflet fibrosis and retraction, together with presence or absence of commissural fusion, determines whether the tricuspid valve will be incompetent, stenotic, or both. Commissural fusion is present in all cases of pure tricuspid stenosis, 95% of cases with stenosis and regurgitation, and 51% of cases with pure tricuspid regurgitation. Leaflet calcification is uncommon in post-rheumatic tricuspid valve disease. Gross inspection is sufficient to establish a diagnosis, especially if typical post-rheumatic mitral or aortic valve lesions are present. In autopsy cases, right atrial dilatation is present.

Other uncommon causes of tricuspid valve stenosis include tricuspid atresia, right atrial tumors, methysergide therapy, and carcinoid heart disease (discussed later).

Tricuspid Valve Insufficiency

Tricuspid insufficiency is much more common than tricuspid stenosis, and in adults, most commonly occurs secondary to left ventricular failure (secondary to ischemic heart disease or any left-sided valve disease), cardiomyopathy, right ventricular infarction, or primary lung disease. In cases of secondary tricuspid insufficiency, the mechanism of regurgitation is tricuspid annular dilatation; the tricuspid valve itself is structurally unremarkable except for focal fibrous leaflet thickening. In autopsy cases,

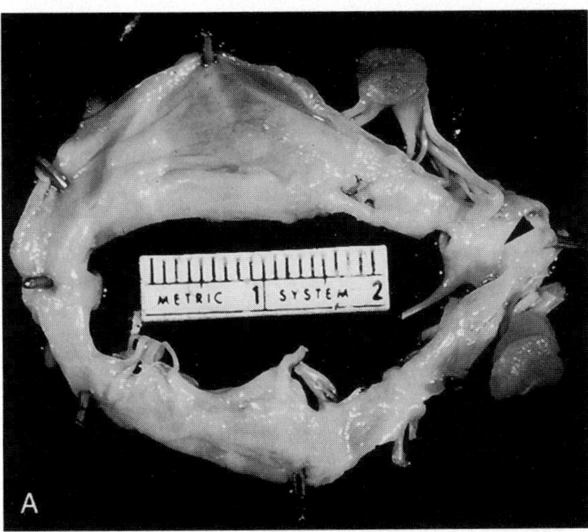

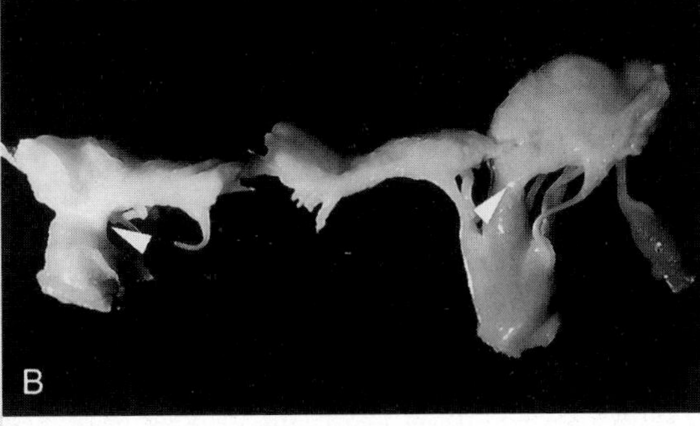

Figure 7–7. Post-rheumatic tricuspid valve scarring. Surgically removed tricuspid valve (*A*) from a patient who also underwent mitral and aortic valve replacement for mitral and aortic stenosis secondary to chronic rheumatic valvular disease. Note thickened, rolled free margins of the valve leaflets and commissural fusion (*arrowhead*). Diffuse tricuspid leaflet thickening with shortened, fused, and thickened chordae (*arrowheads*) is evident in *B*. (From Farb A, Virmani R, Burke AP. Pathogenesis and pathology of valvular heart disease. In: Alpert JS, Dalen JE, Rahimtoola SH (eds): Valvular Heart Disease, p13. Philadelphia: Lippincott Williams & Wilkins, 2000, with permission.)

there is associated right atrial and right ventricular dilatation.

Primary, intrinsic tricuspid valve lesions that are associated with regurgitation include post-rheumatic scarring (discussed earlier), Ebstein's anomaly (discussed below), infective endocarditis[53] (discussed below), valvular clefts as part of the atrioventricular canal defect, papillary muscle dysfunction secondary to infarction, trauma, endomyocardial fibrosis, hypereosinophilic syndrome (discussed below), post-radiation,[54] rheumatoid arthritis,[55] and right ventricular pacemakers. The presence of severe tricuspid regurgitation in patients with rheumatic mitral stenosis is associated with a poor prognosis (35% event-free survival at 4 years).[56] In the surgical series of excised tricuspid valves reported by Hauck et. al., pure tricuspid incompetence was present in 269 (74%), and the underlying etiology was post-rheumatic in 109 (41%), Ebstein's anomaly in 38 (14%), congenital dysplasia or annular dilatation in 49 (18%), pulmonary venous hypertension in 56 (21%), infective endocarditis in 11 (4%), carcinoid syndrome in 2, trauma in 1, iatrogenic damage in 1, and indeterminate causes in 2.[52] Tricuspid valve surgery is relatively uncommon, and surgical approaches have included valve replacement (mechanical and bioprostheses), valve repair, and annuloplasty.[57, 58]

Ebstein's Anomaly

An uncommon congenital abnormality, Ebstein's anomaly accounts for < 1% of congenital heart defects.[59] The pathologic features of Ebstein's anomaly can be divided into anomalies of the valve and abnormalities of the right ventricle.[60] There is downward displacement of the tricuspid valve towards the right ventricle so that part of the right ventricle becomes a functional part of the right atrium (i.e., atrialization) (Fig. 7–8). Mild atrialization may be present in which the downward displacement of the septal and posterior leaflets results in a relatively normal tricuspid valve orifice. Usually, mild tricuspid regurgitation is present, and occasionally, Ebstein's anomaly may go undetected into adulthood. In the most severe form of Ebstein's anomaly, the septal leaflet is plastered to the septum, the posterior leaflet is plastered to the posterior ventricular wall, and the anterior leaflet is enlarged and abnormally attached to a muscular shelf which separates the inlet of the ventricle from the trabecular portion.[61] The anterior leaflet may be large and "sail-like," and the valve cusps may not separate forming a diaphragm with small peripheral openings resulting in a stenotic orifice.

As a result of the downward displacement of the tricuspid valve, the right ventricle becomes divided into an atrialized chamber and a distal "true" ventricular chamber. The proximal right ventricular chamber may be larger or smaller than the distal chamber depending on the extent of downward displacement of the tricuspid valve. The endocardium of the atrialized portion of the right ventricle is usually fibrotic, with poorly developed trabeculations. Often, there is aneurysmal dilatation of the fibrotic posterior wall, which may be devoid of myocytes. The distal true ventricular chamber is located behind the anterior tricuspid valve leaflet. Right ventricular dilatation is present in a majority of cases.

Ebstein's anomaly may exist as an isolated finding, but associated congenital cardiac defects are common including membranous ventricular septal defects, atrial septal defects, and pulmonary stenosis or atresia (with an intact ventricular septum). In patients surviving beyond infancy, exercise intolerance and cyanosis may be observed as a result of right ventricular dysfunction, tricuspid valve insufficiency, and right-to-left shunting.[62]

Myxomatous Degeneration of the Tricuspid Valve (Tricuspid Valve Prolapse)

The morphology of myxomatous degeneration of the tricuspid valve is identical to that found in myxomatous degeneration of the mitral valve. Grossly, there is ballooning and redundancy of leaflet tissue with variable increased lengthening of chordae tendineae. Prolapse most commonly involves the anterior tricuspid valve leaflet, less frequently the septal leaflet, and rarely the posterior leaflet. Histologic findings are similar to those seen in myxomatous degeneration of the mitral valve.

The prevalence of myxomatous degeneration of the tricuspid valve is estimated to be between 0.1% and 5.5% and is found in approximately 37% (range 3–54%) of patients with myxomatous degeneration of the mitral valve;[63] isolated tricuspid valve prolapse is much less frequent.[64] Tricuspid regurgitation is the most frequent physiologic abnormality, is usually mild, and does not correlate with the severity of the prolapse. In surgically excised valves, it may be difficult to make the diagnosis of tricuspid valve prolapse, and therefore one may have to rely

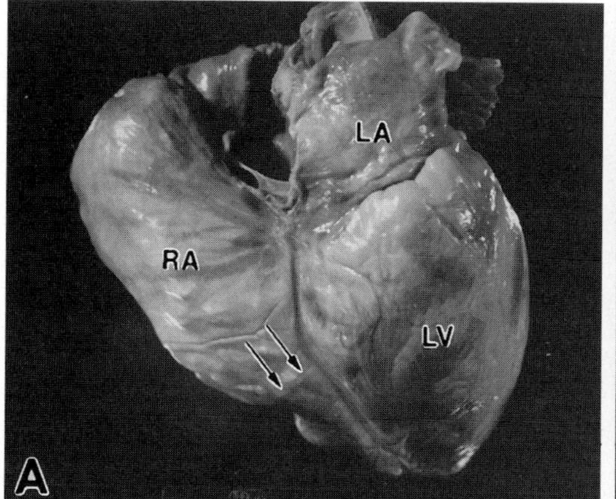

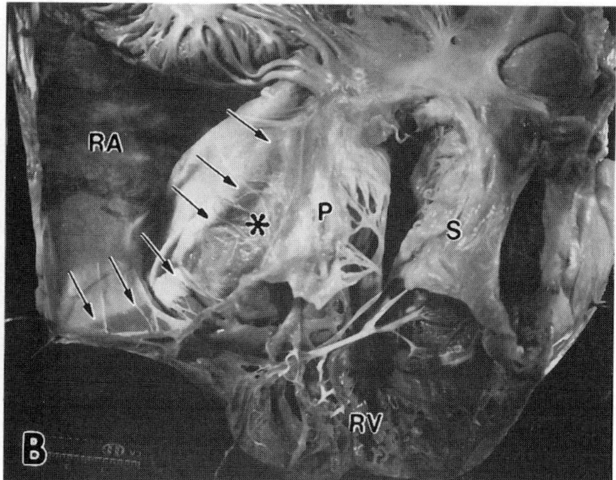

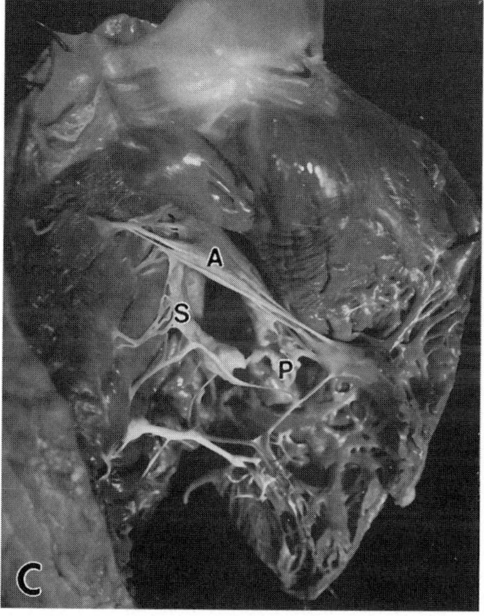

Figure 7–8. Ebstein's anomaly in a 31-year-old man who died suddenly. Posterior surface of the heart (*A*) demonstrates right atrial (*RA*) dilatation, downward displacement of the functional atrioventricular groove (*arrows*) separating the RA (plus atrialized right ventricle) from the distal right ventricle. LA = left atrium, LV = left ventricle. The opened right atrium (*RA*) and right ventricle (*RV*) are shown in *B;* there is downward displacement of the posterior and septal tricuspid leaflets. A portion of the atrialized RV (*) is highlighted (*arrows*). The right ventricular outflow tract with the large anterior tricuspid leaflet (*A*) is shown in *C.* P = posterior leaflet, S = septal leaflet. (From Farb A, Burke AP, Virmani R. Anatomy and pathology of the right ventricle (including acquired tricuspid and pulmonic valve disease). Cardiology Clinics 10 (1):15, 1992, with permission.)

on clinical data (echocardiographic imaging) and the finding of enlarged tricuspid annulus. If the valve area were to be measured, it would be much larger than that of a normal valve or in regurgitant tricuspid valves secondary to ischemic heart disease or pulmonary hypertension. In the series by Hauck et al., tricuspid valve prolapse was not encountered among the surgically excised tricuspid valves.[52] Tricuspid valve prolapse may be a marker of more extensive organ involvement in patients with Marfan syndrome. Additionally, in patients with myxomatous degeneration of the mitral valve, tricuspid valve prolapse is more common in women (3:1 ratio), tend to be older and, more symptomatic, may identify a subset of patients who have a relatively worse prognosis than those in whom the tricuspid valve is normal.[63]

SEMILUNAR VALVES

Aortic Valve

Anatomy of the Aortic Valve

The aortic valve is comprised of three semicircular cusps (left, right, and posterior [noncoronary] cusps) attached to the aorta (Fig. 7–9*A*). The cusps and sinuses of Valsalva are generally equal-sized but mild asymmetry (> 5% difference from the average cusp area) of two or all three cusps may be present in normally functioning valves.[65–67] The commissures are the narrow spaces between each adjacent cusp where they attach to the aorta (three per normal semilunar valve). The line of demarcation between the sinuses of Valsalva and ascending aorta is referred to as the sinotubular junction, which

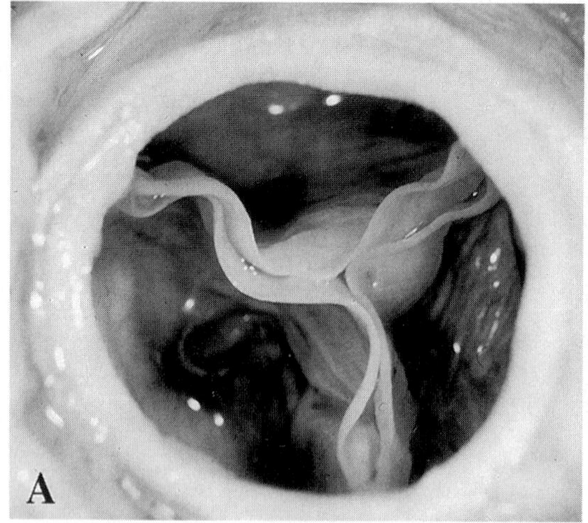

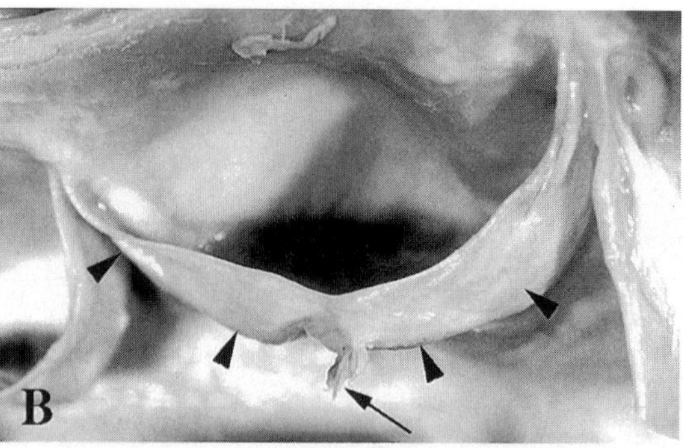

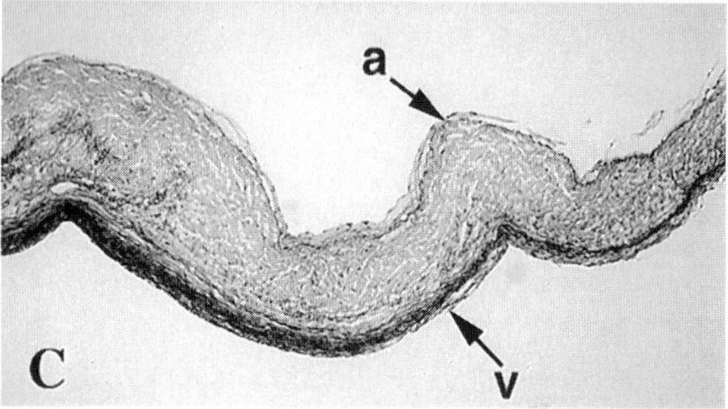

Figure 7–9. Normal aortic valve. The three valve cusps (*A*) show complete coaptation with minor variability of the cusp sizes and three open (nonfused) commissures. An individual aortic valve cusp is shown in *B*. The line of valve closure (*arrowheads*) is below the free edge, and a centrally placed nodule of Arantii with Lambl's excrescence (*arrowhead*) is present. Histologically (*C*, Movat pentachrome stain), the ventricular surface (*v*) has a black-staining elastic layer, a loose connective tissue layer containing proteoglycans, and a dense collagenous layer that extends toward the aortic surface (*a*). (From Farb A, Virmani R, Burke AP. Pathogenesis and pathology of valvular heart disease. In: Alpert JS, Dalen JE, Rahimtoola SH (eds): Valvular Heart Disease, p15. Philadelphia: Lippincott Williams & Wilkins, 2000, with permission.)

is defined as the line joining the superior margin of the three commissures.[68] In the aortic valve, there is a linear relationship among increased cusp area and sinus of Valsalva volume with increased patient age, heart weight, and aortic area at the sinotubular junction.[67] The line of closure of the semilunar valves (aortic and pulmonary) is just below the free edge (Fig. 7–9*B*), the center of which contains a small fibrous nodule (noduli Arantii) from which thin fibrous projections often arise (Lambl's excrescence). The vast majority of fenestrations in the valve cusps have no functional significance because they are above the line of cusp apposition during closure. The histologic structure of the aortic valve cusps (Fig. 7–9*C*) consists of a fibroelastic layer on the ventricular surface (ventricularis), proteoglycan-rich connective tissue in the mid-portion of the cusp, dense collagen extending toward the aortic surface, and a thin fibroelastic layer on the aortic surface (arterialis). The distal two thirds of the semilunar valve cusps are avascular.[68]

Aortic Stenosis

Aortic valve lesions that cause stenosis may be classified as congenital lesions (e.g., unicuspid or bicuspid valves), postinflammatory scarring (usually post-rheumatic), or degenerative changes (e.g., senile calcific aortic stenosis) (Table 7–5). The age at presentation generally correlates with underlying pathologic lesion.[65] Unicuspid aortic stenosis presents in childhood, adolescence, and early adulthood and accounts for only 4–6% of aortic stenosis in older adults. In contrast, in aortic stenosis secondary to congenitally bicuspid valves, patients usually present in fifth and sixth decades. Congenital bicuspid stenotic aortic valves account for 50% of surgical valve replacements in adult patients < 70 years old.[69] In patients ≥ 70 years old, senile tricuspid calcific aortic stenosis is responsible for nearly 50% of surgical valve replacements.[69] With the aging of the general population in the United States and the decline in the incidence of rheumatic fever, the frequency of aortic valve surgery for senile calcific aortic stenosis has increased and the frequency of postinflammatory aortic valve scarring has decreased.[70–72]

The normal aortic orifice valve area is > 2.0 cm^2. A valve area of 1.5–2.0 cm^2 is considered mild aortic stenosis, 0.8–1.5 cm^2 corresponds to moderate stenosis, and < 0.8 cm^2 corre-

Table 7–5. Surgical Pathology of Aortic Stenosis

Etiology	Mayo Clinic (1965)	University of Minnesota (1979–1983)	London (1976–1979)	Mayo Clinic (1990)	AFIP (1990–1997)
Bicuspid	49%	49%	56%	36%	30%
Post-rheumatic	33%	23%	24%	9%	13%
Degenerative	0%	28%	12%	51%	49%
Unicuspid	10%	1%	0%	0%	6%
Other	7%	0%	8%	2%	2%

From Farb A, Virmani R, Burke AP. Pathogenesis and pathology of valvular heart disease. In: Alpert JS, Dalen JE, Rahimtoola SH (eds): Valvular Heart Disease, p 16. Philadelphia: Lippincott Williams & Wilkins, 2000, with permission.

sponds to severe stenosis. The rate of progression from mild to severe stenosis is highly variable among individual patients.[73] In serial cardiac catheterization studies, the presence and extent of aortic valve calcification on initial study was associated with a more rapid progression toward severe aortic stenosis.[74] Despite the presence of severe aortic stenosis suggested by cardiac catheterization or echocardiography, patients may remain asymptomatic for years and require no specific therapy. However, the appearance of cardiovascular symptoms (syncope, cardiac angina, dyspnea, and/or heart failure) in patients with severe aortic stenosis is associated with increased mortality, and valve replacement is indicated irrespective of the underlying valve morphology.[75–77] Even in elderly individuals, quality of life and survival improve following aortic valve replacement once symptoms appear. However, there is no role for prophylactic aortic valve replacement in asymptomatic patients with severe aortic stenosis.[78] It is uncertain whether individuals undergoing coronary artery bypass surgery should undergo simultaneous prophylactic aortic valve replacement if moderate aortic stenosis is present.[77]

Patients who are at increased risk for accelerated calcification of otherwise normal tricuspid aortic valves leading to stenosis include those with disorders of calcium and phosphate metabolism (e.g., end-stage renal disease with dialysis treatment, primary hyperparathyroidism) and abnormalities of bone metabolism (e.g., Paget's disease).[73] Irrespective of the valve morphology, severe aortic stenosis results in a pressure-overloaded left ventricle characterized by concentric left ventricular hypertrophy without dilatation.

Morphology of Aortic Stenosis

Congenital Unicuspid Aortic Valve

Unicuspid aortic valves can be categorized as one of two morphologic subtypes: (1) a domed-shaped acommissural valve containing three aborted commissures (or raphes); or (2) a unicommissural valve with slit-like opening ("exclamation point" orifice) that reaches the aortic wall at its single intact commissure with two raphes present (Figs. 7–10*A* and 7–10*B*). Leaflet dysplasia is common, and the severity of cusp calcification is variable and typically increases following commissurotomy.

Unicommissural unicuspid aortic valves account for 60% of aortic stenosis cases in patients < 15 years old.[79] A pathologic diagnosis of congenital unicuspid aortic valve can be made with gross evaluation alone. Patients with congenital unicuspid valves are at increased risk for infective endocarditis and aortic dissection.

Congenital Bicuspid Aortic Valve (Stenotic and Nonstenotic Variants)

Congenital bicuspid aortic valves are very common (present in 1–2% of general population with a male to female ratio of 1.4–4 to 1), and are the most frequent cause of aortic stenosis in the 50- to 70-year-old age group. Familial studies suggest that congenital bicuspid aortic valves follow autosomal dominant inheritance patterns with reduced penetrance.[80] While some congenital bicuspid aortic valves do not progress to severe stenosis and function normally, valvular stenosis is the most frequent physiologic complication, affecting approximately 80% of valves studied at autopsy[79] or post-valve replacement.[81] Ten percent of congenital bicuspid aortic valves are surgically excised for combined stenosis and insufficiency.[81] Postinflammatory (post-rheumatic) scarring superimposed on a congenital bicuspid valve is associated with an earlier age of presentation for surgical intervention.[82] Aortic root dilatation is associated with normally and abnormally functioning congenital bicuspid aortic valves. Increased aortic cystic medial change, elastic

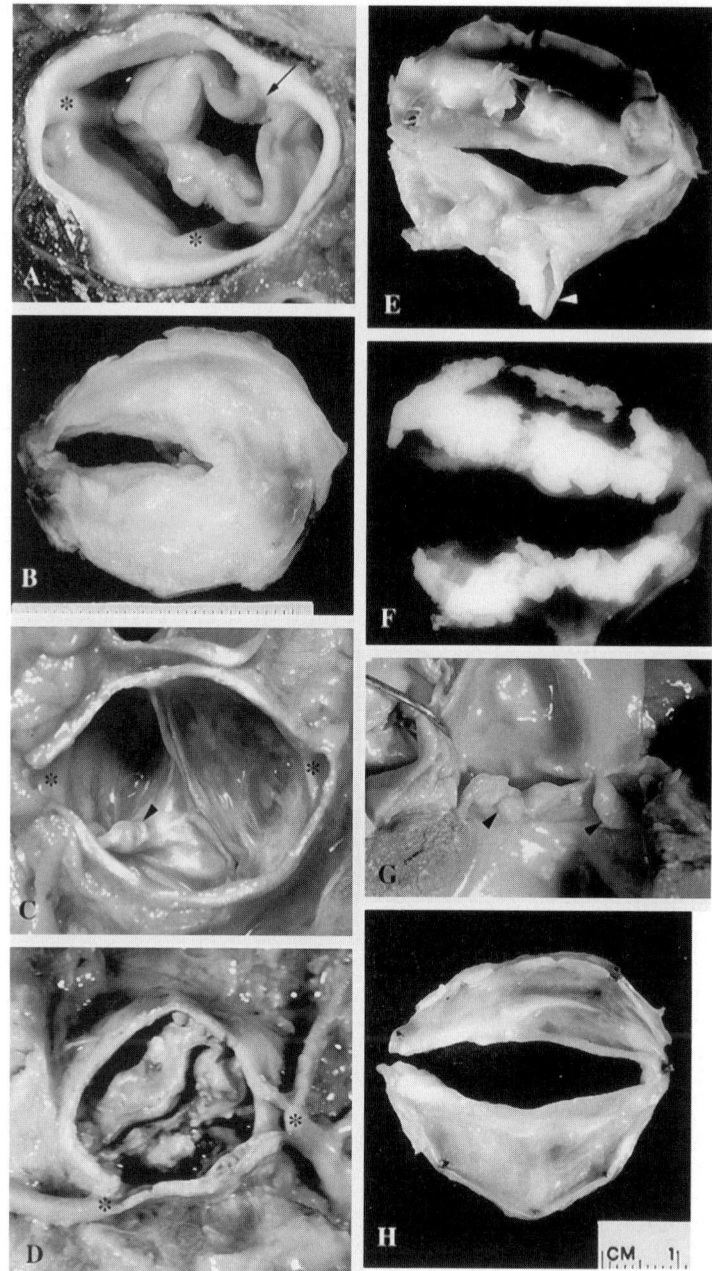

Figure 7–10. Unicuspid and bicuspid aortic valve pathology. Stenotic unicuspid dysplastic aortic valve (*A*) from a 19-year-old woman who died suddenly while dancing. Note the eccentric valve orifice, single commissure (*arrow*), and thickened dysplastic leaflet with rudimentary raphae (*). Surgically excised stenotic congenital unicuspid, unicommissural aortic valve (*B*) with dysplastic leaflet and eccentric valve orifice (''exclamation point''). A nonstenotic, functional normal, mildly calcified congenitally bicuspid valve is shown in *C*. A median raphe is present (*arrowhead*) in the right cusp, and the commissures are located anterior and posteriorly. Coronary arteries are indicated (*). The more typical location of the cusps and commissures in a congenital bicuspid stenotic aortic valve is demonstrated in *D*. The commissures are placed right and left and both the coronary arteries (*) arise from the anterior sinus. Severe cusp calcification is present which obscures the raphe. Surgically excised stenotic congenitally bicuspid aortic valve (*E* with corresponding radiograph *F*) with marked calcification and median raphe (*arrowhead*). A bicuspid dysplastic aortic valve in a child with congenital aortic stenosis is shown in *G* consisting of two thickened and gelatinous cusps (*arrowheads*). Pure aortic insufficiency with a bicuspid valve is presented in *H*. Note the increased annular circumference, nonspecific cusp fibrosis, most pronounced near the line of valve closure, and absence of valve calcification. (*A* from Valvular Heart Disease, p 1.3. Shahbudin H. Rahimtoola (volume ed.). Volume XI of Atlas of Heart Diseases. Eugene Braunwald (series ed.). St. Louis: Mosby, 1997, with permission.) (*B* from Virmani R, Burke AP, Farb A. Atlas of Cardiovascular Pathology, p 53. Philadelphia: W.B. Saunders Co., 1996, with permission.) (*C–H* from Farb A, Virmani R, Burke AP. Pathogenesis and pathology of valvular heart disease. In: Alpert JS, Dalen JE, Rahimtoola SH (eds): Valvular Heart Disease, p18. Philadelphia: Lippincott Williams & Wilkins, 2000, with permission.)

fiber fragmentation, and abnormal smooth muscle cell orientation have been described.[83,84] Similar to patients with unicuspid aortic valves, individuals with congenital bicuspid aortic valves are at increased risk for aortic dissection[85] and infective endocarditis. Interestingly, bicuspid valves with normal function or only mild dysfunction are at greater risk for infective endocarditis compared with calcified stenotic bicuspid valves.[86]

In the most common morphology of congenitally bicuspid aortic valves, there are two cusps of unequal size with the larger conjoint cusp located anteriorly within the aortic root (approximately 80% of excised stenotic bicuspid valves)[81,87] and the smaller cusp found posteriorly; less commonly, the right and noncoronary cusps are conjoint (Fig. 7–10*C*), and the rarest morphology is a conjoint left and noncoronary cusp.[87–89] In the most common form, both the left main and right coronary arteries arise from the sinus of Valsalva of the anterior conjoint cusp (Fig. 7–10*D*). The size of the conjoint cusp is less than two times the size of the nonconjoint cusp, and contains a median raphe (aborted third commissure) in approximately 75% of cases of surgically excised valves.[87] In most cases, the raphe does not reach the free (closing) edge of the conjoint cusp, and there is no evidence of prior separation into two cusp margins (best appreciated by viewing the valve from ventricular aspect). The raphe usually inserts into the aorta below the level of the other two commissures.

Dystrophic calcification begins in the raphe, if present, and extends into the cusp tissue. Severe aortic stenosis secondary to a bicuspid aortic valve is characterized by calcification extending into the tissue of the conjoint and nonconjoint cusps, and calcific nodules may ulcerate the cusp surface (Figs. 7–10*D* to 7–10*F*). When young individuals present with symptomatic stenotic congenital bicuspid valves, the cusps are typically thickened and dysplastic (Fig. 7–10*G*). Unless endocarditis is suspected, a gross diagnosis of a congenital bicuspid valve is sufficient.

Variations of the raphe in congenitally bicuspid aortic valves include raphal ridges that reach the free margin of the cusp and partial separation of the raphe into cusp margins. Sometimes, raphal variants can cause problems in deciding whether a congenitally bicuspid valve is present versus an acquired bicuspid valve (e.g., postinflammatory fusion of one of the three commissures). In cases in which it is difficult to distinguish a congenitally bicuspid valve from an acquired (postinflammatory) bicuspid valve, histologic examination of the median raphe or area of commissural fusion may be performed. A raphe in a congenitally bicuspid valve is rich in elastic fibers; nonelastic fibrous tissue is observed in fused commissures secondary to postinflammatory scarring. However, the sensitivity of this approach is limited because severe raphal calcification may destroy the elastic tissue. Another congenital bicuspid valve variant, accounting for 6% of surgically excised bicuspid aortic valves in one series,[90] is a fenestrated raphe consisting of a fibrous chord of varying thickness that extends from the sinus wall to the free cusp edge. This morphology may be particularly difficult to distinguish by echocardiographic imaging.[90] Occasionally, the bicuspid valve is composed of two cusps of equal size with no median raphe.

Senile Calcific Aortic Stenosis

The most frequent indication for isolated aortic valve replacement, senile calcific aortic stenosis is more common in men than women (male : female is 1.6 : 1). Calcification begins and accumulates in the base of the cusps on the aortic aspect and extends superiorly towards the mid-portion of the cusp with sparing of the free margin (closing edge) (Figs. 7–11*A* to 7–11*C*). Calcification is typically more pronounced in the noncoronary cusp compared with the coronary cusps. The mechanism for this finding may involve the relatively reduced diastolic pressure loads imparted on the coronary cusps due to the presence of the coronary ostia.[91] Typically, nodular calcific deposits are superimposed on a fibrotic cusp.[92] In contrast, calcification occurs diffusely within the cusp spongiosa in congenital bicuspid valve stenosis.[92] Commissural fusion typically is absent in senile calcific aortic stenosis unless there has been an associated inflammatory or infectious disorder. Like congenital unicuspid and bicuspid valves, gross inspection is sufficient for a diagnosis of senile calcific aortic stenosis.

The pathogenesis of calcification of tricuspid aortic valves is uncertain. Mild asymmetry of valve cusps has been suggested as a potential precipitant of the calcification process;[65,66] however, the high prevalence of minor differences in cusp size (> 50% in individuals) makes it unlikely that isolated cusp asymmetry is sufficient to account for severe stenosis in most cases. Calcification is commonly seen in atherosclerotic coronary arteries, and an association

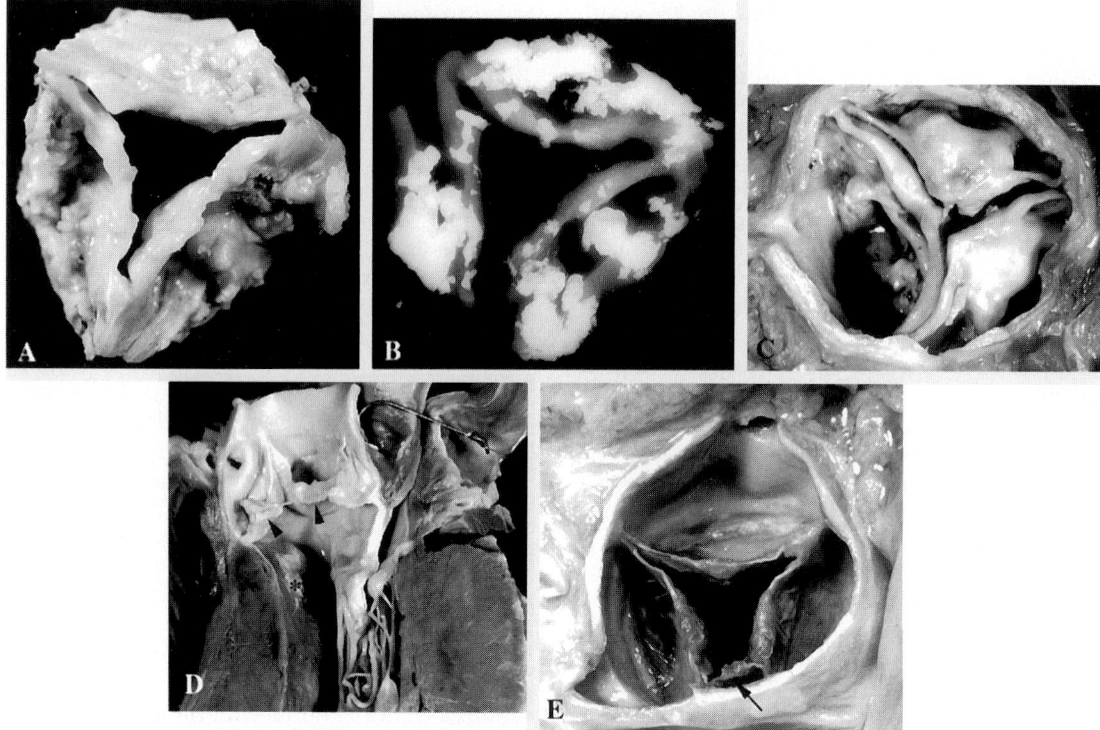

Figure 7–11. A surgically excised stenotic tricuspid aortic valve (*A* with corresponding radiograph in *B*) viewed from the aortic aspect shows nodular calcification which is marked in the cusps and not at the commissures. Tricuspid degenerative aortic valve stenosis (senile calcific aortic stenosis) in an 81-year-old man who died suddenly (*C*). At autopsy, left ventricular hypertrophy was present (heart weight 675 gm). Large nodular calcific deposits are present on the aortic surface of the valve cusps extending in the sinuses of Valsalva; the free edges of the valve cusps are relatively spared. Chronic aortic regurgitation secondary to aortic valve prolapse is shown in *D*. There is fibro-myxomatous thickening of the aortic valve cusps that prolapse toward the left ventricular outflow tract (*arrowheads*), and an endocardial jet lesion of chronic aortic insufficiency is present (*) on the interventricular septum. An incidental quadricuspid aortic valve was found at autopsy in a 53-year-old woman (*E*). The four cusps are dissimilar in size; the right and left sinuses are normal, and the posterior sinus contains two cusps with a smaller left posterior cusp (*arrow*). (*A–D* from Farb A, Virmani R, Burke AP. Pathogenesis and pathology of valvular heart disease. In: Alpert JS, Dalen JE, Rahimtoola SH (eds): Valvular Heart Disease, p19. Philadelphia: Lippincott Williams & Wilkins, 2000, with permission.) (*E* from Virmani R, Burke AP, Farb A. Pathology of valvular heart disease. In: Valvular Heart Disease, p1.3. Shahbudin H. Rahimtoola (volume ed.). Volume XI of Atlas of Heart Diseases. Eugene Braunwald (series ed.). St. Louis: Mosby, 1997, with permission.)

between coronary atherosclerosis (with its epidemiological risk factors) and calcific aortic stenosis has been suggested.[93] In one case-control study, patients with senile calcific aortic stenosis had significantly higher fasting cholesterol levels versus controls.[94] In another study of patients > 40 years old undergoing aortic valve replacement, the presence of at least three of four of the following factors—age > 65 years, total serum cholesterol > 200 mg/dL, body mass index > 29 kg/m^2, and coronary atherosclerosis—was associated with a low probability (10–29%) of a *congenitally* abnormal (unicuspid or bicuspid) aortic valve being present. Conversely, patients lacking three or four of these clinical variables had a high probability of having a congenitally abnormal aortic valve.[95] In other studies, increasing age, smoking, hypertension, increased lipoprotein(a), and increased low density lipoprotein levels—all risk factors for coronary atherosclerosis—have been associated with an increased prevalence of aortic valvular sclerosis.[96–98] The relative increased frequency of simultaneous coronary bypass surgery in patients with tricuspid aortic valve stenosis compared with bicuspid aortic valve stenosis also suggests that coronary atherosclerosis risk factors play a role in the pathogenesis of cusp calcification.[99]

Histologic studies of mildly thickened aortic valves demonstrate subendothelial thickening, intra- and extracellular neutral lipids, fine mineralization, and basement membrane disruption.[100] Inflammatory infiltrates composed of macrophages (foam and nonfoam cells) and scattered T-lymphocytes have been identified in these early aortic valve lesions.[100] Similar, albeit more advanced lesions, have been observed in severely stenotic aortic valves.[100] Of the lymphocytes infiltrating excised stenotic valves, T-helper cells were most frequently seen in the vicinity of calcific deposits, and the valve endothelium has been shown to express receptors for interleukin-2.[101] These data suggest that an active inflammatory process, and not solely age-related degenerative change, may be involved in etiology of senile calcific aortic stenosis. Heavily calcified, nonstenotic valves are more likely to undergo rapid progression to critical stenosis than moderately calcified valves.[102]

Postinflammatory Aortic Stenosis

The etiology of postinflammatory aortic valve scarring and stenosis is presumed to be post-rheumatic, but < 50% of patients have a history of rheumatic fever.[87] Chronic postinflammatory pathologic changes may occur in bicuspid or tricuspid aortic valves, and they occur with equal frequency in men and women. Fusion of one, two, or all three commissures is the most important diagnostic feature of postinflammatory aortic stenosis (Figs. 7–12*A* and 7–12*B*). Fusion of only one commissure results in an acquired bicuspid valve (Fig. 7–12*C*), and fusion of all three commissures produces a dome-shaped valve. Commissures may be completely fused from the aortic wall insertion to the free edge or only partially fused near the aortic wall and remain separate at the free edge. As the number of fused commissures increases, the aortic valve orifice increasingly narrows.[87] Postinflammatory scarring results in diffuse fibrous thickening of the valve cusps. Calcification is variably present and starts in the fused commissures and extends into the body of the cusp; in contrast, in congenital bicuspid valves, calcification occurs in the cusps themselves and largely spares the commissures. Histologic sections are usually not needed to make a diagnosis, but if performed, histology demonstrates fibrotic cusps containing focal calcification, neovascularization (small, thick-walled vessels), myxomatous change, and few chronic inflammatory cells. The fused commissures consist of nonelastic fibrous tissue. Aschoff's nodules are rare but may be seen if there is a recent history of acute rheumatic fever or a documented history of rheumatic carditis. The simultaneous presence of post-rheumatic lesions of the mitral valve provides strong support for the diagnosis of post-rheumatic aortic valve scarring.

Nonvalvular Aortic Stenosis

Congenital supravalvular and subvalvular aortic stenosis are unusual causes of aortic outflow tract obstruction (Fig. 7–13). Dysplasia and thickening of the aortic valve cusps are often present. Typically presenting in childhood, supravalvular aortic stenosis may be secondary to a discrete aortic narrowing (majority of cases) or diffusely involve the aortic root[103] and may occur as part of the Williams syndrome or as an isolated finding. A deletion of the elastin locus on chromosome 7 has been identified in 96% of patients with the Williams syndrome.[104] Most cases of subvalvular stenosis are caused by a discrete fibrous membrane (89% of patients in one series)[105] or a tunnel-like narrowing of the left ventricular outflow tract myocardium. Discrete subaortic stenosis is responsible for 8–20% of cases of congenital left ventricular outflow tract obstruction.[106] The degree of associated left ventricular hypertrophy correlates with the severity of outflow tract impedance to flow. Discrete subaortic membranes can be excised surgically, but the recurrence rate is high. Hypertrophic cardiomyopathy with asymmetric hypertrophy causing subaortic stenosis is discussed in Chapter 6.

Aortic Insufficiency

Aortic insufficiency may be produced by lesions of the aortic valve cusps themselves or lesions of the ascending aorta that result in failure of valve cusps to close effectively (Table 7–6). Currently, ascending aorta abnormalities are the most common causes of pure aortic insufficiency.[107] Postinflammatory scarring of the valve cusps has decreased in incidence as the frequency of acute rheumatic fever has declined.[107] Aortic root dilatation is more common in men, and postinflammatory disease is more common in women. In older individuals (60–80 years old), dilatation of the aorta is most often idiopathic or related to systemic hypertension while in younger persons (20–40 years), Marfan syndrome and congenital heart disease are more frequent.

Clinical Presentation of Aortic Insufficiency

As a result of compensatory left ventricular dilatation, chronic severe aortic regurgitation

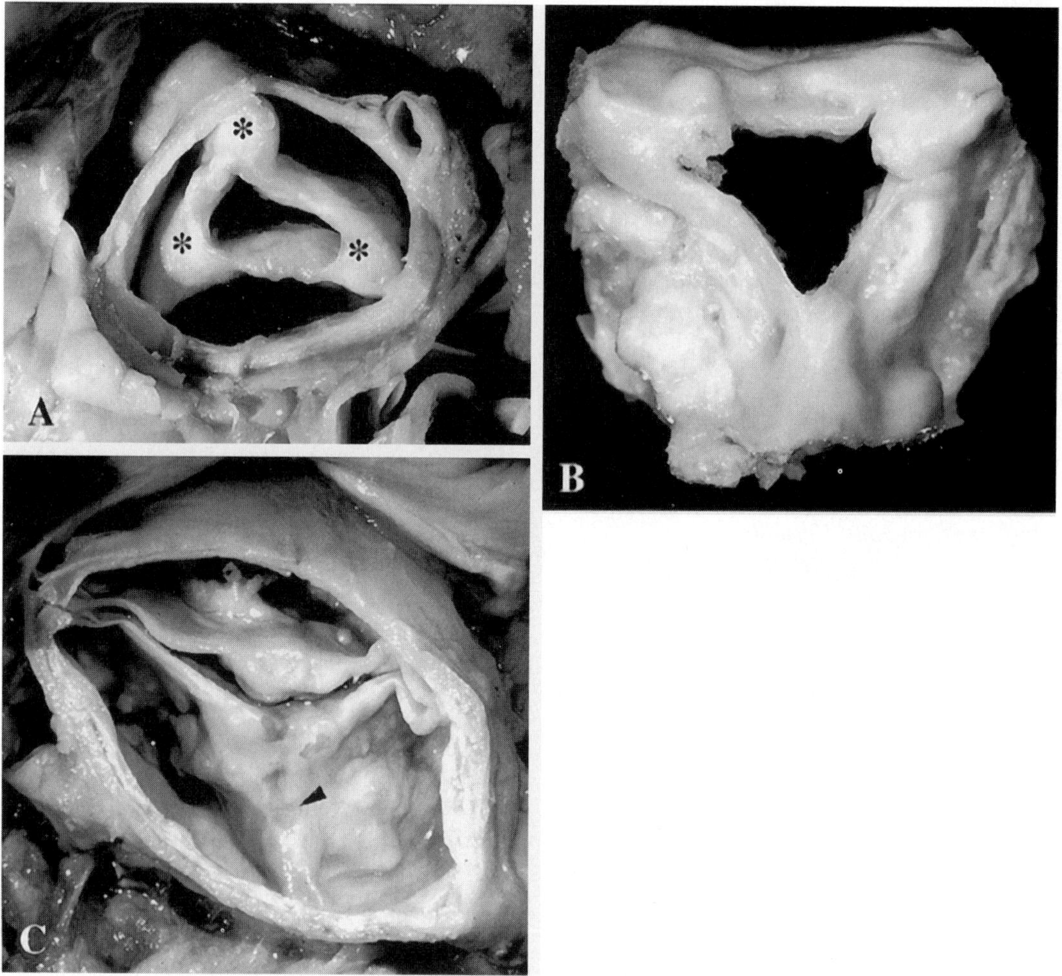

Figure 7–12. Post-rheumatic aortic valve disease. A 44-year-old male with known heart disease was found dead. At autopsy, he had an enlarged heart with severe mitral stenosis and aortic stenosis (*A*). Note fusion of all three aortic valve commissures (*), thickening and fibrosis of all three aortic leaflets, and no calcification. A surgically excised aortic valve (*B*) in a 50-year-old female with mitral and aortic stenosis. All three commissures are fused, and cusp fibrosis and calcification are evident with calcification present both in the commissures and leaflets. An acquired bicuspid stenotic aortic valve (*C*) was found in this 65-year-old man who died while awaiting valve replacement. The anterior commissure is fused (*arrowhead*), and this commissure is at the same level as and equidistant from the other two nonfused commissures. (*A* and *B* from Farb A, Virmani R, Burke AP. Pathogenesis and pathology of valvular heart disease. In: Alpert JS, Dalen JE, Rahimtoola SH (eds): Valvular Heart Disease, p 21. Philadelphia: Lippincott Williams & Wilkins, 2000, with permission.) (*C* from Virmani R, Burke AP, Farb A. Pathology of valvular heart disease. In: Valvular Heart Disease, p1.5. Shahbudin H. Rahimtoola (volume ed.). Volume XI of Atlas of Heart Diseases. Eugene Braunwald (series ed.). St. Louis: Mosby, 1997, with permission.)

may be well-tolerated, and patients often remain asymptomatic for many years. Cardiac compensation involves increases in left ventricular compliance and cavity size to accommodate the regurgitant volume. Stroke volume increases so that forward cardiac output remains in the normal range.[108] With time, however, left ventricular contractility and ejection fraction fall leading to clinical symptoms. In patients with symptoms of left-sided heart failure (dyspnea, orthopnea, and fatigue), surgical intervention for chronic severe aortic regurgitation is indicated.[109, 110] Further, surgery should be strongly considered in asymptomatic patients with a reduced left ventricular ejection fraction or evidence of left ventricular dilatation (left ventricular end diastolic cavity diameter > 75 mm or end-systolic cavity diameter > 55 mm).[108]

Acute severe aortic insufficiency (most commonly caused by infectious endocarditis, aortic dissection, or trauma) is typically extremely

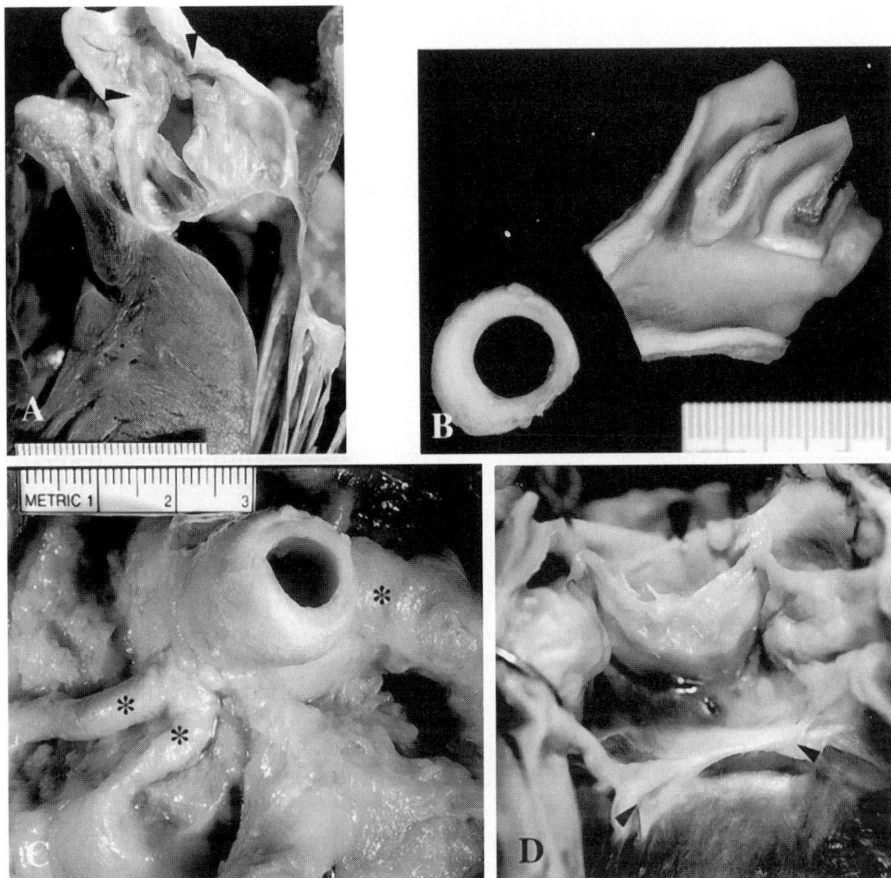

Figure 7–13. Supravalvular and subvalvular aortic stenosis. Supravalvular aortic stenosis (*A, B,* and *C*) was found at autopsy in this 35-year-old male. Note the markedly thickened and narrowed aorta beginning at and extending above the sinotubular junction (*A, arrowheads*). The aortic valve cusps are also thickened. The thickening extends into the aortic arch (*B*), and the epicardial coronary arteries are thickened, dysplastic, and dilated (*C,**). Subaortic stenosis may occur either from a localized fibrous ridge or, less commonly, from a longer diffuse fibrous tunnel. Note a discreet fibrous ridge (*D, arrowheads*) underlying the aortic valve in a 15-year-old boy who died suddenly. The valve has three dysplastic valve cusps. (*A–C* from Farb A, Virmani R, Burke AP. Pathogenesis and pathology of valvular heart disease. In: Alpert JS, Dalen JE, Rahimtoola SH (eds): Valvular Heart Disease, p 21. Philadelphia: Lippincott Williams & Wilkins, 2000, with permission.) (*D* from Virmani R, Burke AP, Farb A. Pathology of valvular heart disease. In: Valvular Heart Disease, p 1.3. Shahbudin H. Rahimtoola (volume ed.). Volume XI of Atlas of Heart Diseases. Eugene Braunwald (series ed.). St. Louis: Mosby, 1997, with permission.)

Table 7–6. Surgical Pathology of Aortic Regurgitation

Etiology	**Mayo Clinic (1965)**	**London (1980)**	**Mayo Clinic (1990)**	**AFIP (1990–1997)**
Post-rheumatic	47%	26%	14%	15%
Aortic dilatation and/or degenerative valve changes*	19%	31%	50%	53%
Bicuspid	17%	26%	14%	19%
Endocarditis	4%	11%	1%	10%
Other	13%	6%	21%	3%

* Degenerative valve changes refers to tricuspid aortic valves with cusp fibrosis or myxomatous degeneration.

From Farb A, Virmani R, Burke AP. Pathogenesis and pathology of valvular heart disease. In: Alpert JS, Dalen JE, Rahimtoola SH (eds): Valvular Heart Disease, p 22. Philadelphia: Lippincott Williams & Wilkins, 2000, with permission.

poorly tolerated as the previously normal left ventricle cannot accommodate the suddenly increased regurgitant volume. Stroke volume does not increase, and as a result, cardiac output drops precipitously.[111] Acute aortic regurgitation commonly causes acute pulmonary edema, often leading to cardiovascular collapse. Patient survival typically requires urgent surgery with aortic valve replacement.

Aortic Valve Pathology in Aortic Insufficiency

Intrinsic abnormalities of the aortic cusps (Figs. 7–11*D* and 7–14) leading to chronic aortic insufficiency are diverse and include congenital cusp lesions (e.g., congenital bicuspid aortic valve), postinflammatory (post-rheumatic) scarring, myxomatous degeneration (aortic valve prolapse), infectious disease (endocarditis), connective tissue disease, and acquired cusp deformity secondary to nonvalvular congenital heart disease. For example, prolapse of the right aortic cusp into the left ventricular outflow tract resulting in valvular regurgitation can occur in membranous ventricular septal defect.

As discussed earlier, congenital bicuspid aortic valves are most often stenotic; however, bicuspid valves account for 7–20% of cases of chronic aortic insufficiency without associated stenosis (Figs. 7–10*H* and 7–14*D*) and may be increasing in incidence.[81, 107, 112] Patients with aortic regurgitation secondary to bicuspid aortic valves undergo valve surgery at an earlier age (mean age 46 years in one recent series) compared with those with bicuspid aortic valve stenosis (mean age 65 years).[81] The valve consists of two cusps of unequal size. A median raphe is frequently present in the conjoint (larger) cusp,[113] and an indentation of the conjoint cusp was a frequent finding (43% of cases) in one surgical series.[114] An uncommon variant is a raphal cord that extends from the sinus wall to the free edge that produces cusp retraction. There have been reports of spontaneous rupture of these fibrous cords producing cusp prolapse and acute severe aortic regurgitation.[115] Regurgitant bicuspid valve cusps show varying degrees of myxoid deposition, fibrous thickening, rolled closing edges, and prolapse of the valve cusp(s) toward the left ventricular outflow tract.[113, 116, 117] Structural abnormalities of the aortic root (cystic medial change) are associated with congenitally bicuspid aortic valves so that regurgitation may be primarily caused by aortic root dilatation rather than intrinsic lesions in the valve cusps. In one surgical series of pure aortic regurgitation, there was a 31% incidence of aortic root dilatation among bicuspid aortic valves,[107] and as noted previously, congenital bicuspid valves are associated with an increased risk of aortic dissection. Of 189 cases of noniatrogenic aortic dissection, congenital aortic valve lesions were present in 16 (8.5%) patients (14 with bicuspid valves and 2 with unicuspid valves), all of whom had an intimal tear in the ascending aorta.[118] Superimposed infective endocarditis may produce aortic regurgitation in nonstenotic bicuspid aortic valves.[116, 119]

A history of rheumatic fever is uncommon (< 10% of cases) in postinflammatory cusp scarring leading to chronic aortic regurgitation. Diffuse fibrosis of valve cusps results in cusp retraction, and calcification is typically mild or absent. If significant commissural fusion is present, mixed valvular stenosis and regurgitation is likely to be the physiologic result.

Myxomatous aortic valves may be seen in Marfan syndrome, associated with myxomatous degeneration of the mitral valve, or as an isolated aortic valve finding.[120] A pathologic study of aortic valves excised for severe regurgitation showed that 13 of 55 (24%) had myxomatous degeneration in the absence of the Marfan syndrome; 85% were males, and 77% had systemic hypertension.[121] The pathology of these valves demonstrates myxomatous thickening and redundancy of the valve cusps (Fig. 7–11*D*). Histologically, there is expansion of the valve cusp spongiosa by proteoglycans that occupy > 50% of the cusp resulting in discontinuity of the zona fibrosa. The pathogenesis of the myxomatous change is not known but may involve an abnormality of collagen synthesis. One hypothesis is that the development of fibrotic, nonredundant, and retracted cusps may represent a later stage of myxomatous degeneration.[122]

Sporadic causes of aortic regurgitation include a quadricuspid valve[123] (Fig. 7–11*E*), large noninfected fenestrations that extend below the line of valve closure (Fig. 7–14*E*),[124] Behçet syndrome,[125] hypereosinophilic syndrome (discussed later in the chapter), mucopolysaccharidoses (Hunter–Hurler phenotype), amyloidosis, and post-methysergide therapy. Rarely, the anatomical cause of chronic aortic insufficiency cannot be determined.

In acute aortic insufficiency secondary to aortic dissection involving the ascending aorta, the dissecting hematoma extends retrograde to the commissural attachments and/or into the valve cusps themselves resulting in cuspal malalign-

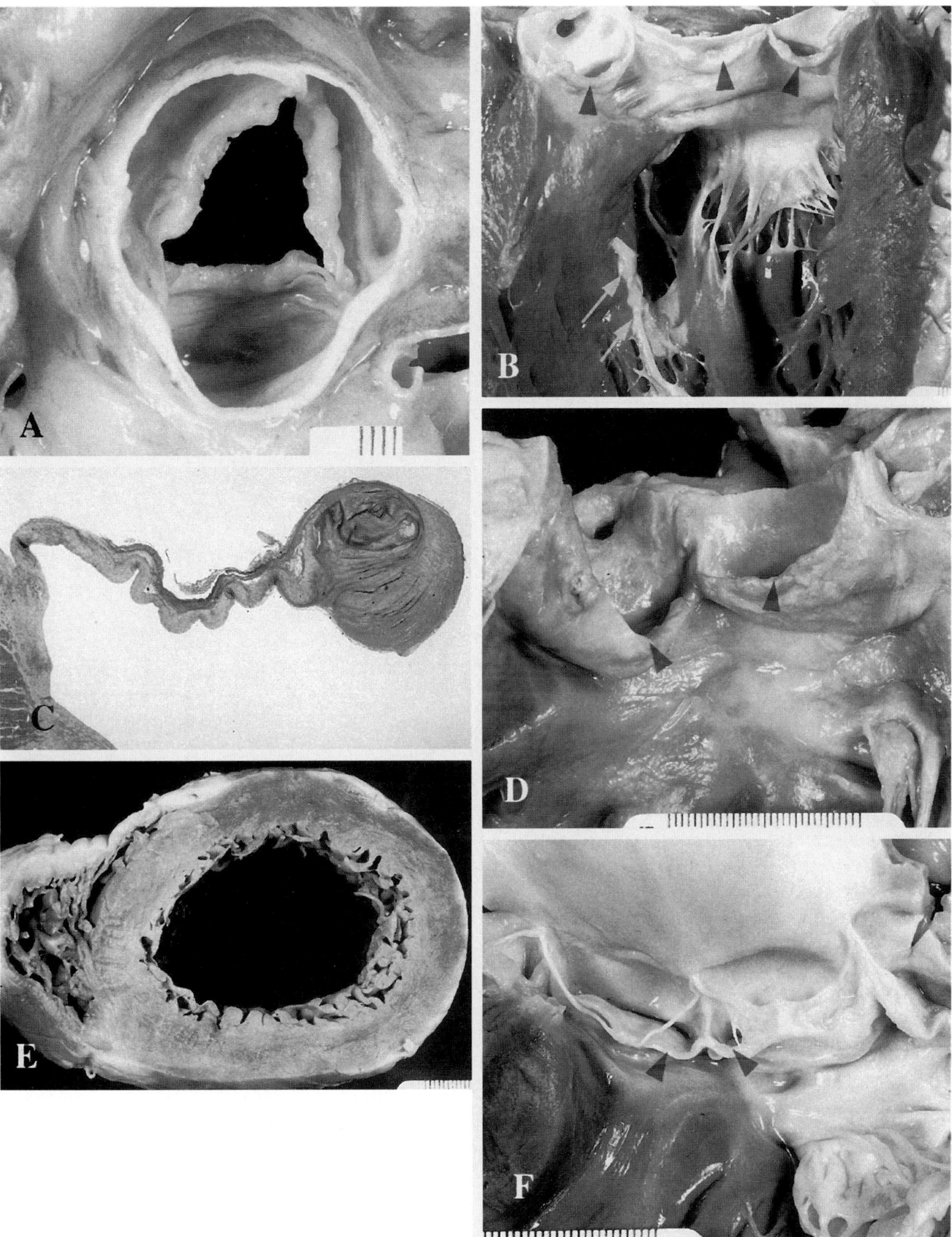

Figure 7–14. Chronic aortic insufficiency. Tricuspid aortic valve (*A–C*) from a 36-year-old man with dyspnea on exertion and nocturnal dyspnea who died suddenly. Note fibrotically thickened aortic valve cusps with nonfused commissures (*A*). There are rolled free edges (*arrows*) and mild prolapse of the aortic valve cusps toward the left ventricular outflow tract (*arrowheads, B*). Arrows indicate an endocardial jet lesion secondary to aortic regurgitation. A histologic section of one of the aortic valve cusps shows marked fibrosis at the closing end (*C*). Severe aortic insufficiency secondary to a congenital bicuspid aortic valve is shown in *D*. The two cusps (*arrows*) are fibrotically thickened and noncalcified. In this case, the heart weighed 720 gm associated with marked left ventricular dilatation (*E*). Abnormally large aortic valve cusp fenestrations (*arrowheads, F*) extending below the line of valve closure are a rare etiology of aortic insufficiency.

ment. In traumatic laceration of the proximal aorta, there may be avulsion of the cuspal attachment to the sinus of Valsalva wall.

Lesions of the ascending aorta that can produce aortic regurgitation are discussed in Chapter 13. In brief, causes of ascending aortic dilatation associated with severe aortic insufficiency include hypertension, aortic dissection, annuloaortic ectasia, traumatic aortic laceration, Marfan syndrome, Ehlers–Danlos syndrome, osteogenesis imperfecta, pseudoxanthoma elasticum, tertiary syphilis, and the various types of aortitis. However, most cases of aortic dilatation (74–90%) are idiopathic (annuloaortic ectasia). In the setting of primary aortic root disease and chronic aortic regurgitation, the aortic valve cusps may be thin and stretched or fibrotically thickened, and the cusp free edges have a rolled appearance. Occasionally, focal chronic inflammation may be present in the valve cusps as an extension of an accompanying aortitis.

In autopsy cases, chronic severe aortic regurgitation is associated with left ventricular dilatation far in excess to left ventricular hypertrophy as a result of left ventricular volume overload (Fig. 7–14*E*). In contrast, in acute aortic regurgitation, there is insufficient time for left ventricular dilatation to occur.

Combined Aortic Stenosis and Regurgitation

Severe combined aortic stenosis and regurgitation is a common indication for valve replacement accounting for approximately 25–30% of aortic valve replacements. Approximately two thirds of patients with calcific aortic stenosis have simultaneous aortic regurgitation of varying degrees of severity.[126] The age range of patients at surgery is broad (40–80 years old) with a male to female ratio of 1.5 to 1. Approximately 70% of cases of combined aortic stenosis and regurgitation are postinflammatory (postrheumatic); however, a definitive history of rheumatic fever is rarely reported. Congenitally bicuspid valves account for 25% of cases, and the remaining cases are due to a variety by miscellaneous lesions (congenital unicuspid valve, infectious endocarditis, and congenitally dysplastic tricuspid aortic valve). Late aortic valve damage requiring valve replacement secondary to external beam radiation, administered to treat malignant disease, has been reported.[127] Symptoms and signs are similar to those of either aortic stenosis or regurgitation, depending on which abnormal physiology dominates. Like isolated aortic stenosis, the appearance of angina, syncope, or heart failure are indications for surgery.

The morphology of mixed aortic stenosis and regurgitation consists of cusp calcification, fibrosis, and commissural fusion that restrict cusp excursion. The degree of calcification is generally less extensive than in postinflammatory valve disease. Regurgitation is further augmented by leaflet fibrosis and retraction that prevents the cusps' closing edges to align properly in diastole. One, two, or all three commissures may be fused. The left ventricle often shows combined left ventricular hypertrophy and dilatation reflecting both volume (secondary to valvular regurgitation) and pressure (secondary to stenosis) overload.

Pulmonary Valve

Anatomy of the Pulmonary Valve

The pulmonary valve consists of three semicircular cusps (left, right, and anterior cusps) and three commissures, and its annulus is approximately 1.5 cm above the level of the aortic annulus.[68] Except for the absence of coronary ostia, the gross and histologic morphology of the pulmonary valve is similar to the aortic valve.[68]

Pulmonary Valve Pathology

A congenital lesion of the pulmonary valve may be an isolated finding (e.g., congenital pulmonary artery stenosis) or may occur in association with other congenital cardiac abnormalities (e.g., tetralogy of Fallot and ventricular septal defect). Pulmonic stenosis is most frequently a congenital lesion, accounts for 7.5–9% of congenital heart defects and occurs equally in males and females.[128] As an isolated cardiac abnormality, congenital pulmonic stenosis is typically associated with survival into adulthood[129, 130] The stenotic pulmonary valve may have three normally placed commissures with dysplastic cusps, two cusps and two commissures (bicuspid valve), one cusp and one commissure (unicuspid, unicommissural valve), or one cusp and no commissure (unicuspid, acommissural dome-shaped valve, Fig. 7–15*A*).[130, 131] The dome-shaped pulmonary valve is the most common morphology accounting for 42% of cases.[131] Thickening of the valve cusps is present to a variable degree and typically involves the entire length of the cusp.[131] Histologically, myx-

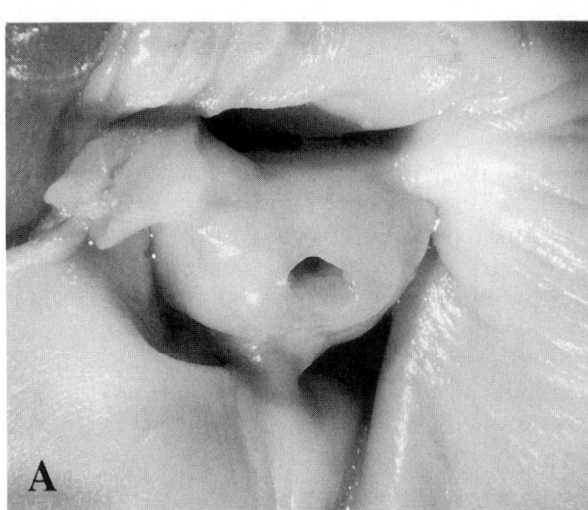

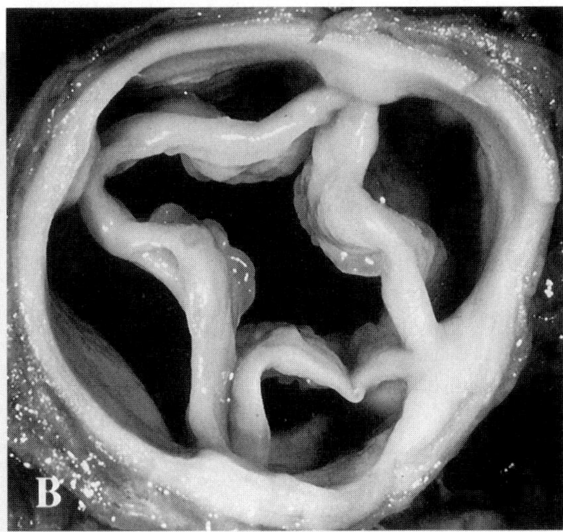

Figure 7–15. Pulmonary valve pathology. Pulmonary stenosis may occur as an isolated congenital anomaly, and the stenosis is either valvular or both valvular and infundibular. The stenotic unicuspid acommissural pulmonary valve shown (*A*) is from a neonate; a dome- or funnel-shaped fibro-myxomatous pulmonary valve with three raphal ridges was present. This quadricuspid pulmonary valve with mild dysplasia (*B*) was found in a 12-year-old girl with tunnel subaortic stenosis. Quadricuspid pulmonary valves are more frequently encountered than quadricuspid aortic valves and are usually an incidental finding. (From Virmani R, Burke AP, Farb A. Pathology of valvular heart disease. In: Valvular Heart Disease, pp 1.19–1.20. Shahbudin H. Rahimtoola (volume ed.). Volume XI of Atlas of Heart Diseases. Eugene Braunwald (series ed.). St. Louis: Mosby, 1997, with permission.)

oid change is present within the cusp with occasional increased collagen and elastic tissue deposition.[131] The right ventricle demonstrates hypertrophy, particularly in the infundibular region, proportionally to the degree of stenosis; right ventricular dilatation is usually mild.[128]

Patients with mild pulmonic stenosis (gradients < 50 mm Hg) typically do not require therapy, while intervention is usually performed on those with higher valve gradients.[128] The current treatment of isolated moderate (gradient 50–79 mm Hg) or severe (gradient ≥ 80 mm Hg) congenital pulmonic stenosis most often is percutaneous balloon valvuloplasty with restenosis occurring in approximately 10% of patients.[128,132,133] Surgical removal of the pulmonic valve is most frequently performed as part of the repair for tetralogy of Fallot;[134] the valve is typically bicuspid and is associated with a hypoplastic annulus.[64] Acquired pulmonic stenosis may occur in carcinoid heart disease (see following). Postrheumatic valve scarring resulting in commissural fusion rarely causes significant pulmonic stenosis.

Similar to the etiology of aortic regurgitation (in which aortic root dilatation is the most common cause), pulmonic regurgitation is most frequently due to dilatation of the pulmonary trunk secondary to the various causes of pulmonary hypertension, idiopathic pulmonary trunk dilatation, or Marfan syndrome.[68] Pulmonic regurgitation secondary to chronic lung disease, thromboembolism, or left-sided heart failure is a marker of poor prognosis.[128] Less commonly, pulmonic regurgitation occurs secondary to pulmonary valve carcinoid plaques, postrheumatic scarring, endocarditis,[134] trauma, congenitally absent or dysplastic leaflets, or surgical treatment of right ventricular and pulmonic valve congenital heart disease.[135]

A quadricuspid pulmonary valve is the most frequent congenital pulmonary valve anomaly seen at autopsy (Fig. 7–15*B*), but is typically an incidental finding without clinical or physiologic consequences.[64]

VALVULAR ABNORMALITIES IN SYSTEMIC DISEASE

Carcinoid Heart Disease and Valve Lesions Associated with Appetite Suppressant Drugs

Carcinoid heart disease occurs in 20–50% of patients with metastatic carcinoid tumors associated with the carcinoid syndrome (flushing, telangiectasias, diarrhea, and bronchconstriction).[136] The pathogenesis of valvular carcinoid plaques is unknown but is believed to be related to endothelial injury caused by vasoactive agents produced by the carcinoid tumor. For example, circulating plasma serotonin levels[137] and urinary 5-hydroxyindoleacetic acid[138] are higher in patients with carcinoid valvular heart disease compared with those with carcinoid tumors but no cardiac involvement. In patients with carcinoid tumors, carcinoid heart disease is an important cause of morbidity and mortality,[136, 139] is associated with a mean survival of 1–2 years,[138, 139] and may be treated with valve replacement or palliative valvotomy in selected cases.[136, 140, 141, 142] In the Mayo Clinic series of 363 surgically excised tricuspid valves, five valves were removed because of carcinoid valvular plaques. Valve replacement in patients > 60 years of age is associated with a high rate of postoperative mortality.[143]

Tricuspid and pulmonic valve carcinoid plaques occur with equal frequency (Figs. 7–16*A* to 7–16*C*). On the tricuspid valve, carcinoid plaque accumulation on the valve surface results in tricuspid regurgitation with or without stenosis; pure tricuspid valve stenosis is rare.[136] Pulmonary valve carcinoid plaques most often cause pulmonic stenosis and less often pulmonic regurgitation.[136] Histologically, carcinoid valve plaques consist of smooth muscle cells within a proteoglycan matrix deposited

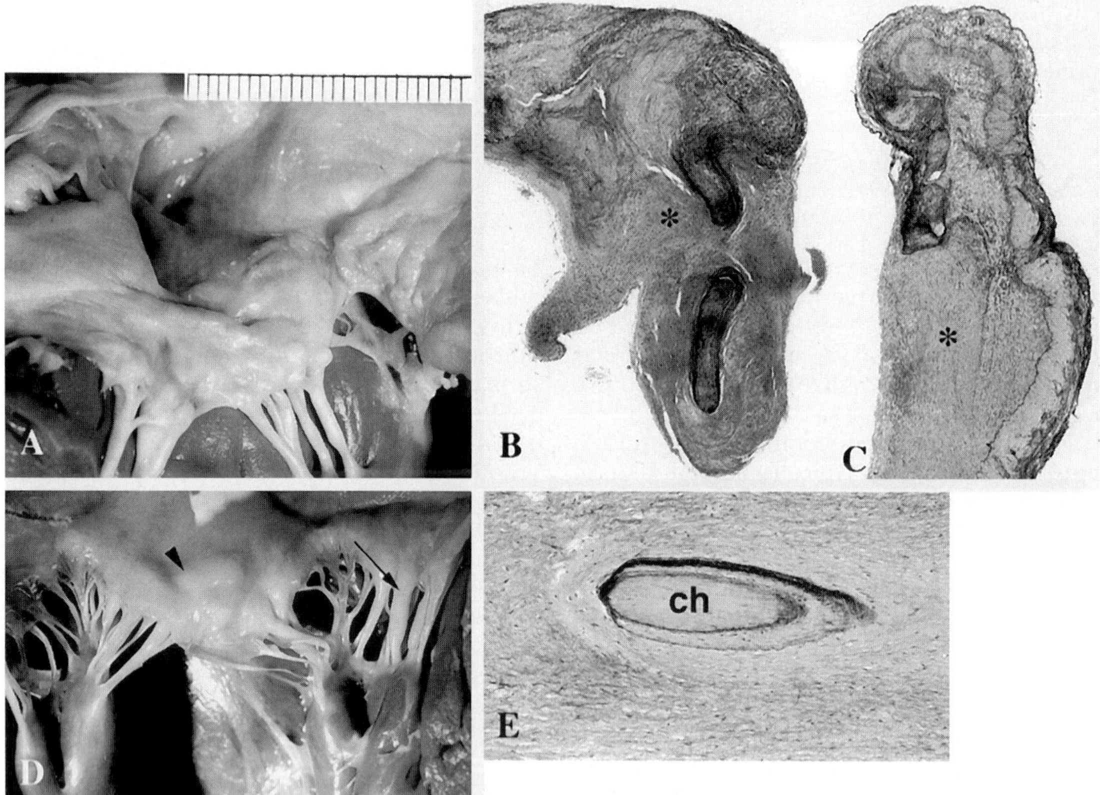

Figure 7–16. Carcinoid and fenfluramine-phentermine associated valve disease. The opened right atrium and tricuspid valve (*A*) show markedly thickened valve leaflets with chordae thickening and fusion. Clinically, the patient had mild tricuspid stenosis and regurgitation in the setting of a small bowel carcinoid tumor with liver metastasis. Grossly, the thickened and fibrotic tricuspid valve resembles post-rheumatic scarring; however, histologically (*B*), the underlying valve structure is well-preserved, but the atrial and ventricular surfaces of the valve are surrounded by carcinoid plaque consisting of smooth muscle cells in a proteoglycan matrix (*). Combined stenosis and regurgitation resulted from carcinoid plaque on the arterial surface of the pulmonary valve cusp (*, *C*). Lesions similar to those associated with the carcinoid syndrome have been described in patients treated by methysergide and ergotamine treatment, and most recently in patients receiving the weight-reducing agents fenfluramine-phentermine. Mitral valve leaflet (*arrowhead*) and chordal (*arrow*) thickening in a 48-year-old woman treated with fenfluramine-phentermine for over 1 year is shown in *D*. Smooth muscle cells in a proteoglycan matrix surrounding a mitral valve chord (*ch*) is shown in *E*. (From Farb A, Virmani R, Burke AP. Pathogenesis and pathology of valvular heart disease. In: Alpert JS, Dalen JE, Rahimtoola SH (eds): Valvular Heart Disease, p 31. Philadelphia: Lippincott Williams & Wilkins, 2000, with permission.)

upon the unremarkable valve endothelium. Plaques on the ventricular endocardial surface of the tricuspid valve result in leaflet and chordal thickening.

Mitral and aortic valve regurgitation, secondary to lesions similar to those seen in the carcinoid syndrome, have been identified in patients taking the combination of fenfluramine and phentermine for weight loss.[3] Connolly et al. found apparently new valvular heart disease in 24 women who had been treated with these agents for approximately one year.[3] Valve abnormalities were severe enough to require surgery in five patients. Pathologic evaluation of excised valves demonstrated plaques consisting of smooth muscle cells in a connective tissue matrix encasing otherwise unremarkable valve structures (Figs. 7–16*D* and 7–16*E*), features identical to those seen in carcinoid or ergotamine valvular heart disease.[3] More recent larger studies have indicated that the overall risk of severe valvular lesions associated with these weight loss agents is low. When valve lesions do occur, the regurgitation is typically mild and primarily affects individuals who have taken the weight loss agents for ≥ 6 months.[144–146]

Systemic Lupus Erythematosus (SLE) and the Antiphospholipid Antibody Syndrome

Cardiac involvement in SLE can involve all structures of the heart resulting in pericarditis, myocarditis, endocardial and valvular lesions, and conduction system abnormalities. First described by Libman and Sacks in 1924, valvular lesions are present at autopsy in 50% of SLE cases[147] but are clinically insignificant in most patients.[148]

Antiphospholipid antibodies associated with SLE were first noted in 1985.[149] In most cases, antiphospholipid antibodies occur with a clinical diagnosis SLE, but the antiphospholipid antibody syndrome in the absence of SLE is increasingly recognized. The antiphospholipid antibody syndrome is characterized by the presence of antiphospholipid antibodies, arterial and venous thrombosis, recurrent miscarriages, and thrombocytopenia. Valve lesions are present in one third of patients with primary antiphospholipid syndrome. In patients with SLE, the frequency of valve lesions is higher when antiphospholipid antibodies are present compared with individuals without antiphospholipid antibodies (48% versus 21%, respectively).[150]

Antiphospholipid antibodies determined by ELISA test, which utilizes the negatively charged phospholipid cardiolipin, are called anticardiolipin antibodies (aCLs).[151] In SLE patients, > 50% of individuals with the highest aCLs levels (> 100 units) have valvular abnormalities, 37% of patients with moderate aCLs levels have valvular defects, and 14% of patients with no elevation of aCLs have valve lesions.[152] Other factors associated with valvulopathy include increasing age, increased duration of SLE or the antiphospholipid syndrome, and a history of arterial thrombosis. In patients with antiphospholipid antibodies, valve lesions are often associated with thromboembolic events.[153] Patients with embolic events are more likely to have elevated aCLs than those without elevated levels, and those with embolic events are typically younger than those without.[154]

Since the introduction of two-dimensional echocardiography, 35% of SLE patients have been shown to have valve lesions with valve thickening in the midportion or base of the posterior mitral leaflet as the most common echo findings.[150] The most common hemodynamic valvular abnormality is mitral regurgitation, which occurs in up to 26% of patients with antiphospholipid antibodies. Aortic regurgitation is less common, occurring in 6 to 10% of patients. Mitral or aortic valve stenosis is rare as is right-sided valvular disease. Superimposed infective endocarditis in patients with SLE-associated valve lesions is uncommon.[155]

Pathologically, valve lesions in SLE (Libman–Sacks endocarditis) appear as pinhead, warty, sessile, fibrinous vegetations, 3 to 4 mm in size, located predominantly near the valve tips (Fig. 7–17*A*) on the ventricular surface of the mitral valve, may be adherent to chordae, and variably extend onto the atrial valve surface.[156] Aortic valve Libman–Sacks vegetations are most commonly found near the commissures. SLE-associated vegetations are firmly attached to the valve surface. Similar vegetations have been described in patients with the antiphospholipid syndrome. Histologically (Fig. 7–17*B*), vegetations are composed of fibrin (at varying stages of organization) associated with neovascularization and mononuclear cell infiltrates. In the absence of steroid treatment, extensive inflammation is present associated with fibrin deposition, granulation tissue, focal necrosis and hematoxylin bodies, the tissue counterpart to lupus erythematosus cells.[147, 157] Healed lesions

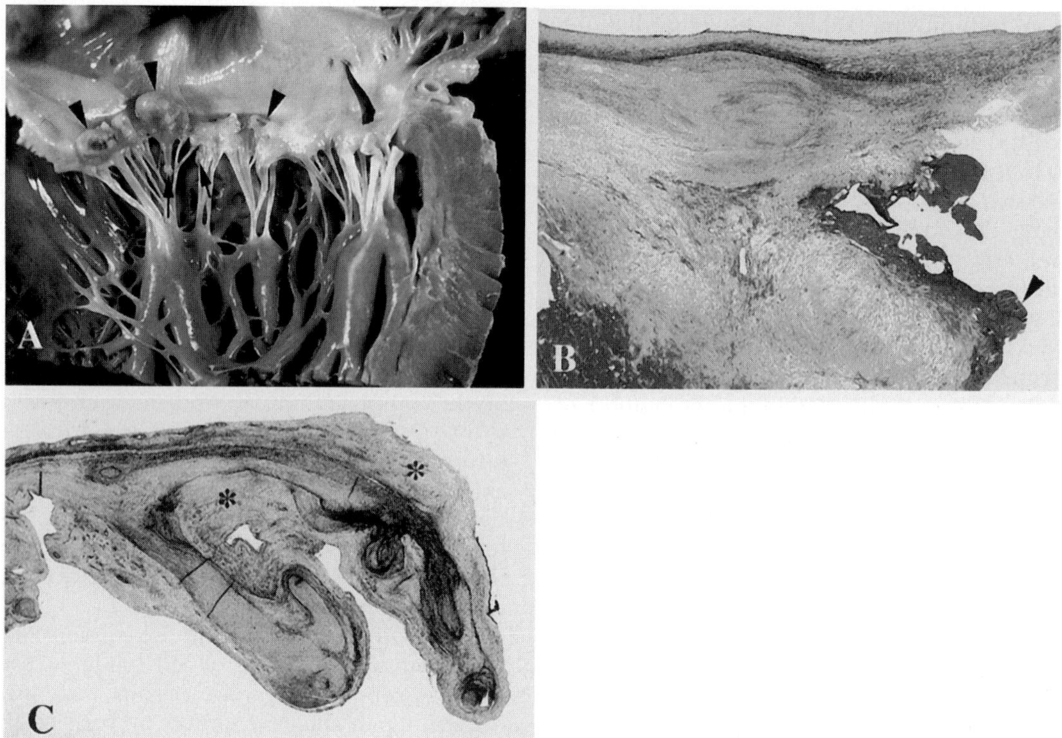

Figure 7–17. Systemic lupus erythematosus (SLE). A 21-year-old women with SLE diagnosed 2 years antemortem developed systemic hypertension and renal failure. At autopsy (*A*), Libman–Sacks verrucous vegetations (*arrowheads*) were evident on the anterior and posterior mitral valve leaflets with a smaller chordal vegetations present (*arrows*). Histologically (*B*), the mitral valve was fibrotic, and an organizing fibrinous vegetation (*arrowhead*) was present on the undersurface of the valve in this field (Movat pentachrome stain). A histologic section of the posterior mitral leaflet from a 42-year-old woman with a long history of SLE treated with immunosuppressive therapy demonstrates healed Libman–Sacks endocarditis characterized by fibrosis (*) on the atrial and ventricular surfaces of the valve (*C*, Movat pentachrome stain). (*A* and *B* from Farb A, Virmani R, Burke AP. Pathogenesis and pathology of valvular heart disease. In: Alpert JS, Dalen JE, Rahimtoola SH (eds): Valvular Heart Disease, p 32. Philadelphia: Lippincott Williams & Wilkins, 2000, with permission.) (*C* from Virmani R, Burke AP, Farb A. Pathology of valvular heart disease. In: Valvular Heart Disease, p 1.14. Shahbudin H. Rahimtoola (volume ed.). Volume XI of Atlas of Heart Diseases. Eugene Braunwald (series ed.). St. Louis: Mosby, 1997, with permission.)

of Libman–Sacks endocarditis consist of fibrous plaques with or without focal calcification.[158] Corticosteroid treatment is believed to be responsible for the healing (fibrosis) of valve lesions.[159] When the lesions are extensive, marked fibrosis (Fig. 7–17*C*), thickening, scarring and retraction of the valve leaflets are typical leading to valvular regurgitation.[158] Valvular stenosis secondary to leaflet fibrosis and calcification is rare. Surgery for SLE-associated valve lesions is rarely performed.

How antiphospholipid antibodies induce valvular damage is unknown, but it has been postulated that they promote thrombus deposition on the injured valve endothelium. Several biologic effects of antiphospholipid antibodies have been shown in *in vitro* studies that may contribute to the increased endothelial cell procoagulant activity: increased production of platelet activating factor, increased tissue factor activity, and inhibition of plasminogen activator release.[160] However, the precise factors that initiate valve damage *in vivo* have not been identified. Immunohistochemical studies have demonstrated valvular immunoglobulin deposition with complement co-localization. Further, valves with adherent immunoglobulins also have been shown to stain positively for aCLs.[161] Therefore, antiphospholipid antibodies probably play an important role in the pathogenesis of SLE-induced valve lesions.

Rheumatoid Arthritis

The classic cardiac lesion is the rheumatoid nodule, which may involve the myocardium, endocardium, and valves.[162] The overall involvement of the heart by rheumatoid granulomas at autopsy is 1–5%. A study of 214 patients with rheumatoid arthritis followed for 18 years demonstrated valvular disease in six (3%) with the mitral valve as the most frequent site of involvement followed by the aortic valve and tricuspid valve.[163] In autopsy studies, rheumatoid nodules may be present in any of the four cardiac valves.[55] Rheumatoid nodules typically do not cause valvular dysfunction, but when present, valvular regurgitation is the functional disturbance produced.[164–166] The frequency of clinical valve involvement correlates with the duration of the rheumatoid arthritis.

Grossly, rheumatoid nodules are located in the center of the valve leaflet, at the base of the valve, near its annular attachment. At the site of the nodule, the valve appears grossly thickened. At the valve annulus, the nodules may bulge into the ventricular cavity. Histologically, the nodules have a central area of necrosis with surrounding palisading histiocytes, giant cells, extensive lymphocyte infiltration, and a variable number of plasma cells. Rheumatoid valve nodule rupture has been reported.[167] Nodules may organize resulting in valve sclerosis and scarring with chronic inflammation. Fibrous scarring and leaflet retraction may result in increased valvular regurgitation.

Seronegative Spondyloarthropathies (HLA-B27-Associated Heart Disease)

Seronegative spondyloarthropathies (ankylosing spondylitis, Reiter syndrome, and psoriatic arthritis) are associated with the HLA-B27 histocompatibility antigen. Aortitis is an extraarticular manifestation of these diseases, which can involve the aortic root and aortic valve cusps to produce significant chronic aortic regurgitation. Pathologically, valve cusps are scarred and fibrotically thickened, particularly in their basal portion, which results in cusp retraction, inward rolling of valve cusp free edges, and focal chronic inflammation.[168] Aortitis secondary to ankylosing spondylitis may extend below the aortic valve and produce a subaortic fibrous ridge.[169] The incidence of aortic regurgitation in ankylosing spondylitis ranges from 10–50% of affected patients and increases with age, disease duration, and presence of peripheral arthritis.[168–172] Mitral valve abnormalities can occur secondary to aortic valve lesions in which the base of the anterior mitral valve leaflet has a hump or ridge of fibrosis and inflammation extending from the aortic valve.[168] The mitral valve typically functions normally unless there is severe dilatation of the left ventricle and mitral annulus secondary to aortic regurgitation.

Aortic valve involvement due to Reiter's disease can produce significant aortic regurgitation. In one study, the prevalence of aortic regurgitation in 164 patients with Reiter's disease was 2.8%.[173] Aortic root dilatation is responsible for severe aortic regurgitation in nearly 80% of patients with relapsing polychondritis, and aortic valve lesions (fibrosis and retraction of valve cusps with elastic tissue loss and cystic degeneration) in the absence of aortic root dilatation is responsible for the remaining 20%.[174]

Hypereosinophilic Syndrome (Loeffler's Endocarditis)

The hypereosinophilic syndrome is defined by chronic eosinophilia of $>$ 1500 eosinophils/mm^2 for $\geq$ 6 months or at the time of death, thromboembolic phenomena, and generalized arteritis.[175] The cause of hypereosinophilia is unknown in most cases; occasionally, it may be secondary to leukemia, parasitic infestation, allergic or hypersensitivity reaction, or neoplasms such as Hodgkin's disease. The hypereosinophilic syndrome has been reported in all ages but most often occurs in middle-aged men in their fourth decade. Morbidity and mortality rates are high secondary to cardiac involvement (seen in $\geq$ 75% of cases), typically causing biventricular dysfunction. In the acute phase of the hypereosinophilic syndrome, cardiomegaly may be present, and there are eosinophil-rich mural thrombi on the endocardium of the ventricular apex, ventricular inflow, and on the ventricular surface of the atrioventricular valves (Fig. 7–18*A*). Portions of the posterior mitral and the tricuspid leaflets may be adherent to the underlying ventricular wall resulting in valvular regurgitation (Fig. 7–18*B*). Thrombi may be seen in small intramyocardial arteries, and eosinophilic myocarditis may be present depending upon the stage of the disease. Charcot–Leiden crystals with surrounding giant cells and macrophages may be seen as a result of degranulation of the eosinophils. Over time in surviving patients, the endocardium becomes markedly thickened, extending from the apex to the papillary muscles; neither eosinophils nor myocarditis is usually present. The disease at this late phase is indistinguishable

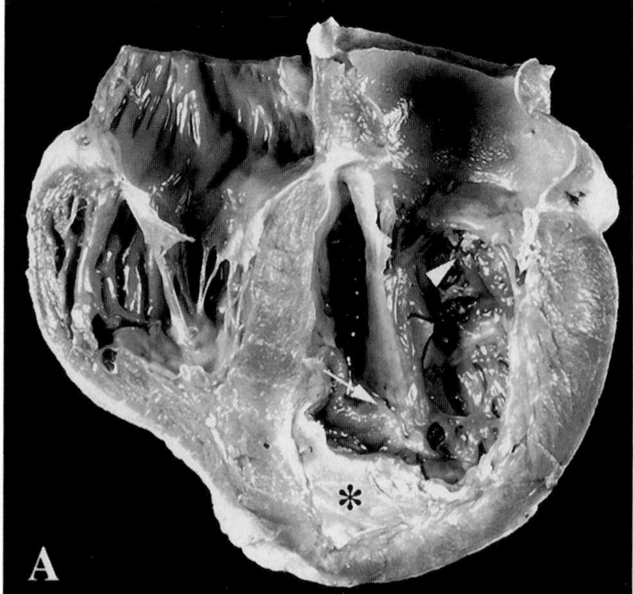

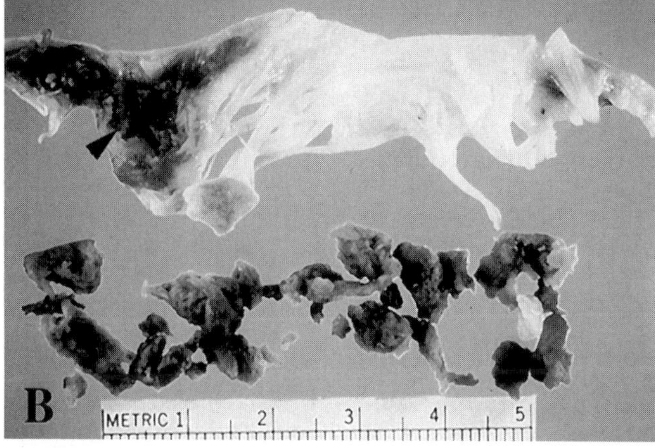

Figure 7–18. Hypereosinophilic syndrome. The heart (*A*) from a 9-year-old boy with eosinophilic leukemia of 9 months' duration shows biventricular dilatation and hypertrophy (four-chamber view). Note the organizing mural thrombus at the apex of the left ventricle (*), enveloping the posteromedial papillary muscle (*arrow*), and extending up and inferior to the posterior mitral valve leaflet (*arrowhead*). Endocardial fibrosis is present in the right ventricular apex extending into the papillary muscle. A surgically removed mitral valve and multiple fragments of endocardial thrombus (*B*) from a patient with hypereosinophilic syndrome shows attached focally organizing thrombus on the ventricular surface of the leaflet (*arrowhead*). (*A* from Virmani R, Burke AP, Farb A. Pathology of valvular heart disease. In: Valvular Heart Disease, p 1.15. Shahbudin H. Rahimtoola (volume ed.). Volume XI of Atlas of Heart Diseases. Eugene Braunwald (series ed.). St. Louis: Mosby, 1997, with permission.) (*B* from Farb A, Virmani R, Burke AP. Pathogenesis and pathology of valvular heart disease. In: Alpert JS, Dalen JE, Rahimtoola SH (eds): Valvular Heart Disease, p 35. Philadelphia: Lippincott Williams & Wilkins, 2000, with permission.)

from endocardial fibrosis (Davies's disease), a disease common in tropical and subtropical Africa (especially Uganda and Nigeria), and also reported in Brazil, Colombia, and Sri Lanka. Treatment of the hypereosinophilic syndrome consists of immunosuppressive therapy; valve surgery is rarely performed.[175, 176]

ENDOCARDITIS

Infective Endocarditis

Infective endocarditis is defined as a microbial infection of the valve endocardial surface often accompanied by disruption or destruction of underlying valvular structures. The median age of patients with infective endocarditis has increased from 30–40 years in the preantibiotic era to 45–65 years in the last few decades. The incidence of infective endocarditis increases after the age of 30 years, increasing to greater than 15–30 cases per 100,000 person–years.[177] Infective endocarditis is more frequent in men with a male to female ratio varying from 1.6–2.5 to 1.

Approximately 55 to 75% of cases of native valve infective endocarditis occur in the setting underlying congenital or acquired valve abnormalities (Table 7–7).[178, 179] In adults, the underlying valve lesions in native valve infective endocarditis is myxomatous degeneration of the mitral valve in 29%, degenerative calcific valve disease in 21%, congenital bicuspid aortic valves or other congenital abnormalities in 13%, and post-rheumatic scarring in 6%. Infective endo-

Table 7–7. Predisposing Conditions and Microorganisms in Native Valve Infectious Endocarditis as a Function of Patient Age

	Children (%)		Adults (%)	
Predisposing Condition	*Neonates*	*2 months–15 years*	*15–60 years*	*>60 years*
RVD	—	2–10	25–30	8
CHD	28	75–90*	10–20	2
MVP	—	5–15	10–30	10
DVD	—	—	Rare	30
IVDA	—	—	15–35	10
Other	—	—	10–15	10
Normal	72**	2–5	25–45	25–40
Microbiology				
Streptococci	15–20	40–50	45–65	30–45
Enterococci	—	4	5–8	15
S. aureus	40–50	25	30–40	25–30
Coagulase-negative staphylococci	10	5	3–5	5–8
GNB	10	5	4–8	5
Fungi	10	1	1	Rare
Polymicrobial	4	—	1	Rare
Other	—	—	1	2
Culture negative	4	0–15	3–10	5

Abbreviations: CHD = Congenital heart disease, DVD = Degenerative valve disease, GNB = gram negative bacteria (frequently *Haemophilus* species, *Actinobacillus actinomycetemitans, Cardiobacterium hominis*), IVDA = Intravenous drug abuse, MVP = mitral valve prolapse, RVD = Rheumatic valve disease.

* 50% of cases follow surgery and may involve implanted devices and foreign material.

** Often tricuspid valve infective endocarditis.

From Karchmer AW. Infective Endocarditis. In: Braunwald E (ed): Heart Disease, 5th Edition, pp 1077–1109. *A Textbook of Cardiovascular Medicine.* Philadelphia: W.B. Saunders, 1997, with permission.

carditis involving structurally normal valves occurs in 31% of cases, and many of these patients have underlying noncardiac conditions that predispose to intravascular infection such as intravenous drug abuse, immunosuppressive therapy, alcohol abuse, and malignancy (particularly colon carcinoma). As the incidence of acute rheumatic fever and chronic rheumatic heart disease have declined, other predisposing conditions such as myxomatous degeneration of the mitral valve, nosocomial endocarditis in the elderly, and endocarditis in intravenous drug abusers have become relatively more common.

The microbiologic agents causing endocarditis have also changed reflecting the alterations in underlying conditions that predispose to endocarditis and the increasing age of the population.[178] A wide range of microorganisms can cause endocarditis, and several of the most common agents will be discussed. Staphylococcus aureus is the most frequent pathogen in intravenous drug abusers, and gram-negative bacilli and Candida species are not uncommon in these individuals. Streptococcus bovis endocarditis is associated with colon carcinoma. Streptococcus pneumoniae endocarditis is associated with chronic alcohol abuse and also occurs in individuals with pneumococcal sepsis. Gram-negative organisms are encountered in diabetics, and fungi most often occur in patients receiving immunosuppressive therapy.[180–182] Streptococcus viridans remains a common organism in subacute cases of infective endocarditis and in post-rheumatic valve disease.[183]

The pathogenesis of infective endocarditis follows a sequence of initial formation of a sterile thrombus on an abnormal valve endocardial surface, followed by colonization, reproduction of microorganisms, and subsequent invasion of the valve tissue.[184] Transient bacteremia is frequently produced by dental extraction procedures; periodontal surgery; and oropharyngeal, gastrointestinal, urologic, or gynecologic invasive diagnostic or surgical procedures.[185] Vegetations in infective endocarditis more often involve left-sided cardiac valves compared with right-sided valves. The aortic valve (39–46%) is slightly more frequently involved than the mitral valve (30–35%), and combined aortic and mitral valve vegetations (18–24%) are not uncommon. Infective endocarditis is more likely to occur with underlying valvular regurgitation, rather than stenosis, due to increase pressure and flow in regurgitant lesions that increase endocardial damage and increase the likelihood of local thrombus deposition. Endocarditis involving the right-sided valves is much less frequent (9–11%) versus left-sided valves, but is particularly common in intravenous drug abuse secondary to repeated venous exposure to nonsterile material; the tricuspid valve is more frequently affected than the pulmonic valve. Right-sided endocarditis is also associated with pulmonary artery (Swan–Ganz) catheterization but the vast majority of the vegetations are sterile.

Presenting cardiac signs and symptoms of infective endocarditis include valvular regurgitation murmurs, congestive heart failure as a result of severe regurgitation, infectious pericarditis, heart block (secondary to annular abscess formation from aortic endocarditis extending to the crest of the interventricular septum), and myocardial infarction secondary to coronary embolization. Noncardiac signs and symptoms include fever, anemia, musculoskeletal pain, glomerulonephritis, peripheral arterial embolization, and septic shock. Significant heart failure, valve annular abscess, heart block, major organ embolization, and persistent bacteremia are indications for urgent valve surgery for acute infective endocarditis. Large, friable vegetations are particularly prone to embolization. Clinically apparent emboli are seen in 15–35% of cases of infective endocarditis,[183, 186] and the incidence of emboli in autopsy series is substantially higher (45–65%).[187]

At surgery, a portion of the vegetation should be cultured to identify microorganisms and to perform antibiotic-sensitivity testing. Histologic examination of the valve is mandatory, and stains for bacteria (Brown and Hopps, and Brown and Brenn tissue Gram stains) and fungi (Gomori methenamine silver or periodic-Schiff stain) are helpful in identifying microorganisms. Brown and Brenn stain is superior for Gram-positive organisms which, upon death, may not stain with Brown and Hopps stain.

In our laboratory, we identified 13 cases of sudden death secondary to acute infectious endocarditis in intravenous drug users seen between 1992–1994 in the State of Maryland, which corresponds to a yearly incidence of infective endocarditis-related sudden unexpected death of 12/100,000.[53] Of these, 11 (85%) cases occurred on otherwise normal valves, and acute drug intoxication was present in 77% of cases. During the same period, the yearly incidence of sudden death due to acute endocarditis in nondrug users was 0.04/100,000. Further, sudden death in all nondrug users occurred on congenitally abnormal valves or prosthetic valves. Thus, intravenous drug users are 300 times more likely to die suddenly secondary to acute infective endocarditis than nondrug users with lesions occurring on previously normal valves.[53] In nonfatal cases of acute endocarditis in drug users, right-sided valve lesions are more common than left sided. However, in lethal cases, left-sided endocarditis occurs two times more frequently than right-sided infective vegetations. Healed endocarditis was more common in right-sided valves than in the left-sided valves (67% vs. 8%).[53]

Pathologically, endocarditis lesions consist of a mass or vegetation containing platelets and fibrin with colonies of microorganisms (Figs. 7–19*A* to 7–19*F*). On gross inspection, infective vegetations are pink, red, or yellow, and change to gray-yellow brown as they organize. Vegetations initially develop along the line of valve closure and are most often located on the atrial surface of the atrioventricular valves and on the ventricular surface of the semilunar valves. Vegetations containing virulent organisms often are associated with valve leaflet erosion or perforation with or without rupture of chordae tendineae. Spread of infection from the closing edge of one valve to its opposite side results in "kissing lesions." Infectious endocarditis usually leads to valvular regurgitation due to leaflet dysfunction or perforation; rarely, valve stenosis occurs secondary to bulky vegetations. Weakening of the leaflet due to surface erosion, without valve perforation, may result in the formation of a leaflet aneurysm, which bulges into the left atrium from the mitral valve, and into the left ventricle from the aortic valve. Valve regurgitation may acutely worsen if the aneurysm perforates.[188] Histologically, the acute vegetation consists of platelets, fibrin, neutrophils, and microorganisms with associated acute and chronic inflammation.

Organizing, healing vegetations contain varying degrees of chronic inflammation, depending on the course of the disease, including lymphocytes, macrophages, plasma cells, and giant cells; neutrophils may be absent or scant in number. In completely healed lesions (Figs. 7–19*G* and 7–19*H*), focal leaflet thickening (which is most marked in the area of previous vegetation), calcification, or leaflet perforation may be observed. The area surrounding a valve perforation is thickened and, within an aneurysm, the valve leaflet is focally attenuated.

At autopsy, evidence of coronary artery embolization should be sought in infective endocarditis cases in epicardial arteries and/or intramyocardial arteries and arterioles. Multifocal areas of myocardial necrosis, larger regions of acute myocardial infarction, and intramyocardial abscesses may be present. In patients with healed infective endocarditis with significant valve deformation or perforation, left- or right-sided atrial and/or ventricular dilatation will be present depending on the valve involved (e.g., left ventricular dilation secondary to chronic aortic regurgitation as a result of a healed aortic valve endocarditis).

Noninfectious Endocarditis (Marantic Endocarditis, Nonbacterial Thrombotic Endocarditis)

Noninfectious valvular vegetations typically occur in the setting of an underlying malignancy, chronic inflammatory disease, disseminated intravascular coagulation, uremia, burns, and intracardiac catheters. At autopsy, noninfectious endocarditis is reported in 1.3% of patients. Although seen at all ages, the frequency of marantic vegetations increases with increasing age. The etiology of these valvular vegetations is unknown but may involve platelet and fibrin deposition on valves that have minor endothelial injury in the setting of a hypercoagulable state (e.g., lupus anticoagulant, antiphospholipid antibodies,[151] underlying adenocarcinoma, disseminated intravascular coagulation) or superficial leaflet trauma (intracardiac catheter placement). In the left heart, aortic valve noninfectious endocarditis is more common than the mitral valve involvement. The tricuspid and the pulmonic valve vegetations often occur secondary to catheter-induced endothelial trauma. Even in patients with nonterminal conditions, surgery is rarely performed unless there is significant embolization.

Pathologically, noninfectious vegetations may be small or large and are gray-pink, friable, soft, or firm masses along the line of valve closure on the atrial surface of the atrioventricular valves and on the ventricular surface of the semilunar valves (Fig. 7–20*A*). On histologic examination, marantic vegetations are composed of platelet fibrin deposits with scant inflammatory cells (Fig. 7–20*B*). The most important diagnostic feature is the absence of associated valve ulceration or perforation; the underlying valve is almost always unremarkable, and no microorganisms are present on special stains.

Whipple's Disease

Cardiac valve disease in Whipple's disease is usually overshadowed by the intestinal symptoms. However, endocarditis in Whipple's disease can occur without gastrointestinal disease.[189, 190] Pathologically, the endocarditis lesions are characterized by infiltration of the valve by macrophages, and interspersed acute inflammatory cells, and valve surface vegetations usually result in valvular regurgitation.[191] Healing of the acute lesions may result in commissural fusion and resultant valve stenosis.[192] The causative organism of Whipple's disease has been identified as a Gram-positive actinomycete (Tropheryma whippeli).[193]

VALVE TUMORS

Cardiac valve papillary fibroelastoma[194] and valve myxoma are rare causes of systemic emboli and are discussed in Chapter 12.

PROSTHETIC HEART VALVES

Prosthetic valves can be broadly classified as either mechanical or biological tissue valves. Based on its tissue of origin, a bioprosthetic valve can be further categorized as a: (1) heterograft (xenograft) (graft from a nonhuman species [e.g., porcine or bovine]), (2) homograft (graft from same species [human-to-human]; allograft refers to a graft originating from different individual [e.g., cadaveric valve]) or (3) autograft (graft within the same individual). Patient age is the most important determinant of which prosthetic valve to implant taking into account: (1) the projected life span of the pros-

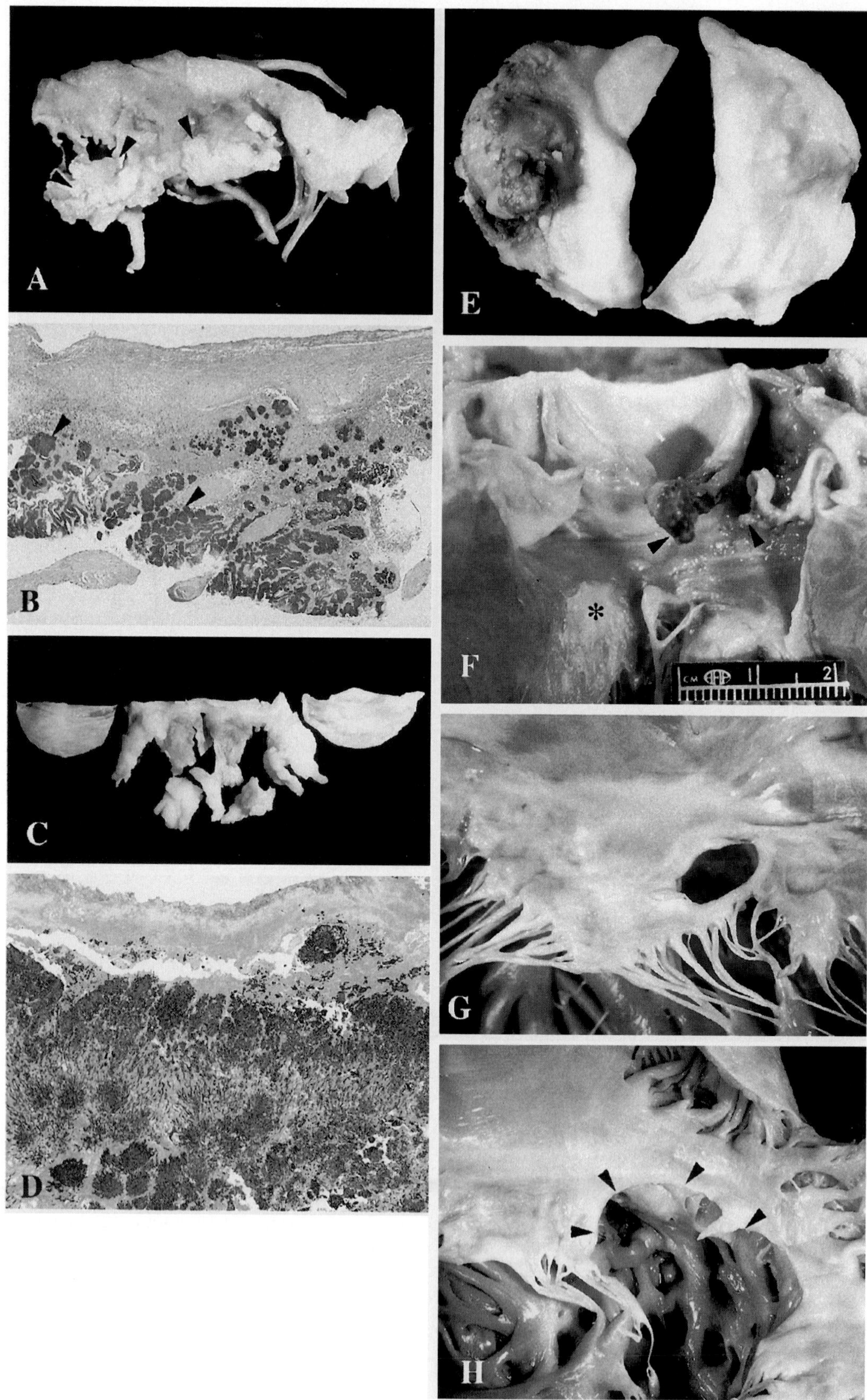

Figure 7–19. *See legend on opposite page*

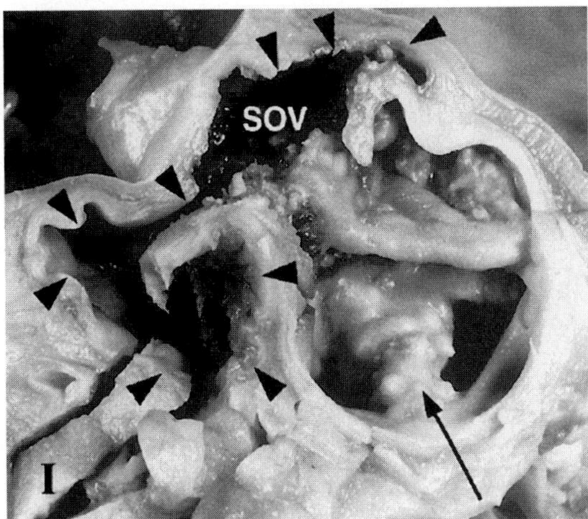

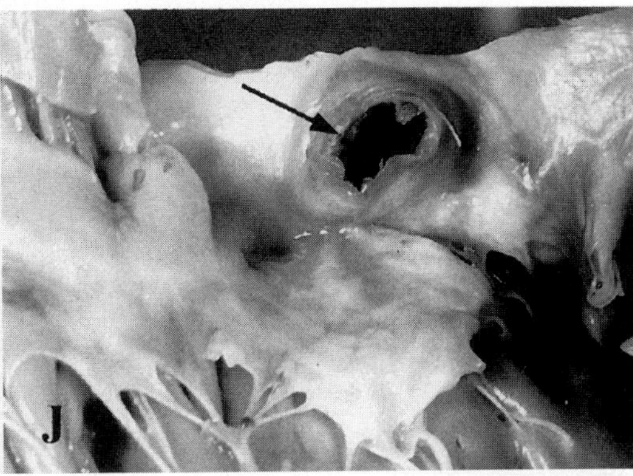

Figure 7–19. Infective endocarditis. A 52-year-old man with mitral regurgitation, low-grade fever, and a mitral valve vegetation demonstrated on echocardiography underwent valve replacement. The excised mitral valve (*A*) demonstrated prolapse, ruptured chordae tendineae, and infective endocarditis characterized by bulky vegetations (*arrowheads*) that partially destroyed the valve leaflet. Histologically (*B,* hematoxylin and eosin stain), the vegetation on the valve surface consisted of fibrin containing bacterial colonies (*arrowheads*) and interspersed acute inflammatory cells. *C* demonstrates the excised aortic valve from a 35-year-old intravenous drug user who presented with acute aortic regurgitation and congestive heart failure. A large vegetation has resulted in multiple perforations of the middle aortic valve cusp. Silver methamine staining of the valve (*D*) revealed numerous microorganism colonies consistent with candida. A large infective vegetation secondary to *S. aureus* resulted in destruction of one cusp of a congenitally bicuspid aortic valve (*E*). Subacute infectious endocarditis resulted in severe aortic regurgitation and sudden death in this 40-year-old man (*F*). The left aortic valve cusp is perforated (*arrowheads*) and the adjacent sinus of Valsalva is dilated. The vegetations are small and organizing, and the chronicity of the aortic regurgitation is indicated by the endocardial thickening (*). Chronic mitral regurgitation secondary to healed mitral valve infective endocarditis is shown in *G*. The valve leaflet surrounding the perforation is thickened. The chordae tendineae are intact, and the remainder of the underlying valve is unremarkable. Healed tricuspid valve endocarditis (*H*) from a 48-year-old intravenous drug user with chronic severe right-sided heart failure secondary to tricuspid regurgitation. Large portions of the anterior and septal leaflets are missing (*arrowheads*), and the margins of the remaining leaflets are mildly thickened. Sinus of Valsalva false aneurysm secondary to *S. aureus* endocarditis from a 47-year-old man is shown in *I*. A calcified congenital bicuspid valve (*arrow,* median raphe) is present with avulsion of the right valve commissure from the aortic wall. The sinus of Valsalva (*sov*) aneurysm is outlined by arrowheads. The false aneurysm ruptured into the right atrial cavity (*J*). (*A–H* from Farb A, Virmani R, Burke AP. Pathogenesis and pathology of valvular heart disease. In: Alpert JS, Dalen JE, Rahimtoola SH (eds): Valvular Heart Disease, p 28. Philadelphia: Lippincott Williams & Wilkins, 2000, with permission.)

thesis and the potential for repeat valve surgery and (2) the need for chronic anticoagulation therapy which is mandatory with mechanical valves and not generally needed with tissue valves (unless atrial fibrillation is present).

The role of the surgical pathologist when faced with most explanted prosthetic valves is to account for the cause of physiologic dysfunction (prosthetic valve thrombosis, stenosis, regurgitation, or combined stenosis/regurgitation). It should be noted, however, that in prosthetic valves explanted for paravalvular leaks (focal dehiscence secondary to late tissue retraction from the sewing ring), the prosthesis itself may be unremarkable. At autopsy, the pathologist should attempt to correlate prosthetic valve pathology with functional antemortem studies. Further, nonvalvular cardiac findings that develop secondary to valvular heart disease (e.g., left ventricular dilatation or hypertrophy) and other cardiac findings that may have contributed to the patient's death (e.g., coronary atherosclerosis) need to be described in detail. The significance of nonvalvular concomitant cardiac lesions was highlighted in a study of 37 patients dying suddenly > 1 month after valve surgery.[195] Of these, 15 (41%) had prosthetic valve lesions that were responsible for the patient's sudden demise (valve thrombosis, thromboembolism, perivalvular regurgitation, left ventricular outflow tract obstruction, strut fracture, and anticoagulation associated hemorrhage). In contrast, the remaining 22 patients (59% of the entire group) had anatomically unremarkable prosthetic valves and died secondary to nonvalvular cardiac conditions such

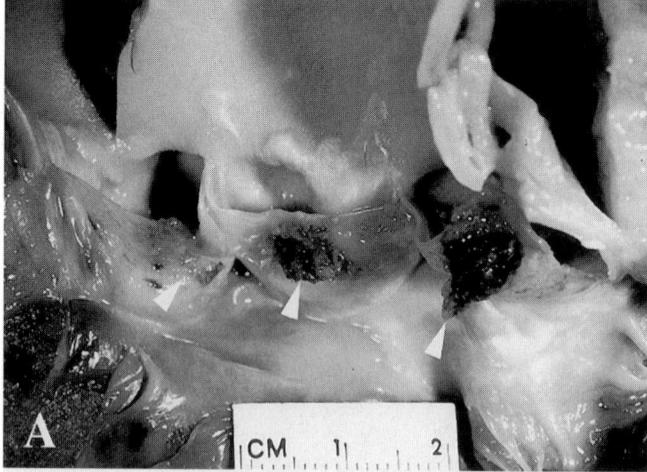

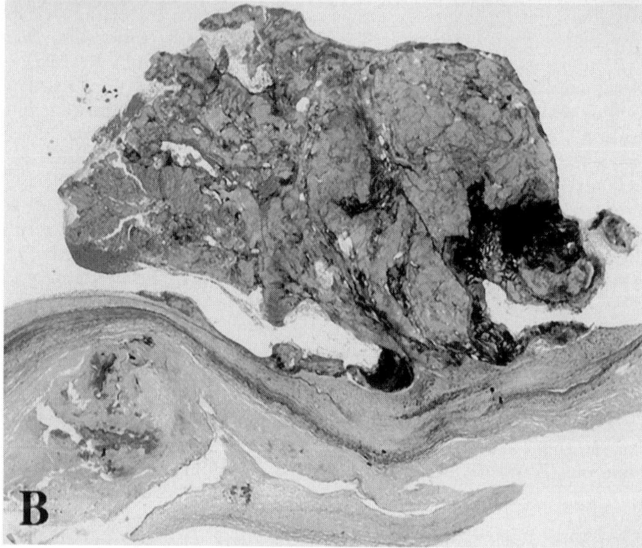

Figure 7–20. Marantic (nonbacterial thrombotic) aortic valve endocarditis characterized by vegetations of varying sizes near the lines of closure on all three cusps (*arrowheads*) is shown in *A*. Histologically (*B*), marantic vegetations consist of fibrin-rich hypocellular thrombi attached to the valve surface in the absence of destruction of the underlying valve. (From Farb A, Virmani R, Burke AP. Pathogenesis and pathology of valvular heart disease. In: Alpert JS, Dalen JE, Rahimtoola SH (eds): Valvular Heart Disease, p 29. Philadelphia: Lippincott Williams & Wilkins, 2000, with permission.)

as severe coronary atherosclerosis and lethal cardiac arrhythmias associated with left ventricular hypertrophy and dilatation.

Findings that should be specifically sought for in cardiac autopsies that apply to all prosthetic valves (Figs. 7–21 and 7–22) include paravalvular leaks, annular abscess, obstruction of coronary ostia (aortic prostheses), long suture knots or chordal remnants that can interfere with valve function, and oversized prostheses that can interfere with ventricular emptying. All prosthetic valves, both autopsy and surgical specimens, need to be inspected for endocarditis. Endocarditis that occurs in the early postoperative period is usually due to perioperative contamination, and endocarditis at ≥ 60 days is usually secondary to bacteremic seeding. The overall rate of prosthetic valve endocarditis is

Figure 7–21. Bioprosthetic valves. Radiograph (*A*) and corresponding excised (*B*) Carpentier–Edwards porcine bioprosthetic valve with severe cusp calcification resulting in functional stenosis. Dehiscence of a porcine bioprosthetic valve cusp from its insertion of the valve strut (*arrow*) is shown in *C*. Pannus ingrowth (*) partially covers the annulus of a porcine Carpentier–Edwards porcine valve (*D*). An infective vegetation resulting in extensive bioprosthetic cusp destruction is shown in *E*. *F* and *G* demonstrate bovine pericardial valves (unremarkable valve in the aortic position in *F*; type II cusp tear in *G*). Aortic wall tear (*arrows, H*) following placement of a bovine pericardial valve in the aortic position in a 78-year-old man with aortic stenosis; adventitial hemorrhage is present (*).

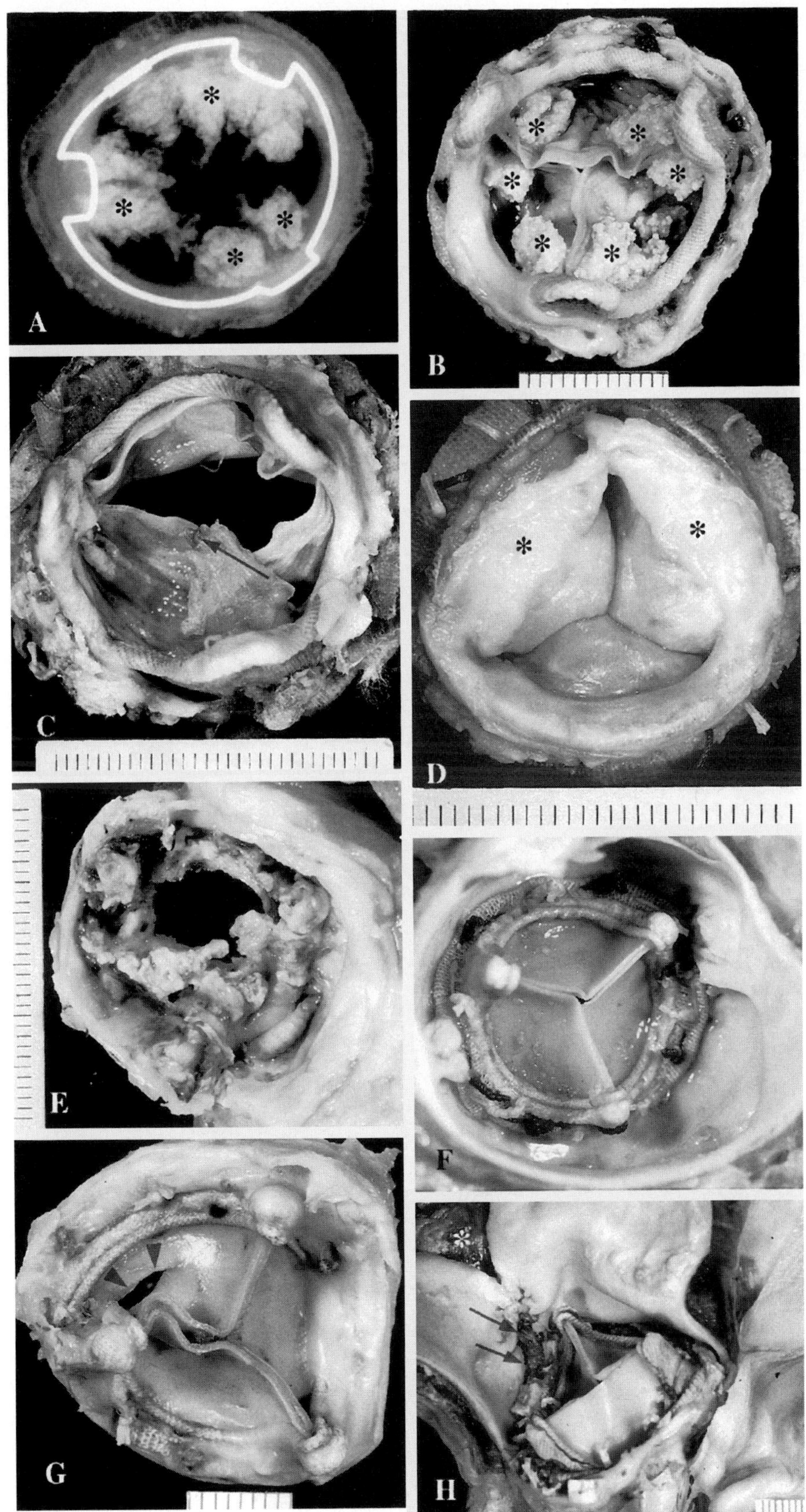

Figure 7–21. *See legend on opposite page*

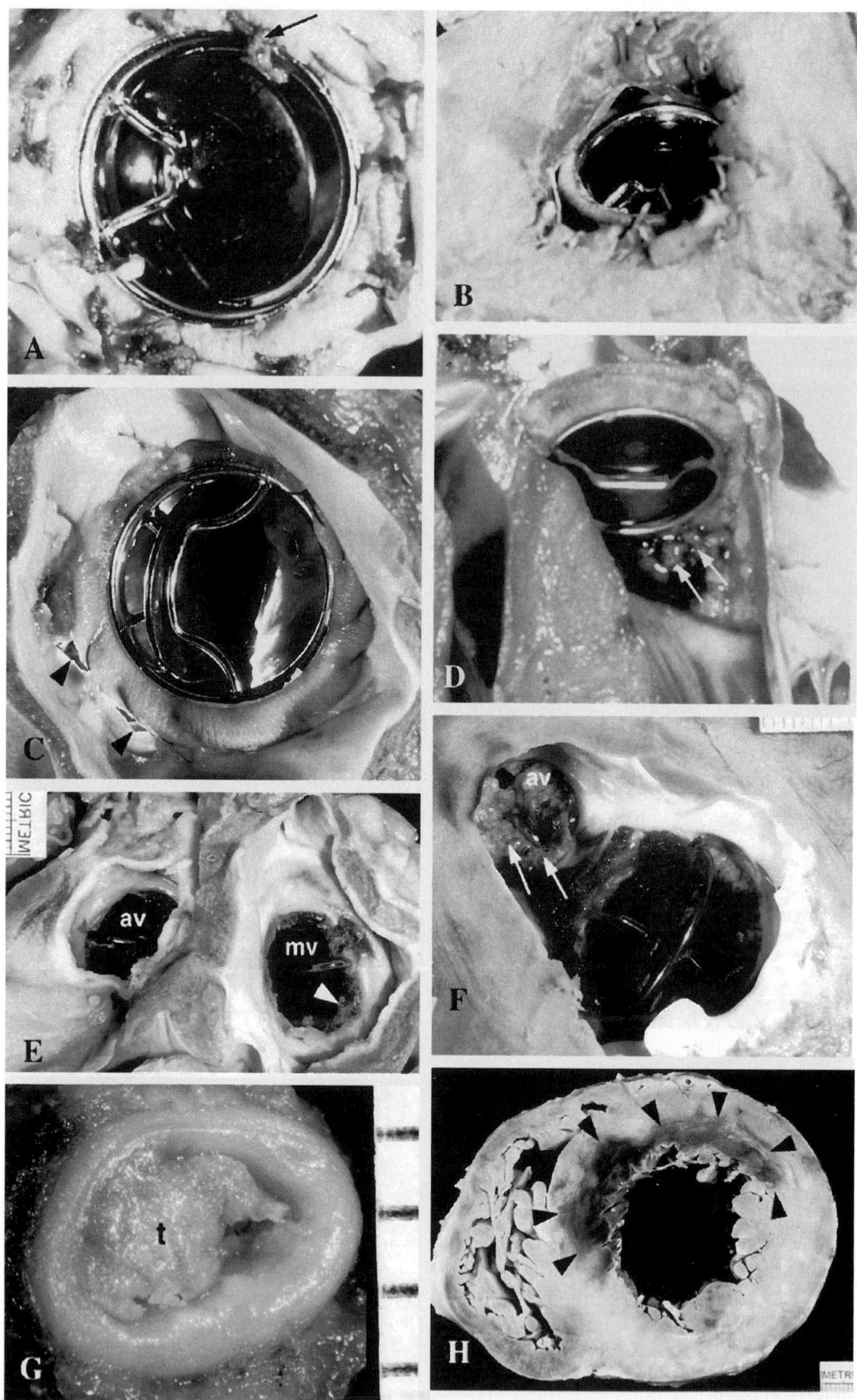

Figure 7–22. Mechanical prosthetic valves. A Bjork–Shiley valve with overhanging suture (*arrow*) that interferes with disc excursion is shown in *A*. Disproportionately large Bjork–Shiley valve in the mitral position obstructs the aortic outflow tract (*B*). Bjork–Shiley prosthetic valve regurgitation due to paravalvular leaks (*arrowheads*) is shown in *C*. An infective vegetation (*arrows*) is present in the aortic annulus containing a Bjork–Shiley valve (*D*). Mechanical prosthetic valve thrombosis is shown in *E* through *H*. Medtronic–Hall mitral (*mv*) and aortic (*av*) valves were placed 8 years antemortem. A small thrombus (*arrowhead*) is present on the atrial surface of the mitral (*mv*) prosthesis (*E*), and a large thrombus covers the ventricular surface of the aortic prosthetic valve (*arrows, F*). An occlusive thromboembolus (*t*) is present within the left anterior descending coronary artery (*G*) resulting in an extensive anterior and septal acute myocardial infarction (*arrowheads, H*).

low (5% incidence at 5 years) with, not surprisingly, an increased frequency in patients undergoing valve replacement for native valve endocarditis.

Bioprosthetic Valves

Two frequently used heterografts derived from porcine aortic valves (Figs. 7–21*A* to 7–21*E*) are the Carpentier–Edwards porcine bioprosthesis and the Hancock bioprosthesis. Both valves are glutaraldehyde-treated with the cusps of the Carpentier–Edwards valve mounted on a slightly noncircular Teflon-covered Elgiloy stent and the cups of the Hancock valve mounted on a circular Dacron-covered polypropylene strut. These bioprosthetic valves offer the advantage of very low thrombosis rates and do not require chronic anticoagulation therapy. The main limitation on use of porcine bioprosthetic valves is the durability of the implant. Structural bioprosthetic valve failure averages 30% by 10 years and reaches as high as 70% at 15 years in some series.[196–199] Thus, bioprosthetic valves are not recommended for implantation in young patients, particularly children in which the calcification process is accelerated. More recently, a new generation of bovine pericardial valves (Figs. 7–21*F* to 7–21*H*) have been introduced (Carpentier–Edwards pericardial bioprosthesis and the Mitroflow pericardial bioprosthesis) that may offer improved durability compared with porcine bioprosthetic valves.[200] Stentless bioprosthetic valves are in clinical trial with encouraging results.[201] Cadaveric homografts and autografts (as part of the Ross procedure) are very resistant to thrombus deposition, and are of particular use in the semilunar position, in young patients with congenital aortic valve disease, and in adults with prosthetic valve endocarditis.

The mechanism of bioprosthetic valve deterioration (Fig. 7–21) involves cusp mineralization and collagen degeneration which progress over time leading to macroscopic cusp tears and prosthetic valve regurgitation.[202] Cusp tears have been classified by location: cuspal tears at the free margin (type I); crescentic tears at the bases of the sinus not involving the free margin (type II); irregular tears in the center of the valve cusp (type III); and multiple small perforations (type IV).[203] Type III tears are associated with infective endocarditis. Large calcific deposits may result in prosthetic valve stenosis. Other pathologic findings that can be seen in bioprosthetic valves are pannus ingrowth that can result in valve orifice stenosis, dehiscence of the commissural insertion from the strut, and endocarditis.

Mechanical Prosthetic Valves

Mechanical valves may be classified by their mechanism of closure and include caged-ball mechanical valves (Starr–Edwards valve), tilting disc valves (Bjork–Shiley, Medtronic–Hall, and Omniscience valves), and bi-leaflet valves (St. Jude, Carbomedics, Sorin Bicarbon, and ATS Open Pivot valves). The major advantage of all mechanical valves is their superior durability compared with bioprosthetic valves. This advantage must be weighed by the significantly increased incidence of thromboembolic events (more common with valves placed in the mitral position versus the aortic position) in patients with mechanical prostheses (Figs. 7–22*E* to 7–22*H*) and the need for chronic anticoagulation. Currently, caged-ball mechanical valves are no longer implanted in the United States due to their large size (profile) and potential complications of ball variance (swelling of the poppet that could obstruct the orifice), hemolysis, and fraying of the cloth covering. The Bjork–Shiley Convexo–Concave valve was found to be susceptible to strut fracture leading to catastrophic disk escape; this valve has been taken off the market. Newer mechanical bileaflet valves have not been shown to have lower complication rates than older models (e.g., St. Jude) in observational (nonrandomized) studies.[204]

REFERENCES

1. Hanson T, Edwards B, Edwards JE. Pathology of surgically excised mitral valves. Arch Pathol Lab Med 109:823–828, 1985.
2. Hendrikx M, Van Dorpe J, Flameng W, et al. Aortic and mitral valve disease induced by ergotamine therapy for migraine: A case report and review of the literature. J Heart Valve Dis 5:235–237, 1996.
3. Connolly HM, Crary JL, McGoon MD, et al. Valvular heart disease associated with fenfluramine-phentermine. N Engl J Med 337:581–588, 1997.
4. Feldman T. Rheumatic heart disease. Curr Opin Cardiol 11:126–130, 1996.
5. Rose AG. Etiology of valvular heart disease. Curr Opin Cardiol 11:98–113, 1996.
6. Olson LJ, Subramanian R, Ackermann DM, et al. Surgical pathology of the mitral valve: A study of 712 cases spanning 21 years. Mayo Clin Proc 62:22–34, 1987.

7. Dare AJ, Harrity PJ, Tazelaar HD, et al. Evaluation of surgically excised mitral valves: Revised recommendations based on changing operative procedures. Hum Patho 24:1286–1293, 1993.
8. Chester E, Gornick CC. Maladies attributed to myxomatous mitral valve. Circulation 83:328–332, 1991.
9. O'Rourke RA. Syndrome of mitral valve prolapse. In: Alpert JS, Dalen JE, Rahimtoola SH (eds): Valvular Heart Disease, pp 157–182. Philadelphia: Lippincott Williams & Wilkins, 2000.
10. Freed LA, Levy D, Levine RA, et al. Prevalence and clinical outcome of mitral-valve prolapse. N Engl J Med 341:1–7, 1999.
11. Perloff JK, Child JS. Clinical and epidemiologic issues in mitral valve prolapse. Am Heart J 113:1324–1132, 1987.
12. Duren DR, Becker AE, Dunning Aj. Long-term follow-up of idiopathic mitral valve prolapse in 300 patients: A retrospective study. J Am Coll Cardiol 17:42–47, 1988.
13. Pocock WA, Bosman CK, Chesler E, et al. Sudden death in primary mitral valve prolapse. Am Heart J 107:378–382, 1984.
14. Kligfield P, Levy D, Devereux RB, et al. Arrhythmias and sudden death in mitral valve prolapse. Am Heart J 113:1298–1307, 1987.
15. Dollar AL, Roberts WC. Morphologic comparison of patients with mitral valve prolapse who died suddenly with patients who died from severe valvular dysfunction or other conditions. J Am Coll Cardiol 17:921–931, 1991.
16. Farb A, Tang AL, Atkinson JB, et al. Comparison of cardiac findings in patients with mitral valve prolapse who die suddenly to those who have congestive heart failure from mitral regurgitation and to those with fatal noncardiac conditions. Am J Cardiol 70:234–239, 1992.
17. La Vecchia L, Ometto R, Centofante P, et al. Arrhythmic profile, ventricular function, and histomorphometric findings in patients with idiopathic ventricular tachycardia and mitral valve prolapse: Clinical and prognostic evaluation. Clin Cardiol 21:731–735, 1998.
18. Burke AP, Farb A, Tang A, et al. Fibromuscular dysplasia of small coronary arteries and fibrosis in the basilar ventricular septum in mitral valve prolapse. Am Heart J 134:282–291, 1997.
19. Enriquez-Sarano M, Orszulak TA, Schaff HV, et al. Mitral regurgitation: A new clinical perspective. Mayo Clin Proc 72:1034–1043, 1997.
20. Popovic Z, Barac I, Jovic M, et al. Ventricular performance following valve replacement for chronic mitral regurgitation: Importance of chordal preservation. J Cardiovasc Surg (Torino) 40:183–190, 1999.
21. Perier P, Stumpf J, Gotz C, et al. Valve repair for mitral regurgitation caused by isolated prolapse of the posterior leaflet. Ann Thorac Surg 64:445–450, 1997.
22. Becker AE, De Wit AP. Mitral valve apparatus. A spectrum of normality relevant to mitral valve prolapse. Br Heart J 42:680–689, 1979.
23. Baker PB, Bansal G, Boudoulas H, et al. Floppy mitral valve chordae tendineae: Histopathologic alterations. Hum Pathol 19:507–512, 1988.
24. Virmani R, Atkinson JB, Byrd BFD, et al. Abnormal chordal insertion: A cause of mitral valve prolapse. Am Heart J 113:851–858, 1987.
25. Chandrashekhar Y, Narula J. Rheumatic fever. In: Alpert JS, Dalen JE, Rahimtoola SH (eds): Valvular Heart Disease, pp 41–74. Philadelphia: Lippincott Williams & Wilkins, 2000.
26. Goldstein I, Halpern B, Robert L. Immunological relationship between streptococcus A polysaccharide and the structural glycoproteins of heart valve. Nature 213:44–47, 1967.
27. Shiffman RN. Guideline maintenance and revision. 50 years of the Jones criteria for diagnosis of rheumatic fever. Arch Pediatr Adolesc Med 149:727–732, 1995.
28. Markowitz M, Gerber MA. The Jones criteria for guidance in the diagnosis of rheumatic fever. Another perspective. Arch Pediatr Adolesc Med 149:725–726, 1995.
29. Stollerman GH. Rheumatic fever. Lancet 349:935–942, 1997.
30. Sanyal SK, Thapar MK, Ahmed SH, et al. The initial attack of acute rheumatic fever during childhood in North India; a prospective study of the clinical profile. Circulation 49:7–12, 1974.
31. Veasy LG, Wiedmeier SE, Orsmond GS, et al. Resurgence of acute rheumatic fever in the intermountain area of the United States. N Engl J Med 316:421–427, 1987.
32. Roberts WC, Virmani R. Aschoff bodies *at necropsy* in valvular heart disease. Circulation 57:803–807, 1977.
33. Narula J, Chopra P, Talwar KK, et al. Does endomyocardial biopsy aid in the diagnosis of active rheumatic carditis? Circulation 88:2198–2205, 1993.
34. Kinare SG. Chronic valvular heart disease. Ann Indian Acad Med Sci 8:48–51, 1972.
35. Dalen JE, Fenster PE. Mitral stenosis. In: Alpert JS, Dalen JE, Rahimtoola SH (eds): Valvular Heart Disease pp 75–112. Philadelphia: Lippincott Williams & Wilkins, 2000.
36. Carabello BA. Indications for valve surgery in asymptomatic patients with aortic and mitral stenosis. Chest 108:1678–1682, 1995.
37. Ben Farhat M, Ayari M, Maatouk F, et al. Percutaneous balloon versus surgical closed and open mitral commissurotomy: Seven-year follow-up results of a randomized trial. Circulation 97:245–250, 1998.
38. Martinez-rios MA, Tovar S, Luna J, et al. Percutaneous mitral commissurotomy. Cardiol Rev 7:108–116, 1999.
39. Yau TM, El-Ghoneimi YA, Armstrong S, et al. Mitral valve repair and replacement for rheumatic disease. J Thorac Cardiovasc Surg 119:53–60, 2000.
40. Hutchison SJ, Tak T, Mummaneni M, et al. Morphological characteristics of the regurgitant rheumatic mitral valve. Can J Cardiol 11:765–769, 1995.
41. Boon A, Cheriex E, Lodder J, et al. Cardiac valve calcification: Characteristics of patients with calcification of the mitral annulus or aortic valve. Heart 78:472–474, 1997.
42. Carpentier AF, Pellerin M, Fuzellier JF, et al. Extensive calcification of the mitral valve anulus: Pathology and surgical management. J Thorac Cardiovasc Surg 111:718–729, 1996.
43. Mazzaferro S, Coen G, Bandini S, et al. Role of ageing, chronic renal failure and dialysis in the calcification of mitral annulus. Nephrol Dial Transplant 8:335–340, 1993.
44. Benjamin EJ, Plehn JF, D'Agostino RB, et al. Mitral annular calcification and the risk of stroke in an elderly cohort. N Engl J Med 327:374–379, 1992.
45. David TE, Bos J, Rakowski H. Mitral valve repair by replacement of chordae tendineae with polytetrafluoroethylene sutures. J Thorac Cardiovasc Surg 101:495–501, 1991.

46. Czer LS, Maurer G, Trento A, et al. Comparative efficacy of ring and suture annuloplasty for ischemic mitral regurgitation. Circulation 86:II46–52, 1992.
47. Warnes CA, Gersh BJ. Pathophysiology, diagnosis, and management of mechanical complications. In: Gersh BJ, Rahimtoola SH, (eds): Acute Myocardial Infarction, pp 259–270. New York: Elsevier Science Publishing, 1991.
48. Hausmann H, Siniawski H, Hetzer R. Mitral valve reconstruction and replacement for ischemic mitral insufficiency: Seven years' follow up. J Heart Valve Dis 8:536–542, 1999.
49. Fasol R, Lakew F, Wetter S. Mitral repair in patients with a ruptured papillary muscle. Am Heart J 139:549–554, 2000.
50. von Oppell UO, Stemmet F, Brink J, et al. Ischemic mitral valve repair surgery. J Heart Valve Dis 9:64–73; discussion 73–74, 2000.
51. Davies MJ. Pathology of Cardiac Valves, pp 124–131. London: Butterworths, 1980.
52. Hauck AJ, Freeman DP, Ackermann DM, et al. Surgical pathology of the tricuspid valve: A study of 363 cases spanning 25 years. Mayo Clin Proc 63:851–863, 1988.
53. Burke AP, Kalra P, Li L, et al. Infectious endocarditis and sudden unexpected death: Incidence and morphology of lesions in intravenous addicts and non-drug abusers. J Heart Valve Dis 6:198–203, 1997.
54. Knight CJ, Sutton GC. Complete heart block and severe tricuspid regurgitation after radiotherapy. Case report and review of the literature. Chest 108:1748–1758, 1995.
55. Roberts WC. Cardiac valvular lesions in rheumatoid arthritis. Arch Intern Med 122:141–146, 1968.
56. Sagie A, Schwammenthal E, Newell JB, et al. Significant tricuspid regurgitation is a marker for adverse outcome in patients undergoing percutaneous balloon mitral valvuloplasty. J Am Coll Cardiol 24:696–702, 1994.
57. Van Nooten GJ, Caes FL, Francois KJ, et al. The valve choice in tricuspid valve replacement: 25 years of experience. Eur J Cardiothorac Surg 9:441–446; discussion 446–447, 1995.
58. Katogi T, Aeba R, Ito T, et al. Surgical management of isolated congenital tricuspid regurgitation. Ann Thorac Surg 66:1571–1574, 1998.
59. Anderson KR, Lie JT. Pathologic anatomy of Ebstein's anomaly of the heart revisited. Am J Cardiol 41:739–745, 1978.
60. Madiwale CV, Deshpande JR, Kinare SG. Ebstein's anomaly—an autopsy study of 28 cases. J Postgrad Med 43:8–11, 1997.
61. Schreiber C, Cook A, Ho SY, et al. Morphologic spectrum of Ebstein's malformation: Revisitation relative to surgical repair. J Thorac Cardiovasc Surg 117:148–155, 1999.
62. Giuliani ER, Fuster V, Brandenburg RO, et al. Ebstein's anomaly: The clinical features and natural history of Ebstein's anomaly of the tricuspid valve. Mayo Clin Proc 54:163–173, 1979.
63. Ewy GA. Tricuspid valve disease. In: Alpert JS, Dalen JE, Rahimtoola SH (eds): Valvular Heart Disease, pp 377–392. Philadelphia: Lippincott Williams & Wilkins, 2000.
64. Farb A, Burke AP, Virmani R. Anatomy and pathology of the right ventricle (including acquired tricuspid and pulmonic valve disease). Cardiol Clin 10:1–21, 1992.
65. Roberts WC. The structure of the aortic valve in clinically isolated aortic stenosis. An autopsy study of 162 patients over 15 years of age. Circulation 42:91–97, 1970.
66. Vollebergh FEMG, Becker AE. Minor congenital variations of cusp size in tricuspid aortic valves. Possible link with isolated aortic stenosis. Br Heart J 39:1006–1011, 1977.
67. Silver MA, Roberts WC. Detailed anatomy of the normally functioning aortic valve in hearts of normal and increased weight. Am J Cardiol 55:454–461, 1985.
68. Waller BF. Morphological aspects of valvular heart disease: Part 1. Curr Prob Cardiol 9:1–65, 1984.
69. Passik CS, Ackerman DM, Pluth JR, et al. Temporal changes in the causes of aortic stenosis: A surgical pathologic study of 646 cases. Mayo Clin Proc 62:119–123, 1987.
70. Davies MJ. Pathology of Cardiac Valves, pp 18–58. London: Butterworths, 1980.
71. Peterson MD, Roach RM, Edwards JE. Types of aortic stenosis in surgically removed valves. Arch Pathol Lab Med 109:829–832, 1985.
72. Dare AJ, Veinot JP, Edwards WD, et al. New observations on the etiology of aortic valve disease: A surgical pathologic study of 236 cases from 1990. Hum Pathol 24:1330–1338, 1993.
73. Faggiano P, Aurigemma GP, Rusconi C, et al. Progression of valvular aortic stenosis in adults: Literature review and clinical implications. Am Heart J 132:408–417, 1996.
74. Davies SW, Gershlick AH, Balcon R. Progession of aortic stenosis: A long-term retrospective study. Eur Heart J 12:10–14, 1991.
75. Ross JJ, Braumwald E. Aortic stenosis. Circulation 38: Suppl V:V61–V67, 1968.
76. O'Keefe JHJ, Vlietstra RE, Bailey KR, et al. Natural history of candidates for balloon aortic valvuloplasty. Mayo Clin Proc 62:986–991, 1987.
77. Carabello BA, Crawford FA, Jr. Valvular heart disease. N Engl J Med 337:32–41, 1997.
78. Pellika PA, Nishimura RA, Bailey KR, et al. The natural history of adults with asymptomatic, hemodynamically significant aortic stenosis. J Am Coll Cardiol 15:1012–1017, 1990.
79. Roberts WC. Morphologic aspects of cardiac valve dysfunction. Am Heart J 123:1610–1632, 1992.
80. Huntington K, Hunter AG, Chan KL. A prospective study to assess the frequency of familial clustering of congenital bicuspid aortic valve. J Am Coll Cardiol 30:1809–1812, 1997.
81. Sabet HY, Edwards WD, Tazelaar HD, et al. Congenitally bicuspid aortic valves: A surgical pathology study of 542 cases (1991 through 1996) and a literature review of 2,715 additional cases. Mayo Clin Proc 74:14–26, 1999.
82. Sadee AS, Becker AE, Verheul JA. The congenital bicuspid aortic valve with postinflammatory disease—a neglected pathological diagnosis of clinical relevance. Eur Heart J 15:503–506, 1994.
83. Nistri S, Sorbo MD, Marin M, et al. Aortic root dilatation in young men with normally functioning bicuspid aortic valves. Heart 82:19–22, 1999.
84. de Sa M, Moshkovitz Y, Butany J, et al. Histologic abnormalities of the ascending aorta and pulmonary trunk in patients with bicuspid aortic valve disease: Clinical relevance to the Ross procedure. J Thorac Cardiovasc Surg 118:588–594, 1999.

85. Burks JM, Illes RW, Keating EC, et al. Ascending aortic aneurysm and dissection in young adults with bicuspid aortic valve: Implications for echocardiographic surveillance. Clin Cardiol 21:439–443, 1998.
86. Arnett EN, Roberts WC. Acute infective endocarditis: A clinicopathologic analysis of 137 patients. Curr Probl Cardiol 1:1–76, 1976.
87. Subramanian R, Olson LJ, Edwards WD. Surgical pathology of pure aortic stenosis: A study of 374 cases. Mayp Clin Proc 59:683–690, 1984.
88. Moore GW, Hutchins GM, Brito JC, et al. Congenital malformations of the semilunar valves. Hum Pathol 11:367–372, 1980.
89. Lerer PK, Edwards WD. Coronary arterial anatomy in bicusspid aortic valve: Necropsy study of 100 hearts. Br Heart J 45:142–147, 1981.
90. Walley VM, Antecol DH, Kyrollos AG, et al. Congenitally bicuspid aortic valves: Study of a variant with fenestrated raphe. Can J Cardiol 10:535–542, 1994.
91. Young ST, Lin SL. A possible relation between pressure loading and thickened leaflets of the aortic valve: A model simulation. Med Eng Phys 16:465–469, 1994.
92. Isner JM, Chokshi SK, DeFranco A, et al. Contrasting histoarchitecture of calcified leaflets from stenotic bicuspid versus stenotic tricuspid aortic valves. J Am Coll Cardiol 15:1104–1108, 1990.
93. Wierzbicki A, Shetty C. Aortic stenosis: An atherosclerotic disease? J Heart Valve Dis 8:416–423, 1999.
94. Wilmshurst PT, Stevenson RN, Griffiths H, et al. A case-control investigation of the relation between hyperlipidaemia and calcific aortic valve stenosis. Heart 78:475–479, 1997.
95. Mautner GC, Mautner SL, Cannon ROD, et al. Clinical factors useful in predicting aortic valve structure in patients > 40 years of age with isolated valvular aortic stenosis. Am J Cardiol 72:194–198, 1993.
96. Nistal JF, Garcia-Martinez V, Fernandez MD, et al. Age-dependent dystrophic calcification of the aortic valve leaflets in normal subjects. J Heart Valve Dis 3:37–40, 1994.
97. Stewart BF, Siscovick D, Lind BK, et al. Clinical factors associated with calcific aortic valve disease. Cardiovascular Health Study. J Am Coll Cardiol 29:630–634, 1997.
98. Gotoh T, Kuroda T, Yamasawa M, et al. Correlation between lipoprotein(a) and aortic valve sclerosis assessed by echocardiography (the JMS Cardiac Echo and Cohort Study). Am J Cardiol 76:928–932, 1995.
99. Davies MJ, Treasure T, Parker DJ. Demographic characteristics of patients undergoing aortic valve replacement for stenosis: Relation to valve morphology. Heart 75:174–178, 1996.
100. Otto CM, Kuusisto J, Reichenbach DD, et al. Characterization of the early lesion of 'degenerative' valvular aortic stenosis. Histological and immunohistochemical studies. Circulation 90:844–853, 1994.
101. Olsson M, Dalsgaard CJ, Haegerstrand A, et al. Accumulation of T lymphocytes and expression of interleukin-2 receptors in nonrheumatic stenotic aortic valves. J Am Coll Cardiol 23:1162–1170, 1994.
102. Bahler RC, Desser DR, Finkelhor RS, et al. Factors leading to progression of valvular aortic stenosis. Am J Cardiol 84:1044–1048, 1999.
103. McElhinney DB, Petrossian E, Tworetzky W, et al. Issues and outcomes in the management of supravalvar aortic stenosis. Ann Thorac Surg 69:562–567, 2000.
104. Joyce CA, Zorich B, Pike SJ, et al. Williams–Beuren syndrome: Phenotypic variability and deletions of chromosomes 7, 11, and 22 in a series of 52 patients. J Med Genet 33:986–992, 1996.
105. Tentolouris K, Kontozoglou T, Trikas A, et al. Fixed subaortic stenosis revisited. Congenital abnormalities in 72 new cases and review of the literature. Cardiology 92:4–10, 1999.
106. Petsas AA, Anastassiades LC, Constantinou EC, et al. Familial discrete subaortic stenosis. Clin Cardiol 21:63–65, 1998.
107. Olson LJ, Subramanian R, Edwards WD. Surgical pathology of pure aortic regurgitation: A study of 225 cases. Mayo Clin Proc 59:835–841, 1984.
108. Bonow RO. Chronic aortic regurgitation. In: Alpert JS, Dalen JE, Rahimtoola SH (eds): Valvular Heart Disease, pp 245–268. Philadelphia: Lippincott Williams & Wilkins, 2000.
109. Turina J, Milincic J, Seifert B, et al. Valve replacement in chronic aortic regurgitation. True predictors of survival after extended follow-up. Circulation 98:II100–106; discussion II106–107, 1998.
110. Dujardin KS, Enriquez-Sarano M, Schaff HV, et al. Mortality and morbidity of aortic regurgitation in clinical practice. A long-term follow-up study. Circulation 99:1851–1857, 1999.
111. Alpert JS. Acute aortic insufficiency. In: Alpert JS, Dalen JE, Rahimtoola SH (eds): Valvular Heart Disease, pp 269–290. Philadelphia: Lippincott Williams & Wilkins, 2000.
112. Roberts WC, Morrow AG, McIntosh CL, et al. Congenitally bicuspid aortic valve causing severe, pure aortic regugitation without superimposed infective endocarditis. Analysis of 13 patients requiring aortic valve replacement. Am J Cardiol 47:206–209, 1980.
113. Yotsumoto G, Moriyama Y, Toyohira H, et al. Congenital bicuspid aortic valve: Analysis of 63 surgical cases. J Heart Valve Dis 7:500–503, 1998.
114. Sadee AS, Becker AE, Verheul HA, et al. Aortic valve regurgitation and the congenitally bicuspid aortic valve: A clinico-pathological correlation. Br Heart J 67:439–441, 1992.
115. Akiyama K, Ohsawa S, Hirota J, et al. Massive aortic regurgitation by spontaneous rupture of a fibrous strand in a fenestrated aortic valve. J Heart Valve Dis 7:521–523, 1998.
116. Mills P, Leech G, Davies M, et al. The natural history of non-stenotic bicuspid aortic valve. Br Heart J 40:951–957, 1978.
117. Stewart WJ, King ME, Gillam LD, et al. Prevalence of aortic valve prolapse with bicuspid aortic valve and its relation to aortic regugitation: A cross-sectional echocardiographic study. Am J Cardiol 54:1277–1282, 1984.
118. Roberts CS, Roberts WC. Dissection of the aorta associated with congenital malformation of the aortic valve. J Am Coll Cardiol 17:712–716, 1991.
119. Turri M, Thiene G, Bortolotti U, et al. Surgical pathology of aortic valve disease. A study based on 602 specimens. Eur J Cardiothorac Surg 4:556–560, 1990.
120. McKay R, Yacoub MH. Clinical and pathological findings in patients with "floppy" valves treated surgically. Circulation 47, 48 (suppl III):III63–75, 1973.
121. Allen WM, Matloff JM, Fishbein MC. Myxoid degeneration of the aortic valve and isolated severe aortic regurgitation. Am J Cardiol 55:439–444, 1985.
122. Lakier JB, Copans H, Rosman HS, et al. Idiopathic degeneration of the aortic valve: A common cause of

isolated aortic regurgitation. J Am Coll Cardiol 5:347–351, 1985.
123. Bortolotti U, Scioti G, Levantino M, et al. Aortic valve replacement for quadricuspid aortic valve incompetence. J Heart Valve Dis 7:515–517, 1998.
124. Kaplan J, Farb A, Carliner NH, et al. Large aortic valve fenestrations producing chronic aortic regurgitation. Am Heart J 122:1475–1477, 1991.
125. Ando M, Okita Y, Sasako Y, et al. Surgery for aortic regurgitation caused by Behcet's disease: A clinical study of 11 patients. J Card Surg 14:116–121, 1999.
126. Paraskos JA. Combined valvular disease. In: Alpert JS, Dalen JE, Rahimtoola SH (eds): Valvular Heart Disease, pp 291–338. Philadelphia: Lippincott Williams & Wilkins, 2000.
127. Beckman DJ, Bandy M, Evans M. Extensive radiation injury of the aortic valve, ascending aorta, left main coronary artery and right ventricle. Cardiovasc Surg 2:117–118, 1994.
128. Rao PS. Pulmonic valve disease. In: Alpert JS, Dalen JE, Rahimtoola SH (eds): Valvular Heart Disease, pp 339–376. Philadelphia: Lippincott Williams & Wilkins, 2000.
129. Kaplan S, Adolf RJ. Pulmonic stenosis in adults. Cardiovasc Clin 10:327, 1979.
130. Waller BF, Howard J, Fess S. Pathology of pulmonic valve stenosis and pure regurgitation. Clin Cardiol 18:45–50, 1995.
131. Gikonyo BM, Lucas RV, Edwards JE. Anatomic features of congenital pulmonary valvar stenosis. Pediatr Cardiol 8:109–116, 1987.
132. Marantz PM, Huhta JC, Mullins CE, et al. Results of balloon valvuloplasty in typical and dyplastic pulmonary valve stenosis: Doppler echocardiographic follow-up. J Am Coll Cardiol 12:476–479, 1988.
133. Sherman W, Hershman R, Alexopoulos D, et al. Pulmonic balloon valvuloplasty in adults. Am Heart J 119:186–190, 1990.
134. Altrichter PM, Olson LJ, Edwards WD, et al. Surgical pathology of the pulmonary valve: A study of 116 cases spanning 15 years. Mayo Clin Proc 64:1352–1360, 1989.
135. Braunwald E. Valvular heart disease. In: Braunwald E (ed): Heart Disease: A Textbook of Cardiovascular Medicine, pp 1007–1076. Philadelphia: W.B. Saunders Co., 1997.
136. Moyssakis IE, Rallidis LS, Guida GF, et al. Incidence and evolution of carcinoid syndrome in the heart. J Heart Valve Dis 6:625–630, 1997.
137. Robiolio PA, Rigolin VH, Wilson JS, et al. Carcinoid heart disease. Correlation of high serotonin levels with valvular abnormalities detected by cardiac catheterization and echocardiography. Circulation 92:790–795, 1995.
138. Himelman RB, Schiller NB. Clinical and echocardiographic comparison of patients with the carcinoid syndrome with and without carcinoid heart disease. Am J Cardiol 63:347–352, 1989.
139. Connolly HM, Nishimura RA, Smith HC, et al. Outcome of cardiac surgery for carcinoid heart disease. J Am Coll Cardiol 25:410–416, 1995.
140. Defraigne JO, Jerusalem O, Soyeur D, et al. Successful tricuspid valve replacement and pulmonary valvulotomy for carcinoid heart disease. Acta Chir Belg 96:170–176, 1996.
141. Konstantinov IE, Peterffy A. Tricuspid and pulmonary valve replacement in carcinoid heart disease: Two case reports and a review of the literature. J Heart Valve Dis 6:193–197, 1997.
142. McDonald ML, Nagorney DM, Connolly HM, et al. Carcinoid heart disease and carcinoid syndrome: Successful surgical treatment. Ann Thorac Surg 67:537–539, 1999.
143. Robiolio PA, Rigolin VH, Harrison JK, et al. Predictors of outcome of tricuspid valve replacement in carcinoid heart disease. Am J Cardiol 75:485–488, 1995.
144. Weissman NJ, Tighe JF, Jr., Gottdiener JS, et al. An assessment of heart-valve abnormalities in obese patients taking dexfenfluramine, sustained-release dexfenfluramine, or placebo. Sustained-Release Dexfenfluramine Study Group. N Engl J Med 339:725–732, 1998.
145. Weissman NJ, Tighe JF, Jr., Gottdiener JS, et al. Prevalence of valvular regurgitation associated with dexfenfluramine three to five months after discontinuation of treatment. J Am Coll Cardiol 34:2088–2095, 1999.
146. Jollis JG, Landolfo CK, Kisslo J, et al. Fenfluramine and phentermine and cardiovascular findings: Effect of treatment duration on prevalence of valve abnormalities. Circulation 101:2071–2077, 2000.
147. Bulkley BH, Roberts WC. The heart in systemic lupus erythematosus and the changes induced in it by corticosteroid therapy: A study of 36 necropsy patients. Am J Med 58:243–264, 1975.
148. Miller CS, Egan RM, Falace DA, et al. Prevalence of infective endocarditis in patients with systemic lupus erythematosus. J Am Dent Assoc 130:387–392, 1999.
149. D'Alton JG, Preston DN, Bormanis J, et al. Multiple transient ischemic attacks, lupus anticoagulant and verrucous endocarditis. Stroke 16:512–514, 1985.
150. Nesher G, Ilany J, Rosenmann D, et al. Valvular dysfunction in antiphospholipid syndrome: Prevalence, clinical features, and treatment. Semin Arthritis Rheum 27:27–35, 1997.
151. Hojnik M, George J, Ziporen L, et al. Heart valve involvement (Libman–Sacks endocarditis) in the antiphospholipid syndrome. Circulation 93:1579–1587, 1996.
152. Nihoyannopoulos P, Gomez PM, Joshi J, et al. Cardiac abnormalities in systemic lupus erythematosus: Association with raised anticardiolipin antibodies. Circulation 82:369–375, 1990.
153. Leung WH, Wong KL, Lau CP, et al. Association between antiphospholipid antibodies and cardiac abnormalities in patients with systemic lupus erythematosus. Am J Med 89:411–419, 1990.
154. Barbut D, Borer JS, Gharavi A, et al. Prevalence of anticardiolipin antibody in isolated mitral or aortic regurgiation, or both, and possible relation to cerebral ischemic events. Am J Cardiol 70:901–905, 1992.
155. Lehmen TJA, Palmeri ST, Hastings C, et al. Bacterial endocarditis complicating systemic lupus erythematosus. J Rheumatol 10:655–658, 1983.
156. Libman E, Sacks B. A hitherto undescribed form of valvular and mural endocarditis. Arch Intern Med 33:701–737, 1924.
157. Mandell BF. Cardiovascular involvement in systemic lupus erythematosus. Semin Arthritis Rheum 17:126–141, 1987.
158. Galve E, Candell-Riera J, Pigrau C, et al. Prevalence, morphologic types, and evolution of cardiac valvular disease in systemic lupus erythematosus. N Engl J Med 319:817–823, 1988.
159. Roberts WC, High ST. The heart in systemic lupus erythematosus. Curr Probl Cardiol 24:1–56, 1999.

160. Kornberg A, Blank M, Kaufman S, et al. Induction of tissue factor-like activity in monocytes by anti-cardiolipin antibodies. J Immunol 153:1328–1332, 1994.
161. Ziporen L, Goldberg I, Arad M, et al. Libman–Sacks endocarditis in the antiphospholipid syndrome: Immunopathologic findings in deformed heart valves. Lupus 5:196–205, 1996.
162. Sokoloff L. Cardiac involvement in rheumatoid arthritis and allied disorders: Current concepts. Mod Conc Cardiov Dis 33:847–850, 1964.
163. Nemchinov EN, Kanevskaia MZ, Chichasova NV, et al. Heart defects in rheumatoid arthritis patients (the results of a multiyear prospective clinico-echocardiographic study). Ter Arkh 66:33–38, 1994.
164. Chand EM, Freant LJ, Rubin JW. Aortic valve rheumatoid nodules producing clinical aortic regurgitation and a review of the literature. Cardiovasc Pathol 8:333–338, 1999.
165. Shimaya K, Kurihashi A, Masago R, et al. Rheumatoid arthritis and simultaneous aortic, mitral, and tricuspid valve incompetence [letter; comment]. Int J Cardiol 71:181–183, 1999.
166. Levine AJ, Dimitri WR, Bonser RS. Aortic regurgitation in rheumatoid arthritis necessitating aortic valve replacement. Eur J Cardiothorac Surg 15:213–214, 1999.
167. Howell A, Say J, Hedworth-Whitty R. Rupture of the sinus of Valsalva due to severe rheumatoid heart disease. Br Heart J 34:537–540, 1972.
168. Bergfeldt L. HLA-B27-associated cardiac disease. Ann Intern Med 127:621–629, 1997.
169. O'Neil TW, Brersnihan B. The heart in ankylosing spondylitis. Ann Rheum Dis 51:705–706, 1992.
170. Graham DC, Smyth HA. The carditis and aortitis of ankylosing spondylitis. Bull Rheum Dis 9:171–174, 1958.
171. Kinsella TD, Johnson LG, Sutherland IR. Cardiovascular manifestations of ankylosing spondylitis. Can Med Assoc J 111:1309–1311, 1974.
172. Roldan CA, Chavez J, Wiest PW, et al. Aortic root disease and valve disease associated with ankylosing spondylitis. J Am Coll Cardiol 32:1397–1404, 1998.
173. Good AE. Reiter's disease: A review with special attention to cardiovascular and neurologic sequelae. Semin Arthritis Rheum 3:263–286, 1974.
174. Lang-Lazdunski L, Hvass U, Paillole C, et al. Cardiac valve replacement in relapsing polychondritis. A review. J Heart Valve Dis 4:227–235, 1995.
175. Corssmit EP, Trip MD, Durrer JD. Loffler's endomyocarditis in the idiopathic hypereosinophilic syndrome. Cardiology 91:272–276, 1999.
176. Imoto Y, Tominaga R, Morita S, et al. Surgical treatment of tricuspid regurgitation caused by Loffler's endocarditis. Jpn J Thorac Cardiovasc Surg 47:570–573, 1999.
177. King JW, Nguyen VQ, Conrad SA. Results of a prospective statewide reporting system for infective endocarditis. Am J Med Sci 295:517–527, 1988.
178. McKinsey DS, Ratts TE, Bisno AL. Underlying cardiac lesions in adults with infective endocarditis. The changing spectrum. Am J Med 82:681–688, 1987.
179. Watanakunakorn C, Burkert T. Infective endocarditis at a large community teaching hospital, 1980–1990. A review of 210 episodes. Medicine (Baltimore) 72:90–102, 1993.
180. MacMahon SW, Roberts JK, Kramer-Fox R, et al. Mitral valve prolapse and infective endocarditis. Am Heart J 113:1291–1298, 1987.
181. Terpenning MS, Buggy BP, Kauffman CA. Infective endocarditis: Clinical features in young and elderly patients. Am J Med 83:626–634, 1987.
182. Danchin N, Voiriot P, Briancon S, et al. Mitral valve prolapse as a risk factor for infective endocarditis. Lancet 1:743–745, 1989.
183. Karchmer AW. Infective endocarditis. In: Braunwald E (ed): Heart Disease: A Textbook of Cardiovascular Medicine, pp 1077–1104. Philadelphia: W.B. Saunders, 1997.
184. Baddour LM, Christensen GD, Lowrance JH, et al. Pathogenesis of experimental endocarditis. Rev Infect Dis 11:452–463, 1989.
185. Durack DT. Current issues in prevention of infective endocarditis. Am J Med 78:149–156, 1985.
186. Mansur AJ, Grinberg M, da Luz PL, et al. The complications of infective endocarditis. A reappraisal in the 1980s. Arch Intern Med 152:2428–2432, 1992.
187. Nakayama DK, O'Neill JA, Jr., Wagner H, et al. Management of vascular complications of bacterial endocarditis. J Pediatr Surg 21:636–639, 1986.
188. Virmani R, Burke AP, Farb A. Atlas of Cardiovascular Pathology, pp 64–68. Philadelphia: W.B. Saunders, 1996.
189. Gubler JG, Kuster M, Dutly F, et al. Whipple endocarditis without overt gastrointestinal disease: Report of four cases. Ann Intern Med 131:112–116, 1999.
190. Elkins C, Shuman TA, Pirolo JS. Cardiac Whipple's disease without digestive symptoms. Ann Thorac Surg 67:250–251, 1999.
191. McAllister HA, Jr., Fenoglio JJ, Jr. Cardiac involvement in Whipple's disease. Circulation 52:152–156, 1975.
192. Rose AG. Mitral stenosis in Whipple's disease. Thorax 33:500–503, 1978.
193. Relman DA, Schmidt TM, MacDermott RP, et al. Identification of the uncultured bacillus of Whipple's disease. N Engl J Med 327:293–301, 1992.
194. Ragni T, Grande AM, Cappuccio G, et al. Embolizing fibroelastoma of the aortic valve. Cardiovasc Surg 2:639–641, 1994.
195. Burke AP, Farb A, Sessums L, et al. Causes of sudden cardiac death in patients with replacement valves: An autopsy study. J Heart Valve Dis 3:10–16, 1994.
196. Hammermeister KE, Sethi GK, Henderson WG, et al. A comparison of outcomes in men 11 years after heart-valve replacement with a mechanical valve or bioprosthesis. Veterans Affairs Cooperative Study on Valvular Heart Disease. N Engl J Med 328:1289–1296, 1993.
197. Grunkemeier GL, Bodnar E. Comparison of structural valve failure among different 'models' of homograft valves. J Heart Valve Dis 3:556–560, 1994.
198. Butany J, Yu W, Silver MD, et al. Morphologic findings in explanted Hancock II porcine bioprostheses. J Heart Valve Dis 8:4–15, 1999.
199. Legarra JJ, Llorens R, Catalan M, et al. Eighteen-year follow up after Hancock II bioprosthesis insertion. J Heart Valve Dis 8:16–24, 1999.
200. Eric Jamieson WR, Marchand MA, Pelletier CL, et al. Structural valve deterioration in mitral replacement surgery: Comparison of Carpentier–Edwards supra-annular porcine and perimount pericardial bioprostheses. J Thorac Cardiovasc Surg 118:297–304, 1999.
201. Walther T, Walther C, Falk V, et al. Early clinical results after stentless mitral valve implantation and comparison with conventional valve repair or replacement. Circulation 100:II78–83, 1999.

202. Schoen FJ, Levy RJ. Bioprosthetic heart valve failure: Pathology and pathogenesis. Cardiol Clin 2:717–739, 1984.
203. Ishihara T, Ferrans VJ, Boyce SW, et al. Structure and classification of cuspal tears and perforations in porcine bioprosthetic cardiac valve implanted in patients. Am J Cardiol 48:665–678, 1981.
204. Grunkemeier GL, Li HH, Naftel DC, et al. Long-term performance of heart valve prostheses. Curr Probl Cardiol 25:73–154, 2000.
205. Farb A, Virmani R, Burke AP. Pathogenesis and pathology of valvular heart disease. In: Alpert JS, Dalen JE, Rahimtoola SH (eds): Valvular Heart Disease, pp 1–39. Philadelphia, Lippincott Williams & Wilkins, 2000.
206. Virmani R, Burke AP, Farb A. Pathology of valvular heart disease. In: Valvular Heart Disease, Rahimtoola SH (volume ed). Volume XI of Atlas of Heart Diseases, Braunwald E (series ed). pp 1.1–1.32. St. Louis, Mosby, 1997.

Chapter

8

THE ENDOMYOCARDIAL BIOPSY: TECHNIQUES AND ROLE IN DIAGNOSIS OF HEART DISEASES

A longstanding doctrine in medicine is that diseases are better understood by knowing the structural alterations of the diseased tissue, and biopsy of organs for microscopic examination remains the diagnostic mainstay. The majority of diagnostic tests available to evaluate cardiovascular diseases emphasize functional physiologic abnormalities and not the underlying pathogenic mechanism. While the diagnostic usefulness of the endomyocardial biopsy is still in evolution, it has several important applications that are well established. This chapter will review techniques and indications for endomyocardial biopsy and summarize diseases that are diagnosed by the endomyocardial biopsy.

TECHNIQUE

The heart biopsy catheter, or bioptome, has undergone several modifications since it was first introduced in 1962.[1] The Stanford bioptome, used primarily in the United States, is relatively short and has hemispherical cutting jaws that remove 1 to 3-mm diameter samples. A disposable bioptome, manufactured by Cordis Corporation, has smaller cutting jaws than the Stanford bioptome and therefore smaller biopsy samples are obtained. Endomyocardial biopsy is usually performed following a standard right-heart catheterization (Fig. 8–1).[2]

Sample Processing

Only careful handling and fixation of the biopsy specimen can provide meaningful information. Four to six pieces of myocardium are routinely obtained. These must be handled carefully to minimize artifacts, and they should be transferred from the bioptome to fixative by use of a sterile needle as soon as possible (within seconds) and in a manner to minimize crushing (Fig. 8–2). Because samples are usually less than 3 mm, they do not require further division. The clinical circumstance under which the biopsy is taken largely determines how the samples are fixed, processed, and stained:

1. Diagnostic biopsies (dilated and restrictive cardiomyopathy, myocarditis): light microscopy—at least four pieces; electron microscopy—one piece (optional); freeze and/or culture—one piece (optional).
2. Cardiac transplant rejection: All pieces are submitted for light microscopy.
3. Anthracycline cardiotoxicity: All pieces are submitted for electron microscopy.

Light Microscopy

For routine light microscopic evaluation of endomyocardial biopsies, a minimum of four pieces of tissue fixed in 10% phosphate-buffered formalin are processed, embedded in

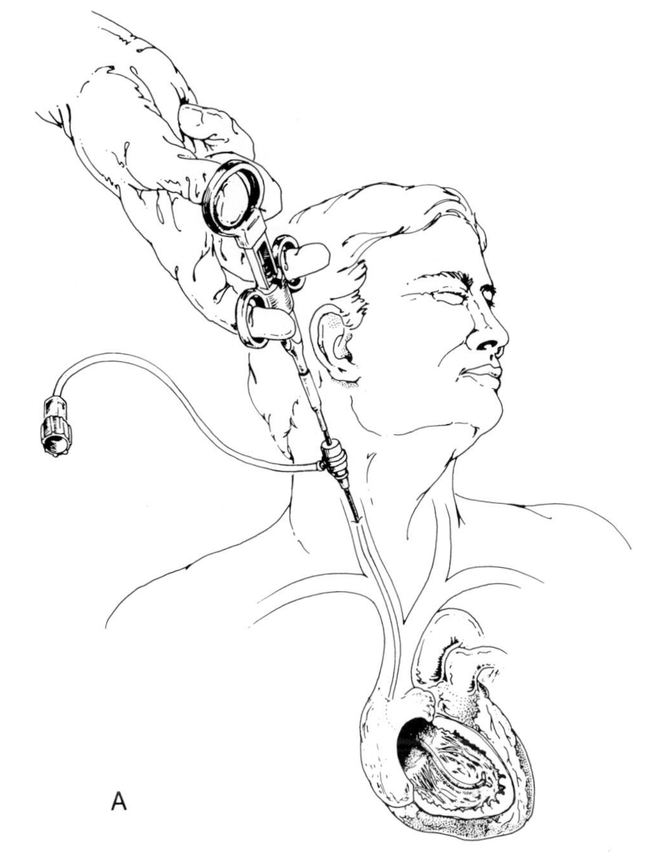

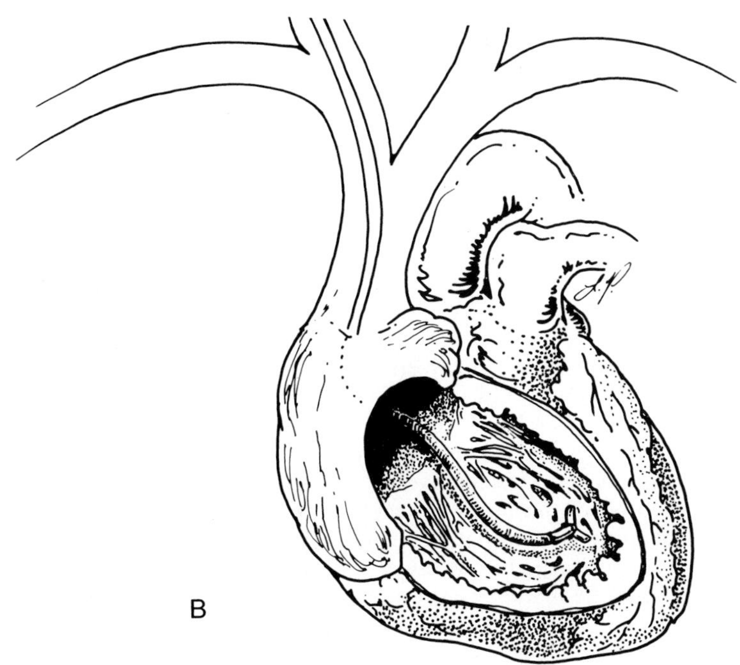

Figure 8–1. Right ventricular endomyocardial biopsy, schematic. *A.* The right internal jugular vein approach is illustrated. *B.* Bioptome is advanced past the tricuspid valve, and the hemispherical cutting jaws are positioned against the apical portion of the septum.

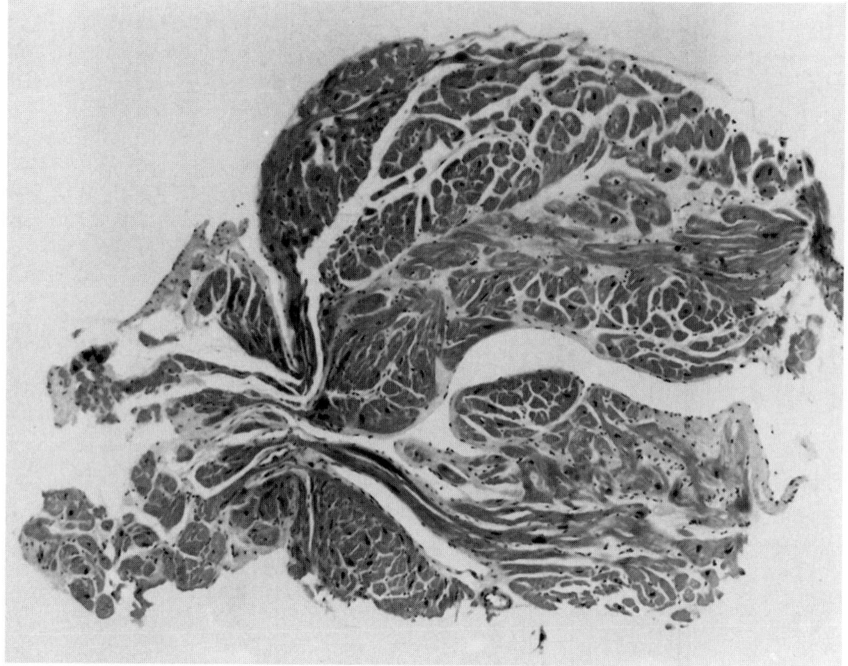

Figure 8–2. Crush artifact. A portion of this specimen was squeezed by forceps prior to fixation, rendering it difficult to interpret.

paraffin, and serial sections are obtained such that the block is exhausted. Slides are stained with H & E, and an additional slide is stained with Masson's trichrome. Special stains—such as the Movat pentachrome stain for connective tissue, Perl's iron stain or Prussian blue for hemochromatosis, and Congo red or thioflavin T for amyloid—are useful in certain circumstances. Multiple levels minimize orientation bias and ensure that focal lesions are not missed (e.g., sarcoid, myocarditis). The Masson trichrome stain aids in evaluating the presence and extent of fibrosis as well as the presence of myocyte necrosis which is important in the grading of acute transplant rejection.

Electron Microscopy

For electron microscopy, enough tissue to make five to ten blocks is fixed in glutaraldehyde and processed by any of a number of established procedures.[3] The biopsy specimen should be placed in a fixative that is at room temperature to minimize contraction artifact.[4] It has been suggested that electron microscopy should be performed on cases in which a diagnosis cannot be made by light microscopy (i.e., cardiomyopathy, storage diseases),[5] although this may not be feasible in all centers. All specimens that are obtained for evaluation of anthracycline cardiotoxicity are submitted for electron microscopy, as the grading system is based on ultrastructure.

Special Studies

Frozen Samples

A piece of myocardium can be snap frozen in OCT-embedding medium and stored at −70°C for potential histochemical, immunohistochemical, or molecular studies. Immunofluorescence is important in the diagnosis of acute vascular (humoral) rejection in the cardiac allograft. While this frozen sample can also be used for routine histology, the pathologist should be aware of certain artifacts that may result, most notably interstitial edema.

Microbiology

If there is a clinical suspicion of viral myocarditis, one biopsy specimen can be placed in Earle's media or modified Eagle's medium for viral culture. Neither viral cultures nor immunofluorescent studies have been rewarding in making the diagnosis of viral myocarditis, however, and polymerase chain reaction (PCR) may be more useful.

Other potential studies that could utilize endomyocardial biopsy samples are biochemical

Table 8–1. Complications of Endomyocardial Biopsy

Cardiac perforation
Hemopericardium
Pneumothorax
Biopsy of tricuspid valve
Air embolism
Arrhythmias (atrial fibrillation, ventricular ectopy)
Transient nerve palsies (right Horner's syndrome, right recurrent laryngeal nerve paralysis, right phrenic nerve palsy)
Cervical soft tissue trauma (hematoma)

From Fowler RE, Mason JW. Role of cardiac biopsy in the diagnosis and management of cardiac disease. Prog Cardiovasc Dis 27:153–172, 1984, with permission.

analysis (enzymes and metabolites), cell culture (to evaluate lymphocytes in cardiac allograft rejection), receptor analysis (e.g., adrenergic receptors in cardiac failure), and molecular biology studies (*in situ* hybridization).[6] Most of these are currently investigational and have no established clinical utility.

Complications

Complications from endomyocardial biopsy are infrequent and have been reported from < 1% to 3.0% (Table 8–1).[7, 8] Premature ventricular contractions are not uncommon, but sustained ventricular arrhythmias are rare, as is atrial fibrillation. The internal jugular vein approach may be complicated by pneumothorax, air embolism, and transient nerve palsies.

Although an attempt is made to obtain the biopsy specimen from the interventricular septum, perforation of the right ventricular free wall can occur. In cardiac transplant patients, this is usually well tolerated and rarely results in cardiac tamponade because the defect is small and the adjacent myocardium is contractile, and there are fibrous adhesions between the epicardium and pericardium. Because the myocardial wall is thin and attenuated in dilated cardiomyopathy, perforation and tamponade may rarely be a cause of mortality.[9, 10] Perforation may manifest as precordial pain or be suspected when mesothelial cells are seen in the biopsy (Fig. 8–3). The presence of fat surrounding a vessel may be suggestive of perforation but is more likely due to the fatty infiltration, which is normally found in the right ventricular myocardium.

Occasionally the bioptome will remove a piece of tricuspid valve or its chordae tendineae, in which case the biopsy will show a sample consisting of fibrous tissue with no myocytes (Fig. 8–4). Because of the presence of numerous chordae and low right-sided pressures, clinically significant right-sided valvular regurgitation is uncommon,[11] although moderate or severe tricuspid regurgitation can be found in as many as one third of patients.[12]

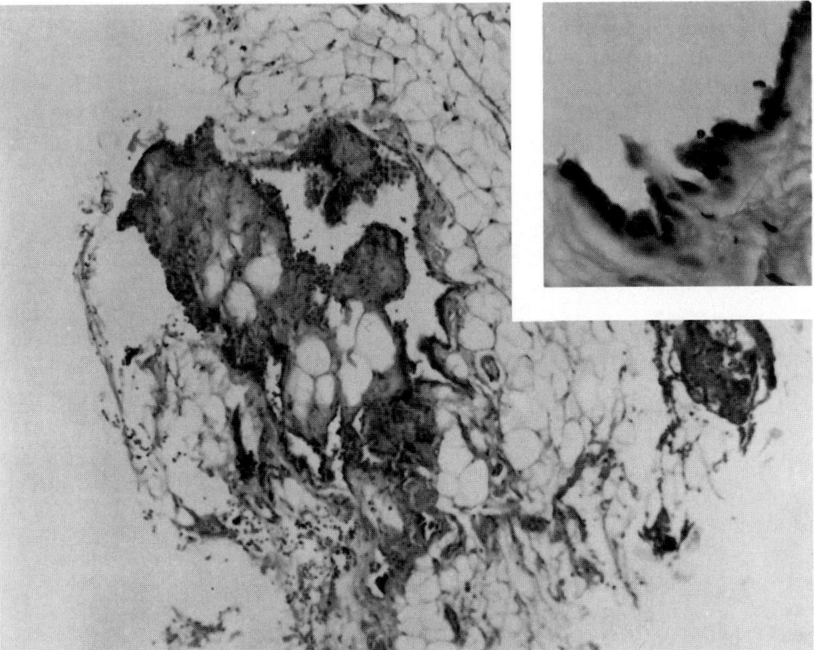

Figure 8–3. Perforation by bioptome. Endomyocardial biopsy specimen consists of fatty tissue and mesothelial cells, seen at higher magnification in the insert, indicative of perforation of the right ventricular free wall.

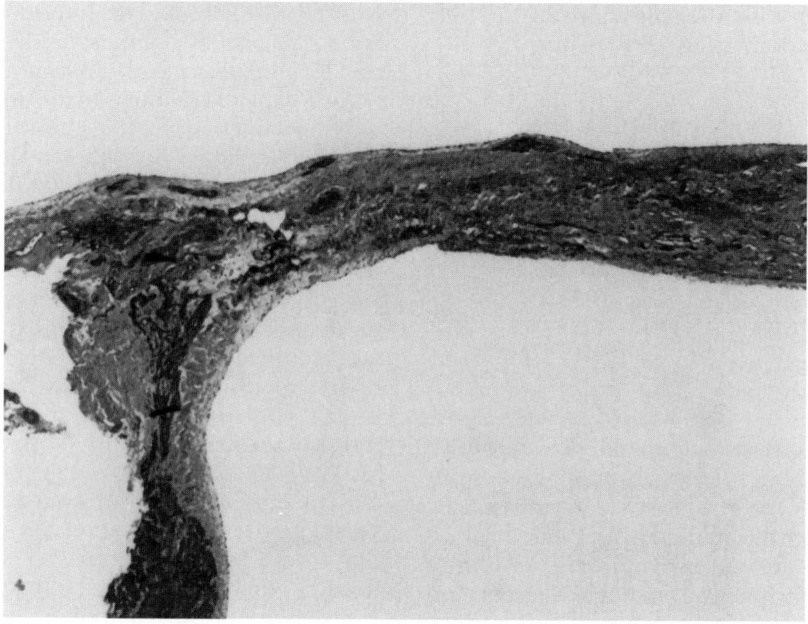

Figure 8–4. Chordae tendineae. A band of fibrous tissue lined by endothelial cells can be seen in continuity with typical myocardium and endocardium.

Artifacts and Nonspecific Findings

In contrast to large sections of often partially autolyzed myocardium from autopsy specimens that the pathologist is accustomed to examining, the endomyocardial biopsy is a small fragment of myocardium that is well-preserved but that has its own peculiar artifacts. The greatest limiting factor in the technique is probably sampling error, as a number of specific heart diseases may be focal in nature (myocarditis, hemochromatosis, sarcoidosis, and myofiber disarray of hypertrophic cardiomyopathy which occurs beyond the usual reach of the bioptome). Myofiber disarray is a normal finding of the right ventricle and should not be taken as evidence of hypertrophic cardiomyopathy (Fig. 8–5). Nonspecific findings also impart limita-

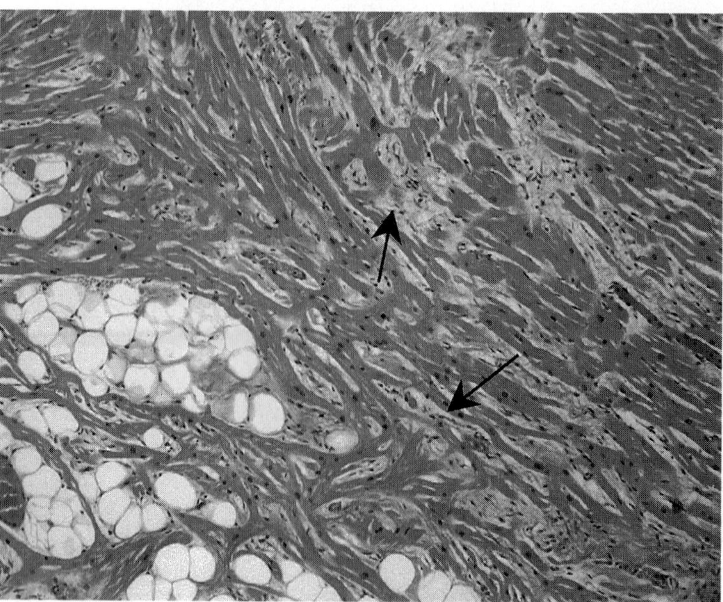

Figure 8–5. Myofiber disarray (*arrows*) is a normal finding in the right ventricle at sites of insertion of the trabeculae carnae into the free wall or septum. Similarly, fat in the right ventricle is almost always seen in most biopsies and does not constitute right ventricular cardiomyopathy. In hypertrophic cardiomyopathy, myofiber disarray occurs in the middle third of the septum and is too deep to access by bioptome. The myofiber disarray of hypertrophic cardiomyopathy, unlike normal right ventricle, is accompanied by a marked increase in cell size.

tions on diagnostic capability. For example, myocyte hypertrophy, atrophy, and interstitial fibrosis (Fig. 8–6) are common but nonspecific findings. While an increase in cell diameter (> 20 μm) is considered indicative of hypertrophy, in dilated cardiomyopathy the myocytes may become stretched (attenuated), resulting in normal cell diameter.[13] For this reason, nuclear changes such as enlargement (which does not regress once hypertrophied), hyperchromicity due to polyploidy, and irregular shapes (box-car shape) are more reliable indicators of myocyte hypertrophy.[13]

The most common artifacts encountered in endomyocardial biopsy are contraction bands (Fig. 8–7), which are due to the biopsy procedure and subsequent handling and processing of the tissue.[2,13,14] These should not be confused with contraction band necrosis, a finding associated with reperfusion injury or catecholamine (pressor) injury,[15] and the attenuated sarcoplasm between the contraction bands should not be mistaken for myocytolysis, which occurs from dilatation of sarcotubular elements.[16] Edema is difficult to diagnose, as variations in fixation and processing may mimic or mask edema. Edema is recognized by separation of myocytes with usually a sparse—almost a naked—nuclear infiltrate, which may be inflammatory in nature within the edematous areas.

A variety of cells exist in the interstitium, such as capillary endothelial cells, pericytes, mast cells, fibroblasts, and nonspecific mesenchymal cells, and these should not be mistaken for inflammatory cells (Fig. 8–8).[13] Also, a small number of lymphocytes may be normally found in the myocardial interstitium.[17,18] Small arteries may undergo intussusception ("telescoping") which should not be mistaken for luminal occlusion. Certain conditions are associated with endocardial thickening (endomyocardial fibrosis, endocardial fibroelastosis), but oblique sections may mimic endocardial thickening (Fig. 8–9.)[13] A fresh thrombus may be found on the endocardial surface and should not be misinterpreted as a mural thrombus, as the bioptome causes endocardial injury during the procedure, resulting in thrombus formation, and the subsequent biopsy may have been taken from or close to a recent previous biopsy site. Due to the architecture of the right ventricle, it is not uncommon for the bioptome to be guided to the same location, and it is important to recognize a previous biopsy site in biopsies especially obtained from cardiac transplant patients.[19] This consists of a focal endomyocardial defect with an overlying organizing fibrin-platelet thrombus, or granulation tissue or fibrosis during the reparative stage, resulting in underlying focal myocyte disarray in the area

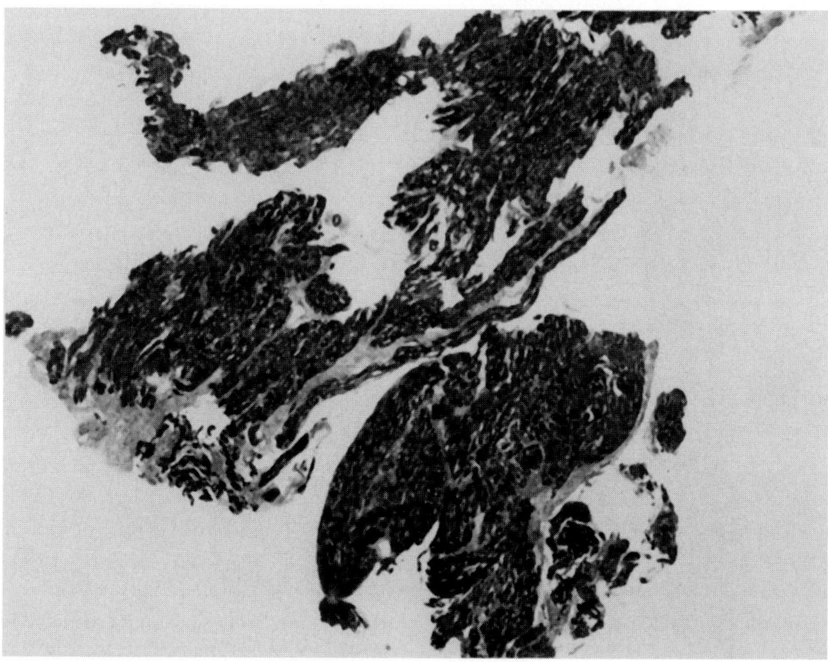

Figure 8–6. Normal heart. This biopsy shows the normal amount and distribution of fibrous tissue that may be present which is not indicative of any specific pathology.

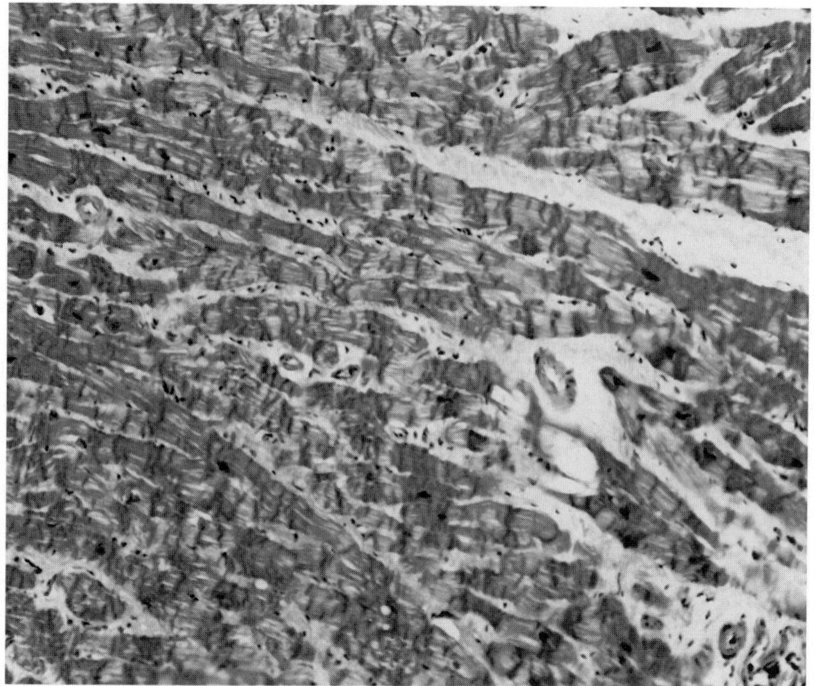

Figure 8–7. Contraction bands. Dark-staining transverse bands with adjacent areas of clear sarcoplasm are seen in individual myocytes.

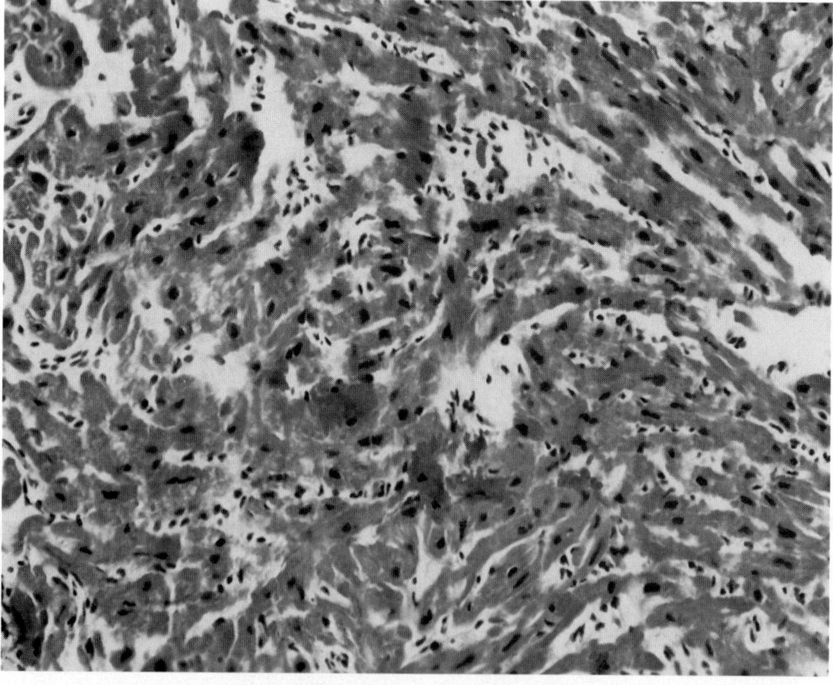

Figure 8–8. Normal biopsy. There is an apparent increase in cellularity in this biopsy. This is accounted for by interstitial cells, which could be mistaken as lymphocytes, leading to an erroneous diagnosis of borderline or myocarditis.

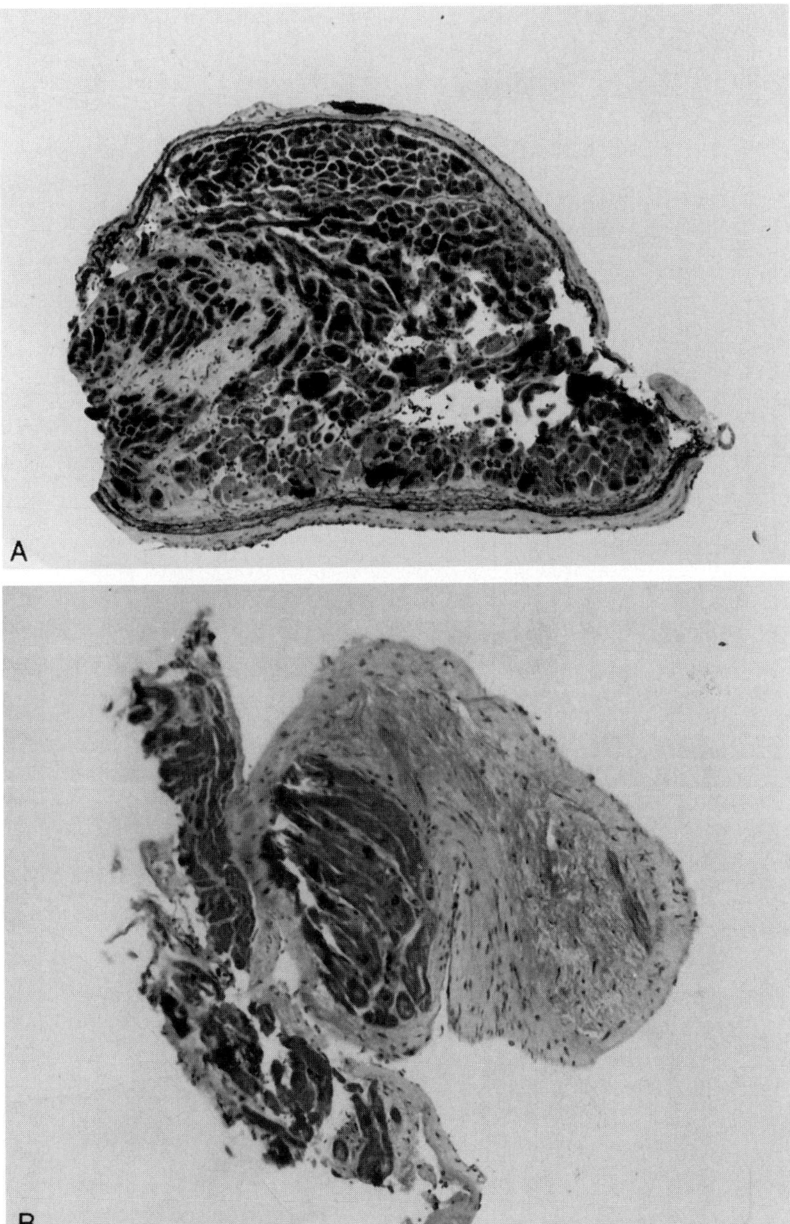

Figure 8–9. Endocardium. *A.* Movat pentachrome-stained section of a normal biopsy, showing normal endocardial thickness and elastic tissue. *B.* Section from the edge of a normal endomyocardial biopsy, showing apparent endocardial thickening due to oblique plane of section. Additional sections and/or reorientation would show a normal endocardium in this specimen.

of the scar (Fig. 8–10). In patients who undergo the procedure repeatedly, as in cardiac transplant evaluation, the chance of obtaining a sample from a previous biopsy site is as high as one of seven. Finally, the procedure of the biopsy itself can induce artifacts. It is not uncommon to find small, focal areas of hemorrhage and thrombus related to the trauma of the biopsy (Fig. 8–10). Improper handling of the biopsy prior to fixation may render some pieces of myocardium difficult to interpret (Fig. 8–2).

INDICATIONS

The diseases that can be diagnosed by endomyocardial biopsy are many and have been grouped by Billingham and Tazelaar[20] into in-

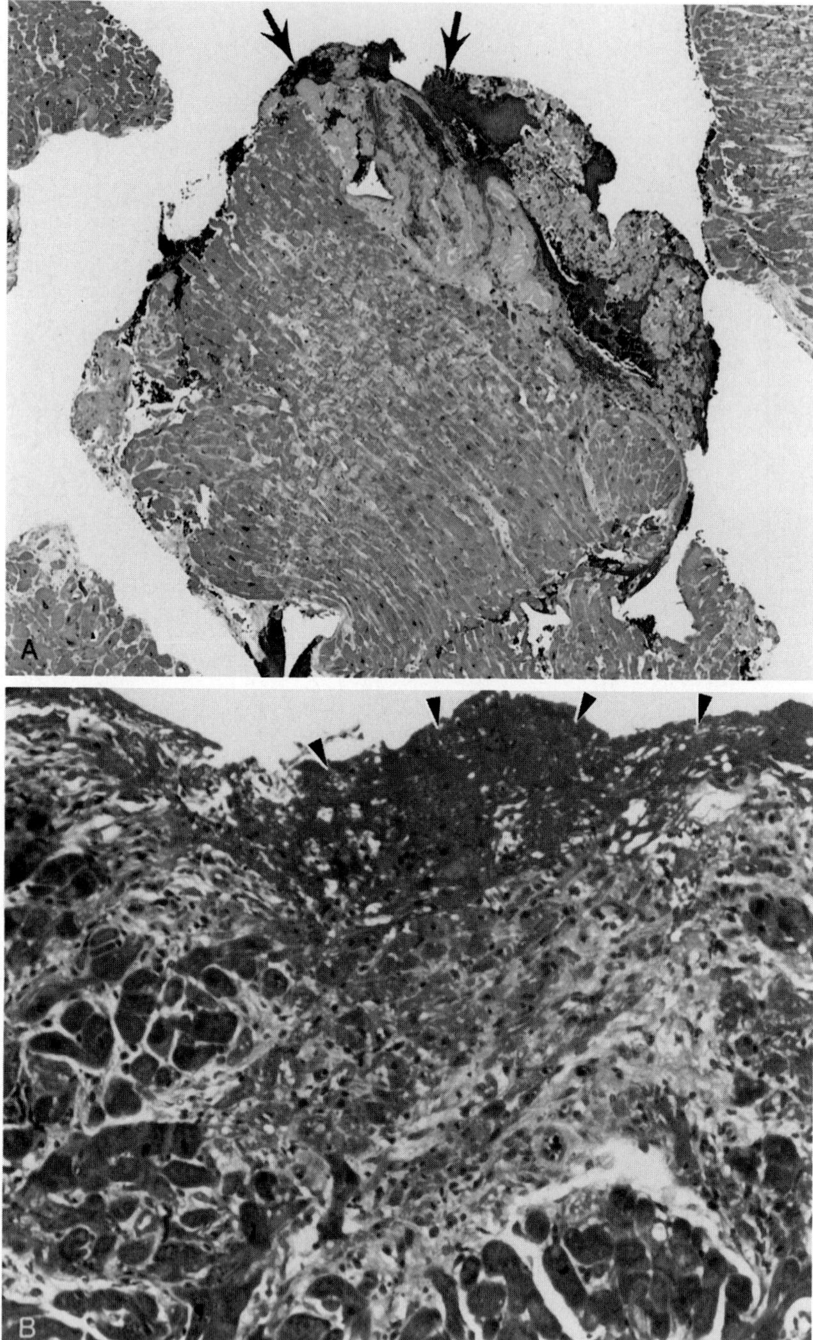

Figure 8–10. Previous biopsy sites. *A.* Low-power photomicrograph, showing recent thrombus overlying endocardium (*arrows*). *B.* A depressed, triangular area representing a recent previous biopsy site, with overlying fibrin deposition along the surface (*arrowheads*), and granulation tissue with a sparse inflammatory infiltrate below.

flammatory, metabolic, endocrine, neuromuscular, toxic, and hematologic infiltrates. The value of endomyocardial biopsy in the management of cardiac allograft rejection is well established and is the mainstay for diagnosis. The endomyocardial biopsy also provides specific information in the assessment of anthracycline cardiotoxicity. Although conditions such as myocarditis and secondary myocardial diseases are relatively rare, they can be readily diagnosed by

Table 8–2. Conditions Diagnosed by Endomyocardial Biopsy

Myocarditis
Idiopathic myocarditis
Giant-cell myocarditis
Hypersensitivity (eosinophilic) myocarditis
Hypereosinophilic myocarditis
Rheumatic myocarditis
Cardiomyopathy
Idiopathic dilated cardiomyopathy
Idiopathic hypertrophic cardiomyopathy
Restrictive cardiomyopathy
Restrictive cardiomyopathy versus pericardial constriction
Specific Heart Muscle Disease
Cardiac amyloidosis
Cardiac sarcoidosis
Hemochromatosis
Metabolic diseases
Glycogen storage diseases
Carnitine deficiency
Fabry's disease
Cardiac tumors
Miscellaneous
Infections of the myocardium (cytomegalovirus, toxoplasmosis, Chagas' disease, Lyme carditis)
Chloroquine cardiomyopathy
Carcinoid disease
Radiation injury
Anthracycline cardiotoxicity

endomyocardial biopsy and help direct specific treatments. Until recently, the role of endomyocardial biopsy in the diagnosis and classification of cardiomyopathies has been controversial. An emerging role for the biopsy in the evaluation of dystrophin and other proteins in familial cardiomyopathies is rapidly evolving and becoming increasingly important.[21] The discussion of idiopathic myocarditis is followed by that of giant-cell myocarditis, hypersensitivity myocarditis, and hypereosinophilic myocarditis. Cardiomyopathies and other specific heart conditions that have been diagnosed by endomyocardial biopsy are also described (Table 8–2).

MYOCARDITIS

Idiopathic Myocarditis

Myocarditis is inflammation of the myocardium that can be caused by bacterial, viral, rickettsial, fungal, or parasitic organisms, or may be autoimmune or idiopathic. Most cases of myocarditis in developed countries are believed to be caused by viruses, as many patients have suffered a recent viral infection or flu-like illness. In order to determine the prevalence of symptomatic myocarditis in patients with congestive heart failure, most authorities agree that recent onset, an ejection fraction of $< 45\%$, and an exclusion of coronary and valvular disease be used as entry criteria into any study of myocarditis. Prior to 1987, there was a wide variation in the incidence of myocarditis in patients with acute onset of congestive heart failure, namely, 15–63%.[22–24] Because the use of immunosuppressive therapy for biopsy-proven myocarditis was a distinct possibility, it was essential that pathologists adopt a more uniform definition. Often, the pathologist mistakes the presence of interstitial fibroblasts or endothelial nuclei of capillaries as lymphocytes. No immunologic markers for the distinction of lymphocytes were in general use in the early 1980s; only hematoxylin- and eosin-stained section were being used to establish presence of myocarditis. A few lymphocytes may be normally present in the interstitium without any destruction of the adjoining myocytes.

Dallas Criteria

Cognizant of the need for establishing reliable diagnostic criteria before a multicenter National Institutes of Health myocarditis treatment trial could be initiated, several cardiac pathologists met in Dallas, Texas in conjunction with the American College of Cardiology meeting in Dallas. Their goal was to define myocarditis from the morphologic standpoint in endomyocardial biopsies. Using these criteria, as outlined below, the incidence of lymphocytic myocarditis on endomyocardial biopsy has varied from 9.1–26%.[25–28] Although the range is smaller than that published prior to the institution of the Dallas criteria, the rate of myocarditis in acute onset congestive heart failure is still dependent upon the criteria used to define the population in which endomyocardial biopsies are being performed.

The Dallas criteria for myocarditis (Table 8–3) are based on inflammation of the myocardium with necrosis and/or degeneration of adjacent myocytes (Figs. 8–11*A* to 8–11*D*). This definition emphasizes the importance of myocyte damage, which may be in the form of necrosis or myocyte vacuolization, manifest by irregular cellular outlines, myocyte disintegration with lymphocytes, or macrophages within the sarcolemma.[29] Contraction bands, which are a very common artifact in endomyocardial biopsies, must not be mistaken for vacuolization or necro-

Table 8–3. Classification of Myocarditis

First Biopsy
Myocarditis with or without fibrosis
Borderline myocarditis (repeat biopsy may be indicated)
No myocarditis
Subsequent Biopsies
Ongoing (persistent) myocarditis with or without fibrosis
Resolving (healing) myocarditis with or without fibrosis
Resolved (healed) myocarditis with or without fibrosis

From Aretz H, Billingham M, Edwards W, et al. Myocarditis: A histologic definition and classification. Am J Cardiovasc Pathol 1:3–14, 1987, with permission.

sis. As mentioned above, the inflammatory infiltrate is primarily lymphocytic, but may contain macrophages or plasma cells, and neutrophils in childhood cases of myocarditis. Occasionally, biopsy may demonstrate the presence of interstitial eosinophilic infiltrates, diagnostic of hypersensitivity myocarditis[30]; this entity should be considered distinct from lymphocytic myocarditis, as the treatment and prognosis are different.

The Dallas investigators used a classification that is based upon whether the first biopsy or subsequent biopsies were examined. Based upon the examination of the first biopsy, the diagnoses that can be rendered are myocarditis with or without fibrosis, borderline myocarditis, and no myocarditis (Table 8–3). Myocarditis can occur in the presence of fibrosis, which is dependent upon the duration of the illness. The diagnosis of borderline myocarditis is rendered when the inflammatory infiltrate is mild and there is absence of myocardial degeneration.

Subsequent biopsies that may be performed in patients with a previous biopsy diagnosis of myocarditis would allow reliable follow-up of myocarditis and the consequence of treatments that may have been rendered. The myocarditis may persist without much change from the previous biopsy and therefore the diagnosis would be "ongoing myocarditis" or "persistent myocarditis" (Fig. 8–12). If the myocarditis is less than the previous biopsy and there are changes of healing identified, then the term "resolving

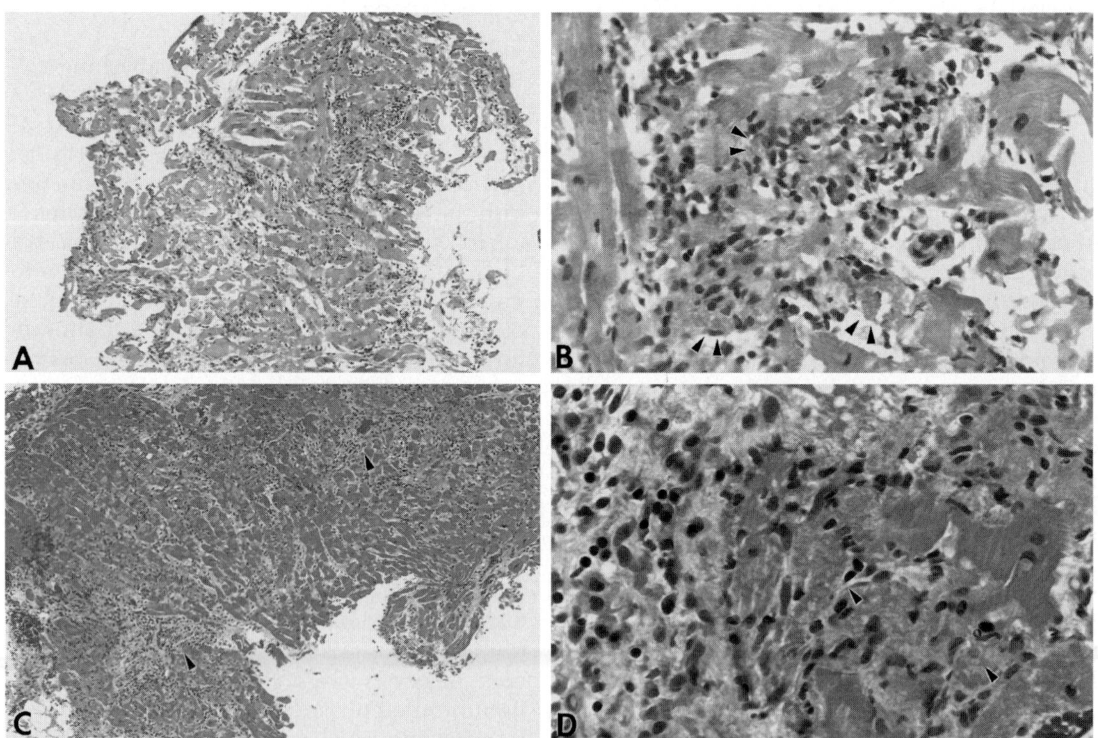

Figure 8–11. Myocarditis. A 45-year-old white woman had sudden onset of dyspnea at rest. Clinical examination revealed congestive heart failure. A right ventricular endomyocardial biopsy was performed. *A.* Low-power view shows diffuse lymphocytic infiltrate. *B.* High-power view shows myocyte necrosis (*arrowheads*) in areas of lymphocytic infiltration. Patient was treated with high doses of corticosteroids and remained on corticosteroid therapy until 2 months before her second presentation, which was 2.5 years after the first biopsy. *C* and *D.* The right ventricular biopsy showed a similar picture as the first biopsy with diffuse lymphocytic infiltration and focal myocyte necrosis (*arrowheads*). (H & E: *A* and *C,* ×75; *B,* ×240; *D,* ×300)

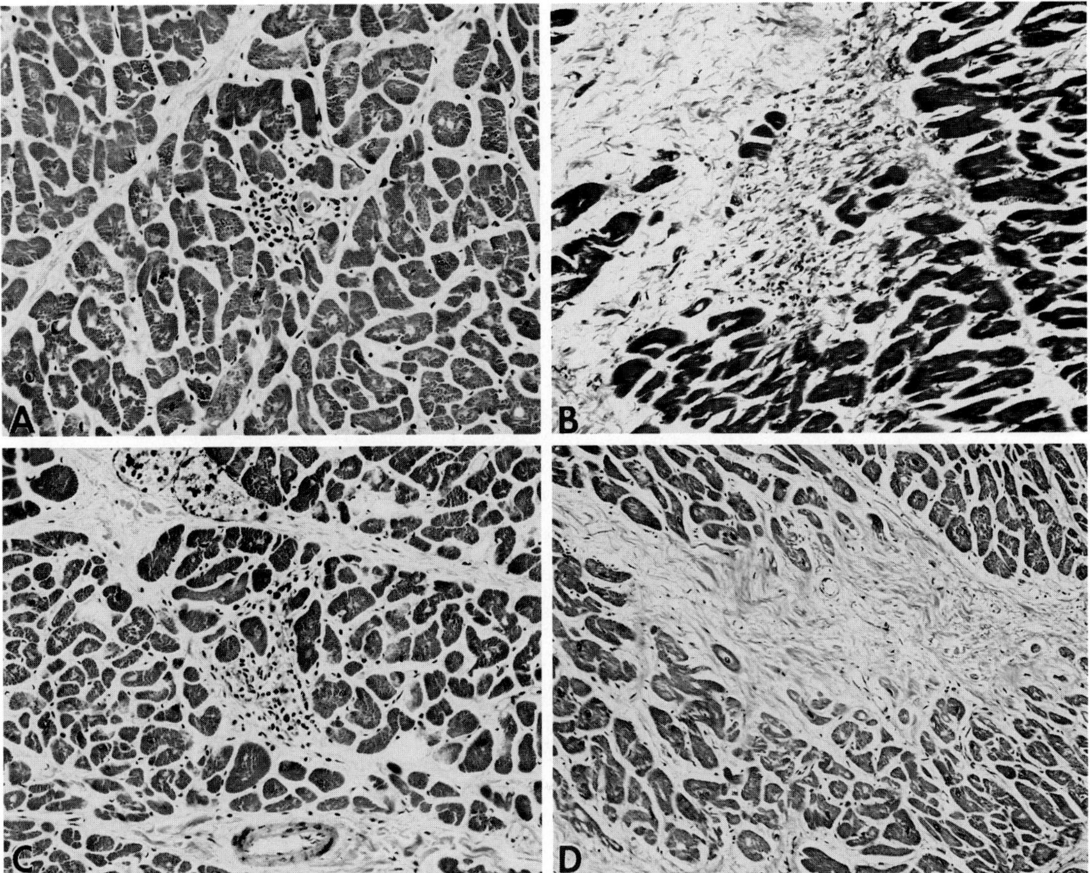

Figure 8–12. Ongoing myocarditis and resolving myocarditis. *A.* Inflammation may be focal and ongoing myocarditis. Note a single focus in this field shows myocyte necrosis with surrounding lymphocytic infiltration. In the same heart, areas of healed and healing myocarditis were seen. Note sparse lymphocytic infiltrate and interstitial fibrosis in *B,* resolving myocarditis. *C* and *D* show other areas in the same heart of borderline myocarditis (*C*) and scarring (*D*); resolved myocarditis with scarring if previous biopsy had shown myocarditis.

myocarditis'' is used. If the myocarditis is fully healed with only areas of fibrosis and absence of inflammation, then the diagnosis is ''healed myocarditis'' or ''resolved myocarditis.'' Following a symptom-free interval and fully resolved myocarditis, the patient may develop another episode of myocarditis; in the biopsy sample this biopsy is now treated as a first biopsy.

As mentioned above, infectious etiologies may masquerade as lymphocytic myocarditis, and should be excluded before Dallas criteria for lymphocytic myocarditis are applied. In addition, the myocyte damage must not be typical of ischemic injury secondary to coronary artery disease. Ischemic infiltrates are often accompanied by hemosiderin deposits (Fig. 8–13). Endocardial and adjoining myocardial involvement is fairly common in myocarditis, whereas in ischemic injury a layer of subendocardial myocytes is spared from ischemic damage.

Inflammatory Cell Typing

With the availability of immunologic markers for determining the nature of the cellular infiltrate, it has been shown that in myocarditis the majority of cells are T-lymphocytes with fewer numbers of macrophages and B-cells. B-lymphocytes and macrophages, along with activated T-lymphocytes, express MHC class II HLA DR molecules, which are also expressed by activated endothelial cells of capillaries and of small intramural vessels. Perivascular and interstitial mast cells may also be increased in cases of lymphocytic myocarditis.[31]

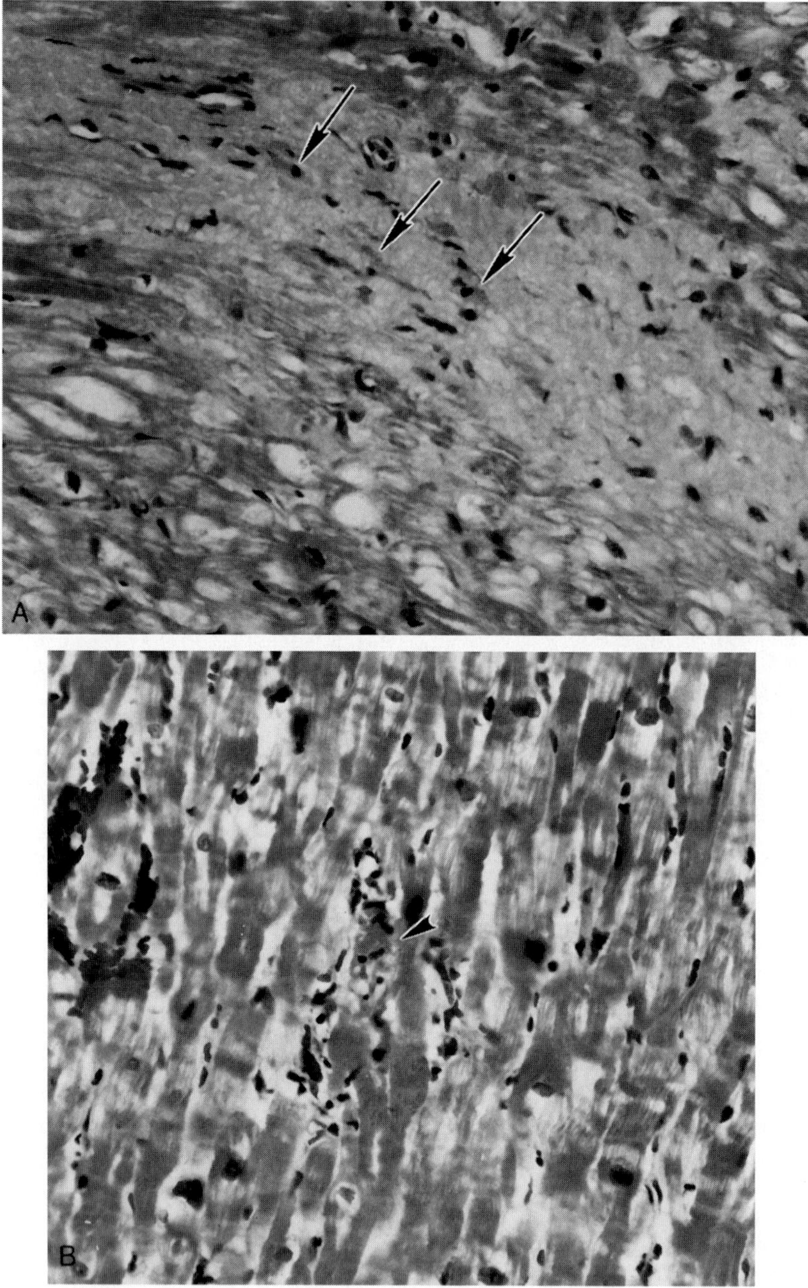

Figure 8–13. Ischemic injury and single cell necrosis. A 57-year-old man presented with sudden onset of congestive heart failure without a prior history of coronary heart disease. Coronary angiography revealed severe coronary atherosclerosis. *A*. Right ventricular biopsy was performed that revealed focal patchy replacement fibrosis with focal presence of macrophages containing hemosiderin pigment (*arrows*), changes consistent with ischemic injury. *B*. Single focus of myocarditis involving a single necrotic myocyte with surrounding inflammation (*arrowhead*) does not constitute myocarditis. (H & E: *A* and *B*, ×300)

Incidence in Heart Biopsies for Idiopathic Heart Failure

Arbustini et al. reported their findings in 601 patients who had undergone endomyocardial biopsy for idiopathic congestive heart failure. In the series the incidence of biopsy-proven myocarditis was only 4.3%. However, 38 of these 601 patients were clinically suspected of having myocarditis on the bases of a recent history of flu-like febrile illness in addition to very recent onset of congestive heart failure, arrhythmias, or conduction disturbances. Corresponding biopsies showed myocarditis in 16 of the 38 cases (42.1%), demonstrating that clinical suspicion of myocarditis may increase the likelihood of myocarditis demonstrated by endomyocardial biopsy.[31]

Treatment and Prognosis

There are many published studies showing that immunosuppressive therapy may be useful in the treatment of myocarditis. However, the most definitive study by Mason and O'Connell failed to show the benefit of azothiaprine and prednisone, cyclosporine and prednisolone versus control group who received conventional drugs for heart failure.[32] All three groups showed a similar improvement in the ejection fraction with time and survival was also not improved with immunosuppressive therapy. It has been suggested that the performance of endomyocardial biopsy in patients suspected of myocarditis is not indicated, as patients with idiopathic dilated cardiomyopathy and myocarditis have identical outcome, possibly because myocarditis progresses to idiopathic dilated cardiomyopathy in many patients.[32] In another study of patients with biopsy-proven myocarditis by Dallas criteria, patients with myocarditis were divided into fulminant myocarditis on the basis of severe hemodynamic compromise, rapid onset of symptoms, fever, and acute myocarditis. Paradoxically, patients with fulminant myocarditis had better survival (93%) compared with those with acute myocarditis (45%),[33] suggesting that fulminant myocarditis is a distinct clinical entity with a good long-term prognosis and response to treatment.

Limitations of Dallas Criteria and Inflammation in "Normal" Hearts

Regardless of the histopathologic criteria used, there is inherent limitation of biopsy size resulting in foci of acute or ongoing myocarditis to be missed. Partly because of small sample size, the authors of the Dallas criteria did not agree on the quantitation of myocarditic lesions, as has been applied to the diagnosis of myocarditis at autopsy,[20] or to the diagnosis of acute allograft rejection on biopsy. In our opinion, the myocarditic lesions should be readily apparent, recognizable at low magnification. Because a single focus of single-cell necrosis in autopsy hearts does not constitute clinically significant myocarditis, it is unclear, despite the small sample, if one focus should constitute myocarditis on biopsy, as per the Dallas criteria. However, in autopsy hearts with known myocarditis, Kubo et al. report that because of sampling error due to small biopsy sample (even if five pieces are submitted), there is only a 50% chance of detecting myocarditic infiltrates.[34]

Our experience in autopsy hearts of myocarditis shows that the inflammatory lesions are usually quite extensive, surrounding at least five to eight myocytes demonstrating a moth-eaten, necrotic appearance. In unquestionable cases of death due to myocarditis, the inflammatory foci are never single, but are diffuse within a given area of myocardium, sometimes involving large areas of the myocardium (> 0.5 mm^2) in the left and right ventricles, with or without atrial involvement. Therefore, the absence of myocarditis on endomyocardial biopsy ("no myocarditis" by Dallas criteria) may be more reliable in ruling out significant clinical myocarditis than previously believed.

In contrast, myocardial lymphocytic infiltration is not unusual in persons dying of noncardiac causes. We have reported that 42% of autopsy hearts (10 of 24 hearts) in patients dying secondary to trauma showed lymphocyte infiltration, and necrosis of more than single cell was documented only in one patient (2%).[35] Using immunohistochemical techniques to identify T-cells, Feeley et al. have shown that the majority of hearts show presence of 0-3 T-lymphocytes/mm^2. When $\geq$14 T-lymphocytes/mm^2 are identified, there is either an underlying myocarditis, allograft rejection, or a lymphoproliferative disorder.[36] These finding are consistent with the recommendations of ISFC (International Society and Federation of Cardiology).[37]

Because of the range of inflammation present in normal hearts, a category of borderline myocarditis is of limited use. The amount of inflammatory infiltrate should be quantitated as being mild, moderate, or severe and focal, confluent, or diffuse. The extent of myocyte necrosis should be described as groups of necrotic myocytes or single-cell necrosis. The amount and distribution of the fibrosis, when present, should be further characterized as endocardial, replacement, or interstitial in location and the extent mentioned.[29]

Viral Agents and Myocarditis

Enteroviruses, especially Coxsackieviruses, are common infections in children, and cause up to 50% of cases of myocarditis.[38, 39] The diagnosis of a viral etiology is problematic. Viral cultures give a low yield because of transient infection, and serologic diagnosis rising serum titers are not entirely specific and require follow-up study. Recently, polymerase chain reaction (PCR) has been used for the detection of viral nucleic acid in endomyocardial biopsies. In a study by Martin et al. on 38 infants and children with suspected acute viral myocarditis, a viral genome was detected in 26 of 38 (68%) biopsies by PCR.[40] The viral types were varied and, surprisingly, enteroviruses were not the most prevalent organism. There were 15 cases of adenoviral infection, 8 enteroviral, 2 herpes simplex virus, and 1 cytomegalovirus (CMV) infection. There was disagreement with the histopathologic finding of myocarditis in 13 of the 26 (50%) PCR positive specimens, and the discrepancy was usually associated with adenovirus, suggesting that the amplification of adenoviral DNA was not necessarily associated with the patient's illness.[40] Nevertheless, the mouse model of coxsackievirus B3 (CB3) myocarditis parallels the human disease. In this model, myocarditis is biphasic, with an initial acute response to the viral infection that does not involve the heart, and a later chronic disease that spreads to the heart. Until recently it has been thought that the myocardial disease is the result of virus-induced immune response directed at infected myocytes or at "mimicked" epitopes shared between viral and cardiac antigens.[41, 42] However, Horwitz et al. have recently shown that murine myocarditis does not occur if there is greater expression of interferon-γ by the pancreatic cells, suggesting that myocarditis is virus-mediated and not an autoimmune phenomenon.[43]

Other viral infections infrequently cause a fatal myocarditis. There have been reports of myocarditis due to influenza, lassa fever (arenavirus), Epstein–Barr virus, poliomyelitis, rubella (German measles), rubeola (measles), varicella (chicken pox), variola, and vaccinia virus. Myocardial involvement in influenza is rare but cardiac symptoms occur in 5 to 10% of cases during an epidemic.[44] Cardiac involvement occurs within 1 to 2 weeks of the onset of the illness.[45] The cellular infiltrate is predominantly lymphocytic with some macrophages and rare neutrophil infiltration. Lassa fever is a major cause of morbidity in West Africa, but cardiac symptoms, although frequent, do not play a significant role in mortality.[46, 47] Childhood viral diseases like mumps, rubeola, rubella, and varicella have all been reported to become complicated rarely by lymphocytic myocarditis.[48–51]

Differential Diagnosis

When the infiltrate is predominately neutrophilic, the process is likely bacterial, an early phase of acute viral myocarditis, or persistent viral myocarditis in children. Ischemic myocardial damage will manifest as groups of myocytes showing necrosis with polymorphonuclear infiltration. Macrophage giant cells are usually a component of well-formed granulomas in sarcoidosis, associated with myocyte necrosis in giant-cell myocarditis, and are rarely present in the interstitium in hearts with hypersensitivity myocarditis (see following). When eosinophils are seen, one must rule out parasitic infections, idiopathic hypereosinophilic syndrome, giant-cell myocarditis, and hypersensitivity myocarditis (Table 8–4).

Table 8–4. Inflammatory Infiltrates and Differential Diagnosis in Myocarditis

Lymphocytic	Neutrophilic	Eosinophilic	Giant Cells
IDIOPATHIC	Bacterial infections	Hypersensitivity	Sarcoidosis
Viral	Ischemic	Parasitic infestations	Giant-cell myocarditis
Sarcoidosis	Idiopathic	Hypereosinophilic syndrome	Hypersensitivity
Toxic	Viral (early, especially children)	Idiopathic	Rheumatoid diseases
Collagen vascular	Pressor agents		Rheumatic fever
Right ventricular dysplasia			Tuberculosis
Kawasaki disease			Fungal infections
Lymphoma			

Adapted from Aretz H, Billingham M, Edwards W, et al. Myocarditis: A histologic definition and classification. Am J Cardiovasc Pathol 1:3–14, 1987, with permission.

Giant-Cell Myocarditis

Giant-cell myocarditis is a rare disease and is considered a subset of idiopathic myocarditis. It usually affects young to middle-aged adults, is rapidly fatal, and is characterized by widespread myocardial degeneration, in the presence of multinucleated giant cells.[52] Giant cells are usually found at the margins of the areas of necrosis. In the largest series reported, the average age of patients with giant cell myocarditis was 43 years; over 88 percent were white, 5 percent were black, 5 percent were Southeast Asian or Indian, and 2 percent were Middle Eastern. Most presented with congestive heart failure (75 percent), ventricular arrhythmia (14 percent), or heart block (5 percent), although in some cases the initial symptoms resembled those of acute myocardial infarction.[53] Nineteen percent had associated autoimmune disorders. The rate of death or cardiac transplantation was 89 percent, and median survival was only 5.5 months from the onset of symptoms. The 22 patients treated with corticosteroids and cyclosporine, azathioprine, or both therapies survived for an average of 12.3 months, as compared with an average of 3.0 months for the 30 patients who received no immunosuppressive therapy (P = 0.001). Of the 34 patients who underwent heart transplantation, 9 (26 percent) had a giant-cell infiltrate in the transplanted heart and 1 died of recurrent giant-cell myocarditis.[53]

The histopathologic features include myocardial necrosis, chronic inflammation consisting of lymphocytes and plasma cells, including prominent eosinophils, and multinucleated giant cells[54] (Fig. 8–14). The giant cells were, at

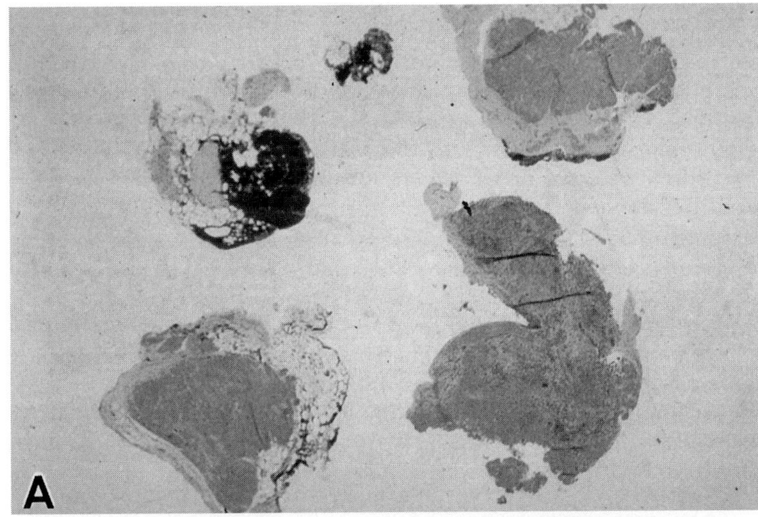

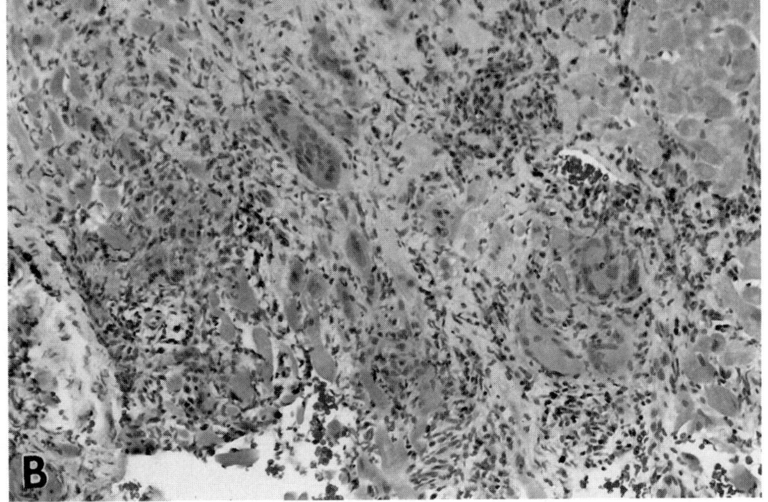

Figure 8–14. Giant-cell myocarditis. A 50-year-old male with 2 weeks' history of congestive heart failure, clinical diagnosis of dilated cardiomyopathy (ejection fraction 35%), underwent right-heart endomyocardial biopsy. *A.* Four pieces of myocardium, one of which shows extensive inflammatory infiltrate. *B.* High power showing a dense inflammatory infiltrate of lymphocytes, macrophages, and large number of giant cells. Also scattered eosinophils are seen within the inflammatory infiltrate.

one time, believed to be entirely myogenic.[55] A histiocytic origin was also suspected, however, and immunohistochemical studies have confirmed that the majority of giant cells are made of macrophages.[52, 56, 57] Myogenic giant cells may also be present in the border zones of necrosis. Chow et al. and Ren et al. have demonstrated that the remainder of the inflammatory infiltrate are composed of macrophages and T lymphocytes; frequently the latter are CD8+ cells.[52, 58, 59] Marboe et al. showed in healed idiopathic myocarditis that the CD8+ to CD4+ ratio is higher than nonhealed cases, suggesting that the phase of lesion may be important in the type of T-cell infiltrate; we have also found that CD8 cells are prominent in the acute phase of giant cell myocarditis.[52]

The major differential diagnosis on endomyocardial biopsy is sarcoidosis. Helpful distinguishing features include the nature and location of the inflammatory infiltrate and the degree of scarring (generally more severe in sarcoid). Well-formed granulomas are not seen in giant-cell myocarditis; also eosinophils are usually plentiful in giant-cell myocarditis and are absent in sarcoidosis. There is often involvement of the epicardium in sarcoidosis, a feature that is absent in giant-cell myocarditis.[52] Other lesions with giant cells include granulomas caused by fungi, mycobacteria, or foreign bodies; the absence of caseation and true granulomas in giant cell myocarditis help establish the diagnosis, and special stains are negative for organisms. In some cases of giant-cell myocarditis, sampling error will result in the lack of giant cells on biopsy, and the histologic features are indistinguishable from severe lymphocytic myocarditis.

Giant-cell myocarditis is localized to the heart but has been reported to be associated with thymoma, systemic lupus erythematosus, and thyrototoxicosis.[60] It appears to be a nonspecific but unique response of the myocardium to an as-yet unidentified agent.

Table 8–5. Drugs Associated With Hypersensitivity Myocarditis

Toxic Myocarditis*	Hypersensitivity Myocarditis†
Anthracyclines	Sulfonamides
Amphetamines	Isoniazid
Antihypertensives	Penicillin
Barbiturates	Tetracyclines
Catecholamines	Phenylbutazone
Paraquat	Thiazide diuretics
Cyclophosphamide	Horse serum
Fluorouracil	Methyldopa
Histamine-like drugs	Cocaine
Lithium compounds	Streptomycin
Phenothiazines	
Theophylline	

* Dose-related lesions of different ages with necrotizing vasculitis.
† Nondose-related lesions of same age with eosinophilic infiltrate.
From Billingham ME, Tazelaar HD. Cardiac biopsy. In: Parmley WW, Chatterjee K (eds): Cardiology, Volume 1, Ch 54. Philadelphia: JB Lippincott, 1987, with permission.

Hypersensitivity Myocarditis

More than 20 drugs have been incriminated as possible etiologic agents in hypersensitivity myocarditis (Table 8–5), with methyldopa, sulfonamides, and penicillin accounting for more than 75% of reported cases. Recently it has been reported that the incidence of hypersensitivity myocarditis is fairly high (22%) in patients undergoing transplantation and most have been attributed to dobutamine.[61, 62] A few case reports describe recurrence of hypersensitivity myocarditis in the donor heart.[63] The diagnosis of hypersensitivity myocarditis should be considered in any patient with an ongoing allergic reaction to a drug, evidence of peripheral eosinophilia, appearance of new electrocardiographic changes, mildly elevated cardiac enzyme (creatine kinase [CK] and MB isoenzyme), mild cardiomegaly, or unexplained tachycardia.[64, 65] The time from initial drug exposure to the development of hypersensitivity myocarditis may vary from hours to months. The patient is usually still taking the drug at the onset of cardiac symptoms and, following discontinuation of the medication, it is unusual for the allergic phenomenon to persist for an extended period. The presumed mechanism is delayed hypersensitivity.[66] Although often asymptomatic, hypersensitivity myocarditis may cause congestive failure, arrhythmias, and even sudden death. Death is presumably due to arrhythmia, and inappropriate sinus tachycardia, conduction delays, or ST-T wave abnormalities may be the only clues.

The histopathologic features of hypersensitivity myocarditis include interstitial chronic inflammatory infiltrate by lymphocytes, plasma cells, and macrophages, with a prominence of eosinophils (Fig. 8–15). Although foci of myocytolysis may be seen, myocyte necrosis is not a prominent feature.[66] The infiltrate is predominantly perivascular, and there is absence of fibrosis or evidence of healing.[66–68] Also, rarely full-blown granulomas may be seen but there is lack of necrosis and a prominence of eosinophils. The inflammation is patchy but usually

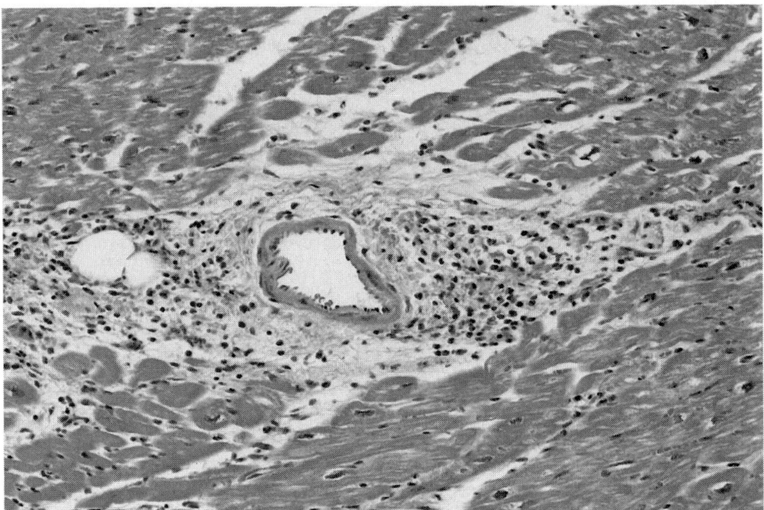

Figure 8–15. Hypersensitivity myocarditis. The inflammation is perivascular and composed of histiocytes, lymphocytes, and eosinophils.

involves all chambers. The diagnostic features are prominence of eosinophils mixed with lymphocytes and plasma cells and absence of extensive necrosis or fibrosis (Table 8–6). The process may be self-limited with little residual cardiac damage, provided the offending agent is withdrawn. In a patient suspected of having hypersensitivity myocarditis, all medications should be withdrawn, corticosteroid therapy instituted, and endomyocardial biopsy performed to confirm the diagnosis.

Hypereosinophilic Myocarditis

Myocarditis may be a manifestation of the hypereosinophilic syndrome, which typically occurs in men in the fourth decade and is characterized by persistent peripheral eosinophilia (1,500 eosinophils per cubic millimeter) for at least 6 months. Cardiac involvement is frequent, occurring in three fourths of the patients. Both sides of the heart are usually involved; therefore, a right ventricular biopsy may be extremely useful. In the early stages, the endocardium and myocardium are heavily infiltrated by eosinophils, but these vary with the stage of the disease. Along with eosinophilic infiltration there is extensive myocyte necrosis resembling myocarditis (Fig. 8–16).[5, 16, 69] The endocardial surface often is involved by a mural thrombus containing eosinophils. Occasionally, the intramyocardial coronary arteries may show thrombosis with or without organization (for greater details, see Chapter 6). Hypereosinophilic myocarditis must be differentiated from hypersensitivity myocarditis, which generally demonstrates little, if any, necrosis, an absence of thrombosis, and different clinical features (see above).

Table 8–6. Differentiating Features of Direct Drug Toxicity and Hypersensitivity Myocarditis

Feature	Direct Toxicity	Hypersensitivity Response
Myocytolysis	Present	Present
Myocyte necrosis	Present	Infrequent
Vasculitis	Necrotizing	Nonnecrotizing
Microthrombi	Occasional	None
Hemorrhage	Occasional	None
Eosinophils	None	Present
Lymphocytes	Normal	Atypical
Giant cells	None	Present
Infiltrate	Nongranulomatous	Granulomatous
Fibroblasts and collagen	Present	Absent
Ages of lesion	Different	Same
Dose-related	Yes	No

Modified from Billingham ME. Morphologic changes in drug-induced heart disease. In: Bristow MR (ed): Drug-Induced Heart Disease, p 127. Amsterdam, Elsevier/North-Holland Biomedical Press, 1980, with permission.

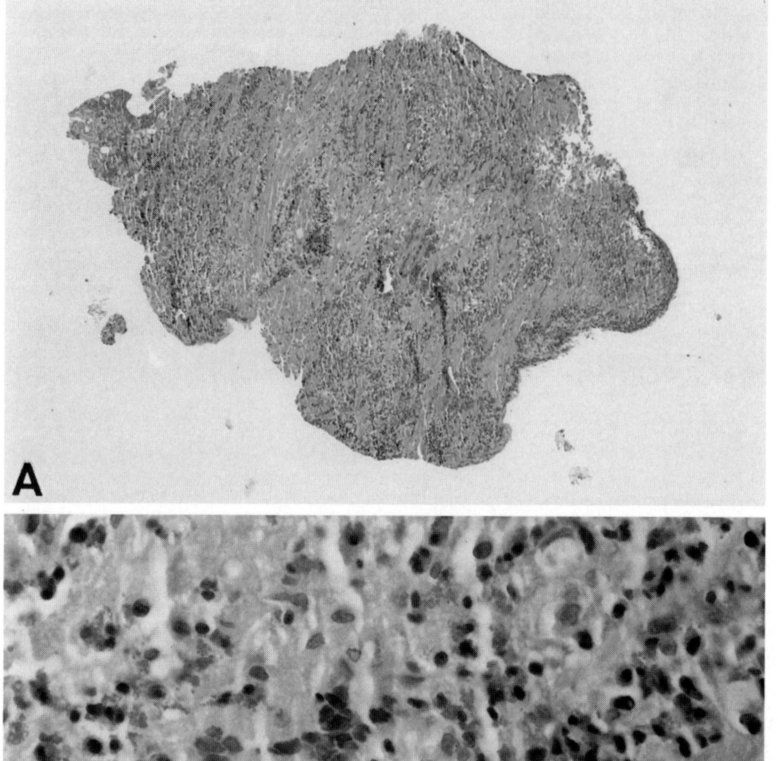

Figure 8–16. Hypereosinophilic syndrome. A 27-year-old man presented with upper respiratory tract infection was found clinically to be in florid congestive heart failure with peripheral eosinophilia. *A.* Note extensive myocardial inflammation along with marked destruction of myocytes. *B.* High-power view showing predominant eosinophilic infiltration, macrophage, and rare giant cell.

Myocarditis in Whipple's Disease

The original description of Whipple's disease affecting the intestine and mesenteric lymphatic tissues appeared in 1907. It was not until 1963 that Enzinger and Helwig described involvement of the heart, characterized by periodic acid-Schiff (PAS)-positive macrophages among the myocardial fibers within areas of interstitial fibrosis.[70] In 1975, MacAllister and Fenoglio reviewed the autopsy findings in 19 patients dying with Whipple's disease.[71] Fifty-eight had clinical cardiac findings, and 79% had gross cardiac lesions. Histologically, they observed PAS-positive macrophages in the pericardium, myocardium, and valves of each patient with cardiac disease. The myocardium showed focal interstitial fibrosis in 89% of cases with interspersed PAS-positive macrophages, scattered lymphocytes, and Anitschkow cells. Occasionally, the areas of fibrosis and macrophage infiltrates were perivascular in location (Fig. 8–17), but no Aschoff nodules were identified. Lie and Davis illustrated a case of Whipple's disease with myocardial lesions consisting of lymphocytes, histocytes, and plasma cells.[72] Southern et al. described a 44-year-old man with a long prodromal period characterized by granulomatous lymphadenitis and progressive lymphedema of the extremities without any gastrointestinal involvement.[73] This patient's clinical condition deteriorated with the onset of lymphocytic myocarditis; at autopsy, a diagnosis of Whipple's disease was made. This case demonstrates that Whipple's disease should be considered in the differential diagnosis of a patient presenting with granulomatous disease. The diagnosis is confirmed by ultrastructural demon-

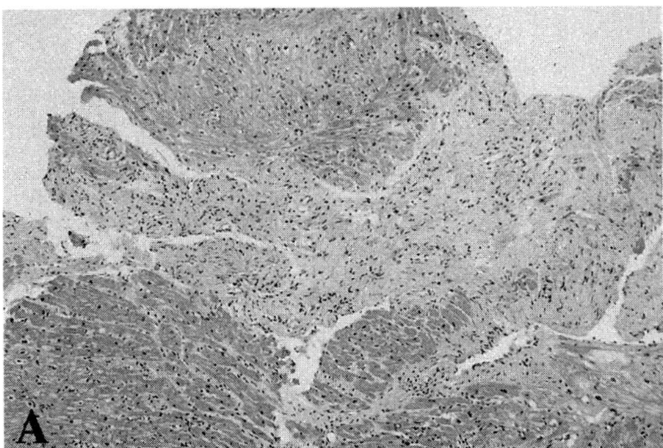

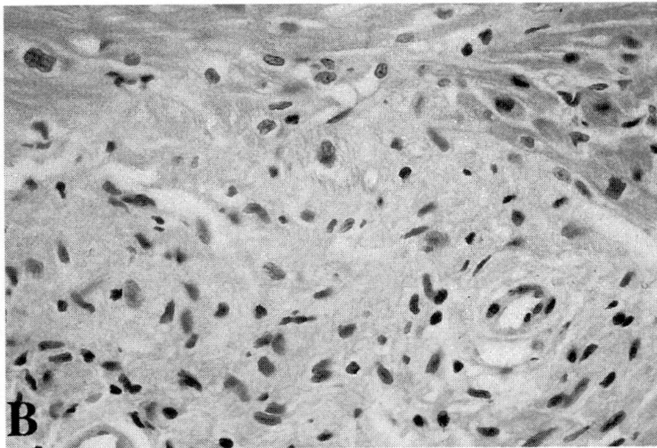

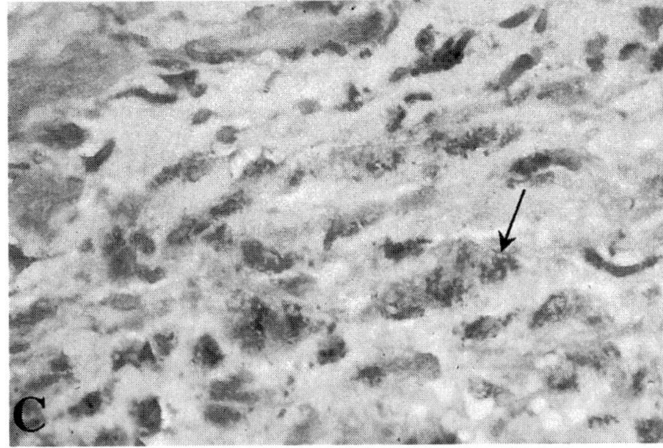

Figure 8–17. Whipple's disease. A patient with malabsorption and restrictive cardiomyopathy underwent endomyocardial and small bowel biopsy. *A.* Endomyocardial biopsy sample demonstrates focal interstitial aggregates of foamy histiocytes. *B.* High-power view demonstrates histiocytic cells with a finely granular homogenous cytoplasm. *C.* A periodic–Schiff stain demonstrated numerous coarse PAS positive granules (*arrow*) representing organisms.

stration of rod-shaped bodies that are 1.5- to 2.0-μm long and 0.2 to 0.4 μm in diameter within macrophages and sometimes in the extracellular tissues. These organisms were identified as *Tropheryma whippelii* in 1992.[74] Currently, the diagnosis may be confirmed by polymerase chain-reaction techniques on tissues or blood.[75]

CARDIOMYOPATHY

Cardiomyopathies are diseases of unknown etiology that affect the myocardium and result in abnormalities in myocardial contractile force or diastolic filling. They are classified as dilated (congestive), hypertrophic, and restrictive (obliterative). Other classification schemes take into account whether cardiomyopathy is idiopathic (primary) or associated with other diseases (secondary cardiomyopathies), or by etiological/pathogenetic factors (see Chapter 6).[37, 76–78] The endomyocardial biopsy—in combination with the clinical history, physical examination, and laboratory studies—can help provide a specific diagnosis in nearly half of patients with "dilated cardiomyopathy," although half of those are classified as "idiopathic."[79]

Dilated (Congestive) Cardiomyopathy

Dilated cardiomyopathy is characterized by dilated ventricles and atria and reduced ejection fraction secondary to primary myocardial disease in the absence of coronary artery, valvular disease, or systemic hypertension.[80–89] The histologic and ultrastructural features in idiopathic dilated cardiomyopathy are nonspecific and can be seen in hearts that fail from other causes, such as coronary artery disease, valvular disease, or systemic hypertension.[24, 80–91] Moreover, the diagnosis is usually not suspected until the disease is well established or far advanced. For these reasons, the endomyocardial biopsy has had rather disappointing success in elucidating the etiopathogenesis of idiopathic dilated cardiomyopathy, as there are no specific pathologic features.[24, 80–91] Nonetheless, the histologic findings, while not diagnostic themselves, can support the diagnosis when combined with the clinical data and also aid in excluding secondary causes of cardiomyopathy.

Light microscopic abnormalities found in idiopathic dilated cardiomyopathy include interstitial fibrosis, variation in myofiber size with hypertrophied (enlarged, hyperchromatic, and irregularly shaped nuclei) as well as atrophic or attenuated myocytes, and myofibrillar loss (Fig. 8–18).[85] The fibrosis is interstitial, may be patchy, and, in advanced cases, may widely separate myofibers from one another. Endocardial and perivascular fibrosis may be seen. While mononuclear inflammatory cells are not a prominent finding, a scant cellular infiltrate (usually lymphocytic) may be seen in end-stage cardiomyopathy.[90] The finding of inflammatory cells has led to the speculation that some cases of idiopathic dilated cardiomyopathy may be preceded by myocarditis. However, most of us do not believe this represents active myocarditis and therefore does not require treatment.[90] Some investigators have attempted to quantitate these changes (i.e., fibrosis, hypertrophy) with the hope of correlating them with the clinical status of the patient.[81, 87–89] While the severity of changes may generally parallel the degree of cardiac dysfunction, this may not always be the case, and at the present time caution is warranted in attempting to clinically prognosticate on the basis of the morphologic findings.

The primary ultrastructural changes in idiopathic dilated cardiomyopathy are those of myocyte degeneration.[80, 81] These include loss of myofilaments, accumulation of glycogen and mitochondria, in areas of myofibrillar loss, dilatation and/or proliferation of sarcotubular elements, aggregation of Z band-like material, and the presence of myelin figures and abnormally shaped mitochondria.[80, 81] Some authors have noted a correlation between the extent of degeneration and severity of the disease; ultrastructural grading has not yet proven to be reliable in predicting clinical status or determining prognosis.[77, 80, 92] A second ultrastructural feature of dilated cardiomyopathy is myocyte hypertrophy, manifest by enlarged myocytes with increased number of mitochondria, large and bizarre-shaped nuclei, accumulation of Z band material, widening of Z bands, increased rough endoplasmic reticulum, and widened and convoluted intercalated disks. Of course, the most reliable criteria for hypertrophy is increased cell size, with the normal human right ventricular

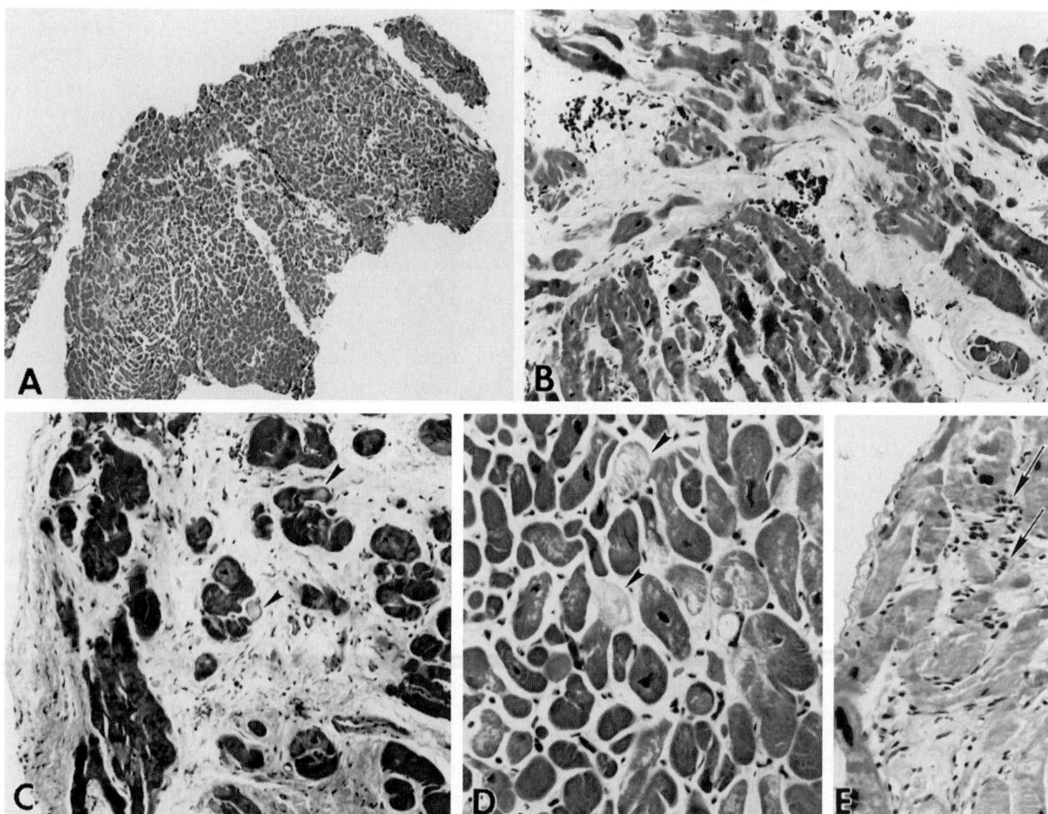

Figure 8–18. Idiopathic dilated cardiomyopathy. *A.* Variation in fiber size. *B.* Interstitial fibrosis. *C.* Focal loss of myofibrils (*arrowheads*) and extensive fibrosis. *D.* High-power view of the myocardium showing loss of myofibrils within myocytes (*arrowheads*). *E.* Focal collection of nuclei probably representing lymphocytes (*arrows*). (H & E: *A,* ×48; *B* and *C,* ×150; *D* ×300; *E* ×240)

myofiber measuring less than 25 μm in diameter.[92] Orientation and sectioning bias may influence accurate measurements of cell diameter. Also, this requires measurement of a sufficiently large sample size and construction of histograms to assess myocyte size.[87, 88]

An unusual cardiomyopathy, termed *histiocytoid cardiomyopathy,* occurs in children and has a unique histopathologic appearance.[93–95] It is characterized by severe, intractable ventricular and supraventricular arrhythmias, and patients die at 6 to 24 months of age. The heart has biventricular hypertrophy and dilatation. Microscopically, multiple clusters of pale-staining myocytes are seen that resemble Purkinje cells (see Chapter 6 for details).

Up to 20% of cases of dilated cardiomyopathy may be familial and include autosomal dominant (most common), autosomal recessive, and X-linked recessive forms.[96, 97] An X-linked dilated cardiomyopathy appears to be due to defects in the dystrophin gene.[98, 99] Affected males present in the late teens and twenties with syncope and rapidly progressive congestive heart failure leading to death or cardiac transplantation within 1 to 2 years. Females are less affected and have a more indolent progression of the disease. Dystrophin is a large cytoskeletal protein that localizes to the inner surface of the plasma membrane or sarcolemma of the skeletal muscle. Although the CK-MM levels are elevated, there may be no overt signs of skeletal myopathy. Because the morphologic characteristics are similar to those of dilated cardiomyopathy, the biopsy evaluation includes dystrophin gene deletion analysis of blood (which has low sensitivity) and dystrophin protein analysis of myocardial biopsy samples (which is the most sensitive and specific test).[21, 98] Such analyses can be performed by immunohistochemical techniques on endomyocardial biopsy samples using antibodies for the C- and N-terminal, and for the rod and midrod domains of dystrophin.[21]

In summary, the role of endomyocardial biopsy in assessing patients with congestive heart failure is rather limited. There may be significant variability in the histologic features of idiopathic dilated cardiomyopathy depending on the stage and severity of the disease. Some authorities advocate use of the endomyocardial biopsy only as a tool to aid in the diagnosis of myocarditis, while others advocate broad use of the technique with the belief that there is meaningful information for effective diagnosis and treatment to be gained by the visualization of myocardial tissue. Continued light and electron microscopic studies as well as potential new analyses, including molecular techniques, will eventually lead to a better understanding of the etiology, pathogenesis, and prognostic indicators of idiopathic dilated cardiomyopathy.

Hypertrophic Cardiomyopathy

The endomyocardial biopsy in hypertrophic cardiomyopathy shows hypertrophied myofibers (> 25 μm in diameter) with hyperchromatic and irregular-shaped nuclei.[100–102] Interstitial fibrosis may be present. Myofiber disarray has been considered by some to be the morphologic hallmark of hypertrophic cardiomyopathy.[103] However, myofiber disarray is patchy and tends to be localized deep in the ventricular septum, usually beyond the reach of the bioptome. Myofiber disarray may be nonspecific and can be seen without hypertrophic cardiomyopathy in the right ventricle at sites of insertion of the trabeculae carnae into the free wall or septum.[13, 16, 20] In patients with a previous biopsy, especially at the site of the previous biopsy or if the biopsy specimen is taken in or close to an area of scarring or fibrosis from some other cause, myofiber disarray is not an uncommon finding. For these reasons, myofiber disarray in a biopsy specimen should not be considered pathognomonic of hypertrophic cardiomyopathy and probably has little specific diagnostic significance. Endomyocardial biopsy may be useful, however, in excluding other diseases that mimic hypertrophic cardiomyopathy.[20] The ultrastructural findings in hypertrophic cardiomyopathy are primarily those of hypertrophy, with myofibrillar disarray that may be seen intracellularly as well.

Up to 55% of cases with hypertrophic cardiomyopathy are familial, and several sarcomeric genes, primarily β-myosin heavy chain, cardiac troponin T, and α-tropomyosin have been identified as having mutations[104] (see Chapter 6). While the endomyocardial biopsy has not yet assumed a major role in diagnosis of familial hypertrophic cardiomyopathy, abnormalities have been identified by endomyocardial biopsy in other forms of hypertrophic cardiomyopathy. For example, defects in oxidative phosphorylation, indicative of mitochondrial disorders, have been found in infants with hypertrophic cardiomyopathy using biopsy samples.[105]

Restrictive Cardiomyopathy

According to the classification of the World Health Organization (WHO), restrictive cardiomyopathy is myocardial disease of unknown etiology in which the ventricular myocardium is stiff during diastole (reduced compliance) but maintains good systolic function.[37] Ventricular filling is impaired, and diastolic volume is normal or decreased.[106] Similar "restrictive" findings can be found in some of the so-called secondary cardiomyopathies, such as amyloidosis and hemochromatosis. By WHO criteria, there are two diseases listed under restrictive cardiomyopathy: endomyocardial fibrosis (Davies' tropical endomyocardial fibrosis) and Loffler's endocarditis parietalis fibroplastica (Loffler's endomyocardial fibrosis with eosinophilia). Both of these will be called endocardial fibrosis because they may be variations of the same disease: the former occurs predominantly in the tropics and is the late form of the disease, and the latter is an early form of the disease occurring in temperate zones. It is often difficult to differentiate the clinical and hemodynamic findings between restrictive myocardial and constrictive pericardial disease without histologic examination of the myocardium. The endomyocardial biopsy can be an extremely useful tool for evaluating patients with restrictive hemodynamics.[107]

The heart is hypertrophied in endocardial fibrosis. The most striking findings are endocardial fibrotic plaques of varying size and thickness in both ventricles, usually along the inflow tracts and the apex. A mural thrombus may overlie these fibrous plaques in over half of the cases. By light microscopy, these fibrous plaques have a characteristic layering. Beneath the relatively acellular plaques are thin-walled sinusoidal vessels and occasional mononuclear cells, forming granulation tissue that may extend focally into the underlying myocardium. In Loffler's endomyocardial fibrosis with eosinophilia, three major stages of evolution have been described by Olsen:[108] a necrotic stage, a thrombotic stage, and a fibrotic stage. The latter is similar to endomyocardial fibrosis.

Idiopathic restrictive cardiomyopathy, a disease that can sometimes be familial, has restrictive hemodynamics without specific histopathologic changes.[106] It is characterized by mild to moderate increase in heart weight, biatrial enlargement, and normal ventricular cavity size. Endomyocardial biopsy may reveal interstitial fibrosis that is severe, but it may be absent, and myofibrillar disarray may be found.[109] As mentioned below, desmin cardiomyopathy may be a relatively common cause of restrictive cardiomyopathy, especially in patients with heart block, and demonstrates characteristic ultrastructural features.

Small-vessel vasculitis, which can be seen on endomyocardial biopsy,[110] may also be associated with restrictive-type hemodynamics that responds to therapy.[110, 111]

Restrictive Cardiomyopathy versus Pericardial Constriction

The differentiation between restrictive cardiomyopathy and constrictive pericarditis may be a major diagnostic dilemma, and noninvasive methods or hemodynamic measurements may not successfully distinguish the two. The differentiation is important because management and prognosis are different. The performance of a thoracotomy in a patient with restrictive heart disease may be associated with significant morbidity and mortality.[13] "Restrictive" myocardial diseases, such as amyloidosis, endomyocardial fibrosis, carcinoid heart disease, generalized myocardial fibrosis, and radiation-induced myocardial fibrosis, can be diagnosed by endomyocardial biopsy.[112] The biopsy may be useful in identifying various types of restrictive cardiomyopathies in patients with suspected pericardial constriction but who lack pericardial calcification radiographically, have no prior history of pericarditis, and no pericardial thickening by echocardiography.[2, 113]

Radiation-Induced Heart Disease

Radiation may affect both myocardium and pericardium, and the clinical differentiation may be impossible. Radiation produces myocardial fibrosis that is interstitial and perivascular and that may be indistinguishable by light microscopy from that seen in idiopathic dilated cardiomyopathy.[114] Although extreme adventitial fibrosis around arterioles may be highly suggestive of radiation-induced damage, the diagnosis can be facilitated by electron microscopy. The ultrastructural changes of radiation-induced cardiomyopathy are thickening of the capillary basement membrane, with replication of basement membrane in the early stages, and fibrosis at the late stages.[115] The basement membrane surrounding myocytes may also become thickened, and this may help to distinguish radiation injury from other diseases that affect capillary basement membranes, such as diabetes mellitus.

Arrhythmogenic Right Ventricular Cardiomyopathy

Arrhythmogenic right ventricular cardiomyopathy is a heart muscle disease characterized by atrophy and fibrofatty replacement of the right ventricular myocardium.[116, 117] It is characterized clinically by abnormalities of conduction, repolarization and depolarization, and ventricular arrhythmias.[118] There is a strong familial disposition,[119] and gene defects have been mapped to chromosomes 14q23-q24 and 1q42-q43.[120, 121] Fibrofatty replacement and myocyte atrophy can occur anywhere in the right ventricle but is most severe in the right ventricular outflow tract.[120] Lymphocytic myocarditis has been reported in up to 80% of hearts and may be indicative of an earlier form of the disease.[118] Arrhythmogenic right ventricular cardiomyopathy (fibrofatty) is distinguished from fatty replacement of the right ventricle by the lack of inflammation, atrophy, and fibrosis in the latter.[118] Endomyocardial biopsy is not useful for establishing the diagnosis of arrhythmogenic right ventricular cardiomyopathy because presence of fat in the right ventricle is seen in normal hearts. However, if there is fat and fibrous tissue replacement and a clinical suspicion with a family history, a diagnosis of right ventricular cardiomyopathy may be suggested (Fig. 8–19). Quantitation of fat in endomyocardial biopsies from patients with idiopathic dilated cardiomyopathy, allograft rejection, and normal and nonspecific conditions varies greatly with considerable overlap with biopsies from patients with right ventricular cardiomyopathy. However, it has been used for confirming the diagnosis of right ventricular cardiomyopathy in appropriate clinical setting when the biopsy shows presence of both fibrosis and fatty tissue in the specimen and when ischemia, valvular, and idiopathic dilated cardiomyopathy have been ruled out.[118, 122]

SPECIFIC HEART MUSCLE DISEASE

Cardiac Amyloidosis

Amyloidosis is characterized by extracellular deposits of proteins that have a beta-pleated sheet conformation.[123] Cardiac amyloid may account for up to 10% of all noncoronary "cardio-

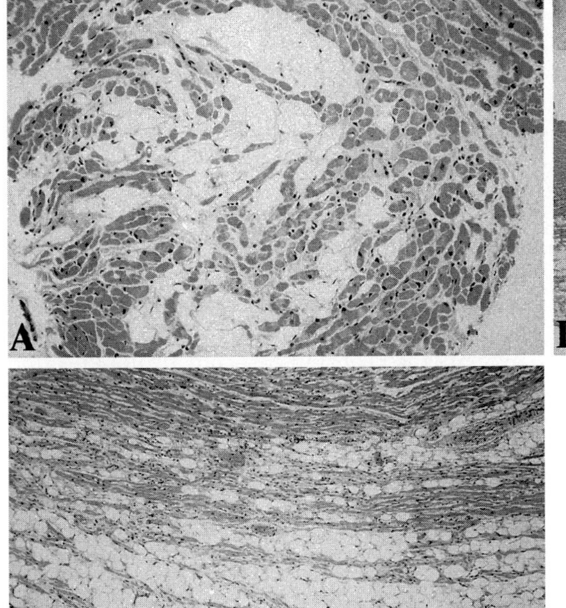

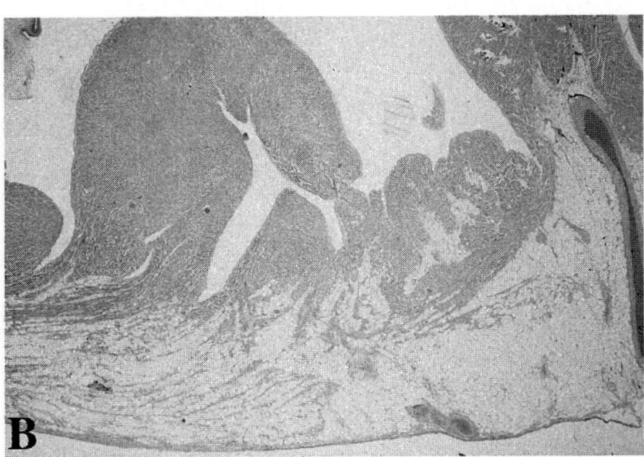

Figure 8–19. Right ventricular cardiomyopathy. A 24-year-old woman underwent endomyocardial biopsy for clinical suspicion of right ventricular cardiomyopathy (*A*): note intermingling of fat and myocytes and with normal amount of fibrous tissue. However, because of progressive disease patient underwent transplantation. The explanted heart showed extensive fat infiltration (*B*) and mild fibrosis with lymphocytic infiltration (*C*), changes consistent with right ventricular dysplasia. (Courtesy of Dr. Henry Tazelaar.)

myopathies."[124] Current classification is based on the biochemistry of the amyloid fibril, and two major groups are recognized: AL, in which fibrils consist of light chains of immunoglobulin, and AA, in which fibrils consist of fragments of serum amyloid A protein. A third group, in which the fibrils are composed predominantly of transthyretin (prealbumin), occurs as senile systemic amyloidosis involving the lung, liver, kidneys, and heart. The AL form, also known as light chain amyloid, is the most common cause of amyloid cardiomyopathy[125] and is associated with plasma cell dyscrasias. The AA form often occurs with inflammatory processes, such as rheumatoid arthritis or chronic infection.[123, 124] Amyloid deposits may be found in the heart of elderly persons with three distinct forms: isolated atrial amyloidosis (derived from atrial natriuretic polypeptide), senile aortic amyloidosis,[125, 126] and senile systemic amyloidosis; the latter can be identified immunohistochemically by using antiserum to transthyretin in myocardial biopsy tissue.[127] Cardiac involvement is the most important prognostic indicator in primary (AL) amyloidosis.[128] Although cardiac involvement in systemic senile amyloidosis (transthyretin) infrequently produces signs and symptoms, it may be responsible for atrial fibrillation, congestive heart failure, and fatal arrhythmia in some elderly subjects.[129]

Amyloid deposits occur in the interstitium; conduction tissue; valves; endocardium; pericardium; and epicardial and intramyocardial coronary arteries, veins, and capillaries.[124, 127, 130, 131] In the myocardium, amyloid may be found surrounding individual myocytes, in the form of focal nodular interstitial deposits that push aside and replace fibers, or both (Fig. 8–20). In coronary vessels, amyloid deposits may involve all vascular layers and even cause luminal obstruction (see Fig. 8–20). The presence of amyloid may be confirmed by the apple-green birefringence under polarized light following Congo red staining, by metachromasia with methyl violet, by green staining of amyloid by sulfated alcian blue stain, or by ultraviolet fluorescence with thioflavin T (the latter may yield false positive results). Amyloid fibrils are most reliably identified by their characteristic ultrastructural appearance as 7- to 10-nm diameter nonbranching fibrils.[123] Amyloid deposits in clinically significant cardiac amyloidosis tend to be extensive (replacement of over 10% of the myocardium) and involve intramyocardial arterioles.[132]

In patients suspected of having cardiac amyloidosis, an endomyocardial biopsy is indicated because biopsy of another site, such as the rectum, yields only 60% to 80% positive results with primary amyloidosis. At least four biopsy specimens should be obtained to minimize the possibility of a false-negative result.[127, 131, 132] If patients do not have a monoclonal protein in serum or urine, the biopsy should be stained by immunohistochemical techniques using antibodies to transthyretin, kappa and lambda light chains, and amyloid A for accurate classification.[129] Patients with known amyloidosis who have typical echocardiographic features do not necessarily need an endomyocardial biopsy, but cardiac amyloidosis cannot be excluded on the basis of a negative extracardiac biopsy.

Desmin Cardiomyopathy

Excessive deposition of the intermediate filament desmin in the skeletal and cardiac muscle has been associated with myopathic effects. The desmin filament is 8 to 10 nm diameters in width and is placed between that of the myosin (14-nm) and the actin (5- to 7-nm) filaments.[133] The desmin filament forms transversely oriented connections linking the Z disks of the myofibrils to those of adjacent myofibrils, the sarcolemma, and the nuclear membrane.[134] Desmin cardiomyopathy is characterized by progressive congestive heart failure. It is often diagnosed as idiopathic restrictive cardiomyopathy and on biopsy shows hypertrophied myocytes with interstitial fibrosis.[133] Electron microscopic examination is necessary for establishing the diagnosis. The diagnostic feature of desmin cardiomyopathy is the presence of granulofilamentous deposits in interfibrillar areas or at the level of the Z bands[135] (Fig. 8–21). By immunohistochemistry, desmin deposits can be seen as localized irregular masses.[133] Desmin cardiomyopathy is reported to occur in families due to missense mutations in the coding region of the desmin gene and less frequently in a sporadic form.[136]

Cardiac Sarcoidosis

Most patients with cardiac sarcoidosis have clinically apparent systemic involvement, but in some patients the heart may be the primary site without significant clinical evidence of other organ involvement. The clinical cardiac mani-

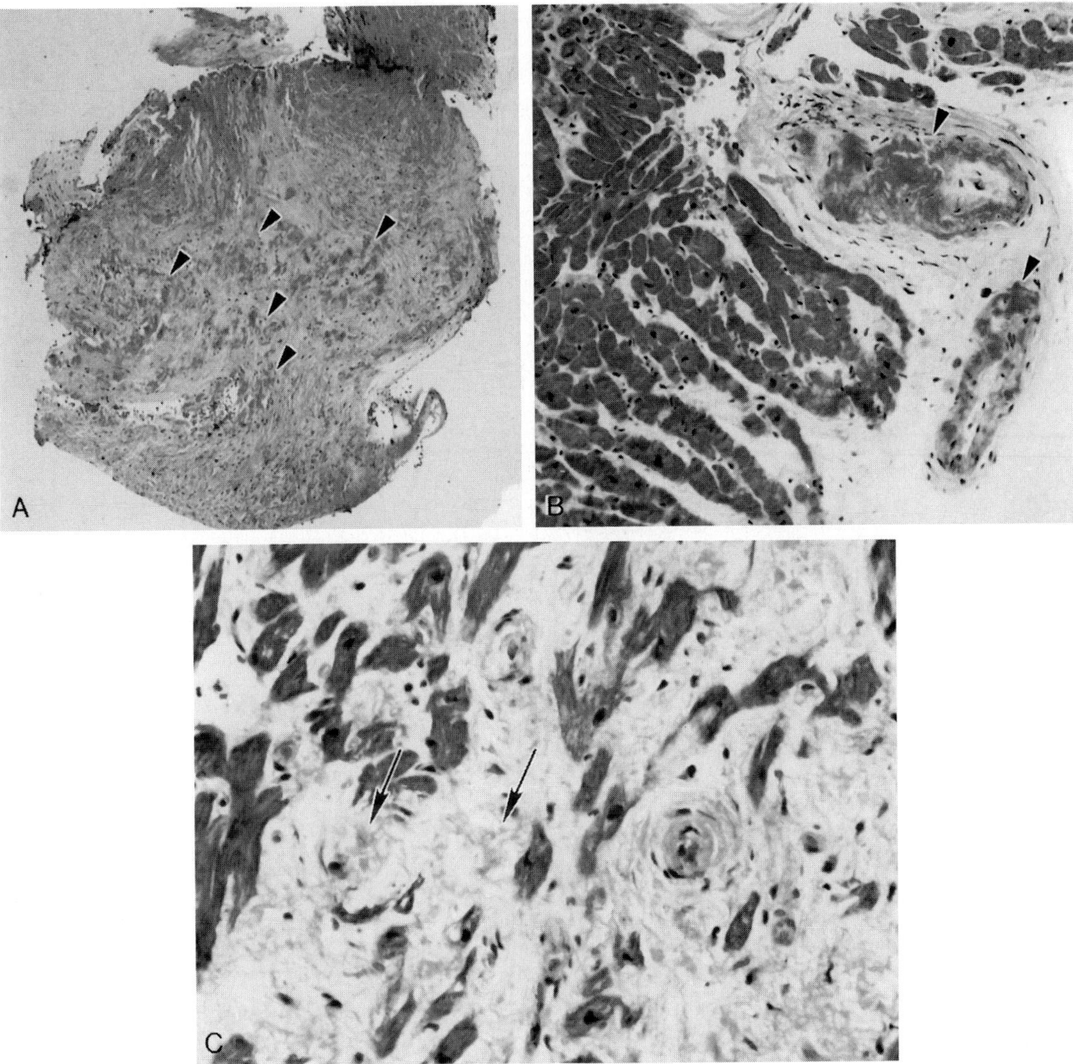

Figure 8–20. Endomyocardial biopsy specimens from a patient with cardiac amyloidosis. *A*. Subendocardial deposits of amyloid (*arrowheads*). *B*. High-power view of amyloid deposits within the wall of arteries (*arrowheads*). *C*. Amyloid deposits in the interstitium (*arrows*) and arteriole. (H & E: *A*, ×60; and Congo red: *B*, ×150; *C*, ×300)

festations are determined by the extent and location of involvement, and these include atrioventricular conduction defects, ventricular arrhythmias, sudden death, congestive heart failure (from widespread myocardial involvement or ventricular aneurysm), or dysfunction of papillary muscles and mitral regurgitation and chest pain. Pericardial abnormalities include pericardial effusion or constrictive pericarditis.[137]

Cardiac sarcoidosis is a focal disease involving the myocardium in decreasing order of frequency: left ventricular free wall, base of interventricular septum, right ventricular free wall, and atrial walls.[137] Therefore, multiple endomyocardial biopsy specimens must be obtained in suspected cases of cardiac sarcoidosis.[138–140] Noncaseating granulomas may be evident in only 20% of patients who undergo endomyocardial biopsy, and the diagnostic yield is greater in those with dilated cardiomyopathy as opposed to those in whom conduction disturbances are the dominant sign.[141] A negative biopsy does not rule out the presence of cardiac sarcoidosis, and patients with clinical evidence of cardiac involvement should be treated de-

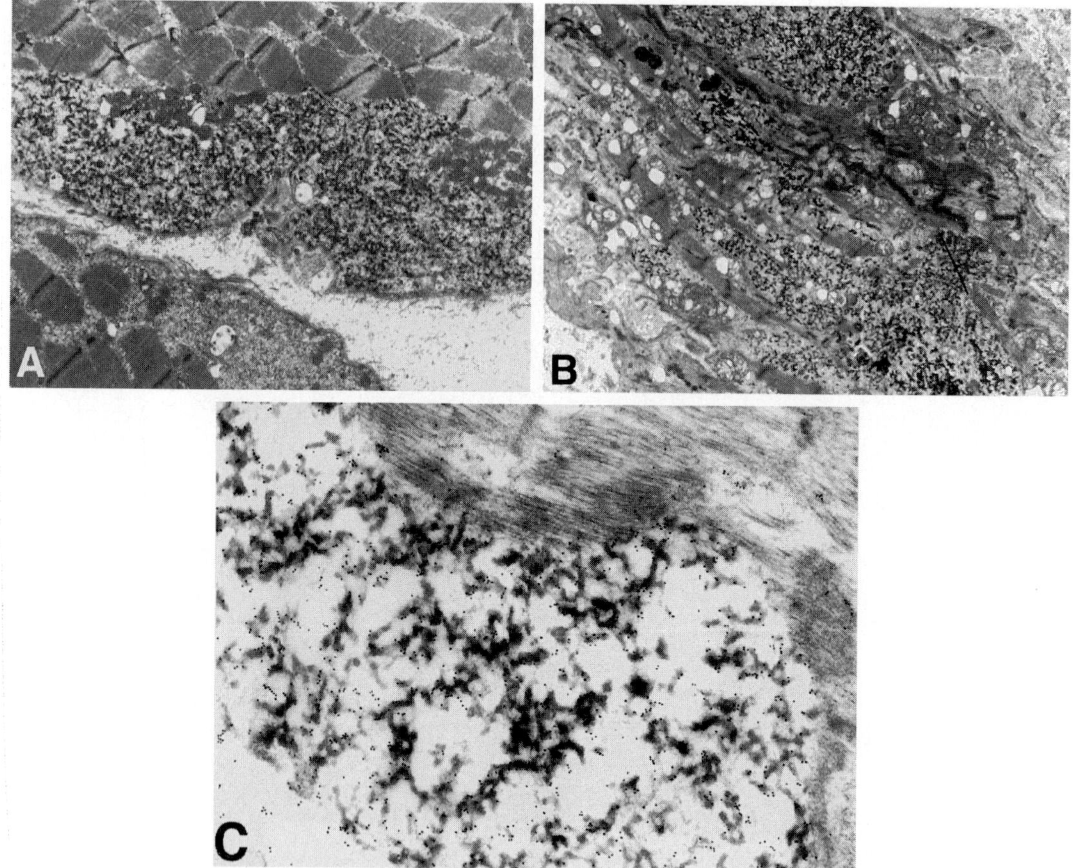

Figure 8–21. Desmin cardiomyopathy. *A.* Skeletal muscle. Typical subsarcolemmal deposition of granulofilamentous material. *B.* Cardiac muscle. Severe diffuse deposition of granulofilamentous material affecting two adjacent myocytes. *C.* Electron microscopy immunostaining with anti-desmin antibody demonstrating the specific immunoreaction of the antibody with the abnormal material. (Courtesy of Dr. Eloisa Arbustini.)

spite a negative biopsy.[141] The lesions in the heart are identical to those described in the lungs, consisting of histiocytes, giant cells, lymphocytes, and plasma cells (Fig. 8–22).[137] Patchy fibrosis and lymphocytic myocarditis may be observed but are nonspecific. While the presence of noncaseating granulomas may be considered diagnostic, special stains must be performed to rule out presence of fungi and acid-fast bacilli. Other conditions associated with giant cells in the heart include idiopathic giant-cell myocarditis, infective endocarditis, rheumatoid arthritis, Takayasu's arteritis, Churg–Strauss syndrome, and Wegener's granulomatosis.

Hemochromatosis/Hemosiderosis

Iron deposits occur in the myocardium in idiopathic (familial) hemochromatosis as well as in hemosiderosis secondary to iron overload (e.g., multiple transfusions, dietary intake).[142,143] The clinical manifestations vary, depending on the extent of myocardial involvement, but patients usually have a dilated, or, uncommonly, restrictive cardiomyopathy.[142,143] The severity of myocardial dysfunction may be proportional to the amount of iron present, and extensive deposits are usually associated with chronic congestive heart failure (occurring in one third of patients), which is usually the cause of death.[16,142] Cardiac failure is progressive and largely refractory to therapy, although serial biopsies may show diminution in stainable iron following therapy.[144–146]

Normally, there is no stainable iron within the myocardium. In hemochromatosis or hemosiderosis, iron deposits are more extensive in the epicardial third, followed by subendocardium and papillary muscle, and are least extensive in the middle third of the ventricular wall.[143] They are typically perinuclear in location ini-

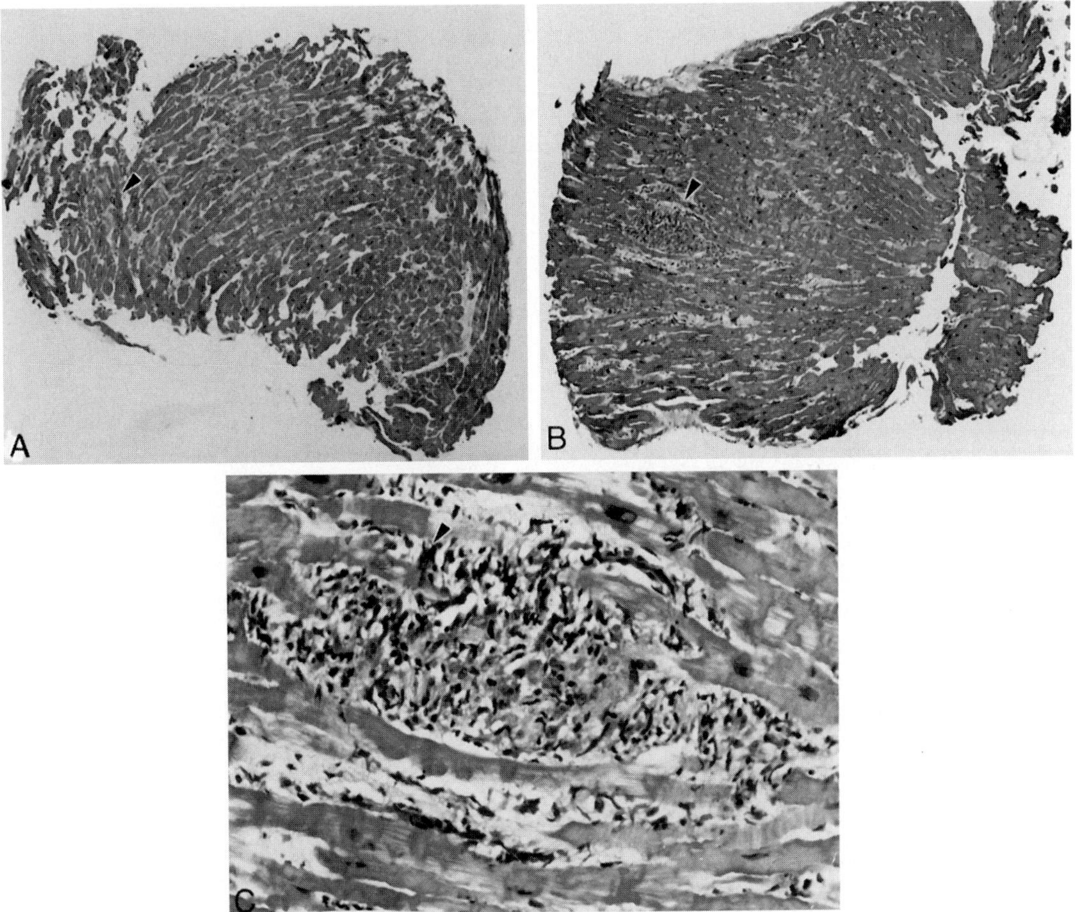

Figure 8–22. Sarcoidosis of the heart. Endomyocardial biopsy specimen from a patient suspected to have cardiac sarcoidosis. *A*. The first few sections failed to reveal any granulomas; however, focal presence of interstitial cells (*arrowhead*) led to deeper cuts in the paraffin block, which revealed the presence of a single focus of a granuloma (*arrowhead in B*). *C*. High-power view of the granuloma showing lymphocytes, histiocytes, and giant cells (*arrowhead*). (H & E: *A* and *B*, ×60; *C* ×300)

tially, but eventually occupy most of the cells (Fig. 8–23). Involvement of the conduction system, coronary arteries, and valves is limited. There may be associated fibrosis, in which case restrictive hemodynamics may be present.[144] When a biopsy is performed, multiple specimens should be obtained to minimize sampling error, as iron deposition may be focal.[13, 145] The diagnostic yield of the endomyocardial biopsy is greatest when performed in patients with impaired left ventricular systolic function, and iron staining has been recommended for all biopsies from patients with idiopathic cardiac dysfunction.[147] In patients with thalassemia major, there was a significant correlation between serum ferritin and endomyocardial biopsy myocardial iron grade. Patients with elevated ferritin levels and poor compliance to chelating therapy are at high risk of severe heart hemochromatosis.[148]

METABOLIC DISEASES

Glycogen Storage Disease

Of the various types of glycogen storage disease, the heart is involved in three: type II (Pompe's disease), due to deficiency of α 1,4 glucosidase (acid maltase); type III (Cori's disease), a deficiency of the debranching enzyme amylo-1,6-glucosidase; and type IV (Andersen's disease), caused by a deficiency of the branching enzyme α 1,4-glucan 6-glucosyl transferase. These diseases are transmitted as autosomal recessive disorders and are manifest by ac-

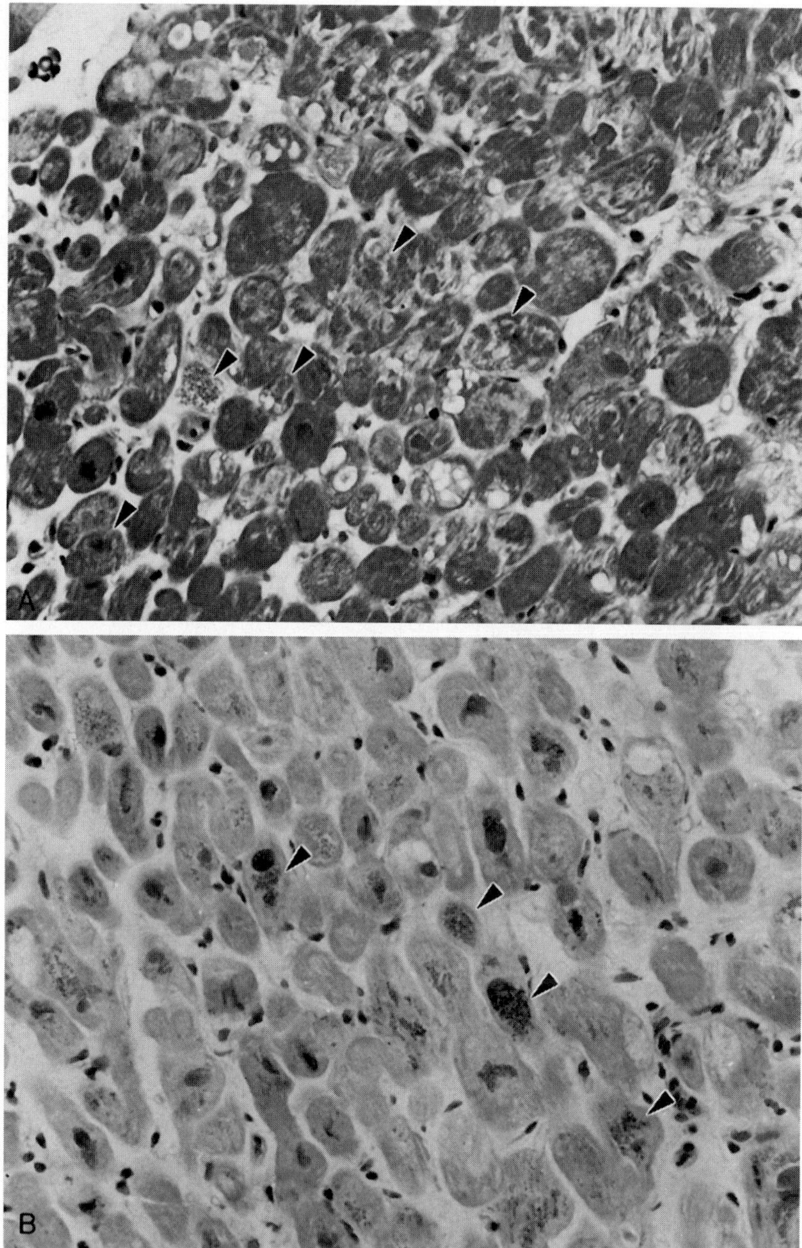

Figure 8–23. Hemochromatosis. Endomyocardial biopsy specimens in a 54-year-old man who presented with severe congestive heart failure of short duration. *A*. Hematoxylin and eosin-stained section of biopsy revealed myocyte hypertrophy and focal brown granular deposits (*arrowheads*) within perinuclear location of the myocytes or occasionally totally replacing myocytes. *B*. Prussian blue stain sowing perinuclear iron deposits (*arrowheads*) in most myocytes consistent with hemosiderin deposits. (*A* and *B*, ×300)

cumulation of glycogen in various tissues. The diagnosis should be based not only on the demonstration of increased glycogen but also on demonstration of the enzyme defect.

Most cases of glycogen storage disease causing cardiomegaly are due to type II glycogenosis. The heart is enlarged, and all chambers have thickened walls and small cavities. Congestive heart failure and/or obstructive cardiomyopathy become evident in the neonatal period (infantile form of Pompe's disease), with failure to thrive, progressive hypotonia, weakness, lethargy, and nonspecific cardiac murmurs. Pompe's disease is fatal within the first year of life.[142] Death is due to cardiac failure or respiratory complications (pneumonia, aspiration).

In histologic sections, there is severe vacuolization within the central areas of the myocytes, giving a lacework appearance to the tissue (Fig. 8–24) due to massive deposits of glycogen that displace myofibrils to the periphery. Cardiac failure is due to myofibrillar loss that can be demonstrated ultrastructurally.[142] If a glycogen storage disease is suspected, the endomyocardial biopsy can be fixed in absolute alcohol to aid in preserving the glycogen, and electron microscopy is usually helpful.[13, 149] The characteristic ultrastructural alteration is large collections of glycogen (in Pompe's disease either free in the cytoplasm in the heart or within lysosomes in other organs). The glycogen may be in a morphologic normal form as granules (type II and III) or in an abnormal form (fibrils, in type IV glycogenosis).[142] Uranyl acetate *en bloc* staining should be omitted in preparing samples for electron microscopy because uranyl acetate extracts glycogen, leaving only large empty spaces ultrastructurally.[142] In type IV glycogenosis, while the clinical manifestations of cardiac disease are uncommon, extensive deposits of glycogen will be found in cardiac cells; these differ from the other glycogenoses in that they are strongly basophilic and the deposits are fibrils measuring 5 to 6 nm in diameter.[142]

Carnitine Deficiency

Carnitine deficiency produces skeletal muscle myopathy and a lipid storage disorder, resulting in accumulation of neutral lipid within skeletal muscle, myocardium, and liver.[150] L-carnitine, a natural substance, is involved in mitochondrial transport of fatty acids and is required in the mitochondrial energy production. The deficiency of L-carnitine may be from carnitine membrane transport defect or from dietary deficiency in otherwise normal infants fed soy formulas unsupplemented with L-carnitine; however, supplementation of all infant formulas has essentially eliminated the cause of secondary deficiency.[151, 152] In patients suspected of having carnitine deficiency, at least a portion of the endomyocardial biopsy should be submitted for electron microscopy. The heart is enlarged, with biventricular hypertrophy and mild endocardial fibrosis. Myocardial fibers contain vacuoles that stain positively for neutral lipid on light microscopy. By electron microscopy, myofibrils are replaced by accumulation of bizarre-shaped mitochondria and the mitochondrial cristae may be disrupted by crystalline inclusions.[150]

Fabry's Disease

Fabry's disease (angiokeratoma corporis diffusum universale) is an X-linked recessive dis-

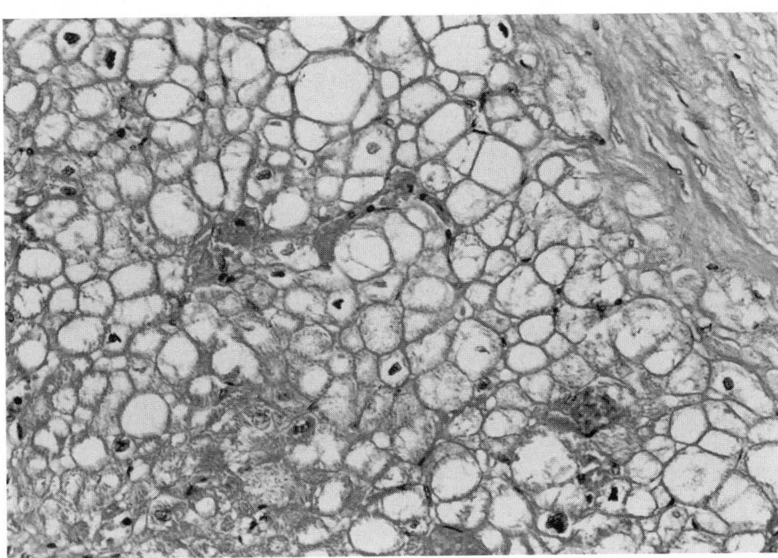

Figure 8–24. Note marked vacuolization of myocytes giving a lacework appearance to myocytes in a patient with glycogen storage disease. (H & E: ×300)

order caused by deficiency of lysosomal α-galactosidase A, resulting in excessive deposits of ceramide trihexoside, particularly in the skin, cornea, kidneys, and heart.[142, 153] Symptoms and signs relative to the heart include congestive heart failure, angina, and hypertension, all of which are due to deposits of ceramide trihexoside in lysosomes in endothelial cells, smooth muscle, and pericytes throughout the vascular system.[142]

Endomyocardial biopsy from patients with Fabry's disease demonstrates a lacework appearance of the myocardial fibers on routine light microscopy, with marked perinuclear vacuolization and displacement of the contractile elements to the periphery (Fig. 8–25).[154, 155] In patients with unexplained cardiac hypertrophy, 3% have been reported to be secondary to Fabry's disease which was diagnosed on endomyocardial biopsy.[156] In frozen sections, the deposits of ceramide trihexoside appear as vacuoles that are sudanophilic, periodic acid-Schiff positive, and birefringent. By electron microscopy, these deposits appear as intralysosomal aggregates of concentric or parallel lamellae composed of alternating dense and light bands (Fig. 8–25).[142]

Mitochondrial Cardiomyopathies

Mitochondrial cardiomyopathies due to mitochondrial (mt)DNA deletions or transfer (t)RNA point mutations in children have most often been associated with hypertrophic cardiomyopathy, atrio-ventricular block, and congestive heart failure[157] with involvement of other organs like the kidney and the endocrine systems. Several clinically distinct subgroups exist, including Kearns–Sayre syndrome; myoclonus epilepsy, and ragged-red fibers (MERRF); and mitochondrial cardiomyopathy, encephalopathy, lactic acidosis, and strokelike episode (MELAS).[157, 158] The mtDNA mutations are most

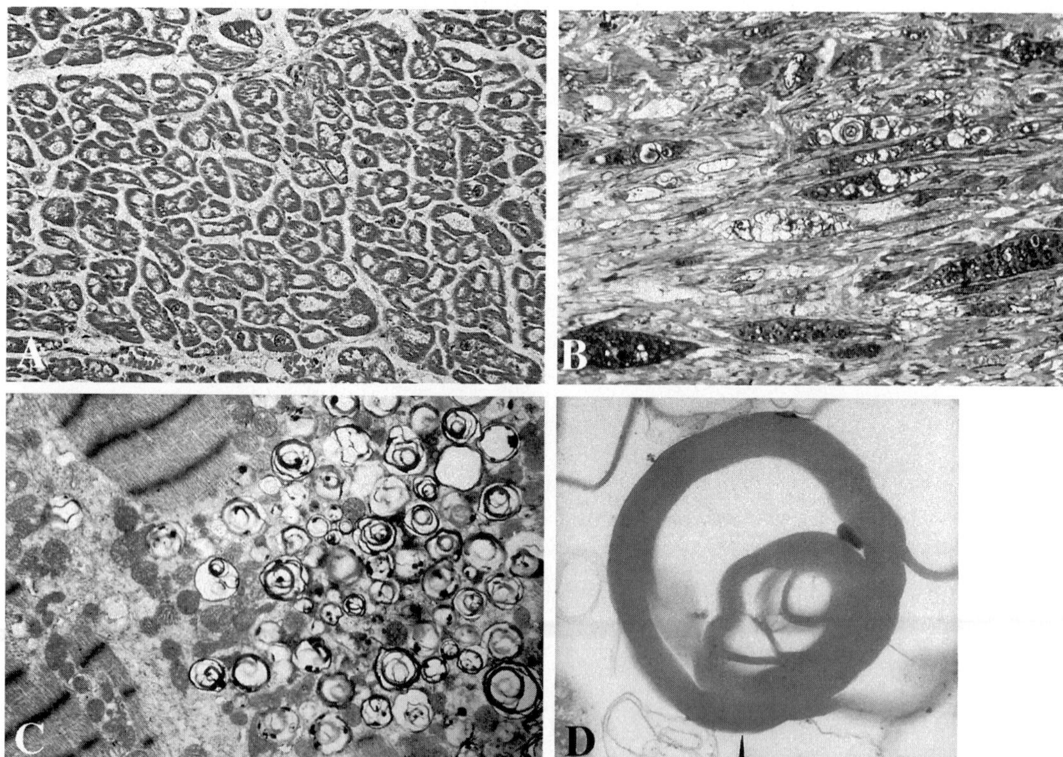

Figure 8–25. Fabry's disease. *A*. Myocardial sections from a 64-year-old man with congestive heart failure. Note marked hypertrophy and extensive vacuolization of myocytes. *B*. One-micron-thick section stained with toluidine blue showing myelin figure within myocytes. Electron photomicrograph showing a myocyte with numerous dense lamellae (*C*) and higher magnification in *D* showing concentric lamellae of alternating light and dark bands. (*A*, H & E: ×300; *B*, ×100,000)

often associated with multisystem syndromes including the heart but others may present as isolated disorders. Morphologic findings in the heart by light microscopy include myocyte hypertrophy, with vacuolization and varying degrees of fibrosis. By electron microscopy there is massive proliferation of the mitochondria and this results in the aggregates of abnormal mitochondria staining red on Gomori modified trichrome on light microscopy. The mitochondria morphologic abnormalities include shape changes, cristae changes—whorled, tubular, angulated, or concentrically arranged, intramitochondrial inclusions of crystalline inclusions or osmiophilic bodies, lipid vacuoles or glycogen, and matrix densities[133] (Fig. 8–26).

Mitochondrial abnormalities of proliferation and variable matrix densities associated with ring-shaped mitochondria; concentric, angulated, and tubular cristae; crystalloid and osmiophilic inclusion bodies; and glycogen or lipid inclusion can often (14%) be seen on ultrastructural examination of endomyocardial biopsies in adult patients presenting with clinical features of dilated cardiomyopathy.[159] These abnormalities were associated in a small group of patients (22%) with mtDNA mutations as well as significant decrease in Cox and in NADH dehydrogenase activity in myocardial tissue.[159]

Cardiac Tumors

Primary cardiac tumors are rare, ranging in incidence at autopsy from 0.0017% to 0.28%, compared with 1% to 22% for metastatic cardiac tumors.[160] The most common primary cardiac tumor is myxoma (42%), followed by angiosarcoma and rhabdomyosarcoma, with these three comprising half of all primary cardiac tumors. Other primary cardiac tumors include papillary fibroelastoma, fibroma and fibrosarcoma, hemangioma, teratoma, and "mesothelioma" of the atrioventricular node (see Chapter 12 for details). Metastatic tumors to the heart include lung and breast carcinoma, hematopoietic-lymphoid neoplasms, and melanomas, with cardiac involvement occurring in about 20% of patients with malignancies. Endomyocardial biopsy has been used in the diagno-

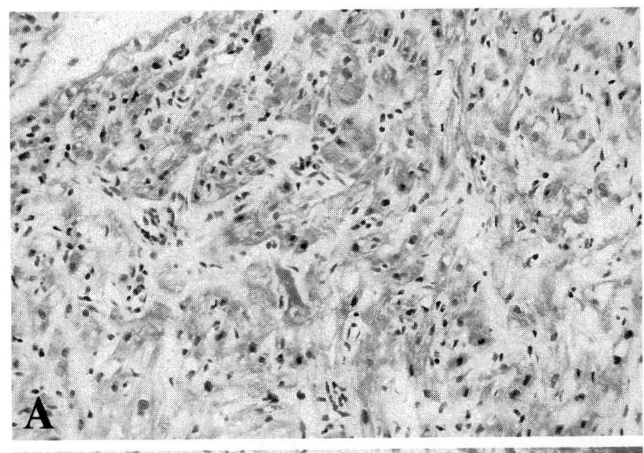

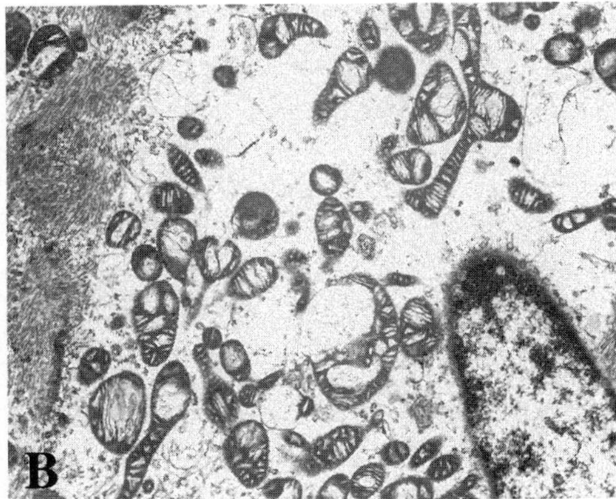

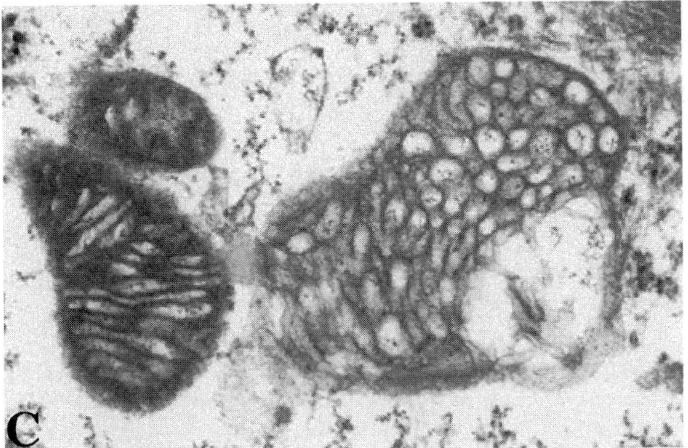

Figure 8–26. Mitochondrial cardiomyopathy. *A.* Light microscopic changes in an infant presenting with dilated cardiomyopathy note vacuolated myocytes without much interstitial fibrosis. *B* and *C.* On electron microscopy there were abnormally shaped and swollen mitochondria with cristae showing membrane fusion and cytolysis (*B*). Most mitochondria were focally devoid of cristae and often showed focal areas of cytolysis and glycogen.

sis of primary and secondary cardiac tumors (Fig. 8–27), and there have been a few reports in which the diagnosis of an intracardiac tumor was made by left or right ventricular transvenous endomyocardial biopsy.[161–166] The procedure is relatively safe, resulting in less discomfort, risk, and expense than an open thoracotomy, especially when no treatment benefit can be demonstrated, and it can be important in differentiating between anthracycline cardiotoxicity and metastasis in patients with heart failure.[165]

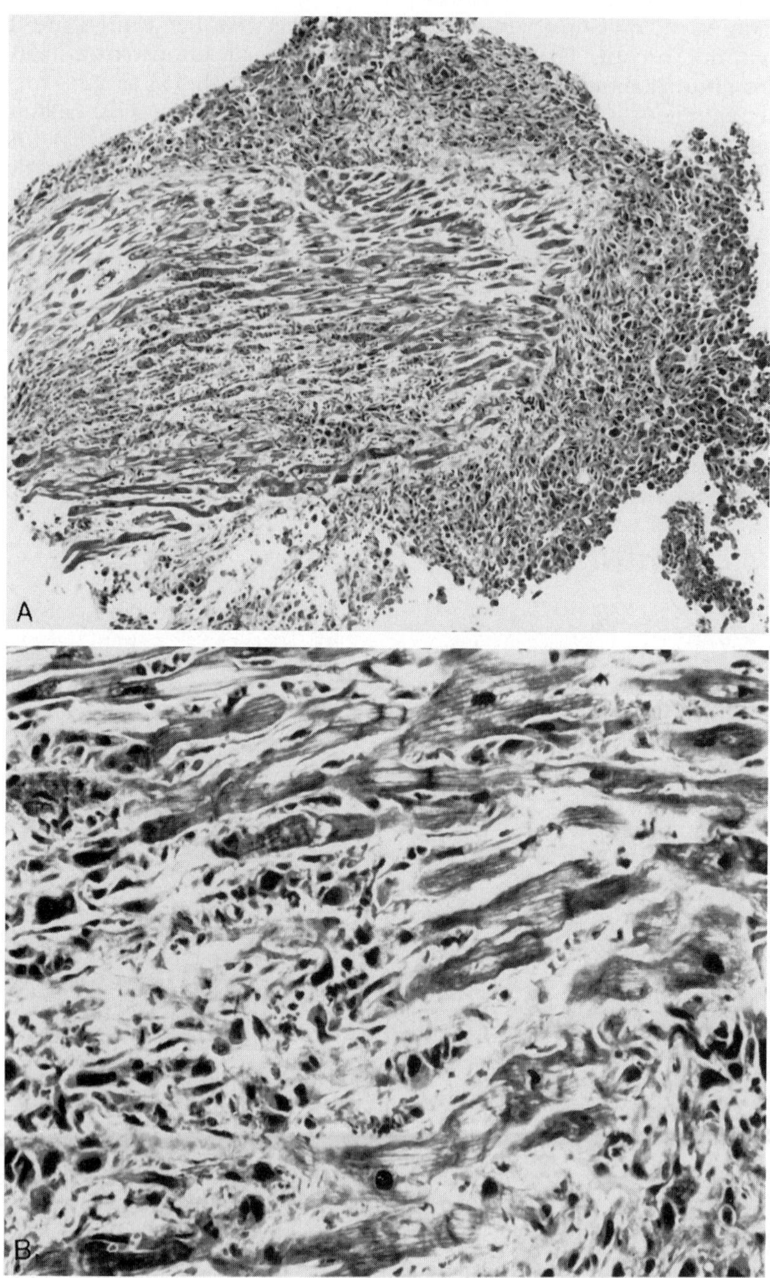

Figure 8–27. Intracardiac metastatic sarcoma. A 26-year-old woman with a known history of soft tissue sarcoma of the thigh was diagnosed by computed tomography and echocardiography to have a right ventricular mass for which an endomyocardial biopsy was performed. The biopsy specimen (*A*) showed focal infiltration of the myocardium by spindle-shaped noncohesive malignant cells (*B,* higher magnification) consistent with the diagnosis of metastatic sarcoma. (Masson's trichrome: *A,* ×30; *B,* ×75)

ANTHRACYCLINE CARDIOTOXICITY

Anthracyclines are antineoplastic drugs that include doxorubicin (Adriamycin) and daunomycin and are effective chemotherapeutic agents for the treatment of numerous solid and hematopoietic malignancies. Cardiac toxicity is a well-recognized complication and is the dose-limiting factor in its use.[167–171] The development of congestive heart failure from anthracycline also depends upon cumulative dose. While the usual practice is to administer these agents up to a maximum total dosage of 500 to 550 mg/m^2, some patients may suffer cardiotoxic effects at lower doses, particularly if they have preexisting cardiac disease (including hypertension), age greater than 70 years or very young, or have had prior irradiation.[167, 168, 172] Prior cyclophosphamide therapy may also potentiate the cardiotoxic effects of anthracyclines. There is significant individual variation in a patient's susceptibility to anthracycline-induced cardiac damage such that limiting dosages to particular levels does not guarantee prevention of cardiotoxicity. A number of noninvasive techniques designed to evaluate cardiotoxicity have yielded equivocal results. Endomyocardial biopsy has allowed the development of a reliable method to evaluate and grade anthracycline cardiotoxicity.[167, 170, 173] A histologic grading scheme of endomyocardial biopsy has been described by Billingham and has proven to be an effective means to monitor patients receiving anthracyclines.[170, 173] It enables patients to receive more drug because of a linear relationship between drug dose and morphologic cardiotoxicity.

Light microscopic evaluation of paraffin-embedded tissue has not proven to be accurate, and therefore all endomyocardial biopsy samples must be submitted for electron microscopy. Sections 1-μm thick stained with toluidine blue should be examined by light microscopy (Fig. 8–28), followed by thin sections to be evaluated by electron microscopy. The morphologic changes due to anthracycline toxicity may be focal or diffuse. Two characteristic lesions can be seen ultrastructurally: sarcotubular dilatation and loss of myofibrils. The extent to which these changes are found form the basis for the grading system described by Billingham and Tazelaar (Table 8–7). Sarcotubular dilatation may progress to sarcotubular coalescence, and eventually the entire myocyte may be vacuolated, at which phase it is possible to appreciate the changes by light microscopy (Fig. 8–28). Mitochondrial swelling can simulate sarcotubular dilatation, and small vacuoles are not uncommon and often found near the intercalated disk.[174] Myofibrillar loss is best detected by electron microscopy consisting of partial or total myofibrillar loss with only peripheral Z band remnants seen.[167, 169, 170] Advanced disease may be recognized by light microscopy as small, shrunken cells with homogeneous, pale cytoplasm. The two types of changes described may be seen in a single cell or separate cells, and only one of them may be seen in a particular biopsy; there is no predictive value to the type of change first seen.[174] It is common to observe contraction bands in endomyocardial biopsies, in which case a portion of a myocyte will be devoid of myofilaments, and these must be distinguished from true myofibrillar loss. In myofibrillar loss, remants of Z bands will be present. Another change that may be observed is the presence of myelin figures, indicating membrane degeneration. Nuclei and mitochondria will appear normal unless overt necrosis is present (which is rare). If cardiotoxicity is severe, the nonspecific finding of interstitial fibrosis may also be seen but it is not included in the grading scheme.

The grading system for anthracycline cardiotoxicity involves three main grades of severity (see Table 8–7). For grade 1, more anthracycline can be given, whereas no further anthracycline is given for a biopsy showing grade 3 changes, regardless of whether hemodynamic parameters are normal or not. Intermediate grades have been designated, such that a biopsy may be classified as 1.5 for borderline grade 1 to 2 changes, and 2.5 for borderline grade 2 to 3 changes. Patients with grades 1.5 and 2 can receive more drug, whereas a grade 2.5 biopsy would indicate only one more dose of anthracycline may be given without further evaluation. To accurately perform this type of grading, it is essential that enough tissue be evaluated (i.e., at least 10 plastic embedded blocks of tissue must be examined at light microscopy level and five further selected for examination by electron microscopy).[167, 170]

The biopsy score has been found to correlate linearly with dosage in a normally distributed population. Previous mediastinal irradiation, even if remote, potentiates anthracycline-induced cardiotoxicity. Data from Stanford University for all patients receiving doxorubicin have shown that in those with the risk factors listed previously (radiation, age, cardiac disease, hypertension), the heart failure incidence was 17%, whereas in the absence of risk factors,

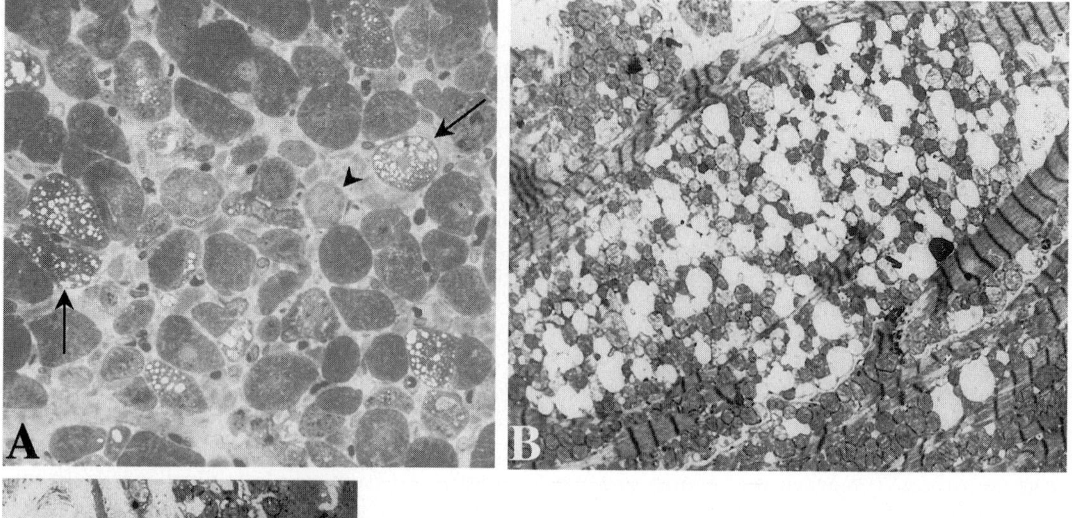

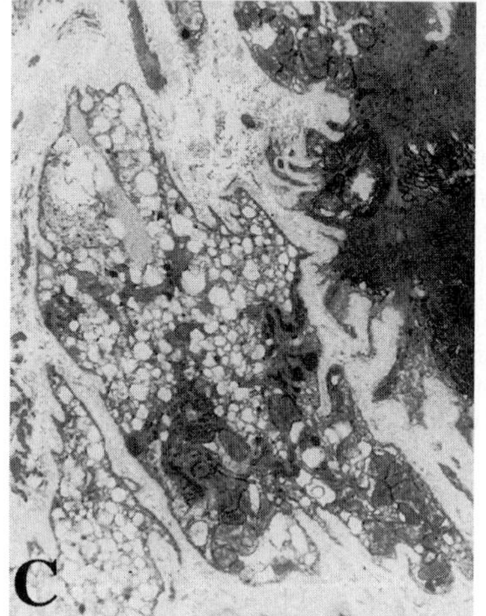

Figure 8–28. Adriamycin cardiotoxicity. *A.* One-micron-thick section showing focal myofibrillar loss (*arrowhead*) and marked vacuolization (*arrows*) of some myocytes. *B.* Electron photomicrograph demonstrating vacuolization of sarcotubular system in an anthracycline-damaged myocyte. *C.* Marked vacuolization of a myocyte, "adria cell." (Courtesy of Dr. M. Billingham)

the incidence was 2%, and at doses less than 450 mg/m^2, no cases of heart failure were found.[170] Thus, endomyocardial biopsy monitoring is indicated only in patients with risk factors or those receiving greater than 550 mg/m^2. Some have recommended the use of baseline biopsy for comparison.

The pathogenesis underlying anthracycline cardiotoxicity is not clear. One postulated mechanism is generation of free radicals.[170] Other possibilities include inhibition of coenzyme Q_{10} (ubiquinone), which is involved in oxidative phosphorylation, increased cellular calcium and/or calcium transport disturbances, diminution of cyclic nucleotides, DNA degradation, release of vasoactive amines, inflammation, and toxicity from metabolites.[172, 175, 176] Recently it has been shown in animal studies and in women with metastatic breast cancer that liposomes-encapsulated doxorubicin chemotherapy regimen, while highly active against metastatic breast cancer, is associated with low cardiac toxicity despite high cumulative doses of doxorubicin.[177, 178] Paclitaxel, another drug used in the treatment of breast cancer, has been reported to have cardiotoxicity. The ultrastructural changes in the myocardium of a fatal case of paclitaxel-induced cardiotoxicity include swelling of the sarcoplasmic reticulum, loss of myofibrils, and accumulation of lipofuschin as well as laminated myeloid figures.[179] Such changes are very similar to those seen in anthracycline-induced cardiotoxicity and may suggest a pathogenetic final common pathway.[179]

The endomyocardial biopsy offers a safe and reliable means of identifying patients at risk for development of anthracycline cardiotoxicity. The morphologic changes in the biopsy appear before the clinical symptoms and can be quantitated by a grading system that correlates with individual patient dosage and is predictive of subsequent functional deterioration. This is

Table 8–7. Grading System for Anthracycline Cardiotoxicity

Grade Morphology	
0	Normal myocardial ultrastructure
1	Isolated myocytes affected by distended sarcotubular system or early myofibrillar loss; damage to fewer than 5% of all cells in ten plastic embedded blocks of tissue
1.5	Changes similar to those in grade 1 but with damage to 6–15% of all cells in ten plastic embedded blocks of tissue
2	Clusters of myocytes affected by myofibrillar loss or vacuolization, with damage to 16–25% of all cells in ten plastic embedded blocks of tissue
2.5	Many myocytes, 26–35% of all cells in ten plastic embedded blocks, affected by vacuolization or myofibrillar loss; only one more dose of anthracycline should be given without further evaluation
3	Severe and diffuse myocytic damage (more than 35% of all cells in ten plastic embedded blocks) affected by vacuolization or myofibrillar loss; no more anthracycline should be given

From Billingham ME, Tazelaar. HD. Cardiac biopsy. In Parmley N, Chatterjee K (eds): Cardiology, Volume 1, Ch 54. Philadelphia: JB Lippincott, 1987, with permission.

one of the unequivocal areas where the endomyocardial biopsy has made a valuable contribution in the treatment of cancer patients.

REFERENCES

1. Sakakibara S, Konno S. Endomyocardial biopsy. Jpn Heart J 3:537, 1962.
2. Fowles RE, Mason JW. Role of cardiac biopsy in the diagnosis and management of cardiac disease. Prog Cardiovasc Dis 27:153–172, 1984.
3. Atkinson JB, Swift LL, Lequire VS. Myotonia congenita. A histochemical and ultrastructural study in the goat: Comparison with abnormalities found in human myotonia dystrophica. Am J Pathol 102:324–335, 1981.
4. Billingham ME. The role of endomyocardial biopsy in the diagnosis and treatment of heart disease. In: Silver MD (ed): Cardiovascular Pathology, Vol. 2, p 205. New York: Churchill Livingstone, 1983.
5. Fenoglio JJ, Jr. Diagnostic approach to the endomyocardial biopsy. In: Endomyocardial Biopsy: Techniques and Applications, p 33. Boca Raton, FL: CRC Press, Inc., 1982.
6. Aretz HT. The endomyocardial biopsy revisited [editorial; comment]. Mayo Clin Proc 65:1506–1509, 1990.
7. Baraldi-Junkins C, Levin HR, Kasper EK, Rayburn BK, Herskowitz A, Baughman KL. Complications of endomyocardial biopsy in heart transplant patients [see comments]. J Heart Lung Transplant 12:63–67, 1993.
8. Fowles RE, Mason JW. Endomyocardial biopsy. Ann Intern Med 97:885–894, 1982.
9. Craven CM, Allred T, Garry SL, Pickrell J, Buys SS. Three cases of fatal cardiac tamponade following ventricular endocardial biopsy. Arch Pathol Lab Med 114:836–839, 1990.
10. Schneiderman H, Hager WD, Gondos B. The endomyocardial biopsy. Ann Clin Lab Sci 16:134–145, 1986.
11. Pophal SG, Sigfusson G, Booth KL, et al. Complications of endomyocardial biopsy in children. J Am Coll Cardiol 34:2105–2110, 1999.
12. Williams MJ, Lee MY, DiSalvo TG, et al. Biopsy-induced flail tricuspid leaflet and tricuspid regurgitation following orthotopic cardiac transplantation. Am J Cardiol 77:1339–1344, 1996.
13. Edwards WD. Pathology of endomyocardial biopsy. In: Waller BF (ed): Pathology of the Heart and Great Vessels, pp 191–275. New York: Churchill Livingston, 1988.
14. Adomian GE, Laks MM, Billingham ME. The incidence and significance of contraction bands in endomyocardial biopsies from normal human hearts. Am Heart J 95:348–351, 1978.
15. Karch SB, Billingham ME. Myocardial contraction bands revisited. Hum Pathol 17:9–13, 1986.
16. Edwards WD. Endomyocardial biopsy and cardiomyopathy. Cardiovasc Rev Rep 4:820, 1983.
17. Edwards WD, Holmes DR, Jr., Reeder GS. Diagnosis of active lymphocytic myocarditis by endomyocardial biopsy: Quantitative criteria for light microscopy. Mayo Clin Proc 57:419–425, 1982.
18. Foley DA, Edwards WD. Quantitation of leukocytes in endomyocardial tissue from 100 normal human hearts at autopsy. Implications for diagnosis of myocarditis from biopsy specimens of living patients. Am J Cardiovasc Pathol 2:145–149, 1988.
19. Rose AG, Novitzky D, Cooper DK, Reichart B. Endomyocardial biopsy site morphology. An experimental study in baboons. Arch Pathol Lab Med 110:622–625, 1986.
20. Billingham ME, Tazelaar HD. Cardiac Biopsy. In: Parmley WW, Chatterjee K (eds): Cardiology. Vol. 1, Ch. 54. Philadelphia: J.B. Lippincott, 1987.
21. Arbustini E, Diegoli M, Morbini P, et al. Prevalence and characteristics of dystrophin defects in adult male patients with dilated cardiomyopathy. J Am Coll Cardiol 35:1760–1768, 2000.
22. Nippoldt TB, Edwards WD, Holmes DR, Jr., Reeder GS, Hartzler GO, Smith HC. Right ventricular endomyocardial biopsy: Clinicopathologic correlates in 100 consecutive patients. Mayo Clin Proc 57:407–418, 1982.
23. Fenoglio JJ, Jr., Ursell PC, Kellogg CF, Drusin RE, Weiss MB. Diagnosis and classification of myocarditis by endomyocardial biopsy. N Engl J Med 308:12–18, 1983.
24. Parrillo JE, Aretz HT, Palacios I, Fallon JT, Block PC. The results of transvenous endomyocardial biopsy can frequently be used to diagnose myocardial diseases in patients with idiopathic heart failure. Endomyocardial biopsies in 100 consecutive patients revealed a substantial incidence of myocarditis. Circulation 69:93–101, 1984.
25. Kasper EK, Agema WR, Hutchins GM, Deckers JW, Hare JM, Baughman KL. The causes of dilated cardiomyopathy: A clinicopathologic review of 673 consecutive patients. J Am Coll Cardiol 23:586–590, 1994.

26. Rizeq MN, Rickenbacher PR, Fowler MB, Billingham ME. Incidence of myocarditis in peripartum cardiomyopathy. Am J Cardiol 74:474–477, 1994.
27. Herskowitz A, Vlahov D, Willoughby S, et al. Prevalence and incidence of left ventricular dysfunction in patients with human immunodeficiency virus infection. Am J Cardiol 71:955–958, 1993.
28. Lieberman EB, Hutchins GM, Herskowitz A, Rose NR, Baughman KL. Clinicopathologic description of myocarditis. J Am Coll Cardiol 18:1617–1626, 1991.
29. Aretz H, Billingham M, Edwards W, et al. Myocarditis: A histologic definition and classification. Am J Cardiovasc Pathol 1:3–14, 1987.
30. Beghetti M, Wilson GJ, Bohn D, Benson L. Hypersensitivity myocarditis caused by an allergic reaction to cefaclor. J Pediatr 132:172–173, 1998.
31. Arbustini E, Gavazzi A, Dal Bello B, et al. Ten-year experience with endomyocardial biopsy in myocarditis presenting with congestive heart failure: Frequency, pathologic characteristics, treatment and follow-up. G Ital Cardiol 27:209–223, 1997.
32. Mason JW, O'Connell JB, Herskowitz A, Rose NR, McManus BM, Billingham ME, Moon TE. A clinical trial of immunosuppressive therapy for myocarditis. N Engl J Med 333:269–275, 1995.
33. McCarthy RE, 3rd, Boehmer JP, Hruban RH, et al. Long-term outcome of fulminant myocarditis as compared with acute (nonfulminant) myocarditis [see comments]. N Engl J Med 342:690–695, 2000.
34. Kubo N, Morimoto S, Hiramitsu S, et al. Feasibility of diagnosing chronic myocarditis by endomyocardial biopsy. Heart Vessels 12:167–170, 1997.
35. Anderson DW, Virmani R, Reilly JM, et al. Prevalent myocarditis at necropsy in the acquired immunodeficiency syndrome. J Am Coll Cardiol 11:792–799, 1988.
36. Feeley KM, Harris J, Suvarna SK. Necropsy diagnosis of myocarditis: A retrospective study using CD45RO immunohistochemistry. J Clin Pathol 53:147–149, 2000.
37. Report of the WHO/ISFC task force on the definition and classification of cardiomyopathies. Br Heart J 44:672–673, 1980.
38. Archard LC, Richardson PJ, Olsen EG, Dubowitz V, Sewry C, Bowles NE. The role of Coxsackie B viruses in the pathogenesis of myocarditis. Biochem Soc Symp 53:51–62, 1987.
39. Kandolf R, Ameis D, Kirschner P, Canu A, Hofschneider PH. In situ detection of enteroviral genomes in myocardial cells by nucleic acid hybridization: An approach to the diagnosis of viral heart disease. Proc Natl Acad Sci U S A 84:6272–6276, 1987.
40. Martin A, Webber S, Fricker F, et al. Acute myocarditis. Rapid diagnosis by PCR in children. Circulation 90:330–339, 1994.
41. Wolfgram LJ, Beisel KW, Rose NR. Heart-specific autoantibodies following murine coxsackievirus B3 myocarditis. J Exp Med 161:1112–1121, 1985.
42. Henke A, Huber S, Stelzner A, Whitton JL. The role of CD8+ T lymphocytes in coxsackievirus B3-induced myocarditis. J Virol 69:6720–6728, 1995.
43. Horwitz MS, La Cava A, Fine C, Rodriguez E, Ilic A, Sarvetnick N. Pancreatic expression of interferon-gamma protects mice from lethal coxsackievirus B3 infection and subsequent myocarditis. Nat Med 6:693–697, 2000.
44. Herskowitz A, Campbell S, Deckers J, et al. Demographic features and prevalence of idiopathic myocarditis in patients undergoing endomyocardial biopsy. Am J Cardiol 71:982–986, 1993.
45. Chan KY, Iwahara M, Benson LN, Wilson GJ, Freedom RM. Immunosuppressive therapy in the management of acute myocarditis in children: A clinical trial. J Am Coll Cardiol 17:458–460, 1991.
46. Cummins D, Bennett D, Fisher-Hoch SP, Farrar B, McCormick JB. Electrocardiographic abnormalities in patients with Lassa fever. J Trop Med Hyg 92:350–355, 1989.
47. Cummins D. Lassa fever. Br J Hosp Med 43:186–188, 190, 192, 1990.
48. Saiman L, Prince A. Infections of the heart. Adv Pediatr Infect Dis 4:139–161, 1989.
49. Ozkutlu S, Soylemezoglu O, Calikoglu AS, Kale G, Karaaslan E. Fatal mumps myocarditis. Jpn Heart J 30:109–114, 1989.
50. Waagner DC, Murphy TV. Varicella myocarditis. Pediatr Infect Dis J 9:360–363, 1990.
51. Frustaci A, Abdulla AK, Caldarulo M, Buffon A. Fatal measles myocarditis. Cardiologia 35:347–349, 1990.
52. Litovsky SH, Burke AP, Virmani R. Giant cell myocarditis: An entity distinct from sarcoidosis characterized by multiphasic myocyte destruction by cytotoxic T cells and histiocytic giant cells. Mod Pathol 9:1126–1134, 1996.
53. Cooper LT, Jr., Berry GJ, Shabetai R. Idiopathic giant-cell myocarditis—natural history and treatment. Multicenter Giant Cell Myocarditis Study Group Investigators. N Engl J Med 336:1860–1866, 1997.
54. Wilson MS, Barth RF, Baker PB, Unverferth DV, Kolibash AJ. Giant cell myocarditis. Am J Med 79:647–652, 1985.
55. Tanaka M, Ichinohasama R, Kawahara Y, et al. Acute idiopathic interstitial myocarditis: Case report with special reference to morphological characteristics of giant cells. J Clin Pathol 39:1209–1216, 1986.
56. Theaker JM, Gatter KC, Heryet A, Evans DJ, McGee JO. Giant cell myocarditis: Evidence for the macrophage origin of the giant cells. J Clin Pathol 38:160–164, 1985.
57. Theaker JM, Gatter KC, Brown DC, Heryet A, Davies MJ. An investigation into the nature of giant cells in cardiac and skeletal muscle. Hum Pathol 19:974–979, 1988.
58. Chow LH, Ye Y, Linder J, McManus BM. Phenotypic analysis of infiltrating cells in human myocarditis. An immunohistochemical study in paraffin-embedded tissue. Arch Pathol Lab Med 113:1357–1362, 1989.
59. Ren H, Poston RS, Jr., Hruban RH, Baumgartner WA, Baughman KL, Hutchins GM. Long survival with giant cell myocarditis. Mod Pathol 6:402–407, 1993.
60. Kloin JE. Pernicious anemia and giant cell myocarditis. New association. Am J Med 78:355–360, 1985.
61. Hawkins ET, Levine TB, Goss SJ, Moosvi A, Levine AB. Hypersensitivity myocarditis in the explanted hearts of transplant recipients. Reappraisal of pathologic criteria and their clinical implications. Pathol Annu 30:287–304, 1995.
62. Spear GS. Eosinophilic explant carditis with eosinophilia: Hypersensitivity to dobutamine infusion [see comments]. J Heart Lung Transplant 14:755–760, 1995.
63. di Gioia CR, d'Amati G, Grillo P, Laurenti A, Gallo P. Eosinophilic infiltration immediately following transplantation: Recurrent hypersensitivity reaction? Cardiovasc Pathol 8:297–299, 1999.

64. Mullick FG, McAllister HA, Jr., Wagner BM, Fenoglio JJ, Jr. Drug related vasculitis. Clinicopathologic correlations in 30 patients. Hum Pathol 10:313–325, 1979.
65. Taliercio CP, Olney BA, Lie JT. Myocarditis related to drug hypersensitivity. Mayo Clin Proc 60:463–468, 1985.
66. Mason JW, O'Connell JB. Clinical merit of endomyocardial biopsy. Circulation 79:971–979, 1989.
67. Billingham ME. Morphologic changes in drug-induced heart disease. In: Bristow M (ed): Drug Induced Heart Disease. Amsterdam: Elsevier/North-Holland Biomedical Press, 1980.
68. McAllister HA, Jr., Mullick FG. The cardiovascular system. In: Riddel RH (ed): Pathology of Drug-Induced and Toxic Disease. New York: Churchill Livingstone, 1982.
69. Fauci AS, Harley JB, Roberts WC, Ferrans VJ, Gralnick HR, Bjornson BH. NIH conference. The idiopathic hypereosinophilic syndrome. Clinical, pathophysiologic, and therapeutic considerations. Ann Intern Med 97:78–92, 1982.
70. Enzinger FM, Helwig EB. Whipple's disease: A review of the literature and report of 15 patients. Virchow Arch A Pathol Anat Histopathol 336:238–269, 1963.
71. McAllister HA, Fenoglio JJ. Cardiac involvement in Whipple's disease. Circulation 52:152–156, 1975.
72. Lie JT, Davis JS. Pancarditis in Whipple's disease: Electronmicroscopic demonstration of intracardiac bacillary bodies. Am J Clin Pathol 66:22–30, 1976.
73. Southern JF, Moscicki RA, Magro C, Dickersin GR, Fallon JT, Bloch KJ. Lymphedema, lymphocytic myocarditis, and sarcoidlike granulomatosis. Manifestations of Whipple's disease. JAMA 261:1467–1470, 1989.
74. Relman DA, Schmidt TA, MacDermott RP, Falkow S. Identification of the uncultured bacillus of Whipple's disease. N Engl J Med 327:293–301, 1992.
75. Mooney EE, Kenan DJ, Sweeney EC, Gaede JT. Myocarditis in Whipple's disease: An unsuspected cause of symptoms and sudden death. Mod Pathol 10:524–529, 1997.
76. Davies MJ. The cardiomyopathies: A review of terminology, pathology and pathogenesis. Histopathology 8:363–393, 1984.
77. Baandrup U, Florio RA, Rehahn M, Richardson PJ, Olsen EG. Critical analysis of endomyocardial biopsies from patients suspected of having cardiomyopathy. II: Comparison of histology and clinical/haemodynamic information. Br Heart J 45:487–493, 1981.
78. Richardson P, McKenna W, Bristow M, et al. Report of the 1995 World Health Organization/International Society and Federation of Cardiology Task Force on the Definition and Classification of cardiomyopathies [news]. Circulation 93:841–842, 1996.
79. Felker GM, Hu W, Hare JM, Hruban RH, Baughman KL, Kasper EK. The spectrum of dilated cardiomyopathy. The Johns Hopkins experience with 1,278 patients. Medicine (Baltimore) 78:270–283, 1999.
80. Baandrup U, Florio RA, Roters F, Olsen EG. Electron microscopic investigation of endomyocardial biopsy samples in hypertrophy and cardiomyopathy. A semiquantitative study in 48 patients. Circulation 63:1289–1298, 1981.
81. Dick MR, Unverferth DV, Baba N. The pattern of myocardial degeneration in nonischemic congestive cardiomyopathy. Hum Pathol 13:740–744, 1982.
82. Ferrans VJ, Massumi RA, Shugoll GI, Ali N, Roberts WC. Ultrastructural studies of myocardial biopsies in 45 patients with obstructive or congestive cardiomyopathy. Recent Adv Stud Cardiac Struct Metab 2:231–272, 1973.
83. Keren A, Billingham ME, Weintraub D, Stinson EB, Popp RL. Mildly dilated congestive cardiomyopathy. Circulation 72:302–309, 1985.
84. Lewis AB, Neustein HB, Takahashi M, Lurie PR. Findings on endomyocardial biopsy in infants and children with dilated cardiomyopathy. Am J Cardiol 55:143–145, 1985.
85. Roberts WC, Ferrans VJ. Pathologic anatomy of the cardiomyopathies. Idiopathic dilated and hypertrophic types, infiltrative types, and endomyocardial disease with and without eosinophilia. Hum Pathol 6:287–342, 1975.
86. Rose AG, Beck W. Dilated (congestive) cardiomyopathy: A syndrome of severe cardiac dysfunction with remarkably few morphological features of myocardial damage. Histopathology 9:367–379, 1985.
87. Schwarz F, Mall G, Zebe H, et al. Quantitative morphologic findings of the myocardium in idiopathic dilated cardiomyopathy. Am J Cardiol 51:501–506, 1983.
88. Schwarz F, Mall G, Zebe H, et al. Determinants of survival in patients with congestive cardiomyopathy: Quantitative morphologic findings and left ventricular hemodynamics. Circulation 70:923–928, 1984.
89. Unverferth BJ, Leier CV, Magorien RD, Unverferth DV. Differentiating characteristics of myocardial nuclei in cardiomyopathy. Hum Pathol 14:974–983, 1983.
90. Tazelaar HD, Billingham ME. Leukocytic infiltrates in idiopathic dilated cardiomyopathy. A source of confusion with active myocarditis. Am J Surg Pathol 10:405–412, 1986.
91. Yonesaka S, Becker AE. Dilated cardiomyopathy: Diagnostic accuracy of endomyocardial biopsy. Br Heart J 58:156–161, 1987.
92. Hammond EH, Menlove RL, Anderson JL. Predictive value of immunofluorescence and electron microscopic evaluation of endomyocardial biopsies in the diagnosis and prognosis of myocarditis and idiopathic dilated cardiomyopathy. Am Heart J 114:1055–1065, 1987.
93. Ferrans VJ, McAllister HA, Jr., Haese WH. Infantile cardiomyopathy with histiocytoid change in cardiac muscle cells. Report of six patients. Circulation 53:708–719, 1976.
94. Gelb AB, Van Meter SH, Billingham ME, Berry GJ, Rouse RV. Infantile histiocytoid cardiomyopathy—myocardial or conduction system hamartoma: What is the cell type involved? Hum Pathol 24:1226–1231, 1993.
95. Ruszkiewicz AR, Vernon-Roberts E. Sudden death in an infant due to histiocytoid cardiomyopathy. A light-microscopic, ultrastructural and immunohistochemical study. Am J Forensic Med Pathol 16:74–80, 1995.
96. Grunig E, Tasman JA, Kucherer H, Franz W, Kubler W, Katus HA. Frequency and phenotypes of familial dilated cardiomyopathy. J Am Coll Cardiol 31:186–194, 1998.
97. Mestroni L, Rocco C, Gregori D, et al. Familial dilated cardiomyopathy: Evidence for genetic and phenotypic heterogeneity. Heart Muscle Disease Study Group. J Am Coll Cardiol 34:181–190, 1999.
98. Beggs AH. Dystrophinopathy, the expanding phenotype. Dystrophin abnormalities in X-linked dilated cardiomyopathy. Circulation 95:2344–2347, 1997.

99. Schwartz K, Carrier L, Guicheney P, Komajda M. Molecular basis of familial cardiomyopathies. Circulation 91:532–540, 1995.
100. Alexander CS, Gobel FL. Diagnosis of idiopathic hypertrophic subaortic stenosis by right ventricular septal biopsy. Am J Cardiol 34:142–151, 1974.
101. Kunkel B, Schneider M, Eisenmenger A, Bergmann B, Hopf R, Kaltenbach M. Myocardial biopsy in patients with hypertrophic cardiomyopathy: Correlations between morphologic and clinical parameters and development of myocardial hypertrophy under medical therapy. Z Kardiol 76:33–38, 1987.
102. Schwartzkopff B, Uhre B, Ehle B, Losse B, Frenzel H. Variability and reproducibility of morphologic findings in endomyocardial biopsies of patients with hypertrophic obstructive cardiomyopathy. Z Kardiol 76Suppl 3:26–32, 1987.
103. Maron BJ, Sato N, Roberts WC, Edwards JE, Chandra RS. Quantitative analysis of cardiac muscle cell disorganization in the ventricular septum. Comparison of fetuses and infants with and without congenital heart disease and patients with hypertrophic cardiomyopathy. Circulation 60:685–696, 1979.
104. Marian AJ, Roberts R. Recent advances in the molecular genetics of hypertrophic cardiomyopathy. Circulation 92:1336–1347, 1995.
105. Rustin P, Lebidois J, Chretien D, et al. Endomyocardial biopsies for early detection of mitochondrial disorders in hypertrophic cardiomyopathies. J Pediatr 124:224–228, 1994.
106. Kushwaha SS, Fallon JT, Fuster V. Restrictive cardiomyopathy. N Engl J Med 336:267–276, 1997.
107. Stamato NJ, O'Connell JB, Subramanian R, Scanlon PJ. Diagnosis of endocardial fibroelastosis by endomyocardial biopsy in an adult with dilated cardiomyopathy. Am Heart J 109:919–920, 1985.
108. Olsen EG. Pathological aspects of endomyocardial fibrosis. Postgrad Med J 59:135–141, 1983.
109. Angelini A, Calzolari V, Thiene G, et al. Morphologic spectrum of primary restrictive cardiomyopathy. Am J Cardiol 80:1046–1050, 1997.
110. Papapietro SE, Rogers LW, Hudson NL, Atkinson JB, Page DL. Intramyocardial coronary arteritis and restrictive cardiomyopathy. Am Heart J 114:175–178, 1987.
111. Frustaci A, Chimenti C, Pieroni M. Idiopathic myocardial vasculitis presenting as restrictive cardiomyopathy. Chest 111:1462–1464, 1997.
112. Schoenfeld MH, Supple EW, Dec GW, Jr., Fallon JT, Palacios IF. Restrictive cardiomyopathy versus constrictive pericarditis: Role of endomyocardial biopsy in avoiding unnecessary thoracotomy. Circulation 75:1012–1017, 1987.
113. Mehta A, Mehta M, Jain AC. Constrictive pericarditis. Clin Cardiol 22:334–344, 1999.
114. Veinot JP, Edwards WD. Pathology of radiation-induced heart disease: A surgical and autopsy study of 27 cases. Hum Pathol 27:766–773, 1996.
115. Niemtzow RC, Reynolds RD. Radiation therapy and the heart. In: Kapoor AS (ed): Cancer and the Heart, pp 232–237. New York: Springer-Verlag, 1986.
116. Corrado D, Basso C, Thiene G, et al. Spectrum of clinicopathologic manifestations of arrhythmogenic right ventricular cardiomyopathy/dysplasia: A multicenter study. J Am Coll Cardiol 30:1512–1520, 1997.
117. Fontaine G, Fontaliran F, Frank R. Arrhythmogenic right ventricular cardiomyopathies: Clinical forms and main differential diagnoses. Circulation 97:1532–1535, 1998.
118. Burke AP, Farb A, Tashko G, Virmani R. Arrhythmogenic right ventricular cardiomyopathy and fatty replacement of the right ventricular myocardium: Are they different diseases?. Circulation 97:1571–1580, 1998.
119. Basso C, Thiene G, Nava A, Dalla Volta S. Arrhythmogenic right ventricular cardiomyopathy: A survey of the investigations at the University of Padua. Clin Cardiol 20:333–336, 1997.
120. Rampazzo A, Nava A, Danieli GA, et al. The gene for arrhythmogenic right ventricular cardiomyopathy maps to chromosome 14q23-q24. Hum Mol Genet 3:959–962, 1994.
121. Rampazzo A, Nava A, Erne P, et al. A new locus for arrhythmogenic right ventricular cardiomyopathy (ARVD2) maps to chromosome 1q42-q43. Hum Mol Genet 4:2151–2154, 1995.
122. Angelini A, Thiene G, Boffa GM, et al. Endomyocardial biopsy in right ventricular cardiomyopathy. Int J Cardiol 40:273–282, 1993.
123. Glenner GG. Amyloid deposits and amyloidosis. The beta-fibrilloses (first of two parts). N Engl J Med 302:1283–1292, 1980.
124. Kyle RA, Greipp PR. Amyloidosis (AL). Clinical and laboratory features in 229 cases. Mayo Clin Proc 58:665–683, 1983.
125. Benson MD. Hereditary amyloidosis and cardiomyopathy. Am J Med 93:1–2, 1992.
126. Cornwell GGD, Westermark P, Murdoch W, Pitkanen P. Senile aortic amyloid. A third distinctive type of age-related cardiovascular amyloid. Am J Pathol 108:135–139, 1982.
127. Olson LJ, Gertz MA, Edwards WD, et al. Senile cardiac amyloidosis with myocardial dysfunction. Diagnosis by endomyocardial biopsy and immunohistochemistry. N Engl J Med 317:738–742, 1987.
128. Arbustini E, Merlini G, Gavazzi A, et al. Cardiac immunocyte-derived (AL) amyloidosis: An endomyocardial biopsy study in 11 patients. Am Heart J 130:528–536, 1995.
129. Kyle RA, Spittell PC, Gertz MA, et al. The premortem recognition of systemic senile amyloidosis with cardiac involvement. Am J Med 101:395–400, 1996.
130. Pomerance A. Senile cardiac amyloidosis. Br Heart J 27:711, 1965.
131. Pellikka PA, Holmes DR, Jr., Edwards WD, Nishimura RA, Tajik AJ, Kyle RA. Endomyocardial biopsy in 30 patients with primary amyloidosis and suspected cardiac involvement. Arch Intern Med 148:662–666, 1988.
132. Smith TJ, Kyle RA, Lie JT. Clinical significance of histopathologic patterns of cardiac amyloidosis. Mayo Clin Proc 59:547–555, 1984.
133. Arbustini E, Morbini P, Grasso M, et al. Restrictive cardiomyopathy, atrioventricular block and mild to subclinical myopathy in patients with desmin-immunoreactive material deposits. J Am Coll Cardiol 31:645–653, 1998.
134. Goebel HH. Desmin-related neuromuscular disorders. Muscle Nerve 18:1306–1320, 1995.
135. Milner DJ, Taffet GE, Wang X, et al. The absence of desmin leads to cardiomyocyte hypertrophy and cardiac dilation with compromised systolic function. J Mol Cell Cardiol 31:2063–2076, 1999.
136. Dalakas MC, Park KY, Semino-Mora C, Lee HS, Sivakumar K, Goldfarb LG. Desmin myopathy, a skele-

tal myopathy with cardiomyopathy caused by mutations in the desmin gene. N Engl J Med 342:770–780, 2000.

137. Roberts WC, McAllister HA, Jr., Ferrans VJ. Sarcoidosis of the heart. A clinicopathologic study of 35 necropsy patients (group 1) and review of 78 previously described necropsy patients (group 11). Am J Med 63:86–108, 1977.
138. Lemery R, McGoon MD, Edwards WD. Cardiac sarcoidosis: A potentially treatable form of myocarditis. Mayo Clin Proc 60:549–554, 1985.
139. Lorell B, Alderman EL, Mason JW. Cardiac sarcoidosis. Diagnosis with endomyocardial biopsy and treatment with corticosteroids. Am J Cardiol 42:143–146, 1978.
140. Ratner SJ, Fenoglio JJ, Jr., Ursell PC. Utility of endomyocardial biopsy in the diagnosis of cardiac sarcoidosis. Chest 90:528–533, 1986.
141. Uemura A, Morimoto S, Hiramitsu S, Kato Y, Ito T, Hishida H. Histologic diagnostic rate of cardiac sarcoidosis: Evaluation of endomyocardial biopsies. Am Heart J 138:299–302, 1999.
142. Ferrans VJ, Boyce SW. Metabolic and familial diseases. In: Silver MD (ed): Cardiovascular Pathology, pp 1153–1167. New York: Churchill Livingstone, 1983.
143. Buja LM, Roberts WC. Iron in the heart. Etiology and clinical significance. Am J Med 51:209–221, 1971.
144. Cutler DJ, Isner JM, Bracey AW, et al. Hemochromatosis heart disease: An unemphasized cause of potentially reversible restrictive cardiomyopathy. Am J Med 69:923–928, 1980.
145. Fitchett DH, Coltart DJ, Littler WA, et al. Cardiac involvement in secondary haemochromatosis: A catheter biopsy study and analysis of myocardium. Cardiovasc Res 14:719–724, 1980.
146. Short EM, Winkle RA, Billingham ME. Myocardial involvement in idiopathic hemochromatosis. Morphologic and clinical improvement following venesection. Am J Med 70:1275–1279, 1981.
147. Olson LJ, Edwards WD, Holmes DR, Jr., Miller FA, Jr., Nordstrom LA, Baldus WP. Endomyocardial biopsy in hemochromatosis: Clinicopathologic correlates in six cases. J Am Coll Cardiol 13:116–120, 1989.
148. Lombardo T, Tamburino C, Bartoloni G, et al. Cardiac iron overload in thalassemic patients: An endomyocardial biopsy study. Ann Hematol 71:135–141, 1995.
149. Olson LJ, Reeder GS, Noller KL, Edwards WD, Howell RR, Michels VV. Cardiac involvement in glycogen storage disease III: Morphologic and biochemical characterization with endomyocardial biopsy. Am J Cardiol 53:980–981, 1984.
150. Gilbert EF. The effects of metabolic diseases on the cardiovascular system. Am J Cardiovasc Pathol 1:189–213, 1987.
151. Helton E, Darragh R, Francis P, et al. Metabolic aspects of myocardial disease and a role for L-carnitine in the treatment of childhood cardiomyopathy. Pediatrics 105:1260–1270, 2000.
152. Winter SC, Buist NR. Cardiomyopathy in childhood, mitochondrial dysfunction, and the role of L-carnitine. Am Heart J 139:S63–S69, 2000.
153. Desnick RJ, Ioannou YA, Eng CM. a-galactosidase A deficiency: Fabry disease. In: Valle D (ed): The Metabolic and Molecular Bases of Inherited Disease. Vol. 7, pp 2741–2784. New York: McGraw-Hill, 1995.
154. Broadbent JC, Edwards WD, Gordon H, Hartzler GO, Krawisz JE. Fabry cardiomyopathy in the female confirmed by endomyocardial biopsy. Mayo Clin Proc 56:623–628, 1981.
155. Matsui S, Murakami E, Takekoshi N, Hiramaru Y, Kin T. Cardiac manifestations of Fabry's disease. Report of a case with pulmonary regurgitation diagnosed on the basis of endomyocardial biopsy findings. Jpn Circ J 41:1023–1036, 1977.
156. Nakao S, Takenaka T, Maeda M, et al. An atypical variant of Fabry's disease in men with left ventricular hypertrophy. N Engl J Med 333:288–293, 1995.
157. Wallace DC. Mitochondrial defects in cardiomyopathy and neuromuscular disease. Am Heart J 139:S70–S85, 2000.
158. Wallace DC. Mitochondrial diseases in man and mouse. Science 283:1482–1488, 1999.
159. Arbustini E, Diegoli M, Fasani R, et al. Mitochondrial DNA mutations and mitochondrial abnormalities in dilated cardiomyopathy. Am J Pathol 153:1501–1510, 1998.
160. Burke A, Virmani R. Tumors of the heart and great vessels. In: Atlas of Tumor Pathology, fascicle 16, Armed Forces Institute of Pathology, 1995.
161. Adachi K, Tanaka H, Toshima H, Morimatsu M. Right atrial angiosarcoma diagnosed by cardiac biopsy. Am Heart J 115:482–485, 1988.
162. Hanley PC, Shub C, Seward JB, Wold LE. Intracavitary cardiac melanoma diagnosed by endomyocardial left ventricular biopsy. Chest 84:195–198, 1983.
163. Hausheer FH, Josephson RA, Grochow LB, Weissman D, Brinker JA, Weisman HF. Intracardiac sarcoma diagnosed by left ventricular endomyocardial biopsy. Chest 92:177–179, 1987.
164. Johnston ID, Popple AW. Right ventricular outflow tract obstruction secondary to small intestinal lymphoma. Br Heart J 43:593–596, 1980.
165. Flipse TR, Tazelaar HD, Holmes DR, Jr. Diagnosis of malignant cardiac disease by endomyocardial biopsy. Mayo Clin Proc 65:1415–1422, 1990.
166. Basso C, Valente M, Poletti A, Casarotto D, Thiene G. Surgical pathology of primary cardiac and pericardial tumors. Eur J Cardiothorac Surg 12:730–737; discussion 737–738, 1997.
167. Billingham ME, Bristow M. Endomyocardial biopsy for cardiac monitoring of patients receiving anthracycline. In: Fenoglio JJ, Jr. (ed): Endomyocardial Biopsy: Techniques and Applications. Boca Raton, FL: CRC Press, 1982.
168. Rowan RA, Masek MA, Billingham ME. Anthracycline cardiotoxicity and dilated cardiomyopathy: Morphometric distinctions. J Am Coll Cardiol 7:121A, 1986.
169. Billingham ME, Bristow MR, Glatstein E, Mason JW, Masek MA, Daniels JR. Adriamycin cardiotoxicity: Endomyocardial biopsy evidence of enhancement by irradiation. Am J Surg Pathol 1:17–23, 1977.
170. Bristow MR, Billingham ME, Mason JW, Daniels JR. Clinical spectrum of anthracycline antibiotic cardiotoxicity. Cancer Treat Rep 62:873–879, 1978.
171. Isner JM, Ferrans VJ, Cohen SR, et al. Clinical and morphologic cardiac findings after anthracycline chemotherapy. Analysis of 64 patients studied at necropsy. Am J Cardiol 51:1167–1174, 1983.
172. Shan K, Lincoff AM, Young JB. Anthracycline-induced cardiotoxicity. Ann Intern Med 125:47–58, 1996.
173. Billingham ME, Bristow M. Evaluation of anthracycline cardiotoxicity: Predictive ability and functional correlation of endomyocardial biopsy. Cancer Treat Symp 3:71, 1984.

174. Mackay B, Ewer MS, Carrasco CH, Benjamin RS. Assessment of anthracycline cardiomyopathy by endomyocardial biopsy. Ultrastruct Pathol 18:203–211, 1994.
175. Boucek RJ, Jr., Dodd DA, Atkinson JB, Oquist N, Olson RD. Contractile failure in chronic doxorubicin-induced cardiomyopathy. J Mol Cell Cardiol 29:2631–2640, 1997.
176. Dodd DA, Atkinson JB, Olson RD, et al. Doxorubicin cardiomyopathy is associated with a decrease in calcium release channel of the sarcoplasmic reticulum in a chronic rabbit model. J Clin Invest 91:1697–1705, 1993.
177. Working PK, Newman MS, Sullivan T, Yarrington J. Reduction of the cardiotoxicity of doxorubicin in rabbits and dogs by encapsulation in long-circulating, pegylated liposomes. J Pharmacol Exp Ther 289:1128–1133, 1999.
178. Valero V, Buzdar AU, Theriault RL, et al. Phase II trial of liposome-encapsulated doxorubicin, cyclophosphamide, and fluorouracil as first-line therapy in patients with metastatic breast cancer. J Clin Oncol 17:1425–1434, 1999.
179. Shek TW, Luk IS, Ma L, Cheung KL. Paclitaxel-induced cardiotoxicity. An ultrastructural study. Arch Pathol Lab Med 120:89–91, 1996.

Chapter

9

PATHOLOGY OF HEART TRANSPLANTATION

In 1953, Downie placed a heterotopic cardiac graft in the neck of a dog, anastomosing the aorta to the carotid artery and pulmonary artery to jugular vein; cardiac function averaged 129 hours.[1] After successful orthotopic transplants in dogs,[2–6] the heart of a chimpanzee transplanted into a dying patient functioned for approximately one hour.[7] In 1967, Barnard performed the first human heart transplant,[8] and as more transplants followed, reports concerning complications emerged.[6, 9–17] The initial enthusiasm for cardiac transplantation decreased when less than optimal results became evident, largely due to rejection, but interest was renewed in the 1980s with the introduction of the immunosuppressive agent, cyclosporine. Cyclosporine therapy has greatly influenced the pathology of cardiac transplantation, both in the early post-transplant period when acute rejection is a potential problem, as well as in long-term survivors.

Cardiac transplantation has evolved from a radical experimental modality to a widely accepted viable therapy for treatment of end-stage heart disease. In 1998, cardiac transplantation was performed in approximately 3,000 patients.[18] Since the early 1970s, the endomyocardial biopsy has become the mainstay for diagnosis and evaluation of rejection, largely as a result of the pioneering work of Billingham and her colleagues at Stanford. With the introduction of cyclosporine as an immunosuppressive agent in the mid 1980s, the role of the biopsy has become even more important, because cyclosporine may mask the clinical manifestations of rejection. Survival has remained constant since the advent of cyclosporine in 1985. Overall 1-year survival is 79%, with a mortality rate of 4% per year after the first year.[18] Risk factors that have a negative effect on mortality include prior cardiac transplantation, use of a ventricular assist device or ventilator support prior to transplantation, and increasing age.[18] The focus of this chapter will be pathology of the native (explanted) heart, early and long-term pathology of the cardiac allograft, and the pathology of rejection.

SURGICAL PATHOLOGY OF THE NATIVE (RECIPIENT) HEART

The indication for cardiac transplantation in the vast majority of adults (90%) is chronic ischemic heart disease and cardiomyopathy, each with approximately equal numbers.[18] Children less than 1 year of age undergo cardiac transplantation for congenital heart disease, while cardiomyopathy as an indication increases in those over the age of 1 year. Other diseases that may be encountered in explanted hearts include hypertrophic cardiomyopathy, storage or infiltrative diseases (amyloid, sarcoid), myocarditis, acute myocardial infarction, and end-stage valvular diseases.

Replacement of the diseased native heart by a cardiac allograft is virtually always orthotopic, versus heterotopic (in which the native heart is left in place). The surgery is straightforward, with four anastomoses: right and left atria, pulmonary artery, and aorta. The explanted heart will therefore contain only remnants of the atria that usually include the appendages.

For the surgical pathology evaluation of ischemic cardiomyopathy in the explanted heart, coronary arteries and bypass grafts should be serially sectioned at 2- to 3-mm intervals. The ventricles are cut through the short axis of the heart, parallel to the atrioventricular sulcus, in a "breadloaf" manner. The location of recent or remote infarcts can be described using standard anatomic frames of reference (i.e., anterior, lateral, inferior/posterior), and the extent of infarction can be described in terms of the circumference of ventricle involved as well as longitudinally (i.e., basal one half, apical two thirds, etc.). The distribution of infarction is described as subendocardial, transmural, focal, or a combination of these.

A four-chamber view is best for evaluation of dilated cardiomyopathies. The heart is sectioned from base to apex, along the margin of the right ventricle and the obtuse margin of the left ventricle, continuing through the remnants of the atria. For evaluation of hypertrophic cardiomyopathies, a long-axis cut through the left ventricular outflow tract is best. The heart is again sectioned from apex to base, but—in contrast to the four-chamber view—the axis is shifted counterclockwise such that the plane of section through the aortic valve leaflets is through the right coronary and the posterior (noncoronary) leaflets.

Congenital heart diseases are best evaluated by dissection along the flow of blood, although explanted hearts with hypoplastic left-heart syndrome and truncus arteriosus can be sectioned using the four-chamber view.

Hypertrophic and dilated cardiomyopathies may be familial, and fresh material may be needed for molecular studies. A specimen should also be placed in glutaraldehyde in the event that a storage disease needs to be evaluated.

In the evaluation of histologic sections from explanted hearts, eosinophilic carditis may occasionally be seen. This can be due to a hypersensitivity reaction to drugs, particularly dobutamine (and specifically the preservative sodium bisulfite that is contained in dobutamine solutions) administered to these end-stage heart failure patients.[19]

EARLY POST-TRANSPLANTATION PATHOLOGY

Changes seen in the early postoperative stages include: (1) immediate graft failure; (2) hyperacute rejection; (3) reperfusion (ischemic) damage; and, (4) acute rejection.[20, 21]

Immediate graft failure usually occurs before the patient leaves the operating room and may be due to surgical problems, prolonged ischemic time, or severe pulmonary hypertension. The myocardium in immediate graft failure may appear normal or exhibit interstitial hemorrhage and diffuse edema.

Hyperacute rejection is usually due to improper cross-matching or major histocompatibility differences and is rare. Predisposing factors include prior blood transfusions, multiple pregnancies, multiple cardiac surgeries, and previous transplantation. The myocardium will have marked diffuse interstitial hemorrhage, with neutrophils marginating in vessels and fibrin thrombi in small vessels (Fig. 9–1). Patients

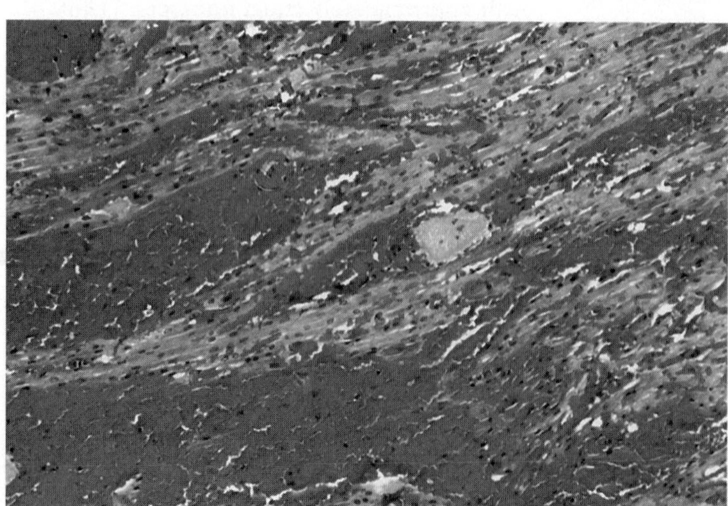

Figure 9–1. Hyperacute rejection. The myocardium of this explanted heart with hyperacute rejection has diffuse interstitial hemorrhage, with a fibrin thrombus in an intramyocardial artery. (H & E)

rarely survive for more than a few hours without emergent retransplantation.

Reperfusion or ischemic injury can be seen in the myocardium of any patient for several weeks following transplantation. It is manifest by focal necrosis (hypereosinophilia, loss of nuclei, loss of cytoplasmic detail), with a heterogeneous inflammatory cell infiltrate consisting of neutrophils, macrophages, and occasional lymphocytes and plasma cells (see following).[22] We have not observed any correlation between the presence of ischemic changes as seen in the first biopsy following transplantation and long-term outcome, although one series reported that extensive perioperative ischemic injury may impact adversely on short-term survival.[22] Ischemic injury may also underlie acute allograft failure (defined as acute graft failure in the early transplant period that is not associated with acute cellular rejection, right ventricular failure from refractory pulmonary hypertension, or technical factors),[23] and total ischemic time greater than 4 hours may be associated with increased mortality.[24] The differential diagnosis between postoperative ischemic injury and acute rejection on endomyocardial biopsy is discussed below.

Acute rejection is unusual within the first 10 days following transplantation. The distinction between acute rejection in the early postoperative period and surgery-related ischemia can be aided by the observation that, in ischemia, myocyte necrosis precedes an acute inflammatory response (which is neutrophilic or mixed and may be less than that associated with rejection), whereas a mononuclear infiltrate is seen first in acute rejection, followed by necrosis.[21]

ACUTE REJECTION

Technical Considerations

The endomyocardial biopsy is the standard by which acute cardiac allograft rejection is evaluated. At least four pieces of myocardium are required to exclude rejection (although some pathologists will make a diagnosis with three pieces). Multiple sections representative of all levels in the paraffin block should be examined by H & E stain. Five "step" levels are usually sufficient, but deeper levels may be needed to distinguish rejection (i.e., focal moderate grade 2) from Quilty lesions (see following). Additionally, vascular (humoral) rejection, which may be prevalent during the first 6 months following transplantation (see below), requires frozen sections for immunofluorescent studies for diagnosis. Frozen sections to make the diagnosis of acute *cellular* rejection should never be performed.

Grading of Acute Rejection

The histopathologic features of acute cardiac rejection are inflammation with or without myocyte damage. The severity of rejection is classified according to the extent and pattern of inflammation and the presence or absence of myocyte necrosis. The inflammatory infiltrate is comprised of large, "activated" (immunoblast-like) T lymphocytes.

Grading acute rejection originally developed by Billingham and colleagues was defined as mild, moderate, and severe. Numerous grading schemes were subsequently utilized by different individual transplant centers, leading to problems in comparing results as patients were seen in different centers and as experimental protocols to investigate new immunosuppressive therapies were initiated. To standardize the grading of acute rejection, a working formulation was developed by the International Society for Heart and Lung Transplantation (ISHLT), and this system is now used widely throughout the world (Table 9–1).[25] It is predicated on the Stanford system of mild, moderate, and severe grades, with the recognition of lower and higher grades within certain categories.

Mild acute rejection is characterized by a sparse endocardial or perivascular infiltrate of mononuclear cells (T lymphocytes). *Grade 1A* rejection is defined by focal perivascular or interstitial lymphocytic inflammation that can involve one or more pieces of the biopsy (Fig. 9–2). *Grade 1B* rejection is characterized by a more diffuse but still sparse lymphocytic infiltrate in one or more pieces (Fig. 9–2). Myocyte necrosis is not seen in mild rejection. Approximately half of patients receiving cyclosporine may progress to a moderate grade of rejection, whereas the rest will exhibit spontaneous resolution on a subsequent biopsy.[23]

In *moderate rejection,* the mononuclear infiltrate spreads into the interstitium, often surrounding individual myocytes, and myocyte necrosis may be evident. Eosinophils are occasionally seen, although infections or hypersensitivity reactions should also be considered when eosinophils are present. Myocyte necrosis is not always evident in moderate rejection, and the

Table 9–1. International Society for Heart and Lung Transplantation Grading of Acute Cardiac Rejection

Grade	Description	Grade	Description
0	No rejection Normal myocardium with no evidence of inflammation or myocyte damage	3A	Multifocal moderate rejection Multifocal lymphocytic inflammatory infiltrates with myocyte damage; eosinophils may be present, and there are areas of normal myocardium between foci of inflammation. These changes can be seen in one or more pieces of myocardium. Grade 3A is distinguished from grade 1A by the presence of multifocal infiltrates in grade 3A, as well as myocyte damage.
1	Mild rejection		
1A	Focal (perivascular or interstitial) lymphocytic infiltration involving one or more pieces and no myocyte damage		
1B	Diffuse, sparse lymphocytic infiltrate involving one or more pieces with no myocyte damage		
2	Focal moderate rejection One focus with an aggressive, sharply circumscribed infiltrate, usually associated with myocyte damage or architectural distortion of the myocardium. The infiltrate is composed of lymphocytes and immunoblasts, with occasional eosinophils.	3B	Diffuse moderate/borderline severe rejection Diffuse inflammation, with myocyte damage; aggressive lymphocytic infiltrates which may contain eosinophils and rare neutrophils. There are fewer areas of normal myocardium separating areas of inflammation than in grade 3A.
		4	Severe rejection Diffuse, aggressive inflammation consisting of lymphocytes, eosinophils, and neutrophils; myocyte necrosis is always present; hemorrhage and vasculitis are also seen.

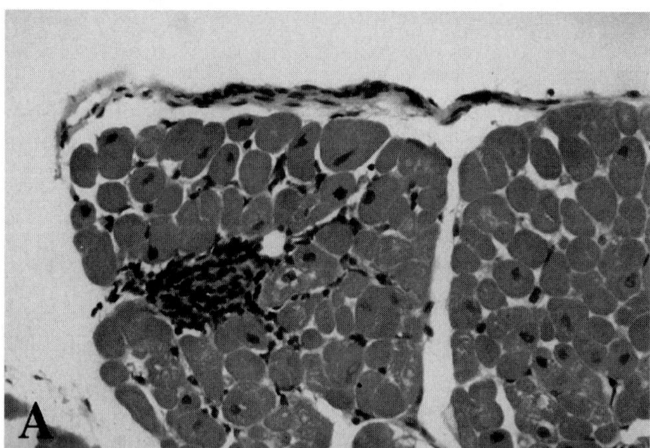

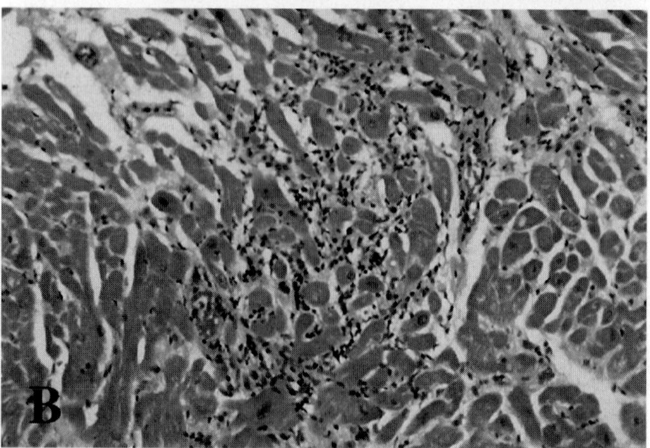

Figure 9–2. Mild acute rejection. *A.* Grade 1A mild rejection: Endomyocardial biopsy with a single focus of lymphocytic inflammation and no myocyte damage. *B.* Grade 1B mild rejection: A sparse but diffuse lymphocytic infiltrate without myocyte damage. (H & E)

amount and distribution of the inflammation can define the diagnostic criteria.[26, 27] Moderate rejection is classified as *focal* (*grade 2*), *multifocal* (*grade 3A*), and *diffuse* (*grade 3B*). In focal moderate rejection (grade 2), an "aggressive," sharply circumscribed infiltrate is present, usually associated with myocyte damage or architectural distortion of the myocardium (Fig. 9–3). Grade 3A rejection is characterized by multifocal lymphocytic inflammation with myocyte damage, seen in one or more pieces of the myocardium (Fig. 9–3). Grade 3A rejection is distinguished from grade 1A by the presence of multifocal inflammatory infiltrates and myocyte damage. In grade 3B rejection, aggressive lymphocytic infiltrates with eosinophils and rare neutrophils are distributed diffusely throughout the myocardium (Fig. 9–3). Grade 3B rejection is distinguished from grade 3A by the extent of inflammation, with fewer areas of normal myocardium separating areas of inflammation.

In *severe acute rejection* (*grade 4*), the inflammatory infiltrate becomes more diffuse and aggressive, as does the extent of myocyte necrosis, which is always evident (Fig. 9–4). The inflammation is perivascular and interstitial, consisting of eosinophils and neutrophils as well as lymphocytes. Interstitial hemorrhage occurs in severe rejection (which is distinguished from biopsy-induced hemorrhage that can be seen in endomyocardial biopsies), and vasculitis may be present. Severe rejection is difficult to reverse but is more likely to do so if the patient is receiving cyclosporine.

After successful treatment of acute rejection, lymphocytes evolve from large, immunoblast-like cells to small lymphocytes. "Resolved" rejection indicates complete resolution and can be graded as "0." "Resolving" acute rejection implies that the degree of inflammation is less than that seen in the previous biopsy and a lesser grade is assigned. "Ongoing" rejection implies that there has been no improvement from the previous biopsy. As acute rejection resolves, small lymphocytes may persist for several weeks, and fibroblasts and hemosiderin-laden macrophages may be seen. In resolved

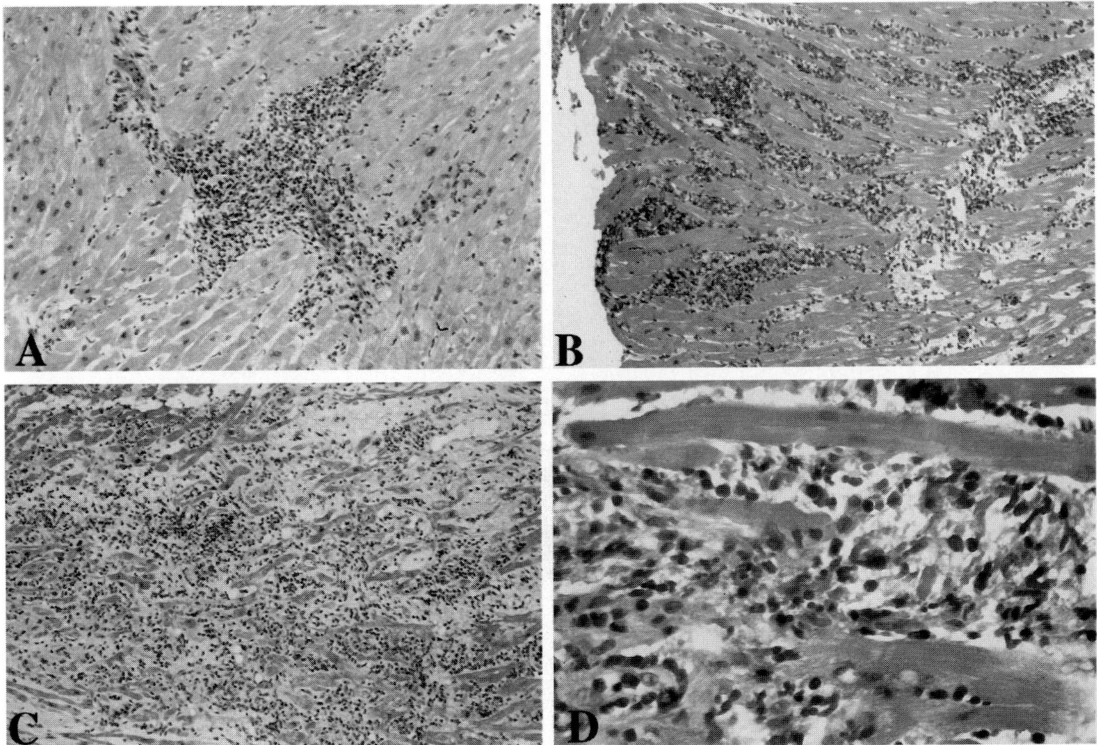

Figure 9–3. Moderate acute rejection. *A.* Grade 2 (focal moderate) rejection: A large perivascular lymphocytic infiltrate displaces adjacent myocytes. *B.* Grade 3A (multifocal) moderate rejection: Multifocal lymphocytic infiltrates involve this piece of myocardium. *C.* Grade 3B (diffuse) moderate rejection: There is diffuse inflammation with little intervening areas of unaffected myocytes. *D.* Grade 3B moderate rejection: Myocyte necrosis and an inflammatory infiltrate consisting of lymphocytes and occasional neutrophils can be seen. (H & E)

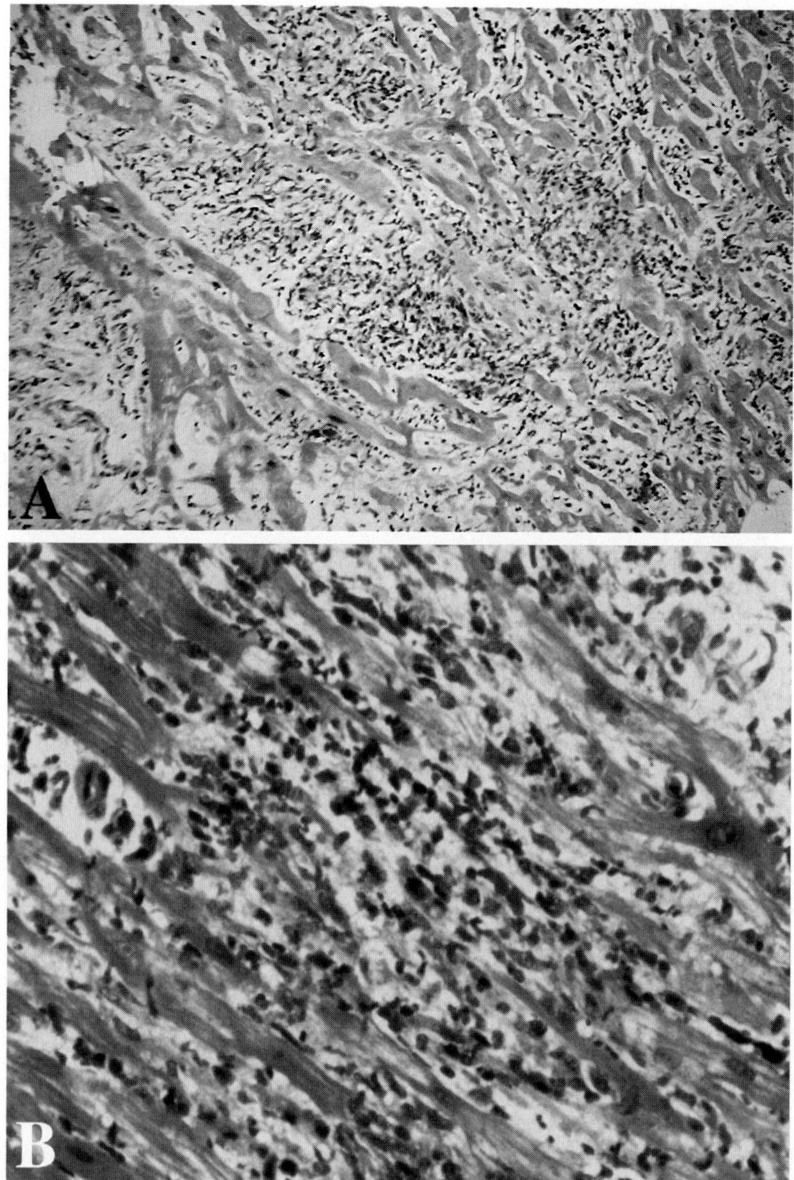

Figure 9–4. Grade 4 severe rejection. *A.* A diffuse inflammatory cell infiltrate with myocyte damage involves the myocardium in this endomyocardial biopsy. *B.* At higher magnification, a mixed lymphocytic and neutrophilic cell infiltrate with scattered erythrocytes are seen. (H & E)

rejection, focal scars can be found in the myocardium. Rare patients may have persistent inflammatory cell infiltrates in biopsies over a prolonged period of time without evidence of graft dysfunction.[28] This may represent a chronic form of continuing cellular rejection, or a state of persistent immunologic activity related to a prior infection.[29]

Myocyte damage may be difficult to identify, and Masson trichrome stain may help facilitate its recognition. Inflammation that is present in scar tissue or in fat is not indicative of acute rejection. In infants and children, the initial (and occasionally only) manifestation of acute rejection may be interstitial edema, with only a sparse inflammatory cell infiltrate. Edema can be an artifact from simply obtaining the biopsy, however, and it only has significance if associated with an inflammatory cell infiltrate. Edema can also be seen in patients with low cyclosporine levels and may portend subsequent rejection. There appears to be no significant difference in outcomes for grade 1A versus grade 1B rejection.

Although the ISHLT grading system has proven to be reproducible among different pathologists, there can be discrepancies that are problematic.[30] Most discrepancies involve differentiating grades 1B from 2, 2 versus 3A, and Quilty effect (see below) versus grade 2 or 3A. Myocyte injury can help in distinguishing grades 1A and 2. Grade 2 is distinguished from grade 3A by the presence of a single focus of inflammation, whereas the focus is less well-defined in grade 3A.

Artifacts and Caveats

Several sources of error in making the diagnosis of acute rejection are possible. Ischemic changes can be seen up to 4 weeks following transplantation. These changes can be particularly prominent in the first biopsy following transplantation. Ischemic changes are recognized by focal myocyte damage or necrosis (Fig. 9–5). There may be a sparse, predominantly neutrophilic, inflammatory infiltrate. Ischemic changes should not be misinterpreted as acute rejection. The distinction between the two may be made by knowing the post-transplant interval, and by recognizing that, with ischemia, myocyte damage precedes the acute inflammatory response. The extent of myocyte damage in ischemia exceeds the degree of inflammation that would be otherwise expected for acute rejection. Coagulation necrosis can be seen with ischemia but does not occur in acute rejection.

One of the most common pitfalls is the misdiagnosis of acute rejection in a previous biopsy site. Evidence of previous biopsies can occur in 16% of those obtained in the immediate postoperative period and is more frequent as the number of biopsies in a patient increases with time.[30] Changes that represent previous biopsy sites range from the presence of fibrin, necrosis, and granulation tissue if recent, to myocyte disarray and fibrosis if remote (healed) (Fig. 9–6). The location and configuration of these changes can provide clues as to their origin. Fibrin, which is not seen with rejection, is a useful marker for a previous biopsy site. Catheter-induced lesions can also look similar to biopsy sites. Catheter lesions are recognized by loose connective tissue with a mild polymorphous inflammatory cell infiltrate.

Quilty Lesion

In 13% to 14% of patients receiving cyclosporine, the biopsy may show a focal, dense

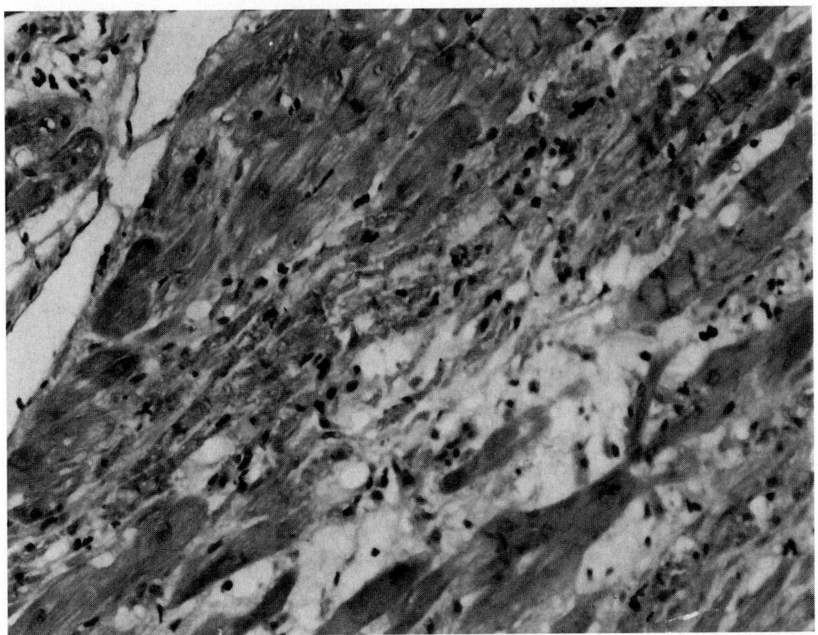

Figure 9–5. Postoperative ischemic injury. Endomyocardial biopsy 7 days after transplantation. Evidence of recent ischemia related to surgery and reperfusion injury can be seen in this endomyocardial biopsy, with edema, focal myocyte damage, and a sparse, predominantly neutrophilic response (H & E)

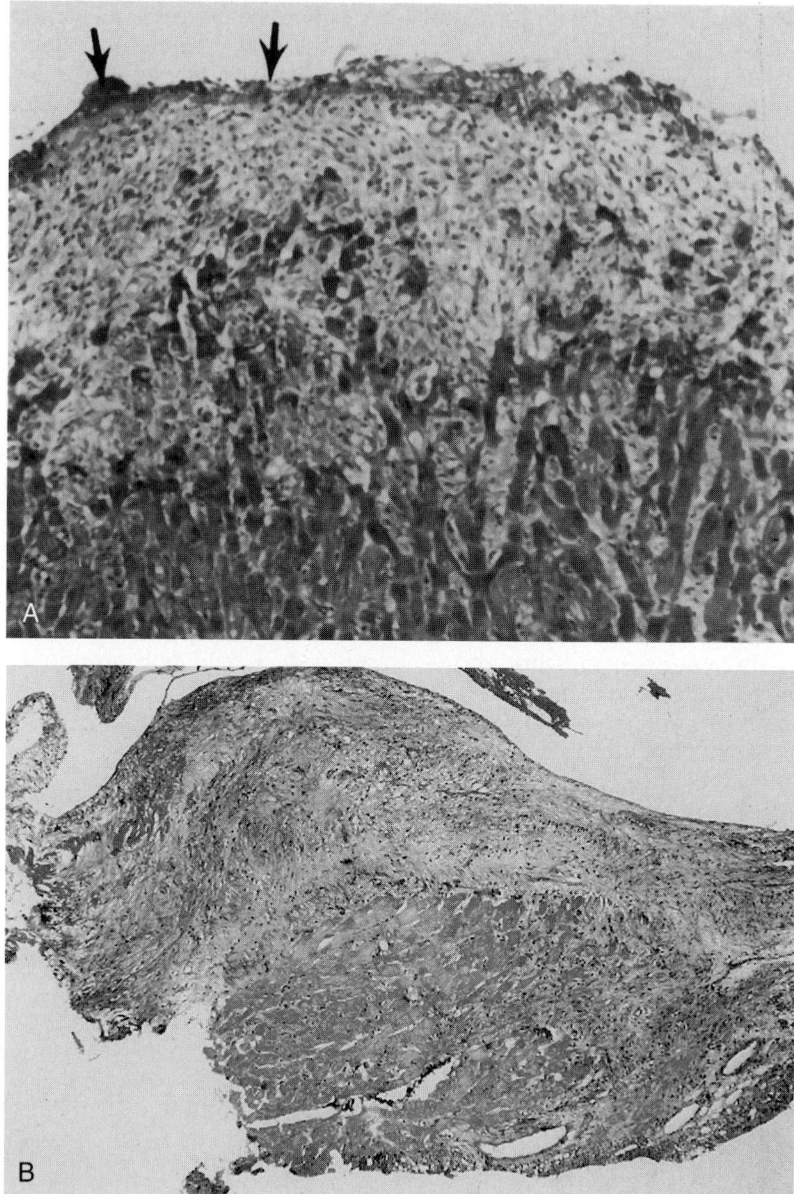

Figure 9–6. Previous biopsy site. *A.* Recent previous biopsy site, with granulation tissue, a sparse inflammatory cell infiltrate, and early fibrosis at the endocardial surface. Fibrin lines the surface of the endocardium. *B.* Remote (healed) biopsy site, with a dense endocardial scar along the endocardial surface (*A,* H & E; *B,* Masson trichrome).

endocardial collection of lymphocytes that can extend into the adjacent subendocardium.[31] These changes have been termed the "Quilty" lesion (effect), named after the first patient at Stanford to show such a lesion. While a possible manifestation of rejection, Quilty lesions do not portend any apparent immediate adverse clinical outcome, although they may occur in patients who have more frequent subsequent episodes of rejection.[32] The Quilty effect is therefore not treated with enhanced immunosuppression and resolves spontaneously, usually within 2 to 3 weeks (although some may persist longer). It has been suggested that the Quilty effect occurs in the setting of low endocardial cyclosporine levels, resulting in a localized endocardial rejection.[33] This infiltrate is comprised primarily of T lymphocytes, with clusters of B cells (unlike the infiltrate in acute rejection) and occasional plasma cells and macrophages at the interface.[34]

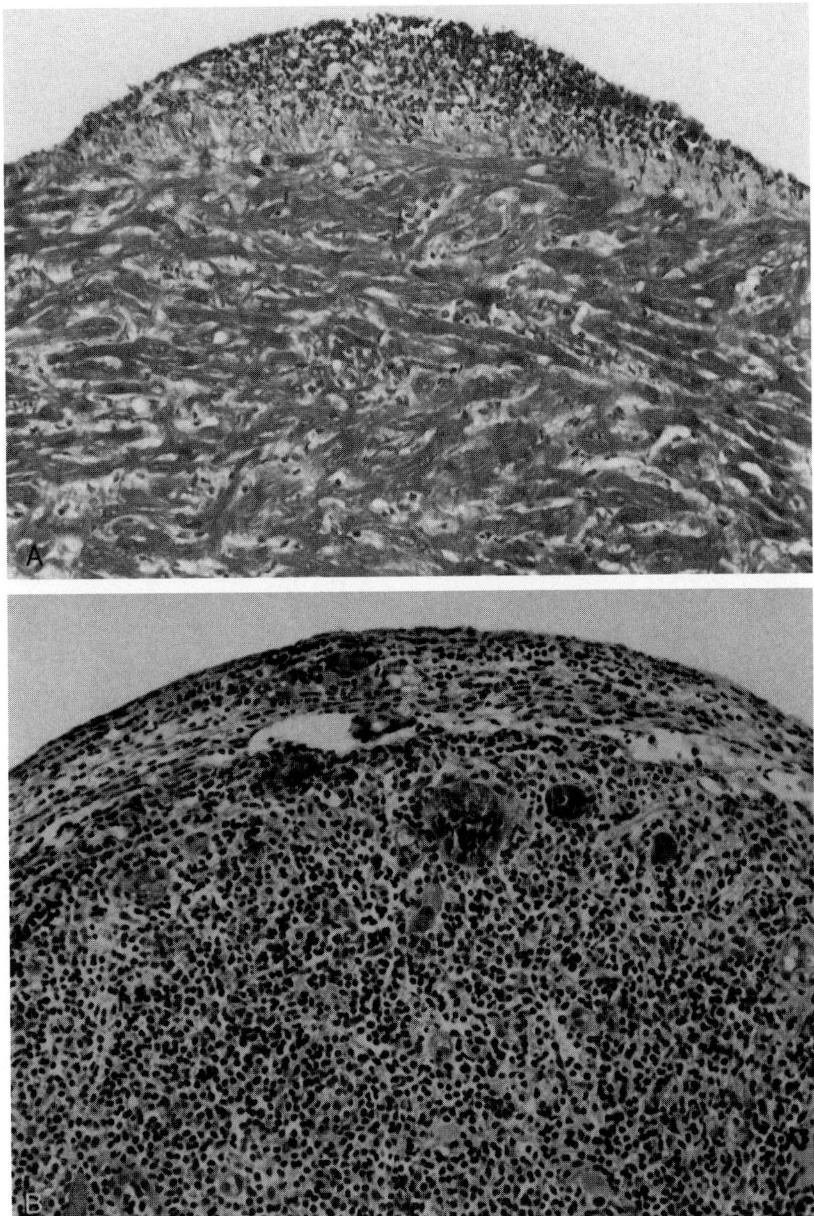

Figure 9–7. Quilty effect. *A.* Quilty A lesion, consisting of a small endocardial infiltrate that is sharply demarcated from the underlying myocardium. *B.* Large Quilty lesion localized along the endocardium, within which are scattered capillaries.

Illustration continued on following page

The distribution may be confined to the endocardium (Quilty A) (Fig. 9–7), or extend into the myocardium (Quilty B) (Fig. 9–7). Quilty lesions are also seen in the epicardial fat of explanted or autopsy hearts as well as diffuse in the myocardium (Fig. 9–7). Quilty lesions can be distinguished from acute rejection (particularly grade 2) by the characteristic presence of small capillaries within the inflammatory cell infiltrate. Also, because 50% of the cells in Quilty lesions are B lymphocytes, immunoperoxidase studies for B- and T-cell markers may occasionally be useful. If endocardial infiltrates typical of Quilty effect are present in other pieces, interpretation of a focus of inflammation within the myocardium as a deep Quilty lesion may be more likely than rejection. Healed Quilty lesions can simulate healed previous biopsy sites; they occur

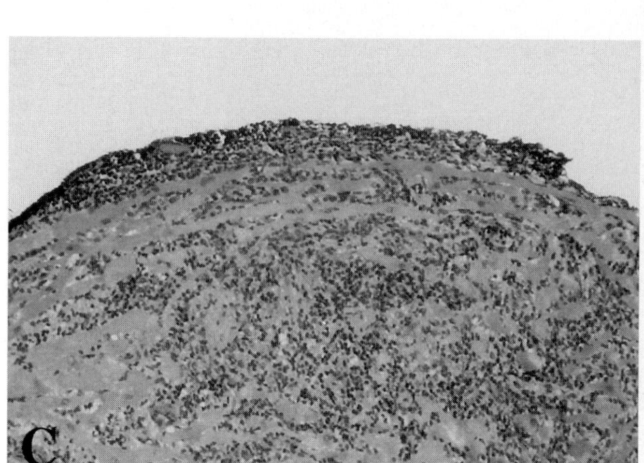

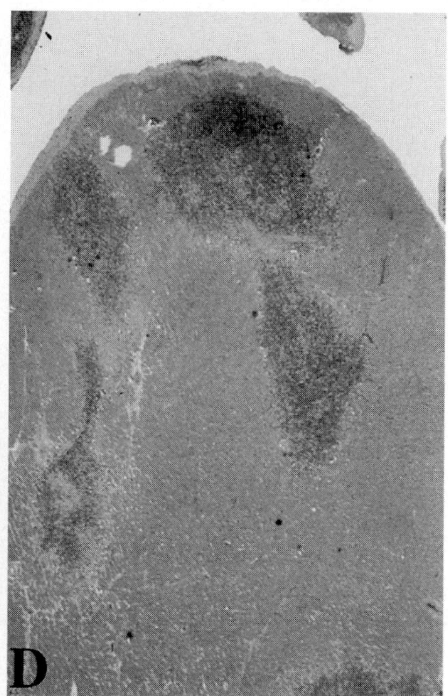

Figure 9–7 *Continued. C.* Quilty B lesion, with extension of the lymphocytic infiltrate away from the endocardium into adjacent myocardium. *D.* Quilty lesions in the papillary muscle of an explanted heart, consisting of large collections of lymphocytes deep within the myocardium. Some foci have associated early fibrosis. (H & E)

as endocardial scars that have an even, linear border, in contrast to a healed biopsy site, which has a more uneven interface.

Myocarditis can occur in the cardiac allograft, and the pathologist should keep in mind the possibility that the inflammatory infiltrate seen in a cardiac biopsy from a transplant patient might represent an acute infection, such as toxoplasmosis or cytomegalovirus (CMV) myocarditis. The inflammatory infiltrate is usually mixed in infectious processes, rather than monomorphic, and necrosis usually exceeds that seen in acute rejection relative to the amount of inflammation. Infectious complications in cardiac allograft recipients is discussed in further detail below. The pathologist should also be aware of an increased risk of malignancy in recipients of organ transplants (see following), particularly lymphoproliferative malignancies that could potentially be initially discovered in a cardiac biopsy.

Some diseases that may recur in the transplanted heart, such as giant-cell myocarditis, sarcoid, or amyloidosis, need to be recognized if present in an endomyocardial biopsy (Fig. 9–8).

Grade 2 (Focal Moderate) Rejection

Grade 2 (focal moderate) rejection may be problematic. Some centers initiate enhanced immunosuppressive therapy with grade 2 rejection, while others do not.[35] Data have been published that suggest many grade 2 lesions actually represent Quilty lesions.[36] Most biopsies with grade 2 rejection do not progress, and no association has been found between grade 2 rejection and survival.[35, 37] Additionally, a large focus of grade 2 rejection may be hard to distinguish from grade 3A rejection, and there appears to be a wide spectrum in the "size" of grade 2 rejection lesions.

Influence of Immunosuppression on Histopathology of Acute Rejection

Although cyclosporine is standard therapy for prevention of allograft rejection in heart transplant recipients, there may be a trend to use less cyclosporine and more azathioprine or other immunosuppressive agents in some patients, particularly those in whom renal function or hypertension become difficult to manage. Thus, it is necessary that the pathologist have some knowledge of the morphologic differences between conventional (azathioprine) and cyclosporine immunosuppressive therapy (Table 9–2).[20] The clinical signs for predicting acute rejection in cyclosporine-treated patients are not so reliable as in those receiving azathio-

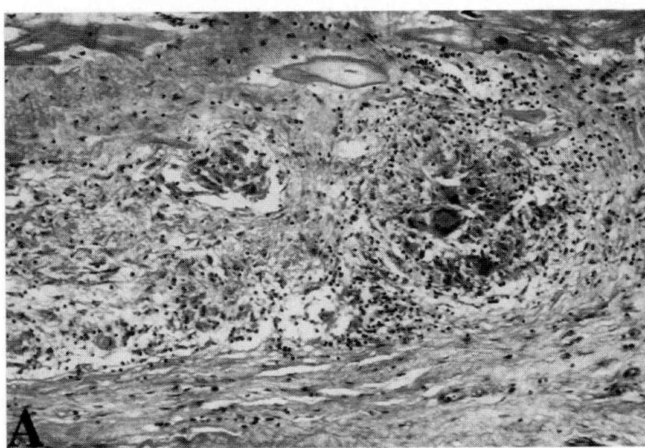
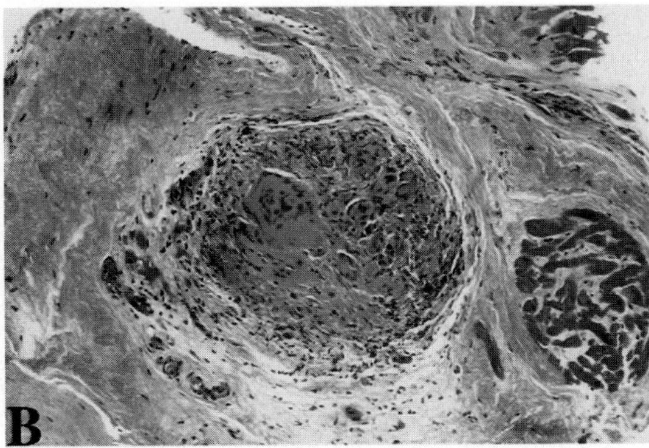

Figure 9–8. *A.* A 41-year-old male underwent orthotopic cardiac transplantation. Histologic sections from the explanted heart showed marked focal fibrosis as well as scattered noncaseating granulomas associated with a sparse lymphocytic infiltrate, diagnostic of sarcoid. *B.* An annual surveillance endomyocardial biopsy 3 years later had noncaseating granulomas, indicative of recurrent sarcoid in the transplanted heart. (H & E)

prine, as the only sign in cyclosporine-treated patients may be fever. Rejection develops much faster in azathioprine-treated patients. Although myocardial fibrosis occurs in all transplant hearts, a fine perimyocytic fibrosis can be observed in cyclosporine-treated patients.

The use of OKT3 monoclonal antibody (a murine antihuman mature T-cell antibody) as an immunosuppressive agent may allow lower doses of cyclosporine. OKT3 may be associated with reduced cellularity of the infiltrates, edema, increased vascular rejection (see below), and increased incidence of the Quilty lesion.[38] To date, use of other newer immunosuppressive agents (tacrolimus, mycophenolate) has not been associated with significant changes in the histology of rejection.

Table 9–2. Cyclosporine versus Azathioprine Immunosuppression

Cyclosporine	Azathioprine
Rejection develops slowly (4–5 days)	Rejection develops rapidly (24–36 hours)
Clinical signs often absent	Clinical signs—fever, gallop, ECG changes
Slow reversal of rejection	Rapid reversal of rejection (2 weeks)
Severe rejection often reversible	Severe rejection often not reversible
Eosinophils common in rejection	Eosinophils rare in rejection
Quilty effect in 5–10% of biopsies	Quilty effect very rare

From Billingham ME. Cardiac transplantation. In: Waller BF (ed): Contemporary Issues in Cardiovascular Pathology, p 185. Philadelphia: FA Davis, 1988, with permission.

Photopheresis is occasionally used as an alternative therapy in some patients for whom standard immunosuppression is contraindicated or who may be refractory to treatment. The procedure involves administration of autologous lymphocytes with 8-methoxypsoralen activated by extracorporally administered ultraviolet-A irradiation. Biopsy samples from patients who receive this therapy may exhibit more extensive inflammatory infiltrates that persist longer, despite clinical resolution of rejection. Other antirejection modalities that have been used in isolated cases of refractory acute rejection include cyclophosphamide and whole-body irradiation. The number of patients who have received these treatments is too low to determine their influence on the histopathology of acute rejection.

Vascular (Humoral) Rejection

While most rejection episodes in cardiac allografts are "cellular," a "vascular" form of rejection may occur in rare patients.[39–41] It has been postulated that endothelial cells stimulated by activated T cells mediate this form of rejection. Because humoral immune responses and B-cell activation are thought to play a role as well, this form of rejection has also been called "humoral" rejection. Vascular rejection can be diagnosed only by immunofluorescence studies on fresh-frozen, unfixed samples using a panel of antibodies against immunoglobulin, components of complement, and fibrinogen.

The diagnosis of vascular rejection may be suggested in paraffin-embedded tissue when endothelial cells appear activated (large, prominent), and perivascular inflammation or edema is present. Confirmation of the diagnosis is made when immune complexes are demonstrated by immunofluorescence (Fig. 9–9). The prevalence (and possibly existence) of vascular rejection and its role in graft coronary artery disease remain to be fully established. Vascular rejection should be considered if the allograft is not functioning optimally, particularly in the immediate postoperative period (first 6 weeks after transplantation), if the classic histopathologic signs of cellular rejection are absent, and if other causes of graft dysfunction (postoperative ischemia, infection) have been excluded. The utility of routine immunofluorescence in heart biopsy specimens for cardiac transplant patients has been questioned, and it has been suggested that positive immunofluorescence is a nonspecific finding in both normal and posttransplantation myocardium.[42]

PATHOLOGY IN LONG-TERM CARDIAC TRANSPLANTS

The causes of morbidity and mortality in long-term (greater than 2 years) heart transplant recipients are predominantly graft vasculopathy, neoplasms, recurrence of pretransplantation diseases, infections, and late acute rejection.[43] Long-term patients are at risk for sudden death due to coronary artery disease with or without associated myocardial fibrosis.[44]

Graft Arteriosclerosis

After approximately 3 months following a cardiac transplant, the frequency of acute rejection decreases, although it still occasionally occurs. Chronic rejection emerges as a complication, and this is currently the major limitation for long-term success of cardiac transplantation. Chronic rejection takes the form of accelerated coronary artery narrowing that involves both small intramyocardial arteries as well as major epicardial arteries.[45] Because the transplanted heart lacks afferent innervation, transplant recipients do not experience angina, and the first manifestation of coronary artery disease may be silent myocardial infarction, congestive heart failure, or ventricular arrhythmia and sudden death. Various terms have been used to describe the coronary artery disease that occurs in cardiac allografts, including allograft vasculopathy, allograft arteriopathy, graft coronary artery disease, chronic rejection, graft vascular disease, and transplant (or graft) arteriosclerosis.

The incidence of coronary artery disease detected by angiography in cardiac transplant recipients is approximately 20% at 1 year and up to nearly 50% at 3 years.[46, 47] Angiographic

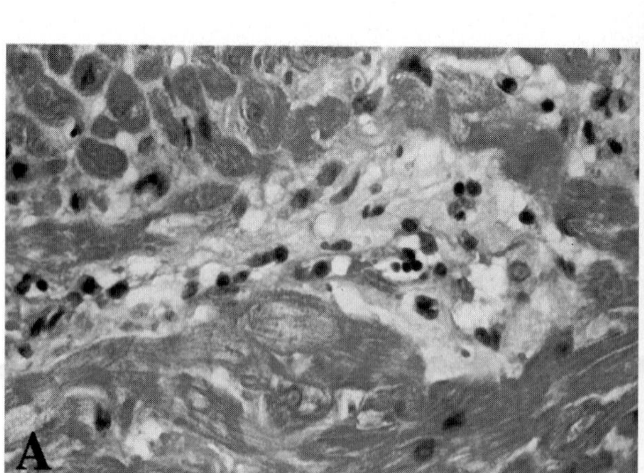

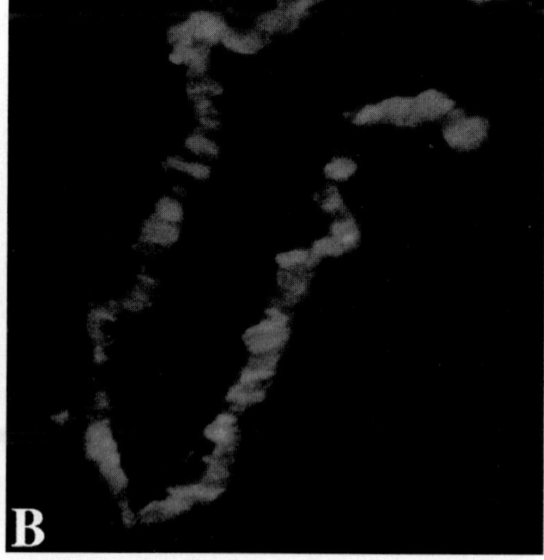

Figure 9–9. Vascular (humoral) rejection. *A*. This endomyocardial biopsy was obtained from a cardiac transplant patient who had echocardiographic signs suspicious for acute rejection. No cellular infiltrates were found in the biopsy. Small arteries, however, were lined by large, swollen endothelial cells, and there was mild endothelialitis. These features were suggestive of vascular rejection, which was confirmed by immunofluorescence on a subsequent biopsy. *B*. This endomyocardial biopsy that was stained by immunofluorescent techniques shows uniform marking of a small blood vessel by IgG, indicative of vascular rejection. (*A*, H & E)

patterns of disease are characterized by diffuse concentric narrowing, most prominent in the middle to distal segments of the arteries, with obliteration of distal vessels; there may be either discreet or tubular narrowings, diffuse concentric narrowing, or irregular narrrowing with occluded branches, and poorly developed collateral vessels.[46] After graft arteriosclerosis is initially detected, survival is dramatically and proportionately dependent upon the number of diseased arteries, with 13% survival at 2 years for triple-vessel disease, compared with 36% survival at 2 years for single-vessel disease.[48]

The vascular lesions that occur in the coronary arteries of transplanted hearts are not unique and can be seen in other long-surviving transplanted organs, including kidney, liver, and lung.[49–51] The histopathologic features correlate with the angiographic findings and consist of uniform, concentric circumferential and longitudinal increases in intimal tissue, comprised of smooth muscle cells and macrophages in an abundant extracellular matrix of fibrous tissue and proteoglycan ground substance (Fig. 9–10).[52] In contrast to conventional atherosclerosis, the internal lamina is intact, and early lesions have minimal lipid deposition (e.g., foam cells, extracellular lipid). Also, unlike conventional atherosclerosis, branch vessels as well as intramyocardial coronary arteries are involved (Fig. 9–10). The thickness of the intima generally correlates with duration of the transplant.

As graft arteriosclerosis progresses over time, particularly in allografts that are older than 5 years, lesions may be more typical of conventional atherosclerosis. They exhibit disruption of internal elastic membrane, intra- and extracellular lipid, necrosis and calcium deposition, and plaque hemorrhage with associated mural or occlusive thrombosis may occur (Fig. 9–10).[53] Active or healed vasculitis can be found in some cases, with a mixed inflammatory cell infiltrate and medial fibrosis.[54]

Although detection of graft vasculopathy in endomyocardial biopsy specimens is uncommon, it is not unusual to see ischemic myocardial changes in these specimens indicative of coronary artery disease. Myocytolysis, characterized by clearing of the sarcoplasm usually of subendocardial myocytes and reflective of reversible ischemic injury, is a marker for coronary artery narrowing and can be recognized in endomyocardial biopsy samples, as can coagulation necrosis secondary to arterial occlusion.[55] Active or healed vasculitis involving intramyocardial coronary arteries may be seen in endomyocardial biopsies or in explanted or autopsy hearts from some cardiac allografts (Fig. 9–10). Vasculitis may be a precursor to occlusive graft vasculopathy and seems to be more common in children. Cellular rejection may occasionally involve vessels as well.

The pathogenesis of accelerated coronary artery disease in transplanted hearts is unknown. The etiology is most likely immunologic, however, with nonimmunologic factors influencing evolution and progression. Immunologic-mediated endothelial injury is the presumed mechanism. However, a correlation has not been observed with the number of acute rejection episodes,[56] or with age of the donor heart, or a prior history of coronary artery disease, although one series did note a correlation between preoperative coronary artery disease and hyperlipidemia following transplantation.[57] Nonetheless, immunologically induced endothelial injury may lead to platelet aggregation, with subsequent release of growth factors and intimal proliferation.[47]

Endothelial cells may be the primary target of both humoral and cell-mediated immunity that initiate graft arteriosclerosis.[58] While major histocompatibility complex (MHC) class I antigens play a role in acute cellular rejection, disparate MHC class II donor–recipient combinations may provide the antigenic stimulus to activate the host immune system and thereby contribute to the genesis of graft arteriosclerosis. MHC class II antigens are not uniformly present during normal conditions, but they are expressed on allograft endothelial cells in experimental conditions leading to arterial narrowing.[59] Transplant arteriosclerosis may represent a sustained allogeneic reaction, which resembles a chronic-delayed hypersensitivity response.[60] While stimulation of the immune system is most likely involved in the initiation of transplant arteriosclerosis, progression of the disease may be modified by traditional risk factors, such as hypertension, hyperlipidemia, and obesity.[61–63] Steroid use[47, 64] and the hyperlipidemia that occurs in transplant recipients[57, 65] have been implicated in the pathogenesis of graft arteriosclerosis, and an association between graft atherosclerosis and CMV infection has been described.[66]

Nonspecific Pathology

In addition to accelerated atherosclerosis, the transplanted heart may exhibit other long-

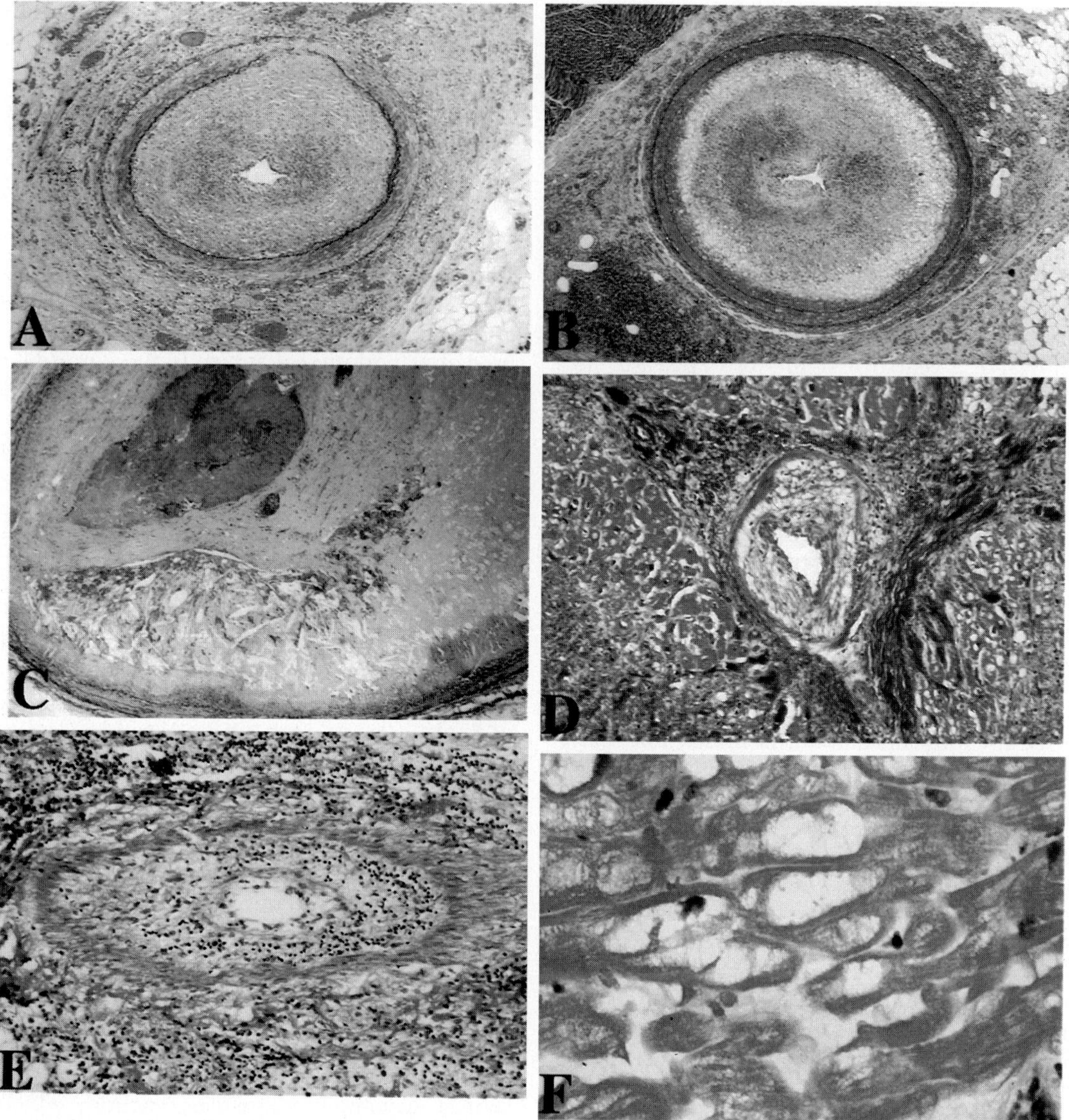

Figure 9–10. Graft arteriosclerosis. *A.* Epicardial coronary artery from an autopsy heart has 95% reduction in cross-sectional area by concentric fibrointimal proliferation, with an intact internal elastic lamina. *B.* A concentric occlusive intimal lesion characteristic for graft arteriosclerosis shows early lipid deposition (foam cells) adjacent to the internal elastic lamina. *C.* Epicardial coronary artery in a patient who died 10 years after cardiac transplantation. The intimal lesion in this older graft has features that are more characteristic of conventional atherosclerosis, with a lipid-rich necrotic core (atheroma) and an overlying fibrous cap. *D.* Intramyocardial coronary artery, with narrowing by fibrointimal proliferation similar to that found in the major epicardial coronary arteries. *E.* Intramyocardial coronary artery from a patient who died suddenly 4 years following cardiac transplantation. The intima is expanded by loose connective tissue with an associated lymphocytic vasculitis, and endothelial cells are large and swollen. Such lesions may be precursors to graft arteriosclerosis. *F.* This routine surveillance endomyocardial biopsy from a cardiac transplant recipient has focal myocytolysis, indicative of reversible ischemia that may be indicative of coronary artery narrowing. (*A, B,* and *C,* Movat pentachrome; *D,* Masson trichrome; *E* and *F,* H & E)

term changes. Myocyte hypertrophy occurs in hearts 3 years after transplantation and appears to have a relationship to the period of ischemia at the time of transplantation, with distantly procured hearts having greater myocyte hypertrophy.[67] Interstitial fibrous tissue may also be increased,[21, 60] the basis of which may be related to either ischemia or cyclosporine therapy.[68, 69] Long-term cyclosporine therapy is also nephrotoxic. Cyclosporine nephrotoxicity includes atrophic tubular damage, interstitial fibrosis, and focal and segmental glomerulosclerosis.[70]

Infections in Cardiac Transplantation

Infections comprise the major cause of death in cardiac transplant patients, particularly in the acute postoperative period (i.e., within 3 months) when immunosuppression and episodes of acute rejection are the greatest.[20, 71, 72] Although bacterial infections are most common,[73] the suppressed immune system allows for infections by viruses, fungi, and protozoa, and it is these latter pathogens that are a challenge.[56, 74, 75] In one series,[72] major infection was documented in 55% of patients within the first year following transplantation, accounting for 59% of the deaths that occurred. The lung comprised the major site, followed by the genitourinary and central nervous systems.[56, 76] Bacteria account for 59% of all infections, while viral, fungal, and protozoal infections have been observed in 64% of fatal infectious cases.[72] Infections may involve the cardiac allograft and can be diagnosed by endomyocardial biopsy. Cardiac infections should be suspected when the inflammatory infiltrate in the cardiac biopsy sample is mixed and not characteristic of acute rejection. *Toxoplasma gondii* and cytomegalovirus (CMV) account for most infections in the early postoperative period.[20]

Cytomegalovirus

CMV infection may occur by transmission from CMV sero-positive donors to sero-negative recipients.[56] In a series of 162 heart and heart–lung transplant recipients, 45% had CMV infection after transplantation, 18.5% of which were considered primary infections and 26.5% of which were reactivation or reinfection.[77] While toxoplasmosis has been diagnosed by endomyocardial biopsy,[72, 78] it is rare that CMV inclusions are found within the myocardium, and myocardial involvement only occurs in primary forms and not reactivation.[79] The diagnosis of CMV infection rests upon serology, such as ELISA for CMV-specific IgM,[77] or the typical histologic findings in other tissues (lung, gastrointestinal tract) (Fig. 9–11). Interpretation of CMV serology in immunocompromised patients may warrant caution, however, due to the high frequency of false-positives and negatives. CMV infections occur most frequently and severely in patients whose transplanted organs are affected by rejection.[80]

Toxoplasmosis

Toxoplasmosis may also be acquired from the donor organ or occur as reactivation of a latent infection. *Toxoplasma gondii* is ubiquitous and as many as 30% of adults may have serologic evidence of a previous infection.[81] Although these individuals are usually asymptomatic, *T. gondii* infections in immunocompromised patients can result in necrotizing encephalitis, myocarditis, or pneumonia.[82] In sero-negative heart and heart–lung transplant recipients who receive organs from sero-positive donors, 57% to 75% have developed primary *T. gondii* infections.[83, 84] In a series from Papworth Hospital in Cambridge describing 217 heart and 33 heart–lung transplant patients who were prospectively studied for evidence of *T. gondii* infection, six patients acquired a primary infection (presumably from the donor organ) and five patients experienced a recrudescence of *T. gondii.*[85] Toxoplasmosis may be life threatening only when acquired from the donor organ, however,[85] and prophylaxis may have a role in mitigating the effects of *T. gondii* infection in this patient population.[84] While the presence of toxoplasmosis can usually be recognized in the myocardium histologically, polymerase chain reaction on endomyocardial biopsies—while not widely used—may enhance diagnostic sensitivity.[86]

Other organisms that have been described in the setting of cardiac transplantation include herpesvirus, *Aspergillus, Nocardia, Petriellidium boudii, Cryptococcus, Pneumocystis carinii,* and mycobacteria.[21, 40] *Staphlococcus aureus* is also beginning to become a problem in some hospitals and may emerge as a significant pathogen in transplant patients in the next few years. The possibility of infection should be borne in mind when interpreting endomyocardial biopsies. It may be difficult to distinguish acute rejection from the necrosis and inflammation associated with viral or parasitic infections; it has been suggested that in *Toxoplasma* myocarditis, small myocyte-sized fibrotic areas may be present, presumably related to previous myocyte necrosis by the parasite.[87]

Neoplasms in Heart Transplant Recipients

Organ transplant recipients carry an increased risk for malignancies.[88] Although tu-

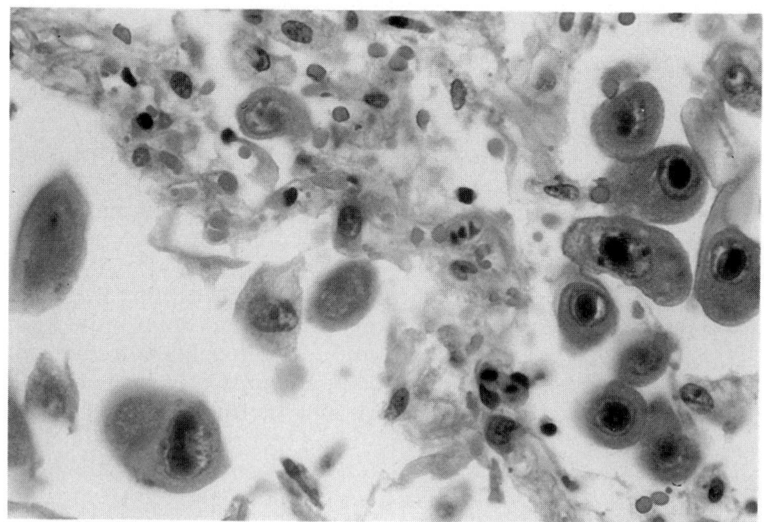

Figure 9–11. Cytomegalovirus. A 54-year-old man who had undergone orthotopic cardiac transplantation 4 years earlier died from pneumonia due to cytomegalovirus infection. Typical CMV inclusions are prominent in this section of lung. (H & E)

mors with low malignant potential, such as squamous cell and basal cell carcinomas, are the most common,[89] of particular concern is the propensity for these patients to develop hematopoietic-lymphoid malignancies.[90–92] Metastasizing carcinomas may also occur with an increased frequency.[43] The incidence of malignant lymphomas in transplant patients may vary with the type of allograft and immunosuppressive regimen. As many as 13% of cardiac transplant recipients who have received cyclosporine have developed malignant lymphomas.[90] Malignant lymphomas in cardiac transplant patients: (1) are usually B cell in origin (and often associated with Epstein–Barr virus, see following); (2) tend to be high-grade, large-cell lymphomas; and (3) show an increased incidence at extranodal sites, such as brain or soft tissues (muscle, fat).

Patients who develop post-transplant lymphomas may initially present with solitary involvement of the central nervous system, an unusual clinical finding, and these may respond to radiation therapy.[93] Young patients who have received transplants for dilated cardiomyopathy appear to be particularly susceptible to lymphoproliferative disorders.[20] The degree of immunosuppression correlates with the development of lymphoma,[90] and clinical recovery has been associated with reduction of immunosuppressive therapy.

Post-transplant Lymphoproliferative Disorders

Post-transplant lymphoproliferative disorders (PTLD) are an aggressive subset of neoplasms that arise as an abnormal polyclonal lymphoid proliferation associated with Epstein–Barr virus infection. They are composed of B lymphocytes in all stages of differentiation, including plasma cells; progression may occur from a polyclonal population of cells to a monoclonal proliferation in association with clonal immunoglobulin gene rearrangements (Fig. 9–12). PTLD involve predominantly lymph nodes and extranodal sites, including central nervous system, gastrointestinal tract, lungs, and soft tissues. Involvement of the cardiac allograft is uncommon (in contrast to allografted lungs).

The etiology and nature of lymphoproliferative lesions in transplant recipients has been controversial. Some have speculated that these are polyclonal B-cell proliferations that may represent virally-induced hyperplasia,[94] and evidence of Epstein–Barr virus has been found in many cells.[95] Extraction of DNA from these tissues has revealed large numbers of cells with uniform, clonal rearrangements of immunoglobulin-gene DNA, suggesting that these lymphoproliferative disorders are indeed neoplastic,[93] and their aggressive clinical course would lend support to that theory. Although there are no known etiologies to explain the development of lymphomas in this setting, various mechanisms may include decreased immune surveillance of neoplastic clones, viral oncogenesis due to immunosuppression, or chronic antigenic stimulation of the host.[90] Perhaps the most likely mechanism for pathogenesis begins with a resting population of B cells that, following Epstein–Barr virus infection, undergoes genetic alteration (e.g., translocation).

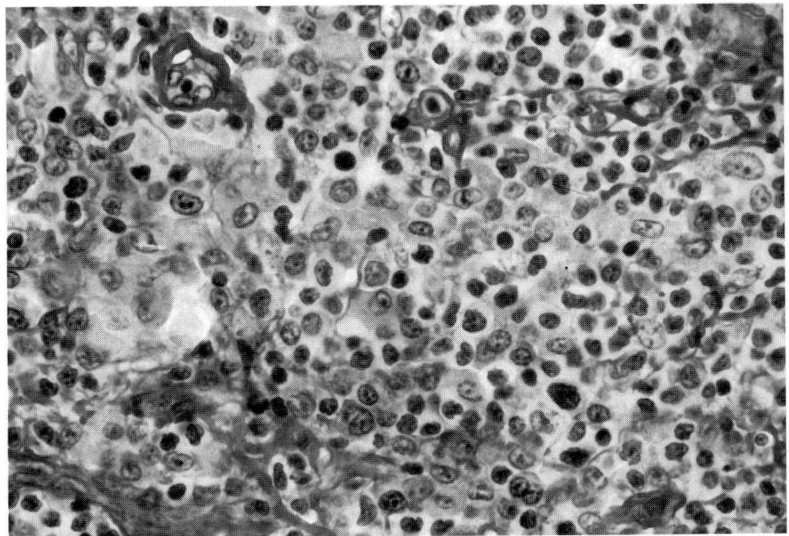

Figure 9–12. Post-transplant lymphoproiliferative disorder. Lymphadenopathy developed in a 21-year-old female 2 years following cardiac transplantation. Lymph-node biopsy showed a polyclonal population of small and transformed B cells, indicative of post-transplant lymphoproliferative disorder. The lymphadenopathy regressed upon decrease in immunosuppression. (H & E)

Due to the normal function of T cells, this population remains latent until immune surveillance is lost by immunosuppressive therapy, resulting in a neoplastic clonal proliferation.[96]

CONCLUSIONS

Heart transplant recipients present clinical problems that are not unusual in the organ transplant population. In addition, they exhibit unique pathology that directly affects therapy. In no other area of practice does the pathologist play a more direct and immediate role in clinical management than in the morphologic and immunologic evaluation of these patients. Heart transplant recipients navigate a fine line between infection and rejection; a misleading diagnosis of rejection can result in over-immunosuppression and fatal infection, while failure to recognize acute rejection in the heart can result in death within hours if appropriate therapy is not promptly instituted.[97] The pathology of heart transplantation is still evolving as more patients survive for longer periods and newer immunosuppressive regimens are instituted. Morphology will continue to complement functional and immunologic parameters used to monitor transplant patients, as well as improve our understanding of the natural history of grafts, and these should lead to improvements in diagnostic capabilities and clinical management.

REFERENCES

1. Downie HG. Homotransplantation of the dog heart. Arch Surg 66:624, 1953.
2. Lower RR, Stofer RC, Shumway NE. Homovital transplantation of the heart. J Thorac Cardiovasc Surg 41:196, 1961.
3. Blumenstock DA, Hechtman HB, Collins JA, et al. Prolonged survival of orthotopic homotransplants of the heart in animals treated with methotrexate. J Thorac Cardiovasc Surg 46:616, 1963.
4. Lower RR, Dong E, Shumway NE. Suppression of rejection process in the cardiac homograft. Ann Thorac Surg 1:645, 1965.
5. Lower RR, Dong E, Shumway NE. Long-term survival of cardiac homografts. Surgery 58:110, 1965.
6. Lower RR, Kontos HA, Kosek JC, et al. Experiences in heart transplantation. Am J Cardiol 22:766, 1968.
7. Hardy JD, Chavez CM, Kurrus FD, et al. Heart transplantation in man: Development studies and a report of a case. JAMA 188:1132, 1964.
8. Barnard CN. A human cardiac transplant. S Afr Med J 49:213, 1967.
9. Thomson JG. Heart transplantation in man—necropsy findings. Br Med J 2:511, 1968.
10. Thomson JG. Production of severe atheroma in a transplanted human heart. Lancet 2:1088, 1969.
11. Bieber CP, Stinson EB, Shumway NE, et al. Cardiac transplantation in man. VII. Cardiac allograft pathology. Circulation 41:753, 1970.
12. Levinsky L, Kessler E, Lurie M, et al. Ultrastructural and histopathologic observation of human cardiac transplant with features of rejection. Am J Clin Pathol 53:811, 1970.
13. Milam JD, Shipkey FH, Lind CJ, et al. Morphologic findings in human cardiac allografts. Circulation 41:519, 1970.
14. Ellis B, Madge G, Kolhatkar M, Still W. Clinical and pathological findings in human cardiac rejection. Arch Pathol 92:58, 1971.

15. Kosek JC, Bieber C, Lower RR. Heart graft arteriosclerosis. Transplant Proc 3:512, 1971.
16. Caves PK, Stinson EB, Billingham ME, Shumway NE. Serial transvenous biopsy of the transplanted human heart. Improved management of acute rejection episodes. Lancet 1:821, 1974.
17. Uys CJ, Rose AG, Barnard CN. The autopsy findings in a case of heterotopic cardiac transplantation with left ventricular bypass for ischemic heart failure. S Afr Med J 49:2029, 1975.
18. Hosenpud JD, Bennett LE, Keck BM, Fiol B, Boucek MM, Novick RJ. The Registry of the International Society for Heart and Lung Transplantation: Sixteenth Official Report—1999. J Heart Lung Transplant 18:611, 1999.
19. Spear GS. Eosinophilic explant carditis with eosinophilia: Hypersensitivity to dobutamine infusion. J Heart Lung Transplant 14:755, 1995.
20. Billingham ME. Cardiac transplantation. In: Waller BF (ed): Contemporary Issues in Cardiovascular Pathology p 185. Philadelphia: FA Davis, 1988.
21. Billingham ME. The postsurgical heart. The pathology of cardiac transplantation. Am J Cardiovasc Pathol 1:319, 1988.
22. Fyfe B, Loh E, Winters GL, Couper GS, Kartashov AI, Schoen FJ. Heart transplantation-associated perioperative ischemic myocardial injury. Morphological features and clinical significance. Circulation 93:1133, 1996.
23. Hauptman PJ, Aranki S, Mudge GH, Couper GS, Loh E. Early cardiac allograft failure after orthotopic heart transplantation. Amer Heart J 127:179, 1994.
24. Pflugfelder PW, Singh NR, McKenzie FM, Menkes AH, Novick RJ, Kostuk WJ. Extending cardiac allograft ischemic time and donor age: Effect of survival on long-term cardiac function. J Heart Lung Transplant 10:394, 1991.
25. Billingham ME, Cary NRB, Hammond ME, et al. A working formulation for the standardization of nomenclature in the diagnosis of heart and lung rejection: Heart rejection study group. J Heart Transplant 9:587, 1990.
26. Sibley RK, Olivari MT, Bolman RM, et al. Endomyocardial biopsy in the cardiac allograft recipient. Ann Surg 203:177, 1986.
27. Winters GL. The pathology of heart allograft rejection. Arch Pathol Lab Med 115:266, 1991.
28. Nakhleh RE, Kubo SH, Olivari MT, McDonald K. Persistent histologic evidence of rejection in a heart transplant recipient without evidence of graft dysfunction. J Heart Lung Transplant 11:37, 1992.
29. Durham JR, Nakhleh RE, Levine A, Levine TB. Persistence of interstitial inflammation after episodes of cardiac rejection associated with systemic infection. J Heart Lung Transplant 14:774, 1995.
30. Zerbe TR, Arena V. Diagnostic reliability of endomyocardial biopsy for assessment of cardiac allograft rejection. Hum Pathol 19:1307, 1988.
31. Kottke-Marchant K, Ratliff NB. Endomyocardial lymphocytic infiltrates in cardiac transplant recipients. Arch Pathol Lab Med 113:690, 1989.
32. Costanzo-Nordin MR, Winters GL, Fisher SG, et al. Endocardial infiltrates in the transplanted heart: Clinical significance emerging from the analysis of 5026 endomyocardial biopsy specimens. J Heart Lung Transplant 12:741, 1993.
33. Freimark D, Czer LSC, Aleksic I, et al. Pathogenesis of Quilty lesion in cardiac allografts: Relationship to reduced endocardial cyclosporine A. J Heart Lung Transplant 14:1197, 1995.
34. Luthringer DJ, Yamashita JT, Czer LSC, Trento A, Fishbein MC. Nature and significance of epicardial lymphoid infiltrates in cardiac allografts. J Heart Lung Transplant 14:537, 1995.
35. Milano A, Caforio ALP, Livi U, Bauce B, Angelini A, Casarotto D, Thiene G. Evolution of focal moderate (International Society for Heart and Lung Transplantation Grade 2) rejection of the cardiac allograft. J Heart Lung Transplant 15:456, 1996.
36. Fishbein MC, Bell G, Lones MA, et al. Grade 2 cellular heart rejection: Does it exist? J Heart Lung Transplant 13:1051, 1994.
37. Winters GL, Loh E, Schoen FJ. Natural history of focal moderate cardiac allograft rejection. Is treatment warranted? Circulation 91:1975, 1995.
38. Kemnitz J, Cremer J, Schaefers H-J, et al. Some aspects of changed histopathologic appearance of acute rejection in cardiac allografts after prophylactic application of OKT3. J Heart Lung Transplant 10:366, 1991.
39. Hammond EH, Yowell RC, Nunoda S, et al. Vascular (humoral) rejection in heart transplantation: Pathologic observations and clinical implications. J Heart Lung Transplant 8:430, 1989.
40. Hammond EH, Hanson JK, Spencer LS, et al. Immunofluorescence of endomyocardial biopsy specimens: Methods and interpretation. J Heart Lung Transplant 12:S113, 1993.
41. Hammond EH, Hansen JK, Spencer LS, et al. Vascular rejection in cardiac transplantation: Histologic, immunopathologic, and ultrastructural features. Cardiovasc Pathol 2:21, 1993.
42. Bonnard EN, Lewis NP, Masek MA, Billingham ME. Reliability and usefulness of immunofluorescence in heart transplantation. J Heart Lung Transplant 14: 163, 1995.
43. Gallo P, Agozzino L, Angelini A, et al. Causes of late failure after heart transplantation: A ten-year survey. J Heart Lung Transplant 16:1113, 1997.
44. Patel VS, Lim M, Massin EK, et al. Sudden cardiac death in cardiac transplant recipients. Circulation 94 (suppl II):II273, 1996.
45. Atkinson JB. Accelerated arteriosclerosis after transplantation: The possible role of calcium channel blockers. Int J Cardiol 62 (suppl 2):S125, 1997.
46. Gao SZ, Alderman EL, Schroeder JS, et al. Accelerated coronary vascular disease in the heart transplant patient: Coronary arteriographic findings. J Am Coll Cardiol 12:334, 1988.
47. Schroeder JS, Gao SZ, Hunt SA, Stinson EB. Accelerated graft coronary artery disease: Diagnosis and prevention. J Heart Lung Transplant 11:S258, 1992.
48. Keogh AM, Valentine HA, Hunt SA, et al. Impact of proximal or midvessel discrete coronary artery stenoses on survival after heart transplantation. J Heart Lung Transplant 11:892, 1992.
49. Mihatsch MJ, Thiel G, Basler V, et al. Morphological patterns in cyclosporine-treated renal transplant recipients. Transplant Proc 17 (suppl 1):101, 1985.
50. Demetris AJ, Zerbe T, Banner B. Morphology of solid organ allograft arteriopathy: Identification of proliferating intimal cell populations. Transplant Proc 21:3667, 1989.
51. Yousem SA, Paradis IL, Dauber JH, et al. Pulmonary arteriosclerosis in long-term human heart-lung transplant recipients. Transplantation 47:564, 1989.

52. Billingham ME. Graft coronary disease: Old and new dimensions. Cardiovasc Pathol 6:95, 1997.
53. Arbustini E, Roberts WC. Morphologic observations in the epicardial coronary arteries and their surroundings late after cardiac transplantation (allograft vascular disease). Amer J Cardiol 78:814, 1996.
54. Atkinson JB. Endomyocardial biopsy of cardiac allografts and transplant atherosclerosis. In: Virmani R, Burke A, Farb A (eds): Atlas of Cardiovascular Pathology, p 24. Philadelphia: WB Saunders, 1996.
55. Winters GL, Schoen FJ. Graft arteriosclerosis-induced myocardial pathology in heart transplant recipients: Predictive value of endomyocardial biopsy. J Heart Lung Transplant 16:985, 1997.
56. Billingham ME, Masek MA, Khanna K, et al. Long-term cardiac allograft pathology in humans. Lab Invest 42:103, 1979.
57. Taylor DO, Thompson JA, Hastillo A, et al. Hyperlipidemia after clinical heart transplantation. J Heart Transplant 8:209, 1989.
58. Chomette G, Auriol M, Cabrol C. Chronic rejection in human heart transplantation. J Heart Lung Transplant 7:292, 1988.
59. Ardehali A, Drinkwater DC, Laks H, et al. Cardiac allograft vasculopathy. Am Heart J 126:1498, 1993.
60. Libby P, Salomon RN, Payne DD, et al. Functions of vascular wall cells related to development of transplantation-associated coronary arteriosclerosis. Transplant Proc 21:3677, 1989.
61. Kobashigawa JA, Katznelson S, Laks H, et al. Effect of pravastatin on outcomes after cardiac transplantation. N Eng J Med 333:621, 1995.
62. Fellstrom B. Transplantation atherosclerosis. J Int Med 240:253, 1996.
63. Ventura HO, Mehra MR, Smart FW, Stapleton DD. Cardiac allograft vasculopathy: Current concepts. Am Heart J 129:791, 1995.
64. Renlund DG, Bristow MR, Crandall BG, et al. Hypercholesterolemia after heart transplantation: Amelioration by corticosteroid-free maintenance immunosuppression. J Heart Transplant 8:214, 1989.
65. Stamler JS, Vaughan DE, Rudd, A, et al. Frequency of hypercholesterolemia after cardiac transplantation. Amer J Cardiol 62:1268, 1988.
66. McDonald K, Rector T, Braunlin E, Olivari MT. Cytomegalovirus infection in cardiac transplant recipients predicts the incidence of allograft atherosclerosis. J Am Coll Cardiol 13:213A, 1989.
67. Imakita M, Tazelaar, HD, Rowan RA, et al. Myocyte hypertrophy in the transplanted heart: A morphometric analysis. Transplantation 43:839, 1987.
68. Stovin PGI, English TAH. Effects of cyclosporine on the transplanted human heart. J Heart Transplant 6:180, 1987.
69. Pickering JG, Boughner DR. Fibrosis in the transplanted heart and its relation to donor ischemic time. Circulation 81:949, 1990.
70. Myers BD, Ross J, Newton L, et al. Cyclosporine-associated chronic nephropathy. N Eng J Med 311: 699, 1984.
71. Mason JW, Stinson EB, Hunt SA, et al. Infections after cardiac transplantation: Relation to rejection therapy. Ann Intern Med 85:69, 1976.
72. Cooper DKC, Lanza RP, Oliver S, et al. Infectious complications after heart transplantation. Thorax 38:822, 1983.
73. Jamieson SW, Oyer PE, Reitz BA, et al. Cardiac transplantation at Stanford. Heart Transplant 1:86, 1981.
74. Hunt SA. Current status of cardiac transplantation. J Am Med Assoc 280:1692, 1998.
75. Fishman JA, Rubin RH. Infection in organ-transplant recipients. N Eng J Med 338:1741, 1998.
76. Graham AR. Autopsy findings in cardiac transplant patients. A 10-year experience. Am J Clin Pathol 97:369, 1992.
77. Wreghitt TG, Hakim M, Gray JJ, et al. Cytomegalovirus infections in heart and heart and lung transplant recipients. J Clin Pathol 41:660, 1988.
78. Pomerance A, Stovin PGI. Heart transplant pathology: The British experience. J Clin Pathol 38:146, 1985.
79. Arbustini E, Grasso M, Diegoli M, et al. Histopathologic and molecular profile of human cytomegalovirus infections in patients with heart transplants. J Clin Path 98:205, 1992.
80. Dummer JS, Monter GC, Griffith BP, et al. Infections in heart–lung transplant recipients. Transplantation 41:725, 1986.
81. Fleck DG. Toxoplasmosis. Public Health 83:131, 1969.
82. Ruskin J, Remington JS. Toxoplasmosis in the compromised host. Ann Intern Med 84:193, 1976.
83. Luft BJ, Naot Y, Araujo FG, et al. Primary and reactivated Toxoplasma infection in patients with cardiac transplants. Ann Intern Med 99:27, 1983.
84. Hakim M, Esmore D, Wallwork J, et al. Toxoplasmosis in cardiac transplantation. Br Med J 292:1108, 1986.
85. Wreghitt TG, Hakim M, Gray JJ, et al. Toxoplasmosis in heart and heart and lung trasnplant recipients. J Clin Pathol 42:194, 1989.
86. Holliman R, Johnson J, Savva D, et al. Diagnosis of toxoplasma infection in cardiac transplant recipients using the polymerase chain reaction. J Clin Path 45:931, 1992.
87. McGregor CGA, Fleck DG, Nagington J, et al. Disseminated toxoplasmosis in cardiac transplantation. J Clin Pathol 37:74, 1984.
88. Penn I. Malignant lymphomas in organ transplant recipients. Transplant Proc 13:736, 1981.
89. Penn I. Tumor incidence in human allograft recipients. Transplant Proc 11:1047, 1979.
90. Weintraub J, Warnke RA. Lymphoma in cardiac allotransplant recipients. Transplantation 33:347, 1982.
91. Cleary ML, Sklar J. Lymphoproliferative disorders in cardiac transplant recipients are multiclonal lymphomas. Lancet 2:489, 1984.
92. Cleary ML, Warnke R, Sklar J. Monoclonality of lymphoproliferative lesions in cardiac-transplant recipients. N Eng J Med 310:477, 1984.
93. Starzl TE, Nalesnik MA, Porter KA, et al. Reversibility of lymphomas and lymphoproliferative lesions developing under cyclosporin steroid therapy. Lancet 1:583, 1984.
94. Frizzera G, Hanto DW, Gajl-Peczalska KJ, et al. Polymorphic diffuse B-cell hyperplasias and lymphomas in renal transplant recipients. Cancer Res 41:4262, 1981.
95. Hanto DW, Frizzera G, Purtilo DT, et al. Clinical spectrum of lymphoproliferative disorders in renal transplant recipients and evidence for the role of Epstein–Barr virus. Cancer Res 41:4253, 1981.
96. Klein G. Lymphoma development in mice and humans: Diversity of initiation is followed by convergent cytogenetic evolution. Proc Natl Acad Sci USA 76:2442, 1979.
97. Atkinson JB. The pathobiology of heart–lung transplantation. Hum Pathol 19:1367, 1988.

Chapter

10

SUDDEN CARDIAC DEATH

OVERVIEW AND CAUSES OF SUDDEN CARDIAC DEATH

Overview

Incidence

Sudden cardiac death occurs in 300,000 to 400,000 individuals annually in the United States. The incidence of sudden death in the entire population is 100–200/100,000 per year.[1-4] In young adults 40 years of age and younger, the incidence is far lower; in Olmsted County, Minnesota, the incidence of sudden death in young adults has been estimated between 5 and 10/100,000 population per year.[5] This incidence in young adults is similar to that reported in Maryland,[6] which has a state-wide medical examiner system (Table 10–1).

Definition

The range in the reported incidence of sudden death is probably due to various definitions of sudden death. Most of the deaths reported as sudden have occurred outside the hospital or in emergency rooms, reflecting their unexpected nature. Clinicians define sudden cardiac death as natural, nonviolent, unexpected, and occurring within one hour of the onset of acute symptoms. A large number of deaths are not witnessed, and the World Health Organization permits symptoms to be present up to 24 hours for its criteria for sudden cardiac death.[7] However, this definition includes many cases of well-established acute myocardial infarction, which many would not consider as sudden cardiac deaths. Kuller et al.[2,3] have shown the influence of the definition of sudden death on the incidence of cardiac causes: When the definition of death was less than 2 hours after onset of symptoms, 12% of deaths were sudden and 88% were due to cardiac causes; when applying a symptom duration of less than 24 hours, 32% of deaths were sudden but cardiac causes of death fell to 75%. In most of our studies, we have defined sudden cardiac death as natural, nonviolent, unexpected, and witnessed within 6 hours of the onset of symptoms from a stable medical condition. For unwitnessed deaths, the definition of sudden death requires that the deceased had been seen in stable condition less than 24 hours before being found dead, and any potentially lethal noncardiac cause must be ruled out.

Epidemiology

The ages at which sudden death is most prevalent are birth to 6 months (sudden infant death syndrome) and between 45 and 75 years. Only 19% of sudden natural deaths in children between 1 and 13 years are cardiac in origin, whereas in the 14–21-year age range, 30% are cardiac.[8] In the adult population, the commonest cause of sudden death is coronary heart disease. The risk of sudden death is greatest in a population with a history of a cardiac arrest or myocardial infarction, and is maximum 6–18 months after the event. The proportion of deaths from heart disease that are sudden declines with advancing age. In the Framingham study, 62% of all coronary heart disease deaths were sudden in men aged 45–54 years, whereas

The opinions or assertions contained herein are the private views of the authors and are not to be construed as official or reflecting the views of the Department of the Army, the Department of the Air Force, or the Department of Defense.

Table 10–1. Population-based Incidence of Sudden Cardiac Death, State of Maryland Population aged 14–40 years, rate/100,000/year

	CAD	HTCM	CM	ALL SUCD
Blacks	4.3	0.8	1.7	9.5
Whites	2.3	0.1	0.5	4.2
Black men	5.6	1.0	3.2	14.5
White men	4.0	0.1	0.9	6.8
Black women	1.2	0.6	0.4	5.1
White women	0.6	0.0	0.1	1.6
Population	2.5	0.3	0.8	5.5

CAD = coronary artery disease; HTCM = hypetensive cardiomyopathy; CM = idiopathic cardiomyopathy (including dilated cardiomyopathy and idiopathic left ventricular hypertrophy); SUCD = sudden unexpected cardiac death

Adapted from Burke AP, Virmani R, Smialek J. Young blacks are at higher risk of sudden cardiac death from all causes than whites. Circulation 86:1–199, 1992.

in the 55–64-year and 65–74-year age groups, the percentage of sudden death fell to 58% and 42%, respectively.[9]

Males are much more prone to sudden death compared with females (Table 10–1), largely because women are protected from coronary heart disease during the premenopausal years. The Framinghan study demonstrated a 3.8-fold higher incidence of sudden cardiac death in men than women.[9] The excess relative risk in men peaked at 55 to 64 years reflected in a male to female ratio of 6.75:1; this ratio fell to 2.17 : 1 in the 65–74-year age group. In women, the risk factors for coronary heart disease are similar to those in men. However, cigarette smoking, diabetes, and use of oral contraceptives are especially strong risk factors in women. Racial differences in the incidence of sudden cardiac death have also been noted, blacks having an increased risk as compared with whites (Table 10–1).

Hereditary factors that contribute to sudden cardiac death are mostly risk factors of coronary heart disease. Genetic factors have been reported in the less common causes of sudden cardiac death, including the congenital prolonged Q-T syndrome, right ventricular dysplasia, and hypertrophic cardiomyopathy.[10]

Causes of Sudden Cardiac Death

Definitions

The *cause* of death is defined as the disease or injury initiating the train of events producing death. Cardiac causes of death are generally related to coronary, valvular, or myocardial diseases. Aortic rupture may result in cardiac tamponade and sudden death, and is occasionally considered part of the spectrum of cardiac death, although the underlying cause is vascular, not cardiac.

The *manner* of death refers to the circumstances of death, and is classified as natural or violent (unnatural or traumatic). Unnatural deaths may be accidental, homicidal, or suicidal. Unnatural deaths are generally not considered in discussions of sudden cardiac death, and violent deaths that result from cardiac trauma are generally easy to distinguish from natural cardiac deaths. However, the distinction between natural and unnatural cardiac death is occasionally difficult. Cardiac rupture may occur secondary to blunt chest trauma that does not necessarily leave marks on the chest. An arrhythmia resulting in a fatal automobile accident may cause multiple internal injuries in the driver; the absence of internal bleeding is the clue that the death was indeed natural and not accidental. The distinction between natural and accidental iatrogenic deaths may be difficult and somewhat arbitrary. Generally, the death is considered natural if the procedure carries a significant risk of a fatal complication, and the condition is life-threatening.

The *mechanism* of death is the terminal physiologic derangement or biochemical disturbance produced by the cause of death. In most cases of cardiac death, the physiologic derangement is a cardiac arrhythmia, although other mechanisms include acute heart failure and obstruction of blood flow (see Table 10–2). A further discussion of the mechanisms of cardiac arrhythmias and their anatomic substrates is found at the end of the chapter.

Spectrum of Disease

Virtually any pathologic process that involves the heart may result in sudden death, by virtue of the wide spectrums of mechanisms that may result in terminal arrhythmias. Acute ischemia, infiltrative diseases (primarily scars or inflammation), cardiac hypertrophy, and cardiac failure are the most common anatomic substrates of ventricular arrhythmias and may have a variety of interrelated causes[8] (Table 10–2).

By far the most common cause of sudden death in adults in Western countries is coronary artery disease. Coronary atherosclerosis may result in sudden death by acute ischemia, arrhythmias secondary to healed infarcts, cardiac rup-

Table 10–2. Causes and Mechanisms of Sudden Cardiac Death

Immediate Cause	Underlying Causes	Mechanisms
Acute ischemia	Coronary atherosclerosis Nonatherosclerotic coronary diseases Aortic stenosis	Ventricular fibrillation Bradycardia Electromechanical dissociation (usually end-stage or post-resuscitation)
Infiltrative diseases	Inflammatory (myocarditis) Scars (healed infarcts, cardiomyopathy)	Ventricular fibrillation Bradyarrhythmias (uncommon[1])
Cardiac hypertrophy	Hypertrophic cardiomyopathy Systemic hypertension Idiopathic concentric left ventricular hypertrophy Aortic stenosis	Ventricular fibrillation Bradyarrhythmias (uncommon)
Cardiac dilatation (congestive failure)	Dilated cardiomyopathy Chronic ischemia Systemic hypertension Aortic insufficiency Mitral insufficiency	Ventricular fibrillation Bradyarrhythmias (uncommon)
Cardiac tamponade	Rupture myocardial infarct Aortic rupture	Electromechanical dissociation
Mechanical disruption of cardiac blood flow	Pulmonary embolism Mitral stenosis Left atrial myxoma	Electromechanical dissociation Ventricular fibrillation
Global myocardial hypoxia	Severe ischemic heart disease Aortic stenosis	Baroreflex stimulation with bradyarrhythmias Ventricular tachyarrhythmias
Acute heart failure	Massive myocardial infarct Rupture papillary muscle Acute endocarditis with chordal or leaflet rupture MVP with chordal rupture	Electromechanical dissociation Ventricular fibrillation
Generalized hypoxia	Pulmonary stenosis Pulmonary hypertension	Bradyarrhythmias
Vasovagal stimulation	Neuromuscular diseases	Baroreflex stimulation with bradycardia
Preexcitation syndrome	Accessory pathways	Atrial fibrillation → ventricular fibrillation
Long Q-T syndrome	Congenital and acquired states	Ventricular fibrillation (torsades de pointes)
Heart block	AV nodal scarring, inflammation, tumor	Bradycardia → ventricular fibrillation

AV = atrioventricular; MVP = mitral valve prolapse
[1] Especially in the presence of infiltrative processes involving the conduction system.

ture, and acute heart failure. The second most common cause of sudden death is intrinsic myocardial diseases, which may be classified as hypertrophic cardiomyopathy, dilated cardiomyopathy, hypertensive cardiomyopathy, and idiopathic left ventricular hypertrophy. The third largest group of deaths are secondary to valvular disease, especially mitral valve prolapse and aortic stenosis. Congenital heart diseases that may result in sudden death include coronary artery anomalies, forms of hypertrophic cardiomyopathy, and forms of aortic stenosis, and are an especially important cause of death in the young (men and women younger than 35 years of age).

A partial list of entities resulting in sudden death in individuals 14–40 years, as well as incidence of occurrence, is presented in Tables 10–3 through 10–6.

Causes of Death in Infants and Children

The age of the patient at time of death greatly affects the likelihood of specific underlying diseases. In neonates and infants, a common cause of sudden unexpected death is the sudden in-

Table 10–3. Causes of Sudden Cardiac Death in Infants and Children

Anatomic Findings	0–1 Years (20 pts)	1–21 Years (50 pts)
Coronary artery anomalies	10 (50%)	12 (24%)
Myocarditis	0	14 (28%)
No finding	7 (35%)	10 (20%)
Other findings	2 (10%)	8 (16%)
Hypertrophic cardiomyopathy	1 (5%)	6 (12%)

Adapted from Steinberger J, Lucas R, Edwards JE, Titus JL. Causes of sudden unexpected cardiac death in the first two decades of life. Am J Cardiol 77:992–995, 1996.

fant death syndrome, which has been defined as the sudden death of an infant under one year of age that remains unexplained after a thorough case investigation, including performance of a complete autopsy, examination of the death scene, and review of the clinical history. A cardiac cause of sudden infant death syndrome has yet to be established.

Steinberger et al.[11] reported their experience in 20 patients less than 1 year old dying suddenly (Table 10–3). In 65% of cases, a cause of death was identified, 80% of which were ectopic aortic origin of one or more coronary arteries. In older infants and young children, up to 75% of sudden unexpected deaths are not attributed to heart disease.[12, 13] Up to 50% of cardiac causes in children dying during exercise are idiopathic arrhythmias with apparently normal heart at autopsy.[14] In 50 cases of sudden cardiac death reported by Steinberger et al. (Table 10–3) in patients aged 1–20 years, cardiac abnormalities were present in 80%. The most common identifiable cause of sudden death in young children is myocarditis and congenital heart disease, including coronary artery anomalies and hypertrophic cardiomyopathy. In young patients with known heart disease who are followed in cardiology clinic, causes of sudden death are generally structural (see congenital heart disease, below).

Table 10–4. Causes of Death, Ages 14–20

Cause of Death	n (%)
No finding	18 (30%)
Myocarditis	8 (13%)
Hypertrophic cardiomyopathy	7 (12%)
Anomalous coronary artery	5 (8%)
Complex congenital heart disease	4 (7%)
Atherosclerosis	3 (5%)
Dilated cardiomyopathy	3 (5%)
Floppy mitral valve	3 (5%)
Idiopathic left ventricular hypertrophy	3 (5%)
Aortic dissection	2 (3%)
Kawasaki	2 (3%)
Tunnel coronary artery	1 (3%)
Hypertensive left ventricular hypertrophy	1 (2%)
TOTAL	60

Adapted from Burke AP, Farb A, Virmani R, Goodin J, Smialek JE. Sports-related and non-sports-related sudden death in young adults. Am Heart J 121:568–575, 1991.

Causes of Death in Adolescents and Adults

In adolescents and young adults, myocarditis, cardiomyopathies (right ventricular dysplasia, hypertrophic, and idiopathic left ventricular hypertrophy), and coronary artery anomalies are the most common causes of sudden cardiac death in individuals with structural heart disease.[14] In developed countries, coronary atherosclerosis is by far the most common finding in cases of sudden cardiac death in patients over 30–35 years of age (Tables 10–1 and 10–6).

Table 10–5. Causes of Death, Ages 21–30

Cause of Death	n (%)
Atherosclerosis	64 (28%)
No finding	49 (21%)
Idiopathic left ventricular hypertrophy	27 (12%)
Hypertrophic cardiomyopathy	16 (7%)
Myocarditis	14 (6%)
Anomalous coronary artery	9 (4%)
Dilated cardiomyopathy	7 (3%)
Tunnel	7 (3%)
Aortic dissection	7 (3%)
Rheumatic mitral stenosis	6 (3%)
Complex congenital heart disease	5 (2%)
Hypertensive left ventricular hypertrophy	4 (2%)
Endocarditis	4 (2%)
Sarcoidosis	3 (1%)
Aortic stenosis	3 (1%)
Floppy mitral valve	2 (1%)
Right ventricular cardiomyopathy	2 (1%)
Coronary aneurysm (congenital)	1 (0.4%)
Amyloid	1 (0.4%)
Pericarditis	1 (0.4%)
TOTAL	229

Adapted from Burke AP, Farb A, Virmani R, Goodin J, Smialek JE. Sports-related and non-sports-related sudden death in young adults. Am Heart J 121:568–575, 1991.

Table 10–6. Causes of Death, Ages 31–40

Cause of Death	n (%)
Atherosclerosis	258 (60%)
No finding	38 (9%)
Hypertensive left ventricular hypertrophy	26 (6%)
Idiopathic left ventricular hypertrophy	18 (4%)
Dilated cardiomyopathy	16 (4%)
Hypertrophic cardiomyopathy	13 (3%)
Myocarditis	12 (3%)
Sarcoidosis	10 (2%)
Aortic stenosis	9 (2%)
Aortic dissection	8 (2%)
Endocarditis	6 (1%)
Floppy mitral valve	6 (1%)
Tunnel coronary artery	3 (1%)
Right ventricular dysplasia	3 (1%)
Rheumatic mitral stenosis	3 (1%)
Anomalous coronary artery	2 (0.5%)
Coronary artery dissection	2 (0.4%)
Congenital heart disease	1 (0.2%)
Lipomatous hypertrophy, atrial septum	1 (0.2%)
TOTAL	432

Adapted from Burke AP, Farb A, Virmani R, Goodin J, Smialek JE. Sports-related and non-sports-related sudden death in young adults. Am Heart J 121:568–575, 1991.

Degrees of Certainty and Causes of Death

There are several problems inherent in assigning a specific cause of death in cases of sudden cardiac death. In cases of ventricular arrhythmias, the underlying substrates may be chronic or subacute conditions, and the specific initiating event for the arrhythmia is obscure. For example, stable but occlusive atherosclerotic plaques, anomalous coronary arteries, cardiac hypertrophy, and ventricular scars predispose to ventricular arrhythmias, but these are chronic conditions that may be found incidentally in deaths clearly due to other causes. Many chronic conditions that predispose to sudden death do so in only a small percentage of patients, further confusing the issue whether the finding is incidental or a cause of death. Some findings are themselves of questionable pathologic significance, such as tunneled coronary arteries or anomalous right coronary arteries. Occasionally, there may be more than one anatomic abnormality that may lead to a lethal arrhythmia, and the exact cause of the terminal event may be difficult to determine.

Causes of sudden cardiac death may be classified as definite, probable, or possible. Definite causes of death are those that result in cardiac tamponade, cardiac rupture, acute heart failure (e.g., ruptured papillary muscle, massive myocardial infarction), and acute coronary thrombi. Probable causes of death include stable coronary plaques (> 75% cross-sectional luminal narrowing), left ventricular hypertrophy, ventricular scars, and cardiomyopathy. These are accepted causes of death but require careful exclusion of a noncardiac cause of death. Possible causes of death include extensively tunnelled coronary arteries, atherosclerotic narrowing between 60–75% of a major epicardial artery, anomalous right coronary artery, narrowing of atrioventricular nodal artery, anomalous connections in the conduction system, and lipomatous hypertrophy of the atrial septum. Mitral valve prolapse, which was previously considered a possible cause of sudden unexpected death, is currently an accepted cause of death in the absence of other findings.

CORONARY CAUSES OF SUDDEN CARDIAC DEATH

Coronary Atherosclerosis

Epidemiological Factors

Coronary atherosclerosis is the overwhelming cause of sudden death in the United States in patients older than 35 years. In patients dying of coronary disease, up to 50% of deaths are sudden. The proportion of deaths from ischemic heart disease that are sudden declines with advancing age, because older patients are more likely to die of complications of heart failure, rather than ventricular arrhythmias.

The major risk factors of sudden coronary death are systemic hypertension and smoking.[9] Complex ventricular ectopy, although relatively benign in the absence of heart disease, identify a group with a high probability of sudden death in patients with coronary artery disease, especially with previous myocardial infarction.

Definition of Severe Narrowing

Based on autopsy studies comparing the degree of luminal narrowing of coronary arteries in patients dying suddenly to other patients dying of other causes, it has been determined that 75–80% cross-sectional luminal narrowing is a useful figure for separating critical stenosis that may result in acute myocardial ischemia, from noncritical stenoses.[15, 16] It must be remembered, however, that this figure is not based on specific hemodynamic factors and does not take into account the presence of collateral circulation, coronary tone, and coronary spasm. Therefore, it is not surprising that many cases of more severe narrowing are incidental findings at autopsy. Of 124 men aged 50–69 years with traumatic or natural noncoronary deaths, the incidence of severe one-vessel disease was 10%; two-vessel disease, 3%; and three-vessel disease, 1%.[16] Therefore, any decision that death is due to coronary atherosclerosis, especially in the presence of a stable plaque, must be supported by rigorous exclusion of other noncardiac causes of death.

Myocardial blood flow is not only governed by the epicardial coronary artery caliber, but also by intramyocardial vascular resistance. With a decrease of vascular resistance and hyperemia at times of vasodilatation, myocardial blood flow is approximately three times baseline levels[17] in normal arteries with < 40% luminal narrowing. At 80% luminal narrowing or greater, coronary vascular dilatory reserve is essentially absent, basal flow and maximal flow being equal.[17] With exercise and other conditions resulting in vasodilation, the pressure gradient across the stenosis increases, which may contribute to collapse or spasm of the vessel at the level of obstruction. Therefore, 60–70% narrowing of one major epicardial artery, especially the left anterior descending in patients with poorly developed collaterals, may occasionally precipitate death especially with exercise or stress.

Extent of Disease in Coronary Sudden Death

In our experience with out-of-hospital sudden coronary deaths, the proportion of hearts with one-vessel disease (single coronary artery cross-sectional lumen area narrowed ≥ 75% by atherosclerotic plaque) is 44%; two-vessel disease, 32%; three-vessel disease, 22%; and four-vessel disease, 1%.[18] In other series of sudden death, in which there are a large number of hospital-based deaths, the proportion of one-vessel disease is as low as 16%, with 27% two-vessel disease, 47% three-vessel disease, and 10% four-vessel disease.[19] In the series of sudden coronary death reported by Thomas et al. one-vessel disease was found in 26% of cases, with 39% having two-vessel disease and 33% three-vessel disease.[20] In the absence of hypertension, the heart weight increases in cases of sudden death as the number of severely narrowed epicardial arteries increases.[21]

In our series, the culprit lesion (area of maximal stenosis or that of acute thrombus) was found in the left anterior descending in 40%, the right coronary in 29%, the left circumflex in 18%, the left obtuse marginal in 5%, left diagonal in 2%, left main in 2%, posterior descending in 2%, and ramus intermedius in 2% of cases of sudden coronary death.[18]

Coronary Plaque Morphology in Sudden Cardiac Death

Incidence of Luminal Thrombi

The frequency of coronary thrombosis in sudden coronary death varies from 20–70%.[18, 22, 23] This wide range is in large part due to the population studied. The time interval between onset of symptoms and death, the presence of acute myocardial infarction, and the type of prodromal symptom (stable angina, unstable angina, no apparent symptoms) all affect the incidence of thrombi in coronary sudden cardiac death. Thrombi are quite common in coronary sudden death associated with acute myocardial infarction; the incidence of thrombi in sudden death with acute infarcts is generally accepted to be 70–80% in angiographic and autopsy studies.[24, 25] The incidence of coronary thrombi in patients with unstable angina and sudden death is clouded by the difficulty in ascertaining an accurate clinical history in out-of-hospital deaths[26]; the preponderance of evidence, however, suggests a major role for thrombi in unstable conditions. The incidence of coronary thrombi in "instantaneous" sudden death occurring in the absence of any chest pain or clinical prodrome ranges from negligible to 50%,[19, 27, 28] suggesting that the terminal arrhythmias may be precipitated by cardiac hypertrophy or healed infarcts. The incidence of acute thrombi in sudden coronary death in patients with systemic hypertension is significantly lower than normotensives, introducing a further factor influencing the frequency of thrombosis in sudden coronary death.[21] Plaque erosion in the absence of plaque fissuring is an important cause of coronary thrombosis in atherosclerotic sudden coronary death, and may be pathogenetically distinct from plaque rupture[29] (Figs. 10–1 and 10–2). Further descriptions of coronary thrombosis in sudden cardiac death and relationship to risk factors are found in Chapter 2.

Incidence of Stable Plaques

In approximately 40% of cases of coronary sudden death, there are no plaque disruptions identified, despite careful postmortem evaluation with angiography, perfusion fixation, and

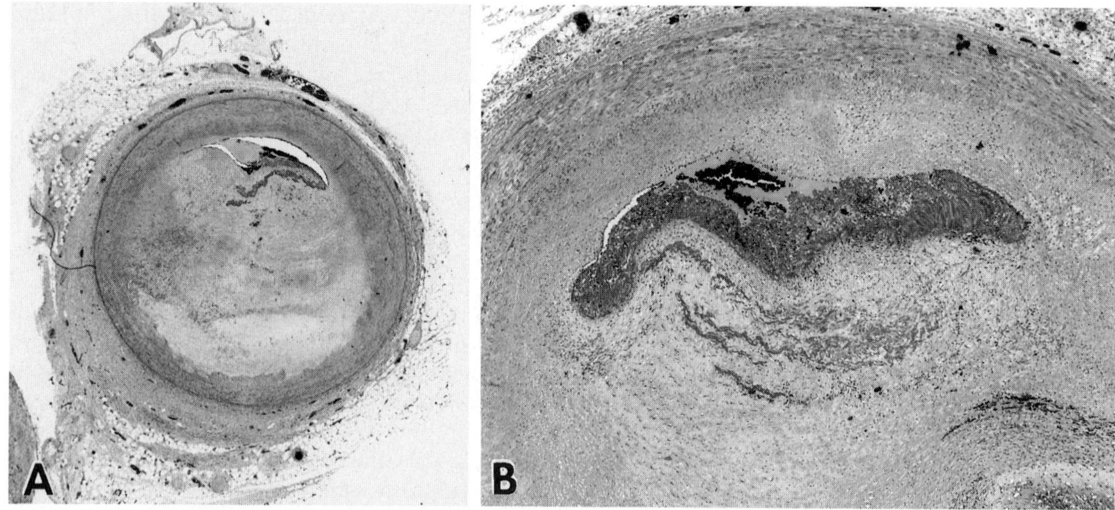

Figure 10–1. Coronary artery thrombosis secondary to eroded plaque. In 60% of sudden coronary deaths, a coronary thrombosis will be found; of these, 40% are erosions. A 28-year-old female had chest pain and dizziness, collapsed, and died within 1 hour of onset of symptoms. She had no significant medical history. At autopsy, the heart weighed 300 grams. *A.* The left anterior descending coronary artery demonstrates a critical narrowing by fibrous plaque with erosion and an occlusive thrombus. *B.* A higher magnification of the plaque demonstrates erosion and thrombosis with layering of fibrin intermingled with smooth muscle cells without evidence of plaque rupture.

serial sectioning. The mechanism of ventricular arrhythmias in these cases is uncertain, but many factors may play a role, including myocardial fibrosis secondary to chronic ischemia, cardiac hypertrophy, and coronary artery spasm. In such cases, noncoronary causes of sudden cardiac death should be carefully excluded, because stable plaques resulting in critical narrowing are common incidental findings. Deep plaque hemorrhage without intraplaque thrombus or plaque fissure is currently considered a form of stable plaque, and is often an incidental finding at autopsy.

Incidence of Plaque Fissures

In most cases of sudden coronary death with plaque fissures, there are superimposed thrombi.[30] Plaque disruption in the absence of luminal thrombus occurs in 3–20% of cases of sudden coronary death,[18, 25, 26, 30] and presumably contributes to acute ventricular ischemia sec-

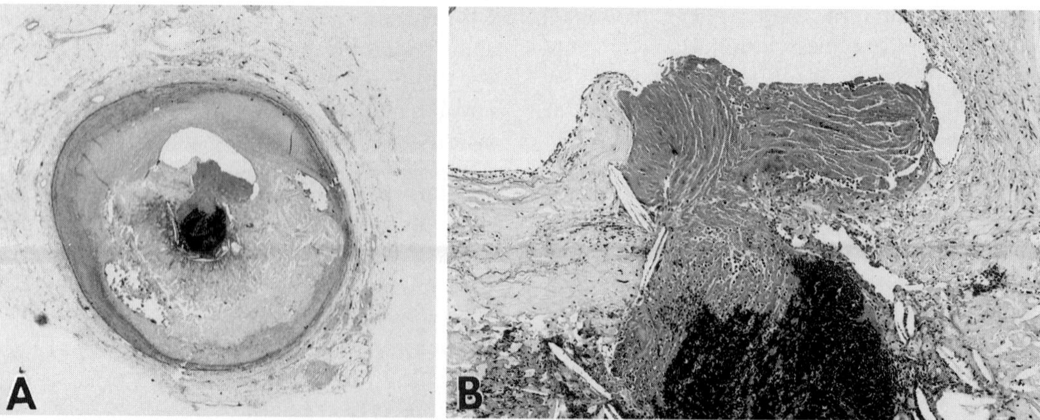

Figure 10–2. Plaque rupture. *A.* Eccentric plaque with hemorrhage into plaque and rupture of thin fibrous cap. The artery was a focal lesion in the mid-left anterior descending coronary artery of a 41-year-old man who died suddenly. *B.* A higher magnification of plaque rupture and fibrin platelet thrombus. The necrotic core is in continuity with the lumen as a result of the tear in the cap.

ondary to sudden coronary narrowing. However, plaque fissures with intraplaque thrombi have been described as incidental findings in up to 9% of hearts in patients with severe coronary artery atherosclerosis.[16] In contrast, plaque fissures with luminal thrombus are found almost exclusively in patients dying from complications of coronary artery disease.

Incidence of Myocardial Infarction

The likelihood of discovering an acute infarction in autopsied cases of sudden coronary death is over 50% in hospital-based studies of sudden death.[23, 24] In out-of-hospital deaths, and cases of instantaneous sudden death with no symptoms or symptoms lasting less than 1 hour, acute infarcts are unusual, and found in less than 25% of cases.[18, 19, 22]

The incidence of healed infarcts in out-of-hospital sudden coronary deaths is greater than that of acute infarcts. We found an acute myocardial infarction in only 21% of sudden coronary deaths, including 11% with both acute and healed infarcts. Healed infarcts in the absence of acute infarction is found in 41% and no infarct in 38% of sudden coronary death.[18] In hearts with acute myocardial infarction, the infarcts are transmural and grossly identifiable in approximately 50% of cases, and subendocardial and identified only by histologic examination in the remainder.

Postinfarction cardiac rupture, when it involves the free wall, is almost uniformly fatal. The incidence of rupture is highest in the elderly, in women, in patients without previous infarction, and in patients with hypertension. The underlying acute infarct is generally transmural, involving at least 20% of the left ventricle. The time interval between infarct and rupture is usually between 1 to 4 days after infarction, but can occur any time between 1 day and 3 weeks.

Coronary Artery Anomalies

Origin from Pulmonary Trunk

The left main coronary artery arises from the pulmonary trunk in 1/50,000 to 1/300,000 autopsies, representing 0.25 to 0.5% of congenital heart disease.[31, 32] There is a female predominance of 2:1. Most cases are identified in the first year of life, and sudden death occurs in approximately 40% of cases. Sudden death usually occurs at rest, but may occur after strenuous activity in older children. The oldest patient with this anomaly in our records was a 17-year-old girl who died suddenly, in whom collateral coronary circulation was extensive.

Pathologically, the aberrant artery arises in the left pulmonary sinus in 95% of cases (Fig. 10–3*A*). Typically, the artery appears thin-walled and vein-like, and the right coronary artery, while normal in location, is tortuous. The heart is typically enlarged, with extensive scarring and thinning of the anterolateral left ventricular wall and anterolateral papillary muscle. Dilatation of the left ventricle with endocardial fibrolelastosis is common, and the gross appearance of the heart may mimic dilated cardiomyopathy. In cases of infantile sudden death, the only significant changes may be abnormal location of the ostium.

Rarely, the right coronary or the left anterior descending coronary artery may arise in the pulmonary trunk. Most patients with this anomaly are asymptomatic. Both coronary arteries arising from the pulmonary sinuses is usually accompanied by other congenital anomalies, and most patients die within days or weeks of birth.

Anomalous Origin of Coronary Arteries in the Aortic Sinuses

Anomalous Left Main

The most common coronary anomaly resulting in sudden death is an aberrant left main arising in the right coronary sinus of Valsalva.[33–35] Over 100 cases have been reported, with a male to female ratio of 4:1–9:1. Sudden death occurs in 50% of these cases, 75% of which occur during exercise.[36] Most patients are adolescents or young adults, although death may occur as young as 1 month of age. There are often premonitory symptoms of syncope or chest pain, but stress electrocardiograms and stress echocardiograms are often negative.[37]

Pathologically, there are several variants to this anomaly. The common feature is the presence of the left main ostium within the right sinus (Fig. 10–3*B*). This ostium is typically near the commissure, and in some cases actually lies above the commissure between the right and left sinuses. Often, the ostium is somewhat malformed and slit-like, and an ostial ridge is present. The proximal artery lies within the aortic media and may be compressed during diastole.

The variants of an anomalous left main coronary artery involve its distal course. In most cases, and virtually all cases of sudden cardiac

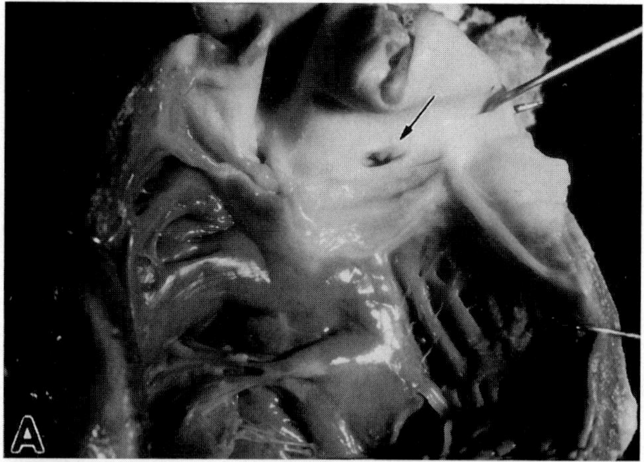

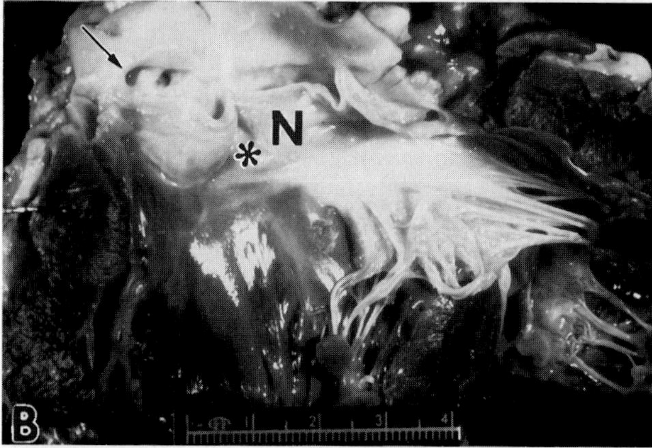

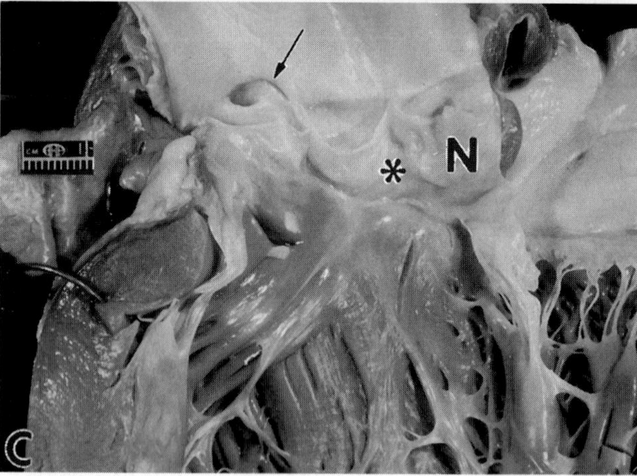

Figure 10–3. Congenital coronary artery anomalies and sudden death. *A.* Anomalous left main coronary artery arising from the pulmonary trunk. Note coronary ostium (*arrow*) and pulmonary valve. The patient was a 7-year-old boy who died suddenly while ice skating; he had a recent history of palpitations attributed to Lyme myocarditis. There was a healed subendocardial infarct in the anterior left ventricle (not shown). *B.* Anomalous left coronary artery arising in right aortic sinus. Note ostial valve-like ridge (*arrow*) of the left coronary artery. The membranous septum (*asterisk*) lies between the right and noncoronary (*N*) cusps. The patient was a previously healthy 22-year-old man who died suddenly while playing soccer. The anomalous left main coursed between the great arteries (not shown). *C.* Anomalous right coronary artery arising in the left aortic sinus. Note the slit-like coronary ostium of the right coronary artery (*arrow*). The membranous septum (*asterisk*) lies between the right and noncoronary (*N*) cusps. The patient was a 19-year-old male who died suddenly while playing football. He had no medical history other than sickle cell trait.

death, the aberrant artery passes between the aorta and the pulmonary trunk. In a minority of cases, the left main travels anterior to the pulmonary trunk, posterior to the aorta, or posterior to the right ventricular outflow tract within the ventricular septum.

The pathophysiology of sudden death in patients with aberrant left main coronary artery is incompletely understood. Theories accounting for acute ischemia in patients with this anomaly involve three proximal segments of the artery. Compression of the left main by the great arteries as it courses between the pulmonary trunk and aorta, diastolic compression of the vessel lying within the aortic media, and poor filling during diastole because of ostial ridges or slit-like ostia have all been proposed as explanations for acute ischemia and ventricular fibrillation. However, it is unusual to detect acute or chronic ischemia in the anterior wall of the left ventricle. In most cases, the mechanism of death is presumed to be a tachyarrhythmia triggered by acute ischemia that has not yet become histologically manifest.

In older patients with this anomaly, there may be superimposed atherosclerosis that may result in sudden death. It is unclear whether the development of atherosclerosis is accelerated in anomalous left main coronary artery. If there is > 75% luminal narrowing, the cause of sudden death is attributed to an atherosclerotic, rather than a congenital cause.

Anomalous Right Coronary Artery

Until recently, an anomalous right coronary artery was considered to be without clinical consequence. In 1982, Roberts et al. described 10 patients with this anomaly, three of whom died suddenly without other significant cardiac findings.[38] We have reported 52 cases, 48 of which were in males, 25% of which apparently resulted in sudden cardiac death.[31] Almost 50% of these deaths were exercise related, and most deaths occurred in young and middle-aged adults under the age of 35 years. Currently, anomalous right coronary artery is considered with anomalous left as a potential cause of sudden death, especially exertional.[37]

Grossly, there are two ostia located in the left sinus of Valsalva (Fig. 10–3*C*). The ostium supplying the right coronary artery may have similar features as anomalous left ostia located in the right sinus. Namely, there may be upward displacement, location near the commissure, and slit-like ostia with ostial ridges. The pathophysiology of sudden death is similar to that of anomalous left coronary artery.

Single Coronary Ostium

Single ostia are rare anomalies, 80% of which are discovered in males. These are generally incidental findings at catheterization or autopsy. We have reported 44 cases, 14% of which were found in patients who died suddenly without other causes of death found at autopsy.[31] Single ostia may be present either within the right or left sinus of Valsalva. Similar to anomalous arteries with two ostia, sudden death is more frequent if the ostium is located in the right sinus of Valsalva.

Multiple Coronary Ostia

These are mentioned only because they are occasionally misinterpreted by the pathologist as possible causes of sudden death. An accessory ostium in the right sinus of Valsalva supplying the conus artery is a normal variant that is found in up to 30% of patients at angiography. Separate ostia for the left anterior descending and left circumflex arteries are found in approximately 10% of individuals and has no pathologic significance.

High Takeoff Coronary Arteries

Location of a coronary ostium above the sinotubular junction is common. Occasionally, with takeoffs greater than 1 cm above the sinotubular junction, there may be associated ostial ridges and downward angulation of the artery, resulting in potential constriction of the artery and myocardial ischemia resulting in sudden death.

Hypoplastic Coronary Arteries

The definition of hypoplastic coronary arteries has not yet been standardized. Postmortem coronary angiograms, which provide the best documentation of hypoperfusion of one area of the heart, are generally not performed in putative cases of hypoplastic coronary arteries. Chronic ischemia to the posterior wall of the heart is evidence of a pathologic condition, but ischemia is often not demonstrated in other, better established types of anomalous coronary arteries.

One definition of hypoplastic coronary arteries, which we currently favor, is a condition in which neither the right nor the left circumflex coronary arteries extends beyond the lateral borders of the heart. In addition, there is no extension of the left anterior descending artery around the apex, nor is there a large obtuse marginal branch supplying the posterior heart. Using this criterion, we have reported 13 adult patients, five of whom died suddenly, three of which were exercise related.[31]

Another form of hypoplastic coronary consists of a diffuse decrease in caliber of the epicardial arteries, without apparent fibrointimal proliferation.[39] The diagnostic criteria for this type of coronary hypoplasia have not yet been established.

When evaluating hearts in cases of sudden death, one must be aware of several normal variants that should not be interpreted as coronary hypoplasia. The left circumflex artery may be quite small or absent in cases of dominant right circulation with extension of the right coronary artery beyond the posterior descending artery. Similarly, the posterior wall of the heart may not be supplied primarily by the posterior descending artery, but from an extension of a wrap-around left anterior descending artery that courses around the apex of the heart, or a large marginal branch of the circumflex.

Tunnel Coronary Arteries

By definition, a tunnel coronary artery is formed by a myocardial bridge that results in a focally intramural coronary artery that is flanked by epicardial segments. The most common location is the middle third of the left anterior descending coronary artery. Tunneled segments of the left anterior descending coronary artery are extremely common, and are found in approximately 30% of hearts at autopsy.[40, 41] At angiography, extensive coronary artery tunneling is demonstrated in only 1% of patients, and is characterized by "milking" of the contrast dye within the tunneled segment.[42]

Strong support for physiologic significance of tunneled coronary arteries in some patients is provided by symptomatic relief of angina after surgical myocardial debridging techniques. Currently, it is difficult to determine in autopsy cases of sudden cardiac death the significance of a tunneled left anterior descending artery, due to the high prevalence of this condition. In cases of sudden death without other apparent cause, we recommend documenting the length and the depth of the tunnel, and carefully evaluating the anterior wall and septum of the left ventricle for ischemic changes. If the tunnel is greater than 5 mm deep, the likelihood of physiologic consequences is high, while tunnels of 3–5 mm depth are of questionable significance (Fig. 10–4). Superficial tunnels are ubiquitous and have no significance. It has been stated that tunnel coronary arteries are an accepted cause of sudden unexpected death only when the dominant left anterior descending coronary artery is involved, and death occurs during strenuous exercise.[40]

Miscellaneous Nonatherosclerotic Coronary Diseases

Spontaneous Coronary Dissection

Coronary artery dissection accounts for approximately 0.5% of sudden deaths in patients 30–40 years old (Table 10–6). Most patients are young women, sometimes in the postpartum period, and one patient with Marfan syndrome has been reported. In cases studied clinically, patients have presented with chest pain, electrocardiographic evidence of acute myocardial infarctions, and contrast dye within the false lumen at catheterization. In patients with coronary dissections who survive after bypass grafting, the involved vessels is usually the right coronary artery.[43]

In autopsy studies of coronary dissections that result in sudden death, over 90% of cases in-

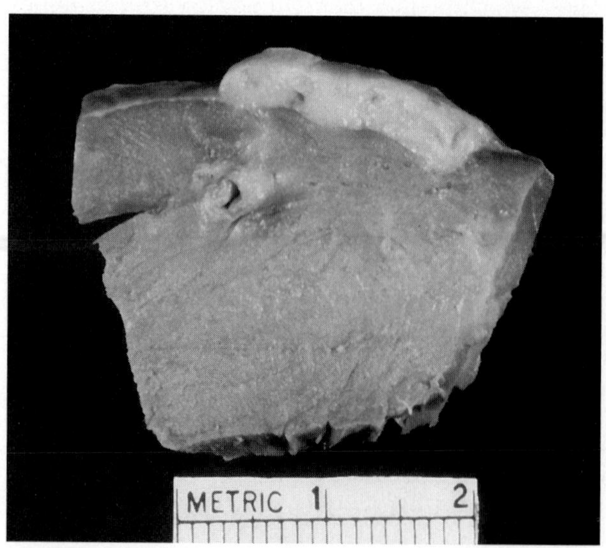

Figure 10–4. Myocardial tunnel. A section of anterior wall of the left ventricular myocardium demonstrates a 4-mm myocardial bridge overlying the left anterior descending coronary artery. The bridge was an incidental finding at autopsy. Occasionally, deep tunnels may be a cause of sudden death during strenuous activity.

volve the left anterior descending coronary artery.[44] Histologically, the dissection plane is in the outer media with infiltrates of eosinophils, lymphocytes, neutrophils, and macrophages in the adventitia[45, 46] (Fig. 10–5). It is unclear whether the inflammatory infiltrate is secondary to the dissection or represents a vasculitis.[1, 45] Underlying disease within the media is unusual, although medial degeneration may be present. Over 50% of cases demonstrate acute and/or healed infarction in the area perfused by the dissected artery, generally the anterior wall of the left ventricle.

Coronary Vasculitis

The majority of sudden deaths secondary to coronary vasculitis occur in children with stage IV Kawasaki disease, when there are healed aneurysms that are occluded by organizing thrombus.[47] These patients are four times more likely to be boys than girls, may not have a documented history of mucocutaneous lymph node syndrome, and are completely asymptomatic at the time of death. At autopsy, the differential diagnosis is congenital aneurysm. The differential diagnosis of Kawasaki disease and congenital aneurysm rests on the identification of in-

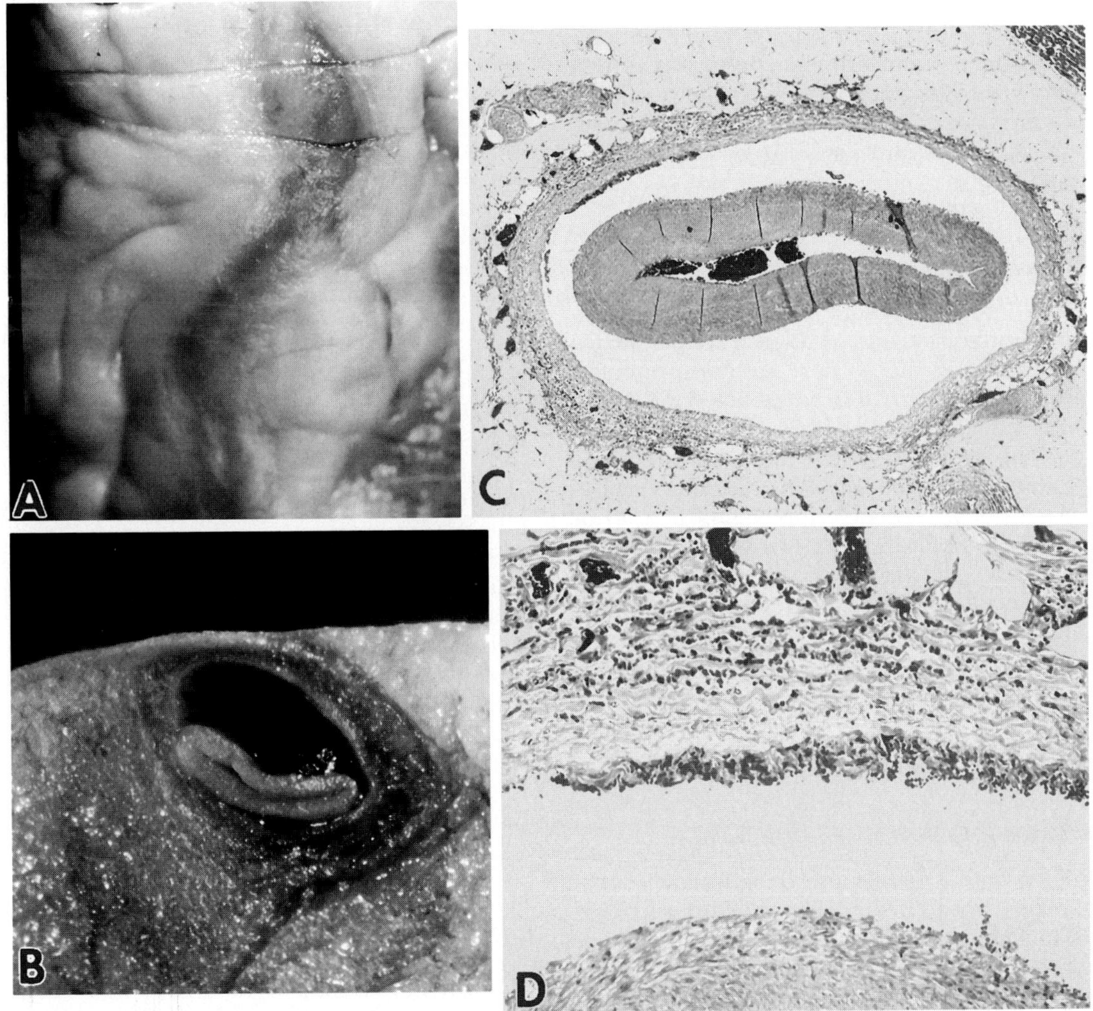

Figure 10–5. Coronary artery dissection. *A.* There is a dark discoloration of the epicardial surface overlying the left anterior descending coronary artery. *B.* A section of the artery demonstrates a hematoma compressing the lumen of the artery. *C.* A histologic section shows separation of the outer media from the adventitia, due to loss of hematoma during processing, which is exaggerated by shrinkage artifact. *D.* A higher magnification of the dissection plane shows an inflammatory infiltrate within the adventitia and focal thrombus lining the dissection plane. The inflammatory infiltrate is composed primarily of eosinophils (not appreciated). The patient was a previously healthy 38-year-old black woman who collapsed after complaining of chest pain.

flammatory destruction of the vessel wall in Kawasaki disease, and the presence of multiple aneurysms, which are more characteristic of inflammatory aneurysms than congenital aneurysms.

Approximately 40% of sudden deaths from coronary complications in Kawasaki disease occur in stage II, characterized by acute coronary thrombosis and acute infarction, or in stage III, in which there are organized coronary thrombi.[47] These patients generally have a recent history of mucocutaneous lymph node syndrome. Most deaths in the acute phase of illness are secondary to heart failure or diffuse myocarditis, occur in acutely ill infants or children, and are usually not classified as sudden.

Fatal coronary vasculitis occurs in septic vasculitis, syphilitic arteritis, polyarteritis nodosa, and collagen vascular disease, particularly rheumatoid arthritis. Patients with coronary vasculitis with these conditions are generally systemically ill and deaths are rarely sudden and unexpected.

Coronary Embolism

A variety of conditions may predispose to coronary embolism and sudden cardiac death. Natural causes of coronary embolism include infectious endocarditis, nonbacterial thrombotic endocarditis, atrial and ventricular mural thrombi, cardiac myxoma, and papillary fibroelastoma.[48] Iatrogenic causes of coronary embolism include cardiac catheterization arteriograms or surgical procedures that dislodge atherosclerotic plaques,[49] foreign bodies (suture, silicon, cloth, air, etc.), and fragments of calcified valves.[48]

Coronary artery emboli have a predilection for left circulation, presumably due to the large caliber and relatively straight course of the left anterior descending artery.

Nonatherosclerotic Coronary Thrombosis

Factors that predispose to epicardial coronary thrombosis in the absence of atherosclerosis include oral contraceptives, chest trauma, coronary aneurysms, hypercoagulable states, thrombocytosis, and cocaine abuse.[50–52] Cigarette smoking and clotting disorders may potentiate the risk of thrombosis in patients taking birth control pills. Epicardial nonatherosclerotic coronary thrombosis as a cause of sudden death accounts for < 1% of deaths in young adults (Tables 10–4 and 10–5).

Diffuse arteriolar thrombosis may occur in patients with disseminated intravascular coagulation, primary thrombocythemia, and thrombotic thrombocytopenic purpura (Fig. 10–6). Occasionally, the presenting symptom of thrombotic thrombocytopenic purpura is sudden death.[53] Typically, there is grossly evident myocardial hemorrhage, often subepicardially and on the endocardial surface. Microscopically, there are diffuse platelet thrombi within arterioles, contraction band necrosis, and interstitial hemorrhage. Immunohistochemical stains for platelet glycoprotein may facilitate diagnosis, as the microthrombi may be overlooked on routinely stained sections.

Small-Vessel Disease

Anecdotally, narrowing of the small arteries supplying the sinoatrial and atrioventricular nodes has been associated with sudden death.[54–57] The etiology of the narrowing in a majority of these cases is a form of arterial dysplasia (Fig. 10–7). Similar changes have been noted in arteries of individuals dying from noncardiac causes, demonstrating that such changes are not a definitive cause of death.

In a series of sudden unexpected deaths from idiopathic cardiac arrhythmias, we found a 35% frequency of dysplasia of the atrioventricular nodal artery, which was significantly greater in individuals dying after trauma (6%).[58] There was no sex predilection in this series, and one third of patients had a familial history of sudden unexpected death.

Small-vessel dysplasia has also been associated with catecholamine-induced sudden death,[59] hypertrophic cardiomyopathy, sickle cell disease, and mitral valve prolapse.[60] Although most cases of small-vessel disease and sudden death have emphasized involvement of arteries supplying the specialized conduction system of the heart, thickened arteries within the wall of the ventricular septum have also been implicated in sudden cardiac death.[61]

MYOCARDIAL CAUSES OF SUDDEN CARDIAC DEATH

Myocardial Ischemia

Mechanisms and Underlying Conditions

The mechanism of sudden death in most cases of ischemic heart disease is ventricular fibrillation; 20–30% of patients die with bradyarrhythmias, and a minority of patients have

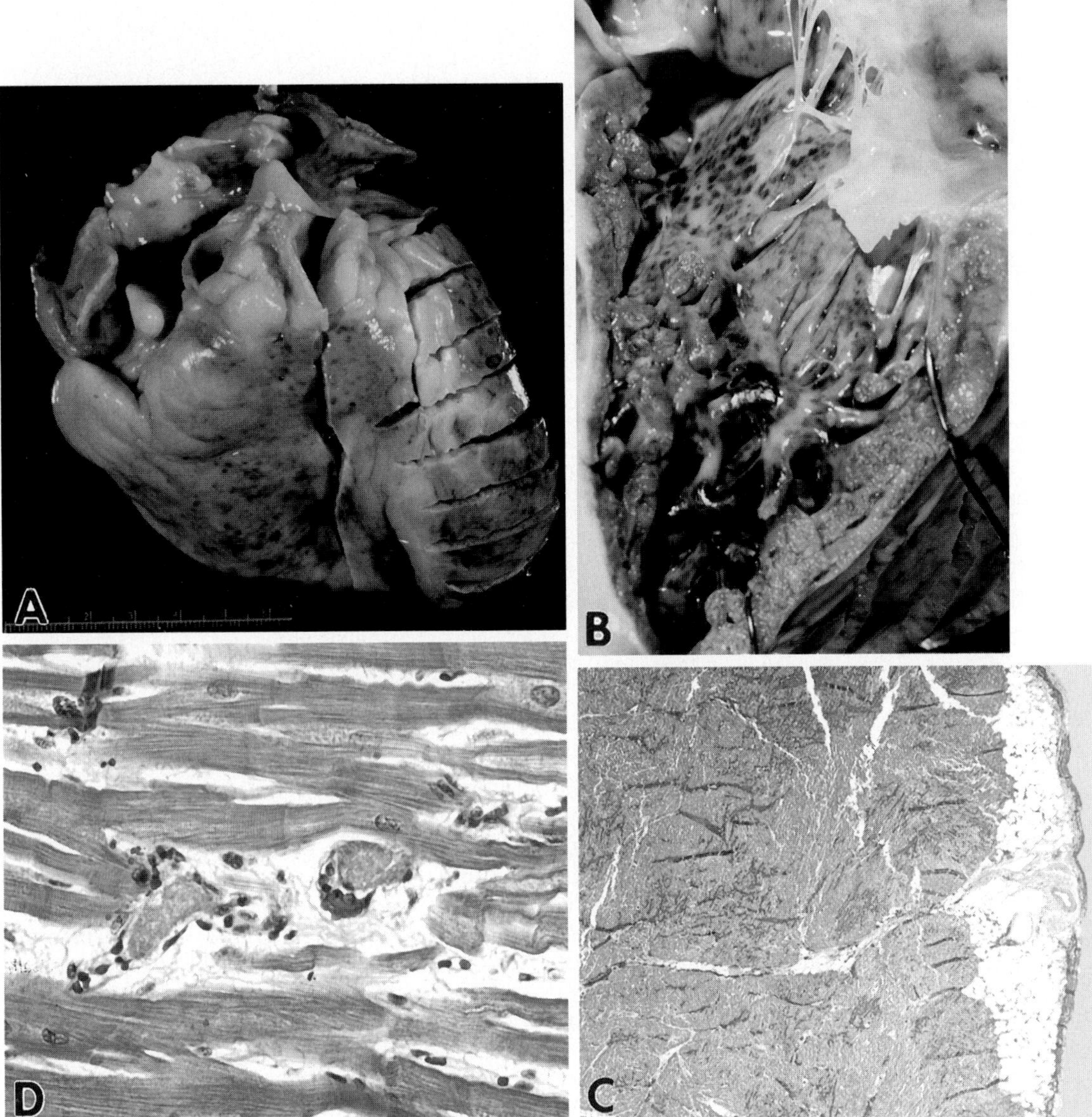

Figure 10–6. Thrombotic thrombocytopenic purpura. *A.* Note petechial hemorrhages over the epicardial surfaces. *B.* The petechial hemorrhages in this case are also prominent on the endocardium. *C.* Histologically, there are small foci of hemorrhage. *D.* A higher magnification demonstrates platelet thrombi within arterioles. The patient was a 37-year-old white woman who had symptoms of acute cholecystitis. While in the emergency room, stat laboratory values demonstrated elevated BUN and creatinine, leukocytosis, marked thrombocytopenia, and normal coagulation studies. The patient died suddenly while being admitted to the hospital ward.

diffuse myocardial damage resulting in acute heart failure or electromechanical dissociation.[8] The mechanisms of ischemia-induced ventricular arrhythmias are most likely related to reentry phenomena. The most common cause of myocardial ischemia in Western countries is atherosclerotic coronary disease, although any of the coronary diseases discussed earlier may result in ventricular ischemia. The incidence of ventricular fibrillation during the first 30 days after acute myocardial infarction is increased in patients with anterior wall infarctions and bundle branch block.[62]

Histologic Demonstration of Ischemia

Acute ischemia resulting in ventricular fibrillation is probably the most common cause of sudden cardiac death in this country; however, the ischemic focus is generally not found at

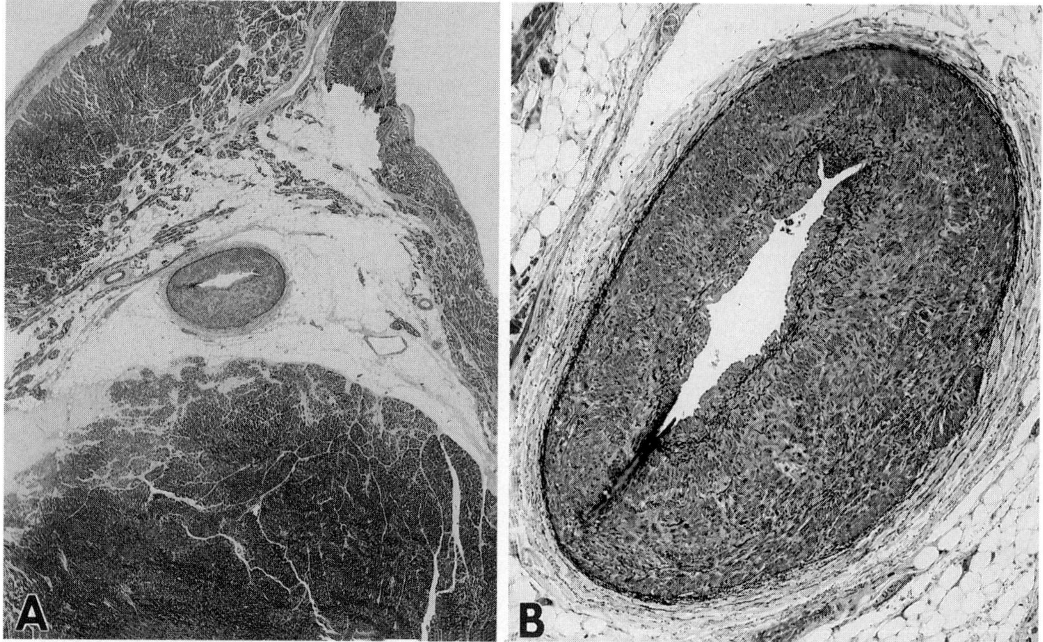

Figure 10–7. Small arterial disease. *A*. There is dysplasia with marked narrowing of the artery to the atrioventricular node. The section is taken posterior to the node, which is not present in this section, the artery lying in the atrioventricular sulcus. *B*. A higher magnification demonstrates medial hypertrophy with marked disorganization of the elastic lamellae (Movat elastic stain). The patient was a 25-year-old man who collapsed and died shortly after exercise.

autopsy. Most lethal arrhythmias occur within minutes or hours after the ischemic episode, before histologic changes are manifest. Acute infarcts are demonstrated by routine techniques in only 20% of sudden cardiac deaths secondary to coronary atherosclerosis. The use of triphenyl tetrazolium chloride staining of gross heart slices can increase the ability to detect early infarction, provided that the postmortem interval is short.[63]

The identification of a critical coronary lesion is sufficient to ascribe it as a cause of death, provided that other causes of death have been excluded. The ischemic focus is presumed to exist within the distribution of the affected artery.

Cardiomyopathies and Sudden Cardiac Death

Assessment of Cardiomegaly

In most cases of cardiomyopathy, it is essential to determine if cardiac hypertrophy exists. It is well known that cardiac mass is physiologically associated with body weight and height. For this reason, heart weight is meaningful only if the patient's body weight or height is taken into consideration. Broad limits of heart weight, such as 400 grams for men and 350 grams for women, as have been used in the past, have little scientific validity. Ninety-five percent confidence intervals of normal heart weight, as based on body weight and body surface area (kg/m^2), are readily available and of extreme importance in the assessment of cardiac hypertrophy.[64] Normal heart weight is approximately 0.45% of the body weight in men, and body weight and body surface area correlate better with heart weight in normals than body height. In some cases of sudden death, the only pathologic finding is concentric left ventricular hypertrophy; cardiac weight based on weight or body surface area of the deceased is the best way to determine this pathologic condition.

Hypertrophic Cardiomyopathy

Sudden death is the mode of presentation for over 50% of patients with hypertrophic cardiomyopathy; for this reason, hypertrophic cardiomyopathy is often a primary consideration in young individuals who die suddenly. In fact, hypertrophic cardiomyopathy accounts for only 5–10% of sudden deaths in young adults, although this frequency is increased to nearly

50% if young athletes constitute the population studied.[65, 66] Patients at risk for sudden death are those with a family history of sudden death and patients with a history of syncope or presyncope. In children with hypertrophic cardiomyopathy, coexistent tunneling of the left anterior descending coronary artery may predispose to sudden death.[67] An increase in the collagen network of the interstitium has been implicated in sudden death due to hypertrophic cardiomyopathy.[68]

The pathologic features of hypertrophic cardiomyopathy are discussed in detail in Chapter 6. Asymmetric left ventricular hypertrophy, small left ventricular chamber cavity, left atrial dilatation, thickening of the anterior leaflet of the mitral valve, and evidence of left ventricular outflow tract obstruction (left ventricular outflow tract plaque) are all gross features of hypertrophic cardiomyopathy (Fig. 10–8). The heart is always enlarged except in occasional cases of apical forms of the disease (Fig. 10–9). Histologic features include myofiber disarray, which should be documented in every case, and intramural myocardial artery thickening. Myofiber disarray is a somewhat subjective finding, but it should encompass 5% or more of the ventricular septal area. "Physiologic" myofiber disarray exists at the junction of the right and left ventricles in the posterior and anterior walls of the heart, but is not associated with marked myocyte hypertrophy. Myofiber disarray may be accompanied by significant interstitial fibrosis, especially in advances stages of disease.

In cases of sudden death with cardiac hypertrophy, we take six transverse sections of ventricular septum, both at the base and towards the apex of the heart, to rule out hypertrophic cardiomyopathy by determining the absence of myofiber disarray.

There are several potential mechanisms of sudden cardiac death in patients with hyper-

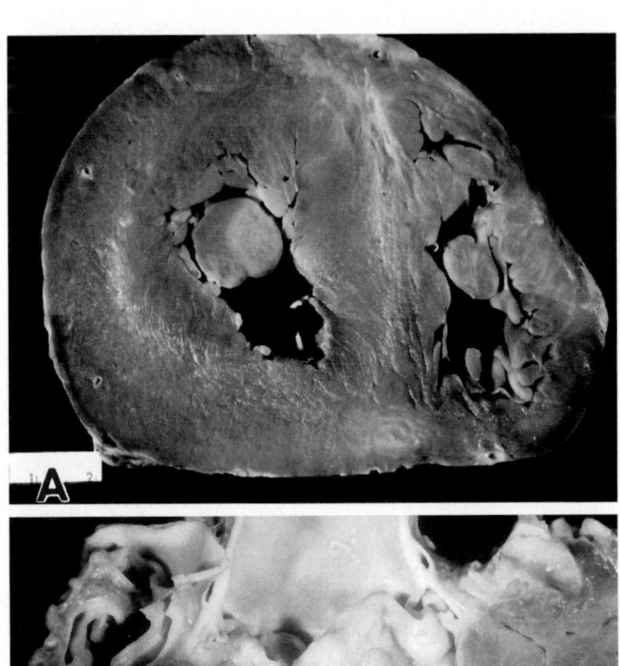

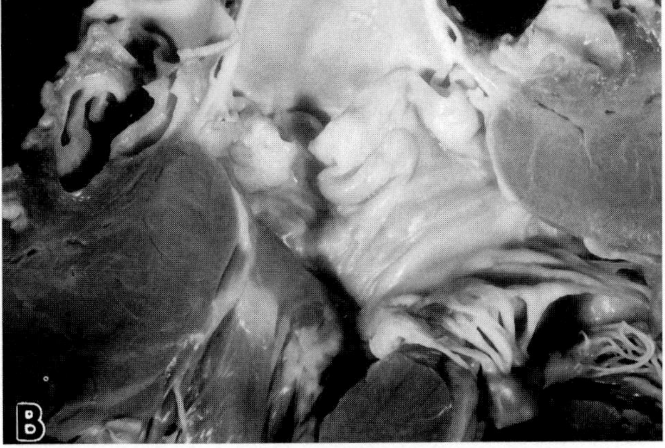

Figure 10–8. Hypertrophic cardiomyopathy. *A*. A cross section of the ventricles towards the base of the heart demonstrates biventricular hypertrophy with asymmetric thickening of the anterior portion of the ventricular septum. *B*. The left ventricular outflow tract demonstrates a discrete plaque (*arrow*) adjacent to the anterior leaflet of the mitral valve, which is thickened. In this patient, who was a 19-year-old man who died suddenly while playing basketball, there was also dysplastic thickening of the aortic valve, as well as an anomalous right coronary artery arising in the left coronary sinus (not shown). The latter two abnormalities are not associated with hypertrophic cardiomyopathy and were presumably coincidental in this patient.

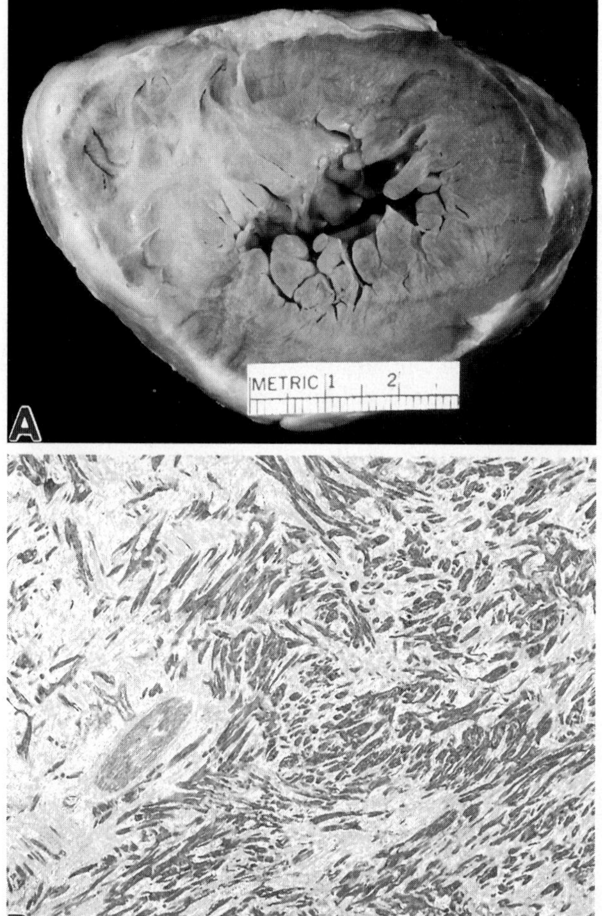

Figure 10–9. Hypertrophic cardiomyopathy, apical type. *A.* A cross section of the ventricles near the cardiac apex demonstrates marked septal scarring with grossly evident muscular disarray. *B.* A histologic section section demonstrates scarring, myocyte disarray, and focal intramural coronary artery thickening. The patient was a 51-year-old white woman in good health who died suddenly. There was a remote history of a heart murmur. At autopsy, the heart was of normal weight (350 grams).

trophic cardiomyopathy. The major possible mechanisms include acute ischemia secondary to subaortic stenosis, ventricular arrhythmias secondary to disordered muscle bundles in the ventricular septum, myocardial ischemia secondary to small-vessel coronary disease, altered autonomic vascular control, and myocardial hypertrophy.[65, 66, 69]

Hypertensive Cardiomyopathy

Left ventricular hypertrophy of any cause is associated with ventricular ectopy and increased risk for ventricular tachyarrhythmias.[70] Patients with hypertension and left ventricular hypertrophy have an increased risk of sudden death. Pathologically, there are no specific features that identify hypertension as the etiology for left ventricular hypertrophy. In the absence of a clinical history, examination of the kidneys for arteriolar thickening is helpful in establishing the presence of systemic hypertension.[71]

As for other causes of cardiomegaly, the diagnosis of concentric left ventricular hypertrophy requires demonstration of increased heart weight as a function of body weight and height. In general, the left ventricular free wall thickness exceeds 1.5 cm, but this value is dependent on the size of the individual and is more subjective than heart weight.

Idiopathic Concentric Left Ventricular Hypertrophy

In 10–40% of sudden deaths in young individuals, especially athletes, concentric left ventricular hypertrophy, as determined by body weight and height, is the only pathologic findings at autopsy.[72, 73] (Fig. 10–10). Some cases of idiopathic concentric left ventricular hypertrophy may represent forms of hypertrophic cardiomyopathy lacking typical morphologic expressions of the disease, especially in patients with a family history of cardiomyopathy. Until

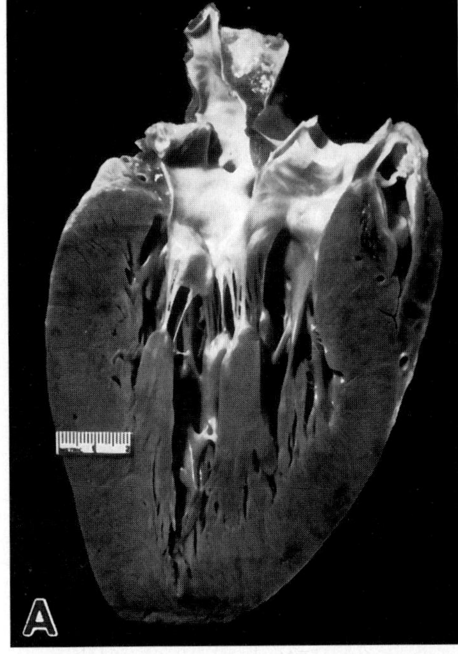

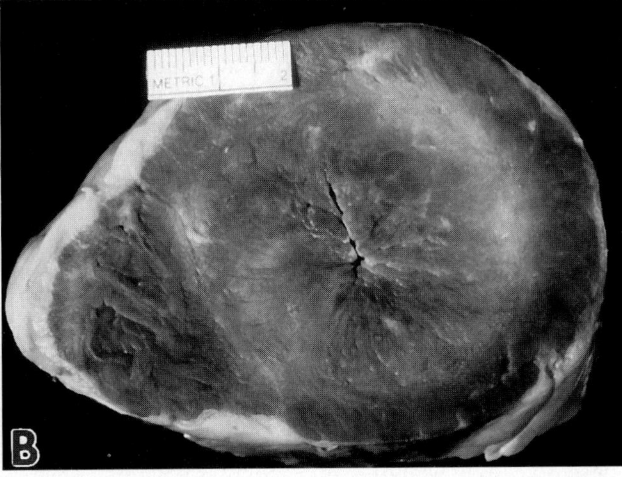

Figure 10–10. Concentric left ventricular hypertrophy. *A*. There is marked left ventricular hypertrophy without asymmetry; no myofiber disarray was noted on microscopic examination. There is mild left ventricular dilatation (chamber cavity 4 cm), suggesting the diagnosis of dilated cardiomyopathy. The patient was a 17-year-old black male who died suddenly while playing basketball; the heart weighed 740 grams. *B*. Cross section of a different heart shows concentric left ventricular hypertrophy and a small left ventricular chamber cavity. The patient was a 35-year-old white male who died suddenly after playing basketball. There was no history of hypertension.

reliable molecular probes for the diagnosis of myosin heavy chain mutations as present in hypertrophic cardiomyopathy are available, the distinction between "idiopathic" concentric left ventricular hypertrophy and hypertrophic cardiomyopathy will remain difficult. The diagnosis of idiopathic concentric left ventricular hypertrophy assumes the absence of systemic hypertension, as determined by history or examination of renal microvasculature.

Dilated Cardiomyopathy

Regardless of etiology, the failing heart is prone to ventricular arrhythmias that potentially may result in sudden death. Ambulatory Holter monitoring in patients with idiopathic dilated cardiomyopathy often demonstrates ventricular arrhythmias including nonsustained ventricular tachycardia. It has not been established that complex or frequent ventricular arrhythmias predict sudden arrhythmic death, although they do confer independent adverse prognosis and a decreased total mortality.[74]

Although patients with dilated cardiomyopathy frequently die sudden arrhythmic deaths, death is generally not unexpected, because illness is often chronic and progressive. However, occasional patients may die suddenly without a history of heart disease, and autopsy findings will demonstrate typical features of dilated cardiomyopathy. In these patients, symptoms of congestive heart failure may not have been elicited by the scene investigator, the patient may have been indigent without access to medical care, the patient may have ignored symptoms and avoided medical care, or a combination of these factors may have been present.

The autopsy diagnosis of dilated cardiomyopathy rests on the identification of cardiac dilatation, in the absence of significant atherosclerotic and valvular disease. In general, the heart is moderately to massively enlarged, there is four-chamber dilatation (ventricles more pronounced than atria), and the left ventricular wall is of normal thickness (generally < 1.5 cm). Although autopsy dimensions of ventricular size are not always reliable, the ventricular cavity is generally > 4 cm at the level of the papillary muscles. Histologic sections are required to rule out specific causes of cardiomyopathy. A history of normotension and an absence of renal arteriolar thickening are required to rule out end-stage hypertensive cardiomyopathy, which is identical grossly and histologically to dilated cardiomyopathy.

Cardiomyopathy of Obesity

The association of obesity and sudden death has been known since ancient times, as illustrated by Hippocrates's adage that "sudden death is more common in those who are naturally fat than in the lean."[75] In a study where morbid obesity was defined as being more than 100% or 100 pounds over desired body weight, the annual sudden cardiac death mortality rate was 65/100,000 versus 1.6/100,000 in normal weight women.[76]

There have been various explanations for sudden death in the morbidly obese, including increased ventricular ectopy, prolonged QT interval, and a chronic increase in cardiac output and arterial pressure resulting in heart failure and sudden death.[76–78] In the massively obese, excessive weight loss, particularly when achieved with ketogenic (high protein, high fat) diets, has been associated with ventricular ectopy, ventricular fibrillation, and sudden death.

Autopsy studies of sudden death in the massively obese have shown an increase in heart weight in proportion to body weight and myocardial hypertrophy.[79–81] An increase in epicardial fat is not consistently found compared with controls. The most common causes of death are dilated cardiomyopathy (45%), severe coronary atherosclerosis (27%), and concentric left ventricular hypertrophy without left ventricular dilatation (18%). Left ventricular cavity size and increased myocyte nuclear area in hearts from the morbid obese are increased compared with normal controls.[79]

Another cause of sudden death in obesity is sleep apnea.[82] In obese persons with sleep apnea dying suddenly, the heart may be normal or enlarged, and there may be right ventricular hypertrophy and dilatation secondary to pulmonary hypertension. In order to assign a cause of death to sleep apnea, there must have been clinical documentation of the syndrome during life, and death must occur during sleep.

Arrhythmogenic Right Ventricular Dysplasia

Arrhythmogenic right ventricular dysplasia accounts for 20% of sudden cardiac death in parts of Italy, and only 1% in this country.[83] In a series of sudden unexpected death from Olmsted County,[5] Minnesota, features of arrhythmogenic right ventricular dysplasia were found in 17% of deaths, but in two thirds of these deaths the right ventricular findings were considered incidental.

Arrhythmogenic right ventricular dysplasia is familial in up to 50% of cases,[84–86] in which cases the mode of inheritance is autosomal dominant with variable penetrance. Most patients are under 40 years at the time of death, and some deaths occur in children. Clinically, patients have frequent and multiform premature ventricular contractions, which may result in ventricular tachycardia.[87] The propensity for arrhythmogenic right ventricular dysplasia to cause sudden death during excercise is well established; over 75% of deaths occur during exercise.[88, 89]

Pathologically, the right ventricule is dilated, and there is usually focal thinning (< 0.5 mm) of the muscular wall of the right ventricle (Fig. 10–11). Histologically, the right ventricle demonstrates areas of scarring and fatty infiltrates, which may be marked. If multiple sections of the ventricles are taken, characteristic fibrofatty areas with vacuolated myocytes will be demonstrated. Occasionally, the gross findings may be minimal.[90] For this reason, we recommend a minimum of three sections of right ventricular myocardium for histologic analysis in cases of exertion-related sudden death, in which the cause of death is not clear.

The distinction between pure fatty infiltration of the right ventricle and arrhythmogenic right ventricular dysplasia is still a matter of debate. We generally restrict the diagnosis of arrhythmogenic right ventricular dysplasia–cardiomyopathy to cases with both fat and fibrosis.[88] Pure fat infiltration of the right ventricle, when marked and involving more than the anterior wall, could be considered a potential cause of sudden death but is probably far less arrhythmogenic than the fibrofatty changes of arrhythmogenic right ventricular dysplasia. There are anecdotal case reports of massive fat infiltration of both ventricles and sudden cardiac death, however.[91]

Muscular Dystrophy

Myotonic form (Steinert's Disease)

Cardiac involvement in muscular dystrophy is characterized by electrocardiographic abnormalities and only rarely overt heart failure.[92] Patients with muscular dystrophy may develop extreme bradycardia and syncope that improves with pacemaker therapy. The cause of bradycardia in patients with muscular dystrophy may be

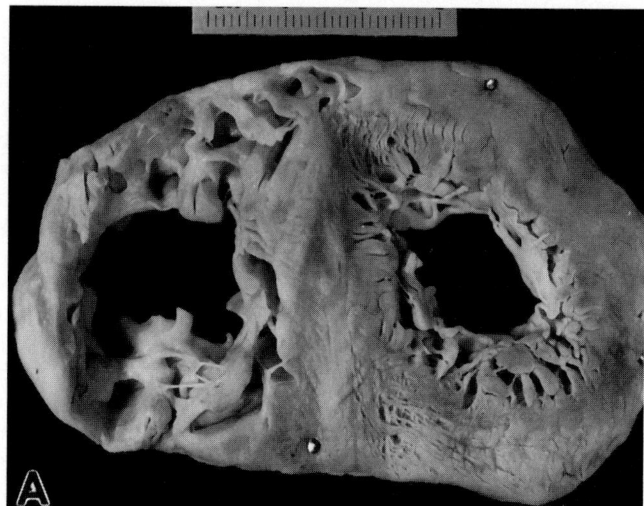

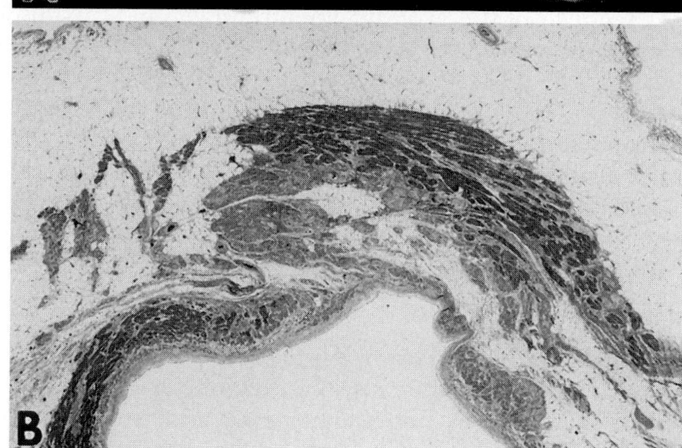

Figure 10–11. Right ventricular dysplasia. *A.* There is marked dilatation of the right ventricle, as demonstrated by this transverse section throughout the ventricles near the base of the heart. *B.* A histologic section demonstrates focal fatty infiltration with scarring. The patient was a 24-year-old man with a history of palpitations who died suddenly after running.

related to increase in vagal tone and diffuse myocardial lesions. Electrophysiologic studies have demonstrated impaired conduction at the level of the atrioventricular node.

Sudden death occurs in 4% of patients.[92] There are a few autopsy reports of fatty and fibrous replacement of sinoatrial and atrioventricular nodes, similar to changes that occur in the working myocardium. The mechanism of death is unknown in most cases, but has generally been attributed to bradyarrhythmias or tachyarrhythmias developing in the dystrophic myocardium, that is, areas of scarring and fatty replacement.

Severe coronary atheroslerosis is found in up to 50% of cardiac deaths in patients with myotonic muscular dystrophy, and must always be excluded, both clinically and at autopsy, in patients with muscular dystrophy and cardiac disease. Coronary involvement is coincidental and not considered related to the myopathy.

Duchenne Type

Duchenne's muscular dystrophy may involve the heart in the form of fibrosis, fat infiltration, and dilated cardiomyopathy. Sudden death may occur in the absence of dilated cardiomyopathy in as many as 27% of patients with Duchenne's muscular dystrophy.[93, 94] The mechanism of sudden death is presumed to be ventricular fibrillation, as these patients have a high prevalence of complex ventricular ectopy, especially those who die suddenly. Pathologic findings in cases of sudden death secondary to Duchenne's muscular dystrophy include myocardial fibrosis and fatty infiltration.[93, 94]

Right Ventricular Hypertrophy and Pulmonary Hypertension

Patients with idiopathic pulmonary hypertension are at an increased risk for sudden death, especially those with a history of syncope.[95] Syncopal episodes and sudden death generally occur at rest, but may be triggered by catheterization procedures and exercise. Sudden death has been reported in various types of primary pulmonary hypertension,[96] and is the initial symptom in up to 5% of cases in large series.[97, 98] For this reason, the pulmonary circulation should be carefully assessed in all cases of sudden unexpected death, especially if there is right ventricular hypertrophy.

Pulmonary hypertension secondary to congenital heart disease and pulmonary disease may also result in sudden death, presumably by a similar mechanism as primary pulmonary hypertension. The mechanism of sudden death in patients with pulmonary hypertension is most likely multifactorial, including the arrhythmogenic effects of the hypertrophied right ventricle complicated by anoxia-induced bradycardia.

Inflammatory Infiltrative and Miscellaneous Myocardial Causes of Sudden Death

Myocarditis

Lymphocytic Myocarditis

Generally considered a viral infection, lymphocytic myocarditis is the cause of sudden cardiac death in 15–20% of children and young adolescents, and somewhat less in young adults.[5, 12, 99, 100] In a study of sudden death in Air Force recruits, myocarditis was the major autopsy finding in 40% of cases.[101] In series of young adults from a general population, this proportion was under 5%.[72] This difference is probably due to the increased incidence of infectious diseases in a closely confined military population studied over a short period of time.

In cases of sudden death due to myocarditis, a preceding history of a flu-like illness is elicited in approximately 50% of cases. Grossly, the heart is generally normal; the classic soft texture is rarely obvious in our experience. In some cases, there may be a degree of cardiac dilatation, especially if there is an antecedent history of congestive heart failure. In cases of chronic myocarditis, areas of congestion or scarring may be present (Fig. 10–12). A pericardial effusion is often found.

Histologically, there is myocyte necrosis with an accompanying lymphocytic infiltrate. Scattered lymphocytes in the interstitium is not enough for the diagnosis; myocyte infiltration with degeneration and necrosis is a requirement. With exhaustive sampling of hearts from trauma victims, rare foci of myocyte necrosis with inflammation may occasionally be found; to make the unequivocal diagnosis of myocarditis, we prefer to identify a minimum of two foci in each section of myocardium examined (anterior, posterior, lateral left ventricle, ventricular septum, and right ventricle).

The degree of infiltration may be especially marked in infants and young children, and there may be scattered neutrophils and histiocytes, in addition to lymphocytes. Areas of scarring are not uncommon,[102] and are indicative of chronicity. Large areas of granulation tissue may be present in cases of extensive myocarditis and healing.

Serologic data suggest that many cases of lymphocytic myocarditis are caused by enteroviruses, especially Coxsackievirus type B3. The presence of virus within the myocardium is transitory; for this reason, viral cultures of pericardial fluid are rarely positive. Molecular biologic studies (RT-PCR) to identify RNA sequences specific for enteroviruses are currently hampered by lack of sensitivity and specificity.[103, 104] *In situ* hybridization for enteroviruses in human cases of myocarditis has been largely unrewarding.

Hypersensitivity Myocarditis

Hypersensitivity myocarditis is a relatively uncommon cause of sudden death, and is most often seen in middle-aged to elderly patients who are taking one or more medications. Clinically, hypersensitivity myocarditis may result in atrial and ventricular tachyarrhythmias, and sudden death has been reported.[105] Pathologically, there are interstitial infiltrates of histiocytes, eosinophils, lymphocytes, and Anitschkow cells. The amount of necrosis is variable, and may be negligible, mild, or moderate. Nonnecrotizing vasculitis of arterioles and arteries is common. Hypersensitivity myocarditis has been associated with a number of drugs, including antibiotics, antileptic drugs, antihistamines, benzodiazepines, antiinflammatory drugs, antimetabolites, diuretics, and antiarrhythmic agents.

Giant-Cell Myocarditis

Giant-cell myocarditis is an especially aggressive form of myocarditis that is characterized by chronic inflammation with numerous giant cells, widespread myocardial necrosis, and scarring (Fig. 10–13). Sudden death may occur sec-

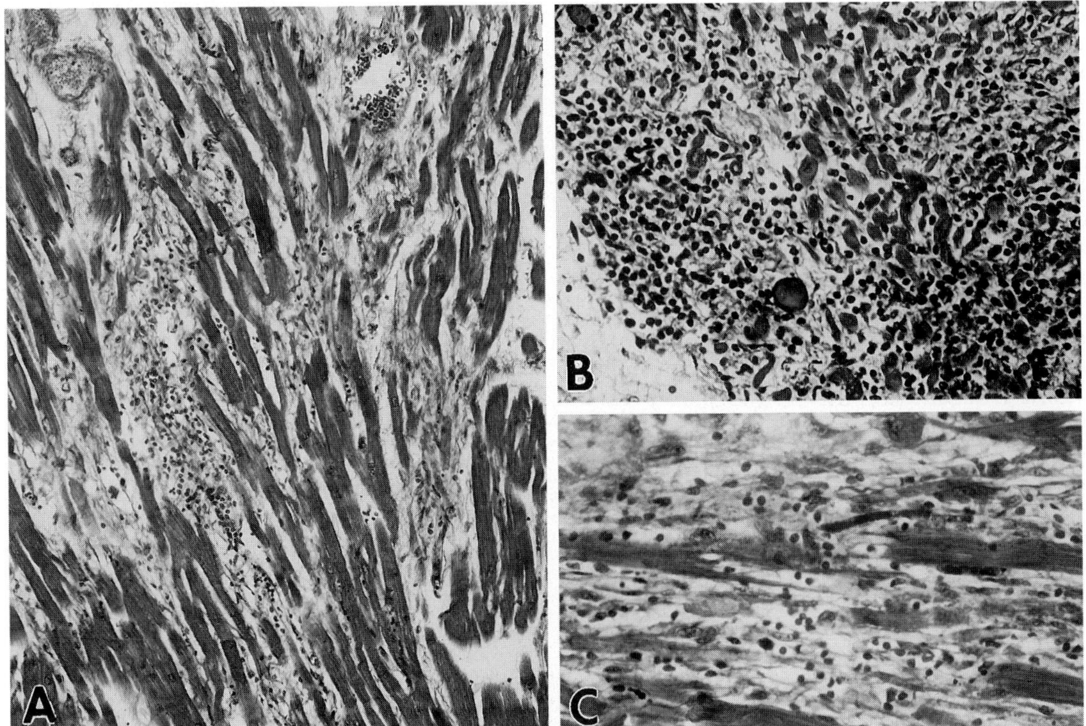

Figure 10–12. Lymphocytic myocarditis, ongoing. *A.* A low magnification of the myocardium demonstrates inflammation with areas of scarring and myocyte replacement. *B.* In areas of active inflammation, there are numerous lymphocytes replacing myocytes. *C.* Areas of myocytes necrosis with early replacement by fibrous tissue and scant lymphocytic infiltration. The patient was an 18-year-old black female who was found dead in bed. Three weeks prior, there was a history of a flu-like illness, with nausea and vomiting. The patient had not received medical attention and was feeling better in the days before death.

ondary to ventricular arrhythmias or acute heart failure.[106] The differential diagnosis is sarcoidosis, which generally involves mediastinal lymph nodes, lacks myocyte necrosis, and demonstrates well-formed granulomas.

Sarcoidosis

Approximately 2% of sudden deaths in young adults are caused by sarcoidosis.[107–110] Of patients who die suddenly with sarcoid, one third have no previous medical history, one third

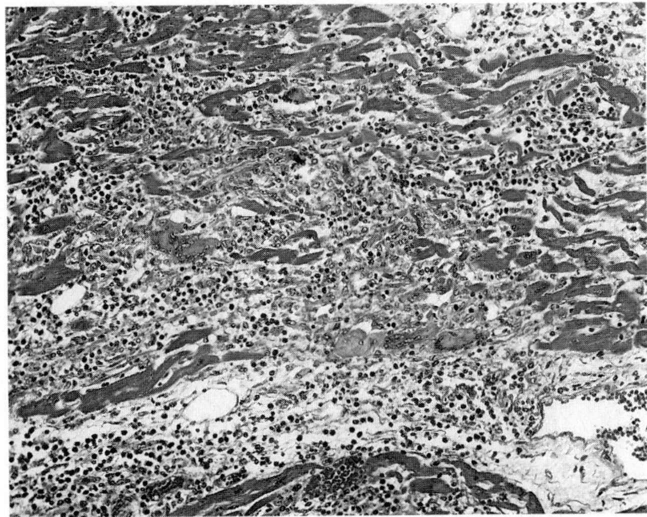

Figure 10–13. Giant-cell myocarditis. The section demonstrates marked inflammation with giant cells and destruction of myocytes. The patient was a 39-year-old woman with a 1-week history of fever, nausea, and generalized abdominal pain who died suddenly.

have a history of cardiac symptoms not attributed to sarcoid, and one third have a previous diagnosis of sarcoidosis.[111] In one large autopsy series of cardiac sarcoidosis, sudden death was the most frequent presenting symptom.[110]

Sarcoidosis affects the heart in 30% of patients with symptomatic pulmonary sarcoidosis, and may result in ventricular premature beats, ventricular tachycardia, and heart block. The left ventricle is involved in 100% of cases with cardiac involvement, and the interventricular septum in 95% of cases (Fig. 10–14). In virtually all cases, the granulomas are grossly evident, although occasionally they may be barely visible to the naked eye. Occasionally, granulomas may become encased by fibrosis, mimicking ischemic scars, and ventricular aneurysms may occur, especially towards the apex.

The differential diagnosis of sarcoidal granulomas includes infectious granulomas, giant-cell myocarditis, and myogenic giant cells surrounding healing infarct. Foreign body granulomas secondary to talc deposits in intravenous drug abusers are not so well-formed as sarcoidal granulomas, and will demonstrate foreign material when viewed with polarized light.

Idiopathic Left Ventricular Scars

Occasionally, the only cardiac finding in cases of sudden cardiac death is ventricular scarring,[102] in the absence of significant coronary artery disease or sarcoidosis. If the scars are subendocardial, it is likely that the scars are due to occult episodes of ischemia. Diffuse ventricular scars are likely related to healed myocarditis; extensive sectioning may reveal areas of ongoing inflammation. Subepicardial scars in the left ventricle are frequent in cases of right ventricular dysplasia,[88] and may also be present in cases of chronic myocardial emboli. Potential sources of emboli, especially on the cardiac

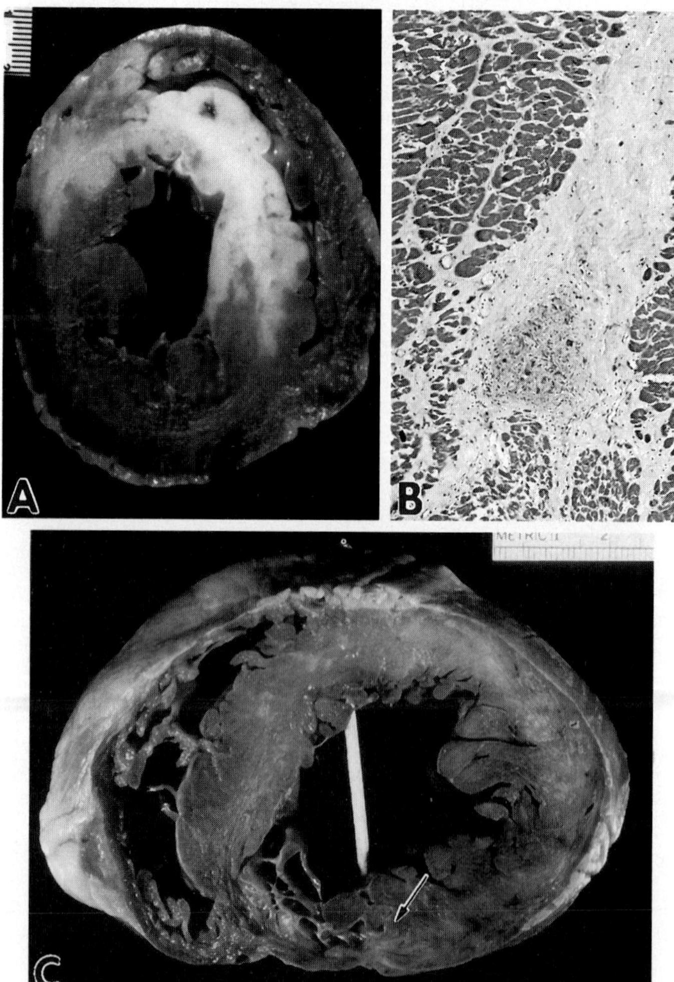

Figure 10–14. Cardiac sarcoidosis. *A.* The typical gross appearance is that of a firm, white area involving the ventricular septum. The patient was a 51-year-old black woman with no known history of sarcoid who died suddenly. Granulomas were noted in the lungs and mediastinal lymph nodes at autopsy. *B.* The histologic findings of cardiac sarcoid include dense scarring with scattered granulomas. *C.* Occasionally, the scarring of sarcoid may result in mural thinning mimicking a healed infarct (*arrow*). The patient was a 57-year-old black male with a history of hypercholesterolemia who died suddenly. At autopsy, the coronary arteries were normal. Histologically, the scar was infiltrated by granulomas (Fig. 10–14*B*); granulomas were also noted in the mediastinal lymph nodes.

valves, should always be excluded in cases of ventricular scarring without apparent etiology. Chronic abuse of cocaine and other drugs may result in ventricular fibrosis in the absence of coronary disease (see following). In a small proportion of remaining cases, the scars are idiopathic despite exhaustive investigation.

Catecholamine Toxicity/Pheochromocytoma

Patients with pheochromocytomas of the adrenal gland and functioning paragangliomas of extraadrenal sites[59,112] may die suddenly secondary to toxic release of catecholamines. Histologic findings in the heart include changes of toxic myocarditis, namely contraction band necrosis associated with areas of neutrophilic infiltrates (Fig. 10–15), and there may be platelet aggregates in the microcirculation. Chronic myocardial changes in patients with pheochromocytoma include small-vessel dysplasia and fibrosis of the conduction system.[59]

Anorexia Nervosa and Weight Reducing Diets

There are several anecdotal reports of sudden death in patients with anorexia nervosa or patients on weight-reducing diets.[113,114] The mechanism of death in most instances is presumed to be ventricular fibrillation, and there is an association between starvation, prolonged QT interval, and low serum potassium. Pathologically, hearts in patients dying from anorexia nervosa are generally small, with marked decrease in epicardial fat demonstrating serous atrophy. There is a decrease in myofibrillar size, and increase in lipofuschin, often imparting a bronze color to the myocardium. Ganglionitis in the epicardial atrial fat has been reported in association with liquid starvation diet.[114]

Cardiac Tumors and Fatty Infiltration

Virtually any cardiac tumor may cause sudden death.[115] There are a variety of mechanisms of sudden death, including rhythm disturbances generated by intramyocardial masses, embolization, and acute heart failure secondary to obstruction of blood flow.

In newborns and infants, cardiac fibromas, rhabdomyomas, and histiocytoid cardiomyopathy (Fig. 10–16) may be a cause of sudden cardiac death secondary to myocardial infiltration. All may result in ventricular arrhythmias, and rhabdomyoma may occasionally project into the chamber cavity causing acute obstruction of blood flow. Cardiac myxomas are generally found in adults, and present as sudden death in approximately 3% of cases[116] due to embolization to the coronary arteries, acute obstruction of the mitral valve, or cerebral embolization. Papillary fibroelastoma may result in transient or permanent coronary ischemia secondary to prolapse into the coronary ostium or embolization into the coronary circulation.[117] Other tumors that may cause sudden death in adults include cardiac hemangioma and cardiac sarcomas. In elderly adults, lipomatous hypertrophy of the atrial septum has been associated with atrial arrhythmias, and rarely sudden death.

Cocaine, Anabolic Steroids, and Sudden Death

The cardiovascular toxicity of cocaine includes acute myocardial infarction with and

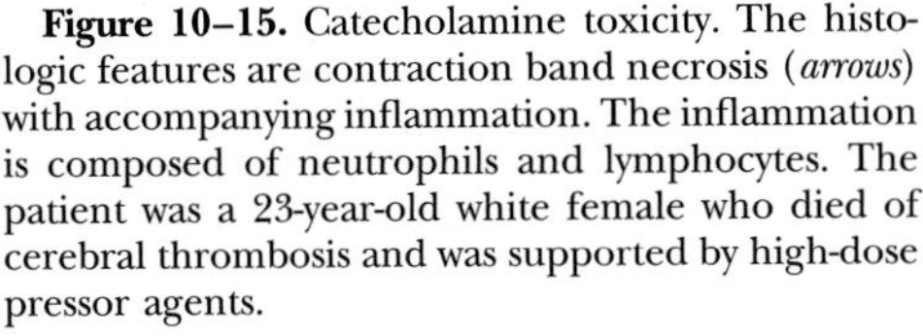

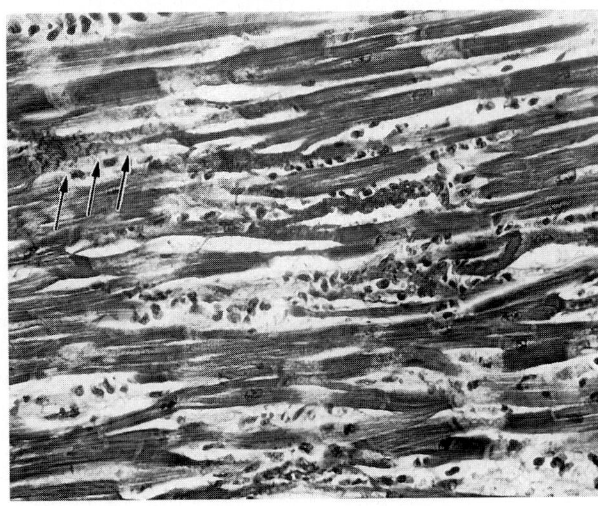

Figure 10–15. Catecholamine toxicity. The histologic features are contraction band necrosis (*arrows*) with accompanying inflammation. The inflammation is composed of neutrophils and lymphocytes. The patient was a 23-year-old white female who died of cerebral thrombosis and was supported by high-dose pressor agents.

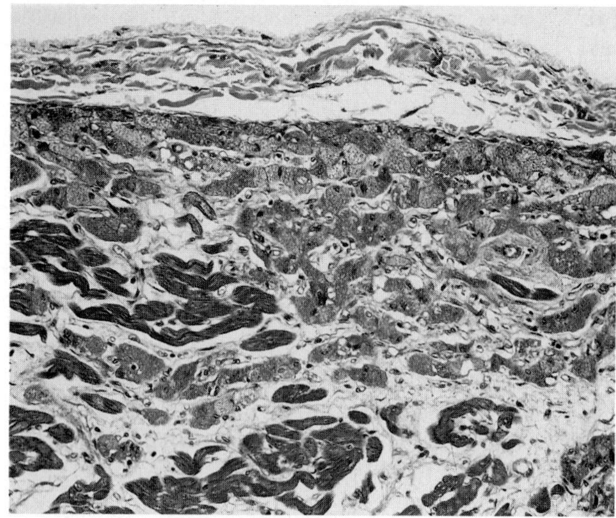

Figure 10–16. Histiocytoid cardiomyopathy. Note aggregates of pale, granular cells interspersed among normal myocytes and concentrated along the endocardium. The patient was a previously well 4-month-old infant who was found dead in his crib.

without atherosclerosis, ischemic or hemorrhage strokes, myocarditis, dilated cardiomyopathy, aortic dissection, cardiac dysrhythmias, and infective endocarditis.[118] The mechanism of cardiac damage includes sympathomimetic actions due to the inhibition of presynaptic reuptake of norepinephrine, coronary vasoconstriction due to alpha–adrenergic receptor activation, and increase in adventitial mast cells.[119] Clinical studies have demonstrated that cocaine increases the heart rate, elevates blood pressure, and results in epicardial vasoconstriction, especially with underlying atherosclerosis. In autopsy studies, the most frequent findings in cocaine-related deaths, in the absence of acute intoxication, are dilated cardiomyopathy, coronary atherosclerosis with thrombosis, and idiopathic scars.[120]

Sudden death has been reported with use of anabolic steroids.[121] Cardiac changes reported include myocardial hypertrophy, toxic myocarditis resembling cocaine cardiomyopathy, and myocardial infarction. There may be elevation of low-density lipoprotein and reduced high-density lipoprotein, platelet hypercoagulopathy, and coronary vasospasm in patients with chronic steroid use.

VALVULAR CAUSES OF SUDDEN CARDIAC DEATH

Mitral Valve Prolapse

Incidence of Sudden Death

While sudden death in patients with mitral valve prolapse and severe mitral regurgitation is not uncommon, the lifetime risk of sudden cardiac death in patients with mitral valve prolapse and competent valves is controversial. In two prospective studies, 1–3% of patients with mitral valve prolapse died from presumed ventricular arrhythmias.[122, 123] Because patients were referred to tertiary centers and were largely symptomatic, these studies exaggerate the true incidence of sudden death in asymptomatic persons with mitral valve prolapse. The percentage of autopsy-diagnosed sudden death cases that are a result of mitral valve prolapse is approximately 2% in young adults (see Tables 10–4 and 10–5). Although the rate of sudden death in patients with mitral valve prolapse is greater if mitral regurgitation is present,[124] most patients with mitral valve prolapse who survive prolonged ventricular tachyarrhythmias do not have significant mitral insufficiency.[125, 126]

Electrophysiologic Abrnomalities in Mitral Valve Prolapse

The patholophysiology of sudden cardiac death in mitral valve prolapse and competent valves is poorly understood. In most patients with mitral valve prolapse without significant mitral regurgitation in whom cardiac rhythms were recorded during successful or unsuccessful resuscitation, ventricular fibrillation was identified.[127, 128] Vectorcardiograms suggest that the majority of ventricular arrhythmias in patients with mitral valve prolapse arise in the posterior basilar septum of the left ventricle.[129] Patients with mitral valve prolapse who die suddenly often demonstrate ventricular premature depolarizations or couplets during life;[129] however, premature depolarizations does not reliably identify a subgroup of patients at increased risk of sudden death.

Bradycardia has also been documented in rare patients with mitral valve prolapse who survive cardiac arrest.[130] The incidence of QTc prolongation in patients with mitral valve prolapse is controversial and ranges from 26–91%; a recent comparison of patients with mitral valve prolapse to normal controls found no difference in the incidence of QTc prolongation or mean QT interval in the two group.[131] Rare conduction system abnormalities that have been demonstrated in patients with mitral valve prolapse include Wolff–Parkinson–White syndrome and atrioventricular block.[132]

In patients with mitral valve prolapse and mitral insufficiency, the mechanism of sudden death may involve heart failure and left ventricular hypertrophy. Epidemiologic and autopsy data suggest that the rate of sudden death in patients with mitral valve prolapse is greater if there is the complication of mitral regurgitation.[126]

Autopsy Studies of Mitral Valve Prolapse and Sudden Cardiac Death

Autopsy studies have provided several theories for sudden death in patients with mitral valve prolapse without mitral insufficiency. Endocardial friction lesions resulting in ventricular arrhythmias,[133] traction of an abnormally inserted valve on the conduction system,[134] and deposition of proteoglycans within the autonomic nerve supply to heart[135] have all been described in hearts from patients with mitral valve prolapse. We have demonstrated a high incidence of dysplasia of the atrioventricular nodal arteries in patients with mitral valve prolapse, and an association between thickened atrioventricular nodal arteries and fibrosis in the ventricular septum.[60] The pathologic features of mitral valve prolapse include elongation and hooding of the valve, especially posterior leaflet, chordal disarray and rupture, left atrial dilatation in cases of regurgitation, and endocardial friction lesions (Fig. 10–17).

In four autopsy series of mitral valve prolapse, the mean age of 68 patients with sudden death (and without evidence of mitral insufficiency) was 37 years, with no sex predilection (34 women, 34 men).[60, 133, 135, 136] Seventeen of these 68 individuals (25%) had a prior history of mitral valve prolapse, and 13 (19%) had a history of ventricular ectopy or syncopal episodes. Seven of these 68 patients (10%) collapsed during or immediately after exercise. We have noted that posterior leaflet length and thickness were greater in mitral valve prolapse heart from patients with symptomatic mitral valve prolapse or sudden death, compared with incidental cases of mitral valve prolapse.[136]

Aortic Stenosis

Incidence of Sudden Death

Sudden death was one of the most common causes of noncoronary sudden death before the advent of valve replacement surgery, and was the most common mode of death in patients with aortic stenosis, accounting for 73% of deaths.[137] Currently, because most patients are treated, aortic stenosis is only a minor cause of sudden death in young adults, accounting for only 2% of deaths (Tables 10–5 and 10–6). However, sudden death still accounts for about 20% of deaths after value surgery, peaking at 3 weeks after operation and plateauing after 8 months.[138] Overall, the rate of sudden death is low, estimated at 0.3% per year.[139] The risk for sudden death is increased in those patients with prior aortic stenosis and left ventricular hypertrophy, and those with multiple valve surgery.

Mechanisms of Sudden Death

The principal mechanism of sudden death in aortic stenosis appears to be due to arrhythmias complicating left ventricular hypertrophy. Other mechanisms include myocardial ischemia due to decreased cardiac output and poor diastolic coronary filling, diastolic compression of intramural coronary arteries,[140] and activation of left ventricular baroreceptors, which causes reflex bradycardia and cardiac arrhythmias. The supravalvar variant of congenital aortic stenosis in children is associated with coronary artery dysplasia,[141] which is an additional cause of myocardial ischemia in aortic stenosis. Rarely, heart block can result from calcification of the bundle of His in senile aortic stenosis.[142] There is an increased risk of aortic dissection and sudden death in patients with aortic stenosis secondary to a congenitally bicuspid or unicuspid aortic valve.

Pathologic Findings

All types of aortic stenosis may result in sudden unexpected death (Fig. 10–18); the patho-

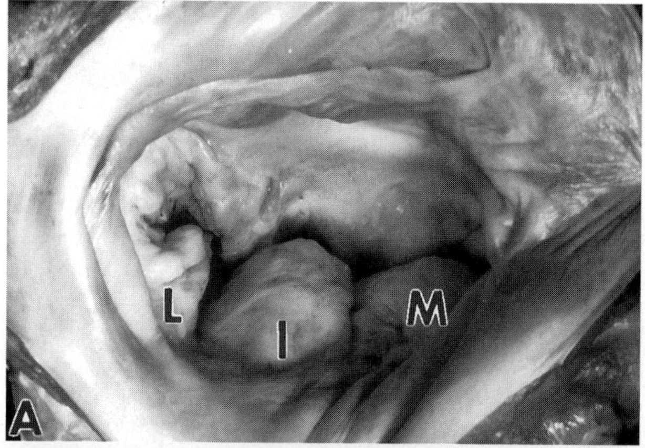

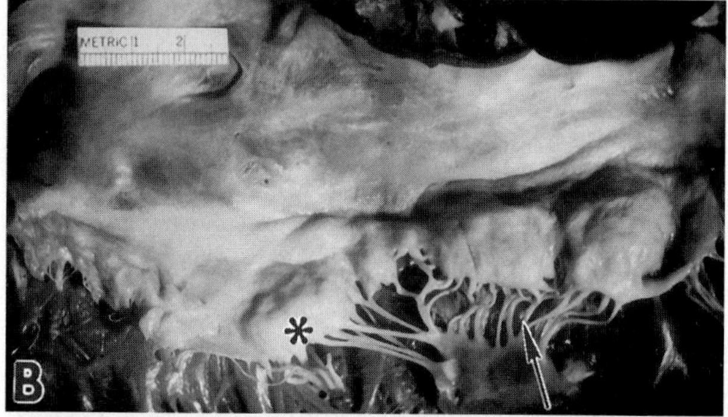

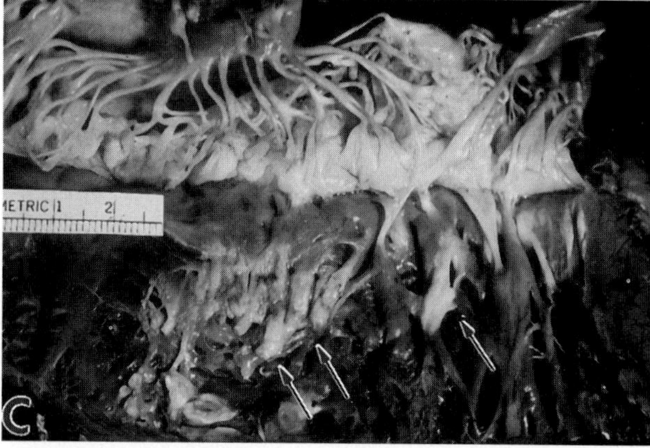

Figure 10–17. Mitral valve prolapse. *A.* The left atrium viewed from above demonstrates billowing and redundancy of the mitral valve, especially the three scallops of the posterior leaflet (*L* = lateral scallop, *I* = intermediate scallop, *M* = medical scallop). *B.* Opening the atrium demonstrates redundancy of the medial portion of the anterior leaflet (*asterisk*) and the posterior leaflet (*arrow*). *C.* Reflecting the valve reveals endocardial friction lesions (*arrows*). The patient was a 30-year-old previously healthy black male who was found dead at home.

logic features are described in Chapter 7. In adult cases of aortic stenosis first diagnosed at autopsy, there is generally marked left ventricular hypertrophy, as well as a critical stenosis of the valve, resulting in a tight opening that does not easily allow passage of a small finger. In cases of mild senile or rheumatic aortic stenosis without significant left ventricular hypertrophy, the valve findings should generally be considered incidental.

Miscellaneous Valvular Causes of Sudden Cardiac Death

Acute Endocarditis

Acute endocarditis may result in sudden cardiac death either by sudden valvular insufficiency and acute heart failure, or by coronary artery embolization. In series of sudden cardiac deaths, endocarditis accounts for approximately 2% of deaths in young adults (Tables

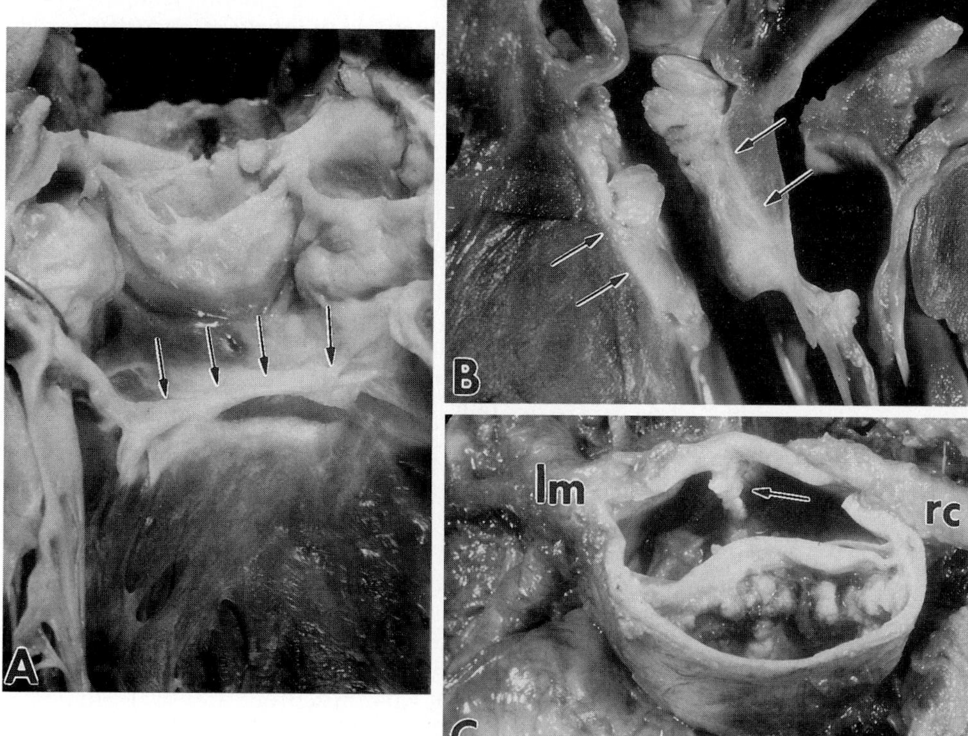

Figure 10–18. Aortic stenosis. Aortic stenosis of any morphologic type may result in sudden death. *A.* A discrete subaortic membrane (*arrows*) is present in this form of subaortic stenosis. The patient was a 15-year-old boy who died suddenly; he had had a resection of a subaortic membrane 9 years prior to death. *B.* The tunnel variety of subaortic stenosis is characterized by dysplasia of the aortic cusps and elongated area of subendocardial thickening (*arrows*). The patient was a 6-year-old boy with Down's syndrome who died suddenly while playing at the gymnasium. *C.* Calcification of a bicuspid aortic valve is a common cause of aortic stenosis in adults. Note the anterior placed raphe (*arrow*) dividing the anterior cusp into two portions containing the ostia of the right coronary (*rc*) and and left main (*lm*) coronary arteries. The patient was a 55-year-old man who died suddenly.

10–5 and 10–6). The most common valve involved is the aortic valve, followed by the mitral and tricuspid valves. A high percentage of patients have a history of intravenous drug abuse, and structurally abnormal valves are frequent in the aortic position (bicuspid, unicuspid valves).[143]

Rheumatic Valve Disease

Rheumatic mitral stenosis is the major cardiac finding in approximately 3% of cases of sudden death in young adults (see Table 10–5). The mechanism of death may involve ventricular arrhythmias secondary to right ventricular hypertrophy or acute heart failure. Aortic stenosis secondary to rheumatic valve disease may also result in sudden cardiac death (see earlier).

Heart Valve Prostheses

Between 7% and 38% of individuals with prosthetic valves die suddenly; the estimated yearly risk for sudden death ranges from 0.2%–0.9%.[144, 145] The causes of death in many cases is unknown because of the unavailability of autopsies. In the few publications with autopsy data on sudden cardiac deaths in patients with valvular prostheses, only 10–25% of deaths were related to malfunction of the prosthetic valve. Long-term clinical results after mitral valve replacement with the Bjork–Shiley prosthesis.[144–146] Valve-related causes of sudden death include valve thrombosis, embolization of valve thrombi, strut fracture, anticoagulation-related hemorrhage, perivalvular fistula, and left ventricular outflow obstruction. In the remaining majority of cases, the causes of death are ventricular arrhythmias secondary to cardiac hypertrophy and severe coronary atherosclerosis.

Congenital Heart Disease and Sudden Cardiac Death

Patients Without Prior Surgery

In children followed in cardiology clinics for known congenital heart disease, nonoperated patients account for 40–82% of sudden cardiac deaths[147,148]; this percentage is likely to decrease as cardiac surgery becomes more commonplace. The most common causes of sudden death in unoperated patients are pulmonary vascular obstructive disease, tetralogy of Fallot and other forms of pulmonary outflow tract obstruction, aortic stenosis, and hypertrophic cardiomyopathy. In infants only a few days old, a common cause of death is physiologic ductal closure in duct-dependent conditions, such as hypoplastic left-heart syndrome or some forms of pulmonary atresia. However, virtually all types of complex congenital heart disease may result in sudden unexpected death. Most children have severe limitation of activity or poor hemodynamic status and are at rest at the time of death.[147,148]

The mechanisms of sudden death in children with congenital heart disease are varied. In most patients, arrhythmias are documented in the year prior to death, although children with Eisenmenger syndrome and tetralogy of Fallot often do not have a prior history of arrhythmias when they die suddenly.[148] Bradyarrhythmias are a likely cause of sudden death in patients with pulmonary hypertension and hypoxic spells may result in bradyarrhythmias in patients with tetralogy and pulmonary outflow obstruction. Ventricular tachyarrhythmias and bradyarrhythmias may occur in patients with aortic stenosis. Patients with L-transposition of the great arteries are prone to develop spontaneous atrioventricular block and supraventricular and ventricular cardiac arrhythmias.[148]

Patients with Ebstein's anomaly have a high incidence of supraventricular and ventricular tachycardias, and Wolff–Parkinson–White syndrome. The incidence of sudden death in patients with Ebstein's anomaly is 20%, and remains high after surgery, necessitating prophylactic antiarrhythmic treatment.[149]

Operated Complex Congenital Heart Disease

The mechanisms of sudden in patients after surgery for congenital heart disease are multifactorial and complex, and may involve ventricular arrhythmias originating from the operative scar, acquired conduction disturbances, heart failure, cardiac hypertrophy, and pulmonary hypertension. If there is postoperative complete heart block, the risk of sudden death was as high as 60–80% before the institution of pacemaker therapy for these patients.[150] Tetralogy of Fallot and pulmonary atresia account for 33% of operated sudden deaths in two combined series,[147,148] followed by ventricular septal defect with pulmonary hypertension, atrioventricular canal defects, transposition of the great arteries, and a variety of other lesions. In a recent study, patients with corrected aortic stenosis, coarctation, transposition of the great arteries, or tetralogy of Fallot had a sudden death rate of 1/454 patients-years, compared with 1/7,154 patient-years for other defects. In this study, the risk of late sudden death increased incrementally 20 years after operation, and the causes of sudden death were arrhythmia in the majority of patients, followed by embolism, aneurysm rupture, and acute heart failure.[151]

The risk of sudden death after repair of tetralogy of Fallot has been extensively studied; sudden death occurs in 2–5% of patients followed for 20 years.[151–153] There is an increased incidence of right bundle branch block, left anterior hemiblock, transient complete atrioventricular block, and premature ventricular contractions in patients with tetralogy and previous surgical repair, but only those patients with premature ventricular contractions appear to be at an increased risk for sudden death.[154,155] Over 40% of patients with surgically corrected tetralogy experience significant ventricular dysrhythmias with treadmill exercise testing, suggesting that exercise may predispose to these arrhythmias. The risk for sudden death is increased if there is residual hemodynamic abnormalities, right ventricular dysfunction, and right ventricular hypertension. Decreased heart rate variability is associated with increased QRS complex duration, autonomic dysfunction, and increased risk of sudden death.[156] Only rarely is there injury to the specialized conduction system.

Supraventricular arrhythmias may degenerate into ventricular fibrillation following atrial surgical procedures. In patients with transposition of the great arteries and atrial switch procedures, there is an extremely high incidence of sick sinus syndrome and atrial arrhythmias, and patients are at increased risk for ventricular tachyarrhythmias. Patients with atrial flutter appear to be at increased risk for sudden death after atrial switch operation for transposition.[150]

PERICARDIAL CAUSES OF SUDDEN CARDIAC DEATH

Cardiac Tamponade

Etiology and Pathophysiology

Sudden death secondary to cardiac tamponade is a dramatic event that is readily diagnosed by the pathologist. The major causes are rupture of the ventricular free wall, ascending aorta, and rarely a coronary artery. Hemopericardium secondary to hemorrhagic pericarditis is generally of relatively gradual onset and does not cause sudden death. Acute cardiac tamponade may occur when there is sudden hemorrhage in a highly vascular pericardial tumors, such as Kaposi sarcoma.[157]

Hemopericardium results in impaired ventricular filling and reduced cardiac output. When massive—such as secondary to rupture of the heart, aorta, or coronary artery—electromechanical dissociation and sudden cardiac death occur.

Myocardial Rupture

Cardiac rupture generally results from acute myocardial infarction. The infarct almost always involves the left ventricular myocardium, although the epicardial rupture site may be located over the right ventricle or left atrium. Rarely, cardiac rupture may result as a complication of cardiac abscess.[158] A case of isolated ventricular rupture has been reported in the absence of myocardial necrosis, possibly precipitated by fatty infiltration.[159]

Direct cardiac rupture secondary to trauma occurs primarily from gunshot wounds and stab wounds, and usually involves the anterior wall of the right or left ventricle. In contrast, blunt trauma results from cardiac compression and affects all four chambers of the heart with equal frequency, and less commonly results in perforation by rib fracture. Because traumatic deaths are not natural, they are not considered in the spectrum of sudden unexpected cardiac death and will not be discussed further.

Iatrogenic forms of traumatic cardiac rupture may result from catheterization procedures, including insertion of pacemakers, and tamponade may be a delayed event.[160, 161] Puncture of the left ventricle or atrium may occur during transvenous approaches to valvoplasty and are often fatal.

Rupture of the Aorta

The most common cause of death from types I and II aortic dissections is cardiac tamponade, because the site of rupture of the false lumen is generally within the pericardial reflection. Less commonly, type III dissections (those with the intimal tear in the aortic arch or descending thoracic aorta) will rupture into the pericardial space; the majority of type III dissections rupture into the left hemothorax.

Rupture of Coronary Arteries

Currently, the most common cause of coronary artery rupture is instrumentation, especially angioplasty or rotational atherectomy.[162] Spontaneous rupture of the coronary artery may complicate myocardial abscess, congenital aneurysm, and dissecting aneurysm.[163–165]

THE CONDUCTION SYSTEM AND SUDDEN DEATH

Dissection of the Specialized Conduction System

Technique

Dissection of the specialized conduction system involves histologic evaluation of the sinoatrial node, atrioventricular node, penetrating bundle, and proximal bundle branches. The sinoatrial node is located, in most hearts, lateral to the anterior junction of the superior vena cava and the right atrial appendage, parallel and superior to the crista terminalis. Often, the artery supplying the sinoatrial node can be grossly visualized, aided by a dissecting microscope; histologically, the node will be present surrounding this artery.

The atrioventricular node is usually approached from the right atrium and ventricle, where the landmarks of the triangle of Koch may be identified. A wedge of tissue, including a portion of the atrial and ventricular septum and the membranous septum, is excised, and the entire tissue is processed and embedded in paraffin with serial sectioning, requiring examination of hundreds of sections. In our laboratory, we evaluate three to five blocks of tissue, and utilize selective and semiserial sectioning to reduce the total number of sections required.

Indications for Histologic Examination of the Conduction System

If examination of the coronary arteries, cardiac valves, and myocardium does not reveal a potential cause of sudden death, an examination of the conduction system should be performed, especially for an witnessed arrest or if there was a history of heart block. In only a small proportion of these cases is a definitive cause of death found on examination of the specialized conduction system.

Pathologic Conditions Involving the Conduction System

Bypass Tracts and Preexcitation Syndromes

Patients with preexcitation syndromes are prone to paroxysmal supraventricular tachycardias that are generally not life threatening. However, if the anomalous tracts have short refractory periods, atrial fibrillation may trigger ventricular fibrillation, especially if there is a familial tendency.[166–168]

The anomalous atrioventricular connections in the Wolff–Parkinson–White syndrome are remote from the atrioventricular node (Kent/Paladino bundles) and may be localized by electrophysiologic testing during life. The incidence of sudden death in patients with Wolff–Parksinon–White syndrome is estimated to be less than 1 per 100 patient-years follow-up; 70% of patients who experience ventricular tachyarrhythmias have a previous history of symptoms.[169] In symptomatic patients, curative ablative therapy prevents recurrent arrhythmias, including atrial fibrillation. In cases of sudden death in patients with known Wolff–Parkinson–White syndrome, histologic confirmation of the bypass tract is tedious, often unrewarding, and unnecessary. Because of the rarity of sudden death in this syndrome, other cardiac and noncardiac causes of death must be carefully ruled out.

Other preexcitation syndromes are characterized by bypass tracts that occur in the vicinity of the atrioventricular node. James fibers, or atriohisian fibers, bypass the atrioventricular node and connect the atrial myocardium to the bundle of His; these were originally described in normal hearts. There is a putative association between James fibers and the Lown–Ganong–Levine syndrome, characterized by short PR interval, normal QRS complex, and tachycardias; anatomic confirmation of these fibers has been lacking, however. Mahaim fibers, or nodoventricular or nodofascicular fibers, connect the atrioventricular node into the left ventricle or right bundle branch. These and accessory tracts between the bundle of His into the ventricle (fasciculoventricular tracts) are a normal finding, in adults as well as infants.[170]

Atrioventricular Nodal Block

Congenital AV Nodal Block

Primary fibrosis of the conduction system in the absence of structural heart disease is commonly associated with intraventricular conduction abnormalities and symptomatic atrioventricular block, and less commonly with sudden cardiac death. Congenital AV block is likely an interplay between hereditary factors (it is often familial) and acquired ones (there is an association with maternal Ro and La antibodies in about 30% of cases). The identification of patients at risk for sudden death is controversial, as well as the efficacy of pacemakers for preventing sudden death. Histologically, there is diffuse scarring of the atrioventricular node and bundle branches, often with a sparse lymphocytic infiltrate.[171–174] In most cases, there is destruction of the AV nodal region, resulting in atrial–axis discontinuity and nodoventricular discontinuity. The defect is rarely limited to the bundle branches, and if bundle branch disease is present, it is associated with nodal disease.

Acquired Fibrosis

Idiopathic bilateral bundle branch fibrosis is referred to as Lev's disease when the branching bundle is involved and Lenegre's disease when middle and distal bundle branches are solely involved.[174, 175] Lev's disease may represent an accelerated form of age-related destruction of the left bundle branch, whereas Lenegre's disease is often associated with cardiomegaly. Patients are usually over 40 years of age, and sudden death is rarely the presenting symptom.

Extension of scarring of the aortic root and aortic valve into the conduction system has been described in seronegative spondyloarthropathies associated with HLA B27. Occasionally, cardiac symptoms, even sudden death, may predate the rheumatologic symptoms.

Acquired heart block may be iatrogenic in patients who have undergone radioablation to the atrioventircular node. Indications for AV junction ablation include atrial fibrillation with poor control of ventricular rate by medical treatment, and other less common atrial arrhythmias; a pacemaker is inserted after the ablation for control of heart rate. There is an increased risk for sudden unexplained death in patients with any form of atrioventricular block,[171, 172] the mechanistic basis of which is not entirely understood. Unexplained sudden death after atrioventricular junction ablation has been estimated at about 1% of patients per year.[176]

Myocarditis

Rarely, myocarditis may be localized to the area of the atrioventricular node, resulting in progressive atrioventricular nodal block and sudden death[173] (Fig. 10–19). Intrauterine atrioventricular nodal block is often a result of antinuclear autoantibodies in maternal lupus and results histologically in inflammation, fibrosis, and calcification of the atrioventricular nodal area. Other autoimmune disorders may result in atrioventricular nodal block in adults, including scleroderma, polyarteritis, and rheumatoid arthritis.

Calcification of the Atrioventricular Node

Atrioventricular nodal calcification may result in atrioventricular nodal block in patients with extensive annular calcification of the mitral valve, calcific aortic stenosis, hypercalcemia with dystrophic calcification, and Paget's disease of bone.[173]

Cystic Atrioventricular Nodal Tumor

This rare lesion, which almost invariably results in atrioventricular block, may present as sudden death (Fig. 10–20). It occurs exclusively in the area of the AV node, tricuspid valve, and inferior atrial septum, and is composed of cysts lined by transitional, cuboidal, squamous, or mixed epithelium. Cystic AV nodal tumors are endodermally derived, and not of mesothelial origin, as previously believed.

Miscellaneous Findings

A variety of nonspecific findings in the conduction system have been associated with unexplained sudden cardiac death. As discussed ear-

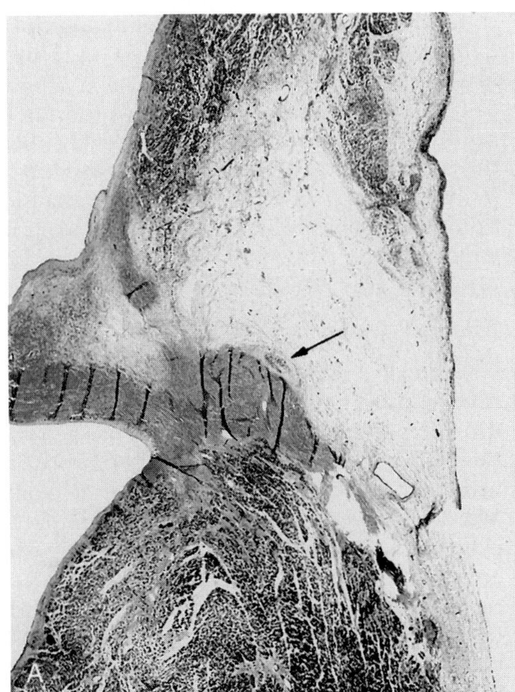

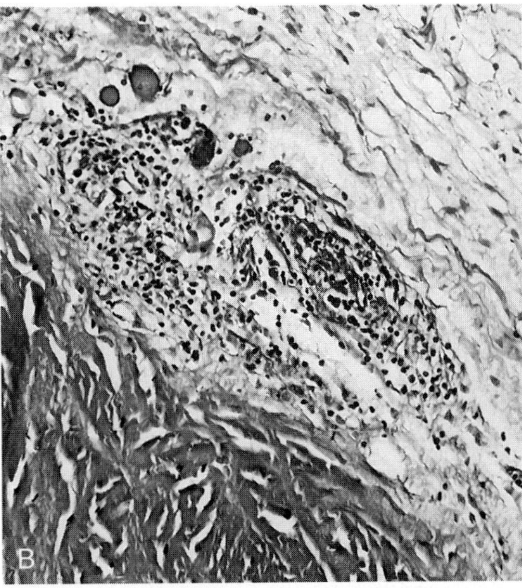

Figure 10–19. Inflammation of the atrioventricular node. *A.* There is extensive fatty replacement of the atrioventricular node, a remnant of which is present at the tip of the *arrow. B.* A higher magnification demonstrates residual nodal tissue with a lymphocytic infiltrate. The atrial approaches to the atrioventricular node were likewise replaced by inflammatory infiltrates. There was no inflammation in five sections of ventricular myocardium sampled. The patient was a 37-year-old schizophrenic on no medications, who was recently diagnosed with complete heart block. She expired suddenly while dancing three days after her doctor's visit.

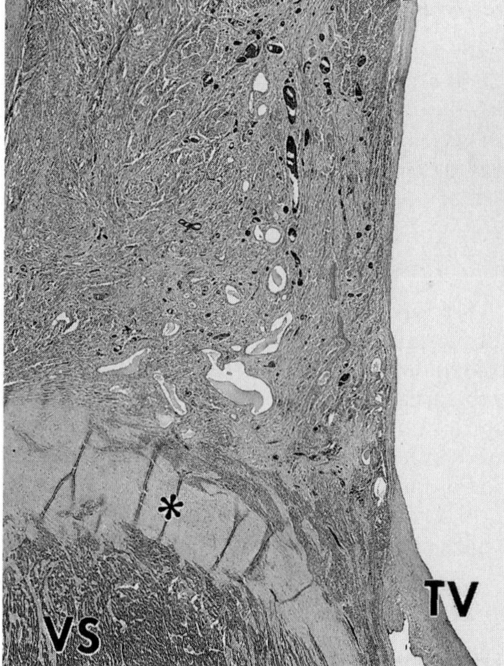

Figure 10–20. Cystic tumor of the atrioventricular node. Note multiple cysts in the area of the atrioventricular node on the atrial aspect of the central fibrous body (*asterisk*). The tricuspid valve (*TV*) is present along the right side of the ventricular septum (*VS*). The patient was a 7-year-old black male who was found dead in bed. He had a history of congenital heart block treated by a pacemaker.

lier, dysplastic narrowing of the atrioventricular nodal artery may be an incidental finding. Because it is more frequent in patients dying unexpectedly with no autopsy findings, it may contribute to sudden death.[58] Other conditions that have been anecdotally seen in conduction systems of patients dying suddenly include ganglionitis of the sinoatrial node,[177] septation and disorganization of the atrioventricular nodal bundles,[178] fatty replacement of the atrioventricular node,[92] hemorrhage within conduction system structures, and increased vascularity of the atrioventricular node.[179] A controlled study has demonstrated that AV nodal septation is seen as frequently in trauma deaths as in unexplained sudden deaths.[170]

Sudden Cardiac Death in the Absence of Autopsy Findings

Idiopathic Ventricular Arrhythmias

In some cases of sudden death, there is no explanation for ventricular tachyarrhythmias despite a thorough cardiac examination and forensic autopsy. It has been suggested that the term "sudden unexpected death syndrome," or SUDS, be used for idiopathic ventricular arrhythmias.[14]

The true nature of idiopathic ventricular arrhythmias will be elucidated only when there is a more complete understanding of the electrophysiologic bases for cardiac arrhythmias and their morphologic substrates. It is possible that a proportion of these deaths are due to coronary spasm and conduction disturbances, that are not readily diagnosed at autopsy. In approximately 10% of patients resuscitated from a cardiac arrest unassociated with myocardial infarct, no identifiable structural heart disease will be found; some of these patients will demonstrate long Q-T intervals, preexcitation, or bradycardia on electrophysiologic studies.[180] Blunt impact to the chest from hockey pucks and baseballs has been implicated as a triggering mechanism of fatal ventricular arrhythmias in apparently normal hearts "commotio cordis."[181]

There are cultural associations with idiopathic sudden death in young people, usually men. Related syndromes include Pokkuri in young Japanese males, Nonlaitai in young Laotian males, and Bangungut in young Filipino males.[182–184]

The forensic pathologist should be aware of a number of mimickers of sudden cardiac death; these include cafe coronaries (obstruction of food in the larynx), drug intoxication, amniotic fluid embolism, pulmonary hypertension, and air embolism.

Long Q-T Syndrome

Clinically, there are two forms of this syndrome: inherited and acquired. The inherited disease is autosomal recessive and has two varieties: the Jervell and Lange–Nielsen syndrome, with associated deafness, and the Romano–Ward syndrome, without deafness. Patients especially at risk of sudden death are female, deaf, and have a prior history of ventricular fibrillation or torsades de pointes. Histologically, a variety of nonspecific findings have been found in the conduction system, including fatty replacement, inflammation, and scarring of the atrioventricular node and bundle branches. The only reason to perform a conduction system in patients dying with known long Q-T syndrome is to exclude other abnormalities, as the heart is usually grossly and histologically normal.

The basic defect in the inherited long Q-T syndrome is related to a mutation coding for one of the cardiac myocyte ion channels. The classification of the syndrome is now largely based on the genotype.[10, 185] At least four genes are involved: KVLQT1, HERG, and Min K encode for cardiac potassium ion channels, and SCN5A encodes for the cardiac sodium ion channel. The altered ion channel function produces prolongation of the action potential and propensity to torsade de pointes ventricular tachycardia.[186] Delayed ventricular repolarization and profound bradycardia are considered to be the substrates for polymorphous ventricular tachycardia and ventricular fibrillation responsible for sudden cardiac death in patients with long Q-T syndrome. Because the measurement of the Q-T interval is not entirely straightforward and must be based on a value corrected for heart rate, the clinical diagnosis may be difficult, and up to 10% of cases may be missed even with electrocardiographic testing. For this reason, and because long Q-T syndrome cannot be diagnosed at autopsy, it is unknown what proportion of sudden deaths with normal cardiac findings are due to the syndrome. Based on clinical evaluation of individuals who survive out-of-hospital arrest, approximately 5% will have no cardiac findings, and of these, only a minority will demonstrate long Q-T syndrome.[187–190]

Acquired long Q-T syndrome may be due to drug idiosyncrasies, especially antiarrhythmics and psychotrophic drugs, including lithium. There are a variety of other predisposing factors, including electrolyte abnormalities, hypothermia, toxic substances, central nervous system injury, weight-reduction programs, liquid protein diets, and anorexia nervosa. There are no histologic features specific to this syndrome, which must be diagnosed by electrocardiography. Ganglionitis has been described in a patient with long Q-T syndrome who had been on a liquid fast diet.[114]

The autopsy diagnosis of long Q-T syndrome may now be accomplished by genetic analysis with sequencing of potential culprit genes, especially the KVLQT1 gene. In selected cases with a strong suspicion, such as unexplained drowning deaths or patients with a family history of unexplained sudden death or long Q-T syndrome, sequencing of the KVLQT1 or other candidate genes may be possible.[191, 192] Technically, sequencing of long fragments of DNA is difficult on formalin-fixed tissues, and frozen tissues are preferred.

Brugada Syndrome

Patients with idiopathic ventricular arrhythmias and idiopathic sudden death form a heterogeneous group. Some patients with unexplained ventricular fibrillation and sudden death demonstrate resting electrocardiograms with right bundle branch block and ST segment elevations in leads V1-3, constituting the Brugada syndrome.[193] It is unclear whether this syndrome is a subset of arrhythmogenic right ventricular dysplasia.[194, 195] The electrocardiographic features of Brugada syndrome is also mimicked by right ventricular ischemia and tricyclic drug overdoses.[196] At this time, the forensic pathologist should, in cases of suspected Brugada syndrome, be careful to rule out right ventricular dysplasia with multiple right ventricular sections, and rule out intoxication with neuroleptic drugs, before ascribing the death to idiopathic ventricular arrhythmia.

EXERCISE AND SUDDEN CARDIAC DEATH

Incidence and Causes of Sudden Death in Athletes

The incidence of sudden death during athletic activity is low, ranging from 1/13,000 man-hours of activity in cross-country skiing to 1 in 396,000 man-hours of activity in jogging.[197–199] The latter figure is approximately seven times the risk of sudden death at rest. In large series of sudden cardiac deaths, the proportion of deaths that occur during exercise is approximately 5% (88), although in a population of recruits, who spend much of their time in strenuous activity, this proportion may be near 75%.[101] In exercising individuals over 35 years of age, atherosclerosis is by far the most frequent finding in sudden cardiac death,[200–203] whereas in individuals under that age, hypertrophic cardiomyopathy, idiopathic left ventricular hypertrophy, right ventricular dysplasia, and coronary artery anomalies are more common.[204–207] In the most recent series of 158 young competitive athletes in the U.S. who died suddenly, the autopsy diagnoses were hypertrophic cardiomyopathy (36%), coronary artery anomalies (19%), idiopathic left ventricular hypertrophy (10%), tunneled coronary artery (5%), rupture aortic aneurysm (5%), aortic stenosis (4%), right ventricular dysplasia (3%), myocarditis (3%), coronary artery disease (2%), and other (11%).[100, 208] In Italy, as noted earlier, right ven-

Table 10–7. Causes of Sudden Cardiac Death in Runners

Pathologic Finding	n	%	Mean Age
Coronary atherosclerosis	96	79%	43
None (idiopathic arrhythmia)	12	10%	—
Hypertrophic cardiomyopathy	6*	4%	32
Tunnel coronary artery	2	2%	44
Idiopathic ventricular scarring	2	2%	—
Myocarditis	1	1%	—
Idiopathic left ventricular hypertrophy	1	1%	—
Mitral valve prolapse	1	1%	27
Aortic stenosis	1	1%	—
TOTAL	122		

* 2 patients had concomitant severe coronary atherosclerosis
—data not available
Adapted from Virmani R, Roberts WC. Sudden cardiac death. Hum Pathol 18:485–492, 1987.

tricular dysplasia is a far more common cause of exercise-related death than in the United States.

In runners, who are often older men who are maintaining fitness, the cause of sudden cardiac death is atherosclerotic coronary disease in nearly 80% of cases (Table 10–7), whereas this proportion is only 40% in sports-related deaths in nonrunners (Table 10–8).[201, 202] This difference largely reflects the older mean age of runners as compared with individuals engaged in other athletic activities (Tables 10–3 and 10–4). Similar to sudden deaths in nonexercising individuals, there is a small but significant proportion of idiopathic ventricular arrhythmias in exercise-related sudden cardiac deaths, especially in children (Tables 10–3 and 10–4).

In approximately 50% of exercise-related deaths in young athletes, there is no prior history of heart disease, arrhythmias, or syncope. Therefore, in many cases of hypertrophic cardiomyopathy, coronary artery anomalies, and arrhythmogenic right ventricular dysplasia, the diagnosis will be suspected first at autopsy. Athletes with any history of syncope or arrhythmias, or family history of premature cardiac death, should be evaluated with electrocardiograms and echocardiography, which will detect most cases of hypertrophic cardiomyopathy and right ventricular dysplasia. Coronary artery anomalies are more difficult to detect, and athletes dying with anomalous left main ostia may have entirely normal echocardiograms and stress electrocardiograms prior to death. Transesophageal echocardiography is a relatively noninvasive technique, short of angiography, to make the diagnosis, although advances in transthoracic echocardiography have led to a high level of success in visualizing the coronary ostia of athletes.[209] Although limited screening of nonsymptomatic athletes without a suggestive family history is justified, the usefulness and cost-effectiveness of 12-lead electrocardiogram and echocardiography has not been established.[208]

Table 10–8. Causes of Sudden Cardiac Death in Sporting Activities Other than Running

Pathologic Finding	n	%	Mean Age
Coronary atherosclerosis	151	41%	45
None (idiopathic arrhythmia)	61	17%	13
Hypertrophic cardiomyopathy	51	14%	32
Idiopathic left ventricular hypertrophy	30	8%	—
Myocarditis	23	6%	16
Anomalous coronary arteries	23	6%	22
Mitral valve prolapse	11	3%	27
Right ventricular dysplasia	11	3%	19
Aortic stenosis	2	0.5%	—
Tunnel coronary artery	1	0.3%	—
Mitral stenosis	1	0.3%	—
TOTAL	365		

—data not available
Adapted from Virmani R, Roberts WC. Sudden cardiac death. Hum Pathol 18:485–492, 1987.

In the differential diagnosis of causes of exertion-related sudden death is heat stroke. Ventricular arrhythmias may be precipitated by hyperthermia, especially in African Americans who are heterozygous for hemoglobin S.[210, 211] In such cases, careful assessment of rectal temperature, ambient humidity and temperature, and presence of sickling on histologic preparations is essential. Other factors that increase the likelihood of heat-related illness is increased body mass index.[212]

The Athlete's Heart

Chronic conditioning may result in both increased left ventricular wall thickness, ventricular dilatation, and a 20–40% increase of cardiac mass.[213–215] Isotonic training results in increased ventricular stroke volume and left end-diastolic volume, with unchanged mass-to-volume ratio, whereas isometric conditioning results in increased left ventricular mass and increased mass-to-volume ratio. It may be difficult to determine whether cardiac hypertrophy in athletes is a physiologic or pathologic process.[216] In general, we consider only severe hypertrophy (> 95% confidence interval by height or weight) as a potential cause of death in athletes. In up to 20% of athletes dying suddenly,[72, 73] there was significant concentric left ventricular hypertrophy that was considered the likely cause of death.

Sinus bradycardia, first-degree atrioventricular block, voltage criteria for left ventricular hypertrophy, and incomplete right bundle branch block can frequently be observed with electrocardiography in athletes.[217, 218] Benign ventricular arrhythmias occur among athletes with the same frequency as in the general population, but they are usually suppressed during exercise-induced increases in sinus rate. These electrophysiologic changes are considered physiologic and do not impart an increased risk of sudden death.

There are several series of atherosclerosis-related-sudden deaths in athletes.[208, 209, 211, 218, 226] Prodromal cardiac symptoms of chest pain and risk factors for coronary artery disease were present in over 50% of these individuals. The cardiac findings at autopsy in exercise-related atherosclerotic sudden death by definition include at least one major epicardial artery narrowed at least 75% in cross-sectional area. A compilation of autopsy studies[72, 200, 201, 203–205, 219, 220] reveals that 48% had healed infarcts; 17%, acute infarcts; 28%, one-vessel disease; 33%, two-vessel disease; 39%, three-vessel disease; 25%, coronary artery thrombi; and 69%, cardiomegaly. Recently, we have shown that in sudden coronary death due to atherosclerosis, acute plaque rupture is much more common than in coronary deaths that occur during rest.[221] The association between acute rupture and exertion is limited to men, especially those with elevated serum cholesterol.

Exercise may provoke sudden death in patients with underlying atherosclerosis,[197, 199] but conditioned individuals have an overall lower risk of sudden death than sedentary individuals.[222] Extreme forms of conditioning, including marathon running, do not prevent severe atherosclerosis and sudden death[223] but may result in coronary artery dilatation.[224]

The Effect of Exertion on Causes of Sudden Cardiac Death

Regardless of physical conditioning, exercise-induced tachycardia may predispose to sudden death in patients with atherosclerotic coronary artery disease,[225] right ventricular dysplasia,[88, 89] hypertrophic cardiomyopathy,[65] and anomalous coronary arteries.[31, 211, 226] The mechanism of tachycardia-induced sudden death involves decrease in threshold for ventricular fibrillation, especially in structurally abnormal hearts, increased levels of catecholamines, and rapid changes in plasma potassium.[227] The association between exercise and sudden death is especially marked in right ventricular dysplasia and aberrant left coronary artery from the right sinus of Valsalva, in which over 50% of deaths are exertion-related. Conditions that are known to predispose to arrhythmias and sudden death during exercise and that are contraindications to strenuous activity include hypertrophic cardiomyopathy, idiopathic left ventricular hypertrophy, Marfan syndrome, coronary artery disease, congestive heart failure, coronary artery anomalies, high-grade ventricular arrhythmias, aortic and pulmonary stenosis, aortic coarctation, acute myocarditis, idiopathic long Q-T syndrome, cyanotic congenital heart disease, and pulmonary hypertension.[215]

ARRHYTHMIAS ASSOCIATED WITH SUDDEN CARDIAC DEATH

Ventricular Tachyarrhythmias

Pathophysiology

A large proportion of sudden cardiac deaths are caused by ventricular tachycardia and fibrillation triggered by focal ventricular lesions. The basic mechanism for the initiation of ventricular arrhythmias is hypothesized to be impulse reentry, although this has yet to be proved.[8] Although a portion of the specialized conduction system, particularly the bundle branches, may be involved, most reentry foci are less than 1.4 cm^2 and are within the ventricular myocardium.[228] The pathophysiologic mechanisms of reentry have been most extensively studied in the setting of ischemic heart disease.[228] Other electrophysiologic mechanisms involved in the initiation of ventricular arrhythmias are automaticity of pacemaker fibers, transformation of nonpacemaker into pacemaker fibers, and injury currents. The pathophysiology of ventricular arrhythmias in diffuse ventricular diseases, such as dilated cardiomyopathy and concentric left ventricular hypertrophy, is poorly understood, and most likely multifactorial.

Acute Ischemia

An increased risk of sudden cardiac death after acute myocardial infarction is well known, and the mechanism of death is usually ventricular fibrillation. Many factors contribute to the development of ventricular fibrillation after ischemia, including size of the ischemic area, presence and extent of previous infarction, left ventricular function, heart rate, and activity of the autonomic nervous system.[229] Experimentally, the effects of ischemia at the cellular level include loss of cell membrane integrity, efflux of potassium ion, influx of calcion ion, acidosis, reductions of transmembrane resting potentials, and enhanced automaticity.[230] The destabilizing effects of acute ischemia are more pronounced in the working myocardium than the specialized conduction tissues, which are relatively resistant to acute ischemia. Reperfusion of ischemic tissue may produce continued influx of calcium ions and formation of superoxide radicals. Topological patterns of ischemic damage may result in reentrant loops; for example, a surviving epicardial layer of tissue or viable islands of myocardium may serve as substrates for reentry tachyarrhythmias.[230] Acute ischemic damage may also result in increased automaticity of the working myocardium, resulting in ventricular tachycardia from a mechanism unrelated to reentry.[184] Tissue healed after previous injury appears to be more susceptible to the electrical destabilizing effects of acute ischemia.[8]

Infiltrative Diseases and Cardiac Hypertrophy

Ventricular tachycardias secondary to reentry arrhythmias may result from microscopic or macroscopic scars. Patients with myocardial scars related to healed infarction, cardiomyopathy, previous cardiac surgery, tumors, and a variety of inflammatory conditions are prone to ventricular tachyarrhythmias. Sudden death in most cases of myocarditis is secondary to ventricular tachyarrhythmias in the absence of congestive heart failure; the mechanism of these arrhythmias is unclear. The mechanism of ventricular fibrillation in patients with ventricular hypertrophy is likewise unclear; the nature of the interaction between myocardial hypertrophy and ventricular fibrillation is incompletely understood.[228] There is likely a diverse group of mechanisms including subendocardial ischemia, reentry secondary to small foci of scarring, and others.

Cardiac Failure

Heart failure of any cause may predispose to a variety of arrhythmias, including ventricular premature beats, ventricular tachyarrhythmias, and left intraventricular conduction defects. Approximately one half of patients with congestive heart failure die suddenly, presumably from a ventricular tachyarrhythmia.[74] The pathophysiology of ventricular arrhythmias in patients with heart failure is undoubtedly multifactorial, and may involve enhanced levels of autonomic sympathetic activation, electrolyte disturbances, conduction disturbances, and foci of ventricular fibrosis or ischemia.

Miscellaneous Factors Predisposing to Ventricular Arrhythmias

A variety of noncardiac factors predispose to ventricular ectopy and ventricular tachycardia or fibrillation.[231] These include hemodynamic failure, hypoxemia, acidosis, electrolyte imbalance, fatty liver, diabetes mellitus, and alcohol intoxication.[232] Other factors facilitating ventricular fibrillation include preexcitation syndromes, long Q-T syndrome, heart block, bradycardia, decreased baroreceptor sensitivity after acute infarction, and electrocution. The central nervous system may increase ventricular ectopy by elevating levels of catecholamines, affinity of receptors, and sympathetic tone.[231]

Medications may have proarrhythmic effects, especially in the setting of cardiac hypertrophy, cardiac dilatation, and ventricular scarring. Delayed afterdepolarizations and reentry rhythms may occur with digitalis toxicity.[228] Exogeneous and endogenous cathecholamines may result in early depolarizations, polymorphous ventricular tachycardias resembling torsades to pointes, and excessive stimulation of the sympathetic nervous system.[231] Antiarrhythmic drugs and other medications may paradoxically result in arrhythmias, especially within the first few days of treatment.[231] The proarrhythmic effect of medications may be enhanced by psychotropic drugs, hypokalemia, hypocalcemia, and hypomagnesemia.

Bradyarrhythmias

Incidence and Prognosis

Although ventricular tachyarrhythmias, especially ventricular fibrillation, are the most common rhythms documented in patients dying suddenly, approximately 20% of patients present with bradyarrhythmias or asystole.[233] Bradyarrhythmias generally have a higher incidence of fatal outcome than tachyarrhythmias.[234] Sudden death secondary to bradyarrhythmias may occur in patients with implanted cardioverter-defibrillators without backup pacing capabilities.[235]

Mechanisms

The basic mechanism of bradycardia is failure of adequate automaticity of subsidiary cardiac pacemaker tissue in the absence of sinus node function.[234] Bradycardia may be initiated by ischemic damage to baroreflex receptors, found most densely in the inferior wall of the left ventricle.[229, 236] Initial bradycardia and hypotension may result in further decrease in coronary blood flow, global anoxic damage, and the withdrawal of sympathetic tone.[236] Bradycardia and decreased baroreflex sensitivity may also increase the risk of ventricular fibrillation and sudden death in the failing myocardium and after acute infarction.[237, 238]

Underlying cardiac conditions resulting in bradycardia include ischemic heart disease, cardiac rupture, aortic stenosis, cardiomyopathies, pulmonary hypertension, athletic heart syndrome, and atrioventricular block.[239, 240] Many patients dying suddenly with bradyarrhythmias have advanced heart disease with diffuse ischemic damage of the subendocardial Purkinje fibers, which would normally establish an idioventricular escape rhythm. However, patients with bradycardic arrests often do not have prominotory events or bundle branch block.[241] Various derangements that decrease automaticity of pacemaker tissues include renal failure, acidosis, anoxia, hyperkalemia, trauma, and hypothermia.[238]

Lethal bradyarrhythmias may reflect disease of the autonomic nervous system, including cardioneurogenic syndrome (hypotension/bradycardia syndrome), diving reflex, and the sleep apnea syndrome. Inflammation of cardiac ganglia in patients with Guillain–Barre syndrome may result in bradycardic sudden death. Rarely, extremes of emotional stress may result in vasovagal syncope and sudden death.[242, 243] Severe asthma,[244] epilepsy,[245] and traumatic irritation to the vagus nerve during chest-tube insertion[246] have also been associated with malignant vasovagal syncope and bradycardia. "Voodoo death," a syndrome studied in underdeveloped countries, is associated with severe bradyarrhythmias, sudden death, and a sense of isolation.[247]

Syncope

Syncope is a nonspecific term denoting transient and sudden loss of consciousness, and may be mediated by neural or cardiac factors. Neurally mediated syncope is a result of bradycardia, with or without hypotension, secondary to diminished systemic venous return. Neurally mediated syncope may be precipitated by exhaustion, peripheral vasodilatation, emotional states, prolonged recumbency, and anorexia nervosa, and can be exacerbated by neurological diseases, anemia, and dehydration. Cardiac syncope resulting in bradycardia is often secondary to sick sinus syndrome, which is due to diseases of the atria. Other forms of cardiac syncope generally do not result from bradyarrhythmias and occur in patients with supraventricular tachycardias, ventricular tachycardias, prolonged Q-T syndrome, and aortic or pulmonary stenosis.[150]

Electromechanical Dissociation (Pulseless electrical activity)

Primary Electromechanical Dissocation

Usually an end-stage event in advanced heart disease, primary electromechanical dissociation is a result of failure of electromechanical coupling. Occasionally, it is seen in sudden cardiac death, either in patients dying from an acute ischemic event, or, more commonly, after electrical resuscitation from a prolonged cardiac arrest. The mechanism of primary electromechanical dissociation is unclear, but is likely related to global ischemia or diffuse disease that results in the abnormal intracellular calcium metabolism, intracellular acidosis, and perhaps adenosine triphosphate depletion.[8, 231]

Secondary Electromechanical Dissociation

Secondary electromechanical dissociation is characterized by pulmonary embolism, acute malfunction of prosthetic valves, exsanguination, and cardiac tamponade. The lack of cardiac contractility in the presence of continued electrical rhythmicity of the heart is secondary to absence of venous return and effective cardiac output.

Role of Molecular Techniques in Sudden Cardiac Death

Diagnosis

Molecular techniques for the detection of mutations in DNA extracted from tissue have recently improved, with the advent of automated sequencers and chip-based screening methods. These techniques have allowed for the diagnosis of the long Q-T syndrome, one of the major causes of sudden death in the absence of morphologic abnormalities, postmortem.[191, 192] Because of the time-intensive nature of molecular diagnosis, however, it has not yet become a routine test in the diagnosis of sudden cardiac death, and must be applied in only very select cases. Furthermore, the ethical and legal implications of genetic diagnosis on surviving family members are complex, and the dissemination of genetic data needs to be carefully orchestrated.

Other than for the long Q-T syndrome, there are no currently available molecular diagnostic tests available for other causes of sudden cardiac death without morphologic abnormality, such as coronary artery spasm and Brugada syndrome. Of course, the primary importance is to rule out occult noncardiac and unnatural causes of death in causes of unexplained sudden death.

Genetic counseling

Establishing a genetic diagnosis results in the necessity for genetic counseling for surviving family members. For example, identification of a specific mutation in a case of long Q-T syndrome at autopsy may direct genetic tests performed on surviving family, in order to identify those persons at risk, as it is known that electrocardiography is not a highly sensitive test. Furthermore, in cases of cardiomyopathy with known genetic basis (primarily hypertrophic cardiomyopathy), identification of a specific mutation may be helpful if genetic testing is contemplated to complement echocardiographic assessment of relatives. Currently, genetic screening for inherited cardiovascular diseases is at an early stage of development, and is primarily the task of clinicians with experience in genetic counseling.

Research

At the time of this writing, the primary role of molecular diagnosis in forensic autopsy is research into the cause of cardiomyopathies and other cardiac diseases. With the linking of specific morphologic entities to gene mutations, a better understanding of these diseases will follow, as the morphologic classification of cardiomyopathies is imprecise. As with any genetic testing, such studies are performed with careful review and prior establishment of guidelines pertaining to the release of any genetic information to surviving family members or clinicians.

REFERENCES

1. Siegel RJ, Koponen M. Spontaneous coronary artery dissection causing sudden death. Mechanical arterial failure or primary vasculitis? Arch Pathol Lab Med 118:196–198, 1994.
2. Kuller LH. Sudden death—definition and epidemiologic considerations. Prog Cardiovasc Dis 23:1–12, 1980.
3. Kuller L, Lilienfeld A, Fisher R. An epidemiologic study of sudden and unexpected death in adults. Medicine 46:341–361, 1967.
4. Virmani R, Roberts WC. Sudden cardiac death. Hum Pathol 18:485–492, 1987.
5. Shen WK, Edwards WD, Hammill SC, Bailey KR, Ballard DJ, Gersh BJ. Sudden unexpected nontraumatic death in 54 young adults: A 30-year population-based study. Am J Cardiol 76:148–152, 1995.
6. Burke AP, Virmani R, Smialek J. Young blacks are at higher risk of sudden cardiac death from all causes than whites. Circulation 86:1–199, 1992.
7. Furberg C, Romo M, Linko E, Siltanen P, Tibblin G, Wilhelmsen L. Sudden coronary death in Scandinavia. A report from Scandinavian coronary heart disease registers. Acta Med Scand 201:553–557, 1977.
8. Myerburg RJ, Castellanos A. Cardiac arrest and sudden cardiac death. In: Braunwald E (ed): Heart Disease.

A Textbook of Cardiovascular Medicine, pp 742–779. Philadelphia: WB Saunders, 1997.

9. Schatzkin A, Cupples A, Heeren T, Morelock S, Kannel WB. Sudden death in the Framingham heart study. Differences in incidence and risk factors by sex and coronary disease status. Am J Epidemiol 120:888–899, 1984.
10. Maron BJ, Moller JH, Seidman CE, Vincent GM, Dietz HC, Moss AJ, Sondheimer HM, Pyeritz RE, McGee G, Epstein AE. Impact of laboratory molecular diagnosis on contemporary diagnostic criteria for genetically transmitted cardiovascular diseases: Hypertrophic cardiomyopathy, long Q-T syndrome, and Marfan syndrome. A statement for healthcare professionals from the Councils on Clinical Cardiology, Cardiovascular Disease in the Young, and Basic Science, American Heart Association. Circulation 98:1460–1471, 1998.
11. Steinberger J, Lucas R, Edwards JE, Titus JL. Causes of sudden unexpected cardiac death in the first two decades of life. Am J Cardiol 77:992–995, 1996.
12. Drory Y, Turetz Y, Hiss Y, Lev B, Fisman EZ, Pines A, Kramer MR. Sudden unexpected death in persons < 40 years of age. Am J Cardiol 68:1388–1392, 1991.
13. Neuspiel DR, Kuller LH. Sudden and unexpected natural death in childhood and adolescence. JAMA 254:1321–1325, 1985.
14. Kelly KL, Titus JL, Edwards JE. Pathology of sudden apparent cardiac death in the young. Leg Med 42:49–86, 1993.
15. Baroldi G. Morphological and functional significance of findings in unstable atherothrombotic plaque underlying acute coronary syndromes: A review. Int J Cardiol 49 Suppl:S3–S9, 1995.
16. Davies MJ. Anatomic features in victims of sudden coronary death: Coronary artery pathology. Circulation 85 (Suppl I):I19–I24, 1992.
17. Uren NG, Melin JA, DeBruyne B, Wijns W, Baudhin T, Camici PG. Relation between myocardial blood flow and the severity of coronary-artery stenosis. N Engl J Med 330:1782–1788, 1994.
18. Farb A, Tang AL, Burke AP, Sessums L, Liang Y, Virmani R. Sudden coronary death. Frequency of active coronary lesions, inactive coronary lesions, and myocardial infarction. Circulation 92:1701–1709, 1995.
19. Warnes CA, Roberts WC. Sudden coronary death: Relation of amount and distribution of coronary narrowing at necropsy to previous symptoms of myocardial ischemia, left ventricular scarring and heart weight. Am J Cardiol 54:65–73, 1984.
20. Thomas A, Knapman P, Krikler D, Davies MJ. Community study of the causes of "natural" sudden death. Br Med J 297:1453–1456, 1988.
21. Burke AP, Farb A, Liang Y-H, Smialek J, Virmani R. The effect of hypertension and cardiac hypertrophy on coronary artery morphology in sudden cardiac death. Circulation 94:3138–3145, 1996.
22. Scott RF, Briggs TS. Pathologic findings in pre-hospital deaths due to coronary atherosclerosis. Am J Cardiol 29:782–787, 1971.
23. Davies MJ, Thomas A. Thrombosis and acute coronary-artery lesions in sudden cardiac ischemic death. N Engl J Med 310:1137–1140, 1984.
24. Davies MJ, Bland JM, Hangartner JR, Angelini A, Thomas AC. Factors influencing the presence or absence of acute coronary artery thrombi in sudden ischemic death. Eur Heart J 10:203–208, 1989.
25. Falk E. Plaque rupture with severe pre-existing stenosis precipitating coronary thrombosis: Characteristics of coronary atherosclerotic plaques underlying focal occlusive thrombi. Br Heart J 50:127–134, 1983.
26. Kragel AH, Gertz D, Roberts WC. Morphologic comparison of frequency and types of acute lesions in the major epicardial coronary arteries in unstable angina pectoris sudden coronary death and acute myocardial infarction. J Am Coll Cardiol 18:801–808, 1991.
27. Corrado D, Basso C, Poletti A, Angelini A, Valente M, Thiene G. Sudden death in the young. Is acute coronary thrombosis the major precipitating factor? Circulation 90:2315–2323, 1994.
28. Friedman M, Manwaring JH, Rosenman RH, Donlon G, Ortega P, Grube SM. Instantaneous and sudden deaths: Clinical and pathological differentiation in coronary artery disease. J Am Med Assoc 225:1319–1328, 1973.
29. Farb A, Burke AP, Tang AL, Liang TY, Mannan P, Smialek J, Virmani R. Coronary plaque erosion without rupture into a lipid core. A frequent cause of coronary thrombosis in sudden coronary death. Circulation 93:1354–1363, 1996.
30. Davies MJ, Thomas AC. Plaque fissuring—the cause of acute myocardial infarction, sudden ischaemic death, and crescendo angina. Br Heart J 53:363–373, 1985.
31. Virmani R, Rogan K, Cheitlin MD. Congenital coronary artery anomalies: Pathologic aspects. In: Virmani R, Forman MB (eds): Nonatherosclerotic Ischemic Heart Disease, p 153. New York: Raven Press, 1989.
32. Roberts WC. Major anomalies of the coronary arterial origin seen in childhood. Am Heart J 111:941–963, 1986.
33. Cheitlin MD, DeCastro CM, McAllister HA. Sudden death as a complication of anomalous left coronary origin from the anterior sinus of Valsalva: A not-so-minor congenital anomaly. Circulation 50:780–789, 1975.
34. Roberts WC. Major anomalies of coronary arterial origin seen in adulthood. Am Heart J 111:941–949, 1986.
35. Taylor AJ, Rogan KM, Virmani R. Sudden cardiac death associated with congenital coronary artery anomalies. J Am Coll Cardiol 20:640–647, 1992.
36. Phelps SE. Left coronary artery anomaly: An often unsuspected cause of sudden death in the military athlete. Mil Med 165:157–159, 2000.
37. Basso C, Maron BJ, Corrado D, Thiene G. Clinical profile of congenital coronary artery anomalies with origin from the wrong aortic sinus leading to sudden death in young competitive athletes. J Am Coll Cardiol 35:1493–1501, 2000.
38. Roberts WC, Siegel RJ, Zipes DP. Origin of the right coronary artery from the left sinus of Valsalva and its functional consequences: Analysis of 10 necropsy patients. Am J Cardiol 49:863–868, 1982.
39. Zugibe FT, Zugibe FTJ, Costello JT, Breithaup MK. Hypoplastic coronary artery disease within the spectrum of sudden unexpected death in young and middle age adults. Am J Forens Med Pathol 14:276–283, 1993.
40. Shotar A, Busuttil A. Myocardial bars and bridges and sudden death. Forensic Sci Int 21:143–147, 1994.
41. Morales AR, Romanelli R, Boucek RJ. The mural left anterior descending coronary artery, strenuous exercise and sudden death. Circulation 62:230–241, 1980.
42. Ishimori T. Clinical significance of myocardial bridges. Am Heart J 106:169–171, 1983.

43. Brody GL, Burton JF, Zawadzki ES, French AJ. Dissecting aneurysm of the coronary artery. N Engl J Med 237:1–6, 1965.
44. Virmani R, Forman MB. Coronary artery dissections. In: Virmani R, Forman MB (eds): Nonatherosclerotic Ischemic Heart Disease, pp 325–354. New York: Raven Press, 1989.
45. Robinowitz M, Virmani R, McAllister HA. Spontaneous coronary artery dissection and eosinophilic inflammation: A cause and effect relationship? Am J Med 72:923–928, 1982.
46. Dowling GP, Buja LM. Spontaneous coronary artery dissection with and without periadventitial inflammation. Arch Pathol Lab Med 111:470–472, 1987.
47. Robinowitz M, Forman MB, Virmani R. Nonatherosclerotic coronary aneurysms. In: Virmani R, Forman MB (eds): Nonatherosclerotic Ischemic Heart Disease, p 277. New York: Raven Press, 1989.
48. Atkinson JB, Forman MB, Virmani R. Emboli and thrombi in coronary arteries. In: Virmani R, Forman MB (eds): Nonatherosclerotic Ischemic Heart Disease, pp 355–385. New York: Raven Press, 1989.
49. Ueda M, Fujimoto T, Ogawa N, Shoji S. An autopsy case of cholesterol embolism following percutaneous transluminal coronary angioplasty and aortography. Acta Pathol Jpn 39:203–206, 1989.
50. Virmani R, Popovsky MA, Roberts WC. Thrombocytosis, coronary thrombosis and acute myocardial infarction. Am J Med 67:498–506, 1979.
51. Penny WJ, Colvin BT, Brooks N. Myocardial infarction with normal coronary arteries and factor XII deficiency. Br Heart J 53:230–234, 1985.
52. Engel HJ, Hundeshagen H, Lichtlen P. Transmural myocardial infarction in young women taking oral contraceptives: Evidence of reduced regional coronary flow in spite of normal coronary arteries. Br Heart J 39:477–484, 1977.
53. Khoo US, Dickens P, Cheung AN. Rapid death from thrombotic thrombocytopaenic purpura following caesarean section. Forensic Sci Int 54:75–80, 1992.
54. James T. Morphologic characteristics and functional significance of focal fibromuscular dysplasia of small coronary arteries. Am J Cardiol 65:12G–22G, 1990.
55. James TN, Marshall TK. De subitaneis mortibus. XVII. Multifocal stenoses due to fibromuscular dysplasia of the sinus node artery. Circulation 53:736–742, 1976.
56. James TN, Hackel DB, Marshall TK. De subitaneis mortibus. V. Occluded A-V node artery. Circulation 49:772–777, 1974.
57. James TN. The spectrum of diseases of small coronary arteries and their physiologic consequences. J Am Coll Cardiol 15:763–774, 1990.
58. Burke AP, Subramanian R, Smialek J, Virmani R. Nonatherosclerotic narrowing of the atrioventricular node artery and sudden death. J Am Coll Cardiol 21:117–122, 1993.
59. James TN. De subitaneis mortibus. XIX. On the cause of sudden death in pheochromocytoma, with special reference of the pulmonary arteries, the cardiac conduction system, and the aggregation of platelets. Circulation 54:348–356, 1976.
60. Burke AP, Farb A, Tang A, Smialek J, Virmani R. Fibromuscular dysplasia of small coronary arteries and fibrosis in the basilar ventricular septum in mitral valve prolapse. Am Heart J 134:282–291, 1997.
61. Burke AP, Virmani R. Intramural coronary artery dysplasia of the ventricular septum and sudden death. Hum Pathol 29:1124–1127, 1998.
62. Lie KI, Leim KL, Schuilenberg RM, David GK, Durrer D. Early identification of patients developing late inhospital ventricular fibrillation after discharge from the coronary care unit. Am J Cardiol 41:674–677, 1978.
63. Piek JJ, Becker AE. Collateral blood supply to the myocardium at risk in human myocardial infarction: A quantitative postmortem assessment. J Am Coll Cardiol 11:1290–1296, 1988.
64. Kitzman DW, Scholz DG, Hagen PT, Ilstrup DM, Edwards WD. Age-related changes in normal human hearts during the first 10 decades of life. Part II (Maturity): A quantitative anatomic study of 765 specimens from subjects 20 to 99 years old. Mayo Clin Proc 63:137–146, 1988.
65. Maron BJ, Roberts WC, Epstein SE. Sudden death in hypertrophic cardiomyopathy: A profile of 78 patients. Circulation 65:1388–1394, 1982.
66. Maron BJ, Lipson LC, Roberts WC, Savage DD, Epstein SE. Malignant hypertrophic cardiomyopathy: Identification of a subgroup of families with unusually frequent premature death. Am J Cardiol 41:1133–1140, 1978.
67. Yetman AT, McCrindle BW, MacDonald C, Freedom RM, Gow R. Myocardial bridging in children with hypertrophic cardiomyopathy—a risk factor for sudden death. N Engl J Med 339:1201–1209, 1998.
68. Shirani J, Pick R, Roberts WC, Maron BJ. Morphology and significance of the left ventricular collagen network in young patients with hypertrophic cardiomyopathy and sudden cardiac death. J Am Coll Cardiol 35:36–44, 2000.
69. Prasad K, Frenneaux MP. Sudden death in hypertrophic cardiomyopathy: Potential importance of altered autonomic control of vasculature. Heart 79:538–540, 1998.
70. Messerli FH. Hypertension, left ventricular hypertrophy, ventricular ectopy, and sudden death. Am J Hypertens 6:335–336, 1993.
71. Tracy RE, Mercante DE, Moncada A, Berenson G. Quantitation of hypertensive nephrosclerosis on an objective rational scale of measure in adults and children. Am J Clin Pathol 85:312–318, 1986.
72. Burke AP, Farb A, Virmani R, Goodin J, Smialek JE. Sports-related and non-sports-related sudden death in young adults. Am Heart J 121:568–575, 1991.
73. Maron BJ, Roberts WC, McAllister HA, Rosing DR, Epstein SE. Sudden death in young atheletes. Circulation 62:218–230, 1980.
74. Braunwald E, Colucci WS, Grossman W. Clinical aspects of heart failure. In: Braunwald E (ed): Heart Disease. A Textbook of Cardiovascular Medicine. Philadelphia: WB Saunders, 1997.
75. Chadwick J, Mann WN. Medical works of Hippocrates, p 154. Oxford: Blackwell, 1950.
76. Alexander JK. The cardiomyopathy of obesity. Prog Cardiovasc Disc 27:325–334, 1985.
77. Messerli FH, Nunez BD, Ventura HO, Synder DW. Overweight and sudden death: Increased ventricular ectopy in cardiomyopathy of obesity. Arch Intern Med 147:1725–1728, 1987.
78. Drenick EJ, Bale GS, Seltzer F, Johnson DG. Excessive mortality and causes of death in morbidly obese men. J Am Med Assoc 243:443–445, 1980.
79. Duflou J, Virmani R, Rabin I, Burke A, Farb A, Smialek J. Sudden death due to heart disease in morbid obesity. Am Heart J 130:306–313, 1995.

80. Kasper EK, Hruban RH, Baughman KL. Cardiomyopathy of obesity: A clinicopathologic evaluation of 43 obese patients with heart failure. Am J Cardiol 70:921–924, 1992.
81. Warnes CA, Roberts WC. The heart in massive (more than 300 pounds or 136 kilograms) obesity: Analysis of 12 patients studied at necropsy. Am J Cardiol 54:1087–1109, 1984.
82. Rossner S, Lagerstrand L, Persson HE, Sachs C. The sleep apnea syndrome in obesity: Risk of sudden death. J Intern Med 230:135–141, 1991.
83. Goodin JC, Farb A, Smialek JE, Field F, Virmani R. Right ventricular dysplasia associated with sudden death in young adults. Mod Pathol 4:702–706, 1991.
84. Virmani R, Robinowitz M, Clark M, McAllister H. Sudden death and partial absence of the right ventricular myocardium. A report of three cases and a review of the literature. Arch Pathol Lab Med 106:163–167, 1982.
85. Nava A, Thiene G, Canciani B, Scognamiglio R, Daliento L, Buja G, Martini B, Stritoni P, Fasoli G. Familial occurrence of right ventricular dysplasia: A study involving nine families. J Am Coll Cardiol 12:1222–1228, 1988.
86. Kullo IJ, Edwards WD, Seward JB. Right ventricular dysplasia: The Mayo Clinic experience. Mayo Clin Proc 70:541–548, 1995.
87. Pawel BR, de Chadarevian JP, Wolk JH, Donner RM, Vogel RL, Braverman P. Sudden death in childhood due to right ventricular dysplasia: Report of two cases. Pediatr Pathol 14:987–995, 1994.
88. Burke AP, Farb A, Tashko G, Virmani R. Arrhythmogenic right ventricular cardiomyopathy and fatty replacement of the right ventricular myocardium. Are they different diseases? Circulation 97:1571–1580, 1998.
89. Thiene G, Nava A, Corrado D, Rossi L, Pennelli N. Right ventricular cardiomyopathy and sudden death in young people. N Engl J Med 318:129–133, 1988.
90. Burke AP, Robinson S, Radentz S, Smialek J, Virmani R. Sudden death in right ventricular dysplasia with minimal gross abnormalities. J Forensic Sci 44:438–443, 1999.
91. Voigt J, Agdal N. Lipomatous infiltration of the heart. An uncommon cause of sudden unexpected death in a young man. Arch Pathol Lab Med 106:497–498, 1982.
92. Moorman JR, Coleman RE, Packer DL, Kisslo JA, Bell J, Hettleman BD, Stajich J, Roses AD. Cardiac involvement in myotonic muscular dystrophy. Medicine 64:371–387, 1985.
93. Risse M, Weiler G. Progressive muscular dystrophy of the Duchenne type. Z Rechtsmed 97:75–81, 1986.
94. Chenard AA, Becane HM, Tertrain F, de Kermadec JM, Weiss YA. Ventricular arrhythmia in Duchenne muscular dystrophy: Prevalence, significance and prognosis. Neuromuscul Disord 3:201–206, 1993.
95. Ackermann DM, Edwards WD. Sudden death as the initial manifestation of primary pulmonary hypertension. Report of four cases. Am J Forensic Med Pathol 8:97–102, 1987.
96. Brown DL, Wetli CV, Davis JH. Sudden unexpected death from primary pulmonary hypertension. J Forensic Sci 26:381–386, 1981.
97. Bjornsson J, Edwards WD. Primary pulmonary hypertension: A histopatholgic study of 80 cases. Mayo Clin Proc 60:16–25, 1985.
98. Burke AP, Farb A, Virmani R. The pathology of primary pulmonary hypertension. Mod Pathol 4:269–282, 1991.
99. Denfield SW, Garson A, Jr. Sudden death in children and young adults. Pediatr Clin North Am 37:215–231, 1990.
100. Maron BJ, Shirani J, Poliac LC, Mathenge R, Roberts WC, Mueller FO. Sudden death in young competitive athletes. Clinical, demographic, and pathological profiles. JAMA 276:199–204, 1996.
101. Phillips M, Robinowitz M, Higgins JR, Boran K, Reed T, Virmani R. Sudden cardiac death in Air Force recruits. J Am Med Assoc 256:2696–2699, 1986.
102. Lecomte D, Fornes P, Fouret P, Nicolas G. Isolated myocardial fibrosis as a cause of sudden cardiac death and its possible relation to myocarditis. J Forensic Sci 38:617–621, 1993.
103. Fujioka S, Koide H, Kitaura Y, Deguchi H, Kawamura K, Hirai K. Molecular detection and differentiation of enteroviruses in endomyocardial biopsies and pericardial effusions from dilated cardiomyopathy and myocarditis. Am Heart J 131:760–765, 1996.
104. Nicholson F, Ajetunmobi JF, Li M, Shackleton EA, Starkey WG, Illavia SJ, Muir P, Banatvala JE. Molecular detection and serotypic analysis of enterovirus RNA in archival specimens from patients with acute myocarditis. Br Heart J 74:522–527, 1995.
105. Burke AP, Saenger J, Mullick F, Virmani R. Hypersensitivity myocarditis. Arch Pathol Lab Med 115:764–769, 1991.
106. Piette M, Timperman J. Sudden death in idiopathic giant cell myocarditis. Med Sci Law 30:280–284, 1990.
107. Kavanagh T, Huang S. Cardiac sarcoidosis: An unforeseen cause of sudden death. Can J Cardiol 11:136–138, 1995.
108. Reuhl J, Schneider M, Sievert H, Lutz FU, Zieger G. Myocardial sarcoidosis as a rare cause of sudden cardiac death. Forensic Sci Int 89:145–153, 1997.
109. Veinot JP, Johnston B. Cardiac sarcoidosis—an occult cause of sudden death: A case report and literature review. J Forensic Sci 43:715–717, 1998.
110. Virmani R, Bures JC, Roberts WC. Cardiac sarcoidosis; a major cause of sudden death in young individuals. Chest 77:423–428, 1980.
111. Roberts WC, McAllister HA, Jr., Ferrans VJ. Sarcoidosis of the heart. A clinicopathologic study of 35 necropsy patients (group I) and review 78 previously described necropsy patients (group II). Am J Med 63:86–108, 1977.
112. Sperry K, Smialek JE. Sudden death due to a paraganglioma of the organs of Zuckerkandl. Am J Forensic Med Pathol 7:23–29, 1986.
113. Isner JM, Sours HE, Paris AL, Ferrans VJ, Roberts WC. Sudden, unexpected death in avid dieters using the liquid-protein-modified-fast diet: Observations in 17 patients and the role of the prolonged QT interval. Circulation 60:1401–1412, 1979.
114. Siegel RJ, Caheen WR, Roberts WC. Prolonged QT interval—ventricular tachycardia syndrome from massive rapid weight loss utilizing the liquid-protein-modified-fast diet: Sudden death with sinus node ganglionitis and neuritis. Am Heart J 102:121–122, 1981.
115. Cina SJ, Smialek JE, Burke AP, Virmani R, Hutchins GM. Primary cardiac tumours causing sudden death: A review of the literature. Am J Forensic Med Pathol 17:271–281, 1996.
116. Burke AP, Virmani R. Cardiac myxomas: A clinicopathologic study. Am J Clin Pathol 100:671–680, 1993.
117. Amr SS, Abu al Ragheb SY. Sudden unexpected death due to papillary fibroma of the aortic valve. Report

of a case and review of the literature. Am J Forensic Med Pathol 12:143–148, 1991.
118. Kolodgie FD, Farb A, Virmani R. Pathobiological determinants of cocaine-associated cardiovascular syndromes. Hum Pathol 26:583–586, 1995.
119. Kolodgie FD, Virmani R, Cornhill JF, Herderick EE, Smialek JE. Increase in atherosclerosis and adventitial mast cells in cocaine abusers: An alternative mechanism of cocaine-associated coronary vasospasm and thrombosis. J Am Coll Cardiol 17:1553–1560, 1991.
120. Mittleman RE, Wetli CV. Cocaine and sudden "natural" death. J Forensic Sci 32:11–19, 1987.
121. Luke JL, Reay DT, Eisele JW, Bonnell HJ. Sudden cardiac death during exercise in a weight lifter using anabolic androgenic steroids and toxicological findings. J Forensic Sci 35:1441–1447, 1990.
122. Nishimura RA, McGoon MD, Shub C, Miller FA, Jr., Ilstrup DM, Tajik AJ. Echocardiographically documented mitral-valve prolapse. Long-term follow-up of 237 patients. N Engl J Med 313:1305–1309, 1985.
123. Duren DR, Becker AE, Dunning AJ. Long-term follow-up of idiopathic mitral valve prolapse in 300 patients: A prospective study. J Am Coll Cardiol 11:42–47, 1988.
124. Kligfield P, Devereux RB. Is the mitral valve prolapse patient at high risk of sudden death identifiable? Cardiovasc Clin 21:143–157; discussion 158–160, 1990.
125. Kligfield P, Hochreiter C, Niles N, Devereux RB, Borer JS. Relation of sudden death in pure mitral regurgitation, with and without mitral valve prolapse, to repetitive ventricular arrhythmias and right and left ventricular ejection fractions. Am J Cardiol 60:397–399, 1987.
126. Kligfield P, Levy D, Devereux RB, Savage DD. Arrhythmias and sudden death in mitral valve prolapse. Am Heart J 113:1298–1307, 1987.
127. Pocock WA, Bosman CK, Chesler E, Barlow JB, Edwards JE. Sudden death in primary mitral valve prolapse. Am Heart J 107:378–382, 1984.
128. Perloff JK, Child JS. Clinical and epidemiologic issues in mitral valve prolapse: Overview and perspective. Am Heart J 113:1324–1332, 1987.
129. Lichstein E. Site of origin of ventricular premature beats in patients with mitral valve prolapse. Am Heart J 100:450–457, 1980.
130. Leichtman D, Nelson R, Gobel FL, Alexander CS, Cohn JN. Bradycardia with mitral valve prolapse: A potential mechanism of sudden death. Ann Intern Med 85:453–457, 1976.
131. Cowan MD, Fye WB. Prevalence of QTc prolongation in women with mitral valve prolapse. Am J Cardiol 63:133–134, 1989.
132. Andre-Fouet X, Tabib A, Jean-Louis P, Anne D, Dutertre P, Gayet C, Huygue de Mahenge A, Loire R, Pont M. Mitral valve prolapse, Wolff–Parkinson–White syndrome, His bundle sclerosis and sudden death. Am J Cardiol 56:700, 1985.
133. Dollar AL, Roberts WC. Morphologic comparison of patients with mitral valve prolapse who died suddenly with patients who died from severe valvular dysfunction or other conditions. J Am Coll Cardiol 17:921–931, 1991.
134. Bharati S, Granston AS, Liebson PR, Loeb HS, Rosen KM, Lev M. The conduction system in mitral valve prolapse syndrome with sudden death. Am Heart J 101:667–670, 1981.
135. Morales AR, Romanelli R, Boucek RJ, Tate LG, Alvarez RT, Davis JT. Myxoid heart disease: An assessment of extravalvular cardiac pathology in severe mitral valve prolapse. Hum Pathol 23:129–137, 1992.
136. Farb A, Tang AL, Atkinson JB, McCarthy WF, Virmani R. Comparison of cardiac findings in patients with mitral valve prolapse who die suddenly to those who have congestive heart failure from mitral regurgitation and to those with fatal noncardiac conditions. Am J Cardiol 70:234–239, 1992.
137. Campbell M. Calcific aortic stenosis and congenital bicuspid aortic valves. Br Heart J 30:606–612, 1968.
138. Blackstone EH, Kirklin JW. Death and other time-related events after valve replacement. Circulation 67:632–639, 1985.
139. Gohlke-Barwolf C, Peters K, Petersen J. Influence of aortic valve replacement on sudden death in patients with pure aortic stenosis. Eur Heart J 9E:139–144, 1988.
140. Cohle SD, Graham MA, Dowling G, Pounder DJ. Sudden death in left ventricular outflow disease. Pathol Annu 23:97–124, 1988.
141. Van Son JA, Edwards WD, Danielson GK. Pathology of coronary arteries, myocardium, and great arteries in supravalvular aortic stenosis. Report of five cases with implications for surgical treatment. J Thorac Cardiovasc Surg 108:21–28, 1994.
142. Thiene G, Ho SY. Aortic root pathology and sudden death in youth: Review of anatomical varieties. Appl Pathol 4:237–245, 1986.
143. Burke AP, Kalra P, Li L, Smialek JE, Virmani R. Infectious endocarditis and sudden unexpected death: Incidence and morphology of lesions in intravenous addicts and non drug abusers. J Heart Valve Dis 6:198–203, 1997.
144. Lindblom D. Long-term clinical results after mitral valve replacement with the Bjork–Shiley prosthesis. J Thorac Cardiovasc Surg 95:321–333, 1988.
145. Rooney SJ, Moreno de la Santa P, Lewis PA, Butchart EG. Sudden death in a large prosthetic valve series based on a single prosthesis: Experience with the Medtronic Hall valve. J Heart Valve Dis 3:5–9, 1994.
146. Burke AP, Farb AF, Sessums L, Virmani R. Sudden cardiac death in patients with heart valve prostheses: An autopsy study. J Heart Valve Dis 10–16, 1994.
147. Lambert EC, Menon VA, Wagner HR, Vlad P. Sudden unexpected death from cardiovascular disease in children. Am J Cardiol 34:89–96, 1974.
148. Garson AS, McNamara DG. Sudden death in a pediatric cardiology population. 1958–1983: Relation to prior arrthythmias. J Am Coll Cardiol 5:134B–137B, 1985.
149. Watson H. Natural history of Ebstein's anomaly of tricuspid valve in childhood and adolescence: An international cooperative study of 505 cases. Br Heart J 36:417–427, 1974.
150. Krongrad E. Syncope and sudden death. In: Emmanouilides GC, Riemenschneider TA, Allen HD, Gutgesell HP (eds): Heart Disease in Infants and Children, and Adolescents, pp 1604–1618. Baltimore: Williams and Wilkins, 1995.
151. Silka MJ, Hardy BG, Menashe VD, Morris CD. A population-based prospective evaluation of risk of sudden cardiac death after operation for common congenital heart defects. J Am Coll Cardiol 32:245–251, 1998.
152. Nollert G, Fischlein T, Bouterwek S, Bohmer C, Klinner W, Reichart B. Long-term survival in patients with repair of tetralogy of Fallot: 36-year follow-up of

490 survivors of the first year after surgical repair. J Am Coll Cardiol 30:1374–1383, 1997.
153. Jonsson H, Ivert T, Brodin LA, Jonasson R. Late sudden deaths after repair of tetralogy of Fallot. Electrocardiographic findings associated with survival. Scand J Thorac Cardiovasc Surg 29:131–139, 1995.
154. Kugler JD. Predicting sudden death in patients who have undergone tetralogy of Fallot repair: Is it really as simple as measuring ECG intervals? J Cardiovasc Electrophysiol 9:103–106, 1998.
155. Berul CI, Hill SL, Geggel RL, Hijazi ZM, Marx GR, Rhodes J, Walsh KA, Fulton DR. Electrocardiographic markers of late sudden death risk in postoperative tetralogy of Fallot children. J Cardiovasc Electrophysiol 8:1349–1356, 1997.
156. McLeod KA, Hillis WS, Houston AB, Wilson N, Trainer A, Neilson J, Doig WB. Reduced heart rate variability following repair of tetralogy of Fallot. Heart 81:656–660, 1999.
157. Steigman CK, Anderson DW, Macher AM, Sennesh JD, Virmani R. Fatal cardiac tamponade in acquired immunodeficiency syndrome with epicardial Kaposi's sarcoma. Am Heart J 116:1105–1107, 1988.
158. Tanaka H, Suzuki H, Kasai T, Kobayashi K. Rupture of the heart in a burn patient: A case report of free wall rupture of the left ventricle. Burns 17:427–429, 1991.
159. Kusano I, Shiraishi T, Morimoto R, Haba K, Yatani R. Cardiac rupture due to severe fatty infiltration of the right ventricular wall. J Forensic Sci 36:1246–1250, 1991.
160. Pan M, Medina A, Suarez de Lezo J, Hernandez E, Romero M, Pavlovic D, Melian F, Segura J, Roman M, Montero A. Cardiac tamponade complicating mitral balloon valvuloplasty. Am J Cardiol 68:802–805, 1991.
161. Byard RW, Bourne AJ, Moore L, Little KE. Sudden death in early infancy due to delayed cardiac tamponade complicating central venous line insertion and cardiac catheterization. Arch Pathol Lab Med 116:654–656, 1992.
162. Nassar H, Hasin Y, Gotsman MS. Cardiac tamponade following coronary arterial rupture during coronary angioplasty. Cathet Cardiovasc Diagn 23:177–179, 1991.
163. Cheung A, Chan CW. Dissecting aneurysm of coronary artery presenting as cardiac tamponade. N Z Med J 103:129–130, 1990.
164. Fan CC, Andersen BR, Sahgal S. Isolated myocardial abscess causing coronary artery rupture and fatal hemopericardium. Arch Pathol Lab Med 118:1023–1025, 1994.
165. Koike R, Oku T, Satoh H, Sawada Y, Suma HTA, Kato Y, Kita Y, Hirota Y, Kawamura K. Right ventricular myocardial infarction and late cardiac tamponade due to right coronary artery aneurysm—a case report. Jpn J Surg 20:463–467, 1990.
166. Vidaillet HJ, Pressley JC, Henke E, Harrell FE, German LD. Familial occurrence of accessory atrioventricular pathways (preexcitation syndrome). N Engl J Med 317:65–69, 1987.
167. Wiedermann CJ, Becker AE, Hopferwieser T, Muhlberger V, Knapp E. Sudden death in a young competitive athelete with Wolff–Parkinson–White syndrome. Eur Heart J 8:651–655, 1987.
168. Klein GJ, Bashore TM, Sellers TD, Pritchett EC, Smith WM, Gallagher JJ. Ventricular fibrillation in the Wolff–Parkinson–White syndrome. N Engl J Med 301:1080–1085, 1979.
169. Teo WS, Klein GJ, Yee R, Leitch J. Sudden cardiac death in the Wolff–Parkinson–White syndrome. In: Akhtar M, Myerburg RJ (eds): Sudden Cardiac Death: Prevalence, Mechanisms, and Approaches to Diagnosis and Managment, pp 215–225. Philadelphia: Williams & Wilkins, 1994.
170. Suarez-Mier MP, Gamallo C. Atrioventricular node fetal dispersion and His bundle fragmentation of the cardiac conduction system in sudden cardiac death. J Am Coll Cardiol 32:1885–1890, 1998.
171. McAnulty JH, Rahimtoola SH, Murphy E, DeMots H, Ritzmann L, Kanarek PE, Kauffman S. Natural history of high-risk bundle-branch block: Final report of a prospective study. N Engl J Med 307:137–143, 1982.
172. Denes P, Dhingra RC, Wu D, Wyndham CR, Amat-y-Leon F, Rosen KM. Sudden death in patients with chronic bifascicular block. Arch Intern Med 137:1005–1010, 1977.
173. Hackel DB. Pathology of congenital complete heart block. Mod Pathol 1:114–128, 1986.
174. Lev M. The pathology of complete atrioventricular block. Prog Cardiovasc Dis 6:317–323, 1964.
175. Lenegre J. Aetiology and pathology of bilateral bundle branch fibrosis in relation to complete heart block. Prog Cardiovasc Dis 6:409, 1964.
176. Darpo B, Walfridsson H, Aunes M, Bergfeldt L, Edvardsson N, Linde C, Lurje L, van der Linden M, Rosenqvist M. Incidence of sudden death after radiofrequency ablation of the atrioventricular junction for atrial fibrillation. Am J Cardiol 80:1174–1177, 1997.
177. James TN, Pearce SN, Givham EG. Sudden death while driving. Role of sinus perinodal degeneration and cardiac neural degeneration and ganglionitis. Am J Cardiol 45:1095–1102, 1980.
178. Bharati S, Dreifus LS, Chopskie E, Lev M. Conduction system in a trained jogger with sudden death. Chest 93:348–351, 1988.
179. Bell MD, Tate LG. Vascular anomaly of the bundle of His associated with sudden death in a young man. Am J Forensic Med Pathol 15:151–155, 1994.
180. DiMarco JP. Sudden death in patients without structural heart disease. In: Akhtar M, Myerburg RJ (eds): Sudden Cardiac Death: Prevalence, Mechanisms, and Approaches to Diagnosis and Managment, pp 202–208. Philadelphia: Williams & Wilkins, 1994.
181. Maron BJ, Poliac LC, Kaplan JA, Muller FO. Blunt impact to the chest leading to sudden death from cardiac arrest during sports activities. N Engl J Med 333:337–381, 1995.
182. Otto CM, Tauxe RV, Cobb LA, Green HL, Gross BW, Werner JA, Burroughs RW, Samson WE, Weaver WD, Trobaugh G.B. Ventricular fibrillation causes sudden an death in Southeast Asian immigrants. Ann Intern Med 101:45–47, 1984.
183. Aponte C. The engima of "bangungut." Ann Intern Med 52:1259–1272, 1960.
184. Sugai M. A pathologic study on sudden and unexpected death, especially on the cardiac death authopsied by medical examiners in Tokyo. Acta Pathol Jpn 9:723–737, 1959.
185. Wang Q, Chen Q, Li H, Towbin JA. Molecular genetics of long QT syndrome from genes to patients. Curr Opin Cardiol 12:310–320, 197.
186. Vincent GM. The molecular genetics of the long QT syndrome: Genes causing fainting and sudden death. Annu Rev Med 49:263–274, 1998.
187. Wever EF, Hauer RN, Oomen A, Peters RH, Bakker PF, Robles de Medina EO. Unfavorable outcome in

patients with primary electrical disease who survived an episode of ventricular fibrillation. Circulation 88:1021–1029, 1993.

188. Roy D, Waxman HL, Kienzle MG, Buxton AE, Marchlinski FE, Josephson ME. Clinical characteristics and long-term follow-up in 119 survivors of cardiac arrest: Relation to inducibility at electrophysiologic testing. Am J Cardiol 52:969–974, 1983.
189. Deal BJ, Miller SM, Scalgiotti D, Prechel D, Gallastegui JL, Hariman RJ. Ventricular tachycardia in a young population without overt heart disease. Circulation 73:1111–1118, 1986.
190. Cobb LA, Baum RS, Alvarez Hd, Schaffer WA. Resuscitation from out-of-hospital ventricular fibrillation: 4 years follow-up. Circulation 52:III223–235, 1975.
191. Ackerman MJ, Tester DJ, Porter CJ. Swimming, a gene-specific arrhythmogenic trigger for inherited long QT syndrome. Mayo Clin Proc 74:1088–1094, 1999.
192. Ackerman MJ, Tester DJ, Porter CJ, Edwards WD. Molecular diagnosis of the inherited long-QT syndrome in a woman who died after near-drowning. N Engl J Med 341:1121–1125, 1999.
193. Brugada J, Brugada P. What to do in patients with no structural heart disease and sudden arrhythmic death? Am J Cardiol 78:69–75, 1996.
194. Corrado D, Nava A, Buja G, Martini B, Fasoli G, Oselladore L, Turrini P, Thiene G. Familial cardiomyopathy underlies syndrome of right bundle branch block, ST segment elevation and sudden death. J Am Coll Cardiol 27:443–448, 1996.
195. Tada H, Aihara N, Ohe T, Yutani C, Hamada S, Miyanuma H, Takamiya M, Kamakura S. Arrhythmogenic right ventricular cardiomyopathy underlies syndrome of right bundle branch block, ST-segment elevation, and sudden death. Am J Cardiol 81:519–522, 1998.
196. Scheinman MM. Is the Brugada syndrome a distinct clinical entity? J Cardiovasc Electrophysiol 8:332–336, 1997.
197. Siscovick DS, Weiss NS, Fletcher RH, Lasky T. The incidence of primary cardiac arrest during vigorous exercise. N Engl J Med 311:874, 1984.
198. Amsterdam EA, Laslett L, Holly R. Exercise and sudden death. Cardiol Clin 5:337, 1987.
199. Thompson PD, Funk EJ, Carleton RA, Sturner WQ. Incidence of death during jogging in Rhode Island from 1975 through 1980. J Am Med Assoc 247:2535–2538, 1982.
200. Thompson PD, Stern MP, Williams P, Duncan K, Haskell WL, Wood PD. Death during jogging or running. J Am Med Assoc 242:1265–1267, 1979.
201. Virmani R, Robinowitz M, McAllister HA. Nontraumatic death in joggers. Am J Med 72:874–881, 1982.
202. Burke AP, Farb A, Virmani R. Causes of sudden death in athletes. Cardiol Clin 10:303–318, 1992.
203. Waller B, Roberts W. Sudden death while running in conditioned runners aged 40 years or over. Am J Cardiol 45:1292, 1980.
204. Maron B, Epstein S, Roberts W. Causes of sudden death in competitive athletes. J Am Coll Cardiol 7:204, 1986.
205. James TN, Froggatt P, Marshall TK. Sudden death in young athletes. Ann Intern Med 67:1013, 1967.
206. McClellan JT, Jokl E. Congenital anomalies of coronary arteries as a cause of sudden death associated with physical exertion. Medicine and Sport 5:91, 1971.
207. Moades TD, Rose AG, Opie LH. Hypertrophic cardiomyopathy associated with sudden death during marathon racing. Br Heart J 41:624–632, 1979.
208. Maron BJ, Thompson PD, Puffer JC, McGrew CA, Strong WB, Douglas PS, Clark LT, Mitten MJ, Crawford MH, Atkins DL, Driscoll DJ, Epstein AE. Cardiovascular preparticipation screening of competitive athletes. A statement for health professionals from the Sudden Death Committee (clinical cardiology) and Congenital Cardiac Defects Committee (cardiovascular disease in the young), American Heart Association. Circulation 94:850–856, 1996.
209. Zeppilli P, dello Russo A, Santini C, Palmieri V, Natale L, Giordano A, Frustaci A. In vivo detection of coronary artery anomalies in asymptomatic athletes by echocardiographic screening. Chest 114:89–93, 1998.
210. Kark JA. Sickle-cell trait as an age-dependent risk factor for sudden death in physical training. N Engl J Med 317:781–787, 1987.
211. Virmani R, Burke AP, Farb A, Kark JA. Causes of sudden death in young and middle-aged competitive athletes. Cardiol Clin 15:439–466, 1997.
212. Gardner JW, Kark JA, Karnei K, Sanborn JS, Gastaldo E, Burr P, Wenger CB. Risk factors predicting exertional heat illness in male Marine Corps recruits. Med Sci Sports Exerc 28:939–944, 1996.
213. Morganroth J, Maron BJ, Henry WL, Epstein SE. Comparative left ventricular dimension in trained athletes. Ann Intern Med 82:5214–5222, 1975.
214. Maron BJ. Structural features of the athlete's heart as defined by echocardiography. J Am Coll Cardiol 7:190–203, 1986.
215. Wright JN, Salem D. Sudden death and the "athlete's heart." Arch Intern Med 155:1473–1480, 1995.
216. Grossman W. Cardiac hypertrophy: Useful adaptation or pathologic process? Am J Med 69:576–580, 1980.
217. Lie H, Erikssen J. Five-year follow-up of ECG aberrations, latent coronary heart disease and cardiopulmonary fitness in various age groups of Norwegian cross-country skiers. Acta Med Scand 216:377–383, 1984.
218. Zehender M, Meinertz T, Keul J, Just H. ECG variants and cardiac arrhythmias in athletes: Clinical relevance and prognostic importance. Am Heart J 119:1378–1391, 1990.
219. Noakes TD, Opie LH, Rose AG, Kleynhans PH. Autopsy-proved coronary atherosclerosis in marathon runners. N Engl J Med 301:86–89, 1979.
220. Northcote RJ, Ballantyne D. Sudden cardiac death in sport. Br Med J 287:1357–1359, 1983.
221. Burke AP, Farb A, Malcom GT, Liang Y-H, Smialek J, Virmani R. Plaque rupture and sudden death related to exertion in men with coronary artery disease. J Am Med Assoc 281:921–926, 1999.
222. Siscovick DS, Ekelund LG, Hyde JS, Johnson JL, Gordon DJ, LaRose JC. Physical activity and coronary heart disease among asymptomatic hypercholesterolemic men (the Lipid Research Clinics Coronary Primary Prevention Trial). Am J Public Health 78:1428–1431, 1988.
223. Opie LH. Sudden death and sport. Lancet 1:263–266, 1975.
224. Haskell WL, Sims C, Myll J, Bort ZWM, St Goar FG, Alderman EL. Coronary artery size and dilating capacity in ultradistance runners. Circulation 87:1076–1082, 1993.
225. Cobb LA, Weaver WD. Exercise: A risk for sudden death in patients with coronary heart disease. J Am Coll Cardiol 7:215–219, 1986.
226. Coplan NL, Gleim GW, Nicholas JA. Exercise and sudden cardiac death. Am Heart J 115:207–212, 1988.

227. Struthers AD, Quigley C, Brown MJ. Rapid changes in plasma potassium during a game of squash. Clin Sci 74:397–401, 1988.
228. Zipes DP. Genesis of cardiac arrhythmias: Electrophysiological considerations. In: Braunwald E (ed): Heart Disease. A Textbook of Cardiovascular Medicine, pp 548–592. Philadelphia: WB Saunders, 1997.
229. Janse MJ. Infarct anatomy, baroreflex sensitivity and sudden death. J Mol Cell Cardiol 497–499, 1993.
230. DeBakken JM, Coronel R, Tasseron S, Wilde AA, Opthof J, Janse MJ, van Capelle FJ, Becker AE, Tambroes G. Ventricular tachycardia in the infarcted Langendorff-perfused human heart: Role of the arrangement of surviving cardiac fibers. J Am Coll Cardiol 15:1594–1607, 1990.
231. Myerburg RJ, Kessler KM, Bassett AL, Castellanos A. A biological approach to sudden cardiac death: Structure, function and cause. Am J Cardiol 63:1512–1516, 1989.
232. Rozin L, Perpe JA, Jaffe R, Drash A. Sudden unexpected death in childhood due to unsuspected diabetes mellitus. Am J Forensic Med Pathol 15:251–256, 1994.
233. Hinkle LE, Thaler HT. Clinical classification of cardiac deaths. Circulation 65:457–462, 1982.
234. Remole S, Hansen R, Bendit DG. Mechanisms of bradyarrhythmic sudden death. In: Akhtar M, Myerburg RJ (eds): Sudden Cardiac Death: Prevalence, Mechanisms, and Approaches to Diagnosis and Management, pp 406–415. Philadelphia: Williams & Wilkins, 1994.
235. Khastgir T, Aarons D, Veltri E. Sudden bradyarrhythmic death in patients with the implantable cardioverter-defibrillator: Report of two cases. Pacing Clin Electrophysiol 14:395–398, 1991.
236. Greenberg HM. Bradycardia at onset of sudden death: Potential mechanisms. Ann NY Acad Sci 427:241–252, 1984.
237. Bissett JK, Watson JW, Scovil JA, De Soyza N, Ohrt DW. Sudden death in cardiomyopathy: Role of bradycardia-dependent repolarization changes. Am Heart J 99:625–629, 1980.
238. La Rovere M, Specchia G, Mortara A, Schwartz PJ. Baroreflex sensitivity, clinical correlates, and cardiovascular mortality among patients with a first myocardial infarction. Circulation 78:816–824, 1988.
239. Panidis IP, Morganroth J. Initiating events of sudden cardiac death. Cardiovasc Clin 15:81–92, 1985.
240. Radhakrishnan S, Kaul U, Bahl VK, Talwar KK, Bhatia ML. Sudden bradyarrhythmic death in dilated cardiomyopathy: A case report. Pacing Clin Electrophysiol 11:1369–1372, 1988.
241. Kempf FC, Josephson ME. Cardiac arrest recorded on ambulatory electrocardiograms. Am J Cardiol 53:1577–1582, 1984.
242. Engel GL. Psychologic stress, vasodepressor vasovagal syncope, and sudden death. Ann Intern Med 89:403–412, 1978.
243. Hartel G. Psychological factors in cardiac arrhythmias. Ann Clin Res 19:104–109, 1987.
244. Grubb BP, Wolfe DA, Nelson LA, Hennessy JR. Malignant vasovagally mediated hypotension and bradycardia: A possible cause of sudden death in young patients with asthma. Pediatrics 90:983–986, 1992.
245. Linzer M, Grubb BP, Ho S, Ramakrishnan L, Bromfield E, Estes NA. Cardiovascular causes of loss of consciousness in patients with presumed epilepsy: A cause of the increased sudden death rate in people with epilepsy? Am J Med 96:146–154, 1994.
246. Ward EW, Hughes TE. Sudden death following chest tube insertion: An unusual case of vagus nerve irritation. J Trauma 36:258–259, 1994.
247. Cannon WB. "Voodoo" death. Psychosom Med 19:182–193, 1957.

Chapter

11

PERICARDIAL DISEASE

GENERAL ASPECTS OF PERICARDIAL DISEASE

Clinical Syndromes

Acute Pericarditis

Acute pericarditis accounts for approximately 1 in 1,000 hospital admissions.[1] As a clinical term, acute pericarditis encompasses all conditions that result in pericardial inflammation, including neoplasia and trauma. Idiopathic or nonspecific pericarditis is the most common cause of acute pericarditis, accounting for 199 of 213 patients admitted for acute pericarditis in a series reported by Permanyer-Miralda et al.[2] The etiology of many cases of idiopathic pericarditis may be infection by entero- and other viruses that elude clinical detection. The most common known etiologies of acute pericardial disease are neoplasms, myocardial infarction, radiation therapy, tuberculosis and other mycobacterial infection, bacterial and fungal pericarditis, viral infections other than enteroviruses, and connective tissue diseases.

The symptoms of acute pericarditis include chest pain, often localized to retrosternal and left precordial regions, dyspnea, and fever. A pericardial friction rub, if present, is pathognomonic. Electrocardiography often demonstrates diffuse ST segment elevations in acute pericarditis.

Specific diagnostic tests to exclude bacterial, mycobacterial, fungal, protozoal, and viral etiologies, and serologic tests to exclude lupus erythematosus, rheumatoid arthritis, and acute rheumatic fever may be performed in selected patients based on history and clinical findings. Echocardiography is performed in patients with chronic symptoms or a suspicion of effusion or tamponade. Chest radiographs are rarely diagnostic, but demonstrate pleural effusions, generally left-sided, in 25% of patients. Occasionally, life-threatening nonpericardial disease, such as aortic dissection, may present as pericarditis, and should be considered in the differential diagnosis.[3]

Pericardial effusions occur in over 50% of cases of acute pericarditis; 35% of patients with pericarditis and large effusions will develop pericardial tamponade. The most common causes of pericardial tamponade secondary to acute pericardial disease are idiopathic and neoplastic pericarditis; tuberculous and purulent pericarditis result in tamponade in a high percentage of cases, but are relatively rare in this country.

The pathologic findings of acute pericarditis vary depending on etiology, and are discussed below. Pericardial biopsies are rarely performed in patients with idiopathic pericarditis in the absence of persistent symptoms, significant effusions, or evidence of pericardial constriction. A common feature of acute pericarditis is the deposition of fibrin in an inflammatory background, which is initially acute; grossly, there is the classic "bread and butter" appearance (Fig. 11–1).

Pericardial Effusion

The normal pericardium (Fig. 11–2) contains up to 50 mL of clear fluid. Small effusions, with a volume of 50–100 mL, are present in up to 15% of asymptomatic subjects. Pericardial effusions are detectable on chest X-ray only if there are >250 mL of fluid. Echocardiography is the most widely used tool to diagnose and quantitate pericardial effusions, and may detect as little as 20 mL of pericardial fluid.

The majority of isolated pericardial effusions result from acute pericarditis of virtually any

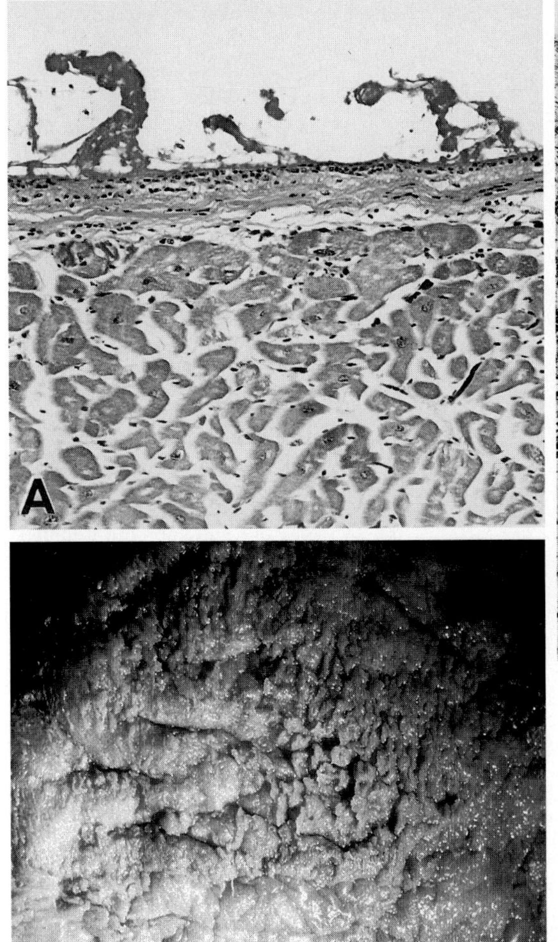

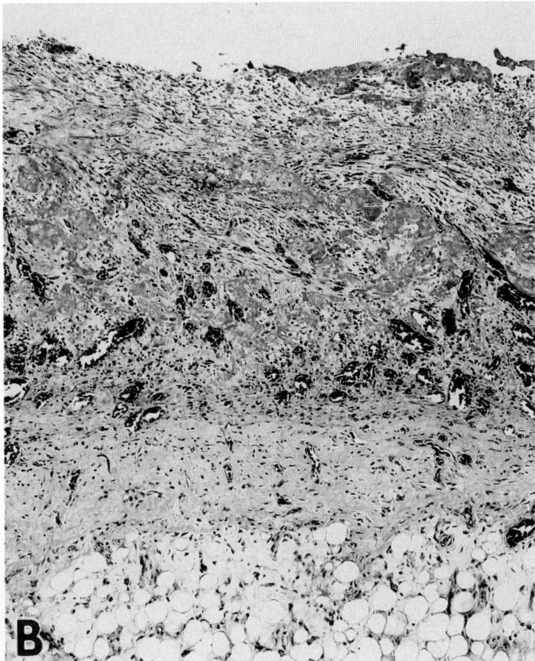

Figure 11–1. Fibrinous pericarditis. *A.* In the acute stage, there is a sparse neutrophilic infiltrate with fibrin exudate on the epicardial surface. The patient died 1 day after acute myocardial infarction. *B.* In the subacute stages of fibrinous pericarditis, the epicardium is thickened, with increased fibrous tissue and vascularity. The patient was an IV drug addict with subacute bacterial endocarditis and sterile pericarditis. *C.* Note shaggy appearance of epicardium which has been likened to buttered bread. Gross specimen of that illustrated in *B.*

etiology. Effusions in patients with bacterial, uremic, and postradiation pericarditis are generally exudates; effusions of collagen vascular and idiopathic pericarditis are either transudates or exudates. Isolated transudative pericardial effusions may also occur as a sympathetic effusion adjacent to mediastinal or pleural infection. Large transudative pericardial effusions commonly accompany pleural effusions and ascites in congestive heart failure, nephrotic syndrome, myxedema, cirrhosis, and other causes of chronic salt and water retention.

In a recent series of hospitalized patients, the most common cause of large pericardial effusion was malignancy, followed by radiation pericarditis, viral pericarditis, collagen vascular disease, uremia, and idiopathic pericarditis.[4] The causes of fetal effusions are congestive heart failure (30%), renal anomalies (16%), hydrops (16%), intrauterine growth retardation (11%), chromosomal abnormalities (11%), idiopathic (11%), and miscellaneous causes (5%).[5]

Pericardial Tamponade

Pericardial tamponade is defined by increased pericardial fluid that results in elevation of intracardiac pressures, limitation of ventricular diastolic filling, and reduction of stroke volume. Factors influencing the progression of tamponade include the volume of pericardial fluid, rapidity of accumulation of fluid, and distensibility of the pericardium. Because of the gradual accumulation of fluid in cases of hypothyroidism, pericardial fluid accumulations of

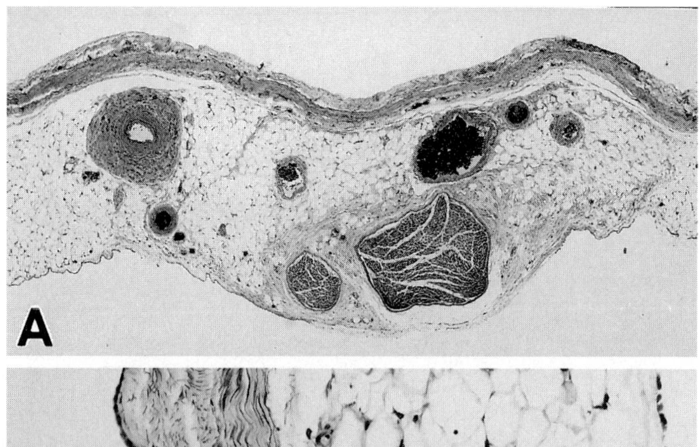

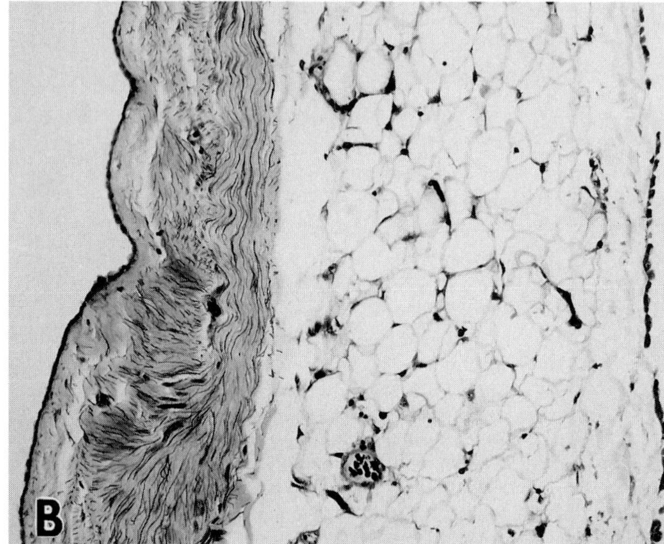

Figure 11–2. Normal pericardium. *A*. The parietal pericardium is at the upper aspect of the photomicrograph; fat accumulates towards the outer aspect of the pericardial sac. Note vascular supply, and phrenic nerve. *B*. A higher magnification demonstrates parietal pericardium (*left*), thin layer of fibrous tissue with elastic fibers, fibrovascular tissue, and pleural mesothelial layer (*right*). In this section, mesothelial cells coat both surfaces (the outer layer at the lower aspect of the field represents parietal pleura). The explanation for the double mesothelial layer is the fact that the anterior pericardium is fused with the pleura on its right and left lateral sides. When a pericardial window is performed, a defect is created allowing direct communication between the right pleura and pericardium. (Movat pentachrome)

greater than one liter may be well tolerated. In contrast, in cases of radiation-induced or granulomatous pericarditis—which results in a stiff, noncompliant pericardium—tamponade may result after the accumulation of less than 100 mL of fluid.

The most common cause of pericardial tamponade in this country is metastatic carcinoma.[4] Pericardial tamponade may result from accumulation of blood secondary to cardiac or aortic rupture, or the accumulation of a large pericardial effusion of any etiology. Patients with pericardial effusions who are on anticoagulants and patients with coagulopathies are at an increased risk for the development of tamponade (Fig. 11–3). The causes of pericardial tamponade are presented in Table 11–1.

Chylopericardium

Rarely, a pericardial effusion may be composed primarily of lymph fluid. The underlying disease in these patients is usually mechanical obstruction of the thoracic duct secondary to surgery, trauma, tuberculosis, or congenital lymphangiomatosis. Radionuclide lymphangiography may be helpful in establishing a connection between the pericardium and lymphatic drainage. Chylous pericardial fluid is grossly milky white with high cholesterol and triglycerides, and fat droplets are identified by Sudan stain of a pericardial fluid aspirate. In rare cases of chylopericardium secondary to lymphangiomatosis, the pericardial fluid may be clear. Pericardiectomy is performed only in rare cases of constriction or tamponade.[6]

Myxedema

Myxedema is associated with pericardial effusions, which occur in up to one third of patients.[7] Because patients with hypothyroidism typically have ascites, pleural effusions, and uveal edema as well, it is believed that pericardial effusions are related to a combination of sodium and water retention, slow lymphatic

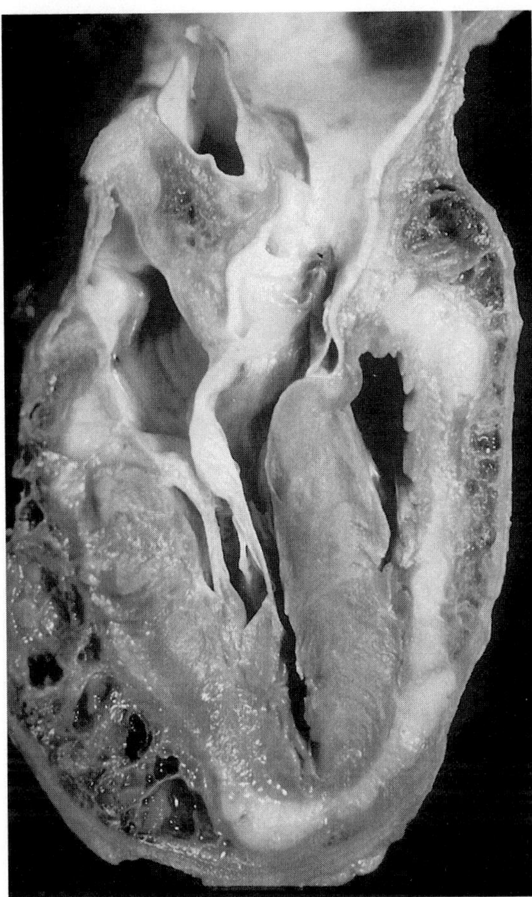

Figure 11–3. Pericardial tamponade. There is a loculated hemorrhagic effusion most evident over the right ventricle and left ventricular free wall. The patient end-stage liver failure, renal failure, and coagulopathy. A similar appearance might be expected from pericardial tamponade secondary to metastatic carcinoma.

drainage, and increased capillary permeability with protein extravasation.

The pericardial fluid in patients with myxedema accumulates slowly and may attain a volume of up to 6 liters. Pericardial tamponade is rare. The fluid may be viscous or clear, and contains a high protein and cholesterol concentration with few blood cells. Pathologic changes in the pericardium are nonspecific. In most cases, the pericardium is normal; however, high cholesterol levels in the pericardial fluid may lead to cholesterol crystal formation and a secondary pericarditis with inflammation and fibrosis.

Constrictive Pericarditis

Constrictive pericarditis is defined by fibrotic thickening of the pericardium that results in obliteration of the pericardial space and restriction of diastolic filling. Virtually any cause of acute pericarditis may result in some degree of scarring (Fig. 11–4), and eventually constrictive pericarditis (Fig. 11–5). Early in this century, tuberculosis was the most common cause of constrictive pericarditis, and remains so to this day in nonindustrialized countries. The most common cause of constrictive pericarditis in developed countries is idiopathic pericarditis, which may be characterized by a protracted clinical course lasting decades.[8] A variety of conditions make up the remaining cases, including radiation pericarditis, postsurgical pericarditis, chronic renal failure treated with hemodialysis, connective tissue diseases, neoplasms, purulent and other forms of infectious pericarditis, and myocardial infarction (Table 11–2).

Constrictive pericarditis in children is uncommon, and is most often caused by tuberculosis. Constrictive pericarditis is a rare complication of childhood viral pericarditis. Other rare congenital conditions may result in pericardial constriction in children.[9, 10]

Constrictive pericarditis results in increased jugular venous pressure, hepatomegaly and liver dysfunction, ascites, and peripheral edema. Rare associations include protein-losing enteropathy[11] and pulmonary artery stenosis.[12] The protein-losing enteropathy associated with constrictive pericarditis is partly a result of obstructed intestinal lymphatics. Pericardiectomy partially corrects associated immunologic defects, presumably by stemming the intestinal loss of lymphocytes.

It may be difficult clinically to distinguish constrictive pericarditis from restrictive cardio-

Table 11–1. Causes of Pericardial Tamponade

Malignancy	58%
Idiopathic pericarditis	14%
Uremia	14%
Cardiomyopathy (receiving anticoagulants)	6%
Bacterial	5%
Systemic lupus erythematosus	2%
Tuberculosis	1%
Other*	<1%

* Includes acute myocardial infarction receiving heparin, iatrogenic, radiation, myxedema, dissecting aortic aneurysm, and postpericardiotomy syndrome.

Modified from Levina MF et al. Implications of echocardiographically assisted diagnosis of pericardial tamponade in contemporary medical patients. J Am Coll Cardiol 17:59, 1991, with permission.

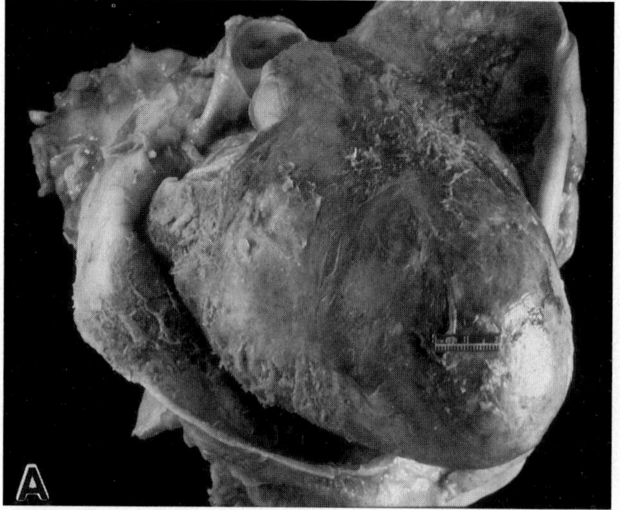

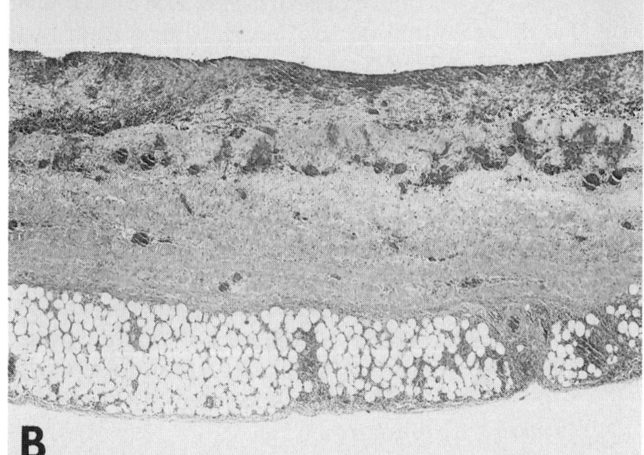

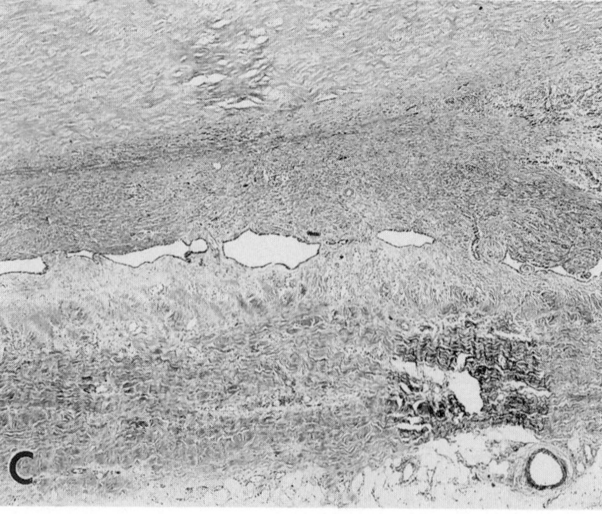

Figure 11–4. Pericardial fibrosis with ongoing inflammation. *A.* Acute pericarditis often results in scarring of the epicardium and pericardium. Note the pericardial thickening and shaggy adhesions over the epicardium from this patient with treated infectious endocarditis. Clinically, there were signs of pericardial constriction. *B.* A histologic section demonstrates pericardial fibrosis, with ongoing hemorrhage and chronic inflammation. *C.* Healed pericarditis. Histologically, there is dense scarring with minimal inflammation. Note islands of entrapped mesothelial cells representing the fused epicardial–pericardial junction.

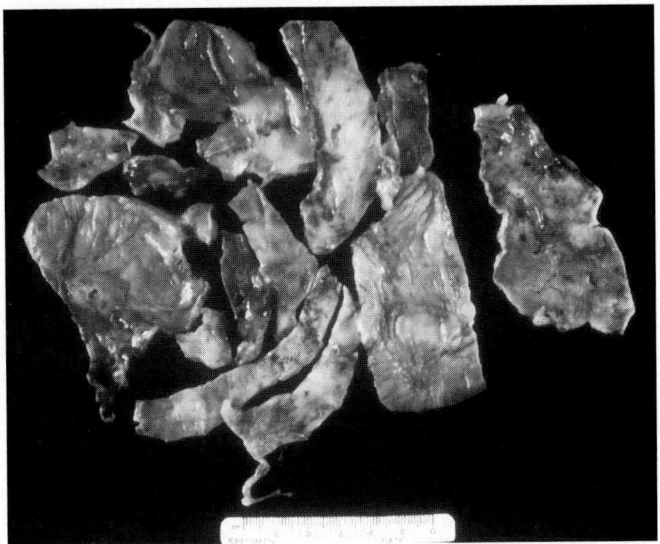

Figure 11–5. Constrictive pericarditis. Pericardial constriction is defined by clinical and hemodynamic criteria, and may be treated surgically. These are strips of thickened, fibrotic pericardium that were removed at surgery from a patient with chronic idiopathic pericarditis and pericardial constriction.

myopathy, because the two conditions share hemodynamic features, and because echocardiography does not reliably detect pericardial thickening.[13, 14] Computed tomography and magnetic resonance imaging have been shown to be helpful in the diagnosis of constrictive pericarditis, in conjunction with hemodynamic data.[15] Transesophageal echocardiography is superior to transthoracic echocardiography in estimating pericardial thickness.[16] In cases of discrepant hemodynamic and imaging data, an endomyocardial biopsy, if positive, establishes the diagnosis of restrictive cardiomyopathy, and, if negative, supports the diagnosis of constrictive pericarditis. Doppler echocardiography shows promise in the clinical differentiation of these two conditions.[17]

Table 11–2. Causes of Constrictive Pericarditis

Idiopathic		42%
Postradiation		31%
Postsurgical		11%
Postinfectious		6%
M. tuberculosis	2%	
S. aureus	1%	
E. coli	1%	
Streptococcus	1%	
Histoplasma	1%	
Connective tissue disease		4%
Rheumatoid arthritis	3%	
Systemic lupus erythematosus	1%	
Neoplastic		3%
Dialysis		2%
Sarcoidosis		1%

From Cameron J, Oesterle SN, Baldwin JC, Hancock EW. The etiologic spectrum of constrictive pericarditis. Am Heart J 113:154–160, 1987, with permission.

Effusive–Constrictive Pericarditis

Effusive–constrictive pericarditis is a form of constrictive pericarditis that is characterized by clinical and hemodynamic signs of pericardial tamponade that are not relieved by pericardiocentesis. The pathologic basis for effusive–constrictive pericarditis is believed to be epicardial fibrosis that involves primarily the visceral pericardium and spares the parietal pericardium and pericardial space. Synonyms include epicarditis and cardiac fibrous constriction.[18–20] The causes are similar to constrictive pericarditis and include tuberculosis, uremia, trauma, radiation, neoplasia, postoperative pericarditis, and bacterial infection. The clinical diagnosis is usually cardiac tamponade, but symptoms and hemodynamic abnormalities do not completely resolve after pericardiocentesis. Definitive treatment is surgical removal of the epicardial fibrous tissue. Localized forms of epicarditis have been described that clinically resemble an epicardial mass.[21] The histologic findings are those of nonspecific inflammation or scarring, unless a granulomatous inflammation or neoplasm is the underlying etiology. The precise etiology of the epicardial fibrosis is unknown, but may be due to organizing blood clot.[18]

Evaluation of Pericardial Disease

Pericardiocentesis and Pericardial Cytology

The indications for pericardiocentesis are generally for diagnostic purposes, especially for chronic effusions without clear etiology, for effusions in patients in whom there is a suspicion of purulent pericarditis, and for effusions in patients with AIDS. Pericardiocentesis may also be performed for therapeutic relief of pericardial tamponade. Percutaneous methods of pericardiocentesis include a subxiphoid needle puncture under ECG guidance, blind needle-guided catheterization, fluoroscopic guided pericardiocentesis with instillation of air or contrast, and guidance with two-dimensional echocardiography. Blind procedures have a low but significant mortality and morbidity that exceed that of cardiac catheterization.[22] The success of the procedure is enhanced if there are large effusions that are not loculated or viscous, as in purulent pericarditis.

The pericardial fluid is analyzed similar to pleural or peritoneal fluid. Frequently ordered tests include red blood cell count, white blood cell count with differential, pH, total protein, glucose, lactic acid dehydrogenase, culture for viruses, bacteria and fungi, gram stain and stain for acid-fast bacilli, and cytologic examination (especially for bloody or recurrent effusions). The sensitivity of cytologic examination in the diagnosis of malignancy has been reported from 50%[23] to 87%.[24] High rates of false negative cytology is associated with pericardial lymphoma and mesothelioma.

Percutaneous Pericardial Biopsy

To increase the diagnostic yield when pericardiocentesis is performed for malignancy and granulomatous disease, percutaneous pericardial biopsy has been advocated.[25] Bioptomes for bronchoscopic and endomyocardial biopsy are passed through 18-gauge pericardial needles and biopsies are taken under fluoroscopic guidance after instillation of air and drainage of pericardial fluid. Pericardioscopy may increase the biopsy sensitivity.[26, 27] Videoscopic visualization has been used to direct biopsy.[28]

Pericardiotomy and Pericardiectomy

The drainage of chronic effusions is accomplished by leaving the pericardial catheter in place for up to several days after catheter-guided pericardiocentesis, or by surgical techniques. *Subxiphoid pericardiotomy* is usually performed under local anesthesia and consists of performing an incision in the apical pericardium, excising a small amount of tissue, and placing a catheter for gravity drainage. *Partial or limited pericardiectomy* is removal at thoracotomy of a portion of anterior pericardium/left parietal pleura, resulting in drainage to the left hemithorax. *Complete pericardiectomy* refers to removal of pericardium under general anesthesia from the right phrenic nerve to the left pulmonary veins, and from the great vessel to the mid-diaphragm. Pericardiectomy may involve both the parietal or visceral pericardial surfaces, or be limited to the parietal pericardium. The term *pericardial* or *pleuropericardial window* is usually applied to partial pericardiectomy, but has also been used for subxiphoid pericardiotomy (*subxiphoid pericardial window*). In general, limited procedures are performed in critically ill patients with limited survival, whereas definitive procedures are reserved for patients requiring long-lasting treatment, in patients with epicarditis, and in patients with loculated effusions.

PERICARDITIS

Infectious Pericarditis

Viral Pericarditis

Etiology

It is generally believed that up to 50% of cases of idiopathic pericarditis are secondary to Coxsackievirus B infection. Other enteroviruses, especially echovirus type 8, are associated with pericarditis. Less common causes of viral pericarditis include mumps, influenza, Epstein–Barr virus, varicella, rubella, hepatitis A, and hepatitis B. Cytomegalovirus is an especially important cause of pericarditis in immunocompromised patients (Fig. 11–6) and in recent reports account for a large proportion of documented viral pericarditis in hospitalized patients.[4] Pericarditis and pericardial effusions are a common finding in patients with AIDS and may, in a minority of AIDS patients, be caused directly by retroviral infection.

Diagnosis

The diagnosis of enteroviral pericarditis depends on serologic testing. Enteroviruses are not cultured from pericardial fluid in patients with acute pericarditis, presumably because of

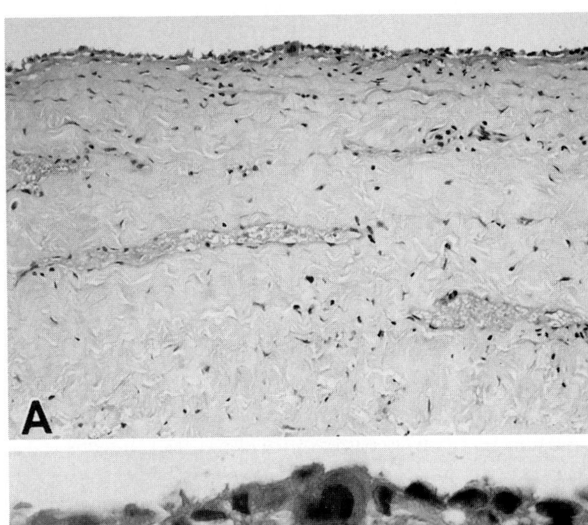

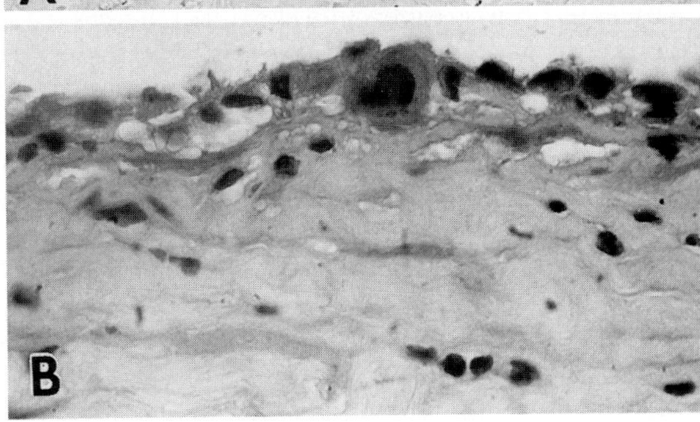

Figure 11–6. Cytomegalic pericarditis. Note typical inclusion within pericardial lining cell. The patient had received an orthotopic transplant and developed effusion with pericardial tamponade. (Courtesy of Dr. Irwin Brun.)

the transient nature of enteroviral infection of the heart. The classic diagnostic test for enteroviral infection is a fourfold rise in serial neutralizing viral antibody titers during the 3 weeks after initial phase of illness.[4] However, in a study of 75 patients with acute pericarditis, no patient had evidence of seroconversion to Coxsackievirus.[4] This finding is in contrast to a 44% prevalence of IgM antibodies in a series of 95 patients with acute myopericarditis.[29]

Pathologic Findings and Clinical Course

Acute enteroviral pericarditis is a short-lived illness that generally resolves within 1–3 weeks, and is often associated with myocarditis. The pericardium is rarely biopsied in the acute phases of illness, which are characterized by a perivascular infiltrate of neutrophils followed by lymphocytes, with fibrin deposition in the pericardial space. Lymphocytic myocarditis is often present in conjunction with acute viral pericarditis. Pericardial fluid in the acute phase is often a transudate, but the appearance may be fibrinous or serosanguinous. Pericardial tamponade occurs in less than 20% of cases. Recurrent pericarditis with multiple relapses may progress to constrictive pericarditis. Chronic pericarditis is characterized by persistent fibrin deposition, a lymphocytic and plasmacytic infiltrate especially in the outer third of the pericardium, and fibrosis. The serosal lining may demonstrate marked proliferation of mesothelial cells with organizing hemorrhage and hemosiderin deposition.

Bacterial Pericarditis

Tuberculous Pericarditis

Tuberculous pericarditis occurs in 1% of patients with active tuberculosis; 50% of patients have active pulmonary disease at the time of diagnosis.[30] Approximately 4% of cases of acute pericarditis are due to tuberculosis. The route of infection in cases without active pulmonary disease is believed secondary to rupture of mediastinal lymph nodes into the pericardial space. Virtually all patients with pericardial tuberculosis develop constrictive pericarditis without treatment; the prevalence of pericardial fibrosis drops to 40% with medical therapy. Because of the high risk of constrictive pericarditis, early pericardiectomy has been recommended in all patients with tuberculous pericarditis, although medical management is effective in many cases. The mortality of tuberculous pericarditis was 100% in the preantibiotic era and was 40% in the years after antibiotic treatment up to 1970.[31]

The diagnosis of tuberculous pericarditis is made by a variety of tests and may be difficult. Thirty to 75% of cultures of pericardial fluid will demonstrate positive growth; the positive culture rate is greater if cultures are taken early in the course of disease and if a portion of pericardial tissue is submitted for culture. Acid-fast stains of pericardial fluid are notoriously unrewarding. Polymerase chain reaction to amplify mycobacterial DNA may be helpful in diagnosis.[32] The diagnosis may be presumed if there is a recently positive tuberculin skin test, if active tuberculosis is present, or if there is a clinical response to antimycobacterial chemotherapy. The tuberculin skin test may be negative in cases of anergy. The demonstration of necrotizing granulomas on pericardial biopsy is virtually diagnostic in the appropriate clinical setting, even in the absence of demonstrable acid-fast bacilli. The pericardial fluid is typically bloody with increased lymphocytes, and an elevated adenosine deaminase activity of >45 units/L is suggestive of tuberculous infection.[1]

Pathologically, necrotizing granulomas may be focal and easily missed if a small biopsy is obtained. The characteristics of the granuloma range from large, necrotic areas of liquefactive necrosis with few poorly formed or no granulomas to compact aggregates of macrophages with little necrosis (Fig. 11–7). Acid-fast bacilli should be aggressively sought if granulomas are identified, although they are not identified in all cases. In a small tissue sample demonstrating granulomas, the distinction between sarcoid and tuberculosis may be difficult. However, the presence of caseation virtually rules out sarcoid. In the differential diagnosis of necrotizing granuloma is necrobiotic rheumatoid granuloma. The latter is generally easily diagnosed by characteristic palisading of histiocytes and by a history of rheumatoid arthritis.

Atypical Mycobacterial Pericarditis

Atypical mycobacterial infections of the pericardium are rare. In a series of 115 autopsies in AIDS, there were no cases of mycobacterial pericarditis[33]; however, in one of 14 AIDS patients with large pericardial effusions, mycobacterium avium-intercellulare was grown from pericardial fluid.[34] Recently, two cases of mycobacterial pericarditis, one due to *M. avium-intercellulare,* and one to *M. chelonei,* were diagnosed in two of 57 patients without AIDS, one of whom had metastatic carcinoma.[4] The diagnosis in these two patients were based on pericardial fluid culture. The histologic features of these cases were not reported, but the pericardium was described as markedly thickened.

Purulent Pericarditis

The most frequent pathogens causing purulent pericarditis are bacteria, generally cocci, and less commonly gram-negative rods. Occasionally, purulent pericarditis may result from fungal infection (see following). Bacterial pericarditis (excluding mycobacteria) represents less than 5% of acute pericarditis. The infecting organism is a streptococcus in up to 50%, most of these are due to *S. pyogenes* or other group A streptococci, and *S. pneumoniae.*[35] Staphylococcal infection represents approximately 25% of purulent pericarditis, and the remainder of cases are caused by meningococci, enterobacteriaciae, and other gram-negative rods. A wide variety of rare pathogens have been isolated from pericardial fluid in immunosuppressed and postoperative patients with pericarditis, including *Corynebacterium acnes*[35] and salmonella.[36] In children, the most common offending organisms are *S. aureus, H. influenzae,* and *N. meningitidis.*[1]

In the preantibiotic era, the majority of cases of purulent pericarditis resulted as a complication of bacterial pneumonia in otherwise healthy patients. Pneumococcal pericarditis is still a recognized complication of pneumococcal pneumonia.[37, 38] Risk factors for the development of bacterial pericarditis are chronic illness and immunocompromised state,[39] postoperative infection, chronic renal failure, malignancy, diabetes mellitus, and myeloproliferative diseases. In over 95% of patients with bacterial pericarditis, a primary infective site is found, most frequently pneumonia with empyema. Other primary infections in patients with bacterial pericarditis include bacterial endocarditis, pleuritis, otitis media, meningitis, and skin infections.

Patients with bacterial pericarditis are usually severely ill and a friction rub and chest pain may be absent. Pericardiocentesis will often demonstrate thick, loculated pus that is difficult to aspirate. Analysis of pericardial fluid is typical of bacterial infection. There is a low glucose level, high protein and high neutrophil count, and elevated lactate dehydrogenase. The key to diagnosis is a positive gram stain with culture.

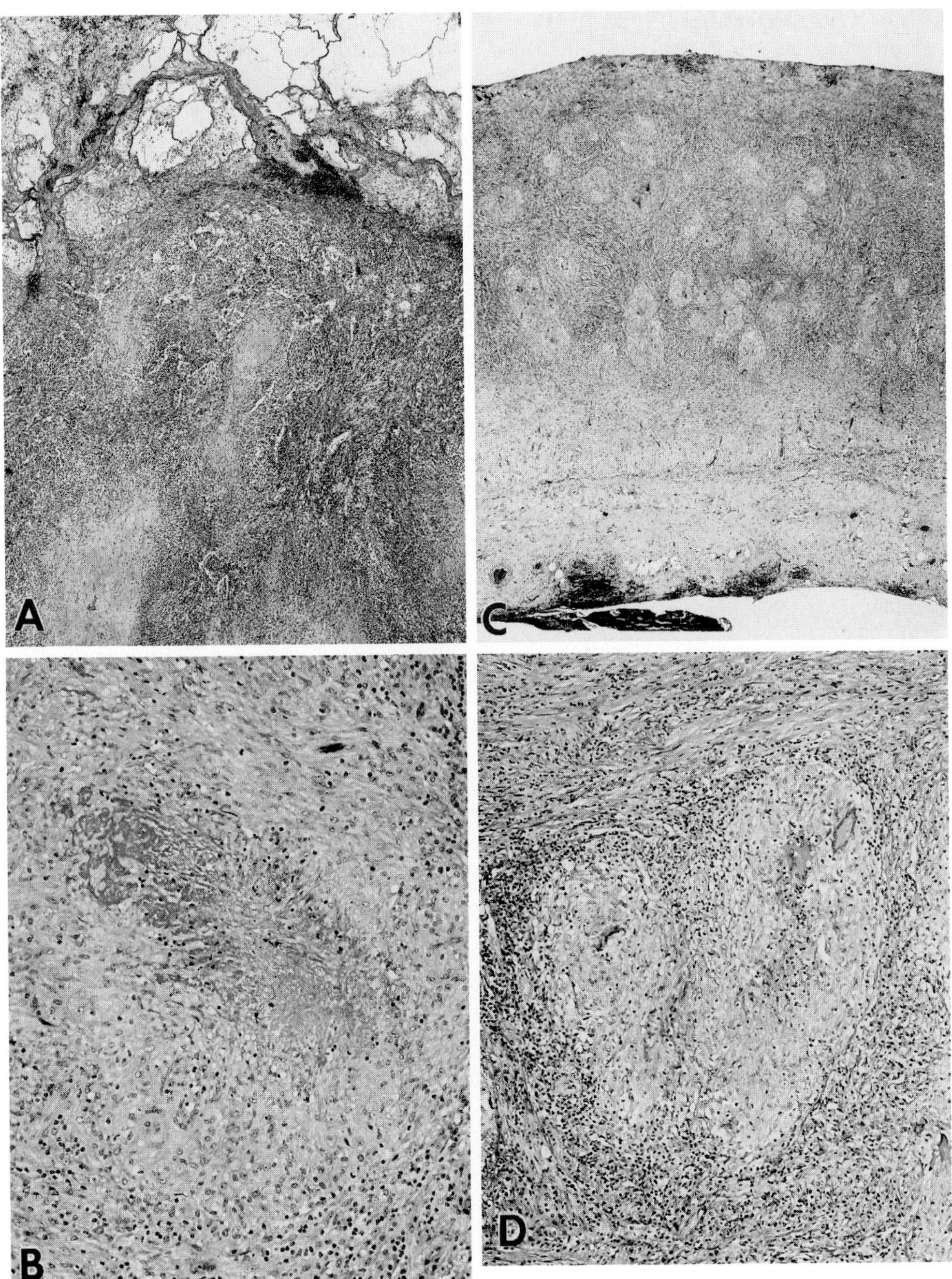

Figure 11–7. Tuberculous pericarditis. *A.* In this example of acute tuberculous pericarditis, there are large areas of necrosis, a layer of fibrinous exudate (*top*) and marked inflammation. *B.* A higher magnification of a different area demonstrated necrotizing granulomas. *C.* A different example of chronic tuberculous pericarditis demonstrates a markedly thickened pericardium with multiple granulomas and little necrosis. *D.* A higher magnification demonstrates granuloma with minimal necrosis, and scattered giant cells, which may be of either the Langerhans or giant-cell type. Chronic tuberculous pericarditis may be difficult to histologically distinguish from sarcoidosis, although with adequate sampling, necrotizing granulomas are generally found.

Diagnostic difficulties arise in patients on antibiotic therapy, in whom bacteria may not be demonstrated in pericardial fluid. In these cases, counterimmunoelectrophoresis or other tests for bacterial antigens may be helpful in diagnosis.[40]

Pathologically, there are usually sheets of neutrophils with abundant fibrin deposition (Fig. 11–8). The degree of neutrophilic infiltration is generally greater than that seen in acute autoimmune or viral pericarditis; a tissue gram stain may demonstrate intracytoplasmic organisms. In chronic organizing purulent pericarditis, the histologic findings are nonspecific, and consist of organizing fibrin, fibrosis, and granulation tissue.

The treatment of purulent pericarditis consists of antibiotic therapy in association with immediate surgical drainage, with early partial or complete pericardiectomy.

Pericarditis Secondary to Zoonotic Bacteria and Parasites

Lyme disease is caused by a tick-borne spirochete (Borrelia burgdorferi) that may cause myocardial disease that manifests as conduction disturbances, arrhythmias, and ventricular dysfunction. Clinically significant pericardial involvement is unusual.[41]

Leptospirosis, a spirochetal infection spread by infected dogs and rodents, may affect heart muscle in the late course of disease. About 5% of patients will demonstrate clinical signs of pericarditis, but large effusions or tamponade has not been reported.[42]

The etiologic agent of tularemia, *F. tularensis,* infects the pericardium in approximately 4% of patients with the disease.[43] Significant effusions or constriction are uncommon, and constrictive pericarditis rare.

Hydatid cysts may occur in the myocardium secondary to infection with echinococcus. If the cysts rupture into the pericardium, acute pericarditis with eventual progression to constrictive pericarditis occurs.[44] Diagnosis rests on the identification of scolices in pericardial fluid or biopsy.

Mycoplasma Pericarditis

Clinical evidence of myocarditis is not uncommon in patients with atypical pneumonia, and pericarditis with effusions are not rare. In contrast to purulent pericarditis, the effusion is generally transitory and does not progress to pericardial constriction.

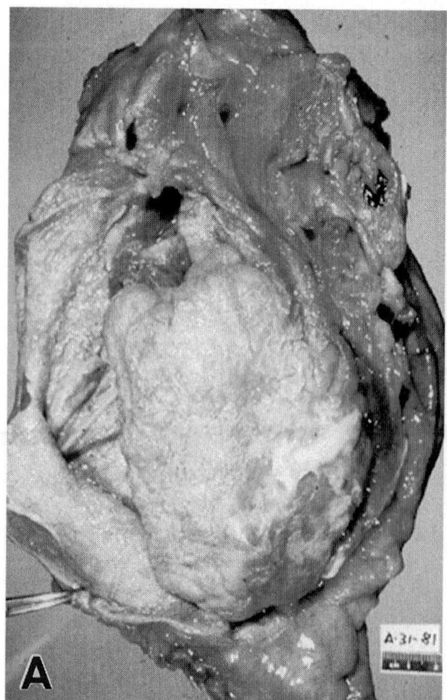

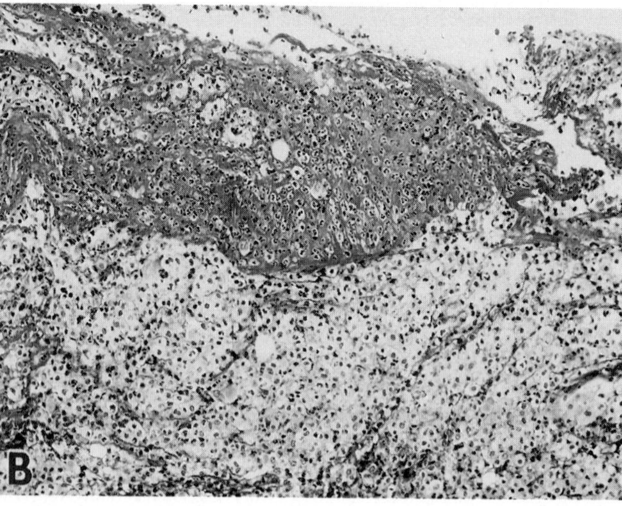

Figure 11–8. Purulent pericarditis. *A.* Note shaggy anterior epicardial surface with glistening white areas corresponding to the purulent exudate. The patient had concomitant pneumonia due to group A streptococcus infection. *B.* A higher magnification of a different area demonstrates sheets of neutrophils and macrophages and a layer of fibrin.

Esophagopericardial Fistula

A rare cause of purulent pericarditis is an acquired connection between the esophagus or stomach and pericardial sac.[45] Benign esophagopericardial fistulas account for 75% of cases and are caused by esophageal ulcers, severe reflux disease, foreign bodies that lodge in the esophagus (e.g., swallowed toothpicks), postoperative injury, trauma, and radiation therapy. Nearly 50% of esophagopericardial fistulas occur in patients with previous surgery. Approximately 25% of cases of esophagopericardial fistula are secondary to malignancies, specifically esophageal carcinomas. The mortality of esophagopericardial fistula is over 80%. The pericarditis results from bacterial or fungal infection that is often polymicrobial, and direct damage to the mesothelial surfaces from acidic gastric contents. Pathologically, there is a purulent pericarditis that may progress to fibrous constriction.

Fungal Pericarditis

Histoplasmosis

Acute infection with *H. capsulatum* generally occurs in young immunocompetent patients, 6% of whom will develop acute pericarditis.[46] The pericardial fluid may be serous or hemorrhagic, with elevated leukocyte counts and protein levels, and may accumulate rapidly. Cardiac tamponade occurs in 40% of patients with acute histoplasmosis and pericarditis. In most cases, organisms are not identified in the pericardial fluid, and fluid accumulates as a response to adjacent infection of mediastinal lymph nodes. Pericardiocentesis is performed for therapeutic considerations, and patients have a good prognosis. Rarely, constrictive pericarditis or epicarditis may develop, requiring surgical intervention.[47] Disseminated histoplasmosis in immunocompromised patients, especially those with AIDS, is frequently complicated by pericarditis.[48]

Aspergillus

Cardiac involvement occurs in 7–22% of disseminated aspergillosis, a disease of immunocompromised patients. The most common manifestation is the presence of multiple cardiac abscesses, which may be associated with endocarditis, epicarditis, and pericarditis; isolated pericarditis is rare. Pathologic findings are thickened, shaggy pericardium, with histologic identification of abscesses and fungal hyphae within acutely inflamed pericardium.[49]

Mucormycosis

Twenty percent of patients with disseminated mucormycosis will have symptomatic cardiac involvement. Typically, fungal infiltration of vessels is present, with occasionally infiltration of the pericardium, endocardial surfaces, and valves. In a series of 17 patients with cardiac mucormycosis, four had fibrinous pericarditis, one with cardiac tamponade.[50]

Candida

Approximately 15 cases of purulent candidal pericarditis have been reported. Most patients are immunocompromised or have had recent surgery involving the mediastinum.[51] Mortality is high; rare survivors have responded to a combination of pericardiectomy and medical treatment (amphotericin or flucytosine), or medical therapy alone.[52] Pathologic features are not well documented, but consist of acute pericarditis with neutrophilic infiltrates, fibrin deposition, and budding yeast forms. Diagnosis generally rests on demonstration of yeast in pericardial fluid, with confirmation by culture.

Coccidioidomycosis

Pericarditis occurs in disseminated coccidioidomycosis in 14% of patients[53]; organisms spread into the pericardium by hematogenous, lymphatic, and contiguous spread from a ruptured epicardial granuloma. Histologically, fibrinous necrotizing pericarditis and chronic fibrosing pericarditis have been described in cases of generalized coccidioidomycosis. Pericarditis complicating localized pulmonary coccidioidomycosis is rare.[54] Constrictive pericarditis may develop in either localized or disseminated disease; histologically there are fibrosis, granulomas, and cocci spherules. Pericardial effusions may be transitory and presumably sympathetic from adjacent pulmonary or endobronchial disease.

Acquired Immune Deficiency Syndrome (AIDS)

Pericardial effusions occur in approximately 14% of AIDS patients seen in the clinic, and up to 100% of hospitalized AIDS patients.[55] In infants and children, pericardial effusions occur in approximately 25% of patients, and are generally sterile overlying a lymphocytic pericarditis.[56] Symptomatic pericardial disease is unusual in HIV-1 infected patients. Pericardial tamponade occurs rarely, and may be related to atypical mycobacterial infection, lymphoma, staphylococcal pericarditis, idiopathic pericarditis, or epicardial Kaposi sarcoma.[57, 58] In an autopsy series of 115 AIDS patients, 59% of hearts demonstrated serous pericardial effusions, 3% fibrinous effusions, and 5% fibrinous pericarditis without effusions; none of these cases had a specific cause (bacterial infection, chronic renal failure, or myocardial infarct) to explain the etiology of the effusion.[33]

Of 14 large pericardial effusions in a series of AIDS patients with pericardiocentesis,[34] eight of 14 (57%) were presumed secondary to mycobacterial infection: four were associated with pulmonary tuberculosis; mycobacteria were demonstrated in pericardial biopsies or pericardial fluid culture in two patients; and in two patients the effusion responded to antituberculous therapy. Other causes of pericardial effusions were idiopathic (four of 14 patients), purulent bacterial pericarditis (one patient), and malignant lymphoma (one case). Tuberculous pericarditis has also been documented at autopsy in AIDS patients.[58–60]

These studies suggest that idiopathic pericarditis is the most common cause of pericardial disease in patients with AIDS. In this population, mycobacterial pericarditis may be increasing in incidence, and purulent pericarditis, lymphoma, and Kaposi sarcoma are relatively uncommon causes of effusions.

Noninfectious Pericarditis

Idiopathic Pericarditis

The cause of most cases of acute pericarditis, and a significant proportion of constrictive pericarditis and tamponade, is never identified. Because of the difficulty in diagnosing enteroviral pericarditis, it is possible that a significant proportion of idiopathic pericarditis results from transient viral infection.

The pathologic findings of idiopathic pericarditis are essentially those of viral pericarditis. Most diagnostic biopsies are taken for the relief of pericardial constriction after chronic changes, including mesothelial proliferation and fibrosis, have occurred. Hemosiderin deposits and cholesterol crystals may also be prominent histologic features.

Tuberculous pericarditis and sarcoidal pericarditis are specific granulomatous diseases that may result in pericardial constriction and should not be overlooked. Because the histologic features of these entities in areas lacking granulomas are nonspecific, the diagnosis may be missed because of sampling error. In cases where these diagnoses are considered, exhaustive sampling of submitted tissue may be necessary.

The major diagnostic problem confronting the surgical pathologist is the distinction between reactive mesothelial hyperplasia in cases of idiopathic pericarditis and metastatic carcinoma. Because there may be florid mesothelial hyperplasia in chronic inflammatory disease of pericardium, this distinction may at times be quite difficult. Aiding the pathologist are stains for mucin, performed for the detection of intracytoplasmic lumina diagnostic of adenocarcinoma, and immunohistochemical stains. The list of antigens that are relatively specific for carcinoma and that are not expressed in mesothelial proliferations is constantly growing. Carcinoembryonic antigen is probably still the most useful antigen whose expression indicates a carcinomatous process. Other antigens that are quite specific for carcinoma (in the differential diagnosis of mesothelial proliferation) are B72.3 antigen and leu-M1. Epithelial membrane antigen and Ber-EP4 expression may be seen in either mesothelial or carcinomatous proliferations.

Uremic Pericarditis

Up to 20% of patients who require chronic dialysis develop uremic pericarditis, either before the institution of dialysis or during the first few months of therapy.[61] The etiology of uremic pericarditis is unknown. It is important to remember that patients with renal failure may develop purulent pericarditis,[36] and pericardial effusions in these patients, although usually a result of uremia, should not be presumed to be sterile.

The major complication of uremic pericarditis is tamponade, which develops in 17% of cases.[61] Uremia is an uncommon cause of constrictive pericarditis.[8] Instillation of steroids during pericardiocentesis has been advocated to minimize the risk of constrictive pericarditis.[1] Constrictive uremic pericarditis is virtually always associated with chronic renal dialysis and recurrent pericarditis.

Pathologically, uremic pericarditis is characterized by shaggy, hemorrhagic exudative surfaces that have been likened to the appearance of buttered bread (Fig. 11–1). Histologically, the findings are nonspecific, and consist of fibrin deposition, organizing hemorrhage, and fibrosis in chronic cases.

Pericarditis Associated with Autoimmune Diseases

Systemic Lupus Erythematosus

Pericardial involvement is common in patients with lupus.[62] Thirty percent of patients with lupus will develop symptomatic pericarditis in the course of illness, 40–50% will have echocardiographic signs of pericarditis,[63] and 80% of autopsy cases of lupus will demonstrate pericarditis.[64] Cardiac tamponade occurs in less than 1% of patients,[65] and constrictive pericarditis is rare.

In 395 consecutive hospital admission for systemic lupus erythematosus, 75 patients (19%) had pericarditis, and 10 (2.5%) had pericardial tamponade.[64] The mean duration of illness in patients with tamponade was 4 years; six of 10 had nephritis, eight of 10 had pleural effusions, and all patients had highly elevated antinuclear antibodies. The volume of pericardial fluid ranged from 300–1400 mL, and there was a wide range of white counts and protein levels. Occasionally, lupus cells (LE cells) are present in the effusion identified on cytologic preparations.

Grossly, lupus pericarditis may be fibrinous, fibrofibrinous, or purely fibrous. The histologic findings of lupus pericarditis are varied and nonspecific. In the early phases of acute lupus pericarditis, there is proliferation and necrosis of endothelial and mesenchymal cells with fibrinoid change and hematoxylin bodies. Vessel walls may be necrotic and obstructed by a granular hyaline material, and neutrophils may be prominent. Eventually, mononuclear infiltrates predominate, and the adipose layer becomes thickened and fibrotic.

Perivascular inflammation has been associated with lupus and other collagen vascular diseases (Fig. 11–9). However, this feature is nonspecific and may be seen in cases of idiopathic pericarditis. Immune complexes have occasionally been demonstrated in pericardial arterioles, but immunofluorescence on frozen tissue is rarely performed and is not generally of diagnostic importance.

Because most patients with lupus pericarditis have been on long-term steroid treatment, purulent pericarditis may complicate autoimmune pericarditis. Pericarditis secondary to staphylococci, salmonella, and candida have been reported in patients with lupus erythematosus.[62] For this reason, culture and gram stain of pericardial fluid, and tissue gram stains in cases of extensive acute inflammation in a pericardial biopsy are indicated.

Rheumatoid Arthritis

Approximately one third of patients with rheumatoid arthritis demonstrate pericardial inflammation at autopsy, 22% of patients demonstrate echocardiographic evidence of peri-

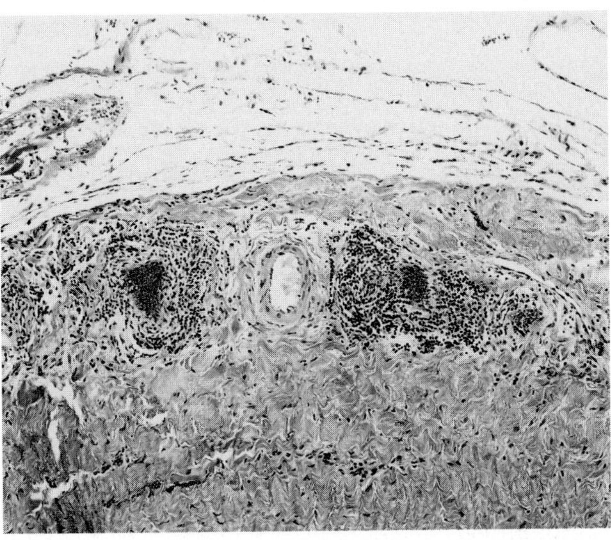

Figure 11–9. Idiopathic pericarditis. Perivascular lymphocytic infiltrates may be present in idiopathic pericarditis and autoimmune pericarditis. Note perivenular cuffing by chronic inflammatory cells. The patient had long-standing idiopathic pericarditis that had progressed to pericardial constriction; there was no history of collagen vascular disease.

cardial disease, and less than 5% of patients have clinical symptoms of pericardial involvement.[66] Only 12 of 960 patients with rheumatoid arthritis were diagnosed with pericarditis in one series,[67] and five of these patients developed tamponade or constrictive pericarditis. Prior to 1990, 121 cases of cardiac tamponade or constriction were reported.[67] Most patients with rheumatoid arthritis and cardiac compression have long duration of illness, are in poor functional class, and have other extraarticular features of the disease.[68, 69]

The characteristics of pericardial fluid in patients with rheumatoid pericarditis are those of an exudate; namely, there is a high cell count with numerous white cells, low glucose, high protein, and elevated lactate dehydrogenase levels.[70] Histologically, rheumatoid granulomas are only occasionally found (Fig. 11–10); more typically, there are nonspecific features of chronic inflammation, fibrosis, and fibrinous pericarditis. Occasionally, cholesterol crystals may be prominent.[71] Perivascular deposits of complement and immunoglobulins may be demonstrated by immunofluorescence, and the majority of the lymphocytes within the pericardial infiltrate type as CD8 suppressor T cells.[72]

Acute Rheumatic Fever

Pericarditis, often with pericardial effusion, is common in acute attacks of rheumatic fever.[73] Acute rheumatic pericarditis is principally an illness of children and young adults, and is rare in the United States. In recent years, however, there has been a resurgence of cases, especially in the Midwest and mountain areas.[74, 75] In developing countries, acute rheumatic fever is a common cause of pericarditis, and is the fourth most frequent cause of pericarditis in Africa.[76] Acute rheumatic pericarditis is associated with clinical stigmata of rheumatic fever, and there is generally valvular insufficiency and cardiac dilatation. Diagnosis is made by serologic tests for recent streptococcal infection, such as antistreptolysin-O, antihyaluronidase, and antistreptokinase titers.

The effusion of rheumatic pericarditis may be transudative or exudative and is generally self-limited. The pericarditis of acute rheumatic fever is likely an extension of underlying myocarditis. Aschoff nodules are uncommonly found in the pericardium in patients with rheumatic fever[73]; histologic findings are usually nonspecific, and consist of a histiocytic and lymphocytic infiltrate with or without a fibrinous pericarditis. Cardiac tamponade, constrictive pericarditis, and extensive pericardial calcification are rare.[73]

Scleroderma and CREST Syndrome

Pericardial disease is present in approximately 50% of patients with scleroderma and related conditions[77] and is generally asymptomatic. Five to 10% of patients have clinical pericarditis during the course of disease, and tamponade and constrictive pericarditis are rare. Tamponade may occur with the accumulation of relatively little fluid because of the poor distensibility of the fibrotic pericardium.

Dermatomyositis–Polymyositis

Pericardial involvement in dermatomyositis–polymyositis is uncommon. In a series of 153

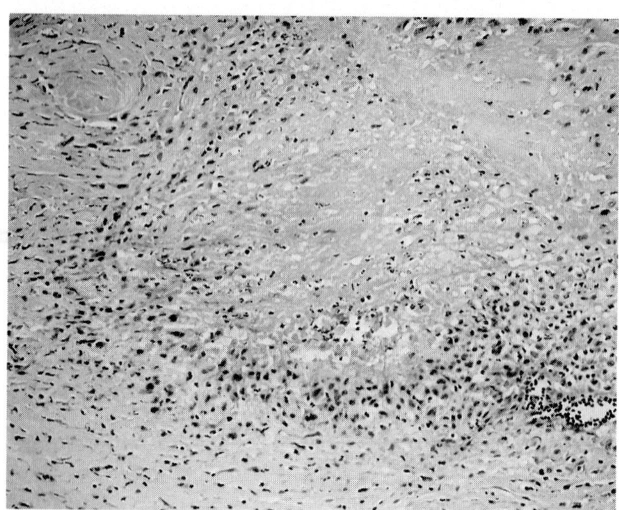

Figure 11–10. Rheumatoid pericarditis, rheumatoid nodule. Rheumatoid nodules are only occasionally identified in cases of rheumatoid pericarditis. In this example, note necrobiotic nodule with surrounding histiocytes; characteristic palisading is not prominent in this example.

patients with dermatomyositis–myocarditis, cardiac involvement was found in 20%, but pericarditis was not described.[78] In a pathologic study of 16 autopsies, there was no pericardial involvement,[79] and the major cardiac manifestations involved the myocardium and conduction system. Pericardial effusion was diagnosed in one of 350 patients,[80] and patients with dermatomyositis and pericardial tamponade has recently been described.[81, 82]

Pericardial Disease Following Myocardial Infarction

Pericarditis and Pericardial Effusions

Pericarditis occurs in virtually all hearts with acute transmural infarcts, and approximately 10% of hearts with acute subendocardial infarcts. Pericardial inflammation is identified by 24 hours, which is initially acute, and organizes by 4–8 days postinfarction.[83] *Clinical* pericarditis is diagnosed in 7–23% of patients after acute infarction,[83] and is generally transient without accumulation of large amounts of pericardial fluid. Postinfarction pericarditis is associated with large infarcts, decreased ejection fraction, congestive heart failure, and atrial arrhythmias,[84] but has little effect on mortality. Echocardiograms demonstrate effusions in 28% of patients after acute infarction, compared with 8% of patients with unstable angina and 5% of control patient.[83] The majority of pericardial effusions and pericarditis following infarction are short-lived and of little clinical significance.

Hemopericardium

The occurrence of hemopericardium after acute infarction is generally related to cardiac rupture. The risks of cardiac rupture include advanced age, female sex, first infarct, and hypertension. It is controversial whether myocardial reperfusion increases the risk of rupture. From a meta-analysis, late reperfusion with thrombolytic therapy was associated with increased frequency of cardiac rupture.[85] However, a more recent study found no correlation between thrombolysis and rupture.[86] Hemopericardium may also result from postinfarction pericarditis, usually within 3 days of infarction. The role of full-dose anticoagulation in the causation of pericardial hemorrhage secondary to postinfarction pericarditis has been debated.[83]

Dressler's Syndrome

Also known as postmyocardial infarction syndrome, Dressler's syndrome occurs in 1–5% of patients after acute infarction, and is characterized by a delayed onset of pericarditis (2–10 weeks after infarct) that is often attributed to autoantibodies against heart muscle. Clinically, the syndrome is marked by fever, elevated sedimentation rate, and leukocytosis. Single episodes are self-limited but recurrences are common. The pericardial fluid may be clear or bloody. A rare complication is pericardial tamponade, which has been associated with heparin treatment and may progress to constrictive pericarditis.[87]

Dressler's syndrome is characterized by fibrinous pericarditis that is not so localized as immediate postinfarction pericarditis.

Recently, it has been suggested that the incidence of Dressler's syndrome has been exaggerated, and that it is best considered within the spectrum of postinfarction pericarditis.[88]

Sarcoidal Pericarditis

Pericardial involvement in sarcoid is uncommon. In echocardiographic studies of patients with sarcoidosis, fewer than 5% of patients have pericardial thickening[89] and up to 10% have pericardial effusions.[90] Pericardial involvement at autopsy is approximately 3%.[91] Sarcoidosis should be considered in patients with constrictive pericarditis, accounting for 1% of cases.[8]

Approximately ten cases of cardiac tamponade secondary to sarcoidosis have been reported.[92] All but one patient were female, and seven of the ten showed hilar adenopathy with or without pulmonary interstitial infiltrates. Pericardial histology in seven patients revealed noncaseating granulomas in six, and nonspecific fibrosis in one. Two of the patients expired within the first week of hospitalization with evidence of myocardial involvement.

Grossly, there is studding of the pericardial surfaces with pericardial adhesions in symptomatic pericardial sarcoidosis (Fig. 11–11). Pericardial granulomas may be demonstrated in grossly normal pericardium in patients with sarcoidosis without clinical pericardial disease. Histologically, noncaseating granulomas must be identified for diagnosis. If there are significant neutrophils or necrosis within the granulomas, mycobacterial infection is more likely. In small biopsies, the distinction between sarcoid and tuberculosis may be impossible, and definitive diagnosis depends on results on culture and other clinical criteria. The use of pericardioscopy has been advocated to increase the yield at biopsy during partial pericardiectomy.[23]

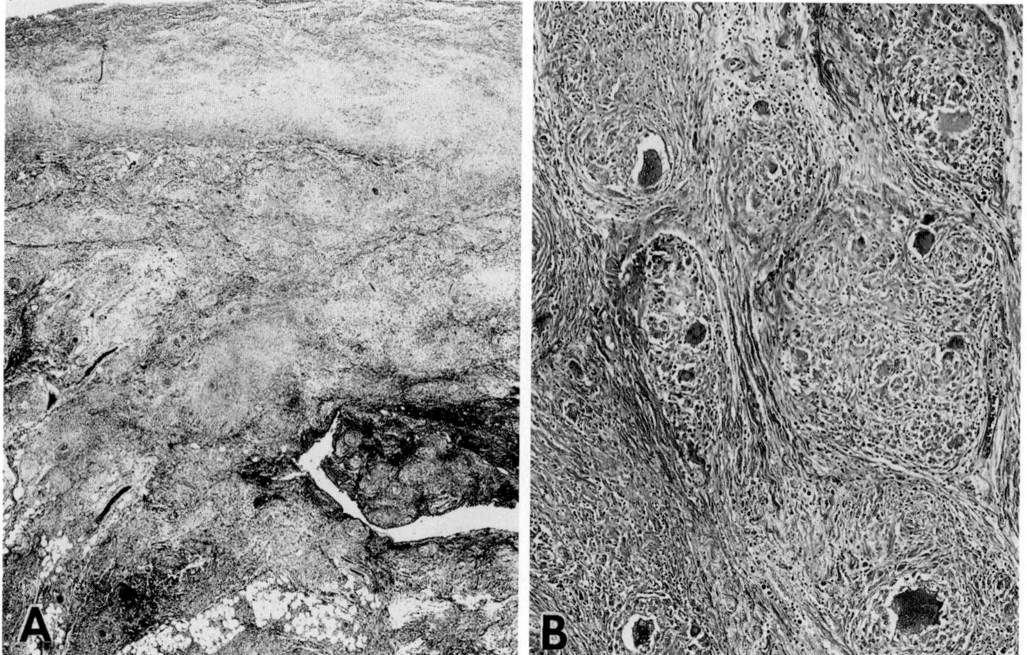

Figure 11–11. Sarcoidal pericarditis, symptomatic. *A.* Note marked thickening of the pericardium. The patient had pulmonary sarcoidosis and pericardial constriction. *B.* A higher magnification demonstrates nonnecrotizing granulomas and giant cells.

Hypereosinophilic Syndrome

The hypereosinophilic syndrome is a heterogeneous group of disorders characterized by peripheral eosinophilia and tissue infiltration of viscera. There are multiple etiologies for the hypereosinophilic syndrome, including hypersensitivity, leukemia, and possibly parasitic infection. The etiology of most cases of hypereosinophilic syndrome is unclear.

Endocardial and myocardial involvement in the hypereosinophilic syndrome result in a restrictive cardiomyopathy (see Chapter 6). Rarely, the pericardium may be the primary cardiovascular manifestation, resulting in effusions and pericardial constriction.[93] Several cases of pericarditis in hypereosinophilic syndrome have been associated with gastrointestinal involvement, typically of the pancreas, gallbladder, and intestinal tract. Some cases of eosinophilic pericarditis are clearly associated with drug sensitivity,[94] and other cases may be associated with a seronegative arthritis.[95]

Pathologically the pericardium is thickened and infiltrated by acute and chronic inflammatory cells, and fibrosis and a fibrinous pericarditis may be present. The diagnosis rests on identifying eosinophils within the pericardium, often forming microabscesses containing masses of eosinophils and their breakdown products (Fig. 11–12), with or without granulomas.

Pericarditis Associated with Pancreatitis

Although serous effusions are common in patients with acute pancreatitis, documented pericarditis is rare.[96] Pericarditis arising in association with acute pancreatitis is partly secondary to increased amylase levels in the pericardial fluid. Pericardial tamponade and pancreatopericardial fistulas may occur as complications of pancreatitis-associated pericarditis.

An additional form of pericardial inflammation in patients with pancreatitis occurs in association with elevated blood eosinophil counts. Peripheral eosinophilia occurs in nearly 20% of patients with acute pancreatitis,[97] of which a majority of cases are associated with pericarditis and tissue damage to other adjacent organs, such as pleural and peritoneal surfaces.

The histologic features of pericarditis associated with pancreatitis are nonspecific, and consist of fibrin deposition, hemorrhage, and chronic inflammation. Occasionally, fat necrosis may be a prominent feature.[98] The histologic features of pancreatitis associated with hypereosinophilia have not been well documented.[97]

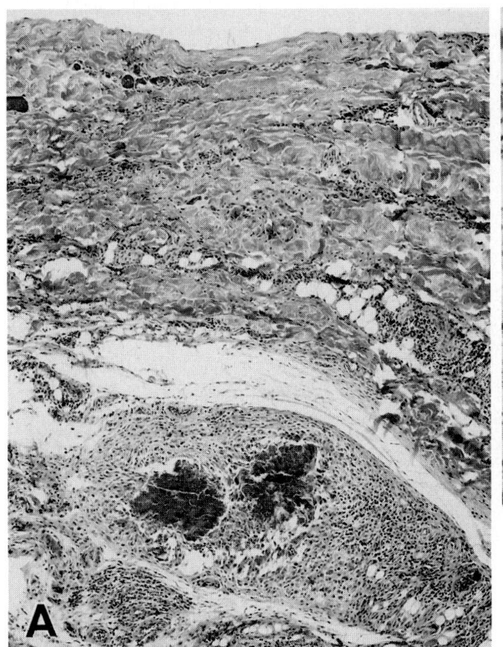

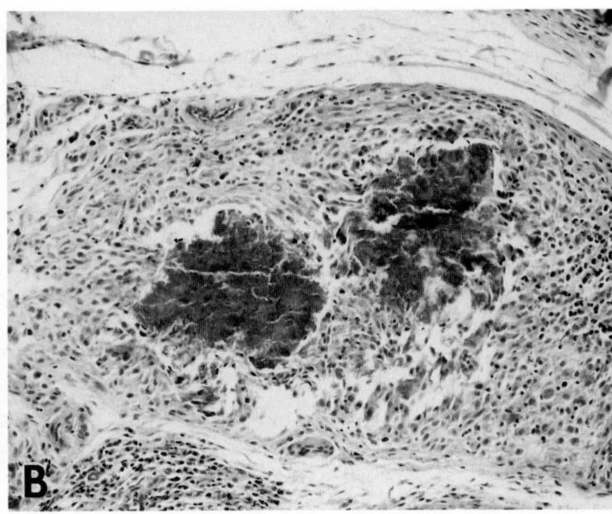

Figure 11–12. Hypereosinophilic syndrome. *A.* Note pericardial fibrosis and necrotic granuloma toward the inner pericardial lining (*bottom*). *B.* A higher magnification demonstrates eosinophilic breakdown products (bright red in original H & E stain) surrounded by histiocytes and lymphocytes. The patient was an 18-year-old man who presented with chest pain and pericardial friction rub with doubling of cardiac silhouette within 1 year. Peripheral eosinophilia was absent.

Cholesterol Pericarditis

Cholesterol pericarditis is a morphologic entity and not a specific disease process.[99] The presence of cholesterol crystals surrounding chronic infiltrates has been described in various types of pericarditis, including tuberculosis, postinfarction, and rheumatoid pericarditis. Patients with hypercholesterolemia may be at increased risk for the development of cholesterol pericarditis. Cholesterol pericarditis is classically associated with the pericardial effusions in patients with myxedema.[7] The majority of patients with cholesterol pericarditis, however, have no known predisposing cause, and suffer from a form of idiopathic pericarditis. Life-threatening complications of cholesterol pericarditis (pericardial tamponade and calcific constrictive pericarditis) are unusual.[100]

The cholesterol crystals in most cases of cholesterol pericarditis are presumed to be secondary to inflammation and cellular breakdown. In myxedema, it has been suggested that the cholesterol crystals form because of increased cholesterol within the effusion.

Pathologically, the pericardial fluid in patients with cholesterol pericarditis has glittering gold appearance.[101] Histologically, the features are that of nonspecific pericarditis. In addition, there are areas of chronic infiltrates with lipid-laden macrophages surrounding cholesterol crystals (Fig. 11–13). The areas of cholesterol deposition are concentrated in the parietal pericardium near the mesothelial surface. The degree of cholesterol crystal deposition may range from small scattered foci in examples of idiopathic pericarditis to widespread diffuse involvement; the latter examples result in the classic gold-dust appearance of the pericardial fluid.

Calcific Pericarditis

In surgical series of pericardial resections for constriction, approximately 40% of patients will demonstrate pericardial calcification.[102] Calcification is demonstrated radiographically in a similar percentage of patients with constrictive pericarditis,[103] and is predominantly located over the right heart chambers and in the atrioventricular grooves, in contrast to left ventricular apical or posterior wall calcification typical of ventricular aneurysms.[104] Although radiographically detected pericardial calcification may be helpful in the clinical diagnosis of constrictive pericarditis, it is not pathognomonic of pericardial constriction.

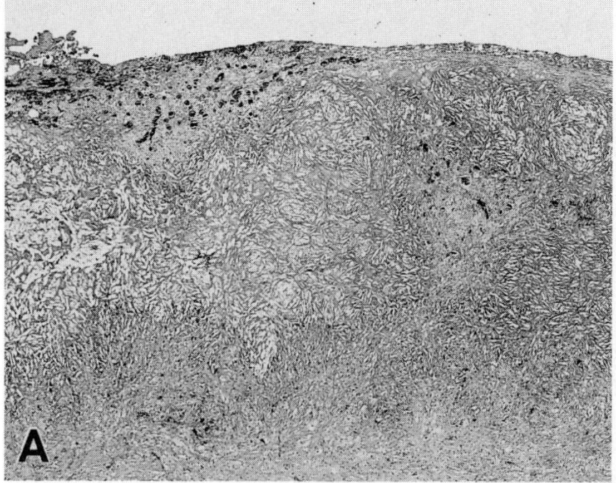

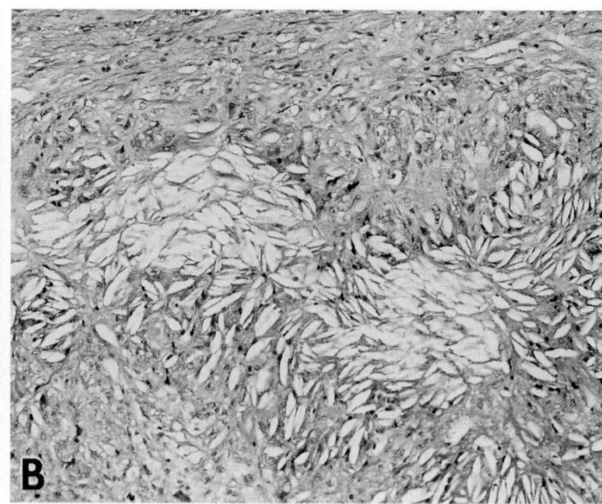

Figure 11–13. Cholesterol pericarditis. *A.* Note the typical appearance of cholesterol clefts. *B.* The spaces left by crystals dissolved during tissue processing are often surrounded by chronic inflammation, predominantly macrophages, suggesting that the cholesterol crystals form as breakdown products. The patient had long-standing chronic pericarditis of uncertain etiology.

Most cases of calcific pericarditis are idiopathic, and are associated with a protracted clinical course.[100] Calcification rarely complicates pericarditis of specific etiology, including rheumatoid pericarditis,[105] postoperative pericarditis,[106] uremic pericarditis in patients on dialysis (Fig. 11–14), and rheumatic pericarditis.[73] Calcific pericarditis as a complication of tuberculous pericarditis is currently rare in developed countries.[107]

In cases of idiopathic calcific pericarditis, the pericardium is markedly thickened due to dense fibrosis, involving both the pericardial and visceral layers.[107] Histologically, there are diffuse layers or nodules of calcification of the parietal pericardium, generally with involvement of the epicardium. In cases of calcific pericarditis secondary to tuberculosis, calcific deposits are not extensive in the early granulomatous stages of the disease, and develop as fibrosis replaces the granulomatous inflammation. Early medical and surgical treatment of tuberculous pericarditis has led to a marked decline in diffuse calcific pericarditis secondary to tuberculosis in the United States.

Pericarditis Following Cardiac Transplantation

Pericardial effusions occur in 5–10% of patients with cardiac allografts.[108] Most effusions occur within the first month of transplant. In most patients, the effusion is sterile, although a variety of organisms, including *Legionella pneumophila* and cytomegalovirus may be cultured.[108] Valantine et al. found a correlation between post-transplant effusions and cardiac rejection, suggesting that many of these effusions represent a manifestation of rejection.[108] However, a correlation between the degree of rejection and post-transplant pericardial effusions was not demonstrated in a different study.[109] Purulent pericarditis, both bacterial and fungal, may occur in transplant patients (cardiac or other allografts), similar to other immunosuppresed individuals.[39, 51, 110]

Pericardial Fat Necrosis

A rare form of pericardial inflammation primarily affects the pericardial fat of the visceral and parietal pericardium. Unlike acute pericarditis, pericardial fat necrosis usually forms a mass, and is often clinically diagnosed as a pericardial cyst or pulmonary tumor.[98] Most cases are idiopathic, and there is an association with obesity and pancreatitis. Histologically, there is hemorrhage and fat necrosis, which develops into a fibrosing panniculitis. The association between pericardial fat necrosis and sclerosing mediastinitis is unclear. The former, by definition, is confined to the pericardial sac.

Iatrogenic Pericarditis and Other Forms of Iatrogenic Disease

Radiation Pericarditis

The risk of developing radiation pericarditis depends upon the proportion of the pericar-

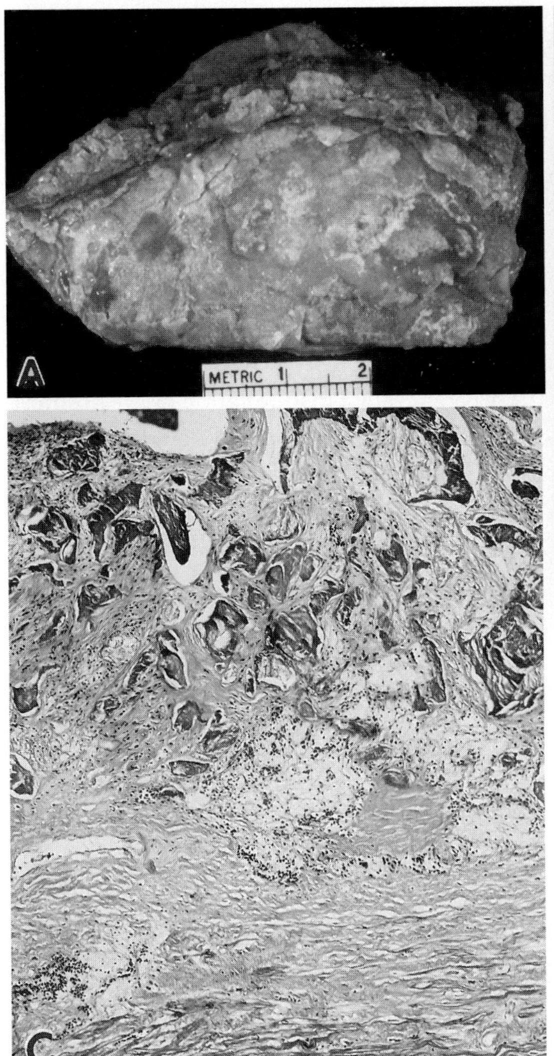

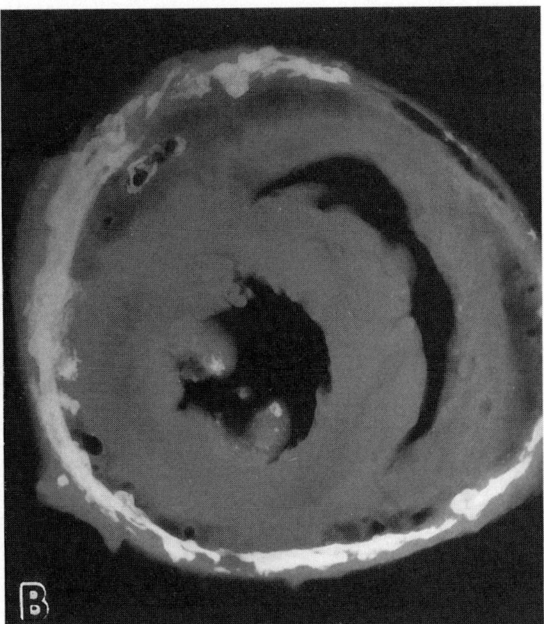

Figure 11–14. Calcific pericarditis. In most cases of pericardial calcification with constriction, there is no underlying etiology identified. *A.* In this surgical specimen, note white calcified areas in the markedly thickened pericardium. The patient had chronic renal failure treated by hemodialysis complicated by constrictive pericarditis. *B.* A radiograph of a section of myocardium taken at autopsy from a patient with idiopathic calcific pericarditis demonstrates nearly concentric epicardial calcification. *C.* A histologic section demonstrates epicardial calcification with focal extension into superficial myocardium.

dium irradiated, the total dose, the fractionation, the time period of radiation, and the technique.[111,112] In a series of patients irradiated for Hodgkin's disease, 20% with total pericardial radiation developed pericarditis, compared with 7% with partial pericardial radiation and 50% with a total radiation dose of >3,000 cGy. An incidence of as low as 3% has been reported with the use of a subcarinal block.[113] In a series of patients studied 5 or more years after radiation for Hodgkin's lymphoma, approximately 40% had echocardiographic evidence of pericardial disease, 50% of whom were symptomatic.[112] Pericardial effusions occur in approximately 20% of patients following radiation therapy, and usually resolve by 16 months.[114] The interval between radiation and onset of symptoms secondary to constrictive pericarditis ranges from several months to 45 years, and averages 7 years. The most common antecedent tumor is Hodgkin's disease, followed by non-Hodgkin's lymphoma, carcinoma of the lung, and a variety of mediastinal malignancies.[8]

The major complication of radiation pericarditis is constriction, which constitutes the most common known cause of constrictive pericarditis in the United States. The treatment of constrictive pericarditis consists of anti-inflammatory therapy and pericardiectomy[115]; the optimal timing of surgery has been debated.[111] Pericardial tamponade is rare following radiation-induced pericarditis.

The pathologic findings of radiation pericarditis vary with the stage of disease.[116] In early stages, there is little difference between radiation pericarditis and idiopathic acute pericarditis (Fig. 11–15*A*); at this stage, the pericardium is rarely biopsied. The effusion may be clear or bloody, typically with increased protein; the white count ranges from 80 to over 1,000, and is predominantly lymphocytic.[114] In patients with chronic effusions, there is fibrosis similar to that seen in idiopathic constrictive pericarditis.

The parietal pericardium is generally affected to a greater degree than the visceral pericardium.[114] Features of acute radiation pericarditis include atypical fibroblasts, endothelial cell proliferation, and fibrinous pericarditis; neutrophilic infiltrates occur in early stages, but are generally replaced by lymphohistiocytic inflammation. In later stages of radiation pericarditis there is vascular thickening which consists primarily of medial hypertrophy and intimal proliferation (Fig. 11–15*B*) and diffuse fibrosis. These features are not diagnostically helpful, however, as they may be superimposed on the findings of recurrent tumor, which is the major differential diagnosis. If pericardial symptoms occur years after radiation in patients with a history of lymphoma or in patients with breast cancer in remission, radiation-induced pericarditis is the likely diagnosis. Recurrent tumor generally causes large effusions, in contrast to fibrosis and constrictive pericarditis, and is usually not isolated to the pericardium. Cytologic examination will demonstrate tumor in over 75% of cases, and the sensitivity increases with concomitant pericardial biopsy.

Postoperative Pericarditis

Pericarditis as a complication of cardiac surgery is generally a manifestation of the postpericardiotomy syndrome. Analogous to Dressler's syndrome, the postpericardiotomy syndrome may be secondary to an autoimmune phenomenon secondary to antiheart autoantibodies, or related to organization of blood in the pericardial space.[18] The incidence of postpericardiotomy syndrome ranges from 10–40% and is higher in children than adults. The onset of symptoms is generally in the second to third postoperative week, and are similar to those of idiopathic acute pericarditis. The syndrome is self-limited in most cases. Approximately 1% of patients with the postpericardiotomy syndrome

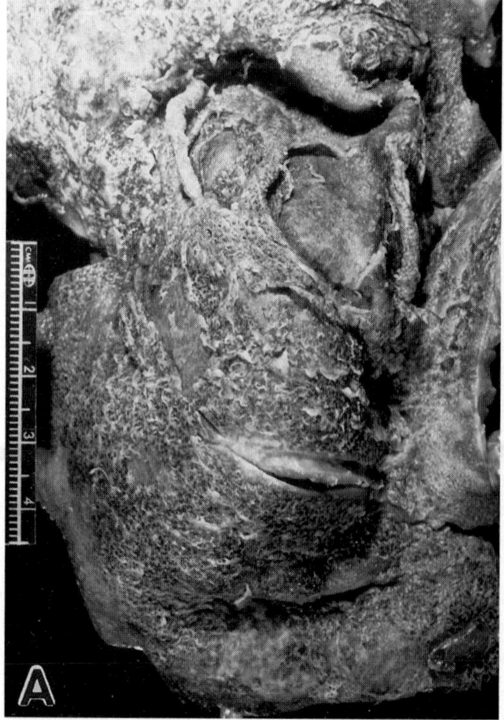

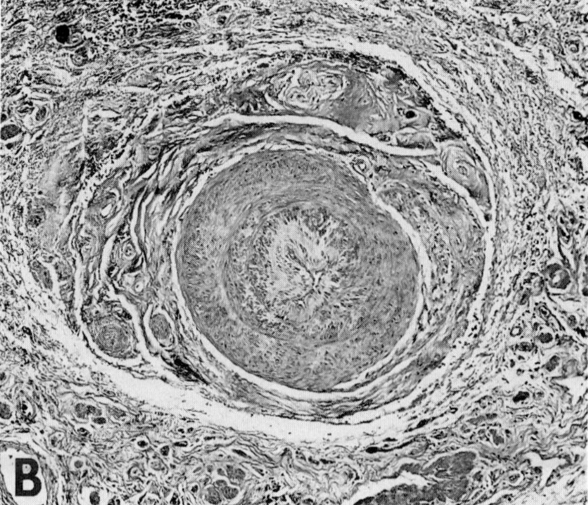

Figure 11–15. Radiation pericarditis. *A.* The gross appearance is that of fibrinous pericarditis. The patient had radiation therapy for Hodgkin's disease 16 months prior to death, which caused cardiac failure; no residual tumor was found at autopsy. *B.* Radiation may result in marked thickening of pericardial arteries, which is secondary to intimal proliferation and medial hypertrophy.

develop cardiac tamponade,[117] an average of 49 days after surgery. A smaller percentage of patients (between 0.2–0.3%) develop constrictive pericarditis after cardiac surgery, an average of 81 days after surgery. In most cases, there is obliteration of the pericardial space, whereas in some patients, the fibrosis is predominantly epicardial.[18] The pathologic findings are nonspecific, but there is generally thickening of the pericardium and histologic changes similar to idiopathic or postinfarction pericarditis.

Effusions occur in 64% of patients after cardiac surgery,[117] and are often asymptomatic and not necessarily associated with the postpericardiotomy syndrome. Seventy percent of postoperative effusions are small by echocardiographic criteria. Postoperative pericardial effusions are often associated with left-sided pleural effusions.[35] The effusion may be clear or bloody, with a wide range of cell counts and protein levels.[118] Postoperative effusions are more common in vein graft surgery than valve replacement surgery, and are more often loculated than diffuse.[117]

Postoperative pericardial constriction has been described anecdotally in patients after intraoperative instillation of povidine–iodine into the pericardial sac[18] and as a consequence of a granulomatous reaction to talc, silicone, or asbestos.[119, 120] The histologic findings in these cases are foreign-body granulomas with the presence of crystalline deposits.

Esophagopericardial Fistulas

Approximately 50% of esophagopericardial fistulas are associated with previous surgery or trauma. These often result in purulent pericarditis (see earlier).

Implantable Cardioverter-Defibrillators

These devices are used for the detection and treatment of ventricular tachycardia and ventricular fibrillation, and consist of an indwelling lead in the vena cava (anode) and a pericardial apical patch serving as a cathode. Scarring occurs in virtually all cases adjacent to the apical patch, and progresses through a stage of acute inflammation, chronic inflammation, and fibrosis.[121] The scarring is localized and does not progress to diffuse fibrosis or pericardial constriction.

Iatrogenic Hemopericardium

Acute pericardial tamponade may result from accumulations of blood in the pericardial space after cardiac surgery. In contrast to pericardial tamponade secondary to the postpericardiotomy syndrome, this complication is generally associated with the use of anticoagulants and occurs usually within the first week of surgery.[117, 118] Hemopericardium has also been reported after cardiac perforation during cardiac catheterization, pacemaker insertion, pericardiocentesis, coronary artery angioplasty, percutaneous aortic and mitral valvuloplasty, sternal bone marrow aspiration, central venous catheterization, esophagoscopy, mediastinoscopy, endomyocardial biopsy, and rotational coronary atherectomy.[122, 123] Treatment is generally open surgical drainage of the pericardial space, although in some patients successful management consists of pericardiocentesis alone.

Drug-Related and Toxic Pericarditis

Drug-Induced Lupus Syndrome

Pericarditis associated with a lupus-like syndrome has been reported after the administration of procainamide, hydralazine, reserpine, methyldopa, isoniazid, and diphenylhydantoin. The incidence of pericarditis in patients with drug-related lupus syndrome ranges from 2–25%. Constrictive pericarditis may develop but is rare.[124]

Hypersensitivity Pericarditis

Hypersensitivity to various drugs may result in a myocarditis characterized by interstitial infiltrates of chronic inflammatory cells and eosinophils. Pericardial inflammation is present at autopsy in at least 5% of cases,[125] but symptomatic pericardial disease is rare. Clinical pericarditis and pericardial tamponade have been reported as hypersensitivity reactions to penicillin and cromolyn sodium. Cephalosporin-associated eosinophilia from a presumed hypersensitivity-related mechanism has been associated with cholecystitis, appendicitis, and pericarditis.[94]

Miscellaneous Forms of Pericarditis

Reports of pericarditis after the administration of 6-amino-9-D-psicofuranosylpurine, minoxidil, dantroelene sodium, and practolol have been reported, occasionally with the development of constrictive pericarditis.[126] The pathologic and etiologic bases for these cases of pericarditis are not well understood.

TUMORS AND CYSTS OF THE PERICARDIUM

Pericardial Cysts

Mesothelial Cyst

The term mesothelial cyst of the pericardium is synonymous with "pericardial cyst." Other synonyms and related terms include pericardial coelomic cyst, hydrocele of the mediastinum, and pericardial diverticulum.[127] Mesothelial cysts are considered to represent pericardial diverticula, in which the site of communication with the pericardium is no longer intact.

Most patients are adults at the time of diagnosis. There is no sex predilection. Sixty percent of patients with mesothelial cysts have no symptoms referable to their cyst. The remaining 40% of patients suffer from precordial or substernal chest pain, dyspnea, cough, palpitations, hemoptysis, pneumothorax, or fever.[128] There may be spontaneous rupture of pericardial cysts with subsequent resolution. Surgical management has been recommended for patients with symptoms of chest pain, dyspnea or airway obstruction, or if the mass is increasing in size.

The most common location for mesothelial cyst of the pericardium is the right cardiophrenic angle, right cardiac border (Fig. 11–16), and the left costophrenic angle. Mesothelial cysts may be located in the anterior, superior, and posterior mediastinum. The gold standards for the radiologic diagnosis of mediastinal cysts are magnetic resonance imaging, computed tomography, and transesophageal echocardiography.

Pathologic Features

Grossly, mesothelial cysts of the pericardium are usually unilocular, thin-walled and translucent (Figs. 11–16*B, C*). Twenty percent are multiloculated and a few are continuous with the pericardial sac (pericardial diverticulum).[128] Mesothelial cysts range in diameter from 2 to 16 cm. The cysts contain clear fluid and are lined by a flattened, single layer of mesothelial cells and, occasionally, hyperplastic mesothelial cells (Figs. 11–16*D, E*). The cyst wall is made up of connective tissue rich in collagen with scattered elastic fibers. Rarely, lymphocytes and plasma cells are present in aggregates, and calcification of the cyst wall may occur.

Bronchogenic Cyst

Bronchogenic cysts are congenital endodermal rests lined by columnar or cuboidal epithelium, usually with a muscular wall. They may be located in the mediastinum, neck, lung, and within the pericardial sac. Synonyms and related terms include inclusion cyst, epithelial cyst, entodermal cyst, heterotopic cyst, gastroenterogenous cyst, and enteric cyst.

Bronchogenic or enteric cysts located within the pericardium are rare.[129] There is an approximate 2 : 1 female predominance for bronchogenic cysts that occur within the pericardium. There may be an association between intrapericardial cyst and multiple gestation, and between bronchogenic cysts and complex congenital heart disease. Approximately one third of patients are infants, and one half are over the age of 15 at the time of presentation. Generally, bronchogenic cysts are located on the epicardial surface over the right side of the heart, with blood supply derived from the root of the ascending aorta.[130] Bronchogenic cysts in infants are often symptomatic, whereas those in adults are generally incidental findings.

Intrapericardial bronchogenic cysts are usually 1 to 3 cm in diameter. Microscopically, the cyst lining is ciliated columnar or cuboidal epithelium (Fig. 11–17), often resembling ciliated respiratory epithelium. Both goblet cells and squamous epithelium may be present, especially if the cyst wall is inflamed. The wall of the cyst generally contains smooth muscle that is often concentric, and there may be cartilage and seromucinous glands similar to normal bronchus. If there is pancreatic tissue, or ectodermal elements, such as hair, teeth, or neural tissue, the diagnosis of teratoma is preferred.

Mesothelial Proliferations

Mesothelial Papilloma

Benign mesotheliomas of cuboidal or epithelioid cells have been reported in the peritoneum, pleural surfaces, and pericardial surfaces. These lesions have been called "benign papillary mesothelioma," "adenomatoid tumors of the omentum," "papillomatosis peritonei," "serosal papillomas," "mesothelial papillomas," "papilloma of the epicardium," and "localized pleural mesothelioma of the epithelial type."[131] Whether these lesions are reactive proliferations, benign neoplasms, or a hetero-

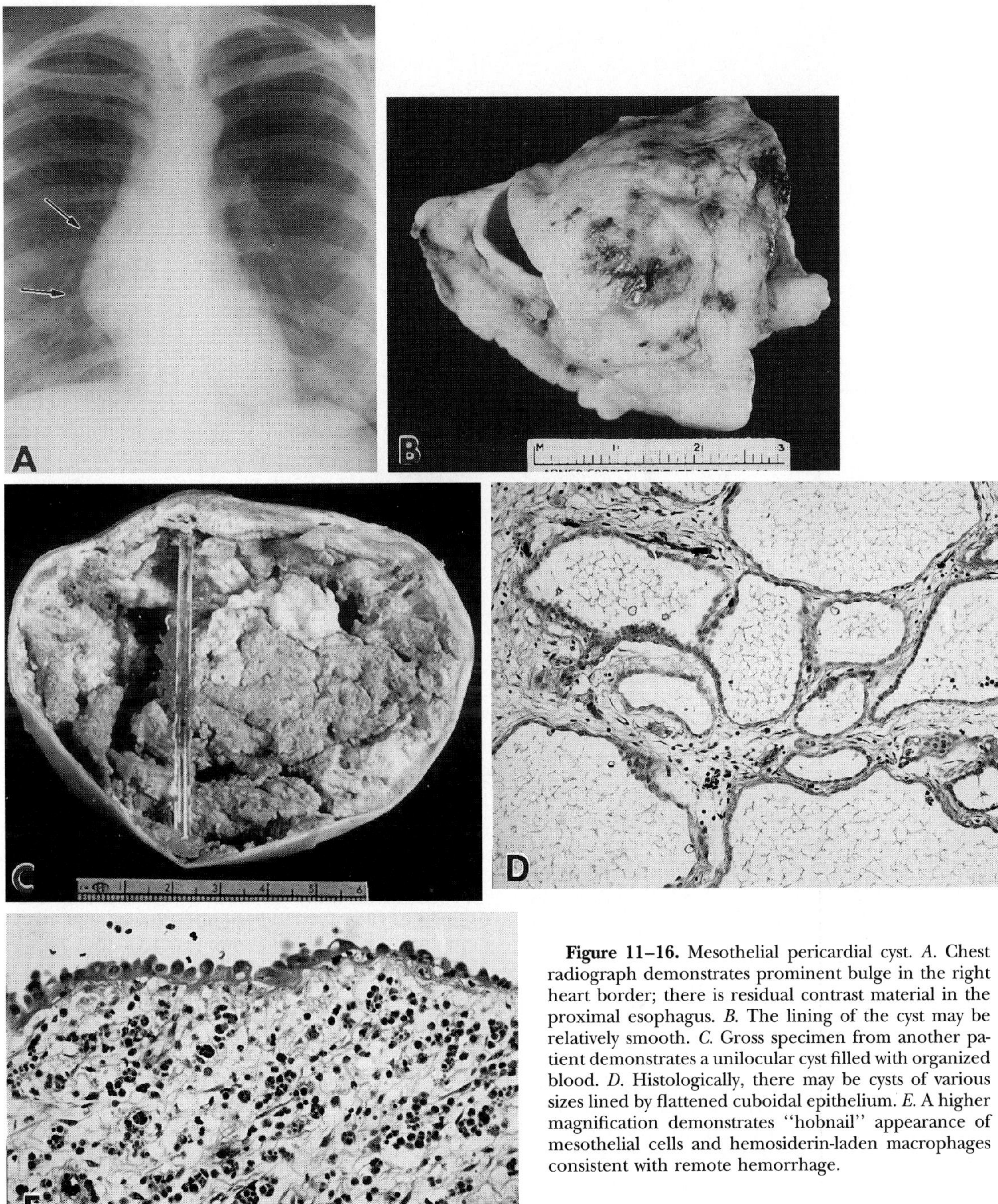

Figure 11–16. Mesothelial pericardial cyst. *A.* Chest radiograph demonstrates prominent bulge in the right heart border; there is residual contrast material in the proximal esophagus. *B.* The lining of the cyst may be relatively smooth. *C.* Gross specimen from another patient demonstrates a unilocular cyst filled with organized blood. *D.* Histologically, there may be cysts of various sizes lined by flattened cuboidal epithelium. *E.* A higher magnification demonstrates "hobnail" appearance of mesothelial cells and hemosiderin-laden macrophages consistent with remote hemorrhage.

geneous group of entities is unknown, largely because too few have been described for precise classification. They are composed of epithelioid mesothelial cells, in contrast to benign fibrous tumors of the serosal surfaces, which are composed entirely of spindle cells that ultrastructurally and immunohistochemically resemble fibroblasts.

Mesothelial papillomas of the pericardium may be incidental findings at autopsy[132] or result

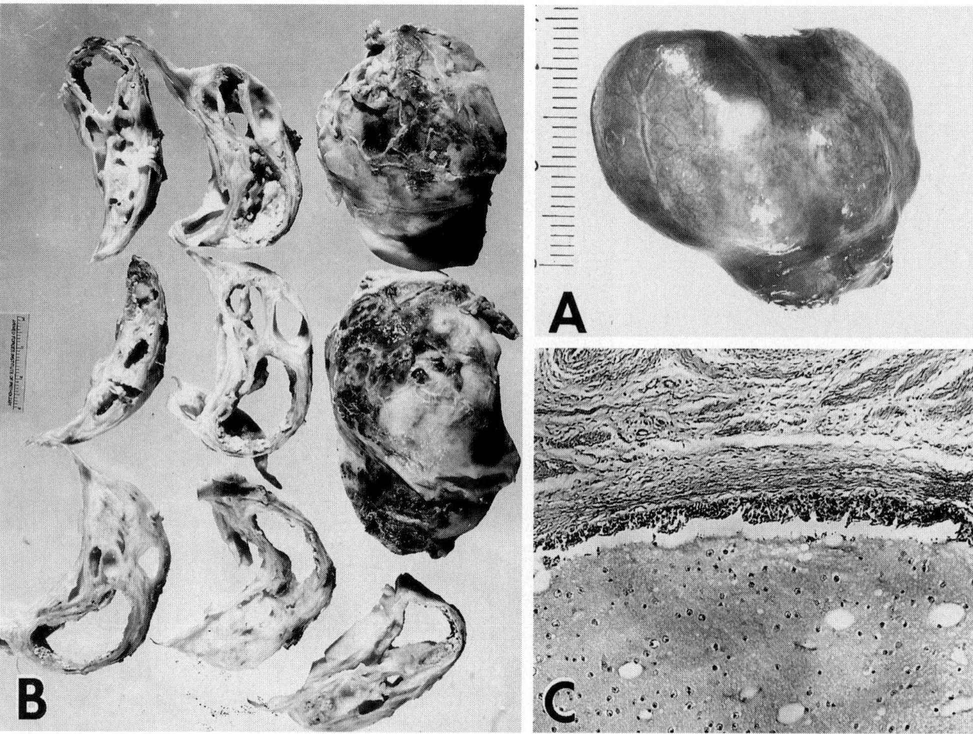

Figure 11–17. Bronchogenic cyst. The cyst was removed from a 6-year-old boy with pericardial mass and effusion. The surface was smooth (*A*), but on section there were multiloculated cysts (*B*). Histologically (*C*), there was a respiratory lining. Neural or other ectodermal tissue indicative of teratoma was not found.

in pericardial effusions. Grossly, mesothelial papillomas are discrete papillary tumors that arise from the epicardial surface via a narrow pedicle. In contrast to reactive mesothelial hyperplasia (Fig. 11–18), there is little inflammation in cytologic specimens or biopsies of the pericardium.

Malignant Mesothelioma

Mesothelioma of the pericardium is a rare tumor. Pericardial mesotheliomas represent approximately 0.7% of malignant mesotheliomas, while pleural and peritoneal tumors represent over 98% of the total.[133] It is currently believed that, like pleural mesotheliomas, some mesotheliomas of the pericardium are caused by asbestosis. There have been several reports of pericardial mesothelioma arising in patients with known exposure to asbestos,[134–136] an association that has been clearly documented for pleural mesotheliomas.

The mean age of patients with pericardial mesothelioma is 46 years, with an age range of 2 to 78 years at the time of presentation and a male:female ratio of 2:1.[137] At the time of presentation, nearly 75% of patients with pericardial mesothelioma are dyspneic and radiographically demonstrate cardiac enlargement. Cardiac tamponade is unusual at the time of presentation, but often develops during the course of disease.[138] Although effusions are the rule, the pericardial cavity may be obliterated by tumor, explaining the lack of fluid at pericardiocentesis in some cases.

Although the diagnosis may be made on the basis of ultrastructural and immunohistochemical evaluation of pericardial fluid,[139] repeated pericardiocentesis may be necessary before the diagnosis of malignancy is made. Hyaluronic acid levels of greater than 800 micrograms/liter is used as diagnostic evidence of pleural mesothelioma. Increased hyaluronic acid in pericardial fluid has been found in a patient with pericardial mesothelioma,[140] indicating that this test may also be useful in the diagnosis of pericardial mesothelioma.

In addition to signs and symptoms of chronic pericarditis, pericardial mesothelioma may cause cerebral ischemia from infiltration of the carotid vessels, superior vena cava syndrome, and acute myocardial infarction.[141] Elaboration

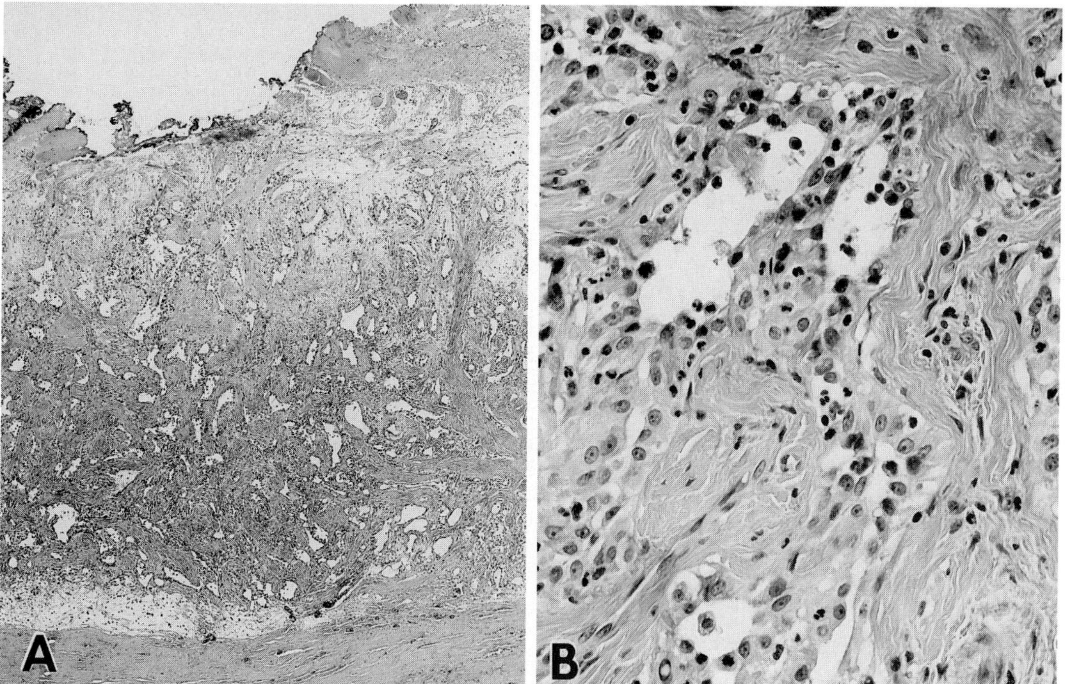

Figure 11–18. Reactive mesothelial hyperplasia. *A.* In cases of chronic pericarditis, there may be organization of the fibrinous exudate with exuberant proliferation of mesothelial cells. *B.* A higher magnification demonstrates cytologically bland cells with inconspicuous nuclei; the lining cells generally do not exceed two to three cells thick.

by the tumor of growth factors, such as granulocyte colony stimulating factor, may result in systemic symptoms of fever and leukocytosis.[142] The prognosis of pericardial mesothelioma is poorer than that of pleural and peritoneal mesothelioma. Fifty percent of patients are dead at 6 months, and an exceptional patient may live as long as 48 months.[133]

Gross Findings

Malignant mesotheliomas of the pericardium form bulky nodules that fill the pericardial cavity, often encircling the heart. Multiple satellite nodules are commonly found, and these may be present along the diaphragmatic and pleural surfaces. Pleural mesotheliomas commonly extend onto the pericardial surfaces; the designation "pericardial mesothelioma" should only be used if the patient's presenting symptoms are referable to the pericardium, and the bulk of tumor is within the pericardial sac.

Pericardial mesotheliomas often encircle the great vessels, and may obstruct the venae cavae. Deep infiltration of the myocardium is rare. The tumor itself is firm and white, although hemorrhagic, cystic, and necrotic areas may be present.

Microscopic Findings

Mesotheliomas may be epithelial, mixed (biphasic), and sarcomatoid. Over 75% of pericardial mesotheliomas are of the biphasic variety. The epithelial component forms tubules, papillary structures, and cords of infiltrating cells that can incite a desmoplastic response (Fig. 11–19). The epithelioid areas generally contain glycogen granules (Fig. 11–20). In biphasic tumors, it may be difficult to separate reactive fibroblasts from malignant spindled-cell components of the tumor. Sarcomatoid mesothelioma may focally resemble malignant fibrous histiocytoma or undifferentiated sarcoma. The sarcomatoid cells have large, oval nuclei, prominent nucleoli, and abundant cytoplasm, and there is usually a subpopulation of cells with a rounded contour. Occasionally, a pattern reminiscent of adenomatoid tumor, a benign mesothelial tumor found predominantly in the genital tract, may be present in malignant mesothelioma of the pericardium.

Staining for hyaluronic acid in mesothelioma has been classically used for diagnosis, but this technique has been largely superseded by immunohistochemical stains. Fewer than 50% of pleural mesotheliomas will reliably demon-

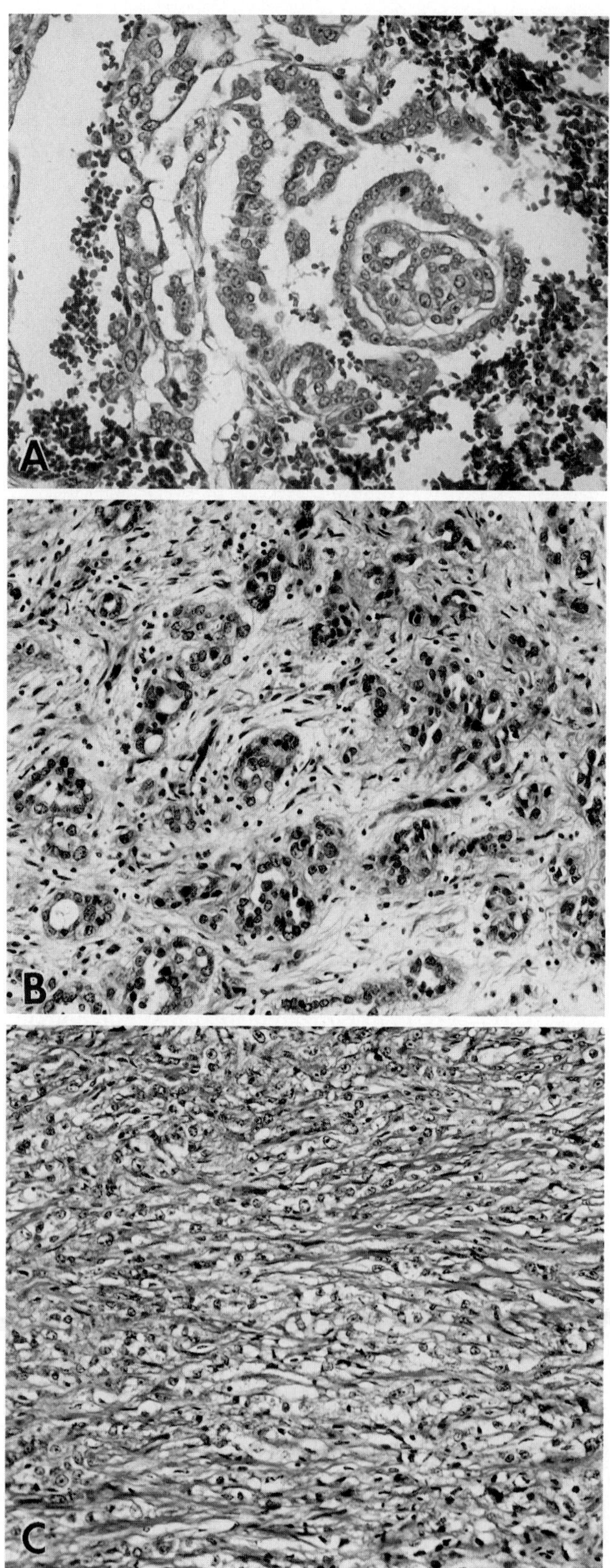

Figure 11–19. Malignant mesothelioma, biphasic type. *A.* In contrast to reactive mesothelium, mesothelioma cells lack cohesion and form complex structures. On the basis of this field, however, the distinction from reactive process would be impossible. *B.* A different area from the tumor illustrated in *A* demonstrates infiltrative growth and cellular pleomorphism. *C.* Another area in the tumor illustrated in *A* and *B* demonstrates sarcomatoid growth pattern.

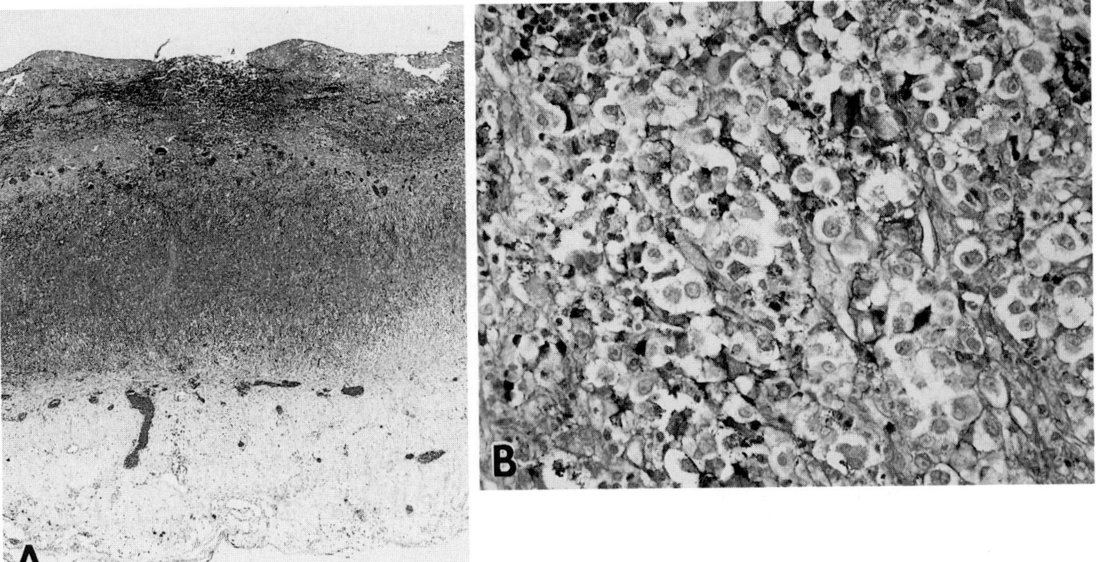

Figure 11–20. Malignant mesothelioma, epithelioid type. *A.* A low magnification demonstrates diffuse thickening of the pericardium by a cellular infiltrate. *B.* A higher magnification demonstrates sheets of epithelioid cells; note fine punctate cytoplasmic droplets of glycogen. (PAS stain)

strate hyaluronic acid digestible colloidal iron or alcian blue vacuoles, and these may also be present in a minority of adenocarcinomas. Immunohistochemically, all mesotheliomas will express cytokeratin, primarily in its high molecular weight form, in epithelioid areas. Sarcomatoid cells express cytokeratin in about 75% of cases, often focally. Epithelial membrane antigen is frequently present in the epithelioid areas of mesothelioma, although expression of this antigen is inconsistent. Mesotheliomas, in general, do not express carcinoembryonic antigen, B72.3 antigen, and leu-M1. Asbestos bodies may be identified within pericardial mesothelioma, supporting the association between asbestos exposure and pericardial mesothelioma.

The distinction between mesothelioma and pleural based lung adenocarcinoma can be quite difficult (Table 11–3). Intracytoplasmic PAS-positive (diastase resistant) vacuoles are rarely if ever present in mesotheliomas, but are present in a majority of adenocarcinomas of the lung. Ultrastructurally, branched, "bushy" microvilli are present in over 75% of mesotheliomas and absent in lung carcinomas. The length-to-diameter ratio of surface microvilli in mesothelioma ranges from 10–16 : 1, and in adenocarcinoma, from 4–7.5 : 1. Carcinoembryonic antigen is expressed in 77–95% of adenocarcinomas, and in 0–22% of mesotheliomas. Leu-M1, a cell membrane-associated glycoprotein, is present in 0–8% of mesothelioma and in 80–100% of adenocarcinomas of the lung. B72.3 antigen and MOC-31 are markers of adenocarcinoma and are negative or only weakly expressed by mesothelioma.

The differential diagnosis between reactive mesothelial proliferations and malignant mesothelioma may be difficult. In general, malignant mesotheliomas can form sheets of cells, infiltrate epicardial fat, and have spindle and sarcomatoid areas—all features lacking in reactive mesothelial processes. Immunohistochemical stains are of limited use in the separation of malignant and benign mesothelial reactions.

Germ Cell Tumors of the Pericardium

Pericardial Teratoma

The majority of pericardial germ cell tumors are teratomas. These tumors are rare. By 1993, approximately 65 cases had been reported.[143, 144] The patient's age at diagnosis ranges from 1 day to 42 years. The majority of patients are infants, and over 75% of cardiac teratomas occur in children under age 15. At least five cases of cardiac teratoma have been positively identified before birth, and intrauterine pericardiocentesis may be successful to avert fetal death.

Table 11–3. Differential Diagnosis of Pericardial Biopsy

	Met. Ca	Benign Meso.	Mal. Meso
Gross features			
Bulky nodules	− or +	−	+
Constriction	− or +	− or (+)	+
Microscopic features			
Intracytoplasmic mucin vacuoles*	+ or −	−	−
Lymphatic nests	+ or −	−	−
Papillae with multiple cell layers	+ or −	−	+ or −
Irregular nucleoli	+	−	+ or −
Biphasic growth	−	−	+ or −
Desmoplasia	− or +	−	+ or −
Hyalinized stroma	−	− or +	+ or −
Immunohistochemical features			
Cytokeratin	+	+	+
CEA	+ or −	−	− or +/−
Leu M-1 (CD15)	+ or −	−	−
B72.3	+ or −	−	−
Ber-EP4	+ or −	− or +	− or +
Thrombomodulin	− or (+)	+	+
ME-1	− or (+)	+	+
Ultrastructural findings			
Long microvilli†	−	+	+‡
Intracytoplasmic lumina	+ or −	−	−

* after diastase pretreatment; † length : diameter ratio >8 : 1; ‡ epithelioid areas

Two thirds of patients are female. Symptoms include respiratory distress, pericardial tamponade, and cyanosis; cardiac murmurs are rarely heard. In adults, pericardial teratomas are usually discovered as an incidental radiographic finding, although chest pain and friction rubs from rapidly growing tumors or from hemorrhage within the tumor have been reported. Pericardial effusion is usually present and is serous, yellow, and clear.

Intrapericardial teratomas may be massive, measuring up to 15 cm. On cut surface, the tumor is multicystic with intervening solid areas. Intrapericardial teratomas are usually located on the right side of the heart, displacing the organs to the left and posteriorly. Similar to pericardial bronchogenic cysts, pericardial teratomas are usually attached by a pedicle to one of the great vessels with arterial supply directly from the aorta.

Germ Cell Tumors of the Pericardium Other than Benign Teratoma

McAllister and Fenoglio[145] reported four malignant pericardial germ cell tumors; the malignant foci were histologically composed of either embryonal carcinoma, squamous cell carcinoma arising in a teratoma, or choriocarcinoma. We have recently encountered a pericardial endodermal sinus tumor in an infant. Although primary seminomas of the mediastinum are not rare, we are unaware of a primary seminoma of the pericardium. Metastatic seminoma to the pericardium, however, may be diagnosed by pericardial biopsy.

Fibrous Tumor of the Pericardium

Benign Fibrous Tumor of the Pericardium

Benign fibrous tumor (solitary fibrous tumor, localized fibrous tumor) is a neoplasm of fibroblasts that arises in close proximity to a mesothelial surface. Most benign fibrous tumors have been described in the pleura and extrapericardial mediastinum and several have been reported in the pericardium.[146, 147]

Grossly, the tumor is white, with a whorled appearance on cut section, and is attached to the pericardial surface either by broad or narrow pedicle. Histologically, the tumor consists of spindle cells with interspersed hyalinized collagen, focally arranged in bundles of collagen fibers. Small foci of calcification may be present. Mitotic figures, necrosis, and cellular atypia are generally absent. Myxoid areas and a vascular pattern reminiscent of hemangiopericytoma may occur. Ultrastructural studies demonstrate cells with the characteristics of fibroblasts.[148] Immunohistochemically, the cells express vimentin and do not express cytokeratin in contrast to mesothelioma. Expression of CD34 is typical of solitary fibrous tumor and a helpful adjunct in diagnosis.

Malignant Fibrous Tumor of the Pericardium

Eight of 14 solitary fibrous tumors of the mediastinum reported by Witkin and Rosai[149] demonstrated cellular areas with mitoses and necrosis. These malignant fibrous tumors may recur and infiltrate surrounding structures. In contrast to sarcomatoid mesotheliomas, solitary fibrous tumors do not express neural or epithelial markers, and are positive for CD34. Because these tumors immunohistochemically and ultrastructurally resemble fibrous tumors, they are believed to originate from submesothelial fibroblasts, and may be considered a type of fibrosarcoma.

Pericardial Sarcoma

Angiosarcoma

The most common sarcoma that arises within the pericardium is angiosarcoma. Patients often undergo a long evaluation for chronic pericarditis before the diagnosis is made.[150] Grossly, angiosarcomas may mimic mesothelioma, with diffuse infiltration of the pericardium.[151] The diagnosis may be missed on repeated pericardial biopsy if adequate tissue is not retrieved,[152] and reactive mesothelial hyperplasia may be present confounding the diagnosis. Histologic features are similar to angiosarcomas of the heart. In practice, it may be difficult to separate primary pericardial angiosarcoma from primary cardiac angiosarcoma because of diffuse infiltration of both structures.

Unclassifiable Pericardial Sarcomas

Rarely, a malignant spindle cell tumor will diffusely infiltrate the pericardium, simulating mesothelioma. Some spindled cell tumors of the pericardium have immunohistochemical features of both sarcoma and mesothelioma and are difficult to classify even after immunohistochemical and ultrastructural studies have been carried out.[153]

Miscellaneous Pericardial Tumors

Pericardial Thymoma

Thymomas involving the heart are usually extensions of primary mediastinal tumors. Approximately 20% of thymomas are locally infiltrative, and pericardial involvement represents a late stage of tumor spread. Occasionally, mediastinal thymomas may present as pericardial effusions, and the diagnosis is first made by examination of pericardial fluid or pericardial biopsy.[154–156]

Rarely, thymomas may be entirely intrapericardial; these tumors are believed to derive from pericardial thymic rests. Histologically, intrapericardial thymomas are generally the epithelial type, with a background of lymphoid cells.

Other Rare Pericardial Tumors

Lipomas of the pericardium are quite rare. Rarely, they may achieve enormous proportions, necessitating surgical excision.[157] Occasionally, massive fat deposits may infiltrate the pericardial space and epicardium. Increased epicardial fat is associated with obesity and steroid therapy.

Several reports of giant lymph node hyperplasia (Castleman's disease) have been reported in the pericardium.[158] Neurofibromas, hemangiopericytomas, and leiomyomas rarely occur in the pericardial sac.[145]

Metastatic Tumors to the Pericardium

Clinical Findings

Pericardial involvement is suspected in patients with malignancy if there is acute pericarditis, rapid enlargement of the heart shadow, low-voltage changes on electrocardiography, serosanguinous or sanguinous effusions, or echocardiographic demonstration of echo-free spaces in pericardial effusions. Pericardial tamponade is a frequent complication and has been reported for a large number of tumor types. Pericardial fluid in patients with malignant tamponade is usually hemorrhagic; accumulations are typically 500 to 1000 mL.[159] Most malignant effusions recur after pericardiocentesis and the mean survival is measured in months, even after surgical drainage. Instillation of sclerosing agents or radiation therapy may retard the reaccumulation of fluid and may slightly extend survival. Pericardial constriction due to desmoplastic fibrosis is relatively rare, and accounts for fewer than 5% of cases of constrictive pericarditis (see Table 11–2).

Effusions in cancer patients may be idiopathic or secondary to radiation or chemotherapy. In patients with breast cancer, small, asymptomatic effusions are likely benign, and of those that are clinically apparent, only 50% are malignant.[160]

Gross Pathologic Findings

At autopsy, pericardial metastases result in hemorrhagic, fibrinous exudates on the mesothelial surfaces. Typically, there are nodular masses that involve the pericardium (Fig. 11–21). Less commonly, the tumor may be grossly evident only as diffuse pericardial thickening resulting in constrictive pericarditis.

The Evaluation of Pericardial Biopsies for Metastatic Tumor

The histologic features of metastatic pericardial tumors, most of which are carcinomas, are similar to their corresponding primaries. Common findings are pericardial thickening with a fibrinous, hemorrhagic exudate (Fig. 11–22). The most common site of origin is the lung; of lung tumors, large cell or adenocarcinomas are the most common histologic types to metastasize to pericardium. A surprisingly high percentage of malignant pericardial biopsies occur in patients in whom the diagnosis of malignancy has not yet been made clinically. Most adenocarcinomas presenting as pericardial metastases originate either in the lung or an undetermined primary site. Breast carcinoma, unlike lung carcinoma, usually manifests as pericardial disease only after the primary site is known.[161]

The histologic diagnosis is generally made on the basis of cytologic examination of pericardial effusion, with pericardial biopsy in a minority of cases. The sensitivity of cytologic examination in the diagnosis of malignant pericardial effusions ranges from 50–95%, and averages 87%. The additional diagnostic sensitivity achieved by biopsy in addition to cytologic examination is small.[24] Pericardial biopsy may be negative in the face of positive cytology, presumably because of tissue sampling error.[162]

The differential diagnosis of pericardial biopsies generally involves metastatic carcinoma, reactive mesothelial hyperplasia, and malignant mesothelioma (Table 11–3). It is preferable to study the cytologic preparations (smears and cell blocks) in conjunction with the pericardial biopsy, if performed. The presence of mucin vacuoles (Fig. 11–23), and positivity for, carcinoembryonic antigen, B72.3 or leu-M1 are supportive of the diagnosis of adenocarcinoma. One can be assured of the diagnosis of meta-

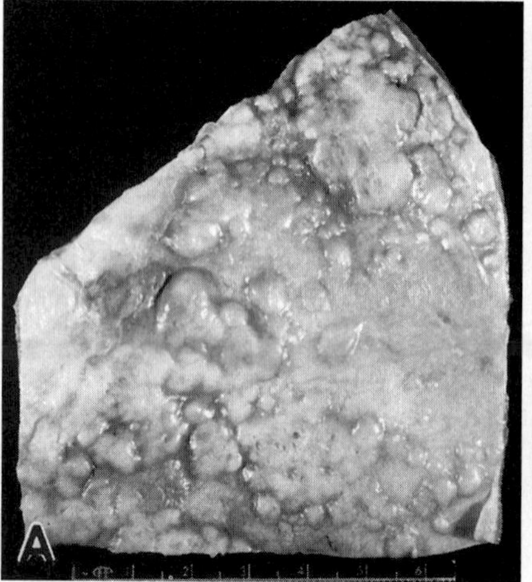

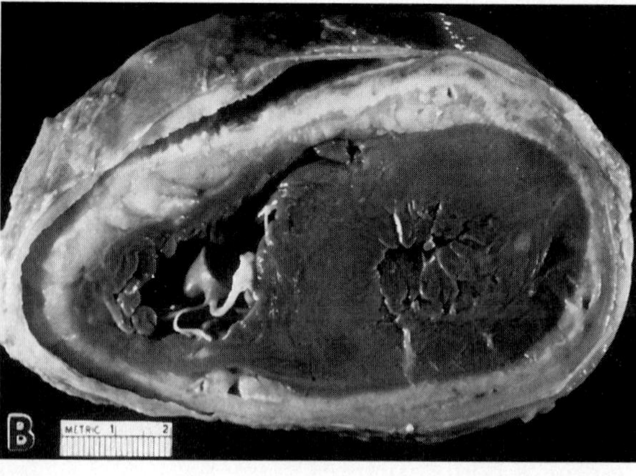

Figure 11–21. Metastatic carcinoma, gross appearance. *A.* Note umbilicated nodules studding the epicardial surface. The patient died with widespread ovarian carcinoma. *B.* Occasionally, metastatic carcinoma may result in pericardial constriction. Note diffuse pericardial thickening and tumor deposits; the patient died with widepread carcinoma of the lung.

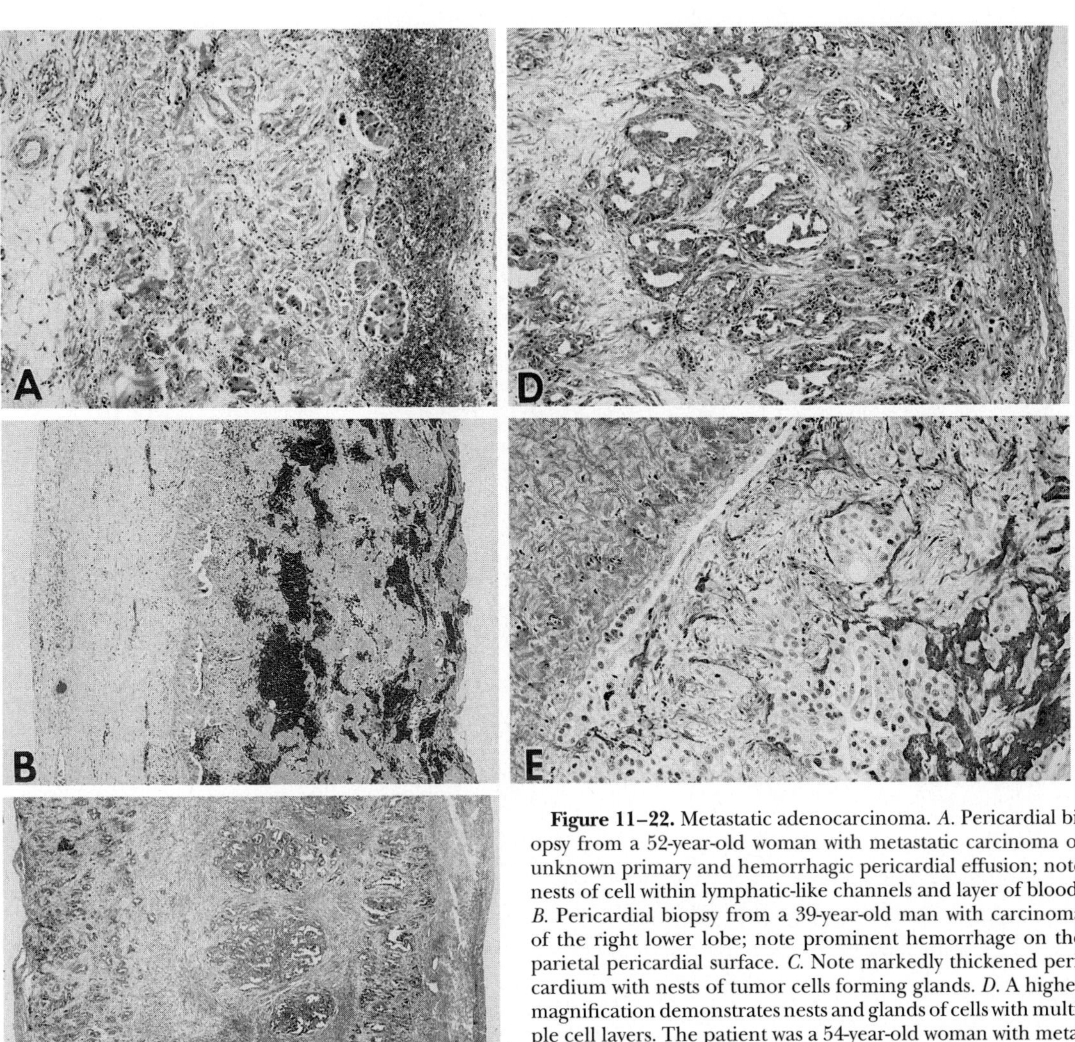

Figure 11–22. Metastatic adenocarcinoma. *A.* Pericardial biopsy from a 52-year-old woman with metastatic carcinoma of unknown primary and hemorrhagic pericardial effusion; note nests of cell within lymphatic-like channels and layer of blood. *B.* Pericardial biopsy from a 39-year-old man with carcinoma of the right lower lobe; note prominent hemorrhage on the parietal pericardial surface. *C.* Note markedly thickened pericardium with nests of tumor cells forming glands. *D.* A higher magnification demonstrates nests and glands of cells with multiple cell layers. The patient was a 54-year-old woman with metastatic adenocarcinoma of unknown primary and pericardial tamponade who underwent partial pericardiectomy. *E.* A higher magnification of *D* demonstrates thick, papillary structures with multiple cell layers.

static carcinoma if a population of malignant cells is clearly discerned from reactive mesothelial cells, both on cytologic preparations and biopsy specimens. False positive reactions for Ber-EP4 in reactive mesothelial proliferations occur, making this marker relatively unreliable in our experience; however, published reports support the use of this marker in the distinction between mesothelial proliferations and carcinoma.[163] Mesothelial markers, such as ME-1, calretinin, and thrombomodulin, which are expressed by mesothelial cells, endothelial cells, and only rarely by epithelial cells, may be helpful in the differential diagnosis. A panel of markers is preferable than reliance on a single immunohistochemical stain.[164]

Metastatic carcinomas rarely found in pericardial biopsies include metastatic carcinoma of the gastrointestinal tract, renal cell carcinoma, transitional cell carcinoma, hepatocellular carcinoma, ovarian carcinoma, prostate carcinoma, parotid gland carcinoma, esophageal carcinoma, and cervical carcinoma.[165, 166] Other neoplasms, including lymphoma, melanoma, multiple myeloma, thymoma, testicular seminoma, and primary sarcomas of the pericar-

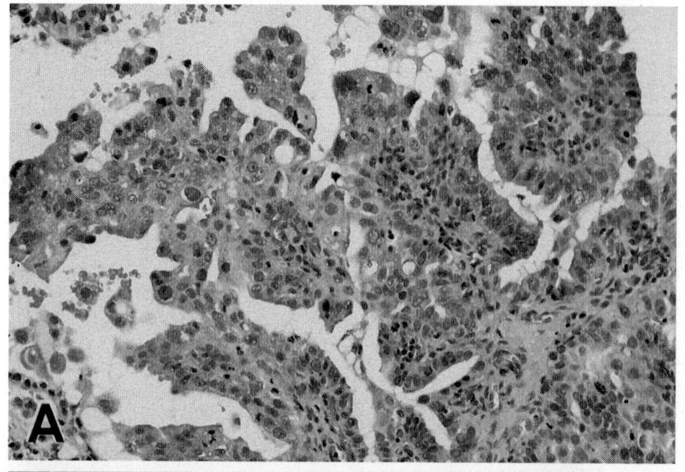

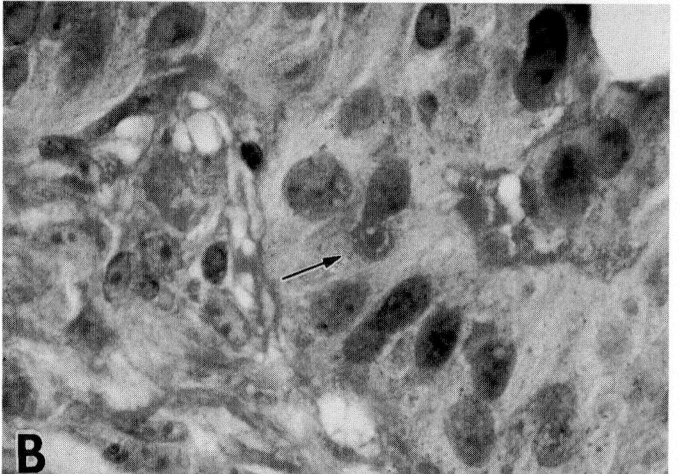

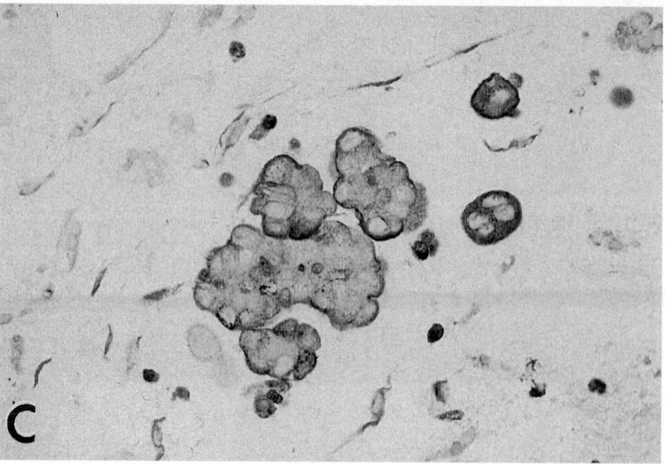

Figure 11–23. Metastatic adenocarcinoma. *A*. Note malignant epithelial proliferation forming papillary structures with multiple layers of atypical pleomorphic cells. The patient was a 54-year-old man who presented with pericardial effusions; CT and MR scans failed to demonstrate a primary site. *B*. Intracytoplasmic mucin vacuole (*arrow*) is virtually diagnostic of metastatic carcinoma. *C*. Immunohistochemical stain for B72.3 antigen demonstrated strong membrane and cytoplasmic staining, supporting the diagnosis of carcinoma and ruling out mesothelioma. After 4 months, a primary lung carcinoma was diagnosed.

dium, should be considered in the differential diagnosis. Replacement of the bone marrow by leukemia may result in pericardial masses of extramedullary hematopoiesis.[167]

REFERENCES

1. Lorell BH, Braunwald E. Pericardial disease. In: Braunwald E (ed): Heart Disease. A Textbook of Cardiovascular Medicine, pp 1465–1516. Philadelphia: WB Saunders, 1992.
2. Permanyer-Miralda G, Sagrista-Sauleda J, Soler-Soler J. Primary acute pericardial disease: A prospective series of 231 consecutive patients. Am J Cardiol 56:623–630, 1985.
3. Saner HE, Gobel FL, Nicoloff DM, Edwards JE. Aortic dissection presenting as pericarditis. Chest 91:71–74, 1987.
4. Corey GR, Campbell PT, Van Trigt P, Kenney RT, O'Connor CM, Sheikh KH, Kisslo JA, T.C. W. Etiology of large pericardial effusions. Am J Med 95:209–213, 1993.
5. Shenker L, Reed KL, Anderson CF, Kern W. Fetal pericardial effusion. Am J Obstet Gynecol 160:1505–1507, 1989.
6. Pereira WM, Kalil RA, Prates PR, Nesralla IA. Cardiac tamponade due to chylopericardium after cardiac surgery. Ann Thorac Surg 46:572–573, 1988.
7. Van Buren PC, Roberts WC. Cholesterol pericarditis and cardiac tamponade with congenital hypothyroidism in adulthood. Am Heart J 119:697–700, 1990.
8. Cameron J, Oesterle SN, Baldwin JC, Hancock EW. The etiologic spectrum of constrictive pericarditis. Am Heart J 113:354–360, 1987.
9. Laxer RM, Cameron BJ, Chaisson D. The camptodactyly-arthroplasty-pericarditis syndrome: Case report and literature review. Arthritis Rheum 29:439–440, 1986.
10. Cotton JB, Rebelle C, Bosnio A. Familial intrauterine nanism with constrictive pericarditis: The Mulibrey syndrome. Pediatrics 43:1978, 1988.
11. Muller C, Wolf H, Gottliche J, Zielinski CC, Eibl MM. Cellular immunodeficiency in protein-losing enteropathy. Predominant reduction of CD3+ and CD4+ lymphocytes. Dig Dis Sci 36:116–122, 1991.
12. Friedman MJ, Gabor GE, Fishman MC, Griepp RB. Bilateral pulmonary artery stenosis associated with pericarditis. Results of surgery and follow-up by magnetic resonance imaging. Chest 93:883–885, 1988.
13. Hinds SW, Reisner SA, Amico AF, Meltzer RS. Diagnosis of pericardial abnormalities by 2D-echo: A pathology-echocardiography correlation in 85 patients. Am Heart J 123:143–150, 1992.
14. Akasaka T, Yoshida K, Yamamuro A, Hozumi T, Takagi T, Morioka S, Yoshikawa J. Phasic coronary flow characteristics in patients with constrictive pericarditis: Comparison with restrictive cardiomyopathy. Circulation 96:1874–1881, 1997.
15. Sechtem U, Tscholakoff D, Higgins CB. MRI of the abnormal pericardium. AJR Am J Roentgenol 147: 245–252, 1986.
16. Ling LH, Oh JK, Tei C, Click RL, Breen JF, Seward JB, Tajik AJ. Pericardial thickness measured with transesophageal echocardiography: Feasibility and potential clinical usefulness. J Am Coll Cardiol 29:1317–1323, 1997.
17. Vaitkus PT, Kussmaul WG. Constrictive pericarditis versus restrictive cardiomyopathy: A reappraisal and update of diagnostic criteria. Am Heart J 122:1431–1441, 1991.
18. Bonchek LI, Burlingame MW, Vazales BE. Postoperative fibrous cardiac constriction. Ann Thorac Surg 45:311–314, 1988.
19. Rasaretnam R, Chanmugam D. Subacute effusive constrictive epicarditis. Br Heart J 44:44–48, 1980.
20. Walsh TJ, Baughman KL, Gardner TJ. Constrictive epicarditis as a cause of delayed or absent reponse to pericardiectomy. J Thorac Cardiovasc Surg 83:126–127, 1982.
21. Dalvi BV, Bisne VV, Khandeparkar JM. Localized epicarditis mimicking cardiac tumor. Chest 98:758–759, 1990.
22. Callahan JA, Seward JB, Nishimura RA, Miller FA, Reeder GS, Shub C, Callahan MJ, Schattenber TT, Tajik AJ. Two-dimensional echocardiographically guided pericardiocentesis: Experience in 117 consecutive patients. Am J Cardiol 55:476–479, 1985.
23. Ziskind AA, Rodriguez S, Lemmon C, Burstein S. Percutaneous pericardial biopsy as an adjunctive technique for the diagnosis of pericardial disease. Am J Cardiol 74:288–291, 1994.
24. Meyers DG, Bouska DJ. Diagnostic usefulness of pericardial fluid cytology. Chest 95:1142–1143, 1989.
25. Uthaman B, Endrys J, Abushaban L, Khan S, Anim JT. Percutaneous pericardial biopsy: Technique, efficacy, safety, and value in the management of pericardial effusion in children and adolescents. Pediatr Cardiol 18:414–418, 1997.
26. Kondos GT, Rich S, Levitsk S. Flexible fiberoptic pericardioscopy for the diagnosis of pericardial disease. J Am Coll Cardiol 7:432–434, 1986.
27. Millaire A, Wurtz A, de Groote P, Saudemont A, Chambon A, Ducloux G. Malignant pericardial effusions: Usefulness of pericardioscopy. Am Heart J 124:1030–1034, 1992.
28. Nataf P, Cacoub P, Regan M, Baron F, Dorent R, Pavie A, Gandibakhch I. Video-thoracoscopic pericardial window in the diagnosis and treatment of pericardial effusions. Am J Cardiol 82:124–126, 1998.
29. Frisk G, Torfason EG, Diderholm H. Reverse immunoassays of IgM and IgG antibodies to Coxsackie B viruses in patients with acute myopericarditis. J Med Virol 14:191–192, 1984.
30. Clifford CP, Davies GJ, Scott J, Shaunak S, Sarvill J, Schofield JB. Tuberculous pericarditis with rapid progression to constriction. Prompt diagnosis and treatment are needed. BMJ 307:1052–1054, 1993.
31. Long R, Younes M, Patton N, Hershfield E. Tuberculous pericarditis: Long-term outcome in patients who received medical therapy alone. Am Heart J 117:1133–1139, 1989.
32. Rana BS, Jones RA, Simpson IA. Recurrent pericardial effusion: The value of polymerase chain reaction in the diagnosis of tuberculosis. Heart 82:246–247, 1999.
33. Lewis W. AIDS: Cardiac findings from 115 autopsies. Prog Cardiovasc Dis 32:207–215, 1989.
34. Reynolds MM, Hecht SR, Berger M, Kolokathis A, Horowitz SF. Large pericardial effusions in the acquired immunodeficiency syndrome. Chest 102: 1746–1747, 1992.
35. Case records of the Massachusetts General Hospital. Weekly clinicopathological exercises. Case 23-1992. A 55-year-old man with recurrent pericardial and pleural

effusions after aortic-valve replacement. N Engl J Med 326:1550–1557, 1992.
36. Sabeel A, Alrajhi A, Alfurayh O. Salmonella pericarditis and pericardial effusion in a patient with systemic lupus erythematosus on haemodialysis. Nephrol Dial Transplant 12:2177–2178, 1997.
37. Kauffman CA, Watanakunakorn C, Phair JP. Purulent pneumococcal pericarditis. A continuing problem in the antibiotic era. Am J Med 54:743–750, 1973.
38. McMechan SR, Cochrane D, Adgey AA. Pneumococcal pericarditis—out of sight, out of mind? Clin Cardiol 19:829–830, 1996.
39. Perez Retortillo JA, Marco F, Richard C, Conde E, Manjon R, Bureo E, Iriondo A, Zubizarreta A. Pneumococcal pericarditis with cardiac tamponade in a patient with chronic graft-versus-host disease. Bone Marrow Transplant 21:299–300, 1998.
40. Starling RC, Yu VL, Shillington D, Galgiani J. Pneumococcal pericarditis. Diagnostic usefulness of counterimmunoelectrophoresis and computed tomographic scanning. Arch Intern Med 146:1174–1176, 1986.
41. Bergler-Klein J, Sochor H, Stanek G, Globits S, Ullrich R, Glogar D. Indium 111-monoclonal antimyosin antibody and magnetic resonance imaging in the diagnosis of acute Lyme myopericarditis. Arch Intern Med 153:2696–2700, 1993.
42. Watt G, Padre L, Tuazon M, Calubaquib C. Skeletal and cardiac muscle involvement in severe, late leptospirosis. J Infect Dis 162:266–269, 1990.
43. Evans ME, Gregory DW, Schaffner W, McGee ZA. Tularemia: A 30-year experience with 88 cases. Medicine 64:251–269, 1985.
44. Umut S, Tosun CA, Mihmanh A. Hydatiodosis with pericardial involvement. Chest 102:1916–1917, 1992.
45. West AB, Nolan N, O'Briain DS. Benign peptic ulcers penetrating pericardium and heart: Clinicopathological features and factors favoring survival. Gastroenterology 94:1478–1487, 1988.
46. Wheat LJ, Stein L, Corya BC. Pericarditis as a manifestation of histoplasmosis during two large urban outbreaks. Medicine 62:110–119, 1983.
47. Wooley CF, Hosier DM. Constrictive pericarditis due to *Histoplasma capsulatum.* N Engl J Med 264:1230–1232, 1961.
48. Wheat J. Histoplasmosis. Experience during outbreaks in Indianapolis and review of the literature. Medicine (Baltimore) 76:339–354, 1997.
49. Atkinson JB, Connor DH, Robinowitz M, McAllister HA, Virmani R. Cardiac fungal infections: Review of autopsy findings in 60 patients. Hum Pathol 15:935–942, 1984.
50. Virmani R, Connors DH, McAllister HA. Cardiac mucormycosis. Am J Clin Pathol 78:42–47, 1982.
51. Canver CC, Patel AK, Kosolcharoen P, Voytovich MC. Fungal purulent constrictive pericarditis in a heart transplant patient. Ann Thorac Surg 65:1792–1794, 1998.
52. Karp R, Meldahl R, McCabe R. Candida albicans purulent pericarditis treated successfully without surgical drainage. Chest 102:953–954, 1992.
53. Forbes WD, Besrebreurije AM. Coccidioidomycosis: A study of 95 cases of disseminated type with special reference to the pathogenesis of the disease. Milit Surg 15:653–719, 1946.
54. Amundson DE. Perplexing pericarditis caused by coccidioidomycosis. South Med J 86:694–696, 1993.
55. Himelman RB, Chung WS, Chernoff DN, Schiller NB, Hollander H. Cardiac manifestations of human immunodeficiency virus infection: A two-dimensional echocardiographic study. J Am Coll Cardiol 13:1030–1036, 1989.
56. Lipshultz SE, Chanock S, Sanders SP, Colan SD, Perez-Atayde A, McIntosh K. Cardiovascular manifestations of human immunodeficiency virus infection in infants and children. Am J Cardiol 63:1489–1497, 1989.
57. Steigman CK, Anderson DW, Macher AM, Sennesh JD, Virmani R. Fatal cardiac tamponade in acquired immunodeficiency syndrome with epicardial Kaposi's sarcoma. Am Heart J 116:1105–1107, 1988.
58. Estok L, Wallach F. Cardiac tamponade in a patient with AIDS: A review of pericardial disease in patients with HIV infection. Mt Sinai J Med 65:33–39, 1998.
59. D'Cruz IA, Sengupta EE, Abraham C, Reddy HK, Turlapati RV. Cardiac involvement including tuberculosis and pericardial effusions complicationg the acquired immune deficiency syndrome. Am Heart J 112:1100–1102, 1986.
60. Mastroianni A, Coronado O, Chiodo F. Tuberculous pericarditis and AIDS: Case reports and review. Eur J Epidemiol 13:755–759, 1997.
61. Rutsky EA, Rostand SG. Treatment of uremic pericarditis and pericardial effusion. Am J Kidney Dis 10:2–8, 1987.
62. Ansari A, Larso PH, Bates HD. Cardiovascular manifestations of systemic lupus erythematosus: Current perspective. Prog Cardiovasc Dis 27:421–434, 1985.
63. Rantapaa-Dahlqvist S, Neumann-Andersen G, Backman C, Dahlen G, Stegmayr B. Echocardiographic findings, lipids and lipoprotein(a) in patients with systemic lupus erythematosus. Clin Rheumatol 16: 140–148, 1997.
64. Kahl LE. The spectrum of pericardial tamponade in systemic lupus erythematosus. Report of ten patients. Arthritis Rheum 35:1343–1349, 1992.
65. Lee IH, Yang SC, Kim TH, Jun JB, Jung SS, Bae SC, Yoo DH, Kim SK, Kim SY. Cardiac tamponade as an initial manifestation of systemic lupus erythematosus—single case report. J Korean Med Sci 12:75–77, 1997.
66. Thould AK. Constrictive pericarditis in rheumatoid arthritis. Ann Rheum Dis 45:89–94, 1986.
67. Escalante A, Kaufman RL, Quismorio FP, Beardmore TD. Cardiac compression in rheumatoid pericarditis. Semin Arthritis Rheum 20:148–163, 1990.
68. Abu-Shakra M, Nicol P, Urowitz MB. Accelerated nodulosis, pleural effusion, and pericardial tamponade during methotrexate therapy. J Rheumatol 21:934–937, 1994.
69. McRorie ER, Wright RA, Errington ML, Luqmani RA. Rheumatoid constrictive pericarditis. Br J Rheumatol 36:100–103, 1997.
70. Hakala M, Pettersson T, Tarkka M, Leirisalo-Repo M, Mattila T, Airaksinen J, Sutinen S. Rheumatoid arthritis as a cause of cardiac compression. Favourable long-term outcome of pericardiectomy. Clin Rheumatol 12:199–203, 1993.
71. Van Offel JF, De Clerck LS, Kersschot IE. Cholesterol crystals and IgE-containing immune complexes in rheumatoid pericarditis. Clin Rheumatol 10:78–80, 1991.
72. Travaglio-Encinoza A, Anaya JM, Dupuy D'Angeac AD, Reme T, Sany J. Rheumatoid pericarditis: New immunopathological aspects. Clin Exp Rheumatol 12:313–316, 1994.
73. Przybojewski JZ. Rheumatic constrictive pericarditis. A case report and review of the literature. S Afr Med J 59:682–686, 1981.

74. Stollerman GH. Rheumatogenic group A streptococci and the return of rheumatic fever. Adv Intern Med 35:1–26, 1990.
75. Veasy LG, Tani LY, Hill HR. Persistence of acute rheumatic fever in the intermountain area of the United States. J Pediatr 124:9–16, 1994.
76. Case records of the Massachusetts General Hospital. Weekly clinicopathological exercises. Case 49-1990. A 47-year-old Cape Verdean man with pericardial disease. N Engl J Med 323:1614–1624, 1990.
77. Sattar MA, Guind RT, Vajcik J. Pericardial tamponade and limited cutaneous systemic sclerosis (CREST syndrome). Br J Rheumatol 29:306–307, 1990.
78. Bohan A, Peter JB, Bowman RL, Pearson CM. A computer-assisted analysis of 153 patients with polymyositis and dermatomyositis. Medicine 56:255–286, 1977.
79. Haupt HM, Hutchins GM. The heart and conduction system in polymyositis–dermatomyositis: A clinipathologic study of 16 autopsied patients. Am J Cardiol 50:998–1006, 1982.
80. Gottdiener JS, Sherber HS, Hawley RJ, Engel WK. Cardiac manifestations in polymyositis. Am J Cardiol 41:1141–1149, 1978.
81. Yale SH, Adlakha A, Stanton MS. Dermatomyositis with pericardial tamponade and polymyositis with pericardial effusion. Am Heart J 126:997–999, 1993.
82. Chraibi S, Ibnabdeljalil H, Habbal R, Bennis A, Tahiri A, Chraibi N. Pericardial tamponade as the first manifestation of dermatopolymyositis. Ann Med Interne (Paris) 149:464–466, 1998.
83. Gregoratos G. Pericardial involvement in acute myocardial infarction. Cardiol Clin 8:601–608, 1990.
84. Tofler GH, Muller JE, Stone PH, Willich SN, Davis VG, Poole WK, Robertson T, Braunwald E. Pericarditis in acute myocardial infarction: Characterization and clinical significance. Am Heart J 117:86–92, 1989.
85. Honan MB, Harrell FE, Reimer KA, Califf RM, Mark DB, Pryor DB, Hlatky MA. Cardiac rupture, mortality and the timing of thrombolytic therapy: A meta-analysis. J Am Coll Cardiol 16:359–367, 1990.
86. Becker RC, Charlesworth A, Wilcox RG, Hampto J, Skene A, Gore JM, Topol EJ. Cardiac rupture associated with thrombolytic therapy: Impact of time to treatment in the Late Assessment of Thrombolytic Efficacy (LATE) study. J Am Coll Cardiol 25:1063–1068, 1995.
87. Cheung PK, Myers ML, Arnold JM. Early constrictive pericarditis and anemia after Dressler's syndrome and inferior wall myocardial infarction. Br Heart J 65:360–362, 1991.
88. Case records of the Massachusetts General Hospital. Weekly clinicopathological exercises. Case 46-1989. A 52-year-old diabetic man with myocardial infarction, pericarditis, and persistent fever. N Engl J Med 321:1391–1402, 1989.
89. Diderholm E, Eklund A, Orinius E, Widstrom O. Exudative pericarditis in sarcoidosis. A case report and echocardiographic study. Sarcoidosis 6:60–62, 1989.
90. Lewin RF, Mor R, Spitzer S, Arditti A, Hellman C, Agmon J. Echocardiographic evaluation of patients with systemic sarcoidosis. Am Heart J 110:116–122, 1985.
91. Pesola G, Teirstein AS, Goldman M. Sarcoidosis presenting with pericardial effusion. Sarcoidosis 4:42–44, 1987.
92. Israel RH, Poe RH. Massive pericardial effusion in sarcoidosis. Respiration 61:176–180, 1994.
93. Virmani R, Chun PKC, Hartman D, McAllister HA. Eosinophilic constrictive pericariditis. Am Heart J 107:803–807, 1984.
94. Felman RH, Sutherland DB, Conklin JL, Mitros FA. Eosinophilic cholecystitis, appendiceal inflammation, pericarditis, and cephalosporin-associated eosinophilia. Dig Dis Sci 39:418–422, 1994.
95. Prattichizzo FA, Bernini L. An idiopathic hypereosinophilic syndrome mimicking seronegative rheumatoid arthritis: 20-year follow-up with clinical and laboratory findings. Clin Exp Rheumatol 10:79–81, 1992.
96. Jones B, Haponik EF, Katz R. Fibrinous pericarditis: An uncommon complication of acute pancreatitis. South Med J 80:377–378, 1987.
97. Tokoo M, Oguchi H, Kawa S, Homma T, Nagata A. Eosinophilia associated with chronic pancreatitis: An analysis of 122 patients with definite chronic pancreatitis. Am J Gastroenterol 87:455–460, 1992.
98. Stephens DA, Kocab F. Pericardial fat necrosis. J Thorac Cardiovasc Surg 95:727–729, 1988.
99. Brawley RK, Vasko JW, Morrow AG. Cholesterol pericarditis: Considerations of its pathogenesis and treatment. Am J Med 41:235–248, 1966.
100. Stanley RJ, Subramanian R, Lie JT. Cholesterol pericarditis terminating as constrictive calcific pericarditis. Follow-up study of patient with 40-year history of disease. Am J Cardiol 46:511–514, 1980.
101. Dempsey JJ, Eissa A, Attia M, Ramzy A. Pericardial effusion of "gold paint" appearance following myocardial infarction. Arch Intern Med 118:246–254, 1966.
102. Anyanwu CH, Umeh BU. Pericarditis: A persisting surgical problem. Cardiovasc Surg 2:711–715, 1994.
103. Nataf P, Cacoub P, Dorent R, Jault F, Fontanel M, Regan M, Bors V, Pavie A, Cabrol C, Gandjbakhch I. Chronic constrictive pericarditis. A retrospective study of a series of 84 patients. Arch Mal Coeur Vaiss 87:241–245, 1994.
104. MacGregor JH, Chen JT, Chiles C, Kier R, Godwin JD, Ravin CE. The radiographic distinction between pericardial and myocardial calcifications. AJR Am J Roentgenol 148:675–677, 1987.
105. Manji H, Raven P. Calcific constrictive pericarditis due to rheumatoid arthritis. Postgrad Med J 66:57–58, 1990.
106. Bewtra C, Schultz RD. Constrictive calcific pericarditis following coronary arterial bypass surgery. Hum Pathol 16:522–525, 1985.
107. Mambo NC. Diseases of the pericardium: Morphologic study of surgical specimens from 35 patients. Hum Pathol 12:978–987, 1981.
108. Valantine HA, Hunt SA, Gibbons R, Billingham M, Stinson EB, Popp RL. Increasing pericardial effusion in cardiac transplant recipients. Circulation 79:603–609, 1989.
109. Vandenberg BF, Mohanty PK, Craddock KJ, Barnhart G, Hanrahan J, Szentpetery S, Lower RR. Clinical significance of pericardial effusion after heart transplantation. J Heart Transplant 7:128–134, 1988.
110. Davies RA, Newton G, Masters RG, Saginur R, Struthers C, Walley VM. Bacterial pericarditis after heart transplantation: Successful management of two cases with catheter drainage and antibiotics. Can J Cardiol 12:641–644, 1996.
111. Coltart RS, Roberts JT, Thom CH, Petch MC. Severe constrictive pericarditis after single 16 MeV anterior mantle irradiation for Hodgkin's disease. Lancet 1(8427):488–489, 1985.

112. Pohjola-Sintonen S, Totterman KJ, Salmo M, Siltanen P. Late cardiac effects of mediastinal radiotherapy in patients with Hodgkin's disease. Cancer 60:31–37, 1987.
113. Carmel RJ, Kaplan HS. Mantle irradiation in Hodgkin's disease. An analysis of technique, tumor eradication, and complications. Cancer 37:2813–2825, 1976.
114. Arsenian MA. Cardiovascular sequelae of therapeutic thoracic radiation. Prog Cardiovasc Dis 33:299–311, 1991.
115. Veeragandham RS, Goldin MD. Surgical management of radiation-induced heart disease. Ann Thorac Surg 65:1014–1019, 1998.
116. Veinot JP, Edwards WD. Pathology of radiation-induced heart disease: A surgical and autopsy study of 27 cases. Hum Pathol 27:766–773, 1996.
117. Pepi M, Muratori M, Barbier P, Doria E, Arena V, Berti M, Celest F, Guazzi M, Tamborini G. Pericardial effusion after cardiac surgery: Incidence, site, size, and haemodynamic consequences. Br Heart J 72:327–331, 1994.
118. Ofori-Krakye SK, Tyuerg TI, Geha AS. Late cardiac tamponade after open heart surgery: Incidence, role of anticoagulants in its pathogenesis and its relationship to the postpericardiotomy syndrome. Circulation 63:1323–1327, 1981.
119. Ratliff NB, McMahon JT, Shirey EK, Groves LK. Silicone pericarditis. Cleve Clin Q 51:185–189, 1984.
120. Fraker TD, Walsh TE, Morgan RJ, Kim K. Constrictive pericarditis late after the Beck operation. Am J Cardiol 54:931–937, 1984.
121. Singer I, Hutchins GM, Mirowski M, Mower MM, Veltri EP, Guarnieri T, Griffith LS, Watkins L, Juanteguy J, Fisher S. Pathologic findings related to the lead system and repeated defibrillations in patients with the automatic implantable cardioverter-defibrillator. J Am Coll Cardiol 10:382–388, 1987.
122. Figuerola M, Tomas MT, Armengol J, Bejar A, Adrados M, Bonet A. Pericardial tamponade and coronary sinus thrombosis associated with central venus catheterization. Chest 101:1154–1155, 1992.
123. Deckers JW, Hare JM, Baughman KL. Complications of transvenous right ventricular endomyocardial biopsy in adult patients with cardiomyopathy: A seven-year survey of 546 consecutive diagnostic procedures in a tertiary referral center. J Am Coll Cardiol 19:43–47, 1992.
124. Browning CA, Bishop RL, Heilpern RJ. Accelerated constrictive pericarditis in procainamide-induced systemic lupus erythematosus. Am J Cardiol 53:376–378, 1984.
125. Burke AP, Saenger J, Mullick F, Virmani R. Hypersensitivity myocarditis. Arch Pathol Lab Med 115:764–769, 1991.
126. Lipworth BJ, Oakley DG. Surgical treatment of constrictive pericarditis due to practolol. A case report. J Cardiovasc Surg 29:408–409, 1988.
127. Feigin D, Fenoglio J, McAllister H, Medwell J. Pericardial cysts. A radiologic–pathologic correlation and review. Radiology 125:15–20, 1977.
128. Santoro MJ, Ford LJ, Chen YK, Solinger MR. Odynophagia caused by a pericardial diverticulum. Am J Gastroenterol 88:943–944, 1993.
129. Deenadayalu RP, Turri D, Dewell RA, Johnson GF. Intrapericardial teratomas and bronchogenic cyst. Review of literature and report of successful surgery in infant with intrapericardial teratoma. J Thorac Cardiovasc Surg 67:945–952, 1974.
130. Shimizu M, Takeda R, Mifune J, Tanaka T. Echocardiographic features of intrapericardial bronchogenic cyst. Cardiology 77:322–326, 1990.
131. Becker SN, Pepin DW, Rosenthal DL. Mesothelial papilloma: A case of mistaken identity in a pericardial effusion. Acta Cytol 20:266–268, 1986.
132. Larsen TE. Serosal papilloma of the epicardium. Report of a case. Arch Pathol 97:271–272, 1974.
133. Hillerdal G. Malignant mesothelioma 1982: Review of 4710 published cases. Br J Dis Chest 77:321–343, 1983.
134. Churg A, Warnock M, Bensch K. Malignant mesothelioma arising after direct application of asbestos and fiber glass to the pericardium. Am Rev Respir Dis 118:419–424, 1978.
135. Beck B, Konetzke G, Ludwig V, Rothi GW, Sturm W. Malignant pericardial mesotheliomas and asbestos exposure: A case report. Am J Ind Med 3:149–159, 1982.
136. Kahn EI, Rohl A, Barrett EW, Suzuki Y. Primary pericardial mesothelioma following exposure to asbestos. Environ Res 23:270–281, 1980.
137. Turk J, Kenda M, Kranjec I. Primary malignant pericardial mesothelioma. Klin Wochenschr 69:674–678, 1991.
138. Coplan N, Kennish A, Burgess N, Deligdish L, Goldman M. Pericardial mesothelioma masquerading as a benign pericardial effusion. J Am Coll Cardiol 4:1307–1310, 1984.
139. Kobayashi Y, Takeda S, Yamamoto T, Goi S. Cytologic detection of malignant mesotheliomas of the pericardium. Acta Cytol 22:344–349, 1978.
140. Takeda K, Ohba H, Hodo H, Shimuzu T, Iwakura H, Hayashi T, Yamamoto H, Yagi S, Take A, Harada M, Hasegawa T. Pericardial mesothelioma: Hyaluronic acid in pericardial fluid. Am Heart J 110:486–488, 1985.
141. Fazeka ST, Ungi I, Tiszlavicz L. Primary malignant mesothelioma of the pericardium. Am Heart J 124:227–231, 1992.
142. Horio H, Nomori-H, Morinaga S, Kikuchi T, Tomonari H, Kuriyama S, Suemasu K. Granulocyte colony-stimulating factor-producing primary pericardial mesothelioma. Hum Pathol 30:718–720, 1999.
143. Garcia-Cors M, Mulet J, Caralps J, Oller G. Fast-growing pericardial mass as first manifestation of intrapericardial teratoma in a young man. Am J Med 89:818–820, 1990.
144. Benatar A, Vaughan J, Nicolini U, Trotter S, Corrin B, Lincoln C. Prenatal pericardiocentesis: Its role in the management of intrapericardial teratoma. Obst Gynecol 79:856–859, 1992.
145. McAllister HA, Fenoglio JJ. Tumors of the Cardiovascular System. Second Series Fascicle. Vol. 15: Armed Forces Institute of Pathology, 62–63, 1978.
146. Bortolotti U, Calabro F, Loy M, Fasoli G, Altavilla G, Marchese D. Giant intrapericardial solitary fibrous tumor. Ann Thorac Surg 54:1219–1920, 1992.
147. Andreani SM, Tavecchio L, Giardini R, Bedini AV. Extrapericardial solitary fibrous tumour of the pericardium. Eur J Cardiothorac Surg 14:98–100, 1998.
148. El-Naggar AK, Ro JY, Ayala AG, Ward R, Ordonez NG. Localized fibrous tumor of the serosal cavities. Immunohistochemical, electron microscopic, and flow cytometric DNA study. Am J Clin Pathol 92:561–565, 1989.
149. Witkin G, Rosai J. Solitary fibrous tumor of the mediastinum. Am J Surg Pathol 13:547–557, 1989.

150. Ananthasubramaniam K, Farha A. Primary right atrial angiosarcoma mimicking acute pericarditis, pulmonary embolism, and tricuspid stenosis. Heart 81:556–558, 1999.
151. Terada T, Nakanuma T, Matsubara T, Suematsu T. An autopsy case of primary angiosarcoma of the pericardium mimicking malignant mesothelioma. Acta Pathol Jpn 38:1345–1351, 1988.
152. Poole-Wilson PA, Farnsworth A, Braimbridge MV, Pambakian H. Angiosarcoma of pericardium. Problems in diagnosis and management. Br Heart J 38:240–243, 1976.
153. Fukuda T, Ishikawa H, Ohnishi Y, Tachikawa S, Oguma F, Kasuya S, Sakashita I. Malignant spindle cell tumor of the pericardium. Evidence of sarcomatous mesothelioma with aberrant antigen expression. Acta Pathol Jpn 39:750–754, 1989.
154. Ileceto S, Quagliara D, Calabrese P, Rizzon P. Visualization of pericardial thymoma and evaluation of chemotherapy by two-dimensional echocardiography. Am Heart J 107:605–606, 1984.
155. Eglen DE. Pericardial based thymoma: Diagnosis by fine needle aspiration. Indiana Med 79:526–528, 1986.
156. Venegas RJ, Sun NCJ. Cardiac tamponade as a presentation of malignant thymoma. Acta Cytol 32:257–261, 1988.
157. Lang-Lazdunski L, Oroudji M, Pansard Y, Vissuzaine C, Hvass U. Successful resection of giant intrapericardial lipoma. Ann Thorac Surg 58:238–234, 1994.
158. Nicolosi AC, Almassi GH, Komorowski R. Cardiac tamponade secondary to giant lymph node hyperplasia (Castleman's disease). Chest 105:637–639, 1994.
159. Reyes CV, Strinden C, Banerju M. The role of cytology in neoplastic cardiac tamponade. Acta Cytologica 265:299–302, 1982.
160. Buck M, Ingle JN, Giuliani ER, Gordon JR, Therneau TM. Pericardial effusion in women with breast cancer. Cancer 60:263–269, 1987.
161. Loire R, Hellal H. Neoplastic pericarditis. Study by thoracotomy and biopsy in 80 cases. Presse Med 22:244–248, 1993.
162. Bardales RH, Stanley MW, Schaefer RF, Liblit RL, Owens RB, Surhland MJ. Secondary pericardial malignancies: A critical appraisal of the role of cytology, pericardial biopsy, and DNA ploidy analysis. Am J Clin Pathol 106:29–34, 1996.
163. Bailey ME, Brown RW, Mody DR, Cagle P, Ramzy I. Ber-EP4 for differentiating adenocarcinoma from reactive and neoplastic mesothelial cells in serous effusions. Comparison with carcinoembryonic antigen, B72.3 and leu-M1. Acta Cytol 40:1212–1216, 1996.
164. Wirth PR, Legier J, Wright GL. Immunohistochemical evaluation of seven monoclonal antibodies for differentiation of pleural mesothelioma from lung adenocarcinoma. Cancer 67:655–662, 1991.
165. Shyu KG, Chiang FT, Kuan PL, Lien WP, Chen CL, How SW. Cardiac metastasis of hepatocellular carcinoma mimicking pericardial effusion on radionuclide angiocardiography. Chest 101:261–262, 1992.
166. Hoda RS, Cangiarella J, Koss LG. Metastatic squamous-cell carcinoma in pericardial effusion: Report of four cases, two with cardiac tamponade. Diagn Cytopathol 18:422–424, 1998.
167. Bradford CR, Smith SR, Wallis JP. Pericardial extramedullary haemopoiesis in chronic myelomonocytic leukaemia. J Clin Pathol 46:674–675, 1993.

Chapter

12

TUMORS AND TUMOR-LIKE LESIONS OF THE HEART AND GREAT VESSELS

CLASSIFICATION AND INCIDENCE

Classification

Three quarters of all primary tumors of the heart and 90% of tumors resected at surgery are benign[1–6] (Table 12–1). Many benign proliferations of the heart have no exact histologic counterpart in extracardiac locations; these proliferations include myxomas, lipomatous hypertrophy, cardiac fibroma, rhabdomyoma, papillary fibroelastoma, and the cystic tumor of the AV node. The histogenesis of many of these entities is still being debated. Most benign proliferations of the heart are not considered true neoplasms, with the exception of cardiac myxoma.

Almost all primary cardiac malignancies are sarcomas; they are classified similarly to sarcomas of extracardiac soft tissue. Rare types of primary cardiac malignancies include lymphomas and malignant paragangliomas. Primary malignancies of the pericardium, which are virtually restricted to mesotheliomas and sarcomas, are discussed with pericardial tumors (Chapter 11); often the distinction between cardiac and pericardial sarcoma is difficult because of tumor extension into both structures.

Incidence

The incidence of cardiac tumors is unknown; estimates from autopsy series vary over 100-fold and range from 0.0017 to 0.28 percent.[7] In autopsy series, one quarter to one half of primary cardiac tumors are myxomas. The proportion of myxomas as the total number of cardiac tumors is much higher in surgical series, and is approximately 80% (Table 12–1). Since the first resection of a cardiac myxoma in 1945, cardiac tumors are now being routinely resected,[1–6] even when asymptomatic.

CLINICOPATHOLOGIC APPROACH TO CARDIAC TUMORS

Clinical Findings

The relative incidence of cardiac tumors is influenced greatly by age at diagnosis, and to a lesser degree, sex of the patient. In general, cardiac rhabdomyomas are tumors of the newborn period; cardiac fibromas usually occur during the first few years of life; other tumors are found in older populations. Primary cardiac tumors in children are extremely rare; in a series of 5,339 autopsies at the University of Minnesota Hospital, there were only 28 tumors in patients younger than 25 years (eight rhabdomyomas, mean age 6 months; five fibromas, mean age 4 years; four rhabdomyosarcomas, mean age 12 years; three atrioventricular nodal tumors, mean age 14 years; and eight myxomas, mean age 16 years).[8] There are few tumors primary to the heart that have a sex predilection; one example is the cystic tumor of the atrioventricular node, which predominates in females in a ratio of 2.5 : 1.

The symptoms that result from cardiac masses are usually related to obstruction of

Table 12–1. Cardiac Tumors, Series of Surgical Resection

	Total (%)	Blondeau et al.	Tazelaar et al.*	Murphy et al.*	Dein et al.	Melo et al.	Verkkala et al.
Myxoma	649 (78%)	444	80	63	27	19	16
Sarcoma	83 (10%)	52†	8	12	8	1	2
Fibroma	27 (3%)	9	9	7	1	1	0
Lipoma	21 (3%)	9	5	4	1	0	2
Angioma	17 (2%)	7	0	3	7	0	0
Rhabdomyoma	14 (2%)	5	0	9	0	0	0
Fibroelastoma	9 (1%)	0	7	0	2	0	0
Hamartoma‡	5 (<1%)	4	0	0	1	0	0
Ectopic thyroid	2 (<1%)	2	0	0	0	0	0
Lymphoma	1 (<1%)	1	0	0	0	0	0
Total	828	533	109	98	47	21	20

* Cases of Purkinje cell hamartoma (histiocytoid cardiomyopathy) reported in these series were excluded from this table.
† Includes two malignant neoplasms that were considered unclassifiable.
‡ Not histologically defined in these series.

blood flow, cardiac failure, pericardial involvement, and embolic phenomena.[9] For example, tumors of the left atrium often present as mitral valve disease (mitral stenosis most commonly), and tumors in the right ventricle can present with syncopal episodes similarly to pulmonic stenosis. Any tumor with extensive myocardial involvement may result in congestive heart failure. If there is pericardial involvement, pericardial effusions and chest pain may dominate the clinical picture, and the cardiac tumor may be diagnosed only after pericardiocentesis. Tumors with luminal involvement (generally myxomas, papillary fibroelastomas, and rarely sarcomas) can present with systemic or pulmonary emboli, depending on the site of origin in the heart. Constitutional symptoms are particularly common in atrial myxoma.

Methods of Tissue Sampling and Evaluation

The surgical treatment of most primary cardiac tumors is complete excision if possible. This may necessitate resection of valve, cardiac muscle, or atrial septum. Therefore, the pathologic specimen may occasionally include resected valve or a portion of normal adjoining ventricular or atrial myocardium that will have to be patched or replaced with a prosthetic valve or graft.

The surgical pathologist will be confronted with evaluating the margins of resection by frozen section when given fresh tissue from a cardiac tumor for intraoperative consultation. Because it has been stated that complete excision of cardiac myxoma results in fewer recurrences, and that complete excision of cardiac sarcomas result in a longer survival, appropriate inking of specimens after orientation of the specimen may be necessary if there is recognizable normal tissue such as atrial septum present.

With the advent of endomyocardial biopsy, it is now possible to make a tissue diagnosis of primary cardiac neoplasm without surgery.[10] The danger of tumor embolization and inadequate tissue sampling may hamper complete evaluation of a small biopsy, and diagnosis occasionally may still rest on subsequent surgical resection.

Electron microscopy and immunohistochemistry are of limited benefit in the diagnosis of cardiac tumors for the institution of therapy. These techniques are of value in the subclassification of cardiac sarcomas, and exclusion of epithelial metastases and of mesothelioma from the diagnosis. Flow cytometry and determination of aneuploidy or S-phase may be of ancillary help as a prognostic feature for cardiac sarcomas, but should not be used for the distinction between benign and malignant processes. Occasionally, cytogenetics can be helpful in the classification of sarcomas; fresh tissue must be immediately grown in culture for this technique. Most sarcomas with typical cytogenetic abnormalities are of the small round-cell variety and synovial sarcomas. These rarely occur in the heart.

NON-NEOPLASTIC PROLIFERATIONS

Cardiac Rhabdomyoma

Definition

Cardiac rhabdomyoma is a congenital hamartoma composed of myocytes that resemble fetal cardiac myocytes. Cardiac rhabdomyomas present in infants and children as multiple myocardial nodules and have a typical histologic appearance. Although there are similarities between cardiac rhabdomyoma and rhabdomyoma of skeletal muscle, the histology and ultrastructure of cardiac rhabdomyoma is distinctive and readily distinguishable from extracardiac rhabdomyomas.

Incidence

Cardiac rhabdomyoma is the most common tumor of the heart in infants and children in autopsy series.[11] The incidence of cardiac rhabdomyoma is difficult to determine because many cases are undetected and regress spontaneously. Cardiac rhabdomyomas are relatively uncommon in surgical series. They are often difficult to resect, occasionally do not cause symptoms, and can be diagnosed clinically if there is a history of tuberous sclerosis, obviating the need for diagnostic biopsy.

Clinical Findings

Most patients with cardiac rhabdomyoma are younger than 5 years of age and there is a slight male predominance.[11, 12] There is a strong association with the tuberous sclerosis, which is characterized by hamartomas of the central nervous system, kidney and skin, as well as pancreatic cysts. It is estimated that 25–50% of patients with cardiac rhabdomyoma have tuberous sclerosis, and that up to 100% of patients with tuberous sclerosis will have cardiac masses demonstrated by echocardiography.[13] Some patients are asymptomatic and the diagnosis is made because of a clinical suspicion in patients with tuberous sclerosis, or on the basis of an incidental murmur.

The severity of symptoms depends on the size of the tumor, its location relative to the conduction system, and its capability to obstruct blood flow. Death from congestive heart failure can occur in utero resulting in the delivery of a hydropic infant. Symptoms are attributable usually to congestive heart failure, which occurs usually in patients with intracavitary tumors or arrhythmias.[14] Intracavitary rhabdomyomas are generally sporadic tumors in patients without tuberous sclerosis.[14] Some individuals with cardiac rhabdomyoma die suddenly without a premortem diagnosis; in these cases, the cause of death is presumed lethal arrhythmia.

Cardiac rhabdomyomas in such patients can be resected with good results. If patients with tuberous sclerosis survive infancy, their cardiac tumors regress spontaneously, are rarely intracavitary, and are rarely surgically resected.

Cardiac rhabdomyomas occasionally occur in association with structural congenital heart disease, including transposition of the great arteries, ventricular septal defect, hypoplastic left heart syndrome, Ebstein's anomaly, double outlet right ventricle, and pulmonary atresia.[12]

Pathology

Gross

Between 70 and 90% of cardiac rhabdomyomas are multiple. They are firm circumscribed whitish-tan nodules that occur anywhere within the cardiac muscle and are especially prevalent in the left ventricle. Nodules of rhabdomyoma range in size from less than 1 mm to several centimeters. Occasionally, they can protrude into the lumen of either ventricle causing obstruction of outflow.

Microscopic

The nodules of rhabdomyoma are composed of vacuolated cells with varying numbers of myofibers (Fig. 12–1*A*). Occasionally the myofibers stream from the center of the cell resulting in so-called spider cells (Fig. 12–1*B*). The ultrastructural features of cardiac rhabdomyoma are similar to fetal myoblasts.[14–16] Invariably, myofibrils are present with identifiable Z-bands, and there is abundant glycogen with sparse mitochondria. Desmosomes and intercalated discs are present around the periphery of the cell, and primitive T-tubules can be identified. There has been immunohistochemical demonstration of intracytoplasmic desmin and myoglobin.

The diagnosis of cardiac rhabdomyoma is usually straightforward. There is a superficial

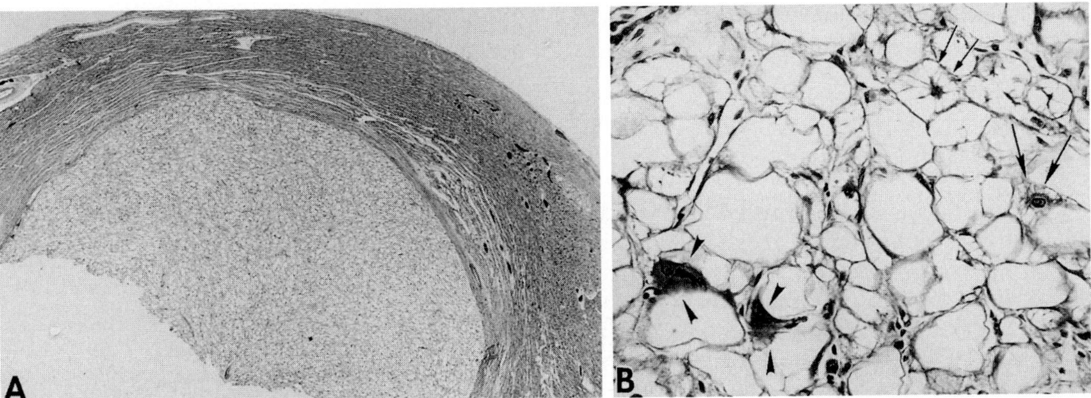

Figure 12–1. Rhabdomyoma. *A.* This figure demonstrates a circumscribed mass of clear cells from a patient with neonatal congestive heart failure and death at age 8 weeks. At autopsy, multiple masses in the myocardium as well as hypoplasia of the left ventricle were found. (H & E × 9.9) *B.* The tumor is composed of altered myocytes, most of which are vacuolated. Some are so-called spider cells with attenuated strands of myofibers (*arrows*); other cells have more abundant cytoplasm (*arrowheads*). (H & E × 300)

resemblance to lipoma because of the extensive cytoplasmic vacuolization. The clinical setting and demonstration of myofibrils easily rule out a diagnosis of lipoma. Rhabdomyomas were once considered forms of glycogen storage disease. However, tumor-like nature of rhabdomyoma and the ultrastructural identification of cardiac myoblasts rule out a form of glycogenosis. The most difficult differential diagnosis is histiocytoid cardiomyopathy. These lesions are always present as microscopic or barely visible nodules that are present diffusely throughout the myocardium. Unlike rhabdomyoma, the cells of histiocytoid cardiomyopathy are finely vacuolated, lack cytoplasmic clearing, and are grouped in microscopic irregular clusters. Histiocytoid cardiomyopathy can be associated with oncocytic change in other organs of the body.

Cardiac Fibroma

Definition

Cardiac fibroma is a discrete, bulging mass in one or more ventricles or atria, that is composed primarily of fibroblasts, collagen, and elastic fibers. Because most cardiac fibromas occur in infants, and histologic findings change with advancing age, cardiac fibromas are considered to be congenital lesions.

Incidence

Fibroma is a rare tumor of infants and children, and is as frequent as rhabdomyoma in surgical series.[1–7] The incidence at autopsy is less than 0.1% in referral centers.[8, 17]

Clinical Findings

Most patients with cardiac fibroma are children, one third of whom are under 1 year of age. They are occasionally first identified in adults as late as the sixth decade. There is no sex or race predominance.

Symptoms related to cardiac fibroma are related primarily to heart failure, arrhythmias, sudden death, and chest pain.[18] Unusual presentations include persistent unexplained pericardial effusion, and pulmonary outflow obstruction with syncope. Incidental lesions are discovered either by the auscultation of cardiac murmurs, diagnosis of an enlarged cardiac silhouette on chest x-ray, or evaluation of Gorlin syndrome, which is characterized by multiple nevoid basal cell carcinomas, jaw cysts, and bifid ribs. An association between cardiac fibroma and Gorlin syndrome has been established.[17]

Unlike fibromatosis of soft tissue, there is little evidence that there is continued capacity for growth, and even patients with incomplete resection do well postoperatively.[19] Therefore, partial resection may be of benefit. Because of the central location of many cardiac fibromas, a total resection is often not possible, and reconstruction or valve replacement is occasionally necessary. Patients with cardiac fibroma who die suddenly are almost always infants; older patients can live for many years without symptoms, and spontaneous regression of cardiac fibroma may occur.[20] For these reasons, some clinicians will choose not to risk surgery in older children with cardiac fibroma.

Pathology

Gross

Cardiac fibromas are whorled masses that bulge on cut section and are grossly reminiscent of uterine leiomyomas (Fig. 12–2). They occur primarily in the ventricles and usually involve the interventricular septum. They can attain a large size and markedly distort the cardiac muscle. Grossly, the margins of cardiac fibroma are well demarcated. Microscopically, however, tongues of tumor typically infiltrate surrounding myocardium.

Microscopic

Cardiac fibromas in newborns and infants are quite cellular and can easily be mistaken for fibrosarcoma (Fig. 12–3*A*). The amount of collagen increases with age, with a concomitant decrease in the cellularity (Fig. 12–3*B*). In older individuals, cardiac fibromas resemble fibromatosis of soft tissue and are composed of bundles of collagen with interspersed fibroblasts. In over 50% of cases, elastic fibers will be present; occasionally they can be quite prominent (Fig. 12–3*C*). Other microscopic features of cardiac fibroma that are variably present include calcification, occasional perivascular aggregates of lymphocytes and histiocytes, and a focal myxoid background.

There are few entities in the differential diagnosis. Fibromas of newborns histologically resemble fibrosarcoma, but cardiac fibrosarcomas essentially do not occur in infants. Although histiocytes and lymphocytes may be present around vessels or at tumor margins, the paucity of these cells contrasts fibroma to inflammatory pseudotumors, which are rare myofibroblastic tumors that may occur in the heart.[10] Also in the differential diagnosis is fibrous histiocytoma, an extremely rare cellular cardiac tumor that is composed of spindle cells and lipid-laden histiocytes. In older patients, the tumor can histologically simulate a scar, but grossly there is always a mass that results in thickening or bulging of the ventricle, in contrast to healed infarcts.

Endocardial Papillary Fibroelastoma

Definition

Papillary fibroelastoma is a benign avascular papilloma of the endocardium. Synonyms include fibroelastic papilloma and giant Lambl's excrescence. There are no gross or microscopic features that reliably distinguish papillary fibroelastoma from Lambl's excrescence.[21] The former term is used if the lesion is unusually

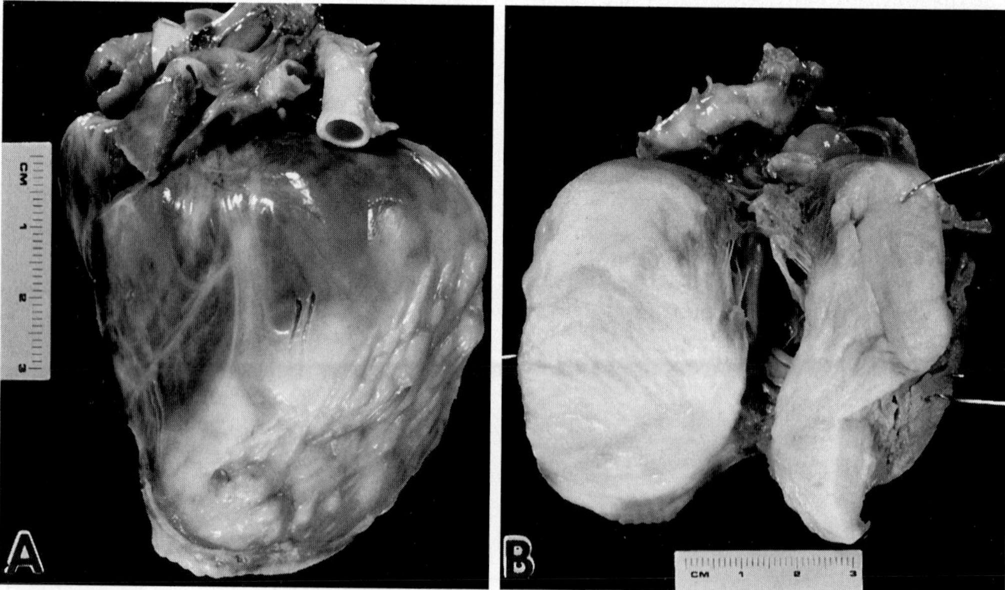

Figure 12–2. Fibroma. Cardiac fibroma is often a large, single tumor and has a propensity to be located in the ventricular septum. These photographs (*A*,*B*) show the heart of a 2-month-old boy who died suddenly without a previous medical history.

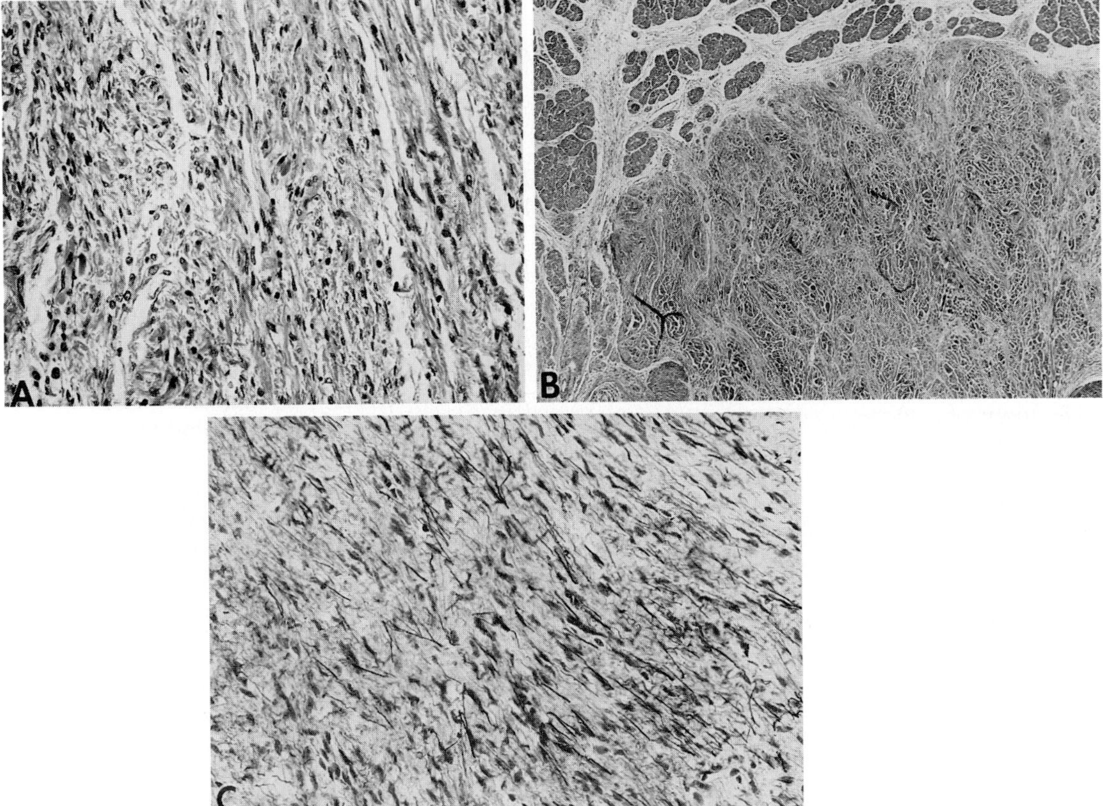

Figure 12–3. Fibroma. *A.* A 3-month-old girl with congestive heart failure had surgical resection of this fibroblastic tumor. (H & E × 300) *B.* In older patients, fibromas are far less cellular than in neonates and are composed of dense collagen and thick-walled vessels. The patient was a 56-year-old man with ventricular fibrillation and sudden death. (Masson's trichrome × 30) *C.* This tumor has abundant elastic fibers. These are present in many cardiac fibromas. (Elastic van Gieson × 300)

large and causes symptoms, or if the location is not typical for Lambl's excrescence, for example, on the ventricular endocardium.

Incidence

The true incidence of papillary fibroelastoma is unknown because they can be easily overlooked at autopsy. They are now being increasingly detected by echocardiography and surgically excised.[22] In recent series of cardiac tumors they are the second most common benign tumors, occurring between three and ten times less often than myxoma.[1–7]

Clinical Findings

Papillary fibroelastomas occur in adults of both sexes equally. The mean age at detection is approximately 60 years.[23, 24] Endocardial scarring secondary to radiation therapy, postinflammatory valve disease and other causes may predispose to the formation of papillary fibroelastomas. Echocardiography demonstrates a mobile, endocardial-based tumor that may attain a large size. Most patients have no symptoms related to the tumor or predisposing conditions.[23, 24] By 1992, there were 22 reports of symptomatic papillary fibroelastoma,[25] all involving the left side of the heart, specifically the mitral valve (ten cases), aortic valve (nine cases), left ventricular papillary muscle (two cases), or free wall (one case); since then more symptomatic papillary fibroelastomas have been reported.[26, 27] Symptoms are caused by coronary occlusion (acute myocardial infarct or sudden death), cerebral vascular occlusion, and, rarely, renal vascular occlusion.

Pathologic Findings

Papillary fibroelastomas are located on the endocardial surface, most often of the aortic valve. Other sites include mitral, tricuspid, and pulmonary valves, the atrial surfaces, and papillary muscles. They are usually located on the atrial aspect of atrioventricular valves and the arterial aspect of the semilunar valves, although any location is possible. They have a characteristic gross appearance that has been likened to that of a sea anemone, which is best appreciated after immersion of the specimen in water. Histologically, normal components of chordae tendineae are present. There is an avascular fibrous core that usually contains proteoglycans, elastic fibers, and occasional stellate mesenchymal cells. A Movat pentachrome stain is especially useful to delineate these components (Fig. 12–4). The papillary core is covered by a single layer of endothelial cells (Figs. 12–4*A*, *B*). Immunohistochemically, lining cells express CD34 and S-100 protein; there are few actin-positive cells in the core, in contrast to cardiac myxoma.[28]

There are few entities that can be mistaken for papillary fibroelastoma. Myxomas are highly vascular tumors (papillary fibroelastomas are avascular) and are rarely located on valve surfaces. There may be superimposed marantic endocarditis or scarring, which may obscure the papillary structures grossly and histologically; multiple levels with elastic stains may be necessary for diagnosis.

Lipomatous Hypertrophy of the Interatrial Septum

Definition

Lipomatous hypertrophy of the interatrial septum is a nonencapsulated proliferation of mature fat, multivacuolated fat, and atypical cardiac myocytes.[29-32] It is exclusively limited to the cardiac atria and is probably a hamartoma. There appears to be an increase in the amount of fat in the interatrial septum as age progresses; it has been suggested that any deposit in excess of 2 cm at the level of the fossa ovalis is abnormal.[33]

Incidence

Lipomatous hypertrophy is a rare lesion; fewer than 120 have been reported.[33-34] The true incidence is difficult to assess because most

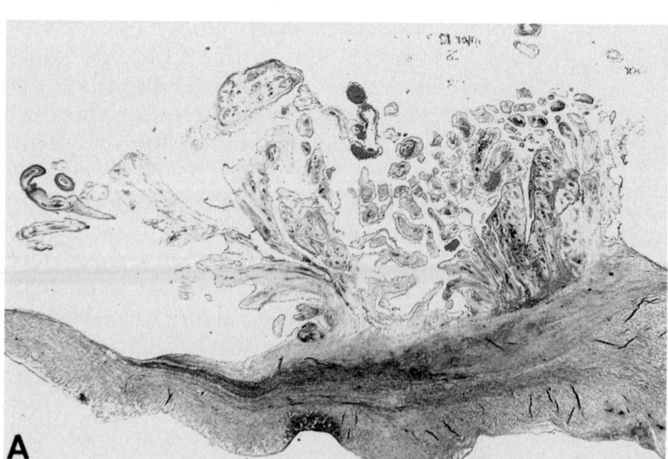

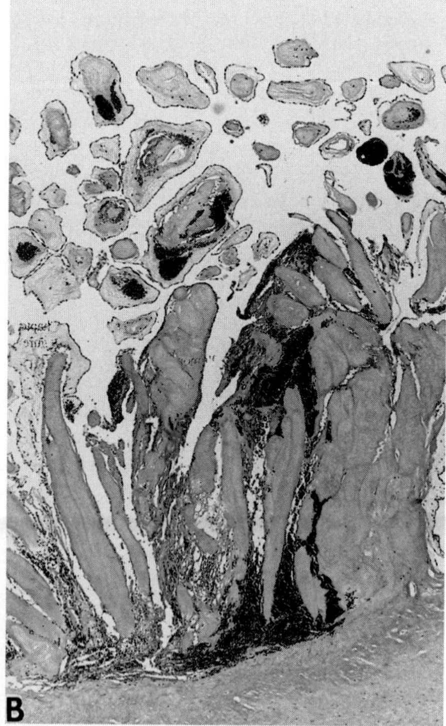

Figure 12–4. Papillary fibroelastoma. *A.* This tumor was present on the mitral valve of a patient who died a traumatic death. On the atrial surface of the valve, there are avascular fronds with variable amounts of elastic tissue. (Movat × 9.9) *B.* Note avascular fronds lined by a single layer of endothelial cells. (Movat pentachrome × 30)

cases are incidental findings and may be overlooked at autopsy.

Clinical Findings

An association between lipomatous hypertrophy of the interatrial septum and supraventricular arrhythmias has long been recognized.[30–31] The first antemortem diagnosis was reported in 1982;[32] since that time, there have been several cases of successful resection. Recent reports of surgical excisions with normalization of cardiac rhythm provide strong support that lipomatous hypertrophy may cause arrhythmias.[35]

There have been several reports of sudden death without pathologic findings at autopsy except for the presence of lipomatous hypertrophy.[7] Although it is impossible to prove that these tumors cause sudden death, lipomatous hypertrophy is generally accepted as a presumptive cause of fatal arrhythmias. Other than arrhythmias or sudden death, lipomatous hypertrophy can cause compression of the superior vena cava[35] and massive tumors may cause congestive heart failure. Most patients with lipomatous hypertrophy of the interatrial septum are elderly, and there is no sex predilection.

Lipomatous hypertrophy may present as a right atrial mass that may be surgically resected.[34] Surgical patients with this tumor may be young or middle-aged adults, and are often slightly or moderately obese, and are often female.[34]

Gross and Microscopic Pathology

Grossly, the atrial septum is thickened up to several centimeters; the normal atrial septum is no wider than 2 cm. These tumors can achieve great dimensions, up to 10 cm. There can be involvement of the entire septum, and bulging is only noted into the right atrium (Fig. 12–5*A*). Occasionally, the bulk of the tumor may be attached to the atrial surface and project into the mediastinum.

Microscopically the lesion is characteristic (Figs. 12–5*B,C*). There is an admixture of fat and cardiac myocytes. At least some of the fat will show vacuolization typical of brown or hibernating fat. In most cases, the interspersed cardiac myocytes will be bizarre and greatly enlarged. Flow cytometric studies in one case with which we are familiar demonstrated aneuploidy, perhaps reflecting the myocyte population. However, mitoses are absent, distinguishing this lesion from a malignancy. We have seen several cases misdiagnosed as sarcoma because of the presence of multivacuolated fat, which has been mistaken for lipoblasts, and bizarre myocytes. Unlike lipoblasts, brown fat cells do not have enlarged, hyperchromatic indented nuclei. Liposarcomas of the heart are extremely rare; this diagnosis should be made with extreme caution, especially for tumors in the atria.

Cardiac Hemangioma and Vascular Malformations

Definition

Hemangiomas are benign tumors composed predominantly of blood vessels. Cavernous hemangiomas (which are composed of multiple dilated thin-walled vessels), capillary hemangiomas (which contain smaller vessels resembling capillaries), and vascular malformations (which are formed of dysplastic, thick-walled vessels) may all occur in the heart. Malformations generally are composed both of arteries and veins (arteriovenous hemangioma). Unicystic blood-filled cysts composed of dilated capillaries or venules, or varices, occur in the atrial septum.[36] Blood cysts are collections of blood that are located in the atrioventricular valves of infants, measure less than 1 mm, and generally regress.

Incidence

Cardiac hemangiomas are quite rare; fewer than 75 cases have been reported.[37] In surgical series, they represent less than 5% of benign cardiac tumors.[38–40]

Clinical Findings

Most cardiac hemangiomas are discovered as incidental findings at autopsy or cardiac surgery. Increasing numbers of asymptomatic cardiac hemangiomas are being discovered with noninvasive means. Cardiac hemangiomas may be detected in patients with murmurs, in patients who are investigated for other cardiac diseases, or as a mass noted on chest x-ray.

In patients who are symptomatic, cardiac hemangiomas can cause arrhythmias,[41] pericardial effusions,[42] congestive heart failure, outflow tract obstruction,[43] and coronary insufficiency.[44] Cardiac hemangiomas that cause symptoms can be resected with good results. Occasionally, the presenting symptom is sudden cardiac death, and the forensic pathologist is the first to diag-

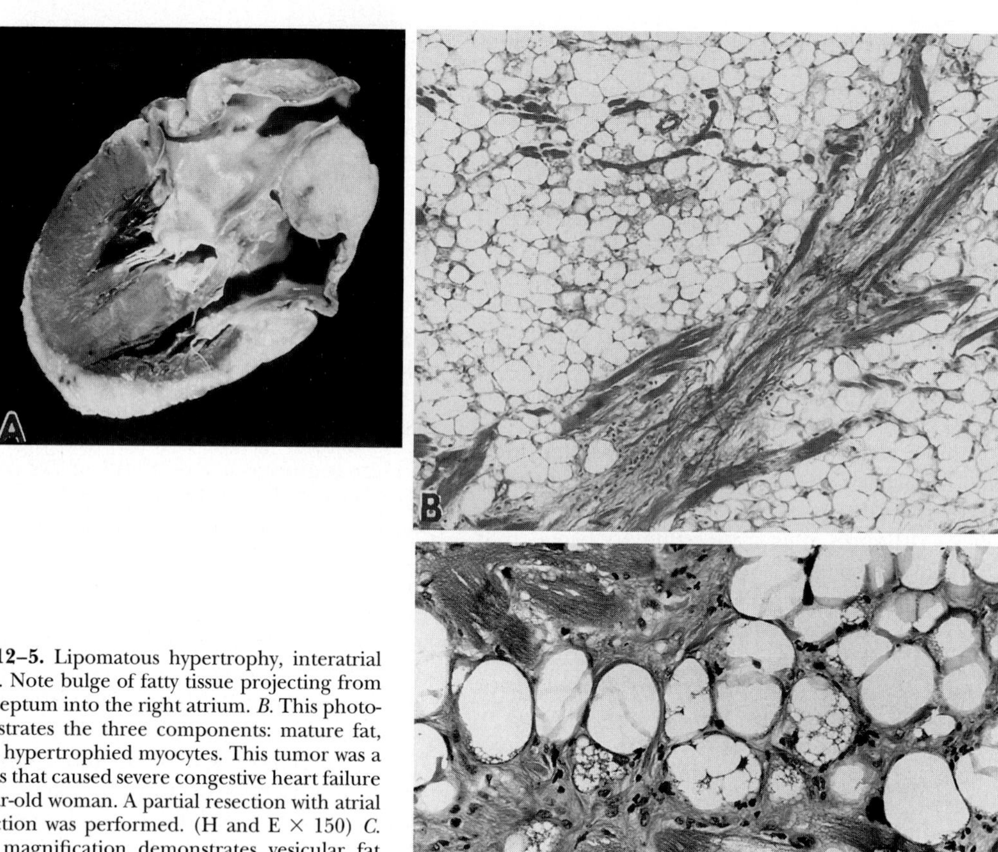

Figure 12–5. Lipomatous hypertrophy, interatrial septum. *A.* Note bulge of fatty tissue projecting from the atrial septum into the right atrium. *B.* This photograph illustrates the three components: mature fat, brown fat, hypertrophied myocytes. This tumor was a 10-cm mass that caused severe congestive heart failure in a 66-year-old woman. A partial resection with atrial reconstruction was performed. (H and E × 150) *C.* A higher magnification demonstrates vesicular fat and myocytes.

nose the tumor. Hemangiomas causing sudden cardiac death may be in the region of the atrioventricular node, or in the ventricles. A rare mechanism of sudden death in individuals with cardiac hemangioma is rupture of the tumor and pericardial tamponade.

There is an occasional association of cardiac hemangioma with extracardiac hemangiomas of the gastrointestinal tract.[41] Giant cardiac hemangiomas can result in thrombosis and coagulopathies (Kasabach–Merritt syndrome).[45]

Several reports have documented the successful surgical resection of cardiac hemangiomas, even if located in relatively inaccessible areas, including the ventricular septum. Because of the infiltrative nature of some cardiac hemangiomas, they are not always completely excised. Reconstruction of ventricular outflow with Dacron grafts may be necessary. There have been reports of a spontaneously resolving cardiac hemangioma,[46] and cardiac hemangiomas in children that respond to steroid therapy.

Pathologic Findings

Hemangiomas can occur in any location of the heart, although there is a predilection for the interventricular septum. Cardiac hemangiomas can be well-demarcated lobulated tumors, or have grossly and microscopically infiltrating margins. The latter features make them difficult to completely resect. The histologic appearance of cardiac hemangiomas is similar to those of extracardiac vascular tumors, and ranges from typical cavernous hemangiomas to arteriovenous malformations with dysplastic arterial and venous type channels (Fig. 12–6). The latter are more likely poorly circumscribed mural tumors and occasionally contain a mixture of fibrous tissue and fat, indicating that they may be variants of intramuscular hemangiomas of soft tissue. Occasional cardiac hemangiomas with epithelioid cells have been reported (Fig. 12–6*D*).[41, 47] Other unusual histologic features of cardiac hemangioma include papillary endothelial hyperplasia,[37] which must not be interpreted as evidence of angiosarcoma.

The differential diagnosis of cardiac hemangioma includes angiosarcoma and myxoma. The former are generally large, infiltrating tumors of the right atrium that extend into the pericardium and demonstrate pleomorphism and mitotic figures. Although intracavitary cardiac hemangiomas of the capillary or cavernous type may resemble myxoma due to prominent vascularity within a myxoid matrix, the inflammatory background and hemosiderin-laden macrophages of myxoma are absent.

Congenital Rests

Cystic Tumor of the AV Node

The existence of a morphologically benign multicystic tumor of the AV nodal region has

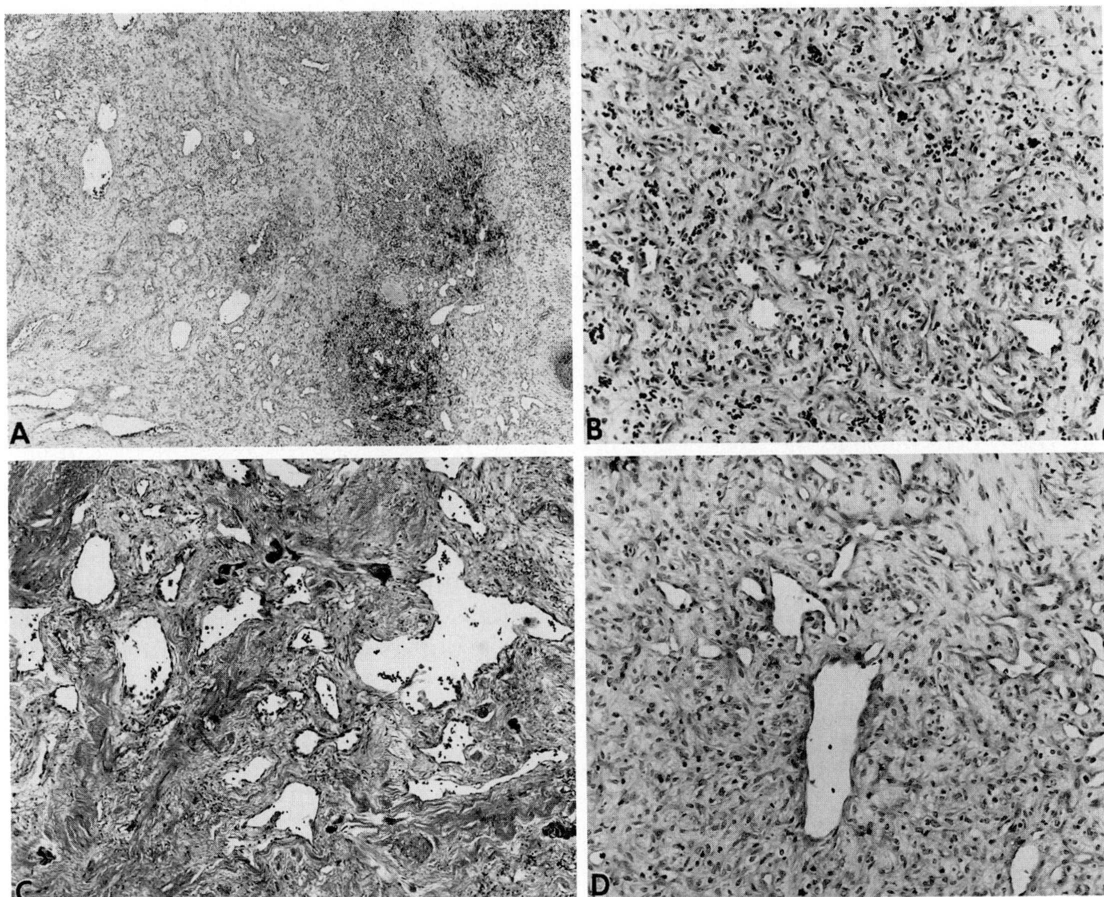

Figure 12–6. Hemangioma. *A.* There is a vaguely lobulated pattern in this example of cardiac hemangioma that suggests pyogenic granuloma. This tumor was excised from a 22-year-old man who presented initially with a cardiac murmur. The tumor was located on the endocardial surface of the anterior wall of the left ventricle. (H & E × 30) *B.* A higher magnification of the tumor demonstrates compact capillary channels. (H & E × 75) *C.* In some examples of cardiac hemangioma, there are areas of fibrous tissue admixed with myocytes suggesting a hamartomatous process. This tumor was resected from the right ventricle of a 41-year-old man with syncopal episodes. (H & E × 75) *D.* There is abundant cytoplasm in the cells forming this hemangioma; such tumors have been called "histiocytoid" or epithelioid hemangiomas. This right atrial mass was resected from a 1-year-old boy with a pericardial effusion. (H & E × 150)

been known since the early 1900s. This lesion has been given a variety of names, including lymphangio(endothelio)ma, mesothelioma, and inclusion cysts. Recent immunohistochemical evidence indicates that the cystic tumor of the AV node is an epithelial lesion of endodermal, not mesothelial origin. It is generally believed that the AV nodal tumor is a congenital rest.

Cystic AV nodal tumors are rare. There have been about 75 reports in the literature.[48] The majority of patients with cystic tumors of the atrioventricular node present with complete heart block. The diagnosis is usually made at autopsy and has been made at all ages, from newborn to the ninth decade. Because of a female predominance, it has been suggested that the diagnosis of atrioventricular nodal tumor be considered in teenage girls with complete heart block. Most cases of death are due to ventricular arrhythmias. There has recently been a report of a successfully resected tumor,[49] in which the clinical diagnosis was facilitated by coronary angiography. The majority of tumors of the atrioventricular node are sporadic. However, these tumors can occur in patients with congenital heart disease or other malformations.

These tumors are located, by definition, in the region of the atrioventricular node. Grossly they may appear as a cyst-like structure in the region of the membranous septum, or an area of thickening with small fluid-filled cysts that are barely perceptible to the naked eye. They range in size from 2 to 20 mm. Often the cysts are first recognized at the time of microscopic examination of the conduction system. Microscopically, the tumor is located in the inferior interatrial septum in the region of the atrioventricular node and proximal His bundles (Fig. 12–7), and respects the boundary of the central fibrous body without extending into ventricular myocardium or into valvular tissues. There are nests of cells that often form cysts of various sizes. The lumens of the cysts contain PAS-positive, diastase-resistant material that occasionally calcifies. The cell nests can replace myofibers within the inferior interatrial septum and are composed of cuboidal, transitional, or squamous cells. The squamous cells may have a clear cytoplasm that resemble sebaceous cells; these can be interspersed among cuboidal cells, forming a two-cell population. The cysts often form two cell layers, a luminal cuboidal single cell layer overlying several layers of transitional-appearing cells. The epithelium can flatten and cysts can assume tortuous shapes, which may account for earlier studies that have mistaken them for endothelial cells. Often there is dense fibrosis surrounding the cysts or cell nests, and a lymphocytic reaction can occur. Cilia are sometimes visible on light microscopy. Endocrine granules have been reported in the epithelial cells of tumors of the atrioventricular nodal region.

Immunohistochemical markers indicate an endodermal derivation for the cells of cystic AV nodal tumors.[50, 51] Most cases are strongly positive for carcinoembryonic antigen as well as B72.3 antigen, and occasionally serotonin and chromogranin.

Other Heterotopias

Simple cysts can occur within the myocardium or pericardium that are lined by cuboidal epithelial cells and are presumably misplaced bronchial structures. Unlike cystic tumors of the AV node, they are generally unilocular, are present anywhere in the heart, and usually are lined by ciliated and sometimes mucin-secreting cells. Such cysts, which are generally assumed to be of bronchogenic origin, are usually detected in infants or children and may be associated with other cardiac malformations.[52, 53] Bronchogenic cysts are generally found within the pericardial space (see Chapter 11).

Thyroid rests are the most common type of ectopic organ to occur within the heart.[54] They can occasionally attain large sizes and cause symptoms in adults, particularly right ventricular outflow tract obstruction. Successful surgical removal has been reported.[54] Less commonly, ectopic thymus tissue has been found within the pericardium; we have seen a case of thymic tissue in association with a cardiac myxoma.

Miscellaneous Proliferations

Histiocytoid Cardiomyopathy

Also known as Purkinje cell hamartoma and oncocytic cardiomyopathy, histiocytoid cardiomyopathy is a multifocal congenital hamartoma. Patients present in infancy and early childhood with tachyarrhythmias, sudden death, or congestive heart failure.[55] Eighty percent of patients are female. Symptoms may respond to surgical removal or local endocardial

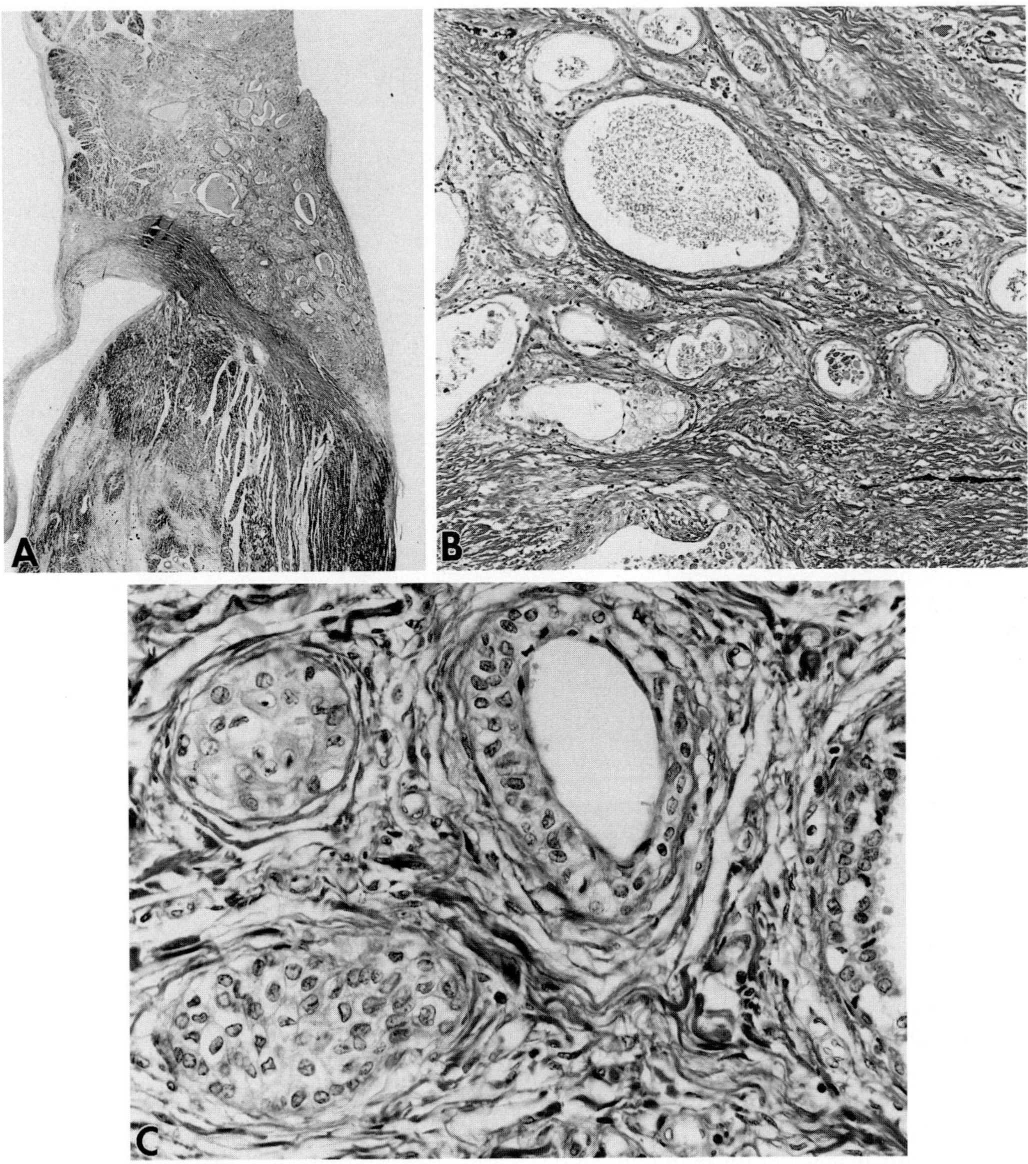

Figure 12–7. Cystic tumor of the AV node. *A.* This tumor was found as the sole pathologic finding of a 43-year-old woman who died suddenly without any medical history. Note inclusions expanding the area superior to the central fibrous body in the area of the AV node and a scar in the basilar portion of the ventricular septum; the mitral valve is seen on the left. (H & E × 10) *B.* Cystic tumor of the AV node. A higher magnification demonstrates cysts of different sizes lined by flattened cuboidal epithelium. (H & E × 75) *C.* The cysts can be lined by two cell layers resembling basal cells and transitional cells. This tumor was found at autopsy of a 48-year-old woman with complete heart block with permanent pacemaker. (H & E × 300)

ablation. Grossly, the tumors are raised yellowish nodules that occur in all areas of the endocardium and myocardium. Histologically, the tumor cells resemble histiocytes on routine stains (Fig. 12–8). Ultrastructurally, the tumors cells resemble modified myocytes with poorly developed intercellular junctions, a marked increase in mitochondria, and few contractile elements.[55]

Hamartomas of Mature Cardiac Muscle

There are several types of cardiac tumors that are often classified as hamartomas and have

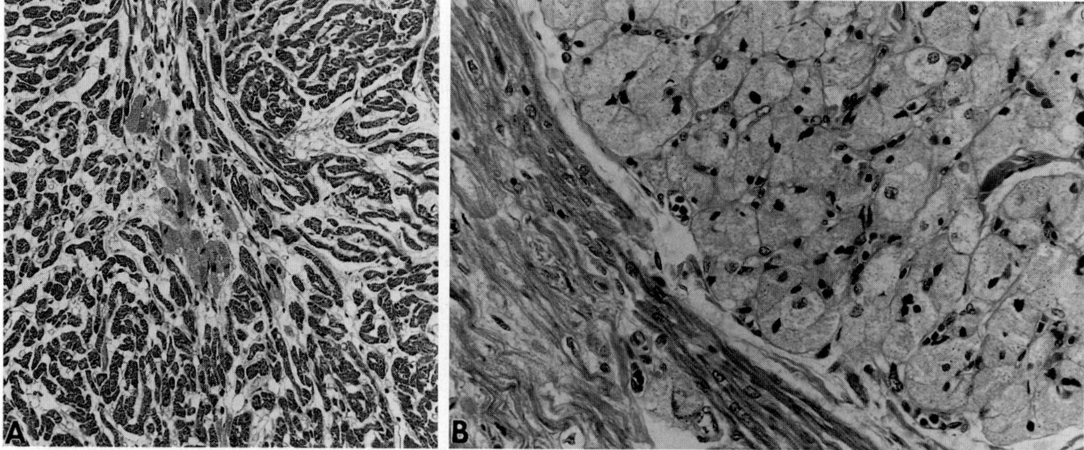

Figure 12–8. Histiocytoid cardiomyopathy. *A*. Note collections of foamy cells surrounded by normal mocytes in an infant. (H & E × 150) *B*. A higher magnification demonstrates the finely granular cytoplasm of the histiocytoid cells; their true nature is unknown. (H & E × 300)

been discussed earlier. These include rhabdomyoma, lipomatous hypertrophy of the interatrial septum, and histiocytoid cardiomyopathy. In addition, many examples of vascular hemangiomas contain fat, cardiac muscle, and vascular elements and are likely hamartomas.

We have seen hamartomas that are composed of mature hypertrophied cardiac myocytes and that do not resemble the entities mentioned earlier. Hamartomas of mature cardiac myocytes are single or multiple, measure up to 6 cm in greatest dimension, are located in either or both ventricles, and occur in children and adults. Unlike rhabdomyoma, the myocytes lack vacuoles and abundant glycogen. These hamartomas are cellular masses composed of hypertrophied myocytes and sparse fibrous tissue that histologically resemble hypertrophic cardiomyopathy (Fig. 12–9). Unlike hypertrophic cardiomyopathy, the masses are focal, demarcated, and are not localized to the ventricular septum. Hamartomas of mature cardiac myocytes may be incidental or cause ventricular outflow obstruction and arrhythmias.

Inflammatory Pseudotumor and Fibrous Histiocytoma

In addition to cardiac fibroma, there are rare examples of fibrous tumors of the heart that resemble inflammatory pseudotumors. Like their counterparts in the lung, they usually occur in children and are histologically composed of fibroblasts, myofibroblasts, lymphocytes, and plasma cells. One case has been reported in association with a systemic vasculitis[56] and another case with spontaneous regression has been reported.[57] It is debated whether inflammatory pseudotumors are reactive proliferations or benign neoplasms of myofibroblasts (inflammatory fibrous histiocytoma). A related fibrous proliferation that may occur in the heart is the benign fibrous histiocytoma. These lesions resemble fibromas in which there are an unusually large number of histiocytic cells. In contrast to malignant fibrous histiocytoma, mitoses and pleomorphism are absent, and patients do well on long-term follow-up.[58]

Mesothelial/Macrophage Incidental Cardiac Excrescences and Other Histiocytoid Lesions of the Heart

In addition to benign or malignant fibrous histiocytomas, there are at least three histiocytoid lesions that have been described in the heart. Histiocytoid cardiomyopathy is a multifocal hamartoma of cardiac myocyte or Purkinje cell origin; the histiocytoid appearance is secondary to oncocytic change. Similar to histiocytoid hemangiomas of soft tissue, cardiac hemangiomas may be composed of endothelial cells, reminiscent of histiocytes, with abundant cleared cytoplasm. In contrast to histiocytes, the endothelial cells of histiocytoid hemangioma form vascular spaces and express endothelial markers. A recently described histiocytic proliferation that may result in an asymptomatic cardiac mass has been given the name cardiac "MICE" (mesothelial/macrophage incidental cardiac excrescence).[59] MICE are distinctive avascular collections of histiocytes, fat, and

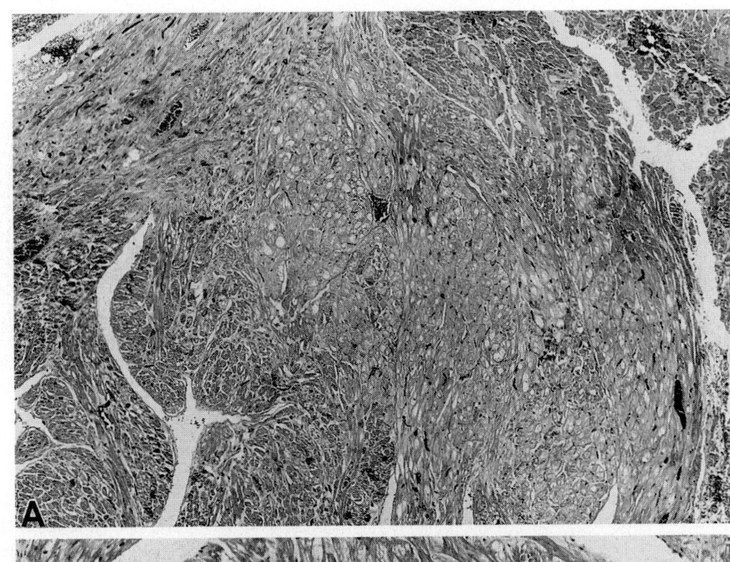

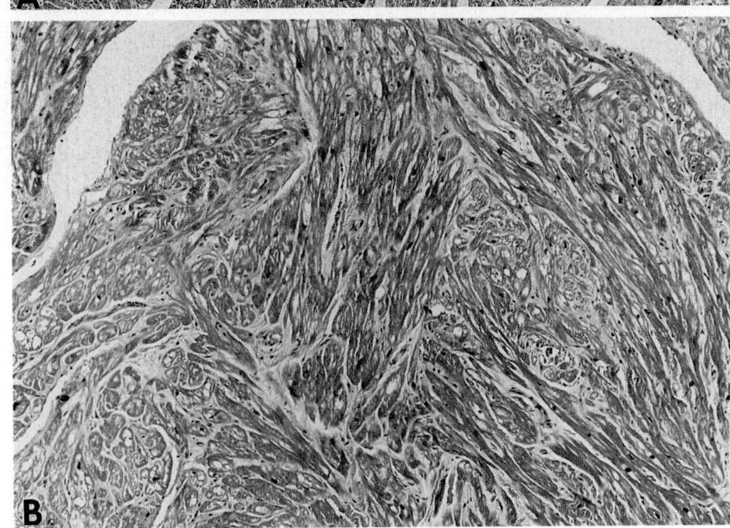

Figure 12–9. Hamartoma of mature cardiac myocytes. *A.* This photomicrograph demonstrates a section of a 5-cm tumor that was resected from the right ventricle of a 28-year-old man with Wolff–Parkinson–White syndrome. The tumor was composed of disorganized, hypertrophied myocytes (H & E × 30) *B.* A higher magnification demonstrates enlarged myocytes that are in disarray, similar to cases of hypertrophic cardiomyopathy. (H & E × 75)

mesothelial cells (Fig. 12–10). MICE have been reported to be artifacts produced by cardiotomy suction[60] and may be found incidentally attached to cardiac myxomas.

BENIGN NEOPLASMS

Cardiac Myxoma

Definition

Cardiac myxoma is a benign proliferation of primitive cells that differentiate primarily along endothelial lines. It occurs exclusively on the endothelial surfaces of the heart, usually the left side of the interatrial septum. The current view is that cardiac myxoma is a benign neoplasm.[61]

Incidence

The incidence of cardiac myxoma in autopsies has been estimated at 0.03 percent.[62]

Clinical Presentation

Series of cardiac myxoma show a slight female predominance.[63] The average age at presentation is 50 years, with a peak age range of 30–60 years. Myxomas occurring in children under age 10 are extremely rare.

The clinical presentation of cardiac myxoma is more varied than any other cardiac tumor. Cardiac myxomas cause symptoms in three ways: by mass effect, embolization, and constitutional effects. Because cardiac myxoma is most often located in the left atrium, the most common presentation secondary to mass effect is

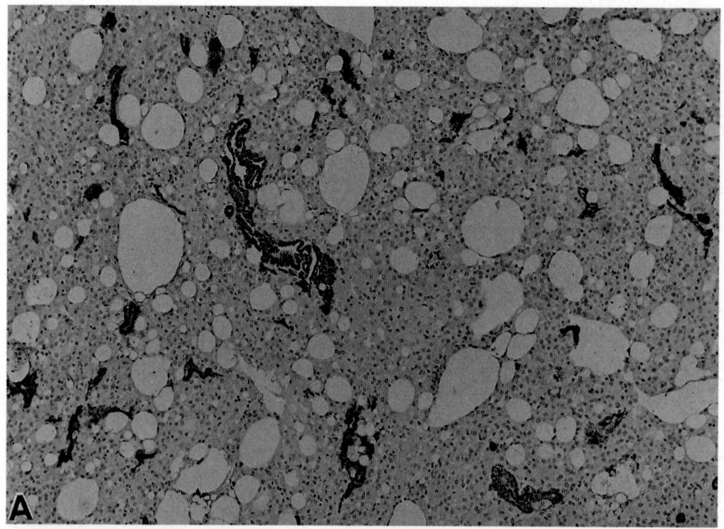

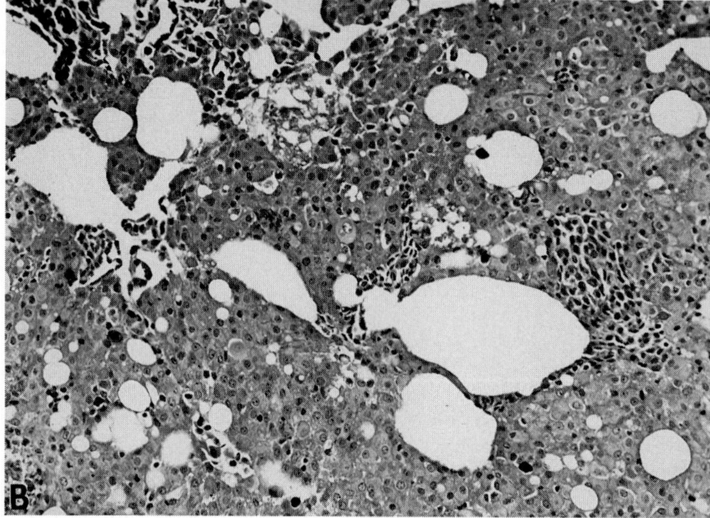

Figure 12–10. Mesothelial/macrophage incidental cardiac excrescence (MICE). *A.* These are collections of histiocytes, fat, and mesothelial cells that are likely artifacts of open heart surgery. This "tumor" was attached to a cardiac myxoma (not shown). The mesothelial cells are prominent because of their cytokeratin content. (Avidin biotin complex anti-cytokeratin × 75) *B.* A higher magnification demonstrates the three components of this lesion. (H & E × 150)

that of mitral stenosis. Embolization is common in patients with myxomas because the tumors are often friable. Symptoms related to embolic phenomena include strokes, transient ischemic attacks, claudication of the extremities, renal insufficiency, myocardial infarction, and pulmonary emboli if the tumor is right-sided. Constitutional symptoms are weakness, malaise, fevers, and are related to hematological abnormalities such as anemia, hypergammaglobulinemia, and increased sedimentation rate. Occasionally, myxomas can become infected, and the presenting symptoms are related to bacterial endocarditis.

The majority of patients with cardiac myxoma are cured with surgical removal. Recurrence is seen in less than 2% of cases[1–4, 64] after excision. Currently, myxomas are resected with a portion of atrial septum, and recurrences are generally at intracardiac sites distant from the original tumor. Patients with recurrent tumors are younger than patients without recurrence and often have familial tumors (see following). Recurrent myxomas are usually extensively myxoid with little fibrosis, and are grossly friable and gelatinous.[65]

The existence of "malignant" cardiac myxoma is controversial,[66] but it is generally agreed that cardiac myxomas are benign lesions. Embolic myxomas have the capacity to grow beyond the vessel wall in embolic sites, and case reports indicate that they can achieve large sizes in bone. Emboli in cerebral arteries typically form fusiform aneurysms that are discovered on angiography; these aneurysms are the result of local vascular infiltration and rarely rupture.

Long-term clinical follow-up in patients with embolic myxoma is lacking. Embolic myxoma can persist as aneurysms in cerebral vessels or as nodules in pulmonary arteries for months or even years after excision of the primary tumor. These deposits tend to remain stable or regress with time and do not behave as typical metastases. Although cardiac myxoma can cause death by embolization to coronary or cerebral arteries, embolic myxomas do not have the histologic characteristics of malignant neoplasms, and do not cause tumor deposits in viscera or lymph nodes.

Myxoma Syndrome

In a small minority of patients, there is a familial constellation of abnormalities that include cardiac myxoma, spotty pigmentation, endocrine overactivity, and myxoid neurofibromas.[67, 68] These patients are much younger than patients with sporadic cardiac myxoma and usually become symptomatic by the third decade. The tumors in these patients are usually multiple, recurrent, friable, and embolic, and may arise in unusual endocardial sites. Autosomal dominant and autosomal recessive modes of inheritance have been described. Occasionally, myxoid lesions in sites outside the heart are encountered, such as skin, breast, and uterus.

Gross Pathology

Seventy-five percent of myxomas are pedunculated left atrial masses attached to the endocardium of the fossa ovalis (Fig. 12–11). Right atrial myxomas, which represent most of the remainder, are less likely attached to the fossa ovalis than left atrial myxomas, although this is still the most common location. About 5% of cardiac myxomas grow on both sides of the fossa and are biatrial tumors that form a single mass. A small proportion of cardiac myxomas are truly multiple. These rare examples, which are typical of the myxoma syndrome, occur in all locations of both atria, and occasionally in the ventricles. Single myxomas occurring in the right or left ventricles are distinctly rare, as are myxomas attached to the atrioventricular valves or chordae tendineae.

The attachment of cardiac myxoma to the interatrial septum can be by a broad base or narrow pedicle. Cardiac myxoma varies from a gelatinous mass with frond-like excrescences to a tumor with a smooth, firm surface. Myxomas with irregular surfaces are more likely to embo-

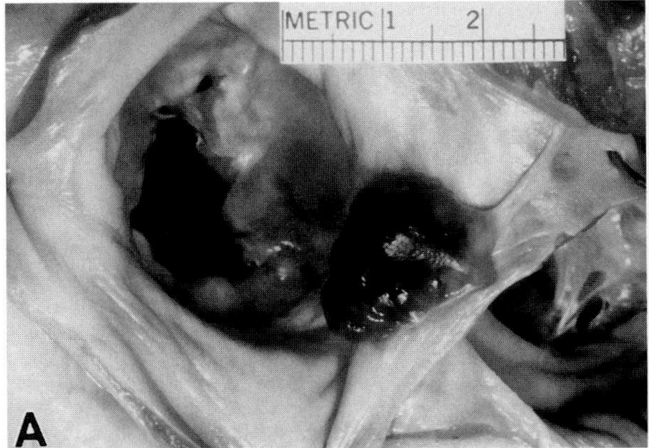

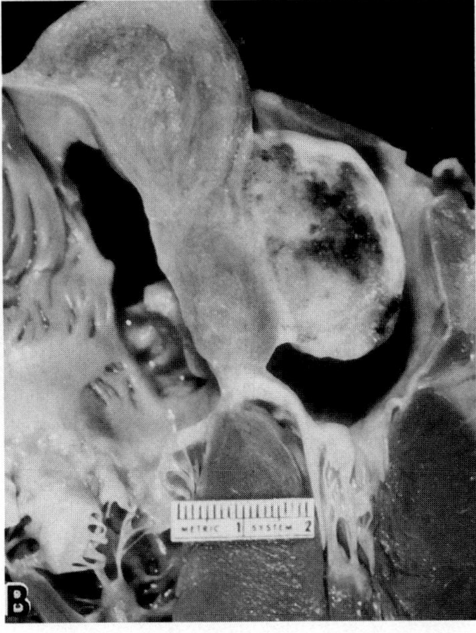

Figure 12–11. Cardiac myxoma. *A.* The majority of cardiac myxomas are located in the left atrium near the fossa ovalis. Note dark-colored tumor attached by a broad base to the left atrial surface at the oval fossa. The mitral valve is intact and not obstructed by this small myxoma, which was an incidental autopsy finding. *B.* The cut section of a different myxoma shows smooth surface and heterogeneous hemorrhage and gritty areas. As is typical, this myxoma projects into the left atrium by a broad attachment at the oval fossa; there is no extension into the septum. Myxomas with smooth surface, such as these, do not embolize.

lize than smooth-surfaced tumors. There is often organized thrombus on the surface. On cut section, tumors are variegated in appearance, and may contain gritty calcified areas.

Microscopic Pathology

The microscopic appearance of cardiac myxoma is distinctive and differs from that of soft-tissue myxomas. In areas of tumor that are not scarred, there is abundant myxoid matrix of mucopolysaccharides and relatively few cells (Fig. 12–12*A*). These cells include myxoma cells, endothelial cells, and inflammatory cells. The nuclei of myxoma cells are ovoid in shape, measure between up to 2 to 4 times the diameter of histiocyte nuclei, have irregular outlines with dense chromatin, and lack prominent nucleoli. Many cells are multinucleated forming syncytia that assume a variety of shapes. Structures formed by multinucleated myxoma cells include cords, rings with multiple cell layers (Figs. 12–12*B,C*), and the flattened lining of the tumor surface. The multinucleated cells may also form ball-like clusters floating within the matrix or lining the surface. The myxoma cells appear to differentiate along endothelial lines, and blood-filled capillaries are present within the rings and cords. If the surface of the tumor is irregular (Fig. 12–12*D*), the tumor is likely to embolize (Fig. 12–12*E*). There is variable expression of endothelial antigens, including Ulex europaeus, factor VIII-related antigen, and CD34. S-100 protein is often expressed in myxoma cells. Other antigens variably expressed by myxoma cells are vimentin, actin, and desmin; cytokeratin is absent unless there are glandular structures.[69, 70]

Secondary changes include scarring, bone formation, organizing thrombi, and inflammation. Abundant hemosiderin, generally within macrophages, is invariably present. In cases of extensive hemosiderin deposition, gamna bodies form; these can rarely form the bulk of the tumor (Fig. 12–12*F*). Calcification is more common than is appreciated radiographically, and is more prevalent in right-sided tumors. Fibrosis is more extensive in tumors from older patients, and is not extensive in embolic myxoma.

At the junction of the tumor and the interatrial septum, there can be smooth muscle proliferation, lymphoid aggregates, thick-walled arteries, and granuloma formation. Extramedullary hematopoiesis is present in less than 10% of cases.

Approximately 1% of cardiac myxomas contain glandular structures lined by mucinous cells that resemble goblet cells of the gastrointestinal tract (Fig. 12–12*G*). The mucin is PAS positive, diastase resistant, and the glands stain for cytokeratin and carcinoembryonic antigen by immunohistochemical techniques. The differential diagnosis of myxoma with glandular structures includes metastatic carcinoma, but there is no nuclear anaplasia or mitotic activity within the glands of myxoma.

There are several entities in the differential diagnosis of cardiac myxoma. Sarcomas of the heart often occur in the left atrium and can be extensively myxoid, so called "myxoid imitators."[71] Myxoid sarcomas are often confused with myxoma both clinically and pathologically. Myxoma cells are absent in sarcoma, and there is a relatively monotonous proliferation of spindle cells with focal mitotic figures. With sufficient sampling of the lesion, areas diagnostic of myxoid fibrosarcoma or myxoid malignant fibrous histiocytoma are found.

Occasionally, surgeons remove embolic fragments from peripheral arteries in patients with occlusive vascular disease. The diagnosis of myxoma is easily made if characteristic myxoma cells are present; thorough sampling of the specimen may be necessary. If a postoperative echocardiogram is normal, the diagnosis of cardiac myxoma is still tenable because the primary tumor can completely dislodge and embolize. Overdiagnosis of embolic myxoma in vascular biopsies occurs when myxoid thrombi or embolic myxoid sarcomas are mistakenly interpreted as myxoma. Again, the identification of the characteristic myxoma cell is critical in the proper diagnosis.

Fibrotic myxomas can histologically resemble fibromas or organized thrombi with scarring. Fibromas generally occur in a much younger age range than fibrotic myxoma, are intramyocardial tumors, and have a predilection for the interventricular septum. Occasionally, the distinction between organized thrombus and myxoma is difficult, and a descriptive diagnosis is all that can be rendered. Because fibrotic myxomas rarely if ever recur,[65] the distinction is probably not critical.

Rare Benign Neoplasms

Granular Cell Tumor

Granular cell tumors of the heart are rare.[7] Histologically and immunohistochemically, granular cell tumors of the heart are identical to those of the breast and gastrointestinal tract (Fig. 12–13). Granular cell tumors are currently

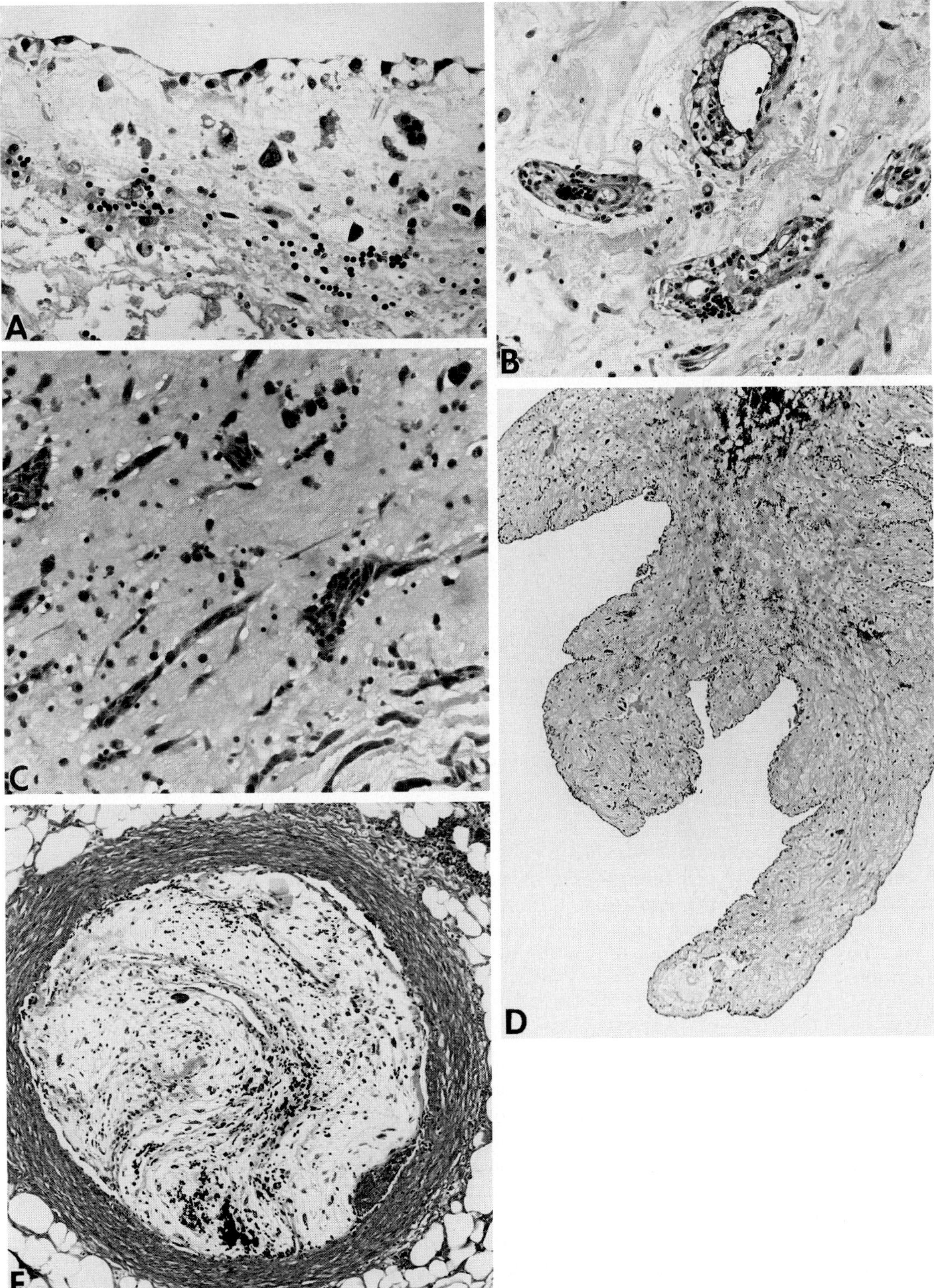

Figure 12–12. Cardiac myxoma. The components of myxoma are free-floating spindle and stellate cells that may form syncytia, mononuclear cells (histiocytes and lymphoid cells), myxoid ground substance, and a surface layer (*A*). This tumor arose in the left atrium of a 72-year-old man with the clinical diagnosis of mitral stenosis. (H & E × 150) Most myxomas in the heart show endothelial differentiation. Myxoma cells form rings that are several layers thick and infiltrated with inflammatory cells (*B*). (H & E × 150) *C.* Myxoma cells can form cord-like vascular structures. In this example, the myxoma cells and histiocytes were heavily laden with hemosiderin. (H & E × 150) *D.* One third to one half of cardiac myxomas have a friable surface that is prone to embolize. This tumor was a 7-cm left atrial mass that was considered on angiogram to represent a sarcoma. (H & E × 30) *E.* Friable myxomas can embolize and cause symptoms related to vascular occlusion. This artery is the epicardial coronary artery of a 45-year-old man who died of myocardial infarction. (H & E × 150)

Illustration continued on following page

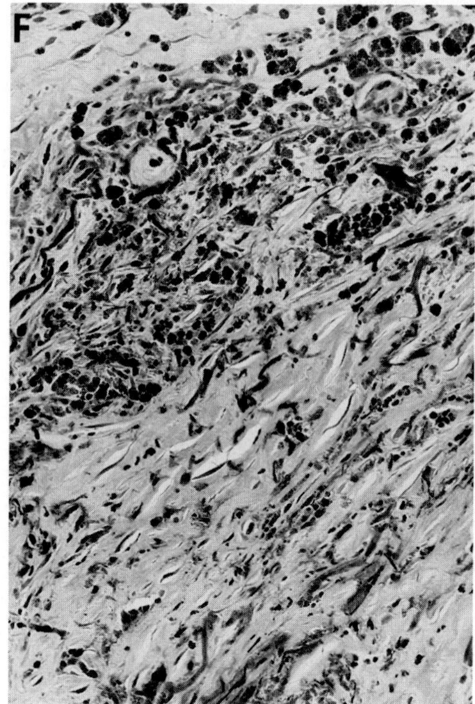

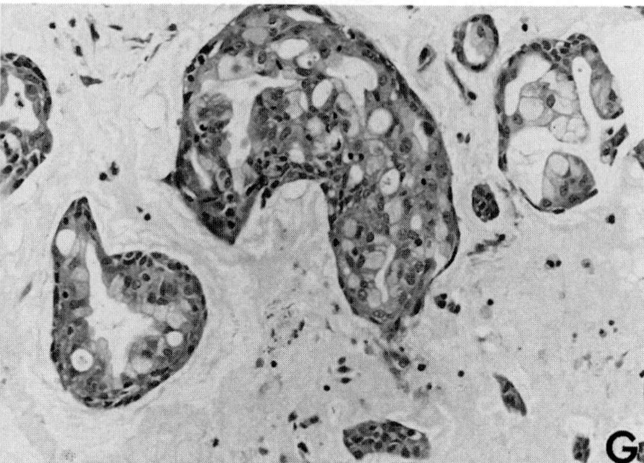

Figure 12–12 (*Continued*). *F.* Degenerative changes of fibrosis, elastic deposition with calcification, and hemosiderin deposition (gamna gandy bodies) are common. (H & E × 150) This tumor arose in a 61-year-old man; the echocardiographic diagnosis was interatrial lipoma; at surgery, a left atrial mass was removed. *G.* One to two percent of myxomas have glandular structures that are lined by goblet cells and that merge imperceptibly with surrounding myxoma cells. (From Burke AP, Virmani R. Cardiac myxomas. Am J Clin Pathol 100:671–680, 1993, with permission.)

believed to be derived from nerve sheath cells. In the heart, granular cell tumors present as incidental nodules on the epicardial surface, often near a coronary artery, or in the atrium. A case has recently been reported in the sinus node.[72]

Lipoma

The most common location of fatty accumulation in the heart is the interatrial septum (see lipomatous hypertrophy of the interatrial septum, earlier). Encapsulated masses of fat, lipomas are similar to benign lipomatous neoplasms of soft issue, but are much rarer. They have been described in various locations in the heart and are most common on the epicardial surface.[7] Lipomas can occur on the mitral valve.[73] Histologically, cardiac lipomas contain mature fat and may be quite vascular.

Teratoma

Intrapericardial teratomas are rare and are histologically similar to teratomas of the gonads and mediastinum. There have been approximately 65 cases reported.[74] Most are benign epicardial masses that present in infancy (see Chapter 11). Only a small number of teratomas have been reported that were within cardiac muscle, that recurred or invaded contiguous structures, or that were first diagnosed in adults. Intracardiac teratomas occur almost exclusively in the right atrium or ventricle. Histologically, teratomas contain all three germ layers, in contrast to bronchogenic cysts, which are exclusively epithelial (Fig. 12–14).

Paraganglioma

Approximately 30 cardiac paragangliomas have been reported.[75–76] Paragangliomas of the heart are similar histologically and immunohistochemically to extracardiac paragangliomas (Fig. 12–15). The majority occur within the atria, are benign,[75–77] and are functional, resulting in systemic hypertension. Functional cardiac paragangliomas have been termed pheochromocytomas[78, 79] and have been successfully removed with remission of symptoms.[80]

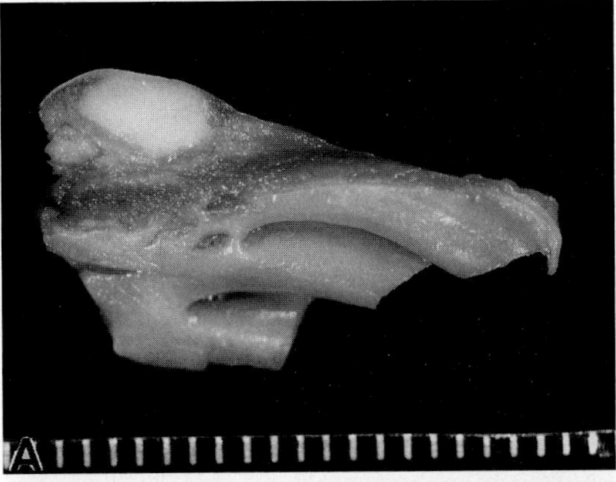

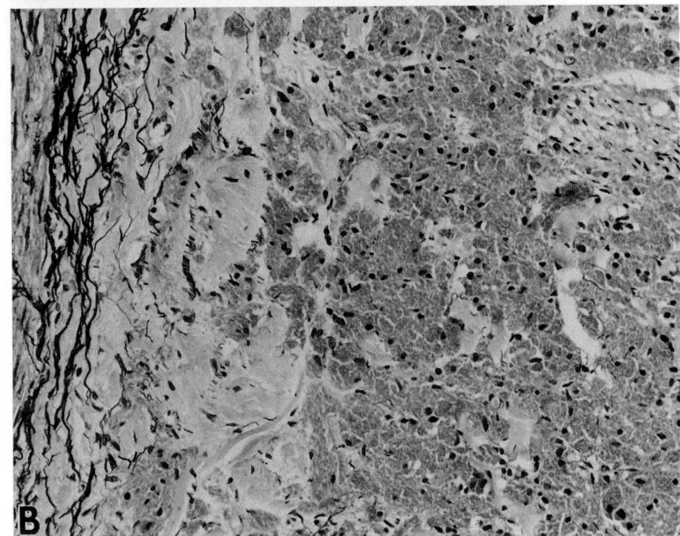

Figure 12–13. Granular cell tumor. Note incidental nodule on the epicardial surface (*A*) (scale in mm). Histologic section demonstrates tumor adjacent to coronary artery (*B*). (Movat × 150)

Neurofibroma

This is an extremely rare tumor of the heart[81–85] that may occur in atria, ventricles, or area of the atrioventricular node. It has been reported in patients with and without neurofibromatosis.[7]

MALIGNANT CARDIAC NEOPLASMS

Sarcomas

Classification

The cell of origin of cardiac sarcomas is presumably an uncommitted mesenchymal cell. Virtually all types of sarcomas have been shown to arise within the cardiac muscle mass, demonstrating the pluripotentiality of the malignant mesenchymal cell. The histologic types are essentially identical to those found in extracardiac soft tissue. Electron microscopy and immunohistochemistry for epithelial, neural, nerve sheath, muscle, and endothelial differentiation are of limited value in determining subtypes of cardiac sarcomas. Desmin is perhaps the most useful immunohistochemical marker in determining striated muscle differentiation.

The histologic classification of cardiac sarcomas is currently of little clinical use. The treatment and survival are not apparently affected by the type of sarcoma. It has been shown that there is especially poor survival in patients with tumors that have a high mitotic rate and areas of necrosis.[86]

Incidence, Clinical Findings, and Prognosis

Primary sarcomas of the heart are rare, and constitute less than 25% of primary cardiac tumors,[1–7] and only 10% of surgically resected cardiac tumors (see Table 12–1).[2–4, 40, 87–89] Of surgically resected tumors in published series, angiosarcomas and malignant fibrous histiocytomas are the most common histologic types (Table 12–2). In a series of cardiac sarcomas

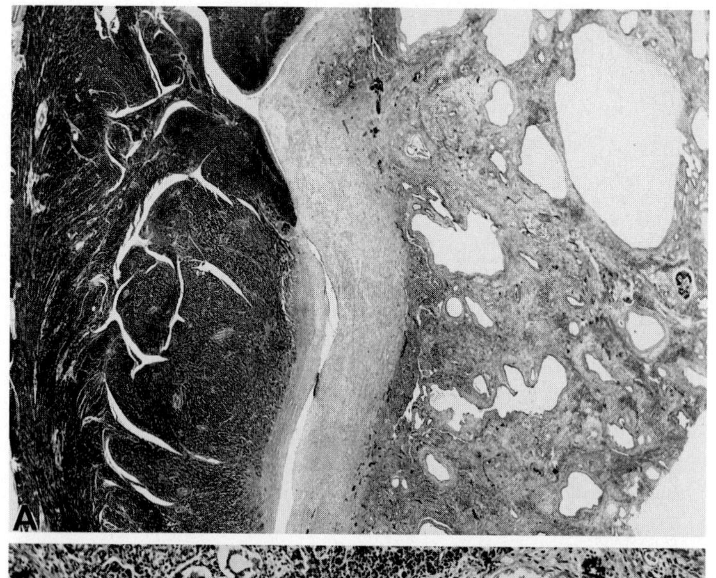

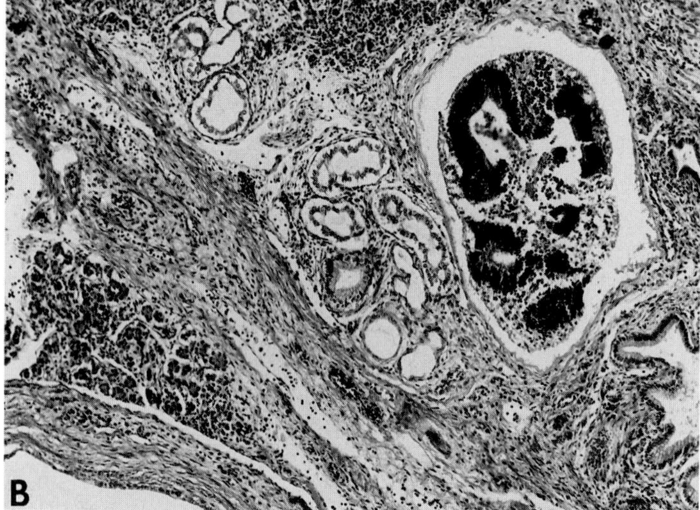

Figure 12–14. Teratoma. Cardiac teratoma located on endocardial surface of left ventricle. Unlike other cysts or rests in the heart, teratomas contain ectodermal, endodermal, and mesodermal elements. *A.* This tumor was found at the autopsy of a premature hydropic infant. (Movat × 7.5) *B.* A higher magnification of the tumor demonstrates neuroectodermal, glandular, and stromal elements. (H & E × 75)

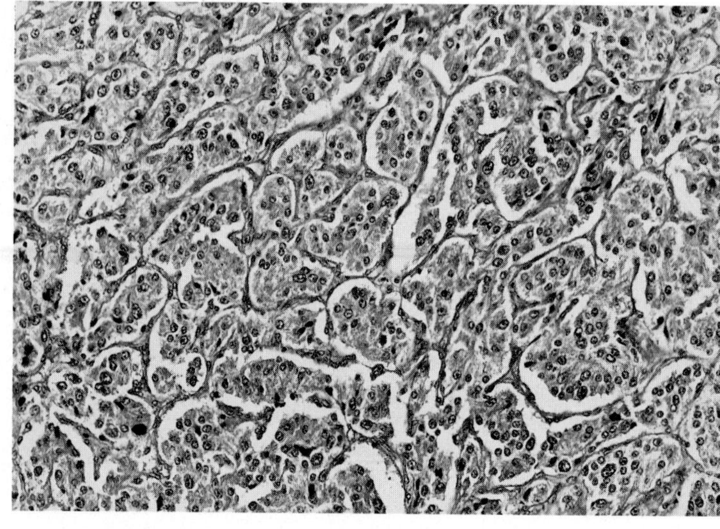

Figure 12–15. Paraganglioma. Most paraganglomas of the heart secrete catecholamines and cause hypertension. This tumor was removed from a 58-year-old woman with hypertension. It was located in the left atrium. The histology of cardiac paraganglioma is identical to that of tumors arising outside the heart. (H & E × 150)

Table 12–2. Primary Cardiac Tumors, AFIP 1976–1993

	n (% Total)	Surgical Cases	< 16 Years*	< 1 Year*
Benign Tumors				
Myxoma	114 (29%)	102	4	0
Papillary fibroelastoma	31 (8%)	8	0	0
Rhabdomyoma	20 (5%)	6	20	19
Fibroma	20 (5%)	18	13	8
Hemangioma	17 (4%)	10	2	1
Lipomatous hypertrophy, atrial septum	12 (3%)	7	0	0
AV nodal tumor	10 (3%)	0	2	1
Granular cell tumor	4 (1%)	0	0	0
Lipoma	2	2	0	0
Paraganglioma	2	2	0	0
Myocytic hamartoma, not further classified	2	2	0	0
Histiocytoid cardiomyopathy	2	0	2	2
Inflammatory pseudotumor	2	2	1	0
Benign fibrous histiocytoma	1	0	0	0
Epithelioid hemangioendothelioma	1	1	0	0
Bronchogenic cyst	1	1	0	0
Teratoma	1	0	1	1
Total Benign Tumors	242	161	45	32
Malignant Tumors				
Sarcoma	137 (35%)	124	11	3
Angiosarcoma	33	22	1	0
Unclassified	33	30	3	1
MFH	16	16	1	0
Osteosarcoma	13	13	0	0
Leiomyosarcoma	12	11	1	1
Fibrosarcoma	9	9	1	0
Myxosarcoma	8	8	1	0
Rhabdomyosarcoma	6	2	3	1
Synovial sarcoma	4	4	0	0
Liposarcoma	2	0	0	0
Malignant schwannoma	1	1	0	0
Lymphoma	7 (2%)	1	0	0
Total Malignant Tumors	144	125	11	3
TOTAL TUMORS	386	286	56	35

* Age of patient at time of diagnosis

seen as referrals at the AFIP, unclassifiable sarcomas are as frequent as angiosarcomas.[86]

The clinical presentation of any primary tumor of the heart depends on its location. Because more than half of cardiac sarcomas are located in the left atrium, the most common presenting symptom is dyspnea secondary to left ventricular inflow obstruction, and the most common clinical diagnosis is myxoma. Other modes of presentation for cardiac sarcoma include pericardial tamponade, especially if there is extensive pericardial involvement, embolic phenomena, chest pain, syncope, fever of unknown origin, and peripheral edema. Rare examples are incidental findings, either at autopsy or cardiac surgery for other causes. Distant metastases commonly develop in patients with primary cardiac sarcoma, and are sometimes the presenting symptom.[86, 90] However, cardiac sarcomas are usually localized to the heart at the time of diagnosis. Occasional examples will present with invasion of contiguous structures, including lungs, diaphragm, and venae cava. Metastatic sites are most commonly lungs, followed by vertebrae, liver, brain, bowel, long bones, spleen, adrenal, and skull.

The prognosis of cardiac sarcomas is poor and generally measured in months (Tables 12–3 and 12–4). Pathologic findings that are associated with increased survival include left-sided tumors, a low mitotic rate, and the absence of necrosis.[86] Even with sarcomas of low mitotic rate that lack necrosis, the long-term outlook is poor, and few patients survive 5 years. Both chemotherapy and radiation therapy have been used for the treatment of cardiac sarcoma, in conjunction with surgical removal.[2–4, 88–90] Protocols generally follow those established for soft tissue sarcomas of the extremities. Although the resection of cardiac sarcomas is rarely curative, the short-term results are generally good, and palliation with extension of life

Table 12–3. Clinical and Morphologic Characterization of Surgically Resected Cardiac Sarcomas, Results of Seven Institutional Series

Histologic Type	Mean Age, Range (yr)	M:F	LA (%)	RA (%)	Other sites	Survival Until Death Mean (mo)	Survival Until Last Follow-up, Mean (mo)
Angiosarcoma (n = 25) (37%)	45 (26–80)	13:12	10%	90%	0%	6.6 (n = 17)	16 (n = 1)
MFH (n = 16) (24%)	44 (24–74)	8:8	86%	0	14%*	14.9 (n = 11)	16 (n = 2)
Leiomyosa (n = 6) (9%)	37 (20–61)	4:2	80%	0	20%†	6.8 (n = 6)	0
Rhabdomyosarcoma (n = 5) (7%)	30 (0–63)	3:2	50%	25%	25%	3 (n = 2)	87‡ (n = 2)
Unclassified (n = 5) (7%)	16 (0–59)	2:3	67%	33%	0	4.5 (n = 2)	21 (n = 3)
Fibromyxosarcoma (n = 4) (6%)	46 (46–56)	0:4	67%	0	33%	4.0 (n = 4)	0
Myxosarcoma (n = 3) (4%)	28 (28–28)	0:3	100%	0	0	8.6 (n = 3)	0
Fibrosarcoma (n = 2) (3%)	43 (26,60)	1:1	0	0	100%	9.5 (n = 2)	0
Osteosarcoma (n = 2) (3%)	25 (18,31)	1:1	100%	0	0	17 days	24 (n = 1) (n = 1)
Totals: (n = 68)	44 (3 mo– 80 yr)	32:36	53%	35%	12% (n = 48)	8 mo (n = 9)	35 mo

Data derived from the following series: Putnam et al. (21 tumors), Murphy et al. (13 tumors), Bear et al. (8 tumors), Tazelaar et al. (7 tumors), Miralles et al. (7 tumors), Dein et al. (7 tumors), Reece et al. (5 tumors). Data were not available for all cases.

* Two tumors in the right ventricle

† Left ventricular tumor

‡ One patient alive 10 years at last follow-up

Abbreviations: M = male; F = female; MFH = malignant fibrous histiocytoma; LA = left atrium; RA = right atrium; mo = months; yr = years

Table 12–4. Clinical and Morphologic Characterization, Sarcomas of the Heart and Pericardium, AFIP 1976–1993

Histologic Type	Mean Age, Range (yr)	M:F	LA (%)	RA (%)	Vent, Diff	Pericardium	Survival Until Death Mean (mo)	Survival Until Last Follow-up, Mean (mo)
Angiosarcoma (n = 37) (26%)	42 (15–70)	29:8	5%	68%	16%	11%	3 (n = 19)	22 (n = 2)
Unclassified (n = 35) (24%)	45 (1–88)	19:16	49%	13%	32%	6%	3 (n = 14)	12 (n = 2)
MFH (n = 16) (11%)	43 (12–86)	5:11	81%	13%	6%	0	5 (n = 9)	8 (n = 2)
Osteosarcoma (n = 13) (9%)	35 (16–67)	6:7	100%*	0	0	0	6 (n = 11)	8 (n = 2)
Leiomyosarcoma (n = 12) (8%)	30 (1–58)	5:7	76%	16%	8%	0	9 (n = 3)	0
Fibrosarcoma (n = 9) (6%)	44 (2–68)	4:5	45%	0	33%	22%†	5 (n = 3)	5 (n = 1)
Myxosarcoma (n = 8) (6%)	42 (2–66)	3:5	76%	12%	12%	0	50 (n = 1)	6 (n = 3)
Rhabdomyosarcoma (n = 6) (4%)	14 (0–24)	2:4	33%	17%	50%	0	4 (n = 3)	0
Synovial sarcoma (n = 5) (3%)	39 (30–48)	4:1	40%	0	40%	20%	56 (n = 2)	8 (n = 1)
Liposarcoma (n = 2) (1%)	67 (64,70)	1:1	0	100%	0	0	9 (n = 2)	nd
MPNST (n = 2) (1%)	52 (48,55)	2:0	0	0	50%	50%	nd	nd
Totals (n = 145)	41 (0–88)	80:65	46%	26%	21%	7%	6.6 (n = 67)	10 (n = 13)

* One tumor arose on the anterior leaflet of the mitral valve
† Alternately classified as malignant fibrous tumor of pericardium (see text)
Abbreviations: diff = diffuse; MFH = malignant fibrous histiocytoma; MPNST = malignant peripheral nerve sheath tumor (malignant schwannoma); nd = no data; vent = ventricles

is often possible. Cardiac transplantation has been attempted in primary cardiac sarcomas that have been localized to the heart.[91]

Angiosarcoma

The largest group of differentiated cardiac sarcomas is comprised by angiosarcoma.[92–96] Unlike all other types of cardiac sarcoma, there is a marked right-sided predominance; 90% of angiosarcomas arise in the right atrium, typically with infiltration of the pericardium. There has been no documented relationship between cardiac angiosarcoma and occupational or toxic exposure. Most cardiac angiosarcomas metastasize to the lungs, and approximately 30% show pulmonary metastases on chest radiograph at the time of diagnosis. Other sites of metastases include bone, liver, adrenal gland, and spleen.

The histologic appearance is similar to extracardiac angiosarcomas (Fig. 12–16). Typically, there are anastomosing endothelial-lined spaces formed by atypical cells that may form papillary structures. Approximately 25% of cardiac angiosarcomas have a prominent spindled cell component; in these tumors, the finding of intracytoplasmic lumina containing red blood cells is a helpful diagnostic feature. Immunohistochemical studies to demonstrate endothelial differentiation are only occasionally useful. Factor VIII-related antigen demonstrates fine granular positivity in those cases that are relatively well differentiated; CD34 lacks specificity for vascular markers; Ulex europaeus is insensitive as a marker for angiosarcoma; CD21 holds promise as a diagnostic marker but has not been extensively studied at this time. The differential diagnosis includes angiomas with papillary endothelial hyperplasia, which can mimic angio-

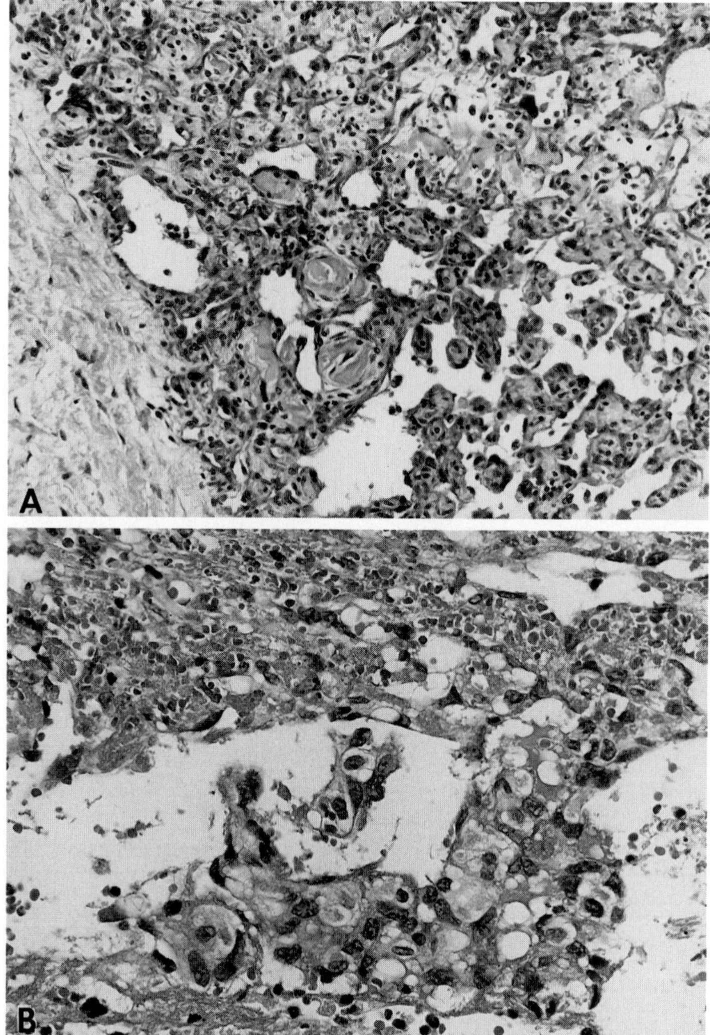

Figure 12–16. Angiosarcoma. When they involve the heart, angiosarcomas are most often right sided and are histologically similar to extracardiac angiosarcomas. *A*. This tumor arose on the epicardial surface of the right ventricle in a 32-year-old man with syncope and pericardial tamponade. (H & E × 150) *B*. Vascular channels can occasionally be difficult to identify in angiosarcoma and the endothelial cells can have abundant cytoplasm similar to epithelial malignancies. (H & E × 300)

sarcoma. In contrast to angiosarcoma, angioma with endothelial hyperplasia will contain areas that are clearly benign.

Rhabdomyosarcoma

Sarcomas with striated muscle differentiation comprise fewer than 10% of cardiac sarcomas in recent series, and are often found in younger adults.[97–102] Unlike sarcomas with fibrous differentiation, there is no predilection for the left atrium. All cardiac rhabdomyosarcomas have been of the embryonal variety, and small round cell areas are typical. The diagnosis requires the identification of rhabdomyoblasts or strap cells, which contain abundant glycogen and express desmin and myoglobin (Fig. 12–17).

Malignant fibrous histiocytoma (MFH)

The relative proportion of cardiac sarcomas diagnosed as MFH has increased in recent years, reflecting changes in the classification of soft tissue sarcomas. The majority of cardiac MFH arise in the left atrium.[103–109] This feature sometimes leads to the erroneous clinical diagnosis of myxoma.[108] There is no male or female predominance. Metastatic sites include lungs, bone, kidney, and pleura. The histologic appearance is similar to MFH in other sites (Fig. 12–18), and myxoid areas are common, occasionally leading to the histologic misdiagnosis of cardiac myxoma. Immunohistochemical findings are nonspecific, and demonstrate diffuse positivity for actin and vimentin; stains for desmin, myoglobin, and neural markers are

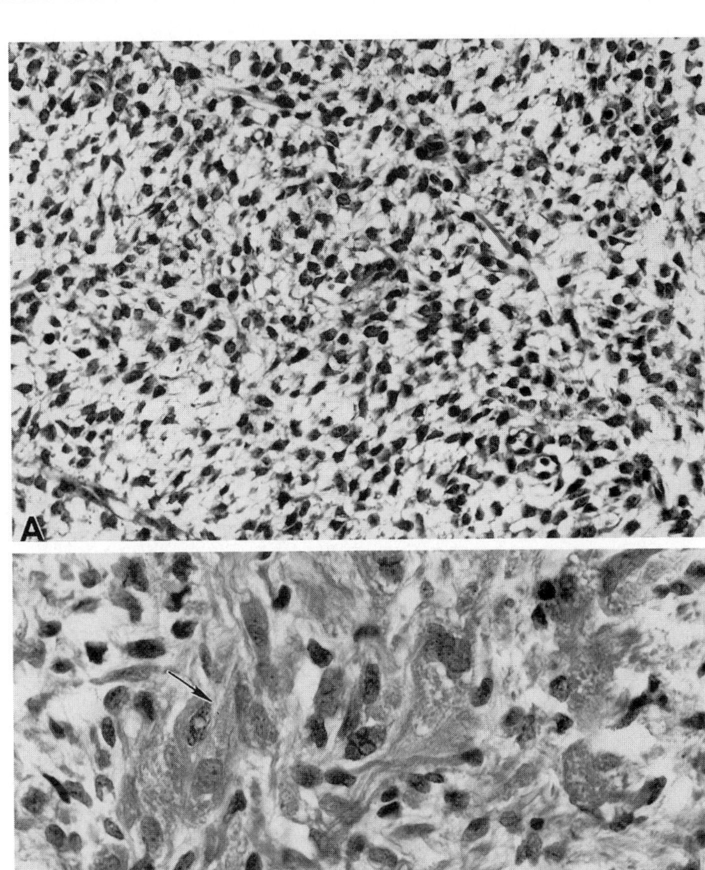

Figure 12–17. Rhabdomyosarcoma. *A.* In this field, the sarcoma appears undifferentiated. The diagnosis depends on detection of rhabdomyoblasts. The patient was an 18-year-old man with dyspnea; the tumor extended from the right ventricle to the right atrium. (H & E × 300) *B.* In this field, rhabdomyoblasts are identified on the basis of cross-striations noted on routine stains. More commonly, immunohistochemical techniques identifying cells that express muscle antigens (myoglobin, desmin) are required for diagnosis. (H & E × 396)

negative. Cytokeratin may rarely show focal positivity.

"Myxosarcoma"

The term *myxosarcoma* is best replaced by the more general term *myxoid sarcoma,* despite its continued use for certain types of cardiac sarcomas.[110,111] At least 10% of cardiac sarcomas, usually occurring in the left atrium, have extensively myxoid areas throughout the tumor, and are clinically, grossly, and microscopically confused with myxoma (Fig. 12–19).[112] We do not believe they represent malignant cardiac myxomas, because there are few if any reliable examples of tumors demonstrating a transition from myxoma to sarcoma. Myxoid sarcomas are composed of spindled or stellate mesenchymal cells that do not form the structures characteristic of myxoma, and do not have the extensive hemosiderin deposition throughout the lesion typical of myxoma. Calcification, fibrosis, and organized thrombus, which are often present in myxoma, are not seen in myxoid sarcomas. With extensive tumor sampling, histologic features characteristic of fibrosarcoma, MFH, rhabdomyosarcoma, or osteosarcoma are generally found in myxoid sarcomas of the heart.

Osteosarcoma

Three to 10% of primary cardiac sarcomas have areas indistinguishable from osteosarcoma of bone (Fig. 12–20).[113–119] Osteoid is usually not present throughout the tumor, and many cardiac osteosarcomas show areas of fibrosarcoma, malignant fibrous histiocytoma, or chondrosarcoma. Rare examples are predominantly

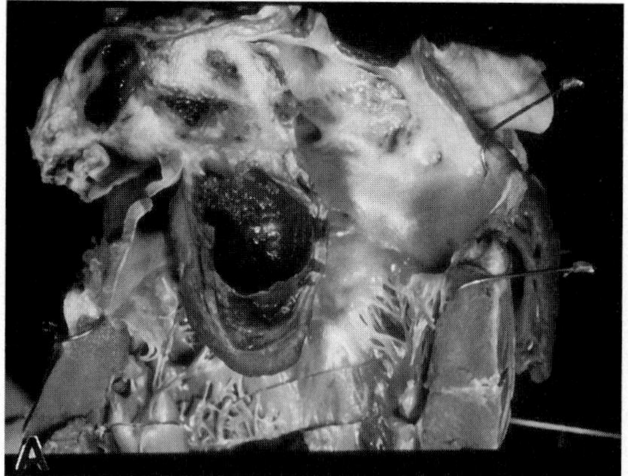

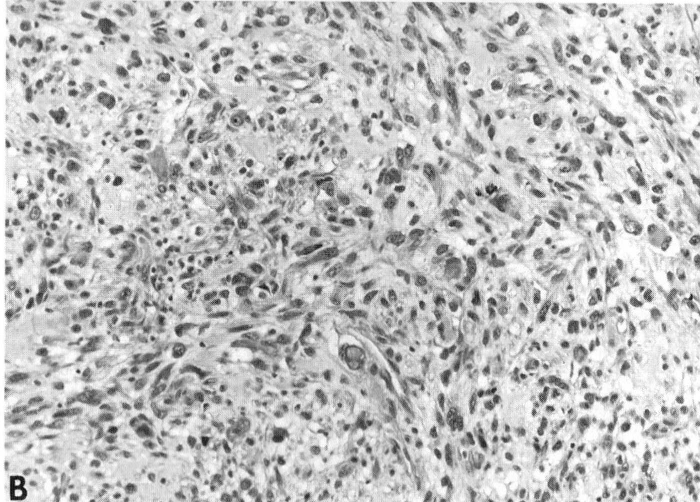

Figure 12–18. Malignant fibrous histiocytoma. *A*. The majority of cardiac sarcomas of fibrohistiocytic differentiation occur in the left atrium. This tumor was clinically diagnosed as myxoma; at autopsy there was an infiltrative left atrial mass covered by laminated thrombus obstructing the mitral valve. *B*. Histologically, there is a "storiform" pattern of malignant fibroblasts and histiocytic cells. The patient was a 63-year-old woman. (H & E × 150)

chondrosarcoma, and have been reported in the literature as such.[120] Like malignant fibrous histiocytoma, osteosarcoma arises almost exclusively in the left atrium, and can therefore be clinically confused with myxoma, as well as at histologic examination, due to extensive myxoid areas.[120] Metastases occur frequently and are occasionally noted before the primary is found in the heart. Sites of metastasis include lung, skin, lymph, nodes, and thyroid.

Synovial Sarcoma

Synovial sarcomas account for fewer than 1% of cardiac sarcomas.[121–123] Their histologic appearance is similar to synovial sarcoma of soft tissue. The diagnosis rests on the demonstration of biphasic growth, lack of gross features of malignant mesothelioma, and, if possible, demonstration of cytogenetic translocations of X-18, which is considered specific for synovial sarcoma.[121]

Liposarcoma

Liposarcomas are extremely rare in the heart[124–129]; several reports of myxoid cardiac liposarcoma are likely undifferentiated sarcomas or malignant fibrous histiocytoma with intracytoplasmic fat droplets. The histologic differential diagnosis includes lipomatous hypertrophy of the interatrial septum and pleomorphic MFH. Although MFH may contain intracytoplasmic fat, as may a variety of sarcomas, lipoblasts are absent. Lipomatous hypertrophy may be confused with liposarcoma, because it infiltrates surrounding structures and contains bizarre myocytes and brown fat cells that may be confused with malignant cells. Liposarcomas, which are much rarer than lipomatous hypertrophy, lack hypertrophied myocytes within the tumor, and contain lipoblasts (Fig. 12–21). Lipoblasts are distinguished from brown fat by the recognition of large, irregular, hyperchromatic nuclei that are indented by fat globules that vary in size and shape. Unlike lipomatous hyper-

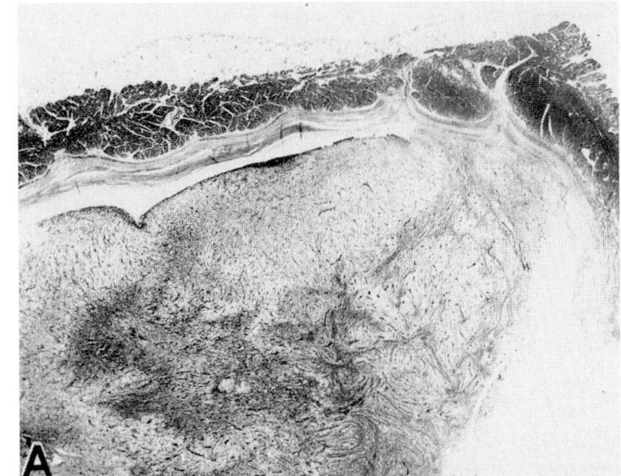

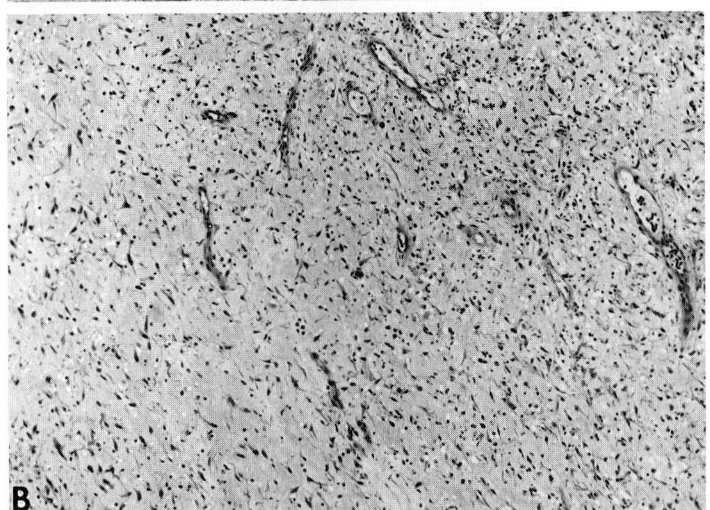

Figure 12–19. "Myxosarcoma." Left atrial sarcomas are occasionally myxoid, fill the lumen of the atrium, and are clinically and pathologically confused with myxomas. *A*. The tumor was in the left atrium of a 55-year-old woman. The majority of the lesion was luminal, reminiscent of sarcomas of the aorta arising in the intima. (H & E × 10) *B*. A higher magnification demonstrates spindle cell proliferation with a prominent myxoid background; strucutres typical of myxoma are absent, however. (H & E × 75) The patient developed multiple recurrences and eventually died of widespread metastases.

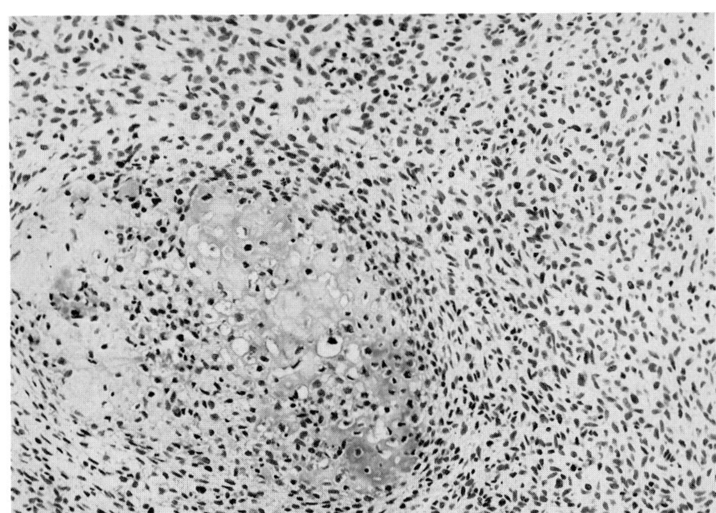

Figure 12–20. Osteosarcoma. Cardiac sarcomas with osteosarcomatous differentiation occur almost exclusively in the left atrium and pathologically resemble skeletal osteosarcomas. The patient was a 16-year-old man with congestive heart failure and a left atrial mass that recurred postoperatively at the suture site. (H & E × 150)

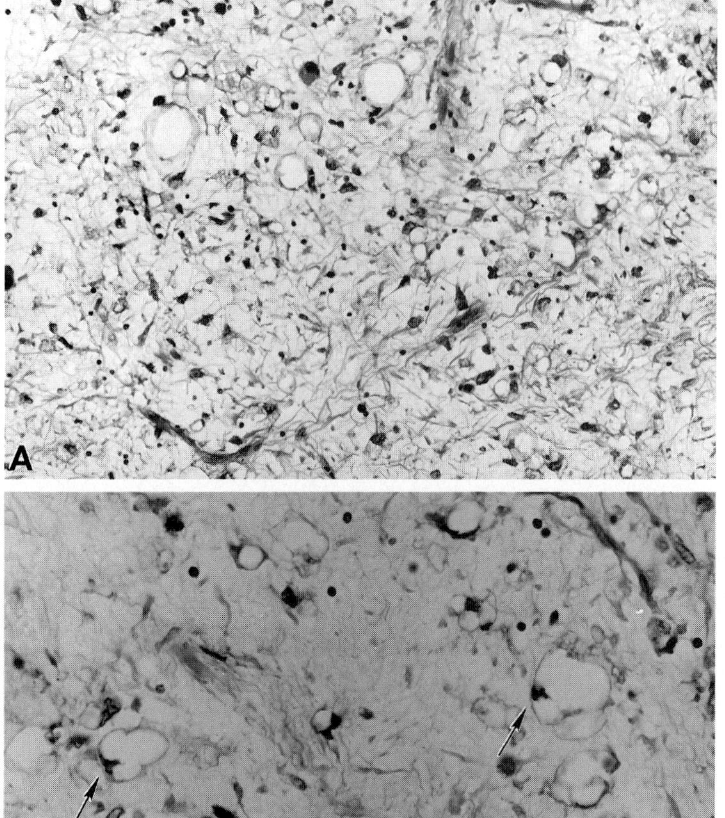

Figure 12–21. Liposarcoma. *A.* There are scattered atypical fat cell with the features of malignant lipoblasts. The tumor was removed from the infundibulum and pulmonary valve of a 60-year-old man with cough and dyspnea. (H & E × 150) *B.* A higher magification demonstrates malignant lipoblasts, which are defined by their irregular, hyperchromatic nuclei that are indented by cytoplasmic fat globules (*arrows*). (H & E × 300)

trophy, liposarcomas of the heart generally contain mitotic figures.

Fibrosarcoma

Only rare cardiac sarcomas are diagnosed as fibrosarcoma,[130, 131] likely because of a recent increase in the use of the term MFH, and the use of myxosarcoma for the myxoid variety of fibrosarcoma (Fig. 12–22). The left atrium is the most common site of cardiac fibrosarcoma. Metastases do not occur so early or so frequently as undifferentiated sarcomas, osteosarcoma or MFH, possibly because fibrosarcomas are generally lower grade tumors.

Leiomyosarcoma

Leiomyosarcomas make up to 10% of cardiac sarcomas; most are located in the left atrium.[132–135] Some examples most likely represent extensions from primary sarcomas of the pulmonary veins or venae cavae. The histologic diagnosis of leiomyosarcoma rests on the presence of intracytoplasmic glycogen, perinuclear vacuoles, blunt-end nuclei, fascicular growth at right angles, and cytoplasmic fuchsinophilia. These features are not always present, and the distinction between pleomorphic leiomyosarcoma and MFH cannot always be made. Immunohistochemical demonstration of desmin, which is quite specific for the diagnosis, is unfortunately not sensitive.

Undifferentiated Sarcoma

Approximately 10% of cardiac sarcomas do not demonstrate histologic features diagnostic of any one subtype. These are often small round

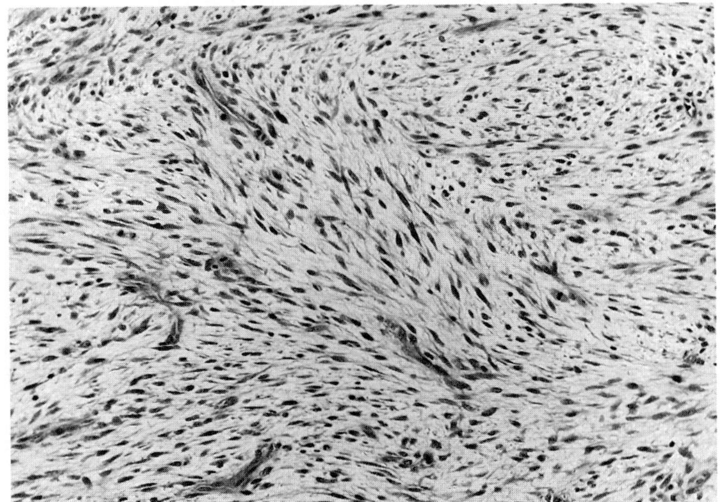

Figure 12–22. Fibrosarcoma, myxoid type. There is a relatively uniform population of spindle cells with mild pleomorphism and occasional mitotic figures. Note the lack of resemblance to myxoma, despite the myxoid background. (H & E × 150)

cell tumors (Fig. 12–23), or pleomorphic sarcomas. The relative proportion of this category depends largely on the degree of strictness with which diagnostic criteria are applied; undifferentiated pleomorphic sarcomas are often designated as MFH.

Neurofibrosarcoma

Although distinctly rare, there are documented cardiac sarcomas with neurofibrosarcomatous differentiation, as documented by immunoreactivity for S-100 protein or other neural markers.[136] We have seen an example of primary cardiac neurofibrosarcoma with rhabdomyosarcomatous differentiation, or so-called "Triton" tumor.

Kaposi's Sarcoma

Kaposi's sarcoma of the heart was extremely rare before the AIDS epidemic.[137] In cases of AIDS, cardiac involvement of Kaposi's sarcoma occurs in about 5% of autopsy cases.[138] It is unresolved whether Kaposi's sarcoma is a true neoplasm or expression of an opportunistic infection. When there is cardiac involvement, Kaposi's sarcoma usually involves the epicardium and pericardium and less frequently the myocardium and coronary arteries. Cardiac Kaposi's sarcoma in AIDS is usually a part of a widely disseminated process and usually does not cause significant clinical symptoms. However, there have been several reports of fatal cardiac tamponade secondary to epicardial Kaposi's sarcoma.

Malignant Mesenchymoma

There are rare reports of cardiac sarcomas with two or more cell types (in addition to fibrohistiocytic); these tumors are designated "malignant mesenchymoma." These tumors contain combinations of two or three of the following: osteosarcoma/chondrosarcoma, rhabdomyosarcoma, angiosarcoma, and liposarcoma, and typically occur in the left atrium or mitral valve.

Cardiac Lymphomas

Incidence and Clinical Findings

Cardiac involvement is relatively common in patients with widespread malignant lymphoma, and generally imparts a grave prognosis. In autopsy series, lymphoma is the second most common type of metastatic malignancy to the heart.[139] However, primary cardiac lymphoma without evidence of extracardiac disease is quite rare. As recently as 1989, only 15 cases had been reported in the literature.[140] The presenting symptoms vary according to the site in the heart, and may be related to conduction system disturbances, pericardial fluid accumulation, valvular obstruction, and congestive heart failure.

The incidence of cardiac lymphoma has increased since the advent of iatrogenic immunosuppression in transplant patients as well as the acquired immune deficiency syndrome; there have been approximately 30 reports of cardiac lymphoma in patients with allografts or AIDS.[141–149] These lymphomas often progress through a histologically benign polymorphous proliferation resulting in a clonal expansion of

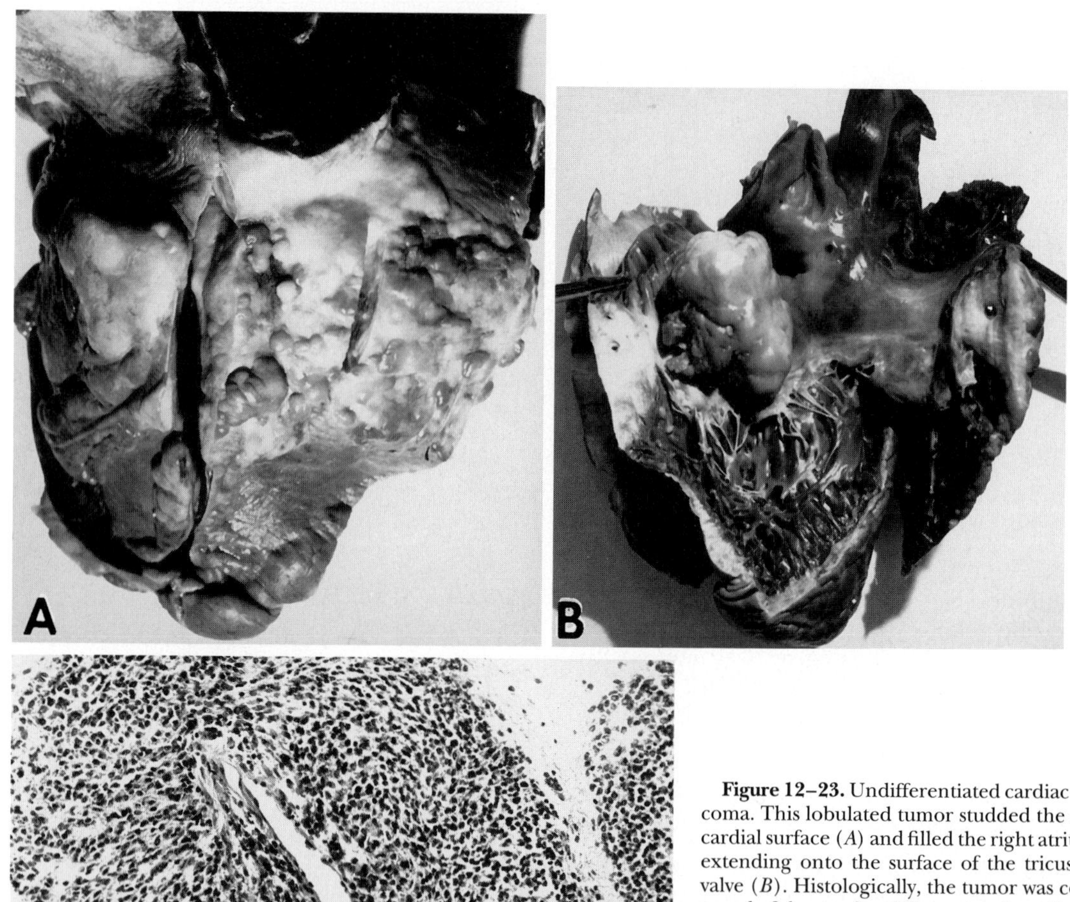

Figure 12–23. Undifferentiated cardiac sarcoma. This lobulated tumor studded the epicardial surface (*A*) and filled the right atrium, extending onto the surface of the tricuspid valve (*B*). Histologically, the tumor was composed of sheets of undifferentiated small cells (*C*) with a perivascular arrangement to the tumor cells. Immunohistochemical stains were compatible with mesenchymal cells; lymphoid and epithelial markers were negative (not shown).

B cells[140–153]; Epstein–Barr virus is implicated in the majority of these cases.[152–153] Lymphomas that arise in immunocompromised patients generally involve extranodal sites such as the liver, the gastrointestinal tract, central nervous system, as well as the heart. Because of the propensity of lymphomas in AIDS patients to involve the pleural and pericardial surfaces, the term AIDS-related body-cavity-based lymphomas has been used.

Although cardiac involvement by lymphoma is usually rapidly fatal, there have been reports of successful treatment of cardiac lymphoma.[154] Early diagnosis with accurate imaging has been emphasized as important in the successful long-term outcome of patients with cardiac lymphoma. Especially in immunocompetent individuals, treatment with chemotherapeutic regimens designed for nodal lymphomas can result in a reduction of tumor mass and a dramatic improvement of cardiac symptoms.

Pathologic Findings

The diagnosis of primary cardiac lymphoma is generally made at autopsy. There are rare reports of surgical excision.[1] In cases of epicardial involvement in patients with mediastinal lymphoma, pericardial fluid cytology may be diagnostic (see Chapter 11).

Lymphomas can involve all areas of the heart, including epicardium, pericardium, ventricles, atria and, rarely, cardiac valves. Rarely, cardiac lymphoma can be localized to one or more coronary arteries, resulting in ischemic symptoms, sudden death, or coronary artery aneurysms. Grossly, cardiac lymphomas are firm whitish masses within the heart that can mimic other infiltrative processes (Fig. 12–24). Sarcoidosis may form well-demarcated, firm, white areas in the myocardium that do not extend into the epicardium or form bulging nodules, typical of lymphoma. The appearance of cardiac lymphoma is somewhat different from the nodular variegated appearance of sarcomas, which are more likely than lymphoma to extend into the cardiac chambers.

Cardiac lymphomas are virtually all of B cell origin.[155–157] A wide variety of histologic patterns have been described, including large cell (Fig. 12–24), nodular small cleaved cell type (poorly differentiated lymphocytic) (Fig. 12–25), large cell immunoblastic, and lymphoplasmacytic types. Cardiac lymphomas form interstitial infiltrates with histologically infiltrating borders.

The differential diagnosis of well differentiated lymphocytic lymphoma is benign lymphoid proliferations. In immunocompromised patients and allograft hearts, lymphoproliferative disorders that are precursors to lymphomas may be associated with myocyte necrosis and giant cells (Fig. 12–26). These proliferations may be difficult to distinguish from severe rejection, are generally polymorphous with a mixed cell infiltrate, and may regress with lowering doses of immunosuppressive agents. Flow cytometric analysis and immunohistochemical stains for light chain restriction may be helpful in these cases in making the distinction between benign lymphoid proliferation and lymphoma, which tend to be more monomorphous. The differential diagnosis of large cell lymphoma includes round cell sarcomas primary in the myocardium, metastatic undifferentiated carcinomas, and metastatic melanoma. Immunohistochemical stains for lymphoid markers, intermediate filaments, epithelial markers, S-100 protein, and melanoma specific antigens are occasionally necessary for the complete evaluation of an undifferentiated malignancy.

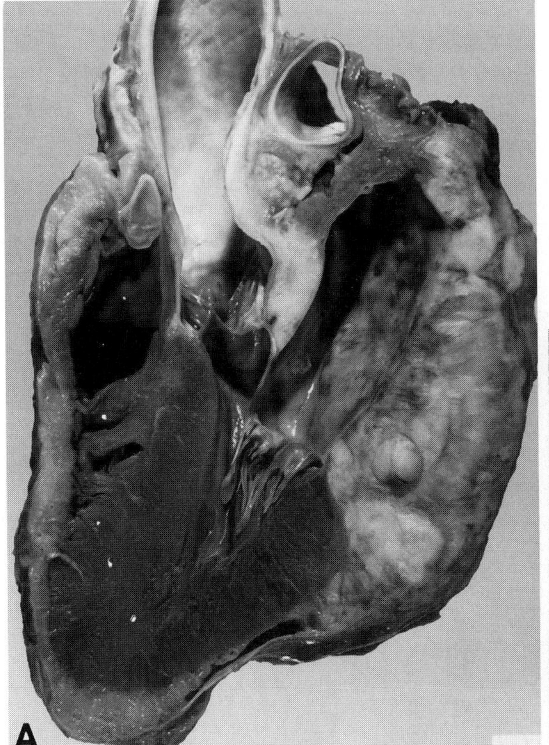

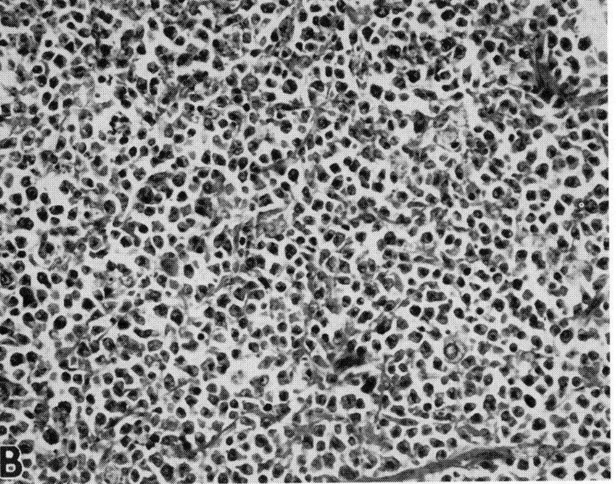

Figure 12–24. Cardiac lymphoma. *A.* This photograph demonstrates the autopsy heart of patient who expired from complications of cardiac lymphoma that was largely confined to the myocardium. Histologic sections (not shown) demonstrated a large cell lymphoma. *B.* Histologic sections of large cell lymphoma diagnosed by open bipsy in an immunocompetent patient with an asymptomatic cardiac mass; phenotyping demonstrated a B-cell lesion.

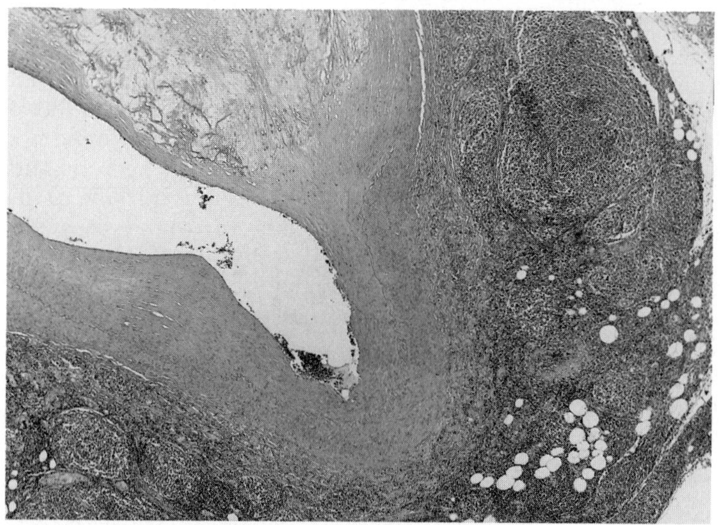

Figure 12–25. Cardiac lymphoma. A 66-year-old man died suddenly; at autopsy, the left anterior descending coronary artery showed a nodular adventitial infltrate of lymphoid cells that was classified as nodular small-cleaved follicular center-cell lymphoma. No lymph node involvement was present at autopsy. (H & E × 30)

Metastatic Cardiac Tumors

Incidence

In a recent review, cardiac metastases were present in 12% of autopsies performed for widespread malignancy.[139] Malignancies that involve the heart secondarily are, in order of incidence, carcinomas of the lung, lymphomas, carcinomas of the breast, leukemia, carcinomas of the stomach, malignant melanoma, hepatocellular carcinoma, and carcinomas of the colon (Table 12–5). The rate of cardiac involvement by metastatic disease has not appeared to change over a 14-year period, indicating that treatment may not have a significant effect on the rate of metastatic malignancy to the heart. The following tumors have an especially high rate of cardiac metastasis if the incidence of the primary tumor is considered: leukemia, melanoma, thyroid carcinoma, extracardiac sarcomas, lymphomas, renal cell carcinomas, carcinomas of the lung, and carcinomas of the breast. These tumors all had a greater than 15% rate of cardiac metastasis in a large autopsy study.[7, 158]

Clinical Findings

The clinical manifestations of cardiac metastasis are, on the whole, similar to those of primary cardiac sarcomas. The site of tumor within

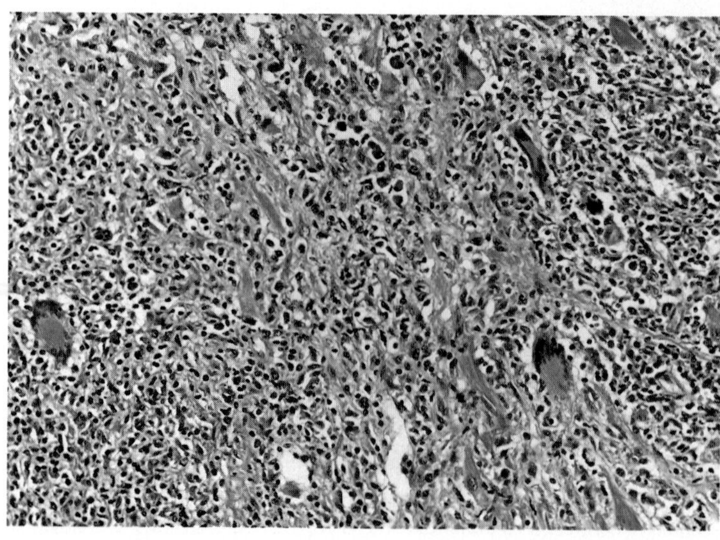

Figure 12–26. Cardiac immunoproliferative disorder. Lymphoid proliferations in immunosuppressed patients are polyclonal B-cell proliferations. This patient, who died of AIDS, had widespread infiltrates in the heart. The interspersed histiocytic giant cells are an unusual feature in this case. The proliferation was polyclonal and typed as a B-cell proliferation. (H & E × 150)

Table 12–5. Tumors Metastatic to the Heart at Autopsy

Primary Tumor	Total Autopsies	Heart* Involvement	Pericardial Involvement†	Total (%)
Melanoma	69	32 (46%)	2 (3%)	34 (49%)
Malignant germ cell tumor	21	8 (38%)	1 (5%)	9 (42%)
Leukemia	202	66 (33%)	2 (1%)	68 (34%)
Carcinoma of lung	1037	180 (17%)	112 (11%)	292 (28%)
Sarcoma	159	24 (15%)	11 (7%)	35 (22%)
Lymphoma	392	67 (17%)	15 (4%)	82 (21%)
Carcinoma of breast	685	70 (10%)	69 (10%)	139 (20%)
Carcinoma of esophagus	294	37 (13%)	13 (4%)	50 (17%)
Carcinoma of kidney	114	12 (11%)	5 (4%)	17 (15%)
Carcinoma of oral cavity + tongue	235	22 (9%)	2 (1%)	24 (10%)
Carcinoma of larynx	100	9 (9%)	2 (2%)	11 (11%)
Carcinoma of thyroid	97	9 (9%)	3 (3%)	12 (12%)
Carcinoma of uterus	451	36 (8%)	5 (1%)	41 (9%)
Carcinoma of stomach	603	28 (5%)	16 (3%)	44 (7%)
Carcinoma of colon and rectum	440	22 (5%)	3 (1%)	25 (6%)
Carcinoma of pharynx	67	1	2	3 (4.5%)
Carcinoma of urinary bladder	128	8 (6%)	0	8 (6%)
Carcinoma of ovary	188	2 (1%)	6 (3%)	8 (4%)
Carcinoma of prostate	171	6 (4%)	0	6 (4%)
Carcinoma of nasal cavity	32	1	0	1 (3%)
Carcinoma of pancreas	185	6 (3%)	0	6 (3%)
Carcinoma liver and biliary tract	325	7 (2%)	0	7 (2%)
Totals‡	6240	654 (10%)	299 (5%)	953 (15%)

* Tumors with pericardial and myocardial involvement
† Bulk of tumor localized to pericardium
‡ Including uncommon tumors not included in table
From McAllister HA, Fenoglio JJ. Tumors of the cardiovascular system. Washington, DC: Fascicles of the Armed Forces Institute of Pathology. 1977, with permission.
From Mykai K, Shinkai T, Tominaga K, Shimosato Y. The incidence of secondary tumors of the heart and pericardium: A 10-year study. Jpn J Clin Oncol 18:195–201, 1988, with permission.

the heart greatly affects the symptoms that the patient will develop. These include pericardial effusions if there is pericardial involvement, arrhythmias if there is involvement of the conduction system, congestive heart failure if ventricular involvement results in decreased contractility or if there is obstruction of the mitral valve, syncope if there is obstruction of the aortic valve, and right-sided heart failure if there is involvement of the right heart and tricuspid valves.

Currently, it is accepted practice to surgically remove metastatic deposits of relatively indolent tumors in order to improve cardiac function. In a recent series of 133 surgically resected cardiac tumors, 19 were metastatic to the heart.[3] The majority of these were metastatic sarcomas and adenocarcinomas. Although long-term prognosis is poor in these patients, it is possible to temporarily improve cardiac function and quality of life by surgical excision.

Tumor Spread and Tumor Types

Malignancies spread to the heart by four paths: direct extension, usually from mediastinal tumor; hematogenous spread; lymphatic spread; and intracavitary extension from the inferior vena cava, or rarely the pulmonary veins. There may be a combination of more than one of these routes. Lymphatic spread is generally accompanied by tumor enlargement of pulmonary hilar or mediastinal lymph nodes, and histologic evidence of pericardial lymphatic infiltration is present. Hematogenous spread is characterized by myocardial metastatic tumors.

Although there are exceptions, epithelial malignancies typically spread to the heart by lymphatics. Melanoma, sarcomas, leukemia, and renal cell carcinoma metastasize to the heart by a hematogenous route. Lymphomas may involve the heart by virtually any path, including direct extension, hematogenous seeding, or lymphatic spread. Melanomas, renal tumors, including Wilms' tumor and renal cell carcinoma, adrenal tumors, liver tumors, and uterine tumors are the most frequent intracavitary tumors.

In general, metastatic cardiac tumors affect the right side of the heart in 20–30% of cases, the left side in 10–33% of cases, bilateral or diffuse involvement in approximately 30–35% of cases, and the endocardium or chamber cavities in 5% of cases.[158] It is extremely uncommon for cardiac metastases to be isolated lesions.

The most common epithelial malignancies to metastasize to the heart are carcinomas of the breast and lung. In most cases there is pericardial involvement with superficial myocardial infiltration. The valves and endocardium are usually spared by metastatic carcinoma.

Leukemic and lymphomatous infiltrates are typically widespread when they occur in the heart, involving the epicardium and myocardium by diffuse infiltrates. The epicardium is involved in 61%, the left ventricle in 55%, and the right atrium in 54% of cases. In cases of melanoma metastatic to the heart, the myocardium is involved in virtually 100% of cases, and there is less frequent infiltration of epi- and endocardium. The four chambers of the heart are involved with approximately equal frequency. Sarcomatous deposits are found within the myocardium (50%), pericardium (33%), or both myocardium and pericardium (17% of cases). Valvular metastases are uncommon.[159] Osteosarcoma, liposarcoma, leiomyosarcoma, unclassifiable sarcomas, rhabdomyosarcoma, neurofibrosarcoma, synovial sarcoma, and MFH have been reported to involve the heart secondarily.

Pathologic Findings

Gross Appearance

Metastatic deposits may be diffuse, multinodular, or consist of a single dominant mass (Fig. 12–27). There may be diffuse studding and thickening of the pericardial surfaces with little infiltration of the heart. This pattern generally occurs in carcinomatous metastases and can grossly be confused with mesothelioma, or benign fibrosing pericarditis (see Chapter 11). Mediastinal lymph nodes are involved in approximately 80% of cases of cardiac metastases, especially if there is pericardial involvement. The presence of melanotic pigment is suggestive of metastatic melanoma (Fig. 12–28). The tumor burden in the heart is the highest with melanoma, as compared with any other malignancy.

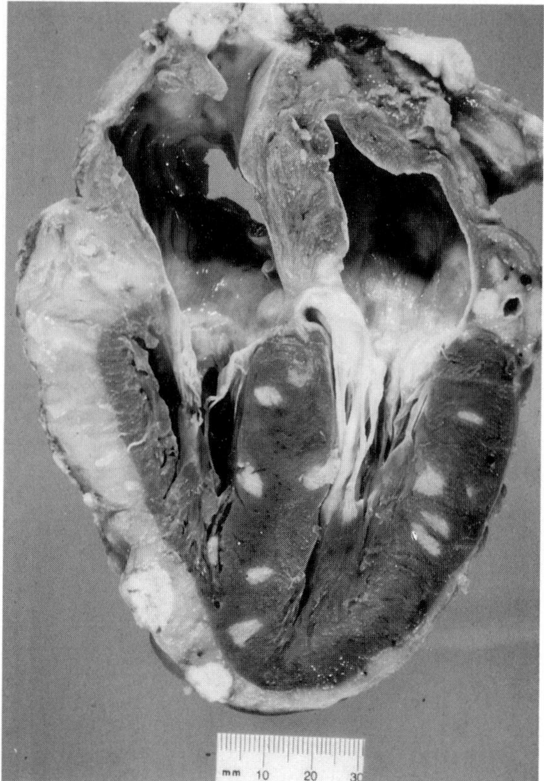

Figure 12–27. Metastatic carcinoma, heart. There are multiple white, focally necrotic masses studding the left ventricle, ventricular septum, and epicardial fat. The patient was a 55-year-old man who died of widespread carcinoma of the lung.

Histologic Findings

The histologic appearance of metastatic tumors to the heart are similar to those of the corresponding primary tumor. Carcinomatous spread in the myocardium is frequently most prominent in subepicardial lymphatics, whereas melanomas, sarcomas, renal cell carci-

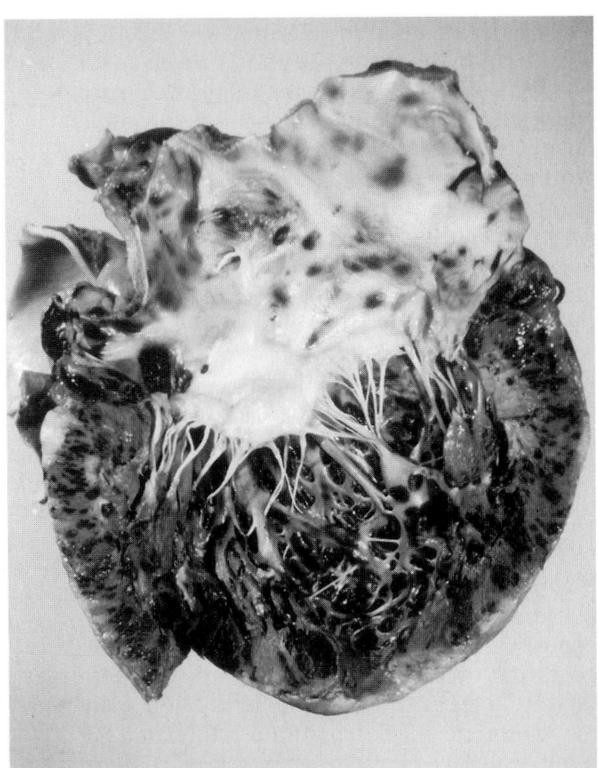

Figure 12–28. Metastatic melanoma, heart. Patients with metastatic melanoma have the highest autopsy incidence of cardiac metastases, which are often quite bulky. Note the multiple black masses virtually replacing the myocardium.

nomas, and lymphoid neoplasms form intramyocardial interstitial tumors. A spindle cell neoplasm of the heart may resemble a primary sarcoma, but with appropriate immunohistochemical stains, these may prove to be epithelial neoplasms metastatic from a remote site.

A histopathologic distinction between primary and metastatic sarcoma may be impossible upon surgical resection of a cardiac tumor. Most sarcomas metastatic to the heart cause symptoms at their primary site before cardiac symptoms are evident.[159] Even though primary sarcomas of the heart are rare, extracardiac sarcomas presenting as cardiac metastases are even rarer.

TUMORS OF ARTERIES AND VEINS

Arterial Neoplasms

Aortic Intimal Sarcomas

Definition

Aortic intimal sarcomas are predominantly luminal neoplasms that are believed to be derived from the aortic intima. The normal aortic intima is composed of endothelial cells and smooth muscle cells. Aortic sarcomas that are derived from intima can differentiate along endothelial, smooth muscle cell, and a variety of other mesenchymal cell types.

Incidence

Primary tumors of the aorta are uncommon. There are fewer than 100 cases of aortic sarcoma reported in the literature.[160–162]

Clinical

Most patients with sarcomas of the aorta are middle aged; in a recent series the mean age was 62 years.[160] There is no sex predilection.[160–162] The most common symptoms are related to embolic phenomena,[163–164] with pain and absent pulses, usually to the lower extremities. Other modes of presentation include back pain, and sequelae of occlusion of the mesenteric vessels, rupture of aneurysm formed by the tumor, and malignant hypertension.[165–169] Most aortic sarcomas occur in the abdominal aorta between the celiac artery to the iliac bifurcation; less often, the descending thoracic aorta is involved. There have been several cases reported of aortic sarcomas arising at the site of a synthetic aortic graft anastomosis.[160, 170] It is not rare for the initial diagnosis to be made on the base of embolectomy material, grossly considered by the surgeon to be a thrombus or myxoma embolus.[164] Treatment is synthetic graft replacement after resection of tumor and segment of the aorta; occasionally, the surgical diagnosis is atherosclerotic aneurysm, and the diagnosis of malignancy is made first at histologic examination. The prognosis of intimal sarcomas of the aorta is generally poor, with death resulting from metastatic disease to various sites including bones, peritoneum, liver, and mesenteric lymph nodes. There are notable exceptions, however, of patients with years of symptom-free follow-up.

Pathologic Findings

Intimal aortic sarcomas are usually poorly differentiated sarcomas of fibroblastic or myofibroblastic differentiation. These sarcomas are composed of mitotically active spindle cells with varying degrees of atypia, necrosis, and pleomorphism; the portion of tumor underlying the luminal surface is often composed of dense fibrous tissue and spindle cells that do not appear malignant or atypical. There can be an epithelioid appearance to tumor cells and a mixture of pleomorphic fibro- and histiocytic cells resembling malignant fibrous histiocytoma (Fig. 12–29).[164]

Approximately 10% of aortic sarcomas demonstrate histologic and immunohistochemical features of angiosarcoma or leiomyosarcoma. We have encountered several epithelioid angiosarcomas arising in the aortic intima; these tumors may coexpress endothelial markers and cytokeratin. The intimal surface of the aorta adjacent to intimal angiosarcomas can demonstrate a lining of atypical cells that has been termed "dysplasia" (Fig. 12–29).[171] Rare examples of aortic intimal sarcomas with osteosarcomatous and chondrosarcomatous differentiation (myxoid chondrosarcomas) have been reported. Embolic deposits of aortic myxoid chondrosarcomas may resemble cardiac myxoma histologically.

Other Aortic Neoplasms

Benign tumors of the aorta are exceedingly rare. We have seen a few examples of benign fibrous histiocytomas and inflammatory pseudotumors of the aortas in young adults and children. These tumors are attached to the aortic adventitia rather than occurring in the lumen, are cured by resection, and usually occur in the proximal aorta.

Sarcomas of Systemic Arteries Other than the Aorta

Muscular arteries can rarely give rise to neoplasms; most of these have been reported as leiomyosarcomas.[172]

Sarcomas of the Pulmonary Artery

Incidence and Terminology

Approximately 75 primary sarcomas of the pulmonary artery have been reported.[160, 161, 173–183] There are several similarities between pulmonary sarcomas and aortic sarcomas: Most pulmonary artery sarcomas are predominantly luminal, present as thromboemboli, and are histologically undifferentiated. It has been recommended that the term intimal sarcoma, as has been applied to aortic sarcomas, be used for pulmonary artery sarcomas as well.[160]

Clinical

Because of the rarity of pulmonary artery sarcomas, it is not uncommon that the histologic diagnosis is made only after a prolonged course of anticoagulants[181] for the presumed clinical diagnosis of pulmonary emboli. Another mode of presentation for pulmonary artery sarcoma is sudden death.[160] Reviews of pulmonary artery sarcomas have shown no sex predilection, despite a male predominance in two large series.[160, 161] Although sarcomas of the pulmonary artery only rarely occur in children,[176] the mean age at presentation (41 years) is younger than that of aortic (62 years) or caval sarcomas (50 years).[160]

Sarcomas of the pulmonary artery are less likely to metastasize to distant sites than are their counterparts in the aorta. However, metastases to the kidney, brain, lymph nodes, and skin have been reported. A clinical course of over 2 years without metastases or treatment is common, but most patients are dead 5 years after diagnosis.[179] Although patients that are operated do better than those without curative procedures, there is no good evidence at this time that chemo- or radiation therapy benefits patients with sarcomas of the pulmonary artery.

Pathology

Grossly, the typical sarcoma of the pulmonary artery distends and fills a proximal pulmonary

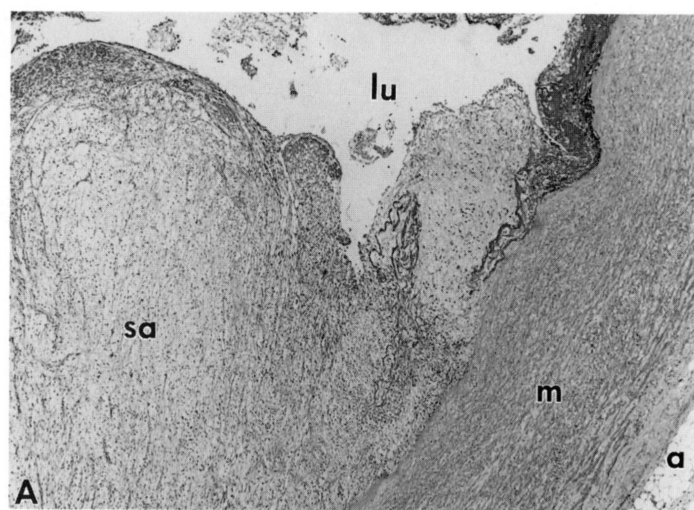

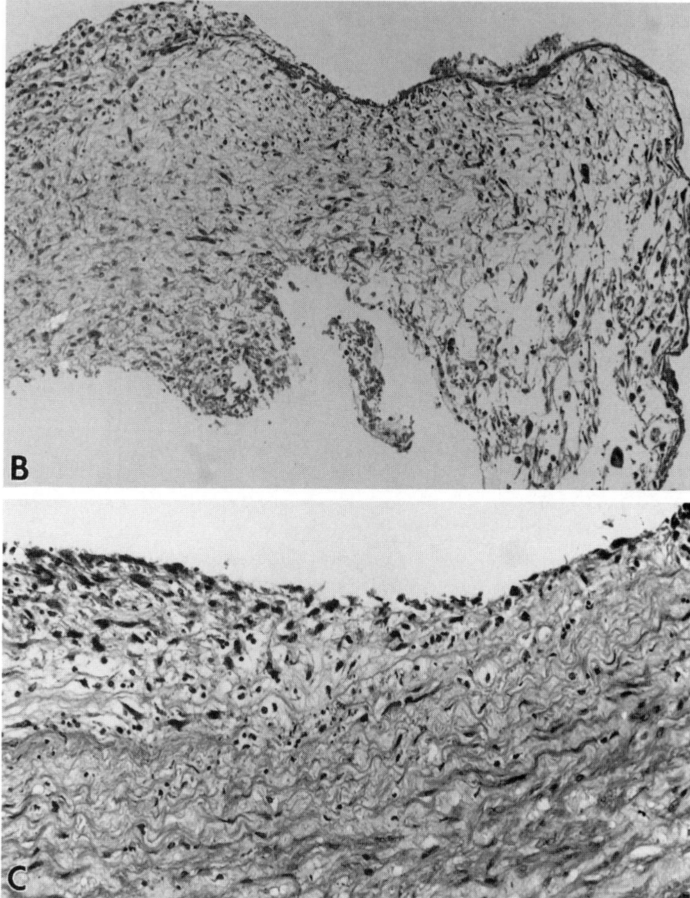

Figure 12–29. Intimal sarcoma, aorta. *A.* In this example, there are atypical myofibroblastic cells with focal myxoid and fibrous background. The patient was a 64-year-old man with mesenteric artery occlusion. (H & E × 150) (sa = sarcoma, *m* = aortic media, *a* = adventitia, *lu* = aortic lumen) *B.* Intimal sarcoma, aorta. Luminal fragments of aortic sarcomas can embolize and be clinically mistaken for clots. Portion of same tumor illustrated in Figure 12–29*A.* (H & E × 150) *C.* Intimal sarcoma, aorta. At the interface between the sarcoma and the uninvolved aorta, there is often a region of atypical cells that either represents lateral tumor growth or *in situ* malignancy, so-called dysplasia. (H & E × 150)

artery or the pulmonary trunk, extending distally within the lumens of the arterial tree and occasionally infiltrating the pulmonary parenchyma. The tumor may be firm and gritty, or resemble a mucoid clot. The pulmonary trunk is usually involved, and, for unknown reasons, extension along the right pulmonary artery is more common than the left.

Microscopically, sarcomas of the pulmonary artery resemble those of the aorta (Fig. 12–30*A*). However, the range of histologic appearances is more varied,[183] and they are more often

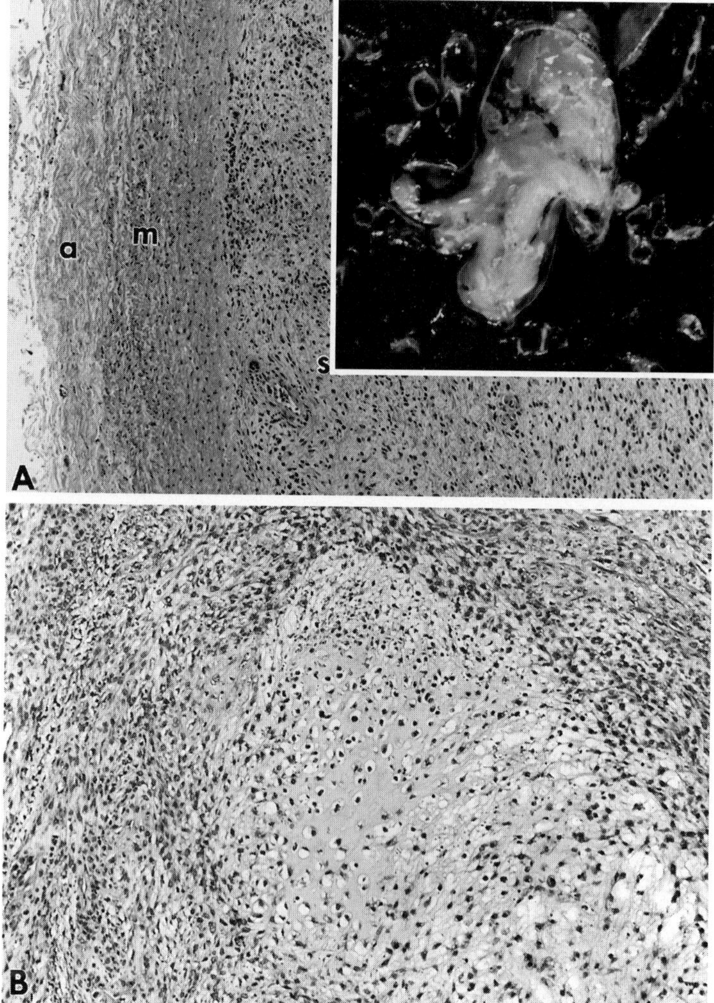

Figure 12–30. Sarcoma, pulmonary artery. *A*. There is a bland proliferation of spindle cells extending from the intimal surface into the lumen of the vessel. The patient was a 47-year-old man with pleuritic chest pain, and a left pulmonary artery tumor that was treated with pneumonectomy. (H & E × 75) (*a* = adventitia; *m* = media, *sa* = sarcoma) The insert demonstrates the gross appearance of the tumor filling the pulmonary artery. *B*. Pulmonary artery sarcomas occasionally have areas of osteosarcoma. The tumor was resected from the lumen as an embolectomy specimen from the left pulmonary artery of a 41-year-old man with recurrent pulmonary emboli. (H & E × 75)

mucoid and contain areas of osteo- or chondrosarcoma (Fig. 12–30*B*). Malignant cell layering over dense collagen is present less often than in aortic sarcomas. Because of the histologic variety, sarcomas of the pulmonary arteries, in contrast to aortic sarcomas, have been given a large number of histologic diagnoses. Although the majority of sarcomas of the pulmonary arteries are undifferentiated "intimal" sarcomas, there have been reports of luminal leiomyosarcomas, rhabdomyosarcomas, angiosarcomas, malignant mesenchymomas, and malignant fibrous histiocytomas.[175, 178, 182] Not all of these reports provided ultrastructural or immunohistochemical documentation of specific differentiation.

Because most sarcomas of the pulmonary arteries involve the pulmonary trunk, it has been hypothesized that they arise from primitive cells of the bulbus cordi.[181] Reports of immunohistochemistry are few,[160, 181, 183] and generally demonstrate positivity for vimentin, smooth muscle, and muscle-specific actin. There are nonspecific staining patterns compatible with myofibroblastic origin.

Neoplasms of Veins

Sarcomas of the Inferior Vena Cava

Clinical

The majority of leiomyosarcomas of the inferior vena cava arise in women, and the average age at presentation is approximately 60 years.[160] The presenting symptom depends on the tumor location: Those at the level of the liver present with Budd–Chiari syndrome and have the worst prognosis; those in the middle portion of the inferior vena cava present with pain, and distal lesions have the best long-term outcome and present typically with the inferior vena cava syndrome.[184, 185] Other modes of presentation include recurring pulmonary emboli and metastatic disease; rarely sarcomas of the inferior vena cava can be incidental findings. Unusual venous sarcomas that have been reported include angiosarcomas of the superior vena cava: synovial sarcomas of the superior vena cava: and leiomyosarcomas of the pulmonary, femoral and iliac veins.[160]

Pathologic Findings

Sarcomas of the inferior vena cava arise in the vessel wall, in contrast to sarcomas of arteries, which are predominantly intraluminal. Sarcomas of the inferior vena cava are usually firmly attached to the wall of the vessel and form discrete masses that extend into the retroperitoneum.

Histologically, most sarcomas of the inferior vena cava are typical leiomyosarcomas (Fig. 12–31). Survival is longer in patients with sarcomas of the inferior vena cava than in patients with sarcomas of the aorta and pulmonary arteries, with an average of about 3 years. Metastases can occur in a variety of sites, including lung, kidney, pleura, chest wall, liver, and bones.[160]

Leiomyomas of Veins

Small, incidental leiomyomas of peripheral veins are quite common and usually present as masses that are often painful. Leiomyomas of the inferior vena cava are much rarer, and are

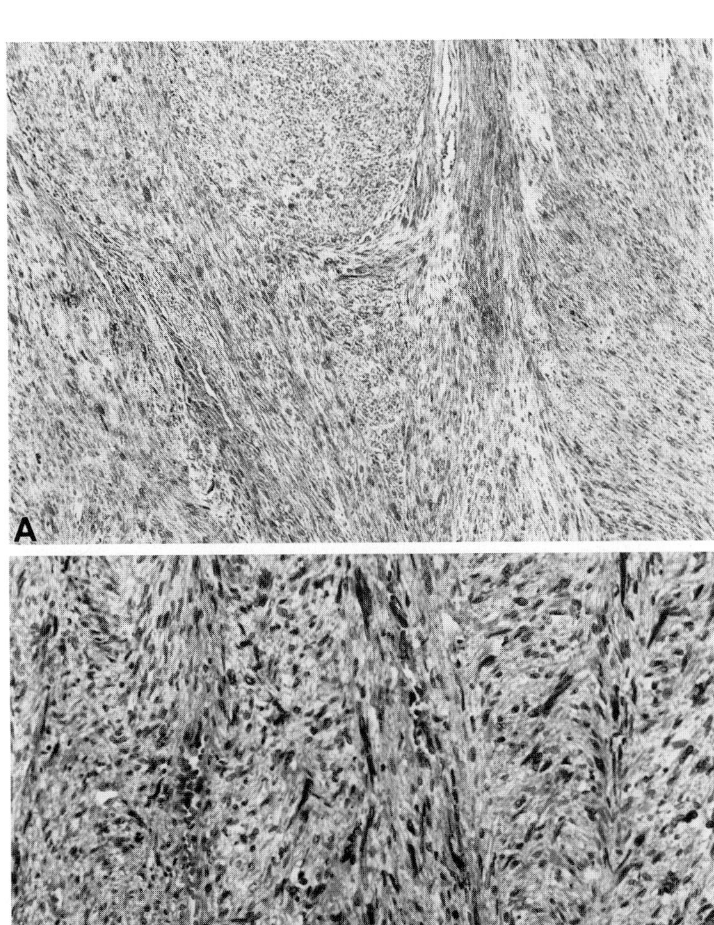

Figure 12–31. Sarcoma, inferior vena cava. These sarcomas are typically well-differentiated leiomyosarcomas (*A*). The patient, a 55-year-old woman, suffered from obstruction of the inferior vena cava at the level of the kidneys. (H & E × 75) *B*. A higher magnification demonstrates fascicular growth of spindled cells with blunt-ended nuclei; the fascicles are focally orientated perpendicularlly one to the other. (H & E × 150)

generally luminal,[186] in contrast to leiomyosarcomas of the vanae cavae, most of which are attached to the vessel wall. The majority of leiomyomas that occur within the lumen of the inferior vena cava are extensions of uterine leiomyomas, and represent so-called intravenous leiomyomatosis.[187] Less often they arise from the lining of the vena cava itself, or are extensions of leiomyomas that originate in the hepatic, femoral, or more distal veins.[188]

REFERENCES

1. Blondeau P. Primary cardiac tumors—French studies of 533 cases. Thorac Cardiovasc Surg 38:192–195, 1990.
2. Tazelaar HD, Locke TJ, McGregor CG. Pathology of surgically excised primary cardiac tumors. Mayo Clin Proc 67:957–965, 1992.
3. Murphy MC, Sweeney MS, Putnam JB, Walker WE, Frazier OH, Ott DA, Cooley DA. Surgical treatment of cardiac tumors: A 25-year experience. Ann Thorac Surg 49:612–617, 1990.
4. Dein JR, Frist WH, Stinson EB et al. Primary cardiac neoplasms. Early and late results of surgical treatment in 42 patients. J Thorac Cardiovasc Surg 93:502, 1987.
5. Melo J, Ahmad A, Chapman R, Wood J, Starr A. Primary tumors of the heart: A rewarding challenge. Am Surg 45:681, 1979.
6. Verkkala K, Kupari M, Maamies T et al. Primary cardiac tumours—operative treatment of 20 patients. Thorac Cardiovasc Surg 37:361, 1989.
7. McAllister HA, Fenoglio JJ. Tumors of the cardiovascular system. Washington DC: Fascicles of the Armed Forces Institute of Pathology, 1977.
8. Burke BA, Edwards JE, Titus JL. Tumors and tumor-like lesions of the heart and great vessels in the young. Adv Pathol Lab Med 5:537–402, 1992.
9. Becker RC, Loeffler JS, Leopold KA, Underwood DA. Primary tumors of the heart: A review with emphasis on diagnosis and potential treatment modalities. Semin Surg Oncol 1:161–170, 1985.
10. Flipse TR, Tazelaar HD, Holmes Dr Jr. Diagnosis of malignant cardiac disease by endomyocardial biopsy. Mayo Clin Proc 65:1415–1422, 1990.
11. Farber S. Congentital rhabdomyoma of the heart. Am J Pathol 7:105, 1931.
12. Burke AP, Virmani R. Cardiac rhabdomyoma, a clinicopathologic study. Mod Pathol 4:70–74, 1991.
13. Diamant S, Sharaz J, Holzman M, Lanaido S. Echocardiographic diagnosis of cardiac tumors in symptomatic tuberous sclerosis patients. Clinical Pediatrics 22:297, 1983.
14. Fenoglio JJ, McAllister HA, Ferrans VJ. Cardiac rhabdomyoma: A clinicopathologic and electron microscopic study. Am J Cardiol 38:241, 1983.
15. Fenoglio JJ, Diana DJ, Bowen TE, McAllister HA, Ferrans VJ. Ultrastructure of a cardiac rhabdomyoma. Hum Pathol 8:700, 1977.
16. Slverman JF, Kay S, McCue CM, Lower RR, Brough AJ, Chang CH. Rhabdomyoma of the heart. Ultrastructural study of three cases. Lab Invest 35:596, 1976.
17. Coffin CM. Congenital cardiac fibroma associated with Gorlin syndrome. Pediatr Pathol 12:255–262, 1992.
18. Parmley LF, Salley RK, Williams JP, Head GB 3d. The clinical spectrum of cardiac fibroma with diagnostic and surgical considerations: Noninvasive imaging enhances management. Ann Thorac Surg 45:455–465, 1988.
19. Ceithaml E, Midgley FM, Perry LW, Dullum MK. Intramural ventricular fibroma in infancy: Survival after partial excision in 2 patients. Ann Thorac Surg 50:471–472, 1990.
20. Lee YC, Singleton RT, Tang CK. Benign mesenchymal tumor of the heart: Spontaneous regression and disappearance of pulmonary artery stenosis. Chest 82:503–505, 1982.
21. Boone SA, Campagna M, Walley VM. Lambl's excrescences and papillary fibroelastomas: Are they different? Can J Cardiol 8:372–376, 1992.
22. Narang J, Neustein S, Israel D. The role of transesophageal echocardiography in the diagnosis and excision of a tumor of the aortic valve. J Cardiothorac Vasc Anesth 6:68–69, 1992.
23. Heath D, Best PV, Davis BT. Papilliferous tumors of the heart valves. Br Heart J 23:20–24, 1961.
24. Fishbein MC, Ferrans VJ, Roberts WC. Endocardial papillary elastofibromas. Arch Pathol 99:335–341, 1975.
25. Valente M, Basso C, Thiene G, Bressan M, Stritoni P, Cocco P, Fasoli G. Fibroelastic papilloma: A not-so-benign cardiac tumor. Cardiovasc Pathol 1:161–166, 1992.
26. Boone S, Higginson LA, Walley VM. Endothelial papillary fibroelastomas arising in and around the aortic sinus, filling the ostium of the right coronary artery. Arch Pathol Lab Med 116:135–137, 1992.
27. Mann J, Parker DJ. Papillary fibroelastoma of the mitral valve: A rare cause of transient neurological deficits. Br Heart J 71:6, 1994.
28. Rubin MA, Snell JA, Tazelaar HD, Lack EE, Austenfeld JL, Azumi N. Cardiac papillary fibroelastoma: An immunohistochemical investigation and unusual clinical manifestations. Mod Pathol 8:402–407, 1995.
29. Bhattacharjee M, Neligan MC, Dervan P. Lipomatous hypertrophy of the interatrial septum: An unusual interoperative finding. Br Heart J 65:49–50, 1991.
30. Prior JT. Lipomatous hypertrophy of cardiac interatrial septum. Arch Pathol 78:11–15, 1964.
31. Hutter AM Jr, Page DL. Atrial arrhythmias and lipomatous hypertrophy of the cardiac interatrial septum. Am Heart J 82:16–21, 1971.
32. Isner JM, Swan CS, Mikus JP, Carter BL. Lipomatous hypertrophy of the interatrial septum: In vivo diagnosis. Circulation 66:470–473, 1982.
33. Shirani J, Roberts WC. Clinical, electrocardiographic and morphologic features of massive fatty deposits ("lipomatous hypertrophy") in the atrial septum. J Am Coll Cardiol 22:226–238, 1993.
34. Burke AP, Dhir S, Tang AL, Virmani R. Lipomatous hypertrophy of the interatrial septum: Surgical and histologic features. Lab Invest 70:27A, 1994.
35. Scully RE, Mark EJ, McNeely WF, McNeely BU. Case Records of the Massachusetts General Hospital. Weekly clinicopathological exercises. Case 10. 320:652–660, 1989.
36. Rose AG. Venous malformations of the heart. Arch Pathol Lab Med 103:18–20, 1979.

37. Abad C, Campo E, Estruch R, Condom E, Barriuso C, Tassies D, Pare JC. Cardiac hemangioma with papillary endothelial hyperplasia: Report of a resected case and review of the literature. Ann Thorac Surg 49:305–308, 1990.
38. Fabian JT, Rose AG. Tumours of the heart. A study of 89 cases. S Afr Med J 16:71–77, 1982.
39. Fine G. Primary tumors of the pericardium and heart. Cardiovasc Clin 5:207–238, 1973.
40. Reece IJ, Cooley DA, Frazier OH, Hallman GL et al. Cardiac tumors. Clinical spectrum and prognosis of lesions other than classical benign myxoma in 20 patients. J Thorac Cardiovasc Surg 88:439–446, 1984.
41. Burke AP, Johns J, Virmani R. Hemangiomas of the heart: A clinicopathologic study of 10 cases. Am J Cardiovasc Pathol 13:283–290, 1991.
42. Chang JS, Young ML, Chuu WM, Lue HC. Infantile cardiac hemangioendothelioma. Pediatr Cardiol 13:52–55, 1992.
43. Reiss N, Theissen P, Feaux de Lacroix W. Right-ventricular hemangioma causing serious outflow-tract obstruction. Thorac Cardiovasc Surg 39:234–236, 1991.
44. Kemme DJ, Rainer WG. Subendocardial arteriovenous malformation in a patient with unstable angina. Clin Cardiol 14:82–84, 1991.
45. Gengenbach S, Ridker PM. Left ventricular hemangioma in Kasabach–Merritt syndrome. Am Heart J 121:202–203, 1991.
46. Palmer TE, Tresch DD, Bonchek LI. Spontaneous resolution of a large, cavernous hemangioma of the heart. Am J Cardiol 58:184–185, 1986.
47. Kuo TT, Hsueh S, Su IJ, Gonzalez-Crussi F, Chen JS. Histiocytoid hemangioma of the heart with peripheral eosinophilia. Cancer 55:2854–2861, 1985.
48. Burke AP, Anderson PG, Virmani R, James TN, Herrera GA, Ceballos R. Tumors of the atrioventricular node. Arch Pathol Lab Med 114:1057–1062, 1990.
49. Balasundaram S, Halees SA, Duran C. Mesothelioma of the atrioventricular node: First successful follow-up after excision. Eur Heart J 13:718–719, 1992.
50. Fine G, Raju U. Congenital polycystic tumor of the atrioventricular node (endodermal heterotopia, mesothelioma): A histogenetic appraisal with evidence for its endodermal origin. Human Pathol 18:791–795, 1987.
51. Linder J, Shelburne JD, Sorge JP, Whalen RE, Hackel DB. Congenital endodermal heterotopia of the atrioventricular node: Evidence for the endodermal origin of so-called mesotheliomas of the atrioventricular node. Hum Pathol 15:1093–1097, 1984.
52. Machens G, Vahl CF, Hofmann R, Wolf D, Hagl S. Entodermal inclusion cyst of the tricuspid valve. Thorac Cardiovasc Surg 39:296–298, 1991.
53. Shimizu M, Takeda R, Mifune J, Tanaka T. Echocardiographic features of intrapericardial bronchogenic cyst. Cardiology 77:332–336, 1990.
54. Polvani GL, Antona C, Porqueddu M, Pompilio G, Cavoretto D, Gherli T, Sala A, Biglioli P. Intracardiac ectopic thyroid: Conservative surgical treatment. Ann Thorac Surg 55:1249–1251, 1993.
55. Malhotra V, Ferrans VJ, Virmani R. Infantile histiocytoid cardiomyopathy: Report of three cases and review of literature. Am Heart J 128:1009–1021, 1994.
56. Stark P, Sandbank JC, Rudnicki C, Zahavi I. Inflammatory pseudotumor of the heart with vasculitis and venous thrombosis. Chest 102:1884–1885, 1992.
57. Pearson PF, Smithson WA, Driscoll DJ, Banks PM, Ehman RL. Inoperable plasma cell granuloma of the heart: Spontaneous decrease in size during an 11-month period. Mayo Clin Proc 63:1022–1025, 1988.
58. Rose AG. Fibrous histiocytoma of the heart. Arch Pathol Lab Med 102:389, 1978.
59. Veinot JP, Tazelaar HD, Edwards WD, Colloy TV, Davy C. Mesothelial/monocytic incidental cardiac excrescences (cardiac MICE). Mod Pathol 7:9–16, 1994.
60. Courtice RW, Stinson WA, Walley VM. Tissue fragments recovered at cardiac surgery masquerading as tumoural proliferations. Evidence suggesting iatrogenic or artifactual origin and common occurrence. Am J Surg Pathol 18:167–174, 1994.
61. Lie JT. The identity and histogenesis of cardiac myxomas. A controversy put to rest. Arch Pathol Lab Med 113:724–726, 1989.
62. Hutchins GM, Bulkley BH. Atrial myxomas: A fifty year review. Am Heart J 97:639, 1979.
63. Markel ML, Waller BF, Armstrong WF. Cardiac myxoma. A review. Medicine 66:114–125, 1987.
64. Larsson S, Lepore V, Kennergren C. Atrial myxomas: Results of 25 years' experience and review of the literature. Surgery 105:695–698, 1989.
65. Burke AP, Virmani R. Cardiac myxomas. Am J Clin Pathol 100:671–680, 1993.
66. Rupp GM, Heyman RA, Martinez AJ, Sekhar LN, Jungries CA. The pathology of metastatic cardiac myxoma. Am J Clin Pathol 91:221–227, 1989.
67. Carney JA, Gordon H, Carpenter PC, Shenoy BV, Go VL. The complex of myxomas, spotty pigmentation, and endocrine overactivity. Medicine 64:270–283, 1985.
68. Atherton DJ, Pitcher DW, Wells RS, MacDonald DM. A syndrome of various cutaneous pigmented lesions, myxoid neurofibromata and atrial myxoma: The NAME syndrome. Br J Dermatol 103:421–429, 1980.
69. Goldman BI, Frydman C, Harpaz N, Ryan SF, Loiterman D. Glandular cardiac myxomas. Histologic, immunohistochemical, and ultrastrucrual evidence of epithelial differentiation. Cancer 15:1767–1775, 1987.
70. Johansson L. Histogenesis of cardiac myxomas. An immunohistochemical study of 19 cases, including one with glandular structures, and review of the literature. Arch Pathol Lab Med 113:735–741, 1989.
71. Attum AA, Johnson GS, Masri Z, Girardet R, Lansing AM. Malignant clinical behavior of cardiac myxomas and "myxoid imitators." Ann Thorac Surg 44:217–222, 1987.
72. Wang J, Dragel AH, Friendlander ER, Cheng JT. Granular cell tumor of the sinus node. Am J Cardiol 71:490–492, 1993.
73. Behnam R, Williams G, Gerlis L, Walker D, Scott O. Lipoma of the mitral valve and papillary muslce. Am J Cardiol 51:1459–1460, 1983.
74. Cox JN, Friedli B, Mechmeche R, Ben Ismail M, Oberhaensli I, Faidutti B. Teratoma of the heart. A case report and review of the literature. Virchows Arch A Pathol Anat Histopathol 402:163–174, 1983.
75. Hui G, McAllister HA, Angelini P. Left atrial paraganglioma: Report of a case and review of the literature. Am Heart J 113:1230–1234, 1987.
76. Abad C, Jimenez P, Santana C, Coello I, Acosta A, Hernandez E, Feijoo JJ, Diaz J, Rodriguez-Parez A. Primary cardiac paraganglioma. Case report and review of surgically treated cases. J Cardiovasc Surg 33:758–772, 1992.

77. Johnson TL, Shapiro B, Beierwalters WH, Orringer MB, Lloyd RV, Sisson JC, Thompson NW. Cardiac paragangliomas. A clinicopathologic and immunohistochemical study of four cases. Am J Surg Pathol 11:827–834, 1985.
78. Aravot DJ, Banner NR, Cantor AM, Theodoropoulos S, Yacoub MH. Location, localization and surgical treatment of cardiac pheochromocytoma. Am J Cardiol 69:283–285, 1992.
79. David TE, Lenkei SC, Marquez-Julio A. Pheochromocytoma of the heart. Ann Thorac Surg 41:98–100, 1986.
80. Orringer MB, Sisson JC, Glazer G, Shapiro B, Francis I, Behrendt DM, Thompson NW, Lloyd RV. Surgical treatment of cardiac pheochromocytomas. J Thorac Cardiovasc Surg 89:753–757, 1985.
81. Betancourt B, Defendini EA, Johnson C, DeJesus M, Pavia-Villamil A, Diaz Cruz A, Medina JC. Severe right ventricular outflow tract obstruction caused by an intracavitary cardiac neurilemoma: Successful surgical removal and postoperative diagnosis. Chest 75:522–524, 1979.
82. Factor A, Turi G, Biempica L. Primary cardiac neurilemoma. Cancer 37:883–890, 1976.
83. Forbes AD, Schmidt RA, Wood DE, Cochran RP, Munkenbeck F, Verrier ED. Schwannoma of the left atrium: Diagnostic evaluation and surgical resection. Ann Thorac Surg 57:743–746, 1994.
84. Jaffe R. Neuroma in the region of the atrioventricular node. Hum Pathol 12:375–376, 1981.
85. Tractos S, Turi G, Bienpica L. Primary cardiac neurilemoma. Cancer 37:883–886, 1976.
86. Burke AP, Cowan D, Virmani R. Cardiac sarcomas. Cancer 69:387–395, 1992.
87. Putnam JB Jr, Sweeney MS, Colon R, Lanza LA, Frazier OH, Cooley DA. Primary cardiac sarcomas. Ann Thorac Surg 51:906–910, 1991.
88. Bear PA Moodie DS. Malignant primary cardiac tumors. The Cleveland Clinic experience, 1956 to 1986. Chest 92:860–862, 1987.
89. Miralles A, Bracamonte L, Soncul H, Diaz del Castillo R, Akhtar R, Bors V, Pavie A, Gandjbackch I, Cabrol C. Cardiac tumors: Clinical experience and surgical results in 74 patients. Ann Thorac Surg 52:886–895, 1991.
90. Herhusky MJ, Gregg SB, Virmani R, Chun PK, Bender H, Gray GF Jr. Cardiac sarcomas presenting as metastatic disease. Arch Pathol Lab Med 109:943–945, 1985.
91. Siebenmann R, Jenni R, Makek M, Oelz O, Turina M. Primary synovial sarcoma of the heart treated by heart transplantation. J Thorac Cardiovasc Surg 3:567–568, 1990.
92. Glancy DL, Morales JB, Roberts WC. Angiosarcoma of the heart. Cancer 21:413–418, 1968.
93. Herrmann MA, Shankerman RA, Edwards WD, Shub C, Schaff HV. Primary cardiac angiosarcoma: A clinicopathologic study of six cases. J Thorac Cardiovasc Surg 103:655–664, 1992.
94. Janigan DT, Husain A, Robinson NA. Cardiac angiosarcomas. A review and a case report. Cancer 57:852–859, 1986.
95. Marafioti T, Castorini F, Gula G. Cardiac angiosarcoma. Histological, immunohistochemical and ultrastructural study. Pathologica 85:103–111, 1993.
96. Masauzi N, Ichikawa S, Nishimura F et al. Primary angiosarcoma of the right atrium detected by magnetic resonance imaging. Int Med 31:1291–1297, 1992.
97. Awad M, Dunn B, al Halees Z, Mercer E. Intracardiac rhabdomyosarcoma: Transesophageal echocardiographic findings and diagnosis. J Am Soc Echocardiogr 5:199–202, 1992.
98. Hajar R, Roberts WC, Folger GM Jr. Embryonal botryoid rhabdomyosarcoma of the mitral valve. Am J Cardiol 57:376, 1986.
99. Hui KS, Green LK, Schmidt WA. Primary cardiac rhabdomyosarcoma: Definition of a rare entity. Am J Cardiovasc Pathol 2:19–29, 1988.
100. Moriarty AT, Nelson WA, McGahey B. Fine needle aspiration of rhabdomyosarcoma of the heart. Light and electron microscopic findings and histologic correlation. Acta Cytol 34:74–78, 1990.
101. Orsmond GS, Knight L, Dehner LP, Micolof FM, Nesbitt M, Bessinger FB. Alveolar rhabdomyosarcoma involving the heart: An echocardiographic, angiographic and pathologic study. Circulation 54:837–843, 1976.
102. Satoh M, Horimoto M, Sakurai K, Funayama N, Igarashi K, Yamashiro K. Primary cardiac rhabdomyosarcoma exhibiting transient and pronounced regression with chemotherapy. Am Heart J 120:1458–1460, 1990.
103. Laya MB, Maillard JA, Bewtra C, Levin HS. Malignant fibrous histocytoma of the heart. A case report and review of the literature. Cancer 59:1026–1031, 1987.
104. Korbmacher B, Doering C, Schulte HD, Hort W. Malignant fibrous histiocytoma of the heart. Case report of a rare left atrial tumor. Thorac Cardiovasc Surg 40:303–307, 1992.
105. Maruki C, Suzukawa K, Koike J, Sato K. Cardiac malignant fibrous histiocytoma metastasizing to the brain: Development of multiple neoplastic cerebral aneurysms. Surg Neurol 41:40–44, 1994.
106. Ovcak Z, Masera A, Lamovec J. Malignant fibrous histiocytoma of the heart. Arch Pathol Lab Med 116:872–874, 1992.
107. Pasquale M, Katz NM, Caruso AC, Bearb ME, Bitterman P. Myxoid variant of malignant fibrous histiocytoma of the heart. Am Heart J 122:248–250, 1991.
108. Shah AA, Churg A, Sbarbaro JA, Sheppard JM, Lamberi J. Malignant fibrous histiocytoma of the heart presenting as an atrial myxoma. Cancer 42:2466–2471, 1978.
109. Terashima K, Aoyama K, Nihei K, Nito T, Imai Y, Takahsahi K, Daidoji S. Malignant fibrous histiocytoma of the heart. Cancer 52:1919–1926, 1983.
110. Harris GJ, Tio FO, Grover FL. Primary left atrial myxosarcoma. Ann Thorac Surg 56:564–566, 1993.
111. Mahar LJ, Lie JT, Groover RV, Seward JB, Puga F, Feldt RH. Primary cardiac myxosarcoma in a child. Mayo Clin Proc 54:261–266, 1979.
112. Johansson L, Kugelberg J, Thulin L. Myxofibrosarcoma in the left atrium orginally presented as a cardiac myxoma with chondroid differentiation. A clinicopathological report (clinical conference). APMIS 97:833–838, 1989.
113. Burke AP, Virmani R. Osteosarcomas of the heart. Am J Surg Pathol 15:289–295, 1991.
114. Lowry WB, McKee EE. Primary osteosarcoma of the heart. Cancer 30:1068–1073, 1972.
115. Marvasti MA, Bove EL, Obeid AK, Bowser MA, Parker FB Jr. Primary osteosarcoma of the left atrium: Complete surgical excision. Ann Thorac Surg 40:402–404, 1985.

116. Reynard JS, Gregoratos G, Gordon MJ, Bloor CM. Primary osteosarcoma of the heart. Am Heart J 109:598–600, 1985.
117. Schneiderman H, Fordham EW, Goren CC, McCall AR, Rosenberg MS, Rozek S. Primary cardiac osteosarcoma: Multidisciplinary aspects applicable to extraskeletal osteosarcoma generally. CA Cancer J Clin 34:110–117, 1984.
118. Seidal T, Wandt B, Lundin SE. Primary chondroblastic osteogenic sarcoma of the left atrium. Case report. Scand J Thorac Cardiovasc Surg 26:233–236, 1992.
119. Yashar J, Witoszka M, Savage DD, Klie J, Dyckman J, Yashar JJ, Reddick RL, Watson KC, McIntosh CL. Primary osteogenic sarcoma of the heart. Ann Thorac Surg 28:594–600, 1979.
120. Hammond GL, Strong WW, Cohen LS, Silverman M, Garnet R, LiVolsi VA, Cornog JL. Chondrosarcoma simulating malignant atrial myxoma. J Thorac Cardiovasc Surg 72:575–580, 1976.
121. Karn CM, Socinski MA, Fletcher JA, Corson JM, Craighead JE. Cardiac synovial sarcoma with translocation (X;18) associated with asbestos exposure. Cancer 73:74–78, 1994.
122. Siebenmann R, Jenni R, Makek M, Oelz O, Turina M. Primary synoval sarcoma of the heart treated by heart transplantation. J Thorac Cardiovasc Surg 3:567–568, 1990.
123. Tak T, Goel S, Chandrasoma P, Colletti P, Rahimtoola SH. Synovial sarcoma of the right ventricle. Am Heart J 121:933–936, 1991.
124. Can C, Arpaci F, Celasun B, Gunham O, Finci R. Primary pericardial liposarcoma presenting with cardiac tamponade and multiple organ metastases. Chest 10-3:328, 1993.
125. Dreyer L, Marik PE, Potgieter AS. Myxoid liposarcoma of the right atrium. S Afr Med J 59:572–574, 1986.
126. Lionarons RJ, Van Baarlen J, Hitchock JF. Constrictive pericarditis caused by primary liposarcoma. Thorax 45:566–567, 1990.
127. Macedo-Davis JA, Queiroz Machado F, Vouga L, Goncalves V, Gomes R. Liposarcoma of the heart. A case report. Am J Cardiovasc Pathol 3:259–263, 1990.
128. Nazyinambaho K, Noel H, Cosyns J, Sonnet J, Chalant C. Primary cardiac liposarcoma simulating a left atrial myxoma. Thorac Cardiovasc Surg 33:193–195, 1985.
129. Paraf F, Bruneval P, Balaton A, Deloche A, Mikol J, Maitre F, Scholl JM, De Saint-Maur PP, Camilleri JP. Primary liposarcoma of the heart. Am J Cardiovasc Pathol 3:175–180, 1990.
130. Knobel B, Rosman P, Kishon Y, Husar M. Intracardiac primary fibrosarcoma. Case report and literature review. Thorac Cardiovasc Surg 40:227–230, 1992.
131. Sethi KK, Nair M, Khanna SK. Primary fibrosarcoma of the heart presenting as obstruction at the tricuspid valve: Diagnosis by cross-sectional echocardiography. Int J Cardiol 24:228–230, 1989.
132. Fox JP, Freitas E, McGiffin DC, Firouz-Abadi AA, West MJ. Primary leiomyosarcoma of the heart: A rare cause of obstruction of the left ventriculr outflow tract. Aust N Z J Med 21:881–883, 1991.
133. Fyfe AI, Huckell VF, Burr LH, Stonier PM. Leiomyosarcoma of the left atrium: Case report and review of the literature. Can J Cardiol 7:193–196, 1991.
134. James CL, Leong AS. Epithelioidleiomyosarcoma of the left atrium: Immunohistochemical and ultrastructural findings. Pathology 21:308–313, 1989.
135. Takamizawa S, Sugimoto K, Tanka H, Sakai O, Arai T, Saitoh A. A case of primary leiomyosarcoma of the heart. Intern Med 31:265–268, 1992.
136. Ursell PC, Albala A, Fenoglio JJ Jr. Malignant neurogenic tumor of the heart. Hum Pathol 13:640–645, 1982.
137. Levinson DA, Semple PD. Primary Cardiac Kaposi's sarcoma. Thorax 31:595–600, 1976.
138. Lewis W. AIDS: Cardiac findings from 115 autopsies. Prog Cardiovascul Dis 32:207–215, 1989.
139. Abraham DP, Reddy V, Gattusa P. Neoplasms metastatic to the heart: Review of 3314 consecutive autopsies. Am J Cardiovasc Pathol 3:195–198, 1990.
140. Gardiner DW, Lindop GB. Coronary artery aneurysm due to primary cardiac lymphoma. Histopathology 15:537–540, 1989.
141. Abu-Farsakh H, Cagle PT, Buffone GJ, Bruner JM, Weibaecher D, Greenberg SD. Heart allograft involvement with Epstein–Barr virus-associated posttransplant lymphoproliferative disorder. Arch Pathol Lab Med 116:93–95, 1992.
142. Andress JD, Polish LB, Clark DM, Hossack KF. Transvenous biopsy diagnosis of cardiac lymphoma in an AIDS patient. Am Heart J 118:421–423, 1989.
143. Balasubramanyam A, Waxman M, Kazal HL, Lee MH. Malignant lymphoma of the heart in acquired immune deficiency syndrome. Chest 90:243–246, 1986.
144. Burtin P, Guerci A, Boman F, Dopff C, Pinelli G, Haberer JP, Villemott MP. Malignant lymphoma in the donor heart after heart transplantation. Eur Heart J 14:1143–1145, 1993.
145. Guarner J, Brynes RK, Chan WC, Birdsong G, Hertzler G. Primary non-Hodgkin's lymphoma of the heart in two patients with the acquired immunodeficiency syndrome. Arch Pathol Lab Med 111:254–255, 1987.
146. Holladay AO, Siegel RJ, Schwartz EA. Cardiac malignant lymphoma in acquired immune deficiency syndrome. Cancer 70:2203–2207, 1992.
147. Kelsey RC, Saker A, Morgan M. Cardiac lymphoma in a patient with AIDS. Ann Intern Med 115:370–371, 1991.
148. Rodenburg CJ, Kluin P, Maes A, Paul LC. Malignant lymphoma confined to the heart, 13 years after a cadaver kidney transplant. N Engl J Med 313:122, 1985.
149. Goldfarb A, King CL, Rosenzweig BP, Feit F Kamt BR, Rumancik WM, Kronzon I. Cardiac lymphoma in the acquired immunodeficiency syndrome. Am Heart J 118:1340–1344, 1989.
150. Cleary ML, Sklar J. Lymphoproliferative disorders in cardiac transplant recipients are multiclonal lymphomas. Lancet 2:489–493, 1984.
151. Cleary ML, Warnke R, Skalar J. Monoclonality of lymphoproliferative lesions in cardiac transplant recipients: Clonal analysis based on immunoglobulin gene rearrangements. N Engl J Med 310:577–482, 1984.
152. Kaplan MA, Ferry JA, Harris NL, Jacobson JO. Clonal analysis of posttransplant lymphoproliferative disorders, using both episomal Epstein–Barr virus and immunoglobulin genes as markers. Am J Clin Pathol 101:590–596, 1994.
153. Purtilo DT, Strobach RS, Okano M, Davis JR. Epstein–Barr virus-associated lymphoproliferative disorders. Lab Invest 67:5–23, 1992.
154. Nand S, Mullen GM, Lonchyna VA, Moncada R. Primary lymphoma of the heart. Prolonged survival with early systemic therapy in a patient. Cancer 68:2289–2292, 1991.
155. Proctor MS, Tracy GP, Von Koch L. Primary cardiac B-cell lymphoma. Am Heart J 118:179–181, 1989.

156. Stein M, Zyssman I, Kantor A, Spencer D, Lewis D, Bezwoda W. Malignant lymphoma with primary cardiac manifestation: A case report. Med Pediatr Oncol 22:292–295, 1994.
157. Pozniak AL, Thomas RD, Hobbs CB, Lever JV. Primary malignant lymphoma of the heart. Antemortem cytologic diagnosis. Acta Cytol 30:662–664, 1986.
158. Mukai K, Shinkai T, Tominaga K, Shimosato Y. The incidence of secondary tumors of the heart and pericardium: A 10-year study. Jpn J Clin Oncol 18:195–201, 1988.
159. Hallahan DE, Vogelzang NJ, borow KM, Bostwick DG, Simon MA. Cardiac metastases from soft-tissue sarcomas. J Clin Oncol 4:1662–1669, 1986.
160. Burke AP, Virmani R. Sarcomas of the great vessels. Cancer 69:387–395, 1993.
161. Fenoglio JJ Jr, Virmani R. Primary malignant tumors of the great vessels. In: Waller B (ed): Pathology of the heart and great vessels, Vol. 12, pp 429–438. New York: Churchill Livingstone, 1988.
162. Becquemin JP, Lebe C, Saada F, Avril MF. Sarcoma of the aorta: Report of a case and review of the literature. Ann Vasc Surg 2:225–230, 1988.
163. Wright EP, Glick AD, Virmani R, Page DL. Aortic intimal sarcoma with embolic metastases. Am J Surg Pathol 9:890–897, 1985.
164. Tajada E, Becker GJ, Waller BF. Malignant myxoid emboli as the presenting feature of primary sarcoma of the aorta (myxoid malignant fibrous histiocytoma): A case report and review of the literature. Clin Cardiol 14, 425–430, 1991.
165. Herzberg AJ, Pizzo SV. Primary undifferentiated sarcoma of the thoracic aorta. Histopathol 13:571–574, 1988.
166. Josen AS, Khine M. Primary malignant tumor of the aorta. J Vasc Surg 9:493–498, 1989.
167. Nishikawa H, Miyakoshi S, Nishimura S, Seki A, Honda K. A case of aortic intimal sarcoma manifested with acutely occurring hypertension and aortic occlusion. Heart Vessels 5:54–58, 1989.
168. Pruszczynski M, Coronel CM, Naudin ten Cate L, Roholl PJ, van der Kley AJ. Immunohistochemical and ultrastructural studies of a primary aortic intimal sarcoma. Pathology 20:173–178, 1988.
169. Taegtmeyer H, Schroth G, Dickerson CA, Farhood AI. A middle-aged woman with dyspnea, cachexia, increased abdominal girth, pericardial effusion, and a continuous murmur. Circulation 89:484–492, 1994.
170. Weinberg DS, Maini BS. Primary sarcoma of the aorta associated with a vascular prosthesis: A case report. Cancer 15:398–401, 1980.
171. Haber LM, Truong L. Immunohistochemical demonstration of the endothelial nature of aortic intimal sarcoma. Am J Surg Pathol 12:798–802, 1988.
172. Leeson MC, Malaei M, Makley JT. Leiomyosarcoma of the popliteal artery. A report of two cases. Clin Orthop 253:225–230, 1990.
173. Baker PB, Goodwin RA. Pulmonary artery sarcomas. Review and report of a case. Arch Pathol Lab Med 109:35–39, 1985.
174. Ceretto AJ, Miller ML, Shea PM, Gregory CW, Vieweg WVR. Malignant mesenchymoma obstructing the right ventricular outflow tract. Am Heart J 101:114–115, 1981.
175. Eng J, Murday AJ. Leiomyosarcoma of the pulmonary artery. Ann Thorac Surg 53:905–906, 1992.
176. Farooki ZQ, Chang CH, Jackson WL, Clapp SK, Hakimi M, Arciniegas E, Pinsky WW. Primary pulmonary artery sarcoma in two children. Pediatr Cardiol 9:243–251, 1988.
177. Fer MF, Greco FA, Haile KL, Rosenblatt PA, Johnson RL, Glick AD, Oldham RK. Unusual survival after pulmonary artery sarcoma. South Med J 74:624–626, 1981.
178. Hagstrom L. Malignant mesenchymoma in pulmonary artery and right ventricle. Acta Pathol Microbiol Scand 51:87–94, 1961.
179. Klinke WP, Gelfand ET, Baron L. Primary sarcoma of the pulmonary trunk: Successful surgical intervention and prolonged survival. Clin Cardiol 8:437–440, 1985.
180. Kruger I, Borowski A, Horst M, de Vivie ER, Theissen P, Gross-Fengels W. Symptoms, diagnosis and therapy of primary sarcomas of the pulmonary artery. Thorac Cardiovasc Surg 38:91–95, 1990.
181. McGlenen RC, Manivel JC, Stanley SJ, Slater DL, Wick MR, Dehner LP. Pulmonary artery trunk sarcoma: A clinicopathological, ultrastructural, and immunohistochemical study of four cases. Mod Pathol 2:486–494, 1989.
182. Van Damme H, Vaneerdeweg W, Schoofs E. Malignant fibrous histiocytoma of the pulmonary artery. Ann Surg 205:203–207, 1987.
183. Nonomura A, Kurumaya H, Kono J, Nakanuma Y, Ohta G, Terahata S, Matsubara F, Matsuda T, Asaka T, Nishino T. Primary pulmonary artery sarcoma. Report of two autopsy cases studied by immunohistochemistry and elecron microscopy, and review of 110 cases reported in the literature. Acta Pathol Jpn 38:883–896, 1988.
184. Griffin AS, Sterchi JM. Primary leiomyosarcoma of the inferior vena cava: A case report and review of the literature. J Surg Oncol 34:53–60, 1987.
185. Bruyninckx CM, Derksen OS. Leiomyosarcoma of the inferior vena cava. Case report and review of the literature. J Vasc Surg 3:652–656, 1986.
186. Payan MJ, Xerri L, Choux R, Gros N, Albrand JJ, Charpin C, Vaillant A, Malmejac C. Giant leiomyoma of the inferior vena cava. Ann Pathol 9:44–46, 1989.
187. Norris HJ, Parmley T. Mesenchymal tumors of the uterus. V. Intravenous leiomyomatosis. A clinical and pathologic study of 14 cases. Cancer 36:2164–2178, 1975.
188. Dunlap HJ, Udjus K. Atypical leiomyoma arising in an hepatic vein with extension into the inferior vena cava and right atrium. Report of a case in a child. Pediatr Radiol 20:202–203, 1990.

Chapter

13

DISEASES OF THE AORTA AND LARGE VESSELS

The aorta is subject to a variety of diseases, both congenital and acquired, inflammatory and neoplastic, degenerative and traumatic, and infectious and idiopathic. The most prevalent disease of the aorta and its major branches is atherosclerosis, which the practicing autopsy pathologist will see on a daily basis. Perhaps even more frequent than atherosclerosis, however, are degenerative changes of aging, which are usually asymptomatic, but may lead to annular dilatation and aortic insufficiency. Aortic dissections, which have various causes including age- and hypertension-related medial degeneration, are less prevalent than atherosclerosis, but are the most common cause of aortic-related death.

This chapter will discuss all types of aortic disease that occur in adults, without discussing congenital diseases of the aorta, with the exception of a few entities (coarctation, sinus of Valsalva aneurysm) that may occur in adults. Neoplastic diseases of the aorta are presented in Chapter 12, and many of the general aspects of atherosclerosis in Chapter 2.

CONGENITAL DISEASES

Coarctation

Congenital coarctation of the aorta occurs exclusively at the level of the left subclavian artery near the ductus arteriosus or ligamentum arteriosum, and may extend proximally for a variable distance to involve the isthmus and the aortic root (tubular hypoplasia of aorta). Atypical acquired coarctation may occur as a result of inflammatory processes (e.g., Takayasu's disease) or fibromuscular dysplasia in other locations of the aorta, such as the aortic arch and abdominal aorta.[1] Congenital coarctation has been historically divided into two groups: an "infantile" type, or preductal type, in which the ductus is wide open and supplies the descending thoracic aorta the majority of its blood supply, and the "adult" type, in which the duct is often closed, and distal circulation is supplied by collateral circulation. In fact, the appearance of the coarctation before or after the duct may in part be due to the stage of the disease in which the lesion is studied. Infantile coarctation is typically associated with complex congenital heart disease which includes ventricular septal defect and left ventricular outflow tract abnormalities. Coarctation that becomes manifest later in life is typically associated with minimal heart defects, with the exception of bicuspid aortic valve (Fig. 13–1), which is commonly present in patients with aortic coarctation.

There are essentially two theories that account for the development of aortic coarctation, and these theories are not necessarily mutually exclusive. The flow hypothesis states that with left-sided obstruction in utero, due to aortic valve or mitral valve defects, there is decreased flow of blood resulting in functional hypoplasia of the distal ascending aorta at the level of the isthmus. A second hypothesis states that there is ectopic ductal tissue within the

---

The opinions or assertions contained herein are the private views of the authors and are not to be construed as official or as reflecting the views of the Department of the Army or Navy or the Department of Defense.

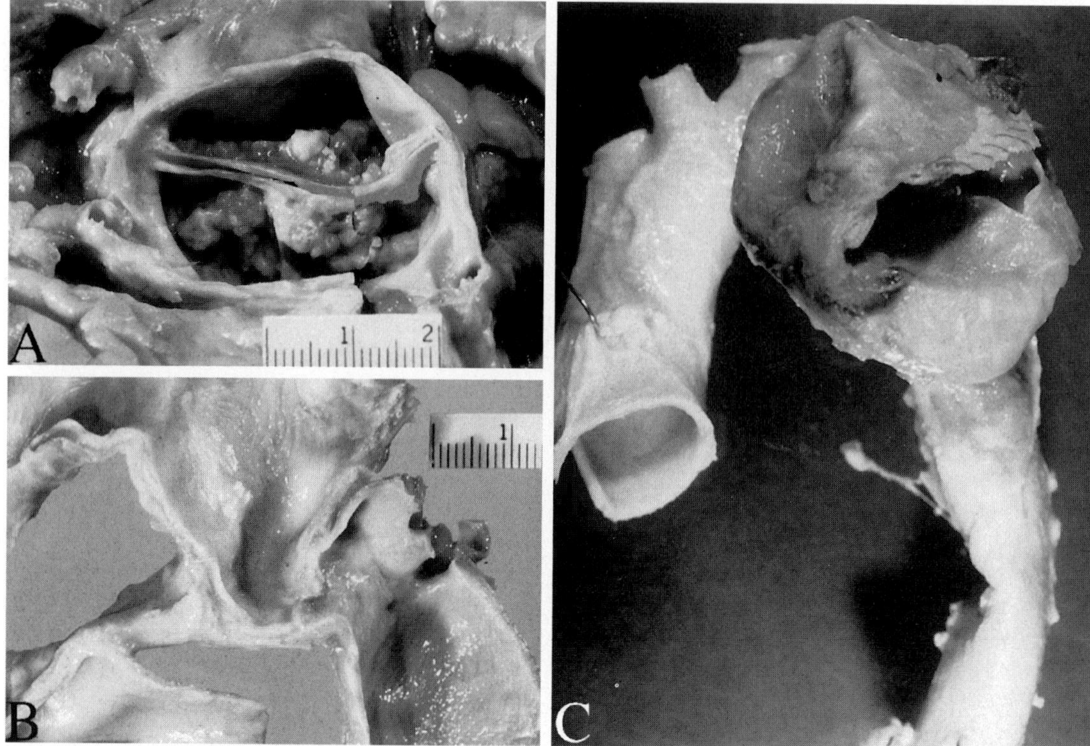

Figure 13–1. Coarctation of aorta. *A.* There is a strong association between congenitally bicuspid aortic valve and aortic coarctation. Note moderate calcification of the aortic valve, which was stenotic. *B.* The aortic arch of the same patient, a 70-year-old man with no history of documented aortic disease, demonstrated a discrete narrowing with contraductal shelf distal to the ligamentum arteriosum, which is seen at the bottom left. *C.* A 34-year-old woman died suddenly 1 week after parturition. She had had a patch repair of the coarctation years prior. An aneurysm had developed at the anastomosis site, which ruptured and resulted in left hemothorax.

aorta, or rather an abnormal extension of ductal tissue that results in constriction and coarctation of the aorta, analogous to normal ductal closure. The latter theory is strengthened by the finding of ductal tissue in histologically examined specimens of coarctation,[2, 3] and accounts for the tendency of most surgeons to excise ductal tissue while repairing coarctation.[4]

In addition to bicuspid aortic valve, which occurs in 35–80% of patients with aortic coarctation, there are several conditions associated with aortic coarctation. *Shone's syndrome* is a complex of supravalvar mitral ring, parachute mitral valve with double orifice, subaortic stenosis, and aortic coarctation. As with other forms of subaortic stenosis, aortic valvar abnormalities are not uncommon in patients with Shone's syndrome. Patients with aortic coarctation are more likely to develop cerebral aneurysms, and coarctation is more prevalent in patients with Marfan syndrome than the general population, in whom the risk is approximately 2 in 10,000 live births. Aortic dissection is more common in patients with aortic coarctation, possibly related to the increased incidence of bicuspid aortic valve. Patients with Turner syndrome (45XO) are likely to have heart defects (approximately 40%); of these, 70% will demonstrate a degree of aortic coarctation, often in combination with bicuspid aortic valve and other features of hypoplastic left-heart syndrome.

The autopsy diagnosis of coarctation of the aorta is generally straightforward, in that there is a severe narrowing of the aorta at the level of the ductus arteriosus. In infants, the duct is generally open, and there is a continuity of the ductus arteriosus with the descending thoracic aorta, which is approximately of the same caliber. The slightly wrinkled, yellowish intima of the duct will allow its recognition and distinguish it from the proximal aorta, as well as its origin from the pulmonary trunk/proximal left pulmonary artery. The duct may be functionally closed, especially in infants with complex congenital heart diseases that are duct dependent, such as variants of the hypoplastic left-heart syndrome.

The diagnosis of coarctation should be suspected if there are conditions that are associated with it, especially left-sided obstructive lesions. It should be kept in mind, however, that the normal caliber of the aortic isthmus is as little as 40% of the ascending aorta, due to normal shunt of blood in utero. Therefore, the diagnosis of the coarctation should be made with care in the absence of other cardiac findings.

There are several types of surgical corrections of aortic coarctation.[5] Surgical repairs include the subclavian flap, which results in sacrifice of the subclavian artery, and is generally performed under one year of age, and techniques of interposition grafts, patch repairs, and end-to-end anastomosis, which may allow for reimplantation of the subclavian artery. The presence of isthmus or tubular hypoplasia of the ascending aorta greatly influence the type of procedure and may necessitate reconstruction of the arch.[6] Complications include recurrent stenoses, especially in infants, persistent left ventricular hypertrophy, and aneurysms at the site of repair, especially with patch aortoplasty. Postsurgical aneurysms may rupture or become infected. Balloon angioplasty with or without stenting is a closed alternative for open repair of aortic coarctation.[7-10] However, dilatation procedures are not effective for cases with isthmus narrowing, and may result in restenosis and postdilatation aneurysms. Dissections and perforations are rare complications of balloon angioplasty. Currently, the primary indication for balloon angioplasty for aortic coarctation is to open postoperative stenosis of repaired coarctation.

Aneurysms of Sinus of Valsalva

Aneurysm of the sinus of Valsalva was first described in 1839.[11] The aneurysm results from a weakness in the wall of the sinus leading to the dilatation or blind pouch (diverticulum) in one of the aortic sinuses, usually the right (Fig. 13–2).

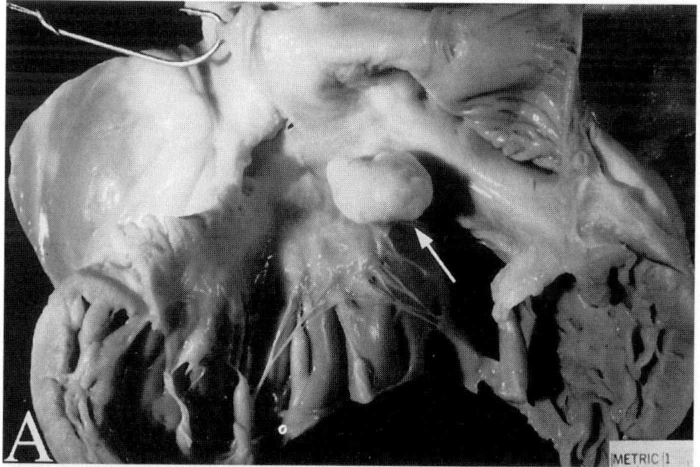

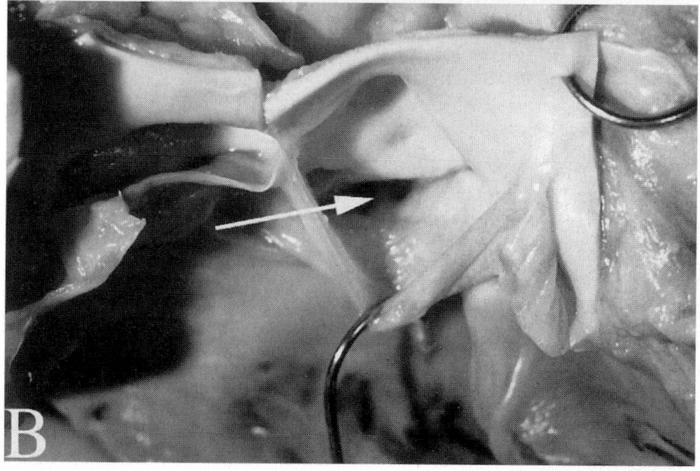

Figure 13–2. Aneurysm of the right sinus of Valsalva. The most obvious feature of a sinus of Valsalva aneurysm at autopsy is the aneurysmal outpouching, which is usually seen in the right atrium or ventricle near the tricuspid valve. *A*. In this case, the aneurysm projected into the right atrium above the septal leaflet of the tricuspid valve (*arrow*). *B*. The aneurysm within the sinus of Valsalva is difficult to see because it is deep within the recess. The gross differential diagnosis of the lesion seen in (*A*) is a spontaneous closure of a ventricular septal defect with windsock deformity; inspection of the aortic root and membranous septum from the left resolves the problem. The patient was an 18-year-old man who died suddenly from a ruptured pseudoaneurysm after remote coarctation repair (similar to Figure 13–1*C*, different patient). The sinus of Valsalva aneurysm was incidental.

Most aneurysms of the sinus of Valsalva are congenital lesions with a strong association with ventricular septal defect. Other congenital anomalies that have been associated with sinus of Valsalva aneurysm are coarctation of aorta and bicuspid aortic valve. The congenital defect may result from a defect of fusion between the aortic media and the heart at the fibrous annulus of the aortic valve. Infective endocarditis and syphilis currently account for the majority of acquired aneurysms of sinus of Valsalva, representing fewer than 20% of total cases.

The age at presentation of congenital aneurysms ranges from 11 to 67 years, with a mean of 34 years. Asians and men appear more susceptible than Caucasians and women.[12] In a recent clinical review of 377 cases, the vast majority were located in the right sinus (81%) and were equally divided between those associated with ventricular septal defect (VSD) (46%) and those without VSD (54%). The next most frequent site is the noncoronary sinus (17%); at this site, only 6% of lesions are associated with VSD. Only 2% have been reported in the left coronary sinus.[13]

The clinical course before rupture is that of a silent lesion. Heart failure and mitral regurgitation may occur in patients with VSD. Rupture results in symptoms that are dependent upon the amount of blood flow through the rupture site and the chamber of flow. In some patients, cardiovascular collapse and even sudden death may occur. In patients who survive the initial rupture, cardiomegaly is usually present.[14] Aortic regurgitation is present in one third of patients and right- or left-sided heart failure is present in 80% of patients with ruptured sinus of Valsalva aneurysm. Chest pain is usually absent. The aneurysmal sac may result in obstruction of the right ventricular outflow tract and (rarely) coronary occlusion; conduction disturbances have also been reported.

The location within the right sinus of Valsalva is predictive of the site of rupture: Those in the left portion of the right sinus of Valsalva protrude towards and rupture into the right ventricular outflow tract near the pulmonary valve. VSDs are frequently associated with this particular anomaly. Those that arise in the middle of the right sinus of Valsalva protrude and rupture into the body of the right ventricle; VSDs are uncommon in this manifestation of the disease. When the aneurysm originates from the posterior portion of the right sinus of Valsalva, it protrudes towards the plane of the tricuspid valve, rupture occurring mostly into the right atrium.[15] Other reported sites of rupture of aneurysms located in the right or left sinuses are the left ventricle and atrium, pericardium, pulmonary artery, and superior vena cava.

The diameter of the rupture site at the base of the sinus of Valsalva aneurysm ranges from 0.4 to 1.1 cm (mean 0.7 cm). The wall of the sinus of Valsalva is thin and consists of smooth muscle cells in a proteoglycan matrix; usually no elastic fibers are identified.

Marfan Syndrome

The Marfan syndrome is an autosomal dominant disorder characterized by abnormalities of the eyes, skeleton, and cardiovascular system.[16] The estimated prevalence rate is approximately 5/100,000 persons, with an estimated average birth rate of 1/10,000 live births.[17] Eye changes include myopia, retinal detachment, elongated globe, and ectopia lentis. Skeletal changes are joint hypermobility, tall stature, pectus excavatum, reduced thoracic kyphosis, scoliosis, arachnodactyly, dolichostenomelia, pectus carinatum, and erosion of the lumbosacral vertebrae from dural ectasia.

The diagnosis of Marfan syndrome is made on clinical criteria, including a close family relative with the syndrome, ectopia lentis, and skeletal changes. Currently, molecular techniques are helpful in the diagnosis, which is supported by mutations in the gene that encodes fibrillin-1 on chromosome 15. Fibrillin-1 is a major component of the 10-12 nm microfibrils, which are thought to play a role in tropoelastin deposition and elastic fiber formation in addition to possessing an anchoring function in some tissues.[18] By the beginning of the year 2000, 137 different fibrillin-1 mutations had been reported.[19] Mutations have been found in almost all of the 65 exons of the fibrillin-1 gene, and most of these mutations have been unique to one affected patient or family. Aside from certain areas in exons 24-27 and 31-32 that are typical of the neonatal Marfan syndrome, there are few morphologic correlates of specific gene mutations.[20] Sporadic cases of Marfan syndrome with the mutation for fibrillin-1 gene have been reported in patients without a family history. To confirm the diagnosis in these patients, there should be documented manifestations in the skeletal system, the cardiovascular system, and one other system. Fibrillin-1 mutations have also been found in patients who do not fulfil clinical criteria for the diagnosis of Marfan syndrome, but have related disorders of connective tissue, such as isolated ectopia lentis, familial aortic aneurysm, and Marfan-like skeletal abnormalities,[21] so that Marfan syndrome may be regarded as one of a range of type 1 fibrillinopathies.[18]

The hallmark histologic manifestation of Marfan syndrome is medial degeneration, or cystic medial necrosis of the aorta (see following) (Fig. 13–3). Medial degeneration, however, is not specific for Marfan syndrome, and may be seen as a consequence of noninflamma-

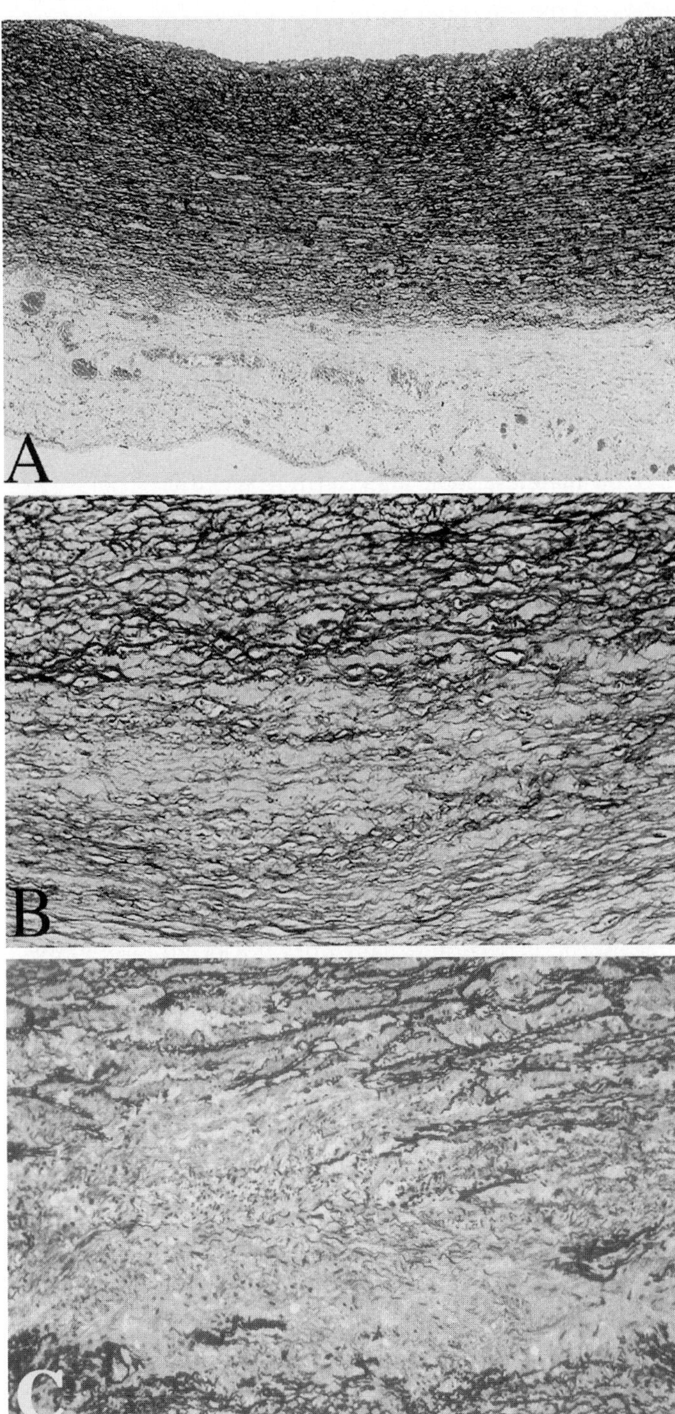

Figure 13–3. Marfan syndrome, histologic appearance of aortic wall. There is variability to the degree of cystic medial necrosis in Marfan syndrome and related diseases. *A* and *B*. Essentially normal and mild medial degeneration, respectively, from the aorta of a 35-year-old man who had been followed since age 4 for Marfan syndrome. At autopsy, a rupture dissection aortic aneurysm was found (not shown). Note the loss of elastic fibers in the lower portion of *B*. *C*. Severe elastic loss with proteoglycan pooling in a different patient with known Marfan syndrome.

tory aortic degeneration in patients with hypertension and bicuspid aortic valve. Cystic medial change tends to be especially prominent and severe in the congenital syndrome, but there are many exceptions to this generalization, as some patients with florid medial degeneration have no familial or known congenital syndrome, and some patients with Marfan and aortic disease have relatively few histologic manifestations.

Cardiovascular abnormalities are detected in the majority of patients with the syndrome; the exact proportion depends on the criteria for diagnosis. The cardiovascular involvement is manifest by aortic root dilatation (39%), aortic dissections (36%), mitral valve prolapse (without other cardiac involvement) (21%), and miscellaneous cardiovascular manifestations. These unusual abnormalities include aneurysms of the sinus of Valsalva and peripheral aneurysms. Although isolated aneurysms of Valsalva are relatively uncommon, aortic root dilatation is believed to begin in the sinuses, and may be manifest soon after birth.[11] Whether there is a significant association between intracranial aneurysms and Marfan syndrome is a matter of debate.[22]

Because of the complications of aortic dissection and aortic insufficiency, patients with Marfan syndrome should be followed for aortic root dilatation. Yearly transesophageal echocardiography is performed. If the aortic root is 1.5 times greater than the expected mean diameter (based on height and weight of patient), more frequent observations are necessary.[23] Aortic regurgitation generally occurs when aortic diameter exceeds 50 mm to 60 mm, but there are no absolute echocardiographic guidelines predicting the onset of symptoms or the onset of dissection. Aortic dissection usually does not occur in adults until the ascending aortic diameter is 55 mm.[24] For this reason, many patients undergo elective composite graft repair of the aorta if the aortic root approaches this diameter.[25] Currently, valve-sparing operations for patients with lesser degrees of dilatation (50 mm) are being offered to patients with Marfan syndrome,[26] although abnormalities of the aortic valve leaflets may theoretically lead to aortic insufficiency.[27]

Mitral valve prolapse in patients with Marfan syndrome occurs with advancing age. Women are more often affected than men. By sensitive two-dimensional echocardiography, as many as 60–80% of women with Marfan syndrome demonstrate mitral insufficiency. The rate of mitral valve prolapse documented at autopsy in patients with Marfan syndrome is probably lower. Gross findings include elongated, redundant anterior and posterior leaflets, with mitral annular calcification in 10%.[28]

Ehlers–Danlos Syndrome

The Ehlers–Danlos syndrome is characterized by hypermobility of the joints, hyperextensibility of the skin, and fragile tissues prone to dystrophic scarring and easy bruising. Body stature and habitus are usually normal, in contrast to Marfan syndrome.

At least nine different forms of the disease have been recognized, many of which show considerable clinical and pathologic overlap. Cardiac complications are limited to type IV Ehlers–Danlos syndrome (vascular type), which is due to defects in the type III procollagen (COL3A1). At the molecular level, the defect is heterogeneous, several different mutations resulting in the clinical phenotype; the types of complications are not associated with specific mutations in COL3A1. Affected patients are at risk for arterial, bowel, and uterine rupture. Complications are rare in childhood, and more than 80% of affected patients have at least one complication by the age of 40. Most deaths resulted from arterial rupture (median age 48 years).[29]

Arterial complications of Ehlers–Danlos syndrome type IV include coronary artery dissections, aortic rupture (Fig. 13–4), iliac and femoral rupture, and coronary and other muscular arterial aneurysms. The most frequently involved sites are the abdominal aorta and its branches, the great vessels of the aortic arch, and the large arteries of the limb.[30] Characteristically, there are multiple rupture sites in the aorta. There are few reports of histologic findings in Ehlers–Danlos syndrome; in our experience, histologic changes may be relatively mild, despite significant transmural tears in the aorta or muscular artery, which may result in fatal hemorrhage or the formation of a pseudoaneurysm.

Osteogenesis Imperfecta

Osteogenesis imperfecta, bearing some clinical overlap with Ehlers–Danlos syndrome, is a heterogeneous disorder of type I collagen affecting approximately one in 60,000 births with a wide range of severity.[31] Clinical manifesta-

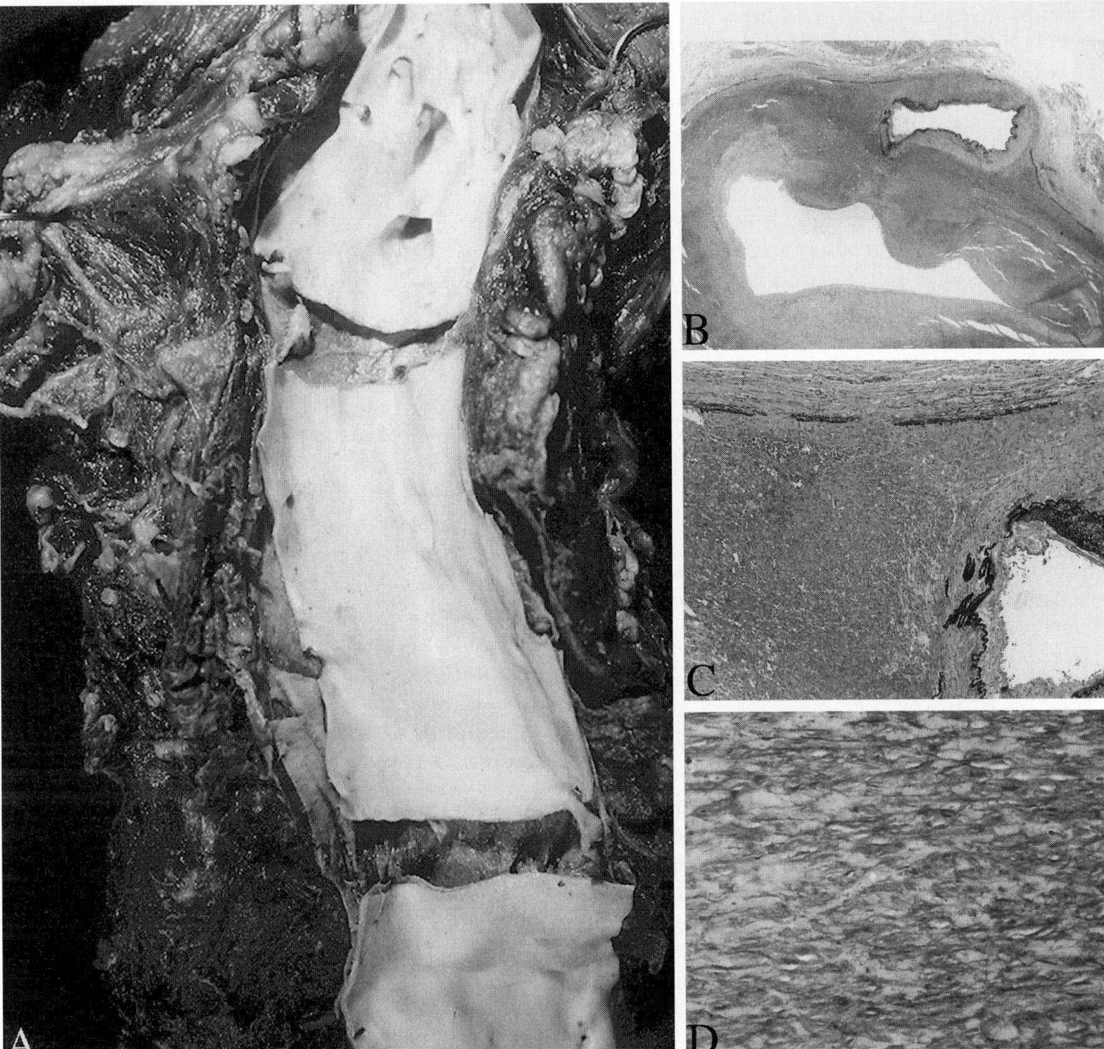

Figure 13–4. Ehlers–Danlos syndrome. *A*. Two transverse lacerations in the aorta of a young man with Ehlers–Danlos syndrome type IV who was found dead. *B* and *C* are photomicrographs (low and high magnification, respectively) from the same section of a splenic artery pseudoaneurysm in a patient with Ehlers–Danlos type IV. *C*. The site of dissection with splitting of the elastic laminae and intervening organizing fibrous tissue. *D*. The aortic media from the ruptured aorta shown in *A*; the histologic features are nonspecific and, often in cases of Ehlers–Danlos syndrome, there is minimal cystic medial change or other recognizable histologic abnormality.

tions include bone fragility with repeated bone fractures, skeletal malformations, and blue sclerae. All forms are the results of mutations in COL1A1 or COL1A2, the genes that encode the proalpha1(I) and proalpha2(I) chains of type I collagen, respectively.[32] The leading cause of death in adults is respiratory insufficiency caused by kyphoscoliosis or (less commonly) compression of the brainstem caused by platybasia of the skull.[33] Cardiac manifestations include aortic root dilatation, aortic insufficiency, and mitral valve prolapse;[34] these complications occur in approximately 7–12% of patients and may result in heart failure.[35] Successful aortic and mitral valve replacements have been performed, although friability of the aorta may make the surgery technically difficult, and aortic dissection may be a complication.[36, 37]

DEGENERATIVE CHANGES

Age-Related Changes

The aorta was called "the greatest artery" by the ancients. This designation is appropriate, as the aorta absorbs the impact of 2.3 to 3 billion heart beats a year while delivering roughly 200 million liters of blood to the various parts of the body.[11] The aorta absorbs the impact of systole by distending. During diastole, the aortic wall recoils, helping to propel the blood distally. Therefore, the elastic properties of the aorta are essential for the maintenance of the pumping function. Because loss of elasticity in soft tissue is a function of senescence, it is not surprising that advanced age results in changes in aortic hemodynamics. The aortic changes in elastic tissue incurred by old age are reflected in gross and microscopic abnormalities, as well as changes in tensile strength. The aorta becomes tortuous because of an increase in length, and its intimal surface doubles between the second and sixth decades. The aortic circumference likewise increases with age, the largest increase occurring in the ascending aorta and the smallest in the abdominal aorta.[38] Medial thickness does not change significantly, whereas the intimal thickness increases with age (the greatest increase occurring in the abdominal aorta). The breaking stress of the human aorta decreases with age, which correlates inversely with collagen recruitment pressure, a measure of stiffness.[39] Histologically, the aging aorta demonstrates fragmentation of elastin with a concomitant increase in collagen, resulting in an increase in collagen to elastic ratio leading to loss in distensibility of the aorta.[40] Degeneration of elastin results in an increase in wall stiffness, leading to an increase in pulse wave velocity. In addition, interruption of the vasa vasorum flow may also lead to an acute decrease in distensibility of the ascending aorta.[41]

Hypertension and atherosclerosis greatly affect the extent of age-related aortic changes. Hypertension results in an accentuation of the age-related increase in the abdominal aortic circumference. Hypertension and atherosclerosis both have a marked effect on the increase in abdominal aortic circumference and intimal thickness.[38]

Medial Degeneration ("Cystic Medial Necrosis")

"Medial degeneration" has been defined as the pooling of proteoglycans and the appearance of cyst-like structures in the media, and "medionecrosis" as an apparent loss of nuclei in the media.[42] These conditions may be present to mild degrees in normal aortas of older people; hence, they are believed to be primarily degenerative in nature. However, there is a genetic predisposition to the development of extensive medial degeneration. The presence of medial degeneration is typically associated with Marfan syndrome,[43] bicuspid aortic valve,[44] idiopathic annuloaortic ectasia,[43] in addition to age-related hypertensive changes. In general, the degree of medial degeneration is greater in the congenital conditions (Marfan and bicuspid aortic valve, and annular ectasia in young patients), as compared with age-related acquired diseases. The pathophysiology of medial degeneration is unknown, although cell cultures of medial smooth muscle cells of affected aortas show evidence of apoptosis.[45] The genetics of medial degeneration that is seen in Marfan syndrome, and possibly other forms of aortic root dilatation, involves mutations in fibrillin-1 (see earlier).

Histologic changes are best evaluated if the aorta is sectioned in the transverse plane and stained for elastic tissue and consist of elastic fragmentation, loss of smooth muscle cells, and pooling of proteoglycans (Fig. 13–5). The site of sectioning is important; we usually section the aorta at or near the site of dissection, as well as remote from the dissection in an area of intact aorta. Although the elastic van Gieson stain demonstrates elastic fibers, the Movat pentachrome stain is preferable, as it stains for proteoglycans (an important component of cystic medial necrosis) and smooth muscle cells (which are lost in areas of degeneration). Immunohistochemical staining for fibrillin using frozen sections demonstrates fragmentation of the elastic in the mid portion of the media which is more prominent in patients with Marfan syndrome and histologic features of severe medial degeneration, as compared to elderly patients with mild medial changes.[27]

Schlatmann and Becker grade the extent of cystic medial necrosis as three grades, based on the extent of cystic change, elastic fragmentation, fibrosis, and "medionecrosis," or loss of nuclei within the media.[40] The most dramatic extent of cystic medial necrosis is seen in patients with Marfan syndrome and forms of idiopathic annuloaortic ectasia. Severe cystic medial necrosis is characterized by pools of proteoglycans in the aortic wall with fragmentation and loss of elastic lamellae. However, in many cases of aortic dissection, including those with Marfan syndrome, only mild medial changes are noted. In these cases there is a minimal increase in proteoglycans with focal mild elastic tissue loss.

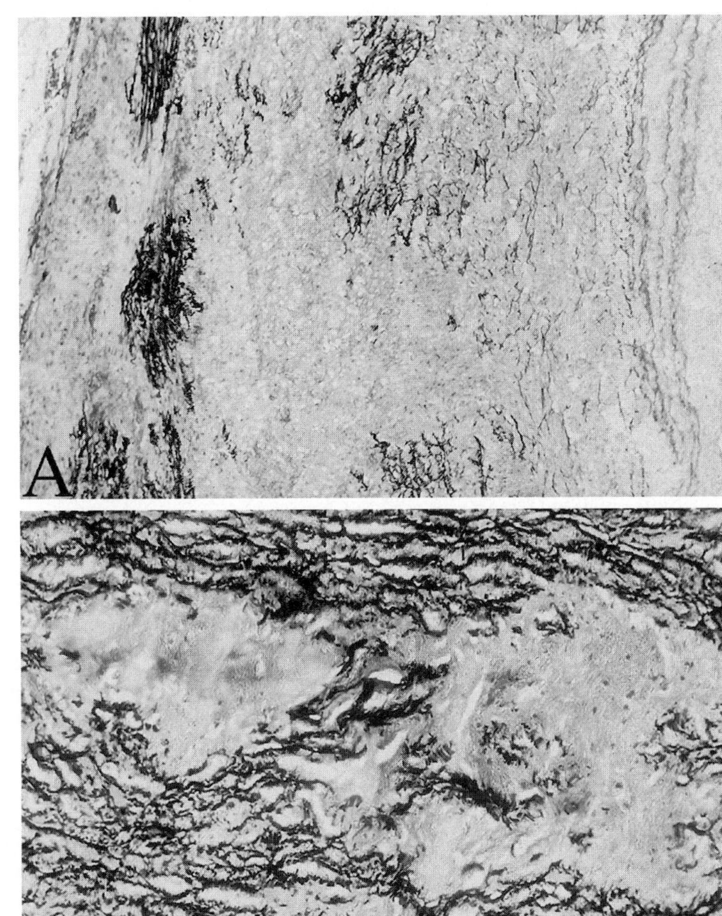

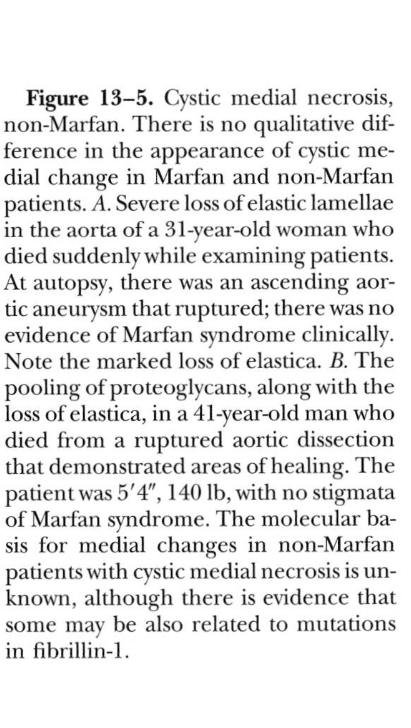

Figure 13–5. Cystic medial necrosis, non-Marfan. There is no qualitative difference in the appearance of cystic medial change in Marfan and non-Marfan patients. *A.* Severe loss of elastic lamellae in the aorta of a 31-year-old woman who died suddenly while examining patients. At autopsy, there was an ascending aortic aneurysm that ruptured; there was no evidence of Marfan syndrome clinically. Note the marked loss of elastica. *B.* The pooling of proteoglycans, along with the loss of elastica, in a 41-year-old man who died from a ruptured aortic dissection that demonstrated areas of healing. The patient was 5′4″, 140 lb, with no stigmata of Marfan syndrome. The molecular basis for medial changes in non-Marfan patients with cystic medial necrosis is unknown, although there is evidence that some may be also related to mutations in fibrillin-1.

INFLAMMATORY DISEASES

Characteristics of Aortitis

Aortitis is defined as inflammation of the wall of the aorta with or without disruption of elastic fibers, aortic wall necrosis, or fibrosis. The definition implies the absence of underlying conditions that may secondarily result in chronic inflammation. The most important of these is atherosclerosis, which is characterized by chronic inflammation of the intima, often with involvement of the media and even adventitia. Because, in addition, atherosclerosis may be superimposed on aortitis, the distinction between atherosclerosis and aortitis as a primary diagnosis is sometimes difficult. This distinction is usually facilitated, however, by considering the distribution of the process and clinical data.

Aortitis is classified into infectious and noninfectious causes. The most important causes are Takayasu's disease (especially in younger patients), syphilis, and giant-cell aortitis (especially in older patients). Because there are no pathognomonic histologic features of the three major types of aortitis, evaluation of clinical and pathologic data is important to arrive at a final diagnosis (Table 13–1).

The connective tissue diseases that may involve the aorta are rheumatoid arthritis, ankylosing spondylitis, Reiter's syndrome, and Behçet's disease; these are discussed below. Tuberculous aortitis is currently rare in developed countries, and involves the thoracic or abdominal aorta with equal frequency and is usually the result of contiguous spread from a tuberculoma from the lung or periaortic lymph node. Extremely rarely, the aorta may be involved by sarcoid, which tends to involve small and medium-sized arteries of the lung. Because tuberculous and sarcoid involvement of the aorta is rare, they will not be further discussed.

Table 13–1. Pathologic Differential Diagnosis of Aortitis

Feature	Giant Cell	Takayasu's	Syphilitic	Collagen-vascular*
Aortic aneurysms	+++	+/−	+++	++
Luminal narrowing	−/+	+++	−	−
Coronary ostial stenosis	+	++	++	+
Aortic valve involvement	−	++	−	+++
Arch involvement	++	+++	++	−/+
Skip areas	−	+++	+/−	+/−
"Tree barking"	+++	+++	+++	+
Site in aorta	throughout	thoracic +/− abd	ascending	ascending +/− abd
Dissection	+/−	−	−	−
Aortic annular dilatation	+	−	++/+++	++
Luminal thrombosis	+/−	+++	+/−	−
Superimposed atherosclerosis	++	+/−	+++	+/−
Endarteritis obliterans	+/−	++	+++	++
Giant cells	+++	+/++	+/−	+
Plasma cells	+	+/++	+++	++
Medial necrosis	+/−	+	+/++	+

* Includes rheumatoid and seronegative spondyloarthropathies (ankylosing spondylitis/Reiter's). In rheumatoid aortitis, characteristic necrobiotic nodules may be present in some cases.
abd = abdominal

Takayasu's Arteritis

Takayasu's arteritis was first described by the Japanese ophthalmologist, Takayasu, in 1908 in a 21-year-old woman with ocular changes.[46] It was not until 1951, however, that Shimizu and Sano[47] detailed the clinical features of this disorder which, in 1954, was termed Takayasu's arteritis. There are numerous syndromes for Takayasu's disease, including aortic arch syndrome, pulseless disease, reversed coarctation, occlusive thromboaortopathy, and young female arteritis. Aortitis in patients without the clinical history of the acute phase of the disease, but with pathologic features of Takayasu's aortitis, is sometimes termed "nonspecific aortoarteritis."

Clinical Manifestations

Takayasu's disease affects women more frequently than men in a ratio of 8:1. The incidence in North American and European populations is approximately 2 per million per year. The majority of the reported cases have been in Asian and African patients, but the disease has a worldwide distribution.[48–50] The age at diagnosis ranges from 3.5 to 66 years, with a mean of 20 to 50 years. There is an association with human histocompatibility haplotypes HLA B52 and HLA B39. These histocompatibility loci are associated with specific sites of involvement: Patients with the HLA B52 histocompatibility allele are more likely to have coronary, pulmonary, and proximal aortic disease, whereas patients with HLA B39 are more likely to have renal and abdominal aortic disease.[51]

The acute phase of the disease is characterized by malaise, weakness, fever, arthralgias, myalgias, weight loss, pleuritic pain, and anorexia. This phase may vary widely in severity and often precedes the occlusive phase by weeks to months, or an asymptomatic period may intervene for up to 6 to 8 years. Coronary artery involvement may result in myocardial infarction and cardiac arrest.[52]

Symptoms of the late phase include diminished or absent pulses in 96% of patients, bruits in 94%, hypertension in 74%, and heart failure in 28%.[49] In addition to stenotic lesions, aneurysmal dilatations may cause palpable pulsatile masses, embolism from mural thrombi, and, rarely sudden death from rupture of a rapidly expanding aneurysm. Although stenotic lesions generally dominate, the incidence of aneurysmal lesions is estimated to be over 30%; indeed, aneurysms may be the sole clinical manifestation.[53] Involvement of the aortic root and aortic valve occurs in 10–20% of patients and may lead to aortic insufficiency.[54] In a series of autopsies from India, the sequelae of chronic hypertension (cardiac hypertrophy, renal failure, and cerebrovascular disease) are especially common; in this series, the unusual manifestation of aortic dissection is reported.[55]

Ueda et al. have subdivided Takayasu's disease into three types.[56] Type I denotes involvement of the aortic arch and the brachiocephalic vessels. In type II, there is involvement of the descending thoracic aorta and abdominal aorta without involvement of the arch. In type III involvement, lesions are located in the arch and in the thoracic and abdominal aorta. Lupi-Herrera has suggested an additional variant (type IV) denoting involvement of the pulmonary arteries as well.[49] In some patients, pulmonary artery involvement may be the primary clinical manifestation, with pulmonary artery obstruction and secondary pulmonary hypertension.[57]

Laboratory abnormalities in Takayasu's disease are most severe in the acute phase of illness, and include elevated sedimentation rate (which is usually normal in the chronic phase), low-grade leukocytosis, and mild normochromic normocytic anemia. Elevated serum IgG and IgM and immune complexes are frequently present. There is an association with HLA B5, Bw52, and Dw12 antigens in patients with severe inflammation and a rapidly progressive course.[58]

Pathology

The acute phase of Takayasu's disease is characterized by edema, patchy necrosis, chronic inflammation, and scattered giant cells in the outer two thirds of the media, adventitia, adventitial fat, and vasa vasorum. The vasa vasorum may show intimal proliferation with obliteration but no fibrinoid necrosis. Because small-vessel involvement of the walls of the elastic arteries is a feature of the disease, which may be accompanied by cutaneous vasculitis and pyoderma gangrenosum, some researchers have suggested that small-vessel inflammation may be involved in the pathogenesis of Takayasu's arteritis.[59] The infiltrates of the acute lesions are primarily composed of T cells and natural killer cells that have been shown by immunohistochemical stains to express perforin.[60]

The late phase is characterized by marked intimal and adventitial thickening of the vessels. Grossly, there are areas of aortic thickening with narrowing of the lumen and stenosis of the arch vessels (Figs. 13–6 and 13–7). In a series of patients from the United States, the most frequently affected arteries after the aorta were the subclavian, 90%; carotid, 45%; vertebral, 25%; and renal, 20%.[61] Autopsies have shown that the subclavian arteries, mesenteric arteries, and abdominal aorta were histologically involved in nearly 80% of patients.[48] In an autopsy study of Indian patients, abdominal aortic involvement was most common, and aneurysms nearly as frequent as stenosis.[55]

Scarring and revascularization give rise to the "tree-bark" appearance characteristic of aortitis. Typically, there are skip areas and segmental areas of stenoses, which may be accompanied by areas of aneurysm.[62] In approximately 30% of patients, the predominant lesions are

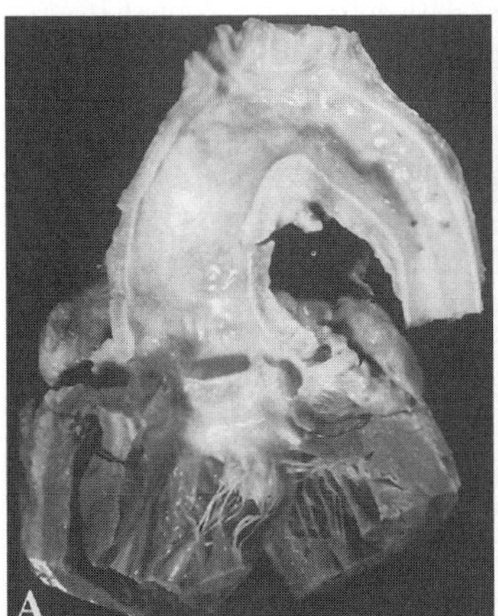

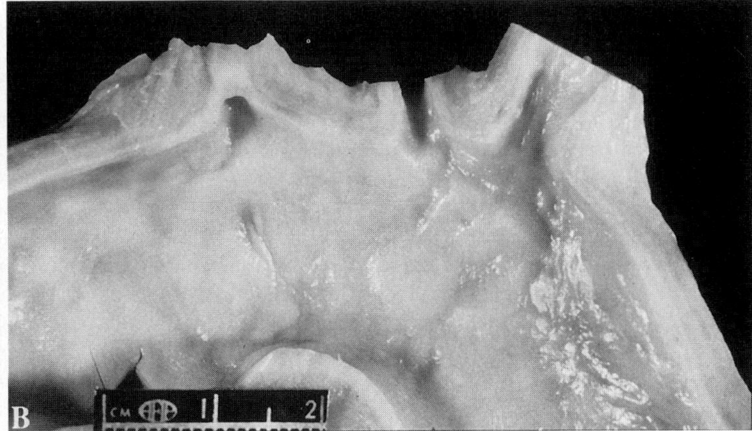

Figure 13–6. Takayasu's aortitis. *A.* The posterior portion of the heart and aorta. Note the intimal fibrosis of the aorta with narrowing of the arch vessels. *B.* A higher magnification of the anterior portion of the aortic arch, the other half of the specimen shown in *A.* Note the thick band of collagen in areas of the adventitia, and ostial narrowing of the arch vessels typical of Takayasu's disease.

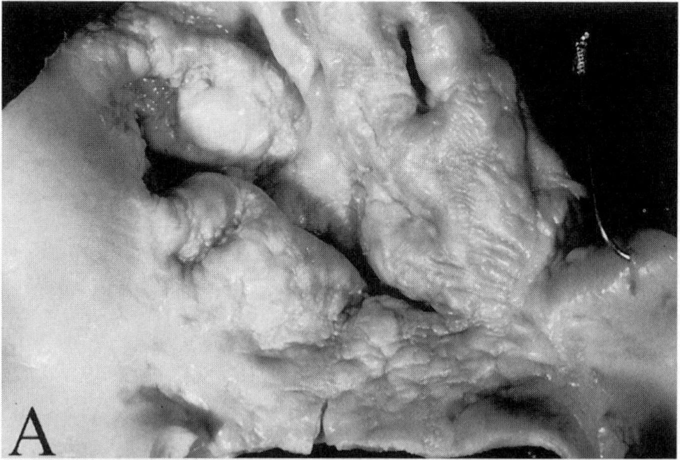

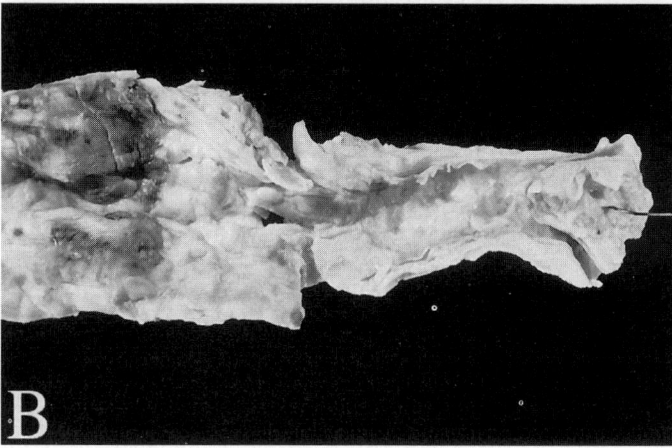

Figure 13–7. Takayasu's aortitis. *A*. Characteristically, there is the "tree-bark" wrinkled appearance of aortitis, with skip areas (note relatively normal intima on the left in this photograph of the aortic arch). *B*. There is narrowing of the abdominal aorta distal to the renal arteries (right is distal in this photograph). Superimposed atherosclerotic changes may complicate gross diagnosis. Abdominal stenoses in Takayasu's disease are especially common in Indian patients.

ectasias or aneurysms of the aorta.[63] The stenotic lesions are produced by a circumferentially thickened intima with a glossy, gray, or myxoid appearance of the cut surface. Multisegmental involvement with areas of normal between affected segments are characteristic, although there may be diffuse involvement of the aorta and isolated disease of individual arteries.

In the chronic phase, the intima is hypocellular with scattered smooth muscle cells and fibroblasts. The medial elastic laminae are disorganized or focally absent and replaced by collagen and granulation tissue. Areas of necrosis with chronic inflammatory infiltrates typically persist into the late phase (Fig. 13–8). The adventitia always demonstrates fibrosis, often with lymphoid aggregates and obliteration of the vasa vasorum. Areas of scarring may demonstrate dystrophic calcification of the media and adventitia.

Coronary artery involvement occurs in 15% of patients, typically limited to the ostia or proximal segments (see Chapter 4). Rarely it is the sole manifestation of the disease, and diffuse involvement of the entire epicardial arteries has been reported.[64–70] Sequelae of coronary artery involvement include angina, myocardial infarction, and even sudden death.

Pulmonary artery involvement in Takayasu's disease is not well studied histologically. In an autopsy series of six cases of typical Takayasu's aortitis, pathohistologic characters of the pulmonary artery were found to be similar to those of the systemic arteries. However, luminal obstruction with recanalized thrombi of the pulmonary elastic arteries were found in four cases and not seen in systemic arteries. Cellular arteritis of muscular pulmonary arteries was seen in two cases, and angiomatoid dilatation of small blood vessels (similar to plexiform lesions) in two cases, suggesting significant pulmonary hypertension.[71]

Treatment of chronic vascular sequela of Takayasu's disease includes bypass and stenting of stenoses, including carotid, abdominal aortic, and renal occlusions,[62, 72–74] bypass or bal-

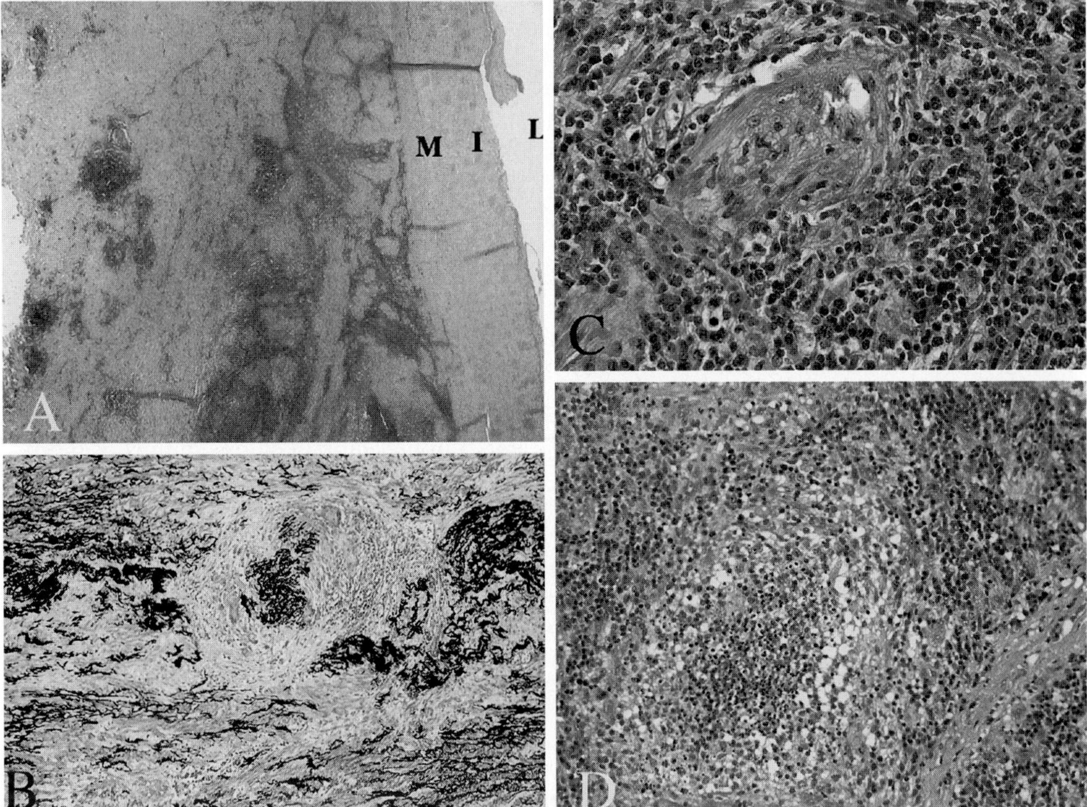

Figure 13–8. Takayasu's aortitis. *A*. The typical appearance of the markedly thickening adventitial with lymphoid aggregates. The media (*M*) and intima (*I*) are at the right, adjacent to the lumen (*L*). *B*. A high magnification of the media, demonstrating fragmentation of the elastic laminae with granulomatous inflammation and scattered giant cells. *C*. There is inflammation of the vasa vasorum. *D*. A focus of acute inflammation, which is relatively unusual in cases of Takayasu disease.

loon angioplasty with stenting of coronary lesions,[75, 76] and aortic root repair for ascending aortic aneurysms.[77]

Giant-Cell Aortitis

Giant-cell arteritis is a systemic panarteritis affecting predominantly elderly patients. It consists of focal granulomatous inflammation of large- and medium-sized arteries, especially the temporal artery. The aorta and its major branches are affected in 15% of the cases. The incidence in the United States is 15 to 30 cases per year per 100,000 persons over the age of 50 years. The disease occurs predominantly in women, with a high incidence in persons of Northern European descent. The etiology of giant-cell arteritis is unknown, but may be a manifestation of autoimmunity or infection. Ten to 15% of patients with known giant-cell arteritis with temporal artery involvement have aortic disease; these patients often have polymyalgia rheumatica.[78–80]

Clinical Manifestations

Symptoms of giant-cell arteritis that suggest aortic involvement are claudication of upper or lower extremities, parasthesias, Raynaud's phenomenon, abdominal angina, coronary ischemia, transient ischemic attacks, and aortic arch and great vessel "steal" syndrome. Aortic aneurysms with aortic valve regurgitation or aortic dissection are being recognized more frequently in patients with giant-cell arteritis. Unlike Takayasu's arteritis, renal artery involvement is rare and hypertension not a characteristic complication of giant-cell aortitis.[81, 82]

Laboratory manifestations of giant-cell arteritis include a very high sedimentation rate, elevated acute phase reactants, hypergammaglobulinemia, and increased serum C_3 and C_4

complement levels, the levels of which often reflect disease activity. Angiography may demonstrate aortic root dilatation, aortic insufficiency, and long, smooth, tapering stenosis with areas of dilatation in the subclavian, axillary, and brachial arteries.

Pathology

The aorta typically demonstrates aortic root dilatation, with medial dissection in occasional cases of aortic rupture. The intima is wrinkled, demonstrating a "tree-bark" appearance similar to that seen in other inflammatory diseases of the aorta (Fig. 13–9). Histologically, the inflammatory infiltrate is mononuclear, consisting of lymphocytes, plasma cells, and histiocytes. There is disruption of the internal elastic lamina with fragmentation and a giant-cell reaction of the Langhan's type. The disruption may be accompanied by a significant degree of necrosis. The finding of a large number of giant cells is helpful but not considered a prerequisite for the diagnosis because, in some cases, only a few such cells are found either in the temporal artery or in the other arteries at autopsy. In healed lesions, intimal fibrosis predominates and minimal cellular reaction remains; however, elastic tissue stains demonstrate extensive disruption of the elastic fibers.

It is usually the combination of the clinical features and the microscopic findings that help separate the giant-cell arteritis from other arteritic diseases.[83] Features of giant-cell aortitis that help distinguish it from Takayasu's disease are patient age greater than 70 years, intimal scarring that is only mild or moderate (Fig. 13–9), a lack of adventitial scarring and inflammation, and the lack of endarteritis obliterans. In some cases, a definitive distinction cannot be made, and a nonspecific diagnosis of aortitis given.

Rheumatoid Aortitis

Rheumatoid involvement of the heart is well recognized to result in symptomatic disease. Histologic features of aortitis are present in approximately 10% of autopsies and are usually not related to clinical symptoms. Gravallese et

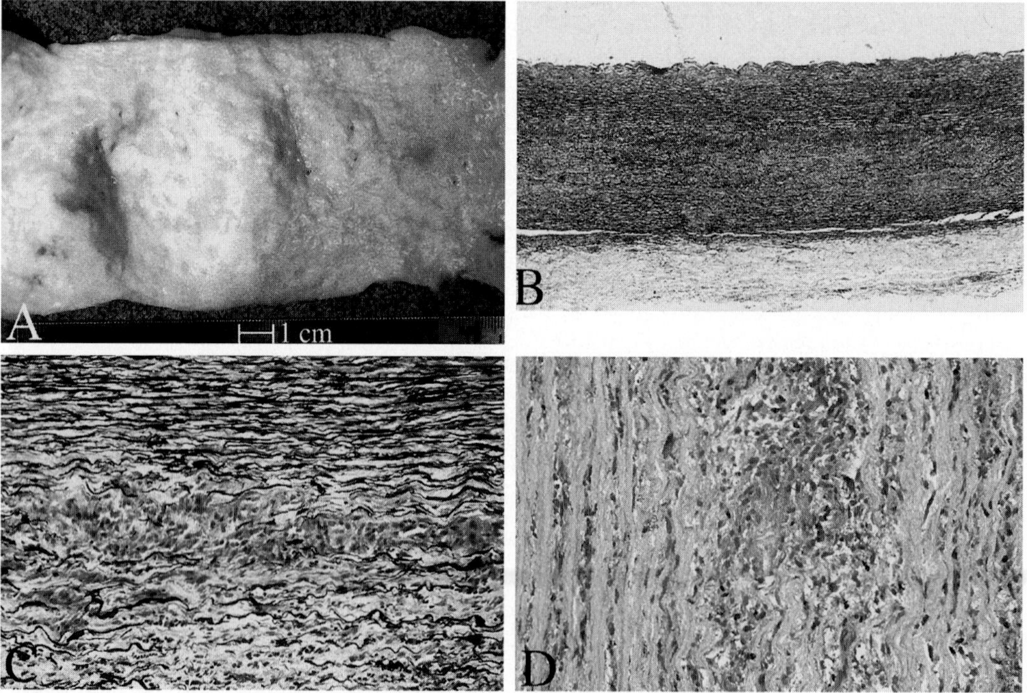

Figure 13–9. Giant cell aortitis. *A.* The wrinkled intimal appearance typical of aortitis of whatever etiology. There is diffuse ectasis of the aorta in this case, which may occur in Takayasu's disease, but which is more typical of giant-cell aortitis. *B.* A histologic section of the specimen; note that the adventitia (bottom pale strip) is relatively spared in giant-cell aortitis, a feature that reliably distinguishes it from Takayasu's disease. *C.* A higher magnification of *B*, showing mild disruption of elastic laminae with giant cells (elastic stain). *D.* A H & E stained section showing the granulomatous inflammation within the media.

al. reported clinically significant aortitis in three of 188 consecutive autopsies of patients with rheumatoid arthritis. Two of these three patients suffered from aortic insufficiency and heart failure, and one from ruptured abdominal aortitic aneurysm.[84, 85]

The mean duration of patients with rheumatoid aortitis is ten years, and there is no sex predilection. Pathologically, the aortic wall is thickened with focal necrosis; aneurysms may develop in the thoracic or abdominal aorta. Microscopically, well-formed rheumatoid nodules are found in approximately 50% of cases; in the remainder, there is a lymphoplasmacytic infiltrate, predominantly in the media and adventitia, accompanied by necrosis of the smooth muscle cells and loss of medial elastic fibers. In the absence of rheumatoid nodules, the histologic features demonstrate considerable overlap with Takayasu's disease, syphilis, and ankylosing spondylitis; a clinical history is generally adequate in establishing the diagnosis. In contrast to ankylosing spondylitis, the severity of aortitis in patients with rheumatoid arthritis appears closely associated with the severity of disease, rather than duration.

Syphilitic Aortitis

Cardiovascular syphilis once accounted for 5 to 10% of all cardiovascular deaths; however, today only an occasional case of syphilis is seen at the autopsy table. Cardiac complications occur in approximately 10% of untreated cases of syphilis. The latent period varies from 5 to 40 years, with the usual being 10 to 25 years.[86–90]

Syphilitic heart disease can be divided into four categories: (1) syphilitic aortitis; (2) syphilitic aortic aneurysm; (3) syphilitic aortic valvulitis with aortic regurgitation; and (4) syphilitic coronary ostial stenosis. Of 126 patients reported by Heggtveit, 42 (33%) had only syphilitic aortitis and 84 (67%) had one or more of the major complications of aneurysm, aortic regurgitation, and coronary ostial stenosis.[88] The clinical diagnosis of syphilis was made in only 20% of his cases.

Pathology

Syphilitic aortitis involves the proximal aorta, and does not extend below the renal arteries, probably because of rich vascular and lymphatic circulation that is limited to the thoracic aorta. However, well-documented cases of syphilitic aneurysms of the abdominal aorta exist.[90] The aortic intima has a "tree-bark" appearance with focal areas of intimal thickening that appears as white and shiny. In late stages, the characteristic gross intimal lesions may be obscured by atherosclerosis. The aortic wall may be thickened in early stages, with subsequent aneurysmal thinning and calcification. Aortic rupture may occur, but dissections are unusual.[89] Because of aortic root involvement and superimposed intimal thickening, there may be coronary ostial narrowing.

Syphilitic aneurysms may be saccular or fusiform (Fig. 13–10), and the frequency of various sites is as follows: sinus of Valsalva, < 1%; ascending aorta, 46%; transverse arch, 24%; descending arch, 5%; descending thoracic aorta, 5%; abdominal aorta, 7%; and multiple sites, 4%. The most common complications of syphilitic aneurysms are aortic insufficiency and rupture. Uncommon complications include superior vena cava syndrome, bony erosion, aortopulmonary fistula, paraparesis, and stroke.[91–93]

The characteristic initial histologic lesion is a multifocal lymphoplasmacytic infiltrate around vasa vasorum of the adventitia with extension into the media (Fig. 13–11). Occasional giant cells may also occur. The lesion is not specific, however, as endarteritis obliterans also occurs in Takayasu's aortitis and ankylosing spondylitis, and plasma cells (and even giant cells) are seen in all types of aortic inflammation including atherosclerosis. The inflammation causes destruction of the media that with time is replaced by scar tissue resulting in wrinkling and scarring. The inflammation may extend into the aortic root resulting in aortic regurgitation from dilatation of the aortic annulus. Microgummas may occur within the aortic media, which consist of a central area of necrosis showing a faint outline of dead cells and surrounding palisading macrophages, lymphocytes, and plasma cells. Organisms are usually scant in these gummas and are difficult to demonstrate.

Differential Diagnosis

Because the histologic appearance of syphilitic aortitis may mimic that of noninfectious aortitis (especially Takayasu's disease and ankylosing spondylitis), we do not advise rendering a diagnosis of syphilitic aortitis based only on histology in the absence of serologic evidence of syphilis. In general, massive aortic root dilatation with thinning of the aortic wall is most

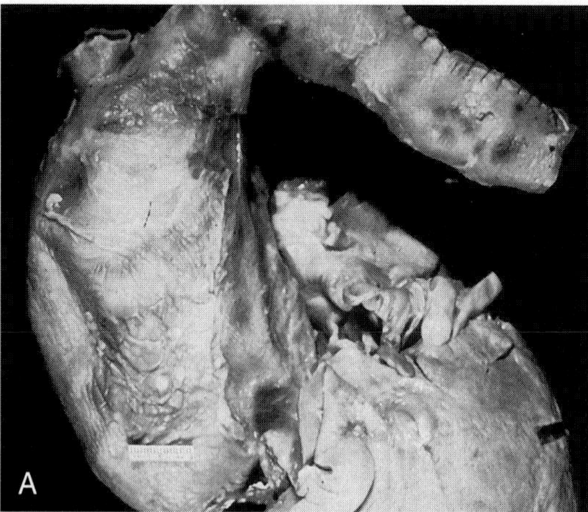

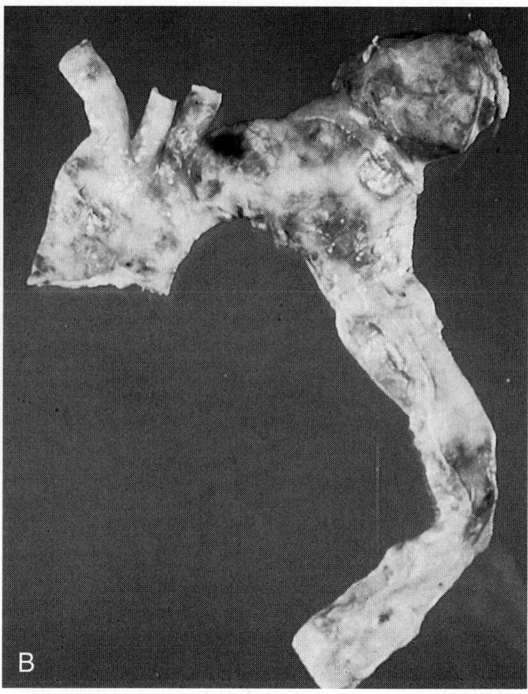

Figure 13–10. Syphilitic aortitis. *A*. The typical location of a syphilitic aneurysm in the ascending aorta. Aneurysms of syphilis tend to be very thin walled and are prone to rupture. *B*. An unusual location of syphilitic aneurysm: the descending thoracic aorta distal to the subclavian artery. In this location, a pseudoaneurysm resulting from latent or occult trauma is a more likely diagnosis. (Courtesy of Dr. William Roberts.)

likely due to syphilis, but lesser degrees of aneurysm formation are currently more typical of Takayasu's aortitis or giant-cell aortitis.

A history of syphilis is necessary for the diagnosis of syphilitic aortitis; other manifestations of tertiary syphilis are seen in 10 to 30% of the patients with cardiovascular syphilis. In the absence of a clinical history, positive serology (which may be performed on postmortem serum) is a prerequisite for the diagnosis. In late stages of tertiary syphilis, nontreponemal tests may be negative, necessitating confirmation with treponemal tests such as treponema pallidum immobilization or fluorescent treponemal antibody (FTA-ABS) absorption. However, it must be remembered that an isolated positive FTA-ABS is not diagnostic for syphilis, as false positives may occur in various conditions, including collagen vascular diseases that may also cause aortitis.[94–97]

Pyogenic Aortitis (Infectious Aneurysm)

Nontreponemal infections of the aorta generally result in saccular or, less commonly, fusiform aneurysms. The original designation "mycotic aneurysm" is gradually being replaced by the more accurate term "infectious aneurysm." There are four routes of invasion of the aorta by bacteria: (1) implantation on intimal surface; (2) embolization of bacteria into vasa vasorum; (3) direct extension of infection from contiguous extravascular site; and (4) traumatic inoculation of contaminated material into vessel wall. Contiguous inoculation is generally a complication of vertebral osteomyelitis, and surface inoculation is often a complication of recent or remote bacterial endocarditis. In some cases of intimal inoculation, the site of infection is an atherosclerotic plaque. The formation of the aneurysm may evolve rapidly, over the course of days, after the initiation of the aortitis.[98–101]

The femoral artery is the most common site of mycotic aneurysms (56%), followed by the abdominal aorta (18%), the thoracic aorta (15%), and mesenteric and peripheral arteries (11%).[102] Before the advent of antibiotics, various coccal species—including pneumococcus, staphylococci, and gonococcal organisms—were the most common pathogens responsible for pyogenic aortitis.[101] More recently, salmonella species have been more frequently isolated from infected aortic aneurysms. Organisms cultured from mycotic aneurysms include *S. aureus* (46%), Salmonella species (15%), streptococci (8%), *E. coli* (8%), no organisms detected (9%), and miscellaneous (13%).[102]

Grossly, infectious aneurysms are often saccular outpouchings measuring up to 5 cm in diam-

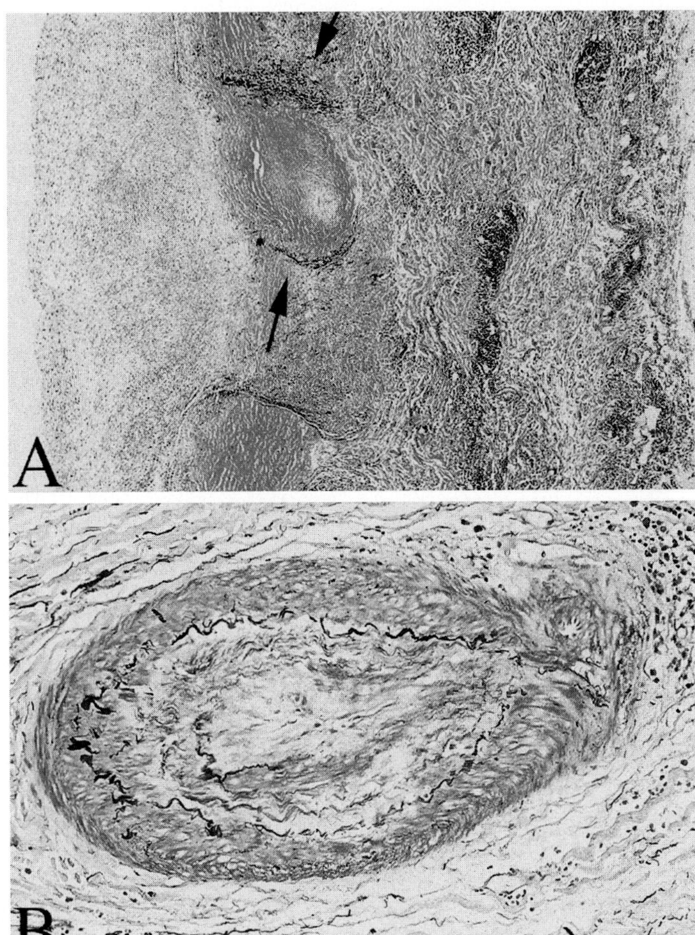

Figure 13–11. Syphilitic aortitis. The histologic features are not specific, and organisms are rarely demonstrated. *A.* There is intimal thickening (*left*), medial destruction (note area of necrosis within the media, *arrows*), and adventitial thickening (*right*). There is lymphoplasmacytic infiltrate especially around vasa vasorum. The histologic features of syphilitic aortitis most closely resemble Takayasu's aortitis; history and serologic testing are critical in separating the two. *B.* Obliteration of the vasa vasorum (endarteritis obliterans), which is typical of syphilis and other aortitis, including Takayasu's disease and Behçet's disease.

eter. There is typically marked edema and inflammation of the adventitia, which results in characteristic soft-tissue swelling on computed tomography or magnetic resonance imaging. Histologically, there are numerous neutrophils with extension into the adventitia. Chronic inflammation with occasional neutrophils are typically seen in atherosclerosis; infected atherosclerotic plaques should only be suspected with a pyogenic reaction and history suggestive of sepsis.

Ankylosing Spondylitis

Ankylosing spondylitis is an idiopathic inflammatory disorder of young men, characterized by progressive bilateral sacroiliitis, peripheral arthritis, and uveitis. The etiology of ankylosing spondylitis is uncertain, although the presence of unusually high frequency of HLA-B27 antigen in up to 95% of affected patients (and in 50% of their first-degree relatives) provides overwhelming evidence of genetic linkage.[103] Aortic disease in patients with ankylosing spondylitis has been described since the 1950s.[104] Symptomatic aortic involvement in ankylosing spondylitis ranges from 1–10% and is related to the duration of the disease, although aortic involvement may precede arthritis. Evidence of aortic insufficiency is found in one third of men with ankylosing spondylitis, and transesophageal echocardiography demonstrates thickened subaortic structures in a high proportion of these patients.[103–106]

Pathologically, there is inflammation and scarring of the sinus of Valsalva and several centimeters of the proximal tubular aorta. In the active phase, there is endarteritis obliterans and perivascular infiltration by lymphocytes and plasma cells. In the chronic phase, there is fibrosis that involves the adventitia, media, and intima; calcification may be present. The coronary ostia may be narrowed and the aortic valve is invariably thickened. Fibrosis extends into the membranous and muscular septum, and onto the anterior leaflet of the mitral valve resulting in a characteristic "bump" seen at autopsy.[106, 107]

The clinical manifestations of aortic involvement in patients with ankylosing spondylitis reflect the pathologic extent of inflammation and fibrosis. Aortic valve disease results in aortic regurgitation, and extension of the fibrotic process in the membranous and muscular septa may result in heart block, conduction defects, and even sudden death.

Reiter's Syndrome

Reiter's syndrome is characterized by the triad of nongonococcal urethritis, conjunctivitis, and polyarthritis. Young men are most often affected, and the arthritis is typically located in the sacroiliac joint. Cardiovascular involvement in Reiter's syndrome is uncommon and is remarkably similar to ankylosing spondylitis. Two to 5% of patients with Reiter's syndrome suffer from aortitis with dilatation of the aortic root and aortic regurgitation. Other cardiovascular manifestations include pericarditis, myocarditis, and various conduction delays.[108] The latter are likely secondary to aortic root inflammation extending into the area of the atrioventricular node. Like ankylosing spondylitis, aortic involvement is limited to the ascending aorta. Microscopically, there is disruption of elastic tissue and infiltration by chronic inflammatory cells.[83]

Behçet's Disease

Behçet's disease is a recurring illness characterized by aphthous stomatitis, genital ulceration, and uveitis.[109] It occurs worldwide but most patients are from the Mediterranean region, Middle East, Japan, and Korea. The etiology of Behçet's disease is unknown, although viral, bacterial, and chemical factors have been suggested.

Involvement of large vessels occurs in 2 to 20% of patients with Behçet's disease.[110, 111] The patients' ages range from 31 to 56 years at presentation and there is a male predominance. The pathologic findings consist of peripheral arterial aneurysms that grossly resemble mycotic aneurysms,[112] aneurysms of the sinus of Valsalva,[113] abdominal aortic aneurysms,[85, 114] arterial occlusions, arterial dissections, and large venous thrombophlebitis. Arterial aneurysms are more frequent than arterial occlusions, although the two may occur together in the same patient. The abdominal aorta is the most common artery involved by aneurysm, followed by the iliac, common femoral, superficial femoral, popliteal, subclavian, carotid, and posterior tibial arteries.[115]

Aortitis in Behçet's disease can be divided into active and scar stages. In active aortitis, intense round cell inflammatory infiltrate occurs in the media and adventitia with predominance of inflammatory cells around proliferating vasa vasorum. Rarely, giant cells may be seen.[111] In the late stages there is fibrous thickening of the intima and adventitia with mild perivascular inflammatory infiltrate and proliferation of vasa vasorum, which may progress to obliteration of the vasa vasorum and endarteritis obliterans. The histologic features are similar to those of Takayasu's disease and ankylosing spondylitis,[116] although granulomas and giant cells are unusual in Behçet's and more typical of Takayasu's aortitis.

AORTIC ANEURYSMS

Thoracic Aortic Aneurysm

Aneurysms of the thoracic aorta comprise five major types: atherosclerotic/degenerative aneurysms, dissecting aneurysms (acute and chronic), annuloaortic ectasia, pseudoaneurysms, and inflammatory aneurysms. The underlying histologic substrate for a large proportion of dissecting aneurysms and annuloaortic ectasia is medial degeneration, although there are a variety of causes. Pseudoaneurysms are generally the result of trauma, but may also result from ruptured atherosclerotic ulcers or infections. Inflammatory aneurysms were historically most frequently due to infections (syphilis and tuberculosis), but are currently only rarely due to infectious agents (so-called mycotic or infectious aneurysms). The majority of inflammatory aneurysms seen today are located in the thoracic aorta and are the result of Takayasu's aortitis in young adults, and giant-cell aortitis in the elderly. The reader is referred to other portions of this chapter for descriptions of the various pathologic processes that give rise to aortic aneurysms.

The relative proportions of etiologic types of thoracic aortic aneurysms are largely unknown, dependent on the patient population and methods of classification, and inclusion criteria. In surgical series, if idiopathic aortic root dilatation is excluded, atherosclerotic aneurysms are most common, followed by chronic dissections.[117] Chronic traumatic pseudoaneurysms account for about 10% of descending thoracic aneurysms, and aortitis approximately 8% of surgically evaluated thoracic aortic aneurysms.[117] In a recent autopsy series,[118] chronic incidental thoracic aneurysms were considered largely (nearly 90%) due to atherosclerosis (degenerative disease), with 10% related to aortitis and less than 2% related to medial degeneration; none were classified as chronic dissections. Ruptured nondissecting aneurysms resulting in death were one third as common than chronic aneurysms, and were the result of atherosclerotic/degenerative process (85%), aortitis (13%), and medial degeneration (3%). Rupture dissections were found as often as incidental thoracic aneurysms, and were the result of medial degeneration in 25% and aortitis in 4%; the histologic features of the remainder were not stated, but presumably these were hypertension related.[118] In this study, there was no male predisposition to aortic aneurysms,[118] unlike abdominal aortic aneurysms, which are two to three times more likely to occur in men than women.

Thoracic aortic aneurysms are uncommon in comparison to abdominal aortic aneurysms. The prevalence of thoracic aneurysms increases with age, ranging from approximately 2/1,000 population at age 60 to approximately 1% of the population by age 80.[118] The etiology of the aneurysm is partly dependent upon the location. Atherosclerotic lesions are most frequent in the descending aorta and and aortic arch, but may involve the proximal aorta in an additional 20% of cases, and extend into the abdominal segment in 5% of cases. Atherosclerotic aneurysms are frequently (30–40%) associated with noncontiguous aneurysms in the abdominal aorta, iliac, or femoral arteries.[118] Aneurysms associated with medial degeneration are almost exclusively in the ascending segment, and dissecting aneurysms may be present either in the proximal or descending portion, depending on etiology (see following). Aneurysms of giant-cell arteritis or Takayasu's aortitis are generally found in the ascending aorta, whereas infectious (mycotic) aneurysms are most frequent in the descending thoracic aorta. Traumatic pseudoaneurysm are typically found near the ligamentum arteriosum.

Many patients with thoracic aneurysms are asymptomatic, although there is often a history of hypertension. The patient may complain of chronic pain that may be pericardial and radiate to the neck and jaw, particularly if the arch is involved. Aneurysms of the descending thoracic aorta often produce back pain between the scapulae, and those in the thoracoabdominal portion of the aorta, lower back pain. Chest radiographs often demonstrate a shadow, which is to the right of the cardiac silhouette in ascending aneurysms, anterior and left-sided if involving the arch, and left-sided and posterior if involving the descending aorta.

Natural history studies of thoracic aortic aneurysm report a 1- and 5-year survival of 39–52% and 13–19%, respectively, but many studies include data on acute type A dissection. Although most mortality in patients with thoracic aortic aneurysm is related to aneurysm rupture, data on the relationship between aneurysm size and rupture risk remains scarce.[119] The early operative mortality for repair of thoracic aortic aneurysms is high, about 15%. The major complications include bleeding, brain damage, paraplegia, and redissection in cases of repair of dissecting aneurysm. Causes for cerebral dysfunction include embolism, cerebral hypoperfusion, and unknown causes. Risk factors for postoperative cerebral complications include advanced age at surgery, preoperative renal failure, aortic arch lesions, atherosclerotic aneurysm, aortic arch procedures, and clamping of the aortic arch. The perioperative mortality is especially high in patients with anoxic brain injury.[120] A variety of surgical techniques has been developed to attempt to minimize the risk of brain damage and paraplegia after descending thoracic aortic aneurysm repair, including a variety of cardiopulmonary bypass procedures, including partial bypass through femoral access and selective cerebral perfusion.[121] Because of the high risk of surgery, patients who are considered high surgical risks are currently evaluated for endoluminal repair with prosthesis constructed from stents covered with polyester fabric.[122] As is the case with endoluminal repair of abdominal aortic aneurysms, complications include migration of the stent, endoleaks, and infections.

Idiopathic Aortic Root Dilatation

Definition

Annuloaortic ectasia is a term (used principally by surgeons) that was introduced in

1961 to denote aneurysmal dilatation of the ascending aorta with pure aortic valve regurgitation.[123] In its broadest sense, the term has been used when specific conditions, such as Takayasu's disease, results in aortic aneurysm with insufficiency.[124] However, the term is generally restricted to cases of idiopathic medial degeneration of the aorta[125] in patients with or without Marfan syndrome. The proportion of patients with extracardiac manifestations of Marfan syndrome varies from 16–22%[126, 127] to over 50%.[128]

Clinical Findings

Idiopathic annuloaortic ectasia is more common in men than women, and typically presents in the fourth, fifth, and sixth decades.[43] Patients with Marfan syndrome are much younger at diagnosis, symptoms of aortic root dilatation often occurring in the third and fourth decades, and are much more likely to have a family history of aortic disease. The tendency to group idiopathic annuloaortic ectasia and Marfan syndrome is due to the difficulty of clearly separating the two entities. It has been demonstrated that annuloaortic ectasia in patients with and without Marfan syndrome forms a continuum, as a family history can often be elicited in patients without Marfan.[127] The prognosis of patients with dilated aortic root is somewhat better in patients without Marfan syndrome, as compared with Marfan patients, with approximately 30% recurrence of cardiac disease after surgery versus 70%, respectively.[43] However, 10-year survival is similar.[43]

Aortic root dilatation accounts for over 50% of aortic valve replacement for pure aortic regurgitation, and, in the majority of patients, the cause is idiopathic (i.e., annuloaortic ectasia).[129] The remaining patients have known defects, such as Marfan syndrome, inflammatory aortic disease, osteogenesis imperfecta, operated congenital heart disease, or intrinsic valve disease.

Pathogenesis and Pathologic Findings

The cause of annuloaortic ectasia is unknown, and may be partly due to age-related degenerative changes. However, inherited genetic defects certainly play a causative role, as demonstrated by the presence of aortic root dilatation in first-degree relatives of over 50% of patients.[127] The precise nature of the genetic defects in patients without Marfan syndrome has yet to be determined.

Grossly, there is dilatation of the proximal aorta, resulting in a pear-shaped, symmetric enlargement (Fig. 13–12). Aortic valve incompetence is secondary to dilation of the aortic wall at the commissural level, which results in the inability of the valve to coapt during systole. The aneurysmal process may involve the entire ascending aorta but generally spares the arch. Dissections may occur within the ectatic aorta, and may be incidentally discovered during surgery. However, the majority of acute aortic dissections occur in the absence of a root aneurysm.[130]

The histologic findings are nonspecific and include cystic medial degeneration of the aortic wall, which may be a causative factor in the aortic weakness. The weak aortic wall is prone to dissections and aortic rupture without dissection.[131]

The elastic composition of aortas in patients with annuloaortic ectasia has been shown to be decreased in some patients, associated with fibrosis and elastin fragmentation histologically. This decrease did not, however, correlate with a family history or the degree of aortic root dilatation.[132]

Pathologic changes in the aortic valve result from the inability of the aortic leaflets to close during diastole. Secondary changes in the aortic valve may follow from an increase in tension and bowing of the valve cusps. These changes include thickening and retraction of the leaflets, which further the inability of the valve to close and intensify the aortic regurgitation. It has been shown that the reduced aortic distensibility may also contribute to the gradual left ventricular dilation and dysfunction in patients with chronic aortic regurgitation.[133]

Abdominal Aortic Aneurysm

Patient Characteristics

The autopsy incidence of abdominal aortic aneurysm is between 1.8 and 6.6% in adults, with a 6% prevalence in the sixth decade, a 10% incidence in the eighth decade,[134] and a 14% prevalence in the ninth decade. There is a male predominance of 3–8:1, which increases for popliteal and femoral artery aneurysms.[135] For reasons that are unknown, Caucasians are more frequently affected than Blacks. Sons of men with abdominal aortic aneurysm demonstrate aortic dilatation at a rate of 20%, suggesting a familial component. Recently,

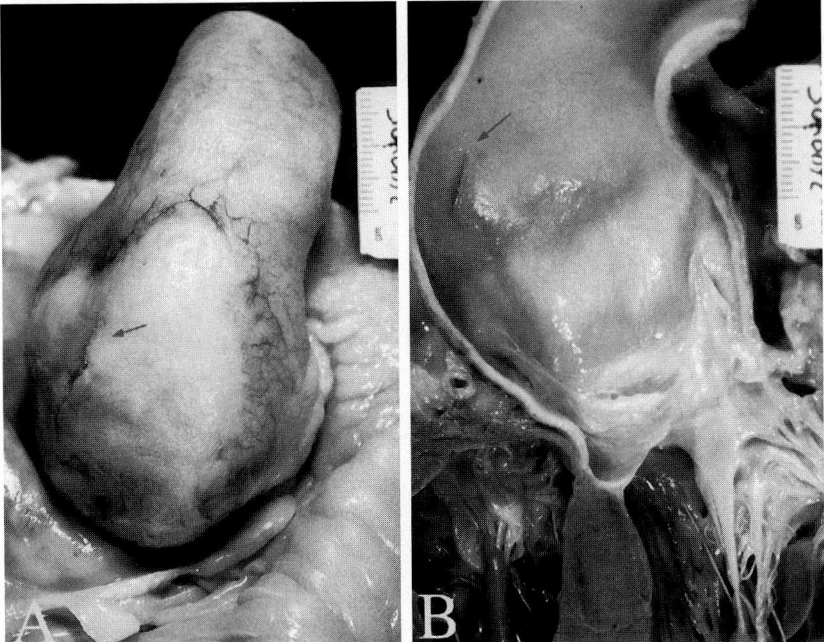

Figure 13–12. Annuloaortic ectasia. Idiopathic aortic root dilatation (annuloaortic ectasia) generally refers to Marfan-like aortic root changes in patients without full-blown Marfan who tend to develop symptoms at a later age. *A.* A pale aneurysmal outpouching in the aortic root of a 300-lb, 73-inch man with no clinical features of Marfan who died suddenly after clutching his throat while driving off the road. The autopsy demonstrated aortic rupture (*arrow*) and hemopericardium. Note the relatively avascular area around the rupture site. Histologically, there was severe medial degeneration (not shown). *B.* The opened aortic specimen with the intimal tear (*arrow*).

there has been a reported increase in the incidence of abdominal aortic aneurysms, with a sevenfold increase between 1951 and 1980 in a Minnesota population.[135] This increase is partly due to improved diagnostic capability and aging of the population.

Most patients with abdominal aortic aneurysm are asymptomatic. Some patients may experience vague abdominal discomfort or lower back pain, and a pulsating abdominal mass may be palpable if the aneurysm is larger than 4.5 cm. Ultrasound examination is most reliable for screening and monitoring growth, but computed tomography is also useful. Ultrasonographic studies have shown that the rate of growth is estimated to be 0.2–0.5 cm/year, and that follow-up is necessary probably at 10-year intervals.[136] The median rate of growth of 0.3 cm per year increases with enlargement of the aneurysm.[137] Symptoms of rupture include abdominal or back pain, hypotension, and a tender abdominal mass; the only symptom may be hypovolemic shock.

Pathologic Features

The majority of abdominal atherosclerotic aneurysms are single, involving the infrarenal aorta above the iliac bifurcation (Fig. 13–13). Fusiform (cylindrical) aneurysms are most common, and affect the entire circumference of the aorta, often extending into iliac arteries distally, or proximally to the celiac trunk or even the thoracic aorta. Less common saccular aneurysms are sharply demarcated, affecting only a portion of the aortic circumference, and are more likely to occur in the thoracic aorta. All aneurysms show laminated yellow-brown thrombus, the caliber of the lumen generally approximating that of the adjoining aorta in fusiform aneurysms. The aorta adjacent to the aneurysms generally shows severe atherosclerosis extending a variable distance into the aneurysm itself, which shows destruction of elastic lamellae by gradual attenuation with smooth muscle cell atrophy and infiltration by macrophages. Elastic stains are helpful in showing loss of media and increase in collagen. Calcification

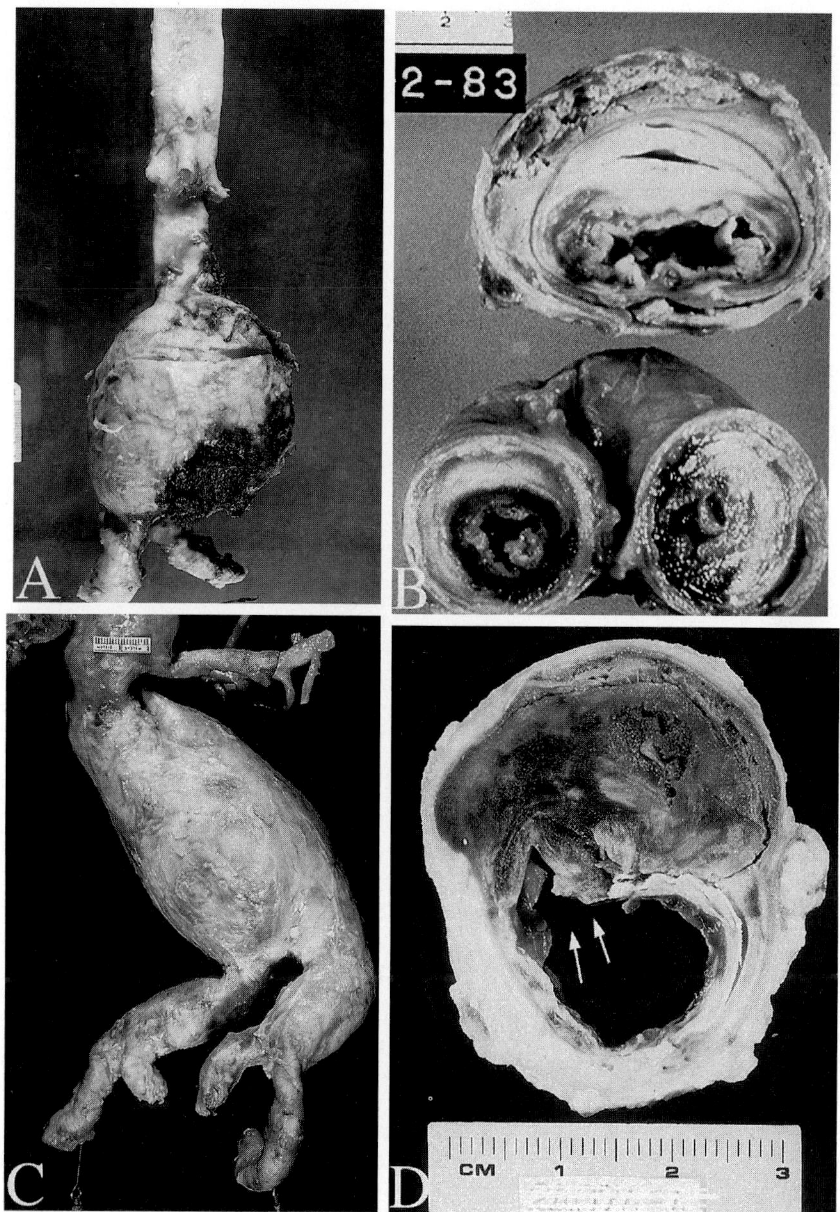

Figure 13–13. Abdominal aortic aneurysm. *A.* The typical location distal to the renal arteries and proximal to the iliac bifurcation. *B.* Cross sections demonstrate luminal thrombosis and extension into the iliac arteries. *C.* A typical infrarenal aneurysm with multiple aneurysm involving the iliac arteries. *D.* There is a pseudoaneurysm that has formed at the anastomosis of a Dacron graft (*arrows*). The pseudoaneurysm is at the top of the field filled with thrombus.

and bony metaplasia are common, and correspond to densities that may be seen on plain radiographs. Old leaks indicative of previous rupture are identified by hemosiderin-laden macrophages in adventitial infiltrates.

Complications

The most feared complication of abdominal aortic aneurysm is rupture, which most commonly occurs into the retroperitoneal space. Rarely, the pleura, gastrointestinal tract, inferior vena cava, or left renal vein may be the sites of rupture. Aneurysms that are smaller than 5 cm have a small risk of rupture, while larger ones have a 25% risk of rupture over 5 years. Other complications include secondary bacterial infection and embolization. Cholesterol emboli may result in renal failure, and cholesterol or thromboemboli may result in ischemia of the lower extremities. Infection is a relatively rare complication; organisms include salmonella, staphylococcus, *Escherichia coli,* and bacteroides, and may be seeded by arterial or venous catheters.

Treatment

The conventional surgical treatment of fusiform aneurysms consists of bypass with Dacron or polytetrafluoroethylene (Gore-Tex) tube grafting, with inclusion of prosthesis and oversewing with aneurysmal tissue. Woven Dacron tube graft placement with inclusion technique often yields relatively little tissue for the surgical pathologist, consisting of tissue obtained at anastomotic sites as well as thrombus. In patients with significant iliac stenosis or aneurysms, bifurcating graft is utilized between the aorta and iliac arteries. Saccular aneurysms may be repaired by a Dacron patch if less than 50% of the aortic circumference is involved. Survival depends on initial risk of patient. High-risk patients are those older than 75 years of age with other life-threatening medical conditions and with aneurysms of larger than 6 cm. Complications of aneurysm repair include infection and pseudoaneurysm at the site of anastomosis (Fig. 13–13). The utility of operating aneurysms detected by screening has been questioned, as the 5-year mortality from myocardial infarction and stroke is approximately 33% in patients who are 75 years of age, similar to patients who are not operated.[134] However, selective operation on patients with larger expanding aneurysms has shown to be beneficial.[137]

Endovascular treatment of abdominal aortic aneurysm with fenestrated grafts is a currently accepted alternative to open surgery. Complications include leakage at the anastomotic site (endoleak), migration of the graft distally, and increased pressure of the excluded aneurysmal sac without obvious leakage.[138] Complications are more often encountered in patients with large aneurysms, advanced age, and if adjuvant procedures are required. In addition, a compromised cardiac and general medical status has adverse effects on the risk of systemic complications, as well as inexperience of the operating team. An 18-month endoleak-free survival is considered a satisfactory mid-term result.[139] In successful endovascular repairs, the size of the aneurysm decreases at a similar rate (3–4 mm/year) as the rate of increase in untreated aneurysms. However, in patients with endoleaks, stented aneurysms may continue to increase in size.[140]

Pathogenesis

Although typically considered atherosclerotic, several facts challenge the atherosclerotic origin of abdominal aortic aneurysms and suggest that at least a portion of the atherosclerotic process is superimposed. Animal models of atherosclerosis that involve high-cholesterol diets do not cause aneurysms. There is increased collagenase and elastase activity and increased levels of cathepsins S and K within tissue extracts of aortic aneurysm walls. Smooth muscle cells in patients with abdominal aortic aneurysms secrete significantly increased amounts of elastase in response to the breakdown products of atherosclerosis.[141] Matrix metalloproteinases that are involved in aneurysm formation are generally derived from macrophages within the aneurysm wall. Some inhibitors of elastolytic cysteine proteases, such as cystatin C, are reduced in aneurysm walls as well as serum from patients with abdominal aortic aneurysms.[142] However, some metalloproteinases inhibitors, such as tissue inhibitor of metalloproteinase-1 (TIMP-1) are actually elevated in patients with abdominal aortic aneurysms, suggesting that there is a compensatory mechanism in response to increased collagen degradation products.[143] There is increased fibrinolytic capacity in aortic aneurysms, which may promote angiogenesis and contribute to local proteolytic degradation of the aortic wall leading to physical weakening and active expansion of the aneurysm.[144]

Other pathogenetic factors that may be active in the development of aortic aneurysms include genetic factors, increased pulse wave reflected at the aortic bifurcation, and alpha-1 antitrypsin deficiency. Genetic factors include increased height with acromegaly and poorly defined X-linked and autosomal inheritance.

Risk Factors

Risk factors for the development of abdominal aortic aneurysms differ somewhat from those for aortic and coronary atherosclerosis. Cigarette smoking is the strongest risk factor, as smokers are three to eight times more likely than nonsmokers to develop abdominal aneurysms.[145–147] A large study of thousands of patients demonstrated that hypercholesterolemia, hypertension, height, positive family history, and the presence of other atherosclerotic disease are also independently associated with abdominal aortic aneurysms[147]; studies with smaller numbers of patients do not show a correlation with hypertension or cholesterol.[146] Characteristics that are negatively associated with abdominal aortic aneurysms are diabetes mellitus and female gender[147] and black race.[145, 147]

In order to determine if there is a difference in risk-factor profiles between men with abdominal aneurysms and abdominal aortic atherosclerosis with iliac stenosis, men operated for aneurysm were compared with those bypassed for stenosis. The stenosis group had significantly lower high-density lipoprotein-cholesterol, a lower incidence of hypertension, and a similar rate of smoking, suggesting that while some risk factors are shared, there is a pathogenetic difference between the two disease processes.[148]

Inflammatory Aneurysms of the Abdominal Aorta

Inflammatory aneurysms of the aorta as a distinct entity was first described by Walker et al. in 1972.[149] It is sometimes considered a variant of abdominal atherosclerotic aneurysm, occurring in a similar location (generally the abdominal aorta).[150] The incidence of inflammatory abdominal aneurysm is 11% of all operated abdominal aortic aneurysms. The male/female ratio is 9:1, similar to atherosclerotic abdominal aneurysm. The etiology of inflammatory aneurysm of the abdominal aorta is unknown, although there may be pathogenetic similarities with retroperitoneal fibrosis.[151] An association with coronary arteritis suggests a localized manifestation of systemic vasculitis or an autoimmune disease.[152] Recently, a genetic risk determinant has been mapped to the HLA-DR B1 locus.[153]

Clinically, patients often present with abdominal pain, a mass, or both. In some patients, there is an elevated erythrocyte sedimentation rate. Computed tomographic and ultrasonographic scans demonstrate an area of soft-tissue density surrounding the atherosclerotic portion of the aneurysmal wall; this density corresponds pathologically to the marked fibrosis and perianeurysmal inflammation.[151] At surgery, this inflamed fibrotic process distinguished inflammatory aneurysms from pure atherosclerotic aneurysms, and is recognized as a thick wall extending into the retroperitoneum (Fig. 13–14). There is occasionally displacement and obstruction of the ureters, duodenum, jejunum and ileum, mesentery, sigmoid colon, renal artery and vein, and the inferior vena cava. Spontaneous rupture is unusual.

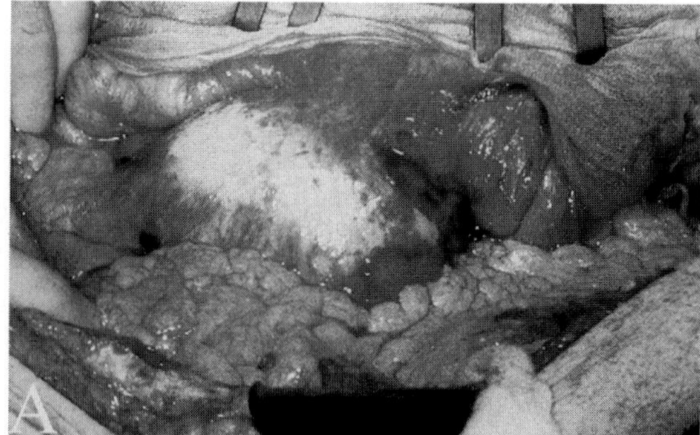

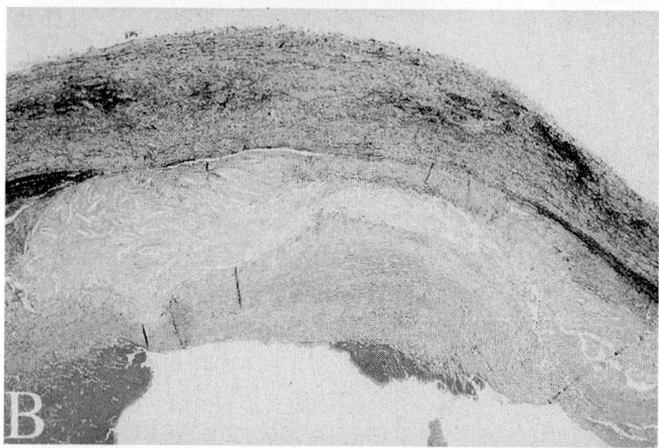

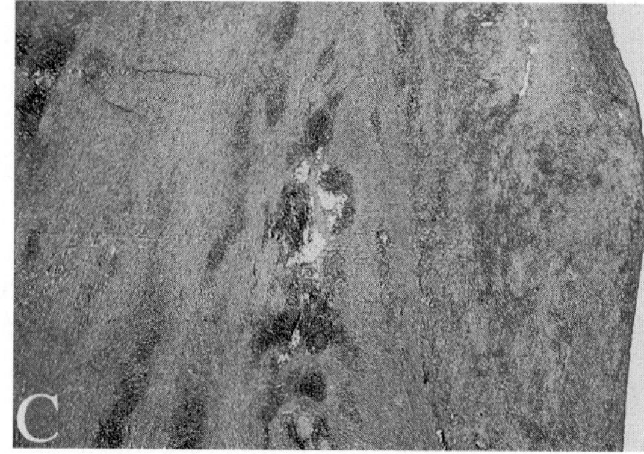

Figure 13–14. Inflammatory aortic aneurysm. Abdominal aortic aneurysms with extensive inflammation are characterized by a white, scarred adventitia (*A*). Histologically, there is extensive luminal atherosclerosis, but, in addition, there is medial destruction (*B*), note absence of dark elastic-rich media in the center) and adventitial scarring. The adventitial scarring is extensive (*C*), and histologically mimics idiopathic retroperitoneal fibrosis, in that there are lymphoid aggregates, scarring, and entrapment of nerves. There is also some resemblance to Takayasu's disease, which, in contrast to inflammatory aneurysm, is more frequently proximal and aneurysmal.

Pathologically, the inner surface of the wall of the aneurysm consists of atherosclerotic plaque. There is no clear demarcation between plaque, attenuated media, and periadventitial fibrous tissue.[83] Microscopically, the aneurysmal aortic wall consists of complex atherosclerotic plaque;

the underlying media is attenuated, fragmented, or replaced by fibrous tissue. The adventitia is replaced by a dense connective tissue almost in direct continuity with the atherosclerotic plaque. The fibrous tissue extends beyond the adventitia, entraps fat, nerves, ganglia, and lymph nodes (Fig. 13–14). There is either focal or diffuse heavy lymphocytic and plasma cell inflammatory infiltrate within the fibrous tissue.

ATHEROSCLEROSIS

Pathologic Progression of Atherosclerotic Aortic Plaques

Characteristics of Aortic Atherosclerosis

The morphologic characteristics and progression of atherosclerotic plaques in the aorta is similar to those of the coronary arteries (see Chapter 2). As a result of the larger vessel diameter and elastic nature of the aorta, however, there are likely to be some differences in the morphologic lesions of aortic plaques. For example, plaque erosion has not been described in the aorta, and some aortic lesions, such as penetrating atherosclerotic ulcer, have not been described in the coronary arteries.

Early Lesions: Fatty Streak (Intimal Xanthoma)

As in the coronary arteries, the fatty streak is a flat or minimally raised lesion that is grossly identified as a yellowish pale area on the intimal surface (Fig. 13–15). The gross appearance is enhanced by the use of lipophilic dyes, such as sudan red, which stains the fat red. Histologically, the hallmark of the fatty streak is the deposition of lipid within macrophages and smooth muscle cells (foam cells) as well as extracellular lipid accumulation (Fig. 13–16). Because we favor the term "intimal xanthoma" for foam-cell accumulations in coronary arteries, as is the case for other organs, "intimal xanthoma" is the preferred term for fatty streaks of the aorta as well. However, the term fatty streak is historically used for early lesions of the human and animal aorta, and is likely to remain in usage for some time.

Although classically the intimal xanthoma (fatty streak) is considered to be formed exclusively of xanthoma cells, there is significant overlap between the fatty streak and intimal thickening. Electron microscopic and cytochemical techniques demonstrate that fat droplets in intimal cells account for approximately half of the increase in intimal thickness in fatty streaks, with nonfat portions of cells and extracellular matrix accounting for the remainder.[154] The difficulty in precisely separating intimal

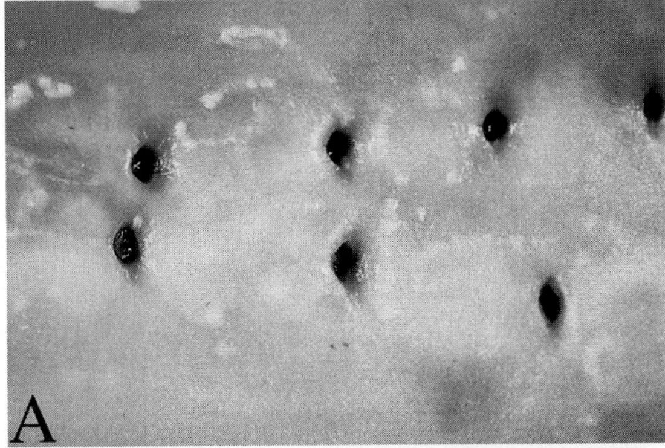

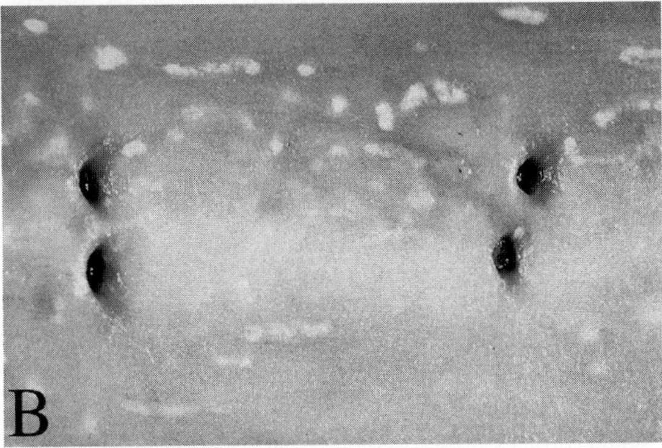

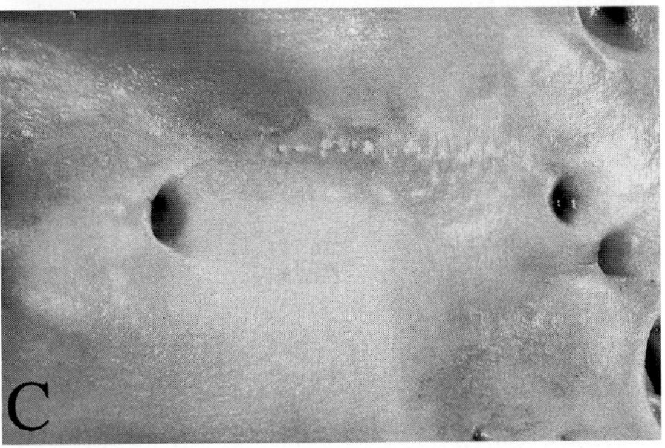

Figure 13–15. Fatty streaks, aorta. In this series of photographs, all from the same 22-year-old man who died of trauma, blood flow occurred from right (proximal) to left (distal). The flow dividers are the crescentic lips at the distal left portions of the intercostal ostia. *A.* Note fatty streaks in the proximal descending thoracic aorta. *B.* Fatty streaks in the distal thoracic aorta. Note the preponderance of lesions near the segmental vessels (dorsal portion of aorta). *C.* The distal abdominal aorta. Note the renal arteries and superior mesenteric ostia on the right, and the inferior mesenteric ostium on the left. In contrast to severe disease, early fatty streaks are less extensive in the abdominal segment.

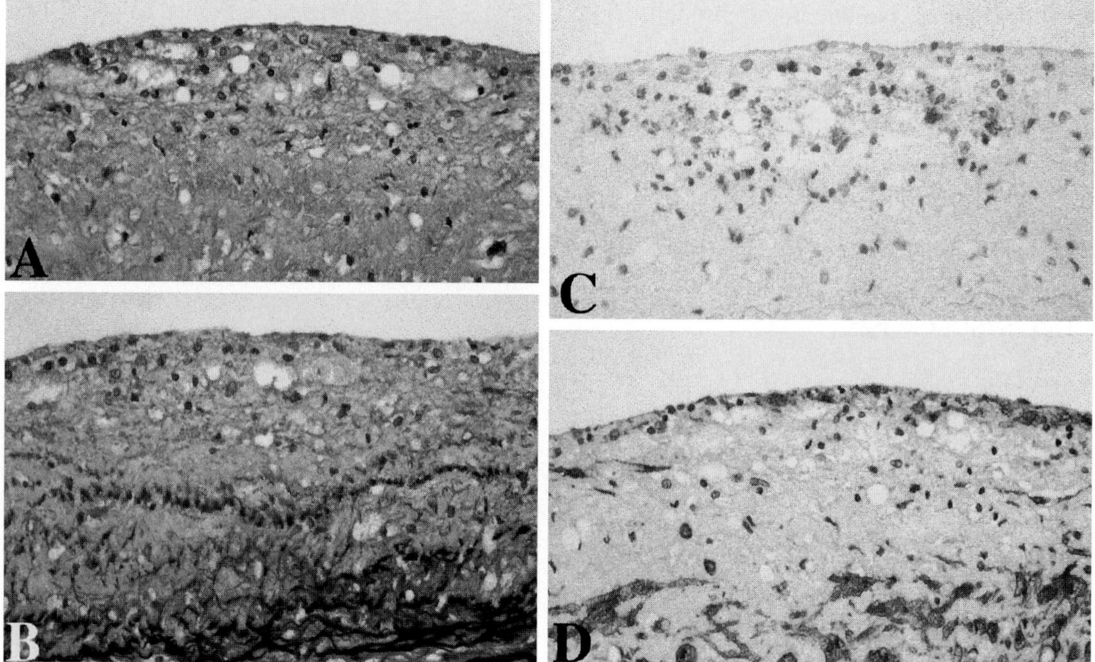

Figure 13–16. Fatty streaks, aorta. Histologic sections of aortic fatty streaks demosntrate foam cells (*A*), reduplication of elastic laminae with elastosis of the lower intima (*B*), accumulation of macrophages (*C*, anti-CD68), and occasional surface smooth muscle cells (*D*, anti-smooth muscle actin).

xanthomas from cellular intimal thickening without lipid undoubtedly accounts for some of the controversy involving the true precursor lesion of symptomatic fibroatheroma.

The extracellular lipids that accumulate within fatty streaks are composed of two types of particle: esterified cholesterol-rich droplets and unesterified cholesterol-rich multilamellar liposomes. The former may result from the direct accumulation of plasma low-density lipoprotein particles, whereas the latter may be derived from the breakdown of foamy macrophages.[155] Glycosphingolipids, especially glucosylceramide, and sphyngomyelin are present in far higher quantities in esterified than nonesterified aortic lipid particles, and have been shown to be involved in aortic smooth muscle cell proliferation and atherogenesis.[156]

Aortic fatty streaks occur earlier than coronary lesions; in general, there is an interval of approximately 10 years between onset and progression of aortic disease and coronary disease. From the early years of the second decade, fatty streaks increase until approximately 35 years of life, and then decline; the progression of lesions is most rapid in the 15- to 34-year age span.[157] In men, fatty streaks occur more prominently in the thoracic aorta, as compared with the abdominal aorta, but the converse is true in women.[158] They begin in the posterior intimal surface, often around ostia of the intracostal arteries.[159] In the thoracic aorta sudanophilia is found in the posterior (dorsal) aspect, with sparing of the anterior surfaces; this distribution continues down the abdominal aorta, but shifts to the ventral (anterior) wall from the ostia of the renal arteries to the origin of the inferior mesenteric artery showing increased probability of fatty streaks.[160, 161]

From 6 to 20 years of life, fatty streaks cover approximately 25% of the aortic intima in the U.S. population and about one half this amount in a Japanese population.[162] Fatty streaks are more frequent in African Americans than Caucasians,[163] and are present in 23% of Ethiopians under the age of 20, and 32% of all adult Ethiopians.[164] In the United States, the extent of fatty streaks correlates with total cholesterol, elevated low-density lipoprotein cholesterol, and ponderal index (a measure of truncal obesity) in men.[158] Smoking is associated with more extensive fatty streaks of the abdominal aorta in young men, particularly in the dorsolateral region of the distal third of the abdominal aorta. Hypertension is not associated with fatty streaks in Caucasians or Blacks.[165]

Early Lesions: Intimal Thickening

As in the coronary arteries, aortic plaques may progress without going through a xanthomatous phase. Intimal thickening without significant intracellular lipid is common in human arteries, including the aorta, at a very early age, even in utero. The definition of pathologic intimal thickening has not been firmly established, but it is valid to consider it an earlier lesion than fatty streak. In the fetus, there is a well-developed internal elastic lamina over which there is a single endothelial layer, the intima being almost negligible. At branch points, the aorta demonstrates focal intimal thickening, composed of reduplicated elastica and occasional smooth muscle cells, as early as 15 weeks in utero. After birth, there is a progressive thickening of the intima, characterized by a superficial edematous zone, and a deeper more elastic zone, composed primarily of smooth muscle cells, proteoglycans, and elastic fibers, most prominent in the infrarenal dorsal abdominal aorta. The innermost elastic layer (internal elastic lamina) becomes indistinct and merges with the lower elastic zone of the intima. These areas may demonstrate gross wrinkling that precedes fatty streaks[166]; this wrinkling has been referred to as "wave lines"[167] or "rhythmic structures"[168] and has an uncertain significance in the progression of atherosclerosis. The definition of pathologic intimal thickening is not firmly established, but over one fifth of the aortic thickness has been designated as abnormal intimal thickening.[166] Eventually, intimal thickening develops a mononuclear cell infiltrate with the accumulation of extracellular lipid and lipid droplets within smooth muscle cells and macrophages. More advanced lesions demonstrate cholesterol clefts and necrotic cores characteristic of fibroatheroma (seen following). The relationship of this sequence of events with classic fatty streaks is a matter of debate.

The intimal smooth muscle cells of early atherosclerotic plaques are composed of several morphologic subtypes. Contractile smooth muscle cells are elongated cells devoid of cell processes, possessing a well-developed contractile apparatus in the form of microfilament bundles with dense bodies, a basal membrane surrounding the cell, and micropinocytotic vesicles along the plasma membrane. Modified smooth muscle cells or synthetic smooth muscle cells differ from the typical smooth muscle cells in that they have fewer contractile structures and are rich in endoplasmic reticulum, and are associated with progressive intimal thickening, deposition of lipids, and increased amount of proteoglycans. Ultrastructurally, some stellate and irregular-shaped cells are utterly devoid of contractile structures, and are difficult to differentiate from macrophages.[169]

The majority of studies of early atherosclerosis in the human aorta have combined intimal thickening with other forms of raised lesions (fibrous plaques). A recent study of intimal thickening of adolescents and young adults has shown some differences in the distribution between intimal thickening and fatty streaks. Intimal thickening is most prominent in the abdominal segment, and is most pronounced in the posterior (dorsal) aspect in the thoracic and distal abdominal aorta, and in the anterior (ventral) aspect in the mid-aorta.[170, 171] Lesions are uncommon in the ventral portion of the descending thoracic aorta in cases of mild atherosclerosis, especially the middle third.[171]

Fibrous Plaque

Raised lesions of the aorta are grossly characterized as fibrous plaques that may become calcified and ulcerated[162] (Fig. 13–17). Histologically, the majority of raised lesions demonstrate extracellular lipid or lipid cores, and are therefore categorized as fibroatheromas. The intermediate category of preatheroma has been used for intemediate lesions with pools of extracellular lipid but without a well-developed lipid-rich necrotic core,[172] and was first described by Stary et al.[173]

Fibrous aortic plaques progress with age, occur later than fatty streaks, and are more frequent in males than females, without a racial predilection.[158] Although they may occur rarely under age 10, fibrous plaques begin to account for a significant surface area of the aortic intima only after age 30, at which time fatty streaks begin to regress. Between ages 40 and 80 fibrous plaques continue to increase, and are associated with hypertension at all ages, and to a lesser extent hypercholesterolemia in older age ranges.[172] A large study of autopsy samples collected with risk-factor data has shown that high low-density lipoprotein cholesterol and low high-density lipoprotein cholesterol concentrations are associated with raised lesions in subjects under age 35, and smoking is associated with raised lesions of the abdominal aorta, particularly in the dorsolateral region of the distal third. Hypertension is associated with more extensive raised lesions in Blacks.[165] In another

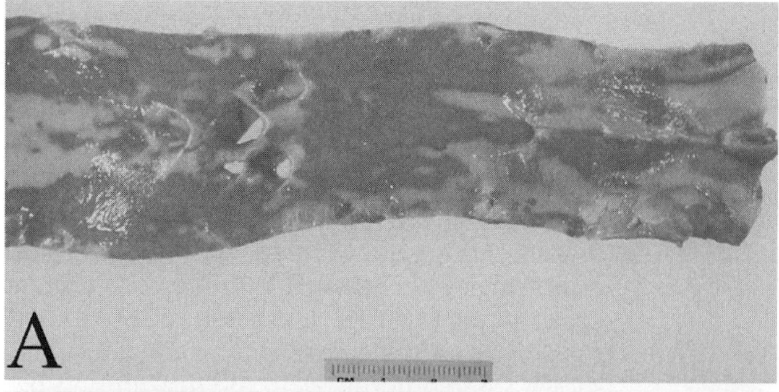

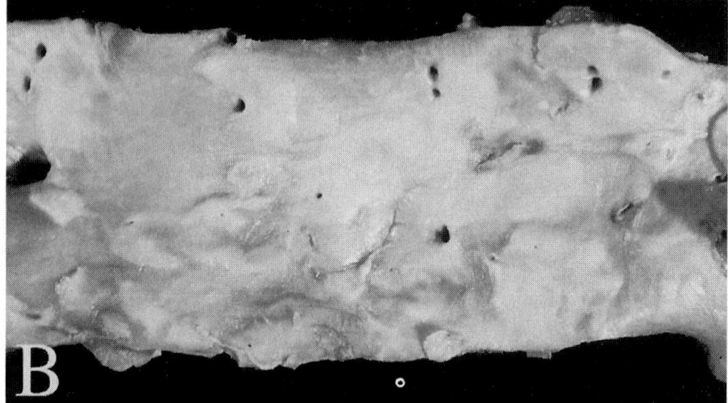

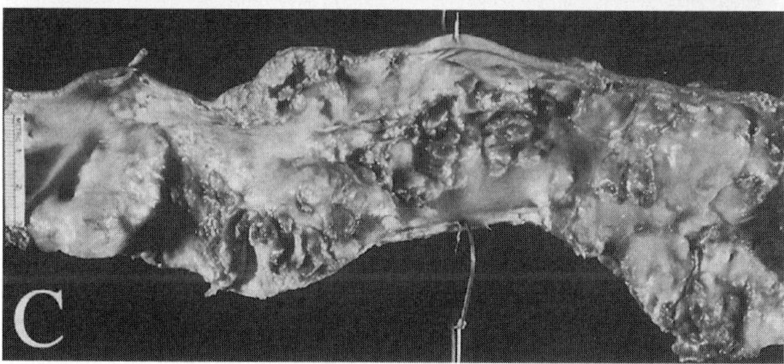

Figure 13–17. Progression of aortic atherosclerosis. *A.* A Sudan stain of the aorta opened along the dorsal (posterior) aspect. The iliac bifurcation is to the right. The predominant lesion is the fatty streak (*dark areas*). Note the relative sparing proximally (*left*, white areas) at the ventral (anterior) portion. *B.* Raised fibrous plaques along the distal aorta; the iliac bifurcation is to the right. *C.* Severe aortic atherosclerosis, with ulcerated thrombosed crater-like atheromas.

study, elevated, fibrous lesions and complicated lesions in the abdominal aorta were more extensive in men with the P1(A2) genotype.[174] The association between this platelet glycoprotein and coronary atherosclerosis has been mentioned in Chapter 2.

As with fatty streaks, there are racial differences in the extent of aortic fibrous plaques. They are less common in Japanese and Ethiopians as compared with American subjects.[162, 164] However, aortic fibrous plaques are common in all races studied, and ethnicity only affects the extent, but not the distribution, of early aortic plaques.[161]

Precursors of the Fibroatheroma

The classification and progression of early atherosclerotic plaques is somewhat controversial, especially regarding the precursor of the fibroatheroma. Intimal thickening and fatty streaks are the earliest atherosclerotic lesions, the former occurring even in neonates, as noted earlier. Although many studies have suggested that the fatty streak progresses to typical fibroatheromatous plaques,[154, 159, 162, 172] there are several features of the fatty streak that make it an unlikely candidate for the precursor to more advanced raised lesions. As noted earlier, risk factors for fatty streaks differ from those for fibrous plaques, fatty streaks may regress, and the distribution of fatty streaks differs from that of fibroatheromas. Intimal thickening, as opposed to xanthomatous lesions, has been shown to occur in a similar distribution of advanced plaques,[170] and there is only a partial overlap between the distribution of fibrous plaques and fatty streaks.[161] However, the possibility that a minority of fatty streaks may develop characteristics of fibrous plaques and fibroatheromas has not been excluded.

Advanced Lesions

The characteristics of advanced aortic plaques are similar to those of the coronary arteries, and include rupture (ulceration), thrombosis, and calcification. By transesophageal echocardiography, aortic plaques are graded as I (normal), II (increased echodensity of the intima without irregularity), III (increased echodensity with defined fibroatheroma), IV (increased echodensity with fibroatheroma > 3 mm), and V (mobile, protruding lesions).[175] Unlike lesions of the coronary artery, ulcerated thrombosed aortic plaques are frequently incidental, without causing clinical symptoms, presumably because of the larger caliber of the aorta. Symptoms may occur from aneurysms, occlusive disease, and embolization. Rarely, occlusion may occur as the result of a calcified mass above the renal arteries.[176] Although ostial occlusion of intercostal and mesenteric arteries occurs with advanced aortic atherosclerosis, more distal disease of branch vessels is unusual, with the exception of the renal arteries and splenic artery, which may demonstrate significant narrowing with calcification. The intercostal arteries are generally free of any significant plaques distal to the ostia.[159] Ostial disease can, however, result in ischemic changes to the spine, including lumbar disc degeneration.[177]

Association with Coronary and Carotid Atherosclerosis

Aortic plaques begin approximately one decade earlier than significant coronary artery disease. There is a significant correlation between the presence of aortic and iliac atherosclerosis and atherosclerosis of the coronary and carotid arteries. By transesophageal imaging, significant thoracic aortic atherosclerosis is highly correlated with angiographically demonstrated coronary disease, being present in over three fourths of patients with coronary lesions, compared with less than one third of patients without coronary disease.[175] A clinical association between carotid atherosclerosis and aortic calcification has also been established. Patients with abdominal aortic calcification as determined by plain radiographs have significantly increased intima to media ratios by ultrasonography of the carotid arteries performed 5 years later.[178] In addition, patients with calcification of aortic arch have higher rates of coronary artery disease and stroke, suggesting an association between aortic, carotid, and coronary atherosclerosis.[179]

Penetrating Atherosclerotic Ulcer

Penetrating atherosclerotic ulcer refers to a crater-like defect in the media of the aorta, usually descending thoracic aorta, which overlies an atherosclerotic plaque[180] (Fig. 13–18). There may be associated intramural hematoma and limited dissection; complications are transmural aortic rupture, embolization, pseudoaneurysm formation, and progressive aneurysmal dilatation.[181] Penetrating atherosclerotic ulcer is diagnosed in approximately 5% of adult patients with aortic disease investigated by transesophageal echocardiography.[182] Patients are usually in the seventh and eighth decades of life, and are virtually always hypertensive. Typical presenting symptoms include back pain and chest pain, and aortic dissection is usually the clinical diagnosis. Another common symptom is distal embolization of atherosclerotic material (atheroembolism).[183] A rare presenting symptom is dyspnea with dysphagia due to compression of the trachea and esophagus.[184] The diagnosis can be made by transesophageal echocardiography in over 75% of patients, and confirmed in the remainder by angiography, computed tomography, or magnetic resonance imaging. Imaging diagnosis is based on the presence of an aortic defect or outpouching that is generally calcified (discrete ulcer crater). Occasionally, there is associated aneurysmal dilatation and intramural hematoma or localized dissection. The location is the descending thoracic aorta in over 75% of patients, the majority of the remainder occurring in the aortic arch or ascending aorta.[185] Rarely, penetrating ulcers may occur in an abdominal aneurysm.[186] A major complication is extension of medial dissection, occasionally to the aortic root, and rarely distally beyond the diaphragm.[187] Other complications include aortic rupture without dissection, which may occur acutely, or after formation of an aortic pseudoaneurysm.

Treatment consists of surgical repair in symptomatic patients with aneurysms or leaking defects. Patients without significant aneurysm or dissection who are not surgical candidates may

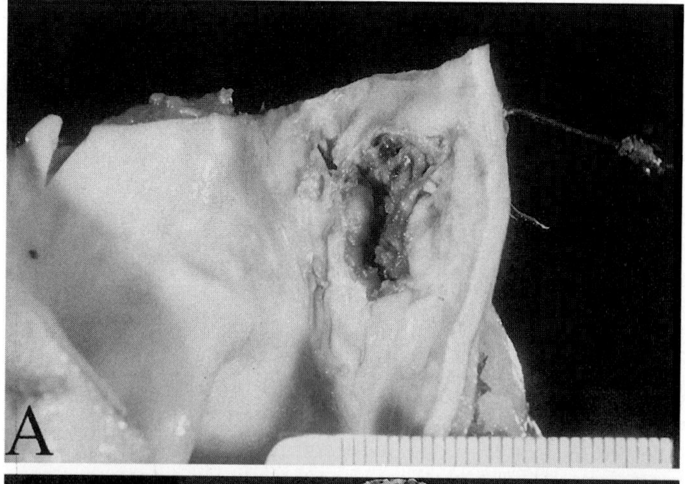

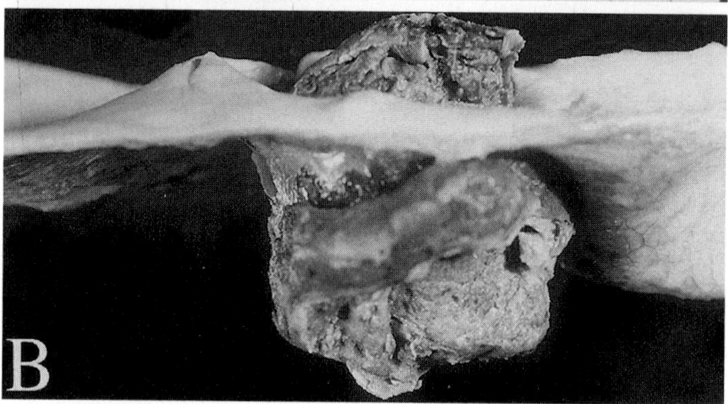

Figure 13–18. Penetrating atherosclerotic ulcer. By definition, a penetrating atherosclerotic ulcer is a crater formed by an atherosclerotic plaque, with intramural hematoma. *A.* The typical gross intimal appearance in the descending thoracic aorta. *B.* The lesion viewed from the side, showing the ulcer crater (*top*) and the hemorrhage and pseudoaneurysm (*bottom*).

be treated medically with antihypertensive therapy. In those patients with leakage and early hemothorax, coil embolization has been attempted to slow hemorrhage and stabilize the patient for surgery.[188] In patients without significant symptoms in whom the diagnosis is an incidental finding, treatment consists of hypertension control and follow-up, with excellent prognosis.[183]

The pathologic diagnosis is generally made at autopsy, although surgical treatment is indicated in patients with aortic diameter enlargement or angiographically demonstrated dissection. Pathologically, there is severe atherosclerosis and the atherosclerotic process erodes into the media, resulting in hemorrhage and some degree of dissection in the outer walls of the media. Fatal cases at autopsy generally demonstrate rupture of the aorta with blood in the adventitial and periaortic soft tissue. The site of rupture is similar to that of dissecting aneurysms, and, because of the location in the descending thoracic aorta, usually leads to left hemothorax. The differential diagnosis includes remote traumatic pseudoaneurysm, which may occur in the same location. However, the presence of atherosclerosis, dissection, and intramural hematoma should help distinguish cases of penetrating atherosclerotic ulcer with partial rupture and healing from traumatic pseudoaneurysm, as well as the clinical history. Infectious (''mycotic'') aneurysms may also occur in the descending thoracic aorta, but, in the absence of severe atherosclerosis and the clinical history of infectious endocarditis or other remote infection, are generally easily distinguished from penetrating ulcer. However, we have seen occasional cases of infected atherosclerotic ulcer with pseudoaneurysm and rupture that are difficult to separate from mycotic aneurysm, and may represent a form of mycotic aneurysm that originated in an atherosclerotic ulcer.

Atheroembolism Syndrome

The atheroembolism syndrome is a systemic disease caused by atheroembolism originating from a severely atherosclerotic aorta and iliofemoral arteries. The primary manifestations are cutaneous lesions, including blue-toe syndrome and livedo reticularis, renal failure, and intestinal ischemia. The diagnosis is suspected in patients with severe atherosclerotic cardiovascular disease and aortic atherosclerosis, and confirmed by skin biopsy, renal biopsy, gastrointestinal biopsy, or fundoscopy for the detection of retinal embolism.[189] Atheroembolism is probably underdiagnosed clinically, and has been estimated to account for up to 10% of cases of acute renal failure[190] and may account for subcapsular renal scars.[191] The syndrome may be precipitated by aortic angiography, cardiac surgery, or abdominal trauma.[192] Iatrogenic atheroembolism imparts a higher risk for renal failure, as opposed to spontaneous atheroembolism which is associated with distal ischemic symptoms.[193] Surgical treatment includes bypass grafts of the aorta, including axillofemoral bypass, amputation of severely affected limbs, and establishment of dialysis access. Other forms of management include endovascular procedures, such as stenting of the iliac and femoral arteries, concurrent with thrombolytic, anticoagulant, or antiplatelet therapy. Mortality ranges from as high as 70% in patients with multiorgan disease[194] to less than 5%[195] in patients with localized ischemia of the extremities.

At autopsy, atheroembolism is seen in 20% of patients dying after coronary artery bypass or valve replacement surgery, and is associated with severe thoracic aortic atherosclerosis. Organs involved include the brain (16%), spleen (11%), kidney (10%), and pancreas (7%), with multiple atheroembolic sites found in the majority of autopsies with atheroembolism.[196] Biopsy diagnosis is made by demonstrating cholesterol clefts within arterioles and small arteries in renal, skin, or colonic biopsy (Fig. 13–19). The cholesterol clefts are typically surrounded by fibrin or organizing thrombus, and may contain calcified material.

AORTIC DISSECTION

Incidence

Aortic dissections occur infrequently, but when they occur they often result in catastrophic consequences. The incidence of aortic dissections in the United States is 2,000 cases per year.[197] Mortality is high, and has been estimated at 1% per hour if untreated. Aortic dissections occur more frequently in males than in females (2–3 : 1), and, in the absence of Marfan syndrome, usually occur in individuals beyond the age of 60 years. There is often a history of long-standing systemic hypertension, explaining its high prevalence in African Americans. The vast majority of dissections, because of an acquired or inherited weakness of the aortic media, manifest by cystic medial necrosis. Rare causes include aortitis and medial dysplasia, which can by diagnosed only by histologic examination. Advanced atherosclerosis is rarely present in patients with aortic dissection, although mild to moderate atherosclerosis may be present. Dissections occurring in patients with atherosclerosis-induced mural hematomas (so-called penetrating atherosclerotic ulcer) are, by definition, limited in extent.

Initiating Event

There is controversy concerning the initial event in aortic dissection. One theory proposes that the intimal tear exposes the medial layer to the driving force of the blood (or pulse pressure), splitting the diseased media into two layers. The blood then passes into the space between the dissection planes, resulting in a false lumen, which distends with blood. The pressure in the false lumen directs blood back into the true lumen, via a reentry tear, or causes the false lumen to rupture the thin layer of outer media and adventitia.

The second theory suggests that the entry of blood into the dissection plane occurs via ruptured vasa vasorum within the aortic media. According to this theory, intimal tears are secondary, or may not occur at all. Although most pathologic studies document the presence of intimal tears in all aortic dissections (which is also our experience), Wilson and Hutchins were unable to detect intimal tears in 13% of 204 cases.[198]

Classification

Of the three major classifications of aortic dissection, the most frequently used is that of DeBakey, which is based upon the site of tear. DeBakey divides aortic dissections into three major groups (Fig. 13–20). In type I dissections, the intimal tear is located in the ascending aorta, with dissection extending to the descending aorta. It is the most frequent, occurring in 54% of cases.[199] In type II dissections (21% of

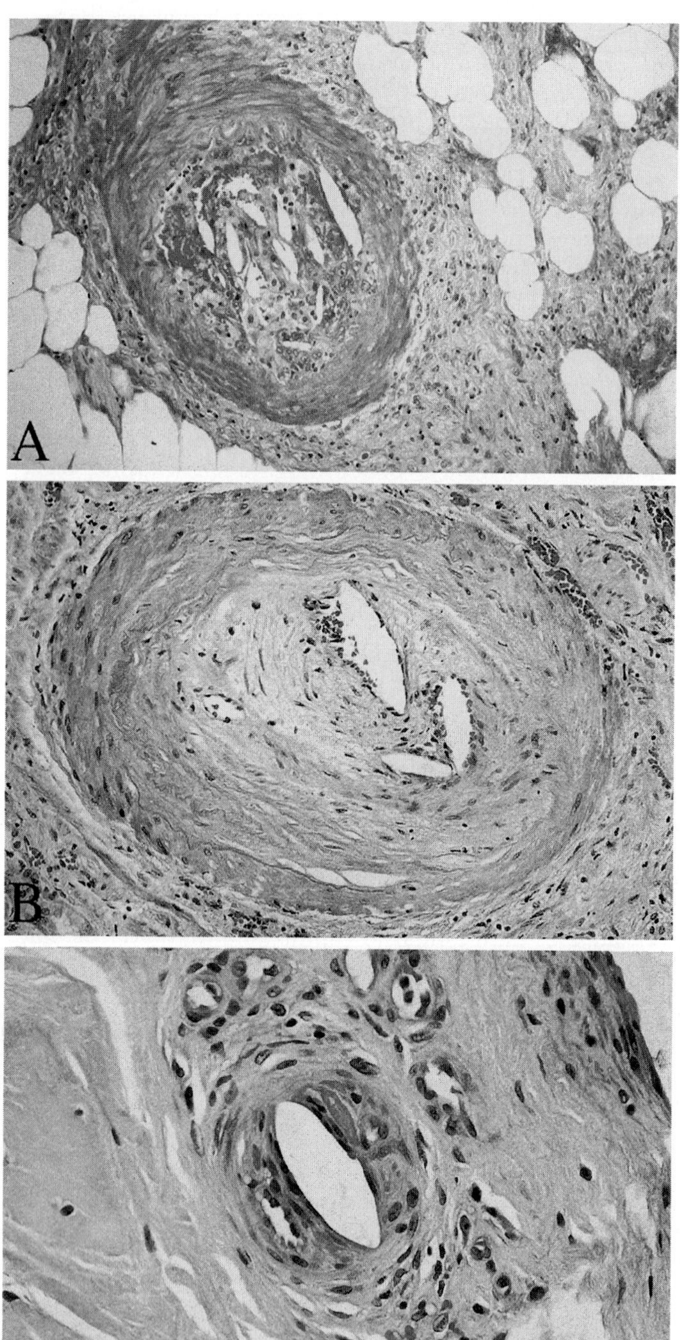

Figure 13–19. Atheroembolism. *A.* A relatively acute atheromatous embolism with cholesterol clefts, red cells, and inflammatory cells within the lumen. *B.* At a later stage, there is fibrosis and occlusion of the lumen; the cholesterol clefts are still evident. *C.* A chronic atheroembolism in the dermis from a patient with severe aortic atherosclerosis and blue toe syndrome.

the total), the intimal tear is also located in the ascending aorta, but the dissection is limited to the ascending aorta. The remaining 25% are comprised of type III dissections, which differ fundamentally from the other types because the intimal tear is in the descending or the transverse aorta, usually in the distal arch or proximal descending aorta. Type III dissections are further classified into type IIIa (dissection extending retrograde into the ascending aorta,

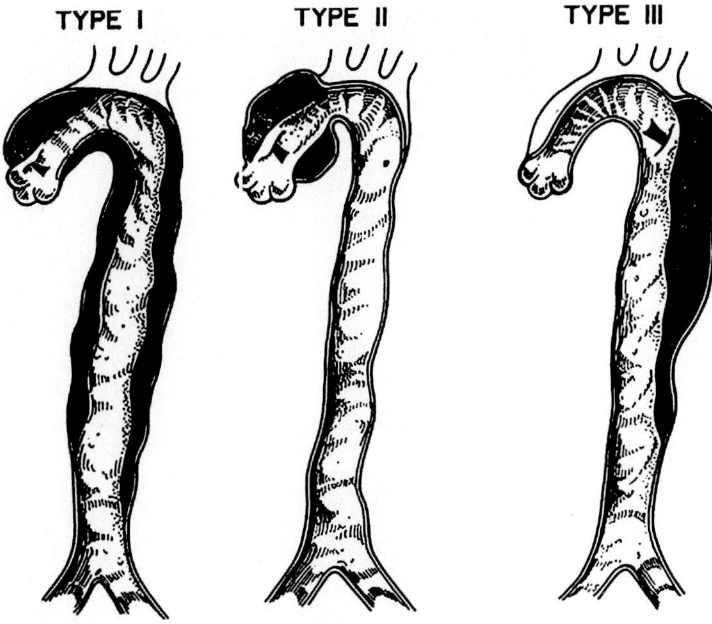

TYPE I TYPE II TYPE III

Figure 13–20. DeBakey classification of aortic dissections. (Reproduced with permission from Isselbacher EM, Eagle KA, Desanctis RW. Diseases of the aorta. In: Braunwald E (ed): Heart Disease. A Textbook of Cardiovascular Medicine, p 1555. Philadelphia, WB Saunders, 1997.)

9% of total) and type IIIb (dissection confined to the transverse arch or the descending aorta, 16% of total).

The Stanford classification is based on the site of dissection. Type A signifies that the dissection involves the ascending aorta irrespective of the site of origin, and type B signifies that the dissection does not involve the ascending aorta. A simplified classification (that is functionally nearly identical to the Stanford) is based simply on the site of intimal tear (proximal versus distal). Because the etiologic bases for aortic dissections vary primarily on the site of intimal tear, this simplified classification is best for discussions of pathogenesis; however, clinically, the DeBakey classification is in widespread use.

Proximal dissections are likely to result in death or life-threatening symptoms, and are therefore usually at an acute stage in autopsy or surgical specimens (Fig. 13–21). Distal dissections are more often chronic, demonstrating organized thrombus within the dissection plane and adventitial scarring.

Associated Conditions and Etiologic Factors

Cystic medial degeneration of the aorta is the common histologic manifestation that underlies most types of aortic dissection. The most common conditions associated with aortic dissection with cystic medial degeneration are hypertension, bicuspid aortic valve, and Marfan syndrome (Table 13–2). Additional miscellaneous associations have also been reported. In approximately 20% of patients, no known associations exist, other than idiopathic aortic root dilatation (annuloaortic ectasia) in patients with proximal dissections.

Hypertension

Hypertension is present in 80% of type III dissection and about one half of types I and II dissections. The mechanism of medial degeneration in hypertensives is unknown. Because hypertension is far more prevalent than aortic dissection, it is likely that there are additional factors predisposing hypertensive patients with aortic dissection to their aortic disease. There appears to be little interrelationship between hypertension and the other major associated conditions, because it is present in only 2–9% of Marfan patients with aortic dissection, and 2–8% of patients with bicuspid aortic valve and aortic dissection. The peak incidence of aortic dissection in hypertensives is in the sixth and seventh decades, with men affected twice as often as women.

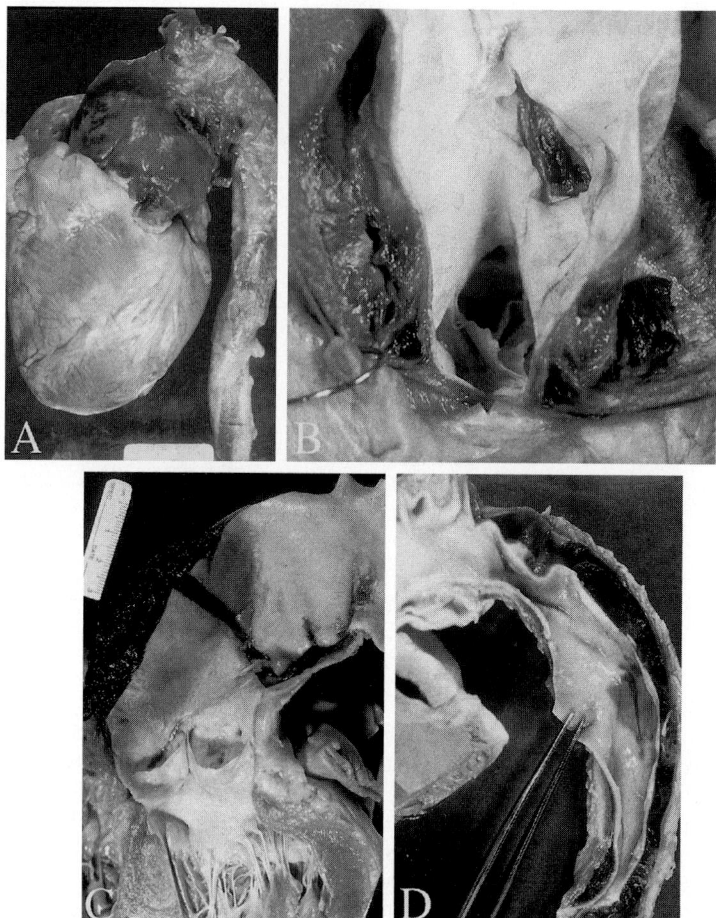

Figure 13–21. Aortic dissection, gross appearance. In *A,* the pericardial sac has been removed, as well as several hundred milliliters of pericardial blood. Adherent blood clots remain at the root of the aorta. *B* shows the opened aortic root demonstrated in *A.* Note a large, diagonal intimal tear and the blood within the outer layers of the aorta. The patient was a 50-year-old woman with a history of hypertension; there were no signs of Marfan syndrome and the aortic valve had three leaflets. Another patient's aorta is demonstrated in *C.* In this case, the tear is nearly circumferential, located above the left and noncoronary cusps. The patient was a 68-year-old man with poorly controlled hypertension who died suddenly while driving a truck. In *D,* there is a distal dissection, with the intimal tear (not shown) occurring distal to the origin of the left subclavian artery. Note the dissection in the outer wall of the aorta. The dissection had ruptured into the left hemithorax. The patient was a 39-year-old white female who was admitted with severe back pain; there was no prior medical history, but the patient was severely hypertensive.

Table 13–2. Frequency of Factors Predisposing to Aortic Dissection

	Hypertension	Marfan Syndrome	Bicuspid AV	None
Type I/II	52%[1]	5%[1]	14–16%[1,3]	27%[1]
Type III	75–83%[1,2]	2%[1]	0–2%[1,3]	15–21%[1,2,6]
Total	63–69%[4,5]	5–9%[4,5]	2–8%[3,4]	26%[4]

[1] Larson and Edwards, Am J Cardiol 53:849, 1984.
[2] Roberts and Roberts, Ann Surg 50:762, 1991.
[3] Roberts and Roberts, J Am Coll Cardiol 17:712–716, 1991.
[4] Nakashima et al., Hum Pathol 21:291, 1990.
[5] Wilson and Hutchins, Arch Pathol Lab Med 106:175, 1982.
[6] Some distal dissections may be precipitated by rupture of calcific atheromas.

Bicuspid and Unicuspid Aortic Valve (Fig. 13–22)

The association between the congenitally malformed aortic valve and aortic dissection was first reported by Abbott in 1927. It has been subsequently demonstrated that this association is only present in type I and type II dissections.[199] Of aortic dissections reported from autopsy series, a bicuspid valve was present in approximately 10%[199–201] which is more than five-fold the rate of bicuspid valve in the general population. A population-based study demonstrated that the relative risk of aortic dissection in patients with congenitally bicuspid valve was nine times normal, and that the relative risk for aortic dissection was 18 times normal in patients with congenitally unicuspid valve.[199] This increased relative risk was reflected in a higher frequency of bicuspid aortic valve (10 times) and unicuspid aortic valve (22 times) in patients with types I and II aortic dissection, compared with the autopsy population. In contrast, the incidence of congenital bicuspid valve in type III dissections was not increased. The mechanism of aortic dissection in patients with bicuspid aortic valve appears to be independent of hemodynamic alterations secondary to aortic stenosis, because significant valvular stenosis was only observed in 38% of patients with aortic dissection and a congenitally bicuspid valve. It remains to be documented if aortic cystic medial change is associated with bicuspid aortic valve in the absence of aortic dissection.

Marfan Syndrome

Marfan syndrome accounts for 6 to 9% of all aortic dissections. Conversely, aortic dissections occur in over one third of patients with Marfan syndrome. In 16 patients with Marfan syndrome in Larson and Edwards' population-based study, seven (44%) had aortic dissections.[199] Of

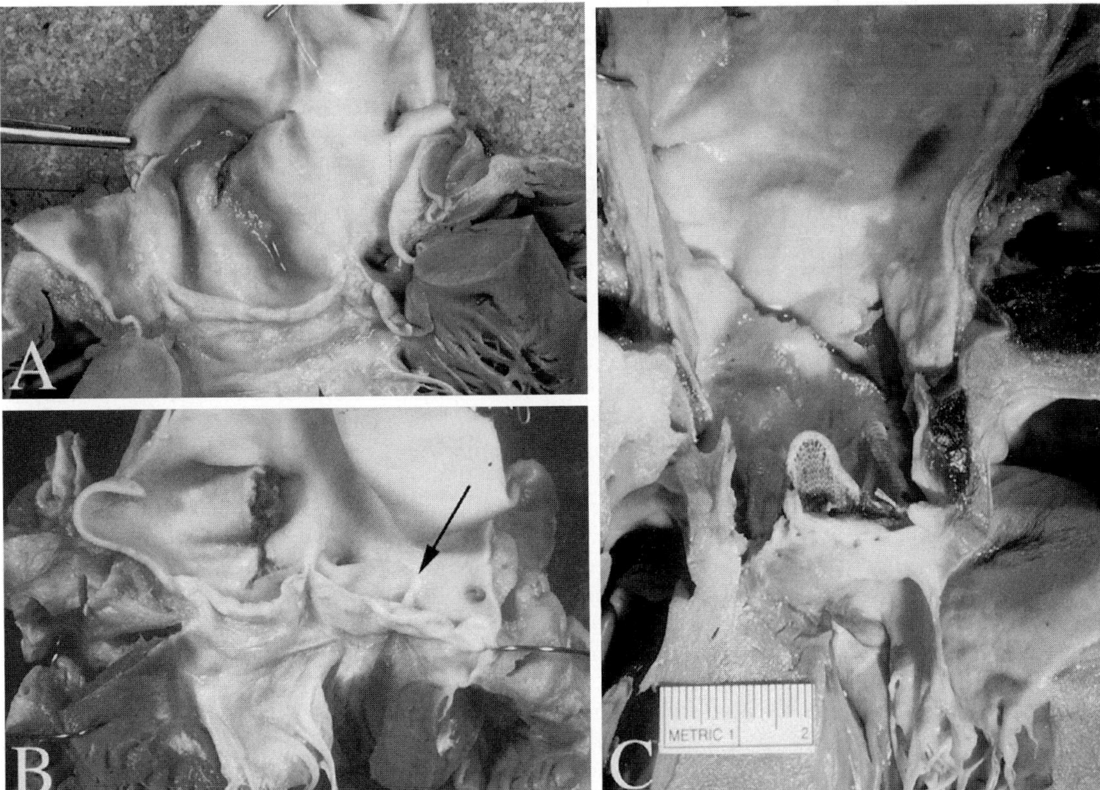

Figure 13–22. Two morphologic associations with aortic dissection include bicuspid aortic valve and associated remote valve repair. *A*. A bicuspid aortic valve; the posterior leaflet is shown, and the anterior leaflet has been cut through. The intimal tear is 1.5 cm above the sinotubular junction. *B*. A raphe (*arrow*) within the conjoint anterior leaflet containing the right and left coronary ostia. The intimal tear is longitudinal over the posterior noncoronary leaflet; note the thick, rolled edges suggesting a degree of premortem valve incompetence. *C*. A porcine bioprosthetic valve that had been in place for 4 years; note the diagonal intimal tear and intramural blood within the aortic wall.

these, three had type I dissection, three had type II dissection, and one had type III dissection.

Miscellaneous Conditions

In addition to hypertension, Marfan syndrome, and congenital malformed aortic valves, there are miscellaneous conditions that underlie or are associated with aortic dissection. A link between pregnancy and aortic dissection has been postulated, but not corroborated in more recent studies.[199] Over half of aortic dissections in women occur 40 years of age or younger, some of which occur during pregnancy (usually in the third trimester) and rarely in the postpartum period. Increase in blood pressure, blood volume, and cardiac output have been implicated as causative factors in dissections during pregnancy. A clear link between pregnancy and aortic dissection has yet to be documented.

Familial dissections in the absence of Marfan syndrome have been reported with increasing frequency.[202–204] To date, it is uncertain if these patients suffer from a forme fruste of Marfan syndrome with a similar genetic defect.

Cardiac surgery is associated with an increased risk of aortic dissection, usually occurring at the anastomotic site (aortotomy or site of saphenous vein grafting) or at the site of cross-clamping. The most common surgical procedure complicated by aortic dissection is aortic valve replacement. A majority of these iatrogenic dissections are discovered at the time of surgery and repaired, but 20% are discovered in the early postoperative period. Few also occur as a late complication (Fig. 13–22). Rarely aortic dissections have been observed following cardiac catheterization and intraaortic balloon pump and are thought to result from direct trauma to the intima. It is unclear if patients with iatrogenic dissections are at an increased risk because of inherent weakness in the aorta. In such cases, careful histologic evaluation for the presence of cystic medial change is warranted.

Uncommon conditions associated with aortic dissection include Noonan and Turner syndromes, as well as coarctation of the aorta. An association with cocaine abuse has been postulated, but it is unclear if this is mediated by catecholamine-induced hypertension. Blunt trauma has also been implicated in aortic dissection, but aortic rupture with pseudoaneurysm is a much more common complication of chest trauma (see following).

Histologic confirmation of aortic dissection is mandatory because, in occasional cases, the cause is inflammatory rather than degenerative. The most common aortitis resulting in dissection is giant-cell aortitis. Other forms of aortitis, such as Takayasu's disease and syphilis, may result in aortic rupture, but dissection is exceptional. Fibromuscular dysplasia (a common etiology of dissections of muscular arteries) rarely involves the aorta resulting in dissection.[205, 206]

Pathologic Findings (Gross)

In most pathologic series, an entry tear is found in virtually all cases.[199, 201, 207–209] An exception to this generalization is the series of Wilson and Hutchins, who found no entry tear in 13%.[198] In clinical series, the absence of an entry tear as documented by imaging studies is relatively common in patients with aortic dissections (so-called intramural hematoma). It is possible that imaging studies are relatively insensitive in the detection of entry tears, explaining the greater frequency of entry tears in autopsy studies. The existence of aortic dissections without entry tears is relevant in the pathogenesis of the disease (see following).

The site of tear in types I and II dissection is usually located 1 to 3 cm above the sinotubular junction (Figs. 13–21 and 13–22). The tear is usually transverse, located over the right and noncoronary cusps, and involves less than 50% of the circumference.[209] However, the tear may be diagonal, irregular, and occasionally involve nearly the entire circumference of the aorta. Most spontaneous dissections of types I and II occur in an area of aneurysmal dilatation, occasionally accompanied by dilatation of the aortic root. The splitting of the wall by the action of the dissection itself results in acute aneurysmal dilatation of the aorta and aortic insufficiency.

In contrast to proximal dissections, type III dissections are frequently silent and show evidence of healing in over 50% of cases. The intimal appearance of a healed dissection differs from that of an acute dissection, and is wrinkled, dull, and whitish-gray secondary to organization of the false luminal surface. The degree of preexisting aneurysmal dilatation is generally minimal in distal dissections, but the false lumen may be markedly dilated. Focally the dissected aortic wall may show residual attachments between torn intima or through organization of the thrombus result in luminal webs connecting the true and false lumens. The webs are anatomic landmarks helpful in the

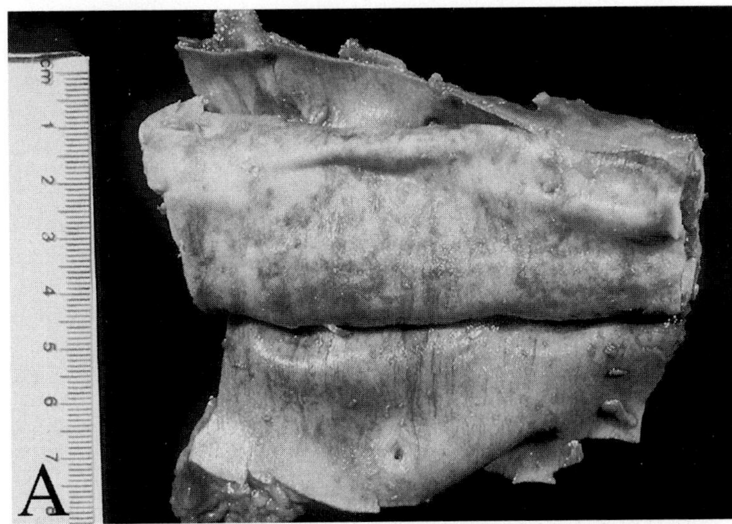

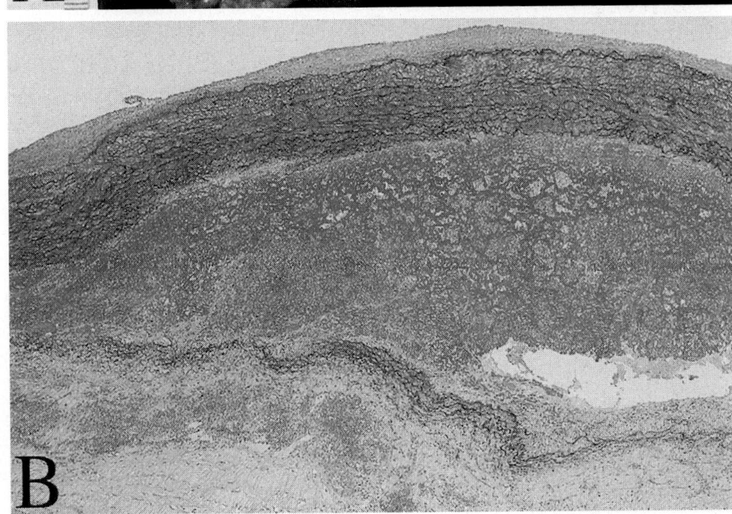

Figure 13–23. Acute aortic dissection. *A.* The false lumen is lined by strands of fibrin. In some cases of acute aortic dissection, portions of the dissected area is without blood (bloodless dissection), and the adventitia and outer media peels away from the remaining aorta. *B.* A histologic section of an acute dissection showing the intima and inner media (above), the blood in the dissection plane, and the adventitia with some elastic lamellae of outer media below.

radiologic diagnosis of acute and chronic dissections.[210] The entry tears are often of different ages; grossly, the appearance of the false lumen's lining may suggest the age of the dissection, acute subacute or chronic, which can be further estimated histologically. The connections between the true or false lumen and the major aortic branches should be documented at autopsy, in order to correlate pathologic findings with clinical history of renal or mesenteric obstruction.

Histologic Findings

The hallmark of histologic change in cases of aortic dissection that are not secondary to aortitis is medial degeneration, so-called cystic medial necrosis. Severe cystic medial necrosis is observed in 44% of Marfan patients, compared with only 18% of patients without the syndrome.[199] It has been suggested that severe medial degenerative changes are more pronounced in patients with Marfan syndrome and proximal type I dissections. In seven aortic dissections in Marfan patients reported by Larson and Edwards, three patients had severe cystic medial necrosis, all of whom had severe medial necrosis. In the four remaining patients, with types II and III dissections, the medial degenerative changes were all mild.[199]

The plane of dissection is usually located between the inner two thirds and the outer one third of the aortic media, or less commonly at the junction between the media and adventitia (Fig. 13–23). The age of the dissection may be estimated by evaluating the presence of granulation tissue and fibrosis in the dissecting plane and adventitial hematoma. In healed dissections, there is organized thrombus with diffuse deposition of fine elastic tissue in the dissection plane (Fig. 13–24).

Ultrastructural Findings

The three-dimensional architecture of the aorta by scanning electron microscopy after hot formic acid or sodium hydroxide digestion demonstrates a decrease in the number of interlaminar elastic fibers, which are irregular in arrangement and shape. The resulting rarefaction of the interconnection between the elastic laminae weakens the aortic wall, leading to the initiation and progression of the dissection.[211]

Clinical Presentation

Severe pain, the most common presenting symptom, is reported by 74 to 90% of patients and typically described as "tearing," "ripping," and "stabbing." Pain that migrates along the lines of dissection is present in 70% of patients.[212] The location of the pain usually coincides with the site of dissection: anterior chest pain corresponds with ascending aortic dissections (type II), and interscapular chest pain corresponds to descending thoracic aortic dissections (types I and III). Less frequent symptoms include congestive heart failure, syncope, cerebrovascular accident, ischemic peripheral neuropathy, paraplegia, and sudden death.

Physical examination can be helpful in establishing the diagnosis and site of dissection. A pulse deficit between the arms, the murmur of aortic insufficiency, and neurologic signs generally indicate a proximal dissection. Hypotension is often indicative of false luminal rupture, caused by cardiac tamponade in most cases of proximal dissections, and intrapleural or retroperitoneal hemorrhage in most cases of distal dissections.

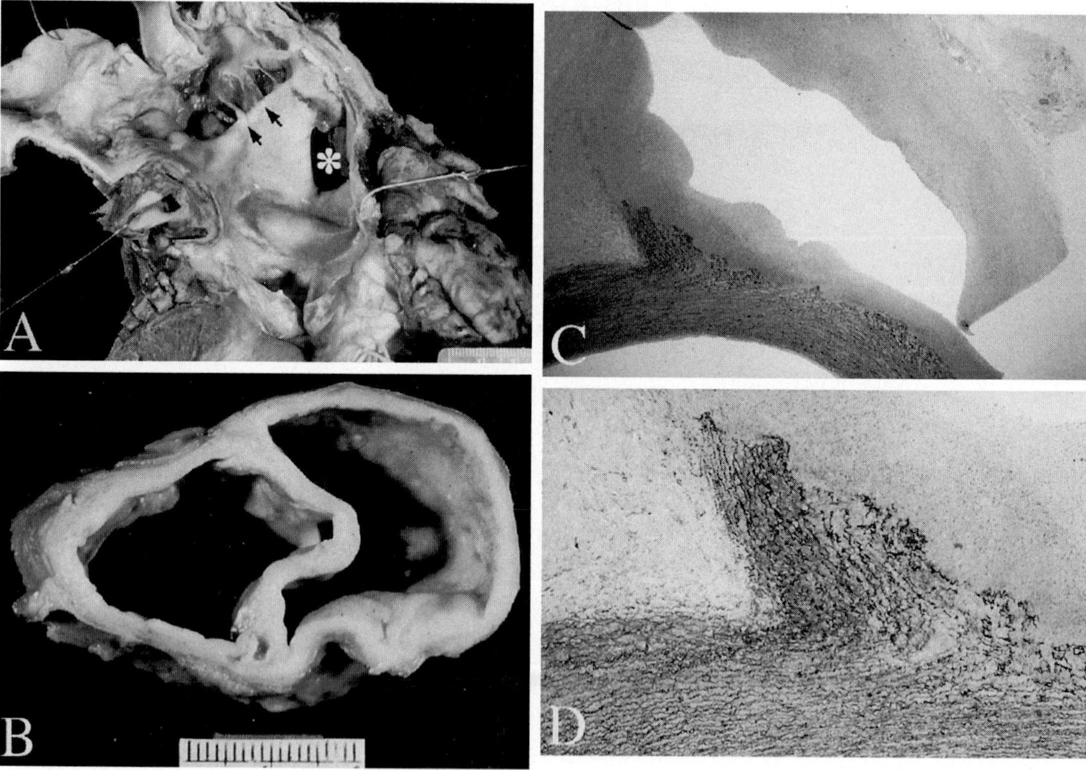

Figure 13–24. Chronic aortic dissection. Chronic aortic dissections result in a false lumen that is lined by fibrous tissue often rich in elastic fibers. *A.* The false lumen communicates with the true lumen in an area of healed intimal tear that is often partly covered with web-like strands of fibrous tissue (*arrowheads*); note an acute intimal tear below and to the right (*asterisk*). *B.* A cross section of a chronic dissection demonstrates the true lumen (*left*) and the false lumen (*right*). *C.* A histologic section of a healed dissection demonstrates the media and true lumen below, and the false lumen above. *D.* A higher magnification demonstrates the splitting of the media with the adventitia to the upper left (*pale area*) and separated media in the center, with the false lumen lining on the upper right.

An enlarged aortic knob or widening of the aortic silhouette on chest X-ray may be helpful in supporting the diagnosis of proximal aortic dissection. Diagnostic techniques include an aortography, contrast-enhanced CT, MRI, and transthoracic or transesophageal echocardiography. Each technique has its advantages and disadvantages in evaluating a patient with suspected aortic dissection, depending upon the site of dissection.

Complications and Cause of Death

The overall in-hospital mortality for acute aortic dissection is approximately 25%.[213] The two major direct complications of aortic dissection are rupture of the false lumen, and compression of the true lumen or arterial branches. The site of rupture of the false lumen in 90% of proximal dissections is the pericardium (Table 13–3). The majority of the remaining 10% of proximal dissections rupture into the left pleural cavity; rare sites of rupture include the mediastinum and right pleural space. In distal dissections, rupture of the false lumen occurs into the left pleural cavity in 60% of patients, and into the right pleural cavity in 24% of patients.[209] Rarely, the false lumen may rupture into the pericardium, mediastinum, or retroperitoneum.

Sustained loss of a peripheral pulse occurs in 24% of patients with aortic dissection, followed by 8% of patients with impaired renal perfusion, 5% of patients with compromised visceral perfusion, 3% of patients with stroke, and 3% of patients with paraplegia.[214] Compression of the coronary ostia, arch vessels, and branches of the abdominal aorta cause myocardial ischemia, stroke, and renal or mesenteric insufficiency, respectively. The mechanism of compression is either due to intimal flaps or webs, or dilatation of the false lumen compressing the true lumen. Repair of aortic dissections that extend into the abdominal aorta may include fenestration of intimal flaps, or replacement of a segment of the aorta with revascularization of renal arteries.[215]

In an autopsy series of 505 dissecting aortic aneurysms from the 1950s, 8% had direct extension into a coronary artery.[216] Both ostia were involved in 18 (46%), the right only in 15 (38%), and the left only in 5 (13%). Rarely, cerebral ischemia may be the presenting symptom in patients with aortic dissection.[217]

The cause of death in hospitalized patients with aortic dissection is rupture of the false lumen (62%), followed by causes unrelated to the dissection (15%), heart failure (9%), renal failure (7%), myocardial infarct (4%), and shock without false luminal rupture (3%).[209] The cause of death in patients dying suddenly with aortic dissection is almost always false luminal rupture. However, in approximately 5% of patients, no rupture of the false lumen is found to explain sudden death.

Treatment

The treatment of proximal aortic dissections includes repair of the aortic root with tube graft, valve replacement, and implantation of the coronary ostia into the tube graft (Bentall's procedure). Complications of this procedure include redissection (Fig. 13–25) at the anastomotic site. Surgical repair of dissections involving the aortic arch are difficult, and in some patients medical management with strict control of blood pressure is advocated.[218]

Most patients with type A dissections (those with involvement of the ascending aorta) are operated. Mortality of patients with type A dissection managed surgically is slightly over 25%;

Table 13–3. Site of False Lumen Rupture, Aortic Dissections

	Types I and II	Type III	All
Pericardium	90%	6%	70%
Mediastinum	2%	6%	3%
Left pleural cavity	6%	59%	19%
Right pleural cavity	2%	23%	7%
Retroperitoneum	0%	6%	1%

Adapted from Nakashima et al. Dissecting aneurysm: A clinicopathologic and histopathologic study of 111 autopsied cases. Hum Pathol 21:291–296, 1990, with permission.

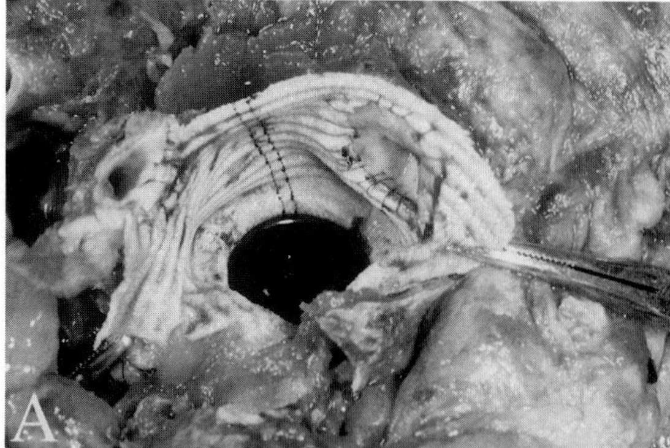

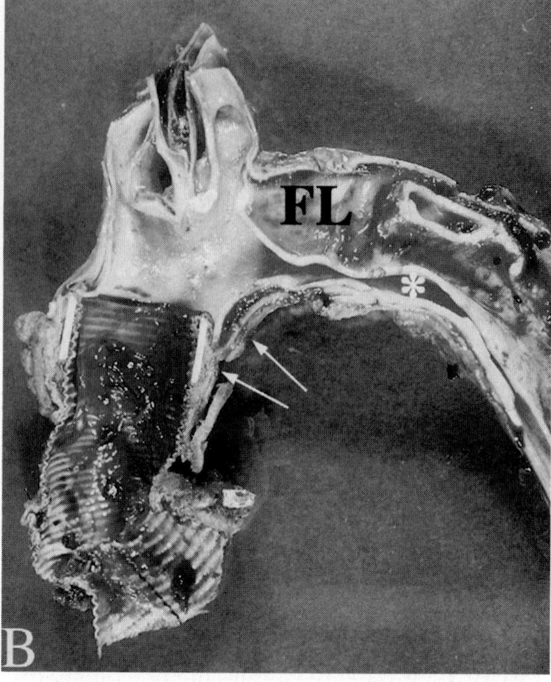

Figure 13–25. Surgical correction, aortic dissection. *A.* A tube graft made of Dacron, in which the coronary arteries have been implanted (upper left and upper right). The black center represents a prosthetic mechanical valve that has been sewn into the conduit. The upper portion of the conduit has been cut away to demonstrate the coronary ostial implantation. One potentially lethal complication of aortic dissection repair is redissection or extension of dissection. *B.* The tube graft is seen below, and there is a plastic sewing ring above at the distal anastomosis (*arrows*). Nevertheless, the dissection has involved this anastomosis (*arrow*), and extends distally; note false lumen above (*FL*), with compressed true lumen (*asterisk*). In this particular patient, a 47-year-old man with no prior history, the continuation of the dissection occurred intraoperatively and the patient did not survive surgery.

mortality is nearly 60% in patients too ill for surgical repair.[213] Type B dissections (distal dissections), however, are treated medically in 80% of cases, partly because of the difficulties involved in arch reconstruction and because the false lumen is less likely to rupture. Direct aortic replacement in the setting of acute descending aortic dissection continues to carry a very high mortality (28–65%) and paraplegia rate (30–35%).[219] Mortality of patients with type B dissection treated medically is approximately 10%, but increases to over 30% if surgical intervention is necessary for impending rupture or ischemic complications.[213] Patients who are followed have a high rate of complications and morbidity. Less than 10% do well, almost one half eventually require operation (including direct replacement of the aorta, thromboexclusion procedures, or fenestration procedures), and the remainder suffer one or more complications of rupture, vascular occlusion, early expansion or extension, and continued pain.[219] Because of the high mortality and morbidity of aortic dissections, endovascular treatments are being aggressively tested.[220] Endovascular stenting with balloon fenestrations of intimal flaps have been used to treat ischemic complications of aortic dissections.[221]

Abdominal Aortic Dissections

Abdominal aortic dissections are extremely rare, accounting for 1% of all aortic dissections.[222] A total of 26 cases with autopsy confirmation have been published. The mean age of these 26 patients (18 of whom were men) was 62 years. The incidence of rupture of the false lumen in abdominal aortic dissections is only 50%, lower than other types of aortic dissection. For this reason, it has been suggested that the chance of healing of the false lumen is directly proportional to the distance of the intimal tear from the aortic root (sinotubular junction).

AORTIC THROMBOSIS

Plaque ruptures are a feature of ulcerated atherosclerotic plaques, and mural thrombi are a constant finding in atherosclerotic abdominal aortic aneurysms. Aortoiliac occlusive disease (Leriche's syndrome) is obstruction of the abdominal aorta and its main branches by atherosclerosis and superimposed thrombosis. It presents as sudden excruciating bilateral lower extremity pain associated with weakness, numbness, and paresthesias. The disease is frequently precipitated by a low flow state secondary to heart failure or dehydration, and treated by intravenous heparin and immediate surgery. The occlusion site is typically distal to the inferior mesenteric artery, but may be between the renal arteries and inferior mesenteric or adjacent to the renal arteries. Magnetic resonance angiography is helpful in evaluating the location of the aortic occlusion, concomitant occlusive disease of the renal and visceral arteries, the type and extent of collateralization, and the level of the most proximal graftable arterial segments.[223] In some patients, the internal mammary artery is the sole source of lower leg perfusion, precluding its use in coronary artery bypass graft surgery.[224, 225]

In some patients, aortic thrombosis may occur in the absence of severe atherosclerosis, and be a result of coagulation disorders or thrombocytosis.[226] Involvement of the proximal branches of the mesenteric arteries is common in aortic thrombosis (Fig. 13–26). Idiopathic thrombosis of the aorta may occur in neonates.[227] Infection is an unusual cause of aortic thrombosis.[228] Intimal sarcomas of the aorta should be considered in the differential diagnosis of aortic mural thrombus (see Chapter 12).

TRAUMATIC PSEUDOANEURYSMS

Blunt trauma to the chest may result in aortic or valvular injury. The most common location of aortic rupture or transsection is the descending thoracic aorta near the ligamentum arteriosum. Other locations of cardiac and aortic damage after blunt trauma include the aortic valve, mitral valve, and aortic root[229–233] (Fig. 13–27).

Rupture of the aorta often results in exsanguination and death, although surgical repair is possible in shock-trauma centers. A minority of aortic ruptures heal, resulting in pseudoaneurysms that may not be diagnosed for years.[234] The most common site of aortic injury after vehicular trauma, seen in 65% of cases, is in the descending aorta within 1 cm of the origin of the subclavian artery at the insertion of the ligamentum arteriosum (65%). A minority are located in the ascending aorta (14%), at the distal descending thoracic aorta (12%), and abdominal aorta (9%).[235] Complete transections occur in two thirds of all cases, and usually occur

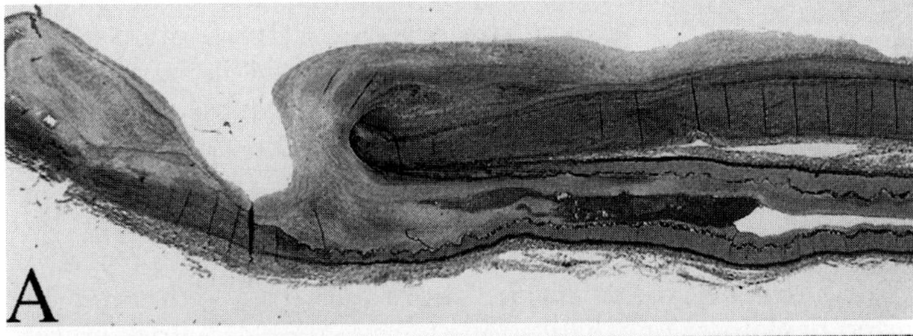

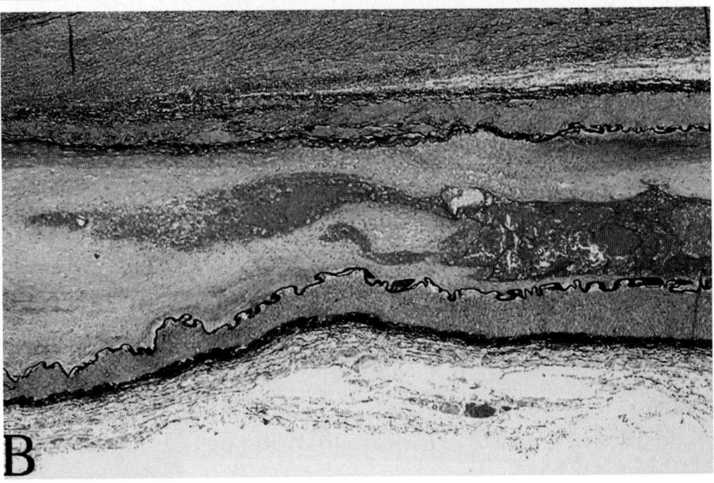

Figure 13–26. Mesenteric thrombosis. Although occlusive thrombosis of the aortic lumen is rare, the major branch may become occluded by embolization or *in situ* thrombosis. *A*. The superior mesenteric artery with total occlusion of the proximal segment by organizing thrombus. *B*. A higher magnification of the muscular artery (mesenteric artery) with occlusive thrombus.

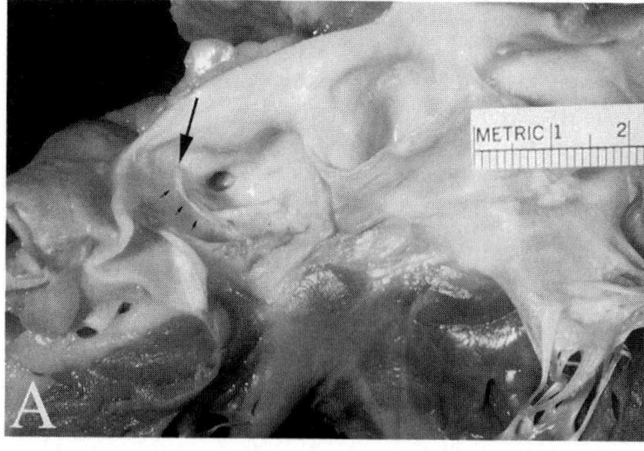

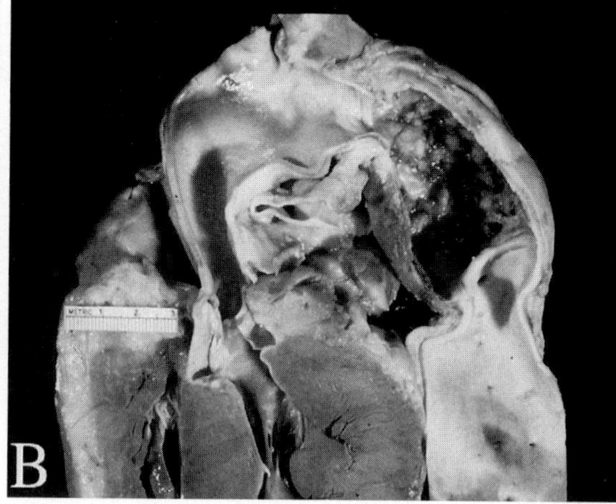

Figure 13–27. Aortic trauma. The major site involvements of aortic trauma are the area adjacent to the ligamentum arteriosum, ascending aorta, and aortic valve. *A.* Acute avulsion (*arrows*) of an aortic cusp secondary to vehicular trauma resulting in acute aortic insufficiency. *B.* There is a chronic aortic rupture at the level of the ligamentum arteriosum in the descending thoracic aorta. This rupture resulted in a pseudoaneurysm that measured over 5 cm and was heavily calcified. These pseudoaneurysms may be stable for years, or gradually expand and rupture.

if the site of tear is adjacent to the left subclavian artery. The remaining third of aortic ruptures are incomplete tears, two thirds of which are in the ascending aorta. The intimal tears are usually transverse, and are multiple in approximately 10% of patients.

It is estimated that 10 to 20% of patients live long enough to undergo surgical repair of a traumatic pseudoaneurysm. Rarely, a pseudoaneurysm is asymptomatic, and the history of chest trauma may be remote or nearly forgotten.[236] In such patients, the aneurysm may be discovered on routine chest x-ray. Occasionally, there may be rupture into an adjacent structure, such as the esophagus.[237] Grossly and histologically, there is a sharp demarcation between the normal media and the fibrous lining of the pseudoaneurysm. With time, the intimal surface shows an organized hematoma or calcification.

DISEASES OF THE LARGE VEINS

Thrombosis of the Superior Vena Cava

Thrombosis of the superior vena cava and its tributaries results in the superior vena cava syndrome, characterized by reduced venous outflow from the head, neck, and upper extremities. Symptoms are facial edema, cyanosis, dyspnea, and prominent neck veins. The most common causes are thoracic neoplasms, including lung carcinomas, lymphomas, and metastatic disease. Unusual causes are fibrosing mediastinitis, indwelling catheters, pacemakers, LeVeen shunts, administration of megestrol acetate,[238] aortic dissections and aneurysms, Behçet's disease,[239] and bronchial artery aneurysm.[240]

Thrombosis of the Inferior Vena Cava

Obstruction of the inferior vena cava is most often a complication of thrombotic occlusion by neoplasms growing within the lumen or causing external compression. The neoplasms implicated are usually renal,[241–243] adrenal, hepatic, or testicular.[244, 245] Idiopathic forms of diffuse thrombosis of the inferior vena cava have been reported.[246] An uncommon complication of orthotopic liver transplant is thrombosis of the inferior vena cava, which can be successfully treated surgically.[247] Tumor-induced thrombosis may be treated with the placement of a filter to prevent pulmonary embolism, similar to treatment for recurrent thromboembolism from leg veins.[248] Neonatal thrombosis of the inferior vena cava may be the result of renal vein thrombosis, and cause fibrous obstruction of the vein and duodenal varices in adulthood.[249]

Thrombosis of the hepatic veins (Budd–Chiari syndrome) may be complicated by obstruction of the inferior vena cava. Symptoms of hepatic vein thrombosis include ascites, jaundice, gastrointestinal bleeding, hepatomegaly, leg edema, varicose veins, and venous collaterals over the abdominal and chest wall. The most common known cause is thrombosis secondary to myeloproliferative diseases.[250] Other causes include abdominal trauma, hepatic tumors, pregnancy, and oral contraceptive use.

Obstruction of distal hepatic veins and inferior vena cava by membranous webs is a form of Budd–Chiari syndrome associated with similar symptoms. Membranous obstruction of the inferior vena cava is sometimes considered congenital, and sometimes considered a sequelae of repeated thrombosis.[251] The simultaneous occurrence of myeloproliferative syndromes and membranous obstruction of the inferior vena cava supports the latter view, and corroborates the link between hepatic vein thrombosis and membranous obstruction.[252]

Mortality is high in the acute phase of hepatic vein obstruction. Prognosis is good if the initial phase is survived, however. Treatment includes anticoagulation, measures to control ascites and bleeding, portal–caval shunts, and orthotopic liver transplants if there is severe liver failure. Membranes in the inferior vena cava may be lysed by percutaneous angioplasty.

Venous Aneurysms

Venous aneurysms are often the result of increased flow and turbulence adjacent to arteriovenous malformations, or as complications of surgery. Congenital venous aneurysms are rare, and have been described in the jugular, portal, superior mesenteric, splenic, femoral, popliteal, saphenous, and axillary veins, as well as the venae cavae.[253–255] Symptoms of aneurysms of the inferior vena cava include deep venous thrombosis, pulmonary embolism, retroperitoneal hemorrhage after rupture, and abdominal mass. Aneurysms of the inferior vena cava may complicate membranous obstruction at the level of the hepatic veins.[256] There are few pathologic descriptions of venous aneurysms; in our experience, the aneurysm wall is composed of focally thinned and disorganized smooth muscle, with luminal thrombosis in some cases.

DISEASE OF THE PROXIMAL PULMONARY ARTERIES

Pulmonary Thromboembolism

Clinical

Thrombosis of elastic arteries is almost always caused by thromboembolism.[257] Clinically, thromboembolism is characterized by chest pain and shortness of breath, although symptoms are notoriously variable. Suspicion for diagnosis is increased with proven leg-vein thrombosis, right-heart strain on electrocardiography, neck-vein distension, and suspicious chest x-ray; diagnosis is confirmed by scintigraphy and, if necessary, angiography.

The pathologist typically encounters pulmonary embolism at autopsy. In fatal cases, a clinical diagnosis was made antemortem in only 28–50% of autopsies demonstrating pulmonary embolism.[258–261] The most important causes of an incorrect diagnosis are failure to suspect pulmonary embolism clinically. The incidence of pulmonary embolism at autopsy in cases of natural sudden death is approximately 5%, the majority of remainder representing coronary artery disease or cardiomyopathy. The initial rhythm diagnosis is usually pulseless electrical activity in 63%; followed by asystole, 32%; and ventricular fibrillation, 5%.[262]

Incidence

The overall incidence of pulmonary embolism is difficult to assess and has been estimated over a large range. This estimate varies from 23 to over 200 per 100,000 population annually, both for fatal and nonfatal cases.[263–265] The rate increases with age, with a cumulative risk of 4% by age 80.[263] It has been estimated that pulmonary embolism is the cause of death of up to 5% of all people,[263] although some studies put this percentage far lower, at approximately 0.2%.[260] The mortality of patients diagnosed with pulmonary embolism is high and has been estimated at over 10%, which increases to 30% after 3 years of hospital discharge.[264] The rate of pulmonary embolism is slightly higher in African Americans as compared to Caucasians, and is higher in women than men over the age of 50. There is no gender predilection at younger ages.[265]

Risk Factors

Pulmonary embolism accounts for at least 1% of hospital admissions.[260] The rate of pulmonary embolism at hospital-based autopsy ranges from 20 to 35%[266–268] and is the cause of death in approximately 3 to 5% of hospitalized patients.[269] The major risk factors for pulmonary embolism are deep venous thrombosis, trauma, postoperative state (accounting for approximately 25% of hospital deaths due to pulmonary embolism),[269] obesity, malignancy, old age, female gender, and chronic heart disease. Among subjects with a malignant neoplasm, patients with pancreatic and gastric cancer, cancer of the large bowel, and women with ovarian cancers had the highest frequency of pulmonary embolism.[268]

Patients with major trauma are at increased risk for the development of pulmonary embolism, with an incidence of approximately 0.3%.[270] After surgical procedures, the risk of pulmonary embolism is approximately 0.4% in patients without major risk factors[271, 272]; the risk for fatal embolism is approximately 0.1%. Death from pulmonary embolism may occur within 24 hours of the procedure and up to 30 days thereafter.[269]

Several genetic risk factors for pulmonary embolism have been investigated. Deficiencies in proteins C and S may be first diagnosed in patients who present with pulmonary embolism at a young age, often postoperatively.[273–279] Affected members of families with protein-S deficiency suffer pulmonary embolism at a high rate, from 7 to 26%, depending on other genetic factors.[280] A much more common inherited hypercoagulable state is resistance to activated protein C (factor V Leiden, caused by a point mutation at amino acid 506, occurring in 3 to 5% of the U.S. population). Although there are anecdotal reports and small series of patients suggesting a relationship between factor V Leiden and pulmonary embolism, larger series show no increased risk or only a slightly increased risk of pulmonary embolism compared with the general population.[281, 282] A large study from a medical examiner has not shown an increased frequency of factor V Leiden in a series of patients dying with unexpected pulmonary embolism,[283] and neither has a retrospective study of medical autopsies.[284] The lack of association between pulmonary embolism and factor V Leiden is perplexing, given the established increased risk for deep venous thrombosis.[285–287] It is possible that resistance to activated protein C is a risk factor for pulmonary embolism only in certain populations, as suggested by a study of young women, which showed that the factor V Leiden mutation is an important risk factor for pulmonary embolism during pregnancy (especially the first trimester), after pregnancy, or during oral contraceptive use.[288] Other thrombophilic factors that have been implicated in pulmonary embolism include a polymorphism of plasminogen activator inhibitor-1, which may increase the risk of pulmonary embolism in protein-S deficient individuals,[280] and polymorphism for factor II (prothrombin G20210A polymorphism).[289, 290]

Pathologic Findings

There are several pathologic features at autopsy concerning pulmonary embolism that are important in pathogenesis and clinical manifestations. Features for the autopsy pathologist to consider are the point of origin, final localization, size and age of thromboemboli, the presence or absence of pulmonary infarction, and the underlying cardiac or other conditions.

The point of origin is usually in the lower veins (legs and abdomen). In a large series, 60% of thrombi were located in the lower venous tree, in 12% in the upper venous tree, and in 28% no source could be detected.[266] A different study demonstrated an originating thrombus in only 53% of cases,[261] the sources in the other 47% being found in the leg veins and inferior vena cava (86%), inferior vena cava extending into the right heart or superior vena cava (8%), right heart alone (3%), and superior vena cava (3%). The most common veins of origin of the thromboembolus are the left femoral vein and the right internal jugular vein. The incidence of upper veins as a source of embolism has increased, possibly because of the increased frequency in indwelling subclavian catheters. The originating thrombi may be overlooked in an attempt to prevent disfigurement of the body, or the entire clot may have dislodged or lysed.

The location of the embolus in the lungs should be described. Although saddle emboli are invariably fatal, pulmonary emboli in cases of sudden death may be segmental, only involving muscular arteries (Fig. 13–28). Often a fatal embolus is relatively small but hardly tolerated because of the underlying cardiopulmonary situation. There is a wide variety of patterns of pulmonary embolism,[261] but there is a predisposition to the right lung and lower lobes, and multiple emboli are the rule.

Dating of pulmonary embolism is impossible based on histologic grounds, but there are several points to consider. Endothelialization of the surface of the clot occurs relatively quickly, but it generally takes more than 1 day for a significant length of clot to demonstrate an endothelial surface. The center of larger clots may be devoid of organization for long periods of time, and care should be taken to make an assessment of an acute lesion on the basis of

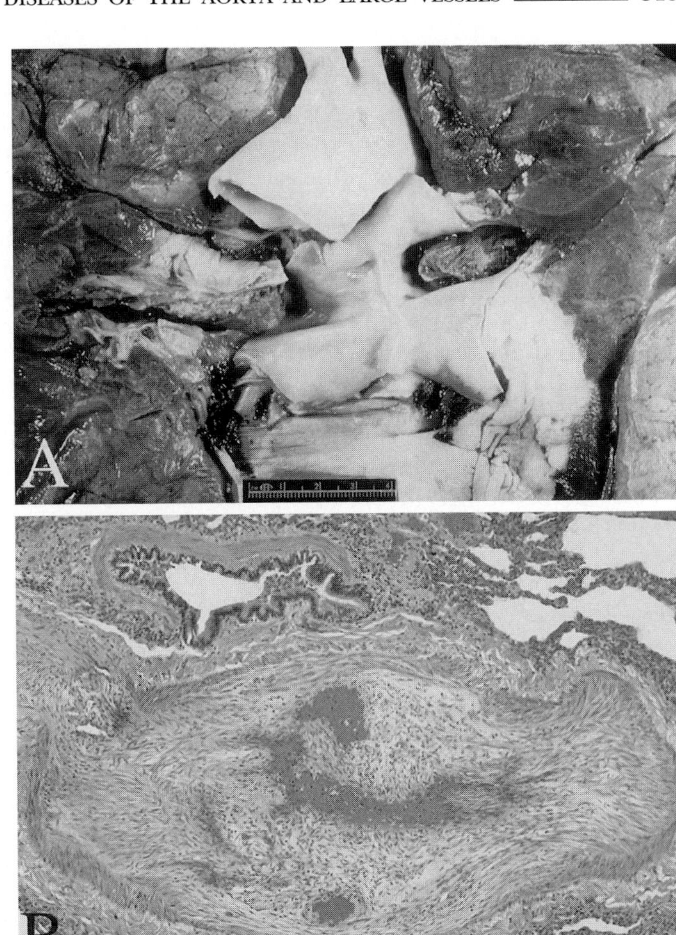

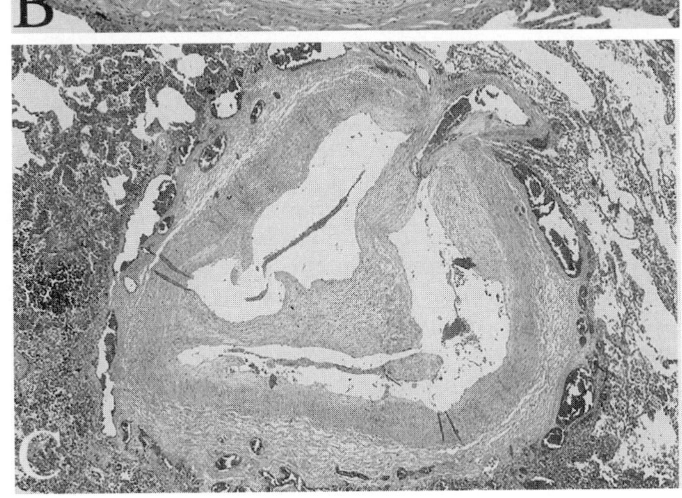

Figure 13–28. Pulmonary embolism. *A.* In this patient who died of massive embolism, there are occlusive thrombi in the right and left main pulmonary arteries. *B.* A recanalized thrombus with cellular intimal proliferation. *C.* An older recanalized thrombus with fibrous webs within the lumen of the artery.

limited sampling. Often, emboli in different vessels will demonstrate various ages, indicating that the patient was showering emboli for some time prior to death. The final stage of pulmonary emboli are recanalized thrombi or vascular webs, which are often overlooked or not well documented at autopsy.

Attention should be called to the frequent autopsy finding of pulmonary infarctions of apparently different age. Because of the dual blood supply of the lungs, infarction occurs only if there is associated heart disease, especially mitral stenosis. Pulmonary infarctions occur in about 15% of the cases, are more common in females, and are rare in patients without underlying cardiac diseases.[291]

Predisposing conditions that contribute to the likelihood of pulmonary embolism at autopsy include malignancies and cardiovascular diseases. Patients with rheumatic heart disease or old myocardial infarction have a significantly higher frequency of pulmonary embolism than patients with acute myocardial infarction.[292] Of pulmonary emboli found at autopsy, approximately 30–40% are considered the cause of death, 25% contribute to death, and the remaining are incidental. Symptomatic deep vein thrombosis or pulmonary embolism are uncommon prior to autopsy-documented pulmonary embolism, partly because these patients are treated with anticoagulation.[266, 267]

Miscellaneous Pulmonary Embolism

Tumors that are likely to embolize to the right heart and proximal pulmonary tree include hepatocellular carcinoma,[293] right atrial myxoma,[294] and renal cell carcinoma, but a variety of others have been reported.[295] Other uncommon sources of embolism are fat embolism after orthopedic surgery, which generally involves smaller arteries,[296] liver tissue following trauma,[297] and herniated nucleus pulposus.[298]

Pulmonary Artery Thrombosis

In situ thrombosis of elastic pulmonary arteries is rare and may be associated with the antiphospholipid syndrome,[299] Behçet's disease,[300, 301] Takayasu's disease,[71] and other forms of vasculitis affecting the pulmonary arteries.[302, 303] Pulmonary artery thrombosis is an uncommon complication of right-heart catheterization.[304] *In situ* thrombosis of medium-sized muscular pulmonary arteries is a frequent finding in pulmonary hypertension; more distal thrombi are usually the result of showering of pulmonary emboli.[257]

Vasculitis of the Main Pulmonary Arteries

The vasculitic syndrome with the most frequent involvement of elastic pulmonary arteries is Takayasu's disease.[71] Abnormalities of pulmonary arteries are seen in up to 70% of patients in whom angiography is performed.[305] Angiographic lesions are occlusions (67%), stenoses (32%) and, rarely, aneurysms (1%). Lesions occur in the entire course of the pulmonary arteries, but are most numerous in segmental and subsegmental branches. Histologically, the elastic arteries show disruption of the elastic layers with thinning of the media and pronounced fibrosis of the adventitia. Occlusions, which are more common distally, are characterized by marked intimal fibrosis and eccentric intimal fibrotic thickening. Chronic inflammation of muscular arteries and small-vessel angiomatoid lesions have also been described.[71]

Behçet's disease involves the pulmonary tree in about 10% of patients, manifesting as aneurysms and thrombosis (see following). Giant-cell arteritis rarely involves the proximal pulmonary arteries, resulting in thrombotic occlusion and medial granulomas.[306, 307]

Pulmonary Artery Aneurysms

Most aneurysms of the pulmonary artery are noninflammatory. They are usually found in patients with severe pulmonary hypertension, either idiopathic or secondary to congenital heart disease, acquired heart disease, or pulmonary disease.[308, 309] Inflammatory pulmonary aneurysms are found in 1% of patients with Behçet's disease[310, 311] and rarely in patients with syphilis.[312] Pseudoaneurysms of the pulmonary artery are usually the result of catheter-induced trauma.[313] Presumed congenital (idiopathic) pulmonary artery aneurysms have been described in patients without predisposing factors.[312, 314] There is an association between pulmonary aneurysm and pregnancy[315] and spontaneous rupture of the pulmonary artery without aneurysm has been reported.[316] Pulmonary artery aneurysm is a rare manifestation of Marfan syndrome.[317]

Grossly, pulmonary artery aneurysms may be fusiform or saccular. Aneurysmal dilatation of the pulmonary trunk is defined as a diameter of 4 cm or greater. The histologic findings of hypertension-induced pulmonary artery aneurysms include medial degeneration in the fusiform types and atherosclerosis in the saccular forms.[308] Behçet's aneurysms show inflammatory infiltrates in all layers of arteries and veins,[309] leading to thrombosis, destruction of the elastic laminae, and arteriobronchial fistula.[301]

The major complication of hypertension-induced pulmonary aneurysms is dissection[315, 318] and rupture.

REFERENCES

1. Janzen J, Vuong PN, Rothenberger-Janzen K. Takayasu's arteritis and fibromuscular dysplasia as causes of acquired atypical coarctation of the aorta: Retrospective analysis of seven cases. Heart Vessels 14:277–282, 1999.
2. Russell GA, Berry PJ, Watterson K, Dhasmana JP, Wisheart JD. Patterns of ductal tissue in coarctation of the aorta in the first three months of life. J Thorac Cardiovasc Surg 102:596–601, 1991.
3. Van Son JA, Lacquet LK, Smedts F. Patterns of ductal tissue in coarctation of the aorta in early infancy. J Thorac Cardiovasc Surg 105:368–369, 1993.
4. Jonas RA. Coarctation: Do we need to resect ductal tissue? Ann Thorac Surg 52:604–607, 1991.
5. Merrill WH, Hoff SJ, Stewart JR, Elkins CC, Graham TPJ, Bender HWJ. Operative risk factors and durability of repair of coarctation of the aorta in the neonate. Ann Thorac Surg 58:399–340, 1994.
6. Zannini L, Gargiulo G, Albanese SB, et al. Aortic coarctation with hypoplastic arch in neonates: A spectrum of anatomic lesions requiring different surgical options. Ann Thorac Surg 56:288–294, 1993.
7. Johnson MC, Canter CW, Strauss AW, Spray TL. Repair of coarctation of the aorta in infancy: Comparison of surgical and balloon angioplasty. Am Heart J 125:464–468, 1993.
8. Thanopoulos BD, Hadjinikolaou L, Konstadopoulou GN, Tsaousis GS, Triposkiadis F, Spirou P. Stent treatment for coarctation of the aorta: Intermediate term follow up and technical considerations. Heart 84:65–70, 2000.
9. Koerselman J, de Vries H, Jaarsma W, Muyldermans L, Ernst JM, Plokker HW. Balloon angioplasty of coarctation of the aorta: A safe alternative for surgery in adults: Immediate and mid-term results. Catheter Cardiovasc Interv 50:28–33, 2000.
10. Suarez de Lezo J, Pan M, Romero M, et al. Immediate and follow-up findings after stent treatment for severe coarctation of aorta. Am J Cardiol 83:400–406, 1999.
11. Isselbacher EM, Eagle KA, Desanctis RW. Disease of the aorta. In: Braunwald E (ed): Heart Disease: A Textbook of Cardiovascular Medicine, pp 1546–1581. Philadelphia: WB Saunders, 1997.
12. Perloff J. Congenital heart disease in adults. In: Braunwald E, (ed): Heart Disease: A Textbook of Cardiovascular Medicine, pp 963–987. Philadelphia: WB Saunders, 1997.
13. Xu Q, Peng Z, Rahko PS. Doppler echocardiographic characteristics of sinus of Valsalva aneurysms. Am Heart J 130:1265–1269, 1995.
14. Boutefeu JM, Moret PR, Hahn C, Hauf E. Aneurysm of the sinus of Valsalva. Report of seven cases and review of the literature. Am J Med 65:18–24, 1978.
15. Sakakibara S, Konno S. Congenital aneurysms of the sinus of Valsalva: Anatomy and classification. Am Heart J 63:405–424, 1962.
16. Pyeritz RE. The Marfan syndrome. Annu Rev Med 51:481–510, 2000.
17. Fuchs J. Marfan syndrome and other systemic disorders with congenital ectopia lentis. A Danish national survey. Acta Paediatr 86:947–952, 1997.
18. Robinson PN, Godfrey M. The molecular genetics of Marfan syndrome and related microfibrillopathies. J Med Genet 37:9–25, 2000.
19. Chikumi H, Yamamoto T, Ohta Y, et al. Fibrillin gene (FBN1) mutations in Japanese patients with Marfan syndrome. J Hum Genet 45:115–118, 2000.
20. Palz M, Tiecke F, Booms P, et al. Clustering of mutations associated with mild Marfan-like phenotypes in the 3' region of FBN1 suggests a potential genotype–phenotype correlation. Am J Med Genet 91:212–221, 2000.
21. Hayward C, Brock DJ. Fibrillin-1 mutations in Marfan syndrome and other type-1 fibrillinopathies. Hum Mutat 10:415–423, 1997.
22. Conway JE, Hutchins GM, Tamargo RJ. Marfan syndrome is not associated with intracranial aneurysms. Stroke 30:1632–1636, 1999.
23. Pyeritz RE. The Marfan syndrome. In: Royce PM, Steinmann B (eds): Connective Tissue and Its Heritable Disorders: Molecular, Genetic, and Medical Aspects, pp 437–468. New York: Wiley-Liss, 1993.
24. Baumgartner WA, Cameron DE, Redmond JM, Greene PS, Gott VL. Operative management of Marfan syndrome: The Johns Hopkins experience. Ann Thorac Surg 67:1859–1860; discussion 1868–1870, 1999.
25. Gott VL, Greene PS, Alejo DE, et al. Replacement of the aortic root in patients with Marfan's syndrome. N Engl J Med 340:1307–1313, 1999.
26. Tambeur L, David TE, Unger M, Armstrong S, Ivanov J, Webb G. Results of surgery for aortic root aneurysm in patients with the Marfan syndrome. Eur J Cardiothorac Surg 17:415–419, 2000.
27. Fleischer KJ, Nousari HC, Anhalt GJ, Stone CD, Laschinger JC. Immunohistochemical abnormalities of fibrillin in cardiovascular tissues in Marfan's syndrome. Ann Thorac Surg 63:1012–1017, 1997.
28. Roberts WC, Honig HS. The spectrum of cardiovascular disease in Marfan syndrome: A clinicopathologic study of 18 necropsy patients. Am Heart J 104:115–135, 1982.
29. Pepin M, Schwarze U, Superti-Furga A, Byers PH. Clinical and genetic features of Ehlers–Danlos syndrome type IV, the vascular type. N Engl J Med 342:673–680, 2000.
30. Byers PH. Disorders of collage biosynthesis and structure. In: Scriver CR, Beaudet AL, Sly WA, Valle D (eds): The Metabolic and Molecular Bases of Inherited Diseases, p 4029. New York: McGraw-Hill, 1995.
31. Shapiro JR, Burn VE, Chipman SD, et al. Pulmonary hypoplasia and osteogenesis imperfecta type II with defective synthesis of alpha I(1) procollagen. Bone 10:165–171, 1989.
32. Slayton RL, Deschenes SP, Willing MC. Nonsense mutations in the COL1A1 gene preferentially reduce nuclear levels of mRNA but not hnRNA in osteogenesis imperfecta type I cell strains. Matrix Biol 19:1–9, 2000.
33. McAllion SJ, Paterson CR. Causes of death in osteogenesis imperfecta. J Clin Pathol 49:627–630, 1996.
34. White NJ, Winearls CG, Smith R. Cardiovascular abnormalities in osteogenesis imperfecta. Am Heart J 106:1416–1420, 1983.
35. Hortop J, Tsipouras P, Hanley JA, Maron BJ, Shapiro JR. Cardiovascular involvement in osteogenesis imperfecta. Circulation 73:54–61, 1986.
36. Isotalo PA, Guindi MM, Bedard P, Brais MP, Veinot JP. Aortic dissection: A rare complication of osteogenesis imperfecta. Can J Cardiol 15:1139–1142, 1999.
37. Zegdi R, D'Attellis N, Fornes P, et al. Aortic valve surgery in osteogenesis imperfecta: Report of two cases

and review of the literature. J Heart Valve Dis 7:510–514, 1998.

38. Virmani R, Avolio AP, Mergner WJ, et al. Effect of aging on aortic morphology in populations with high and low prevalence of hypertension and atherosclerosis. Comparison between occidental and Chinese communities. Am J Pathol 139:1119–1129, 1991.
39. Groenink M, Langerak SE, Vanbavel E, et al. The influence of aging and aortic stiffness on permanent dilation and breaking stress of the thoracic descending aorta. Cardiovasc Res 43:471–480, 1999.
40. Schlatmann T, Becker A. Pathogenesis of dissecting aneurysm of aorta. Comparative histopathologic study of significance of medial changes. Am J Cardiol 39:21–26, 1977.
41. Stefanadis C, Vlachopoulos C, Karayannacos P, et al. Effect of vasa vasorum flow on structure and function of the aorta in experimental animals. Circulation 91:2669–2678, 1995.
42. Sariola H, Viljanen T, Luosto R. Histological pattern and changes in extracellular matrix in aortic dissections. J Clin Pathol. 39:1074–1081, 1986.
43. Ueda T, Shimizu H, Aeba R, et al. Prognosis of Marfan and non-Marfan patients with cystic medial necrosis of the aorta. Jpn J Thorac Cardiovasc Surg 47:73–78, 1999.
44. de Sa M, Moshkovitz Y, Butany J, David TE. Histologic abnormalities of the ascending aorta and pulmonary trunk in patients with bicuspid aortic valve disease: Clinical relevance to the Ross procedure. J Thorac Cardiovasc Surg 118:588–594, 1999.
45. Ihling C, Szombathy T, Nampoothiri K, et al. Cystic medial degeneration of the aorta is associated with p53 accumulation, Bax upregulation, apoptotic cell death, and cell proliferation. Heart 82:286–293, 1999.
46. Takayasu M. Case with unusual changes of the central vessels in the retina. Acta Soc Ophthalmol Jap 112:554–561, 1908.
47. Shimizu K, Sano K. Pulseless disease. J Neuropathol 1:37–47, 1951.
48. Hall S, Barr W, Lie JT. Takayasu's arteritis. A study of 32 North American patients. Medicine 64:89–99, 1985.
49. Lupi-Herrera E, Sanchez-Torres G, Marcushamer J, Mispireta J, Horowitz S, Vela JE. Takayasu's arteritis. Clinical study of 107 cases. Am Heart J 93:94–103, 1977.
50. Morooka S, Saito Y, Nonaka Y, Gyotoku Y, Sugimoto T. Clinical features and course of aortitis syndrome in Japanese women older than 40 years. Am J Cardiol 53:859–861, 1984.
51. Kitamura H, Kobayashi Y, Kimura A, Numano F. Association of clinical manifestations with HLA-B alleles in Takayasu arteritis. Int J Cardiol 66:S121–S126, 1998.
52. Basso C, Baracca E, Zonzin P, Thiene G. Sudden cardiac arrest in a teenager as first manifestation of Takayasu's disease. Int J Cardiol 43:87–89, 1994.
53. Matsumura K, Hirano T, Takeda K, et al. Incidence of aneurysms in Takayasu's arteritis. Angiology 42:308–315, 1991.
54. Ueda H, Sugiura M, Ito I, Saito Y, Morooka S. Aortic insufficiency associated with aortitis syndrome. Jpn Heart J 8:107–120, 1967.
55. Sharma BK, Jain S, Radotra BD. An autopsy study of Takayasu arteritis in India. Int J Cardiol 66:S85–S90; discussion S91, 1998.
56. Ueda H, Morooka S, Ito I, Yamaguchi H, Takeda T, Saito Y. Clinical observations on 52 cases of aortitis syndrome. Jpn Heart J 10:277–288, 1969.
57. Elsasser S, Soler M, Bolliger C, Jager K, Steiger U, Perruchoud AP. Takayasu disease with predominant pulmonary involvement. Respiration 67:213–215, 2000.
58. Numano F, Ohta N, Sasazuki T. HLA and clinical manifestations in Takayasu's disease. Jpn Circ J 46:184–189, 1982.
59. Skaria AM, Ruffieux P, Piletta P, Chavaz P, Saurat JH, Borradori L. Takayasu arteritis and cutaneous necrotizing vasculitis. Dermatology 200:139–143, 2000.
60. Seko Y. Takayasu arteritis: Insights into immunopathology. Jpn Heart J 41:15–26, 2000.
61. Shelhamer JH, Volkman DJ, Parrillo JE, Lawley TJ, Johnston MR, Fauci AS. Takayasu's arteritis and its therapy. Ann Intern Med 103:121–126, 1985.
62. Sparks SR, Chock A, Seslar S, Bergan JJ, Owens EL. Surgical treatment of Takayasu's arteritis: Case report and literature review. Ann Vasc Surg 14:125–129, 2000.
63. Boki KA, Pakas J, Kekatou K, Kataxaki E, Papapavlou E. Takayasu's arteritis-associated aneurysm formation without steno-occlusive lesions. Clin Rheumatol 19:226–228, 2000.
64. Amano J, Suzuki A. Coronary artery involvement in Takayasu's arteritis. Collective review and guideline for surgical treatment. J Thorac Cardiovasc Surg 102:554–560, 1991.
65. Nishimura T, Uehara T, Hayashida K, Kozuka T. Coronary arterial involvement in aortitis syndrome: Assessment by exercise thallium scintigraphy. Heart Vessels Suppl 7:106–110, 1992.
66. Noma M, Sugihara M, Kikuchi Y. Isolated coronary ostial stenosis in Takayasu's arteritis: Case report and review of the literature. Angiology 44:839–844, 1993.
67. Noma M, Kikuchi Y, Yoshimura H, Yamamoto H, Tajimi T. Coronary ectasia in Takayasu's arteritis. Am Heart J 126:459–461, 1993.
68. Panja M, Kar AK, Dutta AL, Chhetri M, Kumar S, Panja S. Cardiac involvement in non-specific aortoarteritis. Int J Cardiol 34:289–295, 1992.
69. Seguchi M, Hino Y, Aiba S, et al. Ostial stenosis of the left coronary artery as a sole clinical manifestation of Takayasu's arteritis: A possible cause of unexpected sudden death. Heart Vessels 5:188–191, 1990.
70. Talwar KK, Kumar K, Chopra P, et al. Cardiac involvement in nonspecific aortoarteritis (Takayasu's arteritis). Am Heart J 122:1666–1670, 1991.
71. Matsubara O, Yoshimura N, Tamura A, et al. Pathological features of the pulmonary artery in Takayasu arteritis. Heart Vessels Suppl 7:18–25, 1992.
72. Ishibashi-Ueda H, Yutani C, Kuribayashi S, Takamiya M, Imakita M, Ando M. Late in-stent restenosis of the abdominal aorta in a patient with Takayasu's arteritis and related pathology. Cardiovasc Intervent Radiol 22:333–336, 1999.
73. Lusic I, Maskovic J, Jankovic S, Cambj-Sapunar L, Hozo I. Endoluminal stenting for subclavian artery stenosis in Takayasu's arteritis. Cerebrovasc Dis 10:73–75, 2000.
74. Teoh MK. Takayasu's arteritis with renovascular hypertension: Results of surgical treatment. Cardiovasc Surg 7:626–632, 1999.
75. Jolly M, Bartholomew JR, Flamm SD, Olin JW. Angina and coronary ostial lesions in a young woman as a presentation of Takayasu's arteritis. Cardiovasc Surg 7:443–446, 1999.
76. Maskovic J, Jankovic S, Lusic I, Cambj-Sapunar L, Mimica Z, Bacic A. Subclavian artery stenosis caused by

non-specific arteritis (Takayasu disease): Treatment with Palmaz stent. Eur J Radiol 31:193–196, 1999.
77. Amano J, Suzuki A, Tanaka H, Sunamori M. Surgical treatment for annuloaortic ectasia in Takayasu arteritis. Int J Cardiol 66:S197–S202; discussion S203–S204, 1998.
78. Hellmann DB. Immunopathogenesis, diagnosis, and treatment of giant cell arteritis, temporal arteritis, polymyalgia rheumatica, and Takayasu's arteritis. Curr Opin Rheumatol 5:25–32, 1993.
79. Huston KA, Hunder GG, Lie JT, Kennedy RH, Elveback LR. Temporal arteritis: A 25-year epidemiologic, clinical, and pathologic study. Ann Intern Med 88:162–167, 1978.
80. Klein RG, Hunder GG, Stanson AW, Sheps SG. Large artery involvement in giant cell (temporal) arteritis. Ann Intern Med 83:806–812, 1975.
81. Costello JJ, Nicholson WJ. Severe aortic regurgitation as a late complication of temporal arteritis. Chest 98:875–877, 1990.
82. Evans J, Hunder GG. The implications of recognizing large-vessel involvement in elderly patients with giant cell arteritis. Curr Opin Rheumatol 9:37–40, 1997.
83. Virmani R, Burke AP. Pathologic features of aortitis. Cardiovasc Pathol 3:205–216, 1994.
84. Gravallese EM, Corson JM, Coblyn JS, Pinkus GS, Weinblatt ME. Rheumatoid aortitis: A rarely recognized but clinically significant entity. Medicine (Baltimore) 68:95–106, 1989.
85. Roeyen G, Van Schil PE, Vanmaele RG, et al. Abdominal aortic aneurysm with lumbar vertebral erosion in Behçet's disease. A case report and review of the literature. Eur J Vasc Endovasc Surg 13:242–246, 1997.
86. Chauvel C, Cohen A, Albo C, Ziol M, Valty J. Aortic dissection and cardiovascular syphilis: Report of an observation with transesophageal echocardiography and anatomopathologic findings. J Am Soc Echocardiogr 7:419–421, 1994.
87. Costa M, Robbs JV. Abdominal aneurysms in a black population: Clinicopathological study. Br J Surg 73:554–558, 1986.
88. Heggtveit HA. Syphilitic aortitis. A clinicopathologic autopsy study of 100 cases, 1950–1960. Circulation 29:346–355, 1964.
89. Kellett MW, Young GR, Fletcher NA. Paraparesis due to syphilitic aortic dissection. Neurology 48:221–223, 1997.
90. Marconato R, Inzaghi A, Cantoni GM, Zappa M, Longo T. Syphilitic aneurysm of the abdominal aorta: Report of two cases. Eur J Vasc Surg 2:199–203, 1988.
91. Fulton JO, Zilla P, De Groot KM, Von Oppell UO. Syphilitic aortic aneurysm eroding through the sternum. Eur J Cardiothorac Surg 10:922–924, 1996.
92. Nakane H, Okada Y, Ibayashi S, Sadoshima S, Fujishima M. Brain infarction caused by syphilitic aortic aneurysm. A case report. Angiology 47:911–917, 1996.
93. Pessotto R, Santini F, Bertolini P, Faggian G, Chiominto B, Mazzucco A. Surgical treatment of an aortopulmonary artery fistula complicating a syphilitic aortic aneurysm. Cardiovasc Surg 3:707–710, 1995.
94. Anderson B, Stillman MT. False-positive FTA-ABS in hydralazine-induced lupus. Jama 239:1392–1393, 1978.
95. Becker GD. Late syphilis. Otologic symptoms and results of the FTA-ABS test. Arch Otolaryngol 102:729–731, 1976.
96. Brauner A, Carlsson B, Sundkvist G, Ostenson CG. False-positive treponemal serology in patients with diabetes mellitus. J Diabetes Complications 8:57–62, 1994.
97. Gibowski M, Neumann E. Non-specific positive test results to syphilis in dermatological diseases. Br J Vener Dis 56:17–19, 1980.
98. Carreras M, Larena JA, Tabernero G, Langara E, Pena JM. Evolution of salmonella aortitis towards the formation of abdominal aneurysm. Eur Radiol 7:54–56, 1997.
99. Molina PL, Strobl PW, Burstain JM. Aortoesophageal fistula secondary to mycotic aneurysm of the descending thoracic aorta: CT demonstration. J Comput Assist Tomogr 19:309–311, 1995.
100. Rubery PT, Smith MD, Cammisa FP, Silane M. Mycotic aortic aneurysm in patients who have lumbar vertebral osteomyelitis. A report of two cases. J Bone Joint Surg. Am 77:1729–1732, 1995.
101. Worrell JT, Buja LM, Reynolds RC. Pneumococcal aortitis with rupture of the aorta. Report of a case and review of the literature. Am J Clin Pathol 89:565–568, 1988.
102. Blebea J, Kempczinski RF. Mycotic aneurysms. In: Yao JST, Pearce WH (eds): Aneurysms. New Findings and Treatments, pp 389–410. Norwalk, CT: Appleton and Lange, 1994.
103. Brewerton DA, James DC. The histocompatibility antigen (HL-A 27) and disease. Semin Arthritis Rheum 4:191–207, 1975.
104. Ansell BM, Bywaters EGL, Doniach I. The aortic lesions of ankylosing spondylitis. Br Heart J 20:507–515, 1958.
105. Arnason JA, Patel AK, Rahko PS, Sundstrom WR. Transthoracic and transesophageal echocardiographic evaluation of the aortic root and subvalvular structures in ankylosing spondylitis. J Rheumatol 23:120–123, 1996.
106. Bulkley BH, Roberts WC. Ankylosing spondylitis and aortic regurgitation. Description of the characteristic cardiovascular lesion from study of eight necropsy patients. Circulation 48:1014–1027, 1973.
107. Virmani R, McAllister HA. Pathology of the aorta and major arteries. In: Lande A, Borkman YM, McAllister HA (eds): Aortitis: Clinical, Pathologic, and Radiographic Aspects, pp 7–53. New York: Raven Press, 1986.
108. Paulus HE, Pearson CM, Pitts W, Jr. Aortic insufficiency in five patients with Reiter's syndrome. A detailed clinical and pathologic study. Am J Med 53:464–472, 1972.
109. Chajek T, Fainaru M. Behçet's disease. Report of 41 cases and a review of the literature. Medicine (Baltimore) 54:179–196, 1975.
110. Hamza M. Large artery involvement in Behçet's disease. J Rheumatol 14:554–559, 1987.
111. Matsumoto T, Uekusa T, Fukuda Y. Vasculo-Behçet's disease: A pathologic study of eight cases. Hum Pathol 22:45–51, 1991.
112. Bastounis E, Maltezos C, Giambouras S, Vayiopoulos G, Balas P. Arterial aneurysms in Behçet's disease. Int Angiol 13:196–201, 1994.
113. Koh KK, Lee KH, Kim SS, Lee SC, Jin SH, Cho SW. Ruptured aneurysm of the sinus of Valsalva in a patient with Behçet's disease. Int J Cardiol 47:177–179, 1994.
114. Tuzuner A, Uncu H. A case of Behçet's disease with an abdominal aortic aneurysm and two aneurysms in the common carotid artery. A case report. Angiology 47:1173–1180, 1996.

115. Tuzun H, Besirli K, Sayin A, et al. Management of aneurysms in Behçet's syndrome: An analysis of 24 patients. Surgery 121:150–156, 1997.
116. Seo JW, Park IA, Yoon DH, et al. Thoracic aortic aneurysm associated with aortitis—case reports and histological review. J Korean Med Sci 6:75–82, 1991.
117. Kirklin JW, Barratt-Boyes BG. Chronic thoracic and thoracoabdominal aortic aneurysm. In: Kirklin JW, Barratt-Boyes BG (eds): Cardiac Surgery, pp 1749–1779. New York: Churchill Livingstone, 1993.
118. Svensjo S, Bengtsson H, Bergqvist D. Thoracic and thoracoabdominal aortic aneurysm and dissection: An investigation based on autopsy. Br J Surg 83:68–71, 1996.
119. Pitt MP, Bonser RS. The natural history of thoracic aortic aneurysm disease: An overview. J Card Surg 12:270–278, 1997.
120. Okita Y, Takamoto S, Ando M, et al. Predictive factors for postoperative cerebral complications in patients with thoracic aortic aneurysm. Eur J Cardiothorac Surg 10:826–832, 1996.
121. Galloway AC, Schwartz DS, Culliford AT, et al. Selective approach to descending thoracic aortic aneurysm repair: A ten-year experience. Ann Thorac Surg 62:1152–1157, 1996.
122. Semba CP, Mitchell RS, Miller DC, et al. Thoracic aortic aneurysm repair with endovascular stent-grafts. Vasc Med 2:98–103, 1997.
123. Ellis RP, Cooley DA, DeBadey ME. Clinical considerations and surgical treatment of annulo-aortic ectasia. J Thorac Cardiovasc Surg 42:363–369, 1961.
124. Shimokawa H, Koiwaya Y, Kaku T. Annuloaortic ectasia in a case of Takayasu's arteritis associated with Hashimoto's disease. Br Heart J 49:94–97, 1983.
125. Cooley DA. Annuloaortic ectasia. Ann Thorac Surg 28:303–304, 1979.
126. Savunen T, Aho HJ. Annulo-aortic ectasia: Light and electron microscopic changes in aortic media. Virchows Arch (A) 407:279–288, 1985.
127. Savunen T. Cardiovascular abnormalities in the relatives of patients operated upon for annulo-aortic ectasia. A clinical and echocardiographic study of 40 families. Eur J Cardiothorac Surg 1:3–9; discussion 9–10, 1987.
128. Painvin GA, Weisel RD, David TE, Scully HE, Goldman BS, Baird RJ. Surgical treatment of annuloaortic ectasia. Can J Surg 23:445–449, 1980.
129. Dare AJ, Veinot JP, Edwards WD, Tazelaar HD, Schaff HV. New observations on the etiology of aortic valve disease: A surgical pathologic study of 236 cases from 1990. Hum Pathol 24:1330–1338, 1993.
130. Kirklin JW, Barratt-Boyes BG. Aortic valve disease. In: Kirklin JW, Barratt-Boyes BG (eds): Cardiac Surgery, pp 491–571. New York: Churchill Livingstone, 1993.
131. Savunen T, Inberg M, Niinikoski J, Rantakokko V, Vanttinen E. Composite graft in annulo-aortic ectasia. Nineteen years' experience without graft inclusion. Eur J Cardiothorac Surg 10:428–432, 1996.
132. Halme T, Savunen T, Aho H, Vihersaari T, Penttinen R. Elastin and collagen in the aortic wall: Changes in the Marfan syndrome and annuloaortic ectasia. Exp Mol Pathol 43:1–12, 1985.
133. Wilson RA, McDonald RW, Bristow JD, et al. Correlates of aortic distensibility in chronic aortic regurgitation and relation to progression to surgery. J Am Coll Cardiol 19:733–738, 1992.
134. Ogren M, Bengtsson H, Bergqvist D, Ekberg O, Hedblad B, Janzon L. Prognosis in elderly men with screening-detected abdominal aortic aneurysm. Eur J Vasc Endovasc Surg 11:42–47, 1996.
135. Reilly JM, Tilson MD. Incidence and etiology of abdominal aortic aneurysms. Surg Clin N Am 69:705–717, 1989.
136. Lederle FA, Johnson GR, Wilson SE, et al. Yield of repeated screening for abdominal aortic aneurysm after a 4-year interval. Aneurysm Detection and Management (ADAM) Veterans Affairs Cooperative Study Investigators. Arch Intern Med 160:1117–1121, 2000.
137. Bengtsson H, Bergqvist D, Ekberg O, Ranstam J. Expansion pattern and risk of rupture of abdominal aortic aneurysms that were not operated on. Eur J Surg 159:461–467, 1993.
138. White GH, May J, Petrasek P, Waugh R, Stephen M, Harris J. Endotension: An explanation for continued AAA growth after successful endoluminal repair. J Endovasc Surg 6:308–315, 1999.
139. Buth J. Endovascular repair of abdominal aortic aneurysms. Results from the EUROSTAR registry. EUROpean collaborators on stent-graft techniques for abdominal aortic aneurysm repair. Semin Interv Cardiol 5:29–33, 2000.
140. Wolf YG, Hill BB, Rubin GD, Fogarty TJ, Zarins CK. Rate of change in abdominal aortic aneurysm diameter after endovascular repair. J Vasc Surg 32:108–115, 2000.
141. Cohen JR, Sarfati I, Danna D, Wise L. Smooth muscle cell elastase, atherosclerosis, and abdominal aortic aneurysms. Ann Surg 216:327–330; discussion 330–332, 1992.
142. Shi GP, Sukhova GK, Grubb A, et al. Cystatin C deficiency in human atherosclerosis and aortic aneurysms. J Clin Invest 104:1191–1197, 1999.
143. Nakamura M, Tachieda R, Niinuma H, et al. Circulating biochemical marker levels of collagen metabolism are abnormal in patients with abdominal aortic aneurysm. Angiology 51:385–392, 2000.
144. Schneiderman J, Bordin GM, Engelberg I, et al. Expression of fibrinolytic genes in atherosclerotic abdominal aortic aneurysm wall. A possible mechanism for aneurysm expansion. J Clin Invest 96:639–645, 1995.
145. Auerbach O, Garfinkel L. Atherosclerosis and aneurysm of aorta in relation to smoking habits and age. Chest 78:805–809, 1980.
146. Lee AJ, Fowkes FG, Carson MN, Leng GC, Allan PL. Smoking, atherosclerosis and risk of abdominal aortic aneurysm. Eur Heart J 18:671–676, 1997.
147. Lederle FA, Johnson GR, Wilson SE, et al. Prevalence and associations of abdominal aortic aneurysm detected through screening. Aneurysm Detection and Management (ADAM) Veterans Affairs Cooperative Study Group. Ann Intern Med 126:441–449, 1997.
148. Louwrens HD, Adamson J, Powell JT, Greenhalgh RM. Risk factors for atherosclerosis in men with stenosing or aneurysmal disease of the abdominal aorta. Int Angiol 12:21–24, 1993.
149. Walker DI, Bloor K, Williams G, Gillie I. Inflammatory aneurysms of the abdominal aorta. Br J Surg 59:609–614, 1972.
150. Rose AG, Dent DM. Inflammatory variant of abdominal atherosclerotic aneurysm. Arch Pathol Lab Med 105:409–413, 1981.
151. Feiner HD, Raghavendra BN, Phelps R, Rooney L. Inflammatory abdominal aortic aneurysm: Report of six cases. Hum Pathol 15:454–459, 1984.

152. Cohle SD, Lie JT. Inflammatory aneurysm of the aorta, aortitis, and coronary arteritis. Arch Pathol Lab Med 112:1121–1125, 1988.
153. Rasmussen TE, Hallett JWJ, Metzger RL, et al. Genetic risk factors in inflammatory abdominal aortic aneurysms: Polymorphic residue 70 in the HLA-DR B1 gene as a key genetic element. J Vasc Surg 25:356–364, 1997.
154. Guyton JR, Klemp KF. Transitional features in human atherosclerosis. Intimal thickening, cholesterol clefts, and cell loss in human aortic fatty streaks. Am J Pathol 143:1444–1457, 1993.
155. Chao FF, Amende LM, Blanchette-Mackie EJ, et al. Unesterified cholesterol-rich lipid particles in atherosclerotic lesions of human and rabbit aortas. Am J Pathol 131:73–83, 1988.
156. Mukhin DN, Chao FF, Kruth HS. Glycosphingolipid accumulation in the aortic wall is another feature of human atherosclerosis. Arterioscler Thromb Vasc Biol 15:1607–1615, 1995.
157. Natural history of aortic and coronary atherosclerotic lesions in youth. Findings from the PDAY Study. Pathobiological Determinants of Atherosclerosis in Youth (PDAY) Research Group. Arterioscler Thromb 13:1291–1298, 1993.
158. Berenson GS, Wattigney WA, Tracy RE, et al. Atherosclerosis of the aorta and coronary arteries and cardiovascular risk factors in persons aged 6 to 30 years and studied at necropsy (The Bogalusa Heart Study). Am J Cardiol 70:851–858, 1992.
159. Cluroe AD, Fitzjohn TP, Stehbens WE. Combined pathological and radiological study of the effect of atherosclerosis on the ostia of segmental branches of the abdominal aorta. Pathology 24:140–145, 1992.
160. Cornhill JF, Herderick EE, Stary HC. Topography of human aortic sudanophilic lesions. In: Liepsch DW (ed): Blood Flow in Large Arteries: Applications to Atherogenesis and Clinical Medicine, pp 13–19. Monogr Atheroscler. Vol. 15. Basel, Switzerland: Karger, 1990.
161. Tanganelli P, Biancardi G, Simoes C, Attino V, Tarabochia B, Weber G. Distribution of lipid and raised lesions in aortas of young people of different geographic origins. Arterioscler Thromb 13:1700–1710, 1993.
162. Ishii T, Hosoda Y, Tsugane S, et al. Natural history of aortic and coronary atherosclerosis in Tokyo. Mod Pathol 1:205–211, 1988.
163. Strong JP, Malcom GT, McMahan CA, et al. Prevalence and extent of atherosclerosis in adolescents and young adults: Implications for prevention from the Pathobiological Determinants of Atherosclerosis in Youth Study. J Am Med Assoc 281:727–735, 1999.
164. Maru M. Prevalence of atherosclerosis of the aorta in Ethiopians: A postmortem study. East Afr Med J 69:214–218, 1992.
165. McGill HC, Jr., McMahan CA, Herderick EE, et al. Effects of coronary heart disease risk factors on atherosclerosis of selected regions of the aorta and right coronary artery. PDAY Research Group. Pathobiological Determinants of Atherosclerosis in Youth (PDAY). Arterioscler Thromb Vasc Biol 20:836–845, 2000.
166. Stehbens WE. Atherosclerosis and degenerative diseases of blood vessels. In: Stehbens WE, Lie JT (eds): Vascular Pathology, pp 175–269. London: Chapman & Hall Medical, 1995.
167. Tanimura A, Cho T, Saito Y, Nakashima T. Role of "wave line" (Doerr; Wellenlinie) of aorta in atherosclerosis. Angiology 37:272–280, 1986.
168. Vikhert AM, Sternby NH, Livshits AM, Duskova J. Rhythmic structures and atherosclerosis in the aorta. Atherosclerosis 106:129–137, 1994.
169. Orekhov AN, Andreeva ER, Krushinsky AV, et al. Intimal cells and atherosclerosis. Relationship between the number of intimal cells and major manifestations of atherosclerosis in the human aorta. Am J Pathol 125:402–415, 1986.
170. Agerbaek M, Kristensen IB, Pedersen EM. A histomorphometric method for evaluating topographic differences in degree of early atherosclerosis within the human aorta. APMIS 107:863–868, 1999.
171. Svendsen E, Eide TJ. Distribution of atherosclerosis in human descending thoracic aorta. A morphometric study. Acta Pathol Microbiol Scand [A] 88:97–101, 1980.
172. Homma S, Ishii T, Tsugane S, Hirose N. Different effects of hypertension and hypercholesterolemia on the natural history of aortic atherosclerosis by the stage of intimal lesions. Atherosclerosis 128:85–95, 1997.
173. Stary HC, Chandler AB, Glagov S, et al. A definition of initial, fatty streak, and intermediate lesions of atherosclerosis. A report from the Committee on Vascular Lesions of the Council on Arteriosclerosis, American Heart Association. Arterioscler Thromb 14:840–856, 1994.
174. Mikkelsson J, Perola M, Kauppila LI, et al. The GPIIIa Pl(A) polymorphism in the progression of abdominal aortic atherosclerosis. Atherosclerosis 147:55–60, 1999.
175. Acarturk E, Demir M, Kanadasi M. Aortic atherosclerosis is a marker for significant coronary artery disease. Jpn Heart J 40:775–781, 1999.
176. Qvarfordt PG, Reilly LM, Sedwitz MM, Ehrenfeld WK, Stoney RJ. "Coral reef" atherosclerosis of the suprarenal aorta: A unique clinical entity. J Vasc Surg 1:903–909, 1984.
177. Kauppila LI, Penttila A, Karhunen PJ, Lalu K, Hannikainen P. Lumbar disc degeneration and atherosclerosis of the abdominal aorta. Spine 19:923–929, 1994.
178. Bots ML, Witteman JC, Grobbee DE. Carotid intima-media wall thickness in elderly women with and without atherosclerosis of the abdominal aorta. Atherosclerosis 102:99–105, 1993.
179. Iribarren C, Sidney S, Sternfeld B, Browner WS. Calcification of the aortic arch: Risk factors and association with coronary heart disease, stroke, and peripheral vascular disease. JAMA 283:2810–2815, 2000.
180. Movsowitz HD, Lampert C, Jacobs LE, Kotler MN. Penetrating atherosclerotic aortic ulcers. Am Heart J 128:1210–1217, 1994.
181. Braverman AC. Penetrating atherosclerotic ulcers of the aorta. Curr Opin Cardiol 9:591–597, 1994.
182. Vilacosta I, San Roman JA, Aragoncillo P, et al. Penetrating atherosclerotic aortic ulcer: Documentation by transesophageal echocardiography. J Am Coll Cardiol 32:83–89, 1998.
183. Harris JA, Bis KG, Glover JL, Bendick PJ, Shetty A, Brown OW. Penetrating atherosclerotic ulcers of the aorta. J Vasc Surg 19:90–98; discussion 98–99, 1994.
184. Primack SL, Mayo JR, Fradet G. Perforated atherosclerotic ulcer of the aorta presenting with upper airway obstruction. Can Assoc Radiol J 46:209–211, 1995.
185. Yano K, Makino N, Hirayama H, et al. Penetrating atherosclerotic ulcer at the proximal aorta complicated with cardiac tamponade and aortic valve regurgitation. Jpn Circ J 63:228–230, 1999.

186. Moriyama Y, Yamamoto H, Hisatomi K, et al. Penetrating atherosclerotic ulcers in an abdominal aortic aneurysm: Report of a case. Surg Today 28:105–107, 1998.
187. Benitez RM, Gurbel PA, Chong H, Rajasingh MC. Penetrating atherosclerotic ulcer of the aortic arch resulting in extensive and fatal dissection. Am Heart J 129:821–823, 1995.
188. Williams DM, Kirsh MM, Abrams GD. Penetrating atherosclerotic aortic ulcer with dissecting hematoma: Control of bleeding with percutaneous embolization. Radiology 181:85–88, 1991.
189. Gittinger JW, Jr., Kershaw GR. Retinal cholesterol emboli in the diagnosis of renal atheroembolism. Arch Intern Med 158:1265–1267, 1998.
190. Mayo RR, Swartz RD. Redefining the incidence of clinically detectable atheroembolism. Am J Med 100:524–529, 1996.
191. Jorgensen L, Nordal EJ, Eide TJ, et al. The relationship between atherosclerosis of the thoracic aorta and renal scarring in an autopsy material. Acta Pathol Microbiol Immunol Scand [A] 93:251–255, 1985.
192. Baumann DS, McGraw D, Rubin BG, Allen BT, Anderson CB, Sicard GA. An institutional experience with arterial atheroembolism. Ann Vasc Surg 8:258–265, 1994.
193. Sharma PV, Babu SC, Shah PM, Nassoura ZE. Changing patterns of atheroembolism. Cardiovasc Surg 4:573–579, 1996.
194. Applebaum RM, Kronzon I. Evaluation and management of cholesterol embolization and the blue toe syndrome. Curr Opin Cardiol 11:533–542, 1996.
195. Jenkins DM, Newton WD. Atheroembolism. Am Surg 57:588–590, 1991.
196. Blauth CI, Cosgrove DM, Webb BW, et al. Atheroembolism from the ascending aorta. An emerging problem in cardiac surgery. J Thorac Cardiovasc Surg 103:1104–1111; discussion 1111–1112, 1992.
197. Wheat MW, Jr. Acute dissecting aneurysms of the aorta. Diagnosis and treatment—1979. Am Heart J 99:373–387, 1980.
198. Wilson SK, Hutchins GM. Aortic dissecting aneurysms: Causative factors in 204 subjects. Arch Pathol Lab Med 106:175–180, 1982.
199. Larson EW, Edwards WD. Risk factors for aortic dissection: A necropsy study of 161 cases. Am J Cardiol 53:849–855, 1984.
200. Gore I, Seiwert VJ. Dissecting aneurysm of the aorta: Pathologic aspects. An analysis of eighty-five fatal cases. Arch Pathol 53:121–141, 1952.
201. Roberts CS, Roberts WC. Dissection of the aorta associated with congenital malformation of the aortic valve. J Am Coll Cardiol 17:712–716, 1991.
202. Nicod P, Bloor C, Godfrey M, et al. Familial aortic dissecting aneurysm. J Am Coll Cardiol 13:811–819, 1989.
203. Hanley WB, Jones NB. Familial dissecting aortic aneurysm. A report of three cases within two generations. Br Heart J 29:852–858, 1967.
204. Toyama M, Amano A, Kameda T. Familial aortic dissection: A report of rare family cluster. Br Heart J 61:204–207, 1989.
205. Gatalica Z, Gibas Z, Martinez-Hernandez A. Dissecting aortic aneurysm as a complication of generalized fibromuscular dysplasia. Hum Pathol 23:586–588, 1992.
206. Heggtveit HA. A case of fibromuscular dysplasia and aortic dissection. Hum Pathol 23:1438–1440, 1992.
207. Edwards WD, Leaf DS, Edwards JE. Dissecting aortic aneurysm associated with congenital bicuspid aortic valve. Circulation 57:1022–1025, 1978.
208. Roberts WC. Aortic dissection: Anatomy, consequences, and causes. Am Heart J 101:195–214, 1981.
209. Nakashima Y, Kurozumi T, Sueishi K, Tanaka K. Dissecting aneurysm: A clinicopathologic and histopathologic study of 111 autopsied cases. Hum Pathol 21:291–296, 1990.
210. Williams DM, Joshi A, Dake MD, Deeb GM, Miller DC, Abrams GD. Aortic cobwebs: An anatomic marker identifying the false lumen in aortic dissection—imaging and pathologic correlation [see comments]. Radiology 190:167–174, 1994.
211. Nakashima Y, Shiokawa Y, Sueishi K. Alterations of elastic architecture in human aortic dissecting aneurysm. Lab Invest 62:761–760, 1990.
212. Spittell PC, Spittell JA, Jr., Joyce JW, et al. Clinical features and differential diagnosis of aortic dissection: Experience with 236 cases (1980 through 1990). Mayo Clin Proc 68:642–651, 1993.
213. Hagan PG, Nienaber CA, Isselbacher EM, et al. The International Registry of Acute Aortic Dissection (IRAD): New insights into an old disease. JAMA 283:897–903, 2000.
214. Fann JI, Sarris GE, Mitchell RS, et al. Treatment of patients with aortic dissection presenting with peripheral vascular complications. Ann Surg 212:705–713, 1990.
215. Laas J, Heinemann M, Schaefers HJ, Daniel W, Borst HG. Management of thoracoabdominal malperfusion in aortic dissection. Circulation 84:III20–24, 1991.
216. Hirst AE, Johns VJ, Kime SW. Dissecting aneurysm of the aorta: A review of 505 cases. Medicine 37:217–239, 1958.
217. Veyssier-Belot C, Cohen A, Rougemont D, Levy C, Amarenco P, Bousser MG. Cerebral infarction due to painless thoracic aortic and common carotid artery dissections. Stroke 24:2111–2113, 1993.
218. Karmy-Jones R, Aldea G, Boyle EM, Jr. The continuing evolution in the management of thoracic aortic dissection. Chest 117:1221–1223, 2000.
219. Elefteriades JA, Lovoulos CJ, Coady MA, Tellides G, Kopf GS, Rizzo JA. Management of descending aortic dissection. Ann Thorac Surg 67:2002–2005; discussion 2014–2019, 1999.
220. Dake MD, Kato N, Mitchell RS, et al. Endovascular stent-graft placement for the treatment of acute aortic dissection. N Engl J Med 340:1546–1552, 1999.
221. Slonim SM, Nyman U, Semba CP, Miller DC, Mitchell RS, Dake MD. Aortic dissection: Percutaneous management of ischemic complications with endovascular stents and balloon fenestration. J Vasc Surg 23:241–251; discussion 251–253, 1996.
222. Roberts CS, Roberts WC. Aortic dissection with the entrance tear in abdominal aorta. Am Heart J 121:1834–1835, 1991.
223. Ruehm SG, Weishaupt D, Debatin JF. Contrast-enhanced MR angiography in patients with aortic occlusion (Leriche syndrome). J Magn Reson Imaging 11:401–410, 2000.
224. Arnold JR, Greenberg JD, Clements S. Internal mammary artery perfusing Leriche's syndrome. Ann Thorac Surg 69:1244–1246, 2000.
225. Arnold JR, Greenberg J, Reddy K, Clements S. Internal mammary artery perfusing Leriche's syndrome in association with significant coronary arteriosclerosis: Four case reports and review of literature. Catheter Cardiovasc Interv 49:441–444, 2000.
226. Josephson GD, Tiefenbrun J, Harvey J. Thrombosis of the descending thoracic aorta: A case report. Surgery 114:598–600, 1993.

227. Kawahira Y, Kishimoto H, Lio M, et al. Spontaneous aortic thrombosis in a neonate with multiple thrombi in the main branches of the abdominal aorta. Cardiovasc Surg 3:219–221, 1995.
228. Sanchez-Gonzalez J, Garcia-Delange T, Martos F, Colmenero JD. Thrombosis of the abdominal aorta secondary to Brucella spondylitis. Infection 24:261–262, 1996.
229. Baillot R, Dontigny L, Verdant A, et al. Intrapericardial trauma: Surgical experience. J Trauma 29:736–740, 1989.
230. Chang JP, Lin PJ, Chu JJ, Chang CH, Lee MC, Shieh MJ. Acute mitral regurgitation secondary to blunt chest trauma: Report of a case. Taiwan I Hsueh Hui Tsa Chih 88:173–175, 1989.
231. Chang JP, Chu JJ, Chang CH. Aortic regurgitation due to aortic root intimal tear as a result of blunt chest trauma. J Formos Med Assoc 89:41–43, 1990.
232. Loeb T, Matuszczak Y, Petit J, Bessou JP, Pinsard M, Oksenhendler G. Aortic valve rupture—an unsuspected cause of acute cardiac failure after chest trauma. Intensive Care Med 22:714–715, 1996.
233. Munshi IA, Barie PS, Hawes AS, Lang SJ, Fischer E. Diagnosis and management of acute aortic valvular disruption secondary to rapid-deceleration trauma. J Trauma 41:1047–1050, 1996.
234. Prat A, Warembourg H Jr, Watel A, et al. Chronic traumatic aneurysms of the descending thoracic aorta (19 cases). J Cardiovasc Surg (Torino) 27:268–272, 1986.
235. Williams JS, Graff JA, Uku JM, Steinig JP. Aortic injury in vehicular trauma. Ann Thorac Surg 57:726–730, 1994.
236. Jensen BT. Fourteen years' survival with an untreated traumatic rupture of the thoracal aorta. Am J Forensic Med Pathol 9:58–59, 1988.
237. Swanson S, Gaffey M. Traumatic false aneurysm of descending aorta with aortoesophageal fistula. J Forensic Sci 33:816–822, 1988.
238. Abulafia O, Sherer DM. Recurrent transient superior vena cava-like syndrome possibly associated with megestrol acetate. Obstet Gynecol 85:899–901, 1995.
239. Tunaci A, Berkmen YM, Gokmen E. Thoracic involvement in Behçet's disease: Pathologic, clinical, and imaging features. AJR Am J Roentgenol 164:51–56, 1995.
240. Hoffmann V, Ysebaert D, De Schepper A, Colpaert C, Jorens P. Acute superior vena cava obstruction after rupture of a bronchial artery aneurysm. Chest 110:1356–1358, 1996.
241. Ashleigh RJ, Sambrook P. Case report: Unilateral hydronephrosis following obstruction of the inferior vena cava by tumour thrombus. Clin Radiol 44:130–131, 1991.
242. Federici S, Galli G, Ceccarelli PL, Rosito P, Sciutti R, Domini R. Wilms' tumor involving the inferior vena cava: Preoperative evaluation and management. Med Pediatr Oncol 22:39–44, 1994.
243. Leder RA. Genitourinary case of the day. Angiomyolipoma of the kidney with fat thrombus in the inferior vena cava. AJR Am J Roentgenol 165:198–199, 1995.
244. Adsan O, Muftuoglu YZ, Suzer O, Beduk Y. Thrombosis of the inferior vena cava by a testicular tumour. Int Urol Nephrol 27:179–182, 1995.
245. Ohwada S, Tanahashi Y, Kawashima Y, et al. Surgery for tumor thrombi in the right atrium and inferior vena cava of patients with recurrent hepatocellular carcinoma. Hepatogastroenterology 41:154–157, 1994.
246. Arao M, Ogura H, Ino T, et al. Unusual inferior vena cava obstruction causing extensive thrombosis: An intravascular endoscopic observation. Intern Med 32: 861–864, 1993.
247. Brouwers MA, de Jong KP, Peeters PM, Bijleveld CM, Klompmaker IJ, Slooff MJ. Inferior vena cava obstruction after orthotopic liver transplantation. Clin Transplant 8:19–22, 1994.
248. Brenner DW, Brenner CJ, Scott J, Wehberg K, Granger JP, Schellhammer PF. Suprarenal Greenfield filter placement to prevent pulmonary embolus in patients with vena caval tumor thrombi. J Urol 147:19–23, 1992.
249. Zhou H, Janssen D, Gunther E, Pfeifer U. Fatal bleeding from duodenal varices as a late complication of neonatal thrombosis of the inferior vena cava. Virchows Arch A Pathol Anat Histopathol 420:367–370, 1992.
250. Valla D, Benhamou JP. Obstruction of the hepatic veins or suprahepatic inferior vena cava. Dig Dis 14:99–118, 1996.
251. Kage M, Arakawa M, Kojiro M, Okuda K. Histopathology of membranous obstruction of the inferior vena cava in the Budd–Chiari syndrome. Gastroenterology 102:2081–2090, 1992.
252. Sevenet F, Deramond H, Hadengue A, Casadevall N, Delamarre J, Capron JP. Membranous obstruction of the inferior vena cava associated with a myeloproliferative disorder: A clue to membrane formation? Gastroenterology 97:1019–1021, 1989.
253. Levesque H, Cailleux N, Courtois H, Clavier E, Milon P, Benozio M. Idiopathic saccular aneurysm of the inferior vena cava: A new case. J Vasc Surg 18:544–545, 1993.
254. Sweeney JP, Turner K, Harris KA. Aneurysms of the inferior vena cava. J Vasc Surg 12:25–27, 1990.
255. van Ieperen L, Rose AG. Idiopathic aneurysm of the inferior vena cava. A case report. S Afr Med J 77:535–536, 1990.
256. Augustin N, Meisner H, Sebening F. Combined membranous obstruction and saccular aneurysm of the inferior vena cava. Thorac Cardiovasc Surg 43:223–226, 1995.
257. Wagenvoort CA. Pathology of pulmonary thromboembolism. Chest 107:10S–17S, 1995.
258. Ryu JH, Olson EJ, Pellikka PA. Clinical recognition of pulmonary embolism: Problem of unrecognized and asymptomatic cases. Mayo Clin Proc 73:873–879, 1998.
259. Patriquin L, Khorasani R, Polak JF. Correlation of diagnostic imaging and subsequent autopsy findings in patients with pulmonary embolism. AJR Am J Roentgenol 171:347–349, 1998.
260. Stein PD, Henry JW. Prevalence of acute pulmonary embolism among patients in a general hospital and at autopsy. Chest 108:978–981, 1995.
261. Morpurgo M, Schmid C. The spectrum of pulmonary embolism. Clinicopathologic correlations. Chest 107: 18S–20S, 1995.
262. Kurkciyan I, Meron G, Sterz F, et al. Pulmonary embolism as a cause of cardiac arrest: Presentation and outcome. Arch Intern Med 160:1529–1535, 2000.
263. Hansson PO, Welin L, Tibblin G, Eriksson H. Deep vein thrombosis and pulmonary embolism in the general population. "The Study of Men Born in 1913." Arch Intern Med 157:1665–1670, 1997.
264. Anderson FA, Jr., Wheeler HB, Goldberg RJ, et al. A population-based perspective of the hospital inci-

dence and case-fatality rates of deep vein thrombosis and pulmonary embolism. The Worcester DVT Study. Arch Intern Med 151:933–938, 1991.
265. Stein PD, Huang H, Afzal A, Noor HA. Incidence of acute pulmonary embolism in a general hospital: Relation to age, sex, and race. Chest 116:909–913, 1999.
266. Diebold J, Lohrs U. Venous thrombosis and pulmonary embolism. A study of 5039 autopsies. Pathol Res Pract 187:260–266, 1991.
267. Lindblad B, Eriksson A, Bergqvist D. Autopsy-verified pulmonary embolism in a surgical department: Analysis of the period from 1951 to 1988. Br J Surg 78:849–852, 1991.
268. Bussani R, Cosatti C. Pulmonary embolism: Epidemiologic analysis of 27,410 autopsies during a 10-year period. Medicina (Firenze) 10:40–43, 1990.
269. Hauch O, Jorgensen LN, Khattar SC, et al. Fatal pulmonary embolism associated with surgery. An autopsy study. Acta Chir Scand 156:747–749, 1990.
270. Owings JT, Kraut E, Battistella F, Cornelius JT, O'Malley R. Timing of the occurrence of pulmonary embolism in trauma patients. Arch Surg 132:862–866; discussion 866–867, 1997.
271. Wroblewski BM, Siney PD, Fleming PA. Fatal pulmonary embolism and mortality after revision of failed total hip arthroplasties. J Arthroplasty 15:437–439, 2000.
272. Ansari S, Warwick D, Ackroyd CE, Newman JH. Incidence of fatal pulmonary embolism after 1,390 knee arthroplasties without routine prophylactic anticoagulation, except in high-risk cases. J Arthroplasty 12:599–602, 1997.
273. Degan TA. Thrombolysis in pulmonary embolism: An adolescent with protein S deficiency. J Am Board Fam Pract 7:523–525, 1994.
274. Kam RM, Tan AT, Chee TS, Wong J. Massive acute pulmonary embolism in protein S deficiency—a case report. Ann Acad Med Singapore 23:396–399, 1994.
275. Girolami A, Simioni P, Sartori MT, Caenazzo A. Intracardial thrombosis with systemic and pulmonary embolism as main symptoms in a patient with protein S deficiency. Blood Coagul Fibrinolysis 3:485–488, 1992.
276. Delalande JP, Sauvanaud D, Abgrall JF, Rea D, Egreteau JP. Disclosure of protein C deficiency with pulmonary embolism followed by cardiac arrest during the recovery period. Ann Fr Anesth Reanim 11:96–99, 1992.
277. Sternberg TL, Bailey MK, Lazarchick J, Brahen NH. Protein C deficiency as a cause of pulmonary embolism in the perioperative period. Anesthesiology 74:364–366, 1991.
278. Sandin KJ, Smith BS. Above-knee amputation with insidious pulmonary embolism and hypercoagulability secondary to protein C deficiency. Arch Phys Med Rehabil 70:699–701, 1989.
279. Fortin F, Jude B, Caron C, Gosset D, Soots J, Lafitte JJ. Severe pulmonary embolism disclosing a deficiency in protein C. Rev Mal Respir 4:269–271, 1987.
280. Zoller B, Garcia de Frutos P, Dahlback B. A common 4G allele in the promoter of the plasminogen activator inhibitor-1 (PAI-1) gene as a risk factor for pulmonary embolism and arterial thrombosis in hereditary protein S deficiency. Thromb Haemost 79:802–807, 1998.
281. Kuismanen K, Savontaus ML, Kozlov A, Vuorio AF, Sajantila A. Coagulation factor V Leiden mutation in sudden fatal pulmonary embolism and in a general northern European population sample. Forensic Sci Int 106:71–75, 1999.
282. Desmarais S, de Moerloose P, Reber G, Minazio P, Perrier A, Bounameaux H. Resistance to activated protein C in an unselected population of patients with pulmonary embolism. Lancet 347:1374–1375, 1996.
283. Rulon JJ, Cho CG, Guerra LL, Bux RC, Gulley ML. Activated protein C resistance is uncommon in sudden death due to pulmonary embolism. J Forensic Sci 44:1111–1113, 1999.
284. Slovacek KJ, Harris AF, Greene JJ, Rao A. Fatal pulmonary embolism: A study of genetic and acquired factors. Mol Diagn 5:53–58, 2000.
285. Turkstra F, Karemaker R, Kuijer PM, Prins MH, Buller HR. Is the prevalence of the factor V Leiden mutation in patients with pulmonary embolism and deep vein thrombosis really different? Thromb Haemost 81:345–348, 1999.
286. Martinelli I, Cattaneo M, Panzeri D, Mannucci PM. Low prevalence of factor V:Q506 in 41 patients with isolated pulmonary embolism. Thromb Haemost 77:440–443, 1997.
287. Vandenbroucke JP, Bertina RM, Holmes ZR, et al. Factor V Leiden and fatal pulmonary embolism. Thromb Haemost 79:511–516, 1998.
288. Hirsch DR, Mikkola KM, Marks PW, et al. Pulmonary embolism and deep venous thrombosis during pregnancy or oral contraceptive use: Prevalence of factor V Leiden. Am Heart J 131:1145–1148, 1996.
289. Ordonez AJ, Carreira JM, Alvarez CR, Rodriguez JM, Alvarez MV, Coto E. Comparison of the risk of pulmonary embolism and deep vein thrombosis in the presence of factor V Leiden or prothrombin G20210A. Thromb Haemost 83:352–354, 2000.
290. Reuner KH, Ruf A, Litfin F, Patscheke H. The mutation G20210 A in the prothrombin gene is a strong risk factor for pulmonary embolism. Clin Chem 44:1365–1366, 1998.
291. Awotedu AA, Igbokwe EO, Akang EE, Aghadiuno PO. Pulmonary embolism in Ibadan, Nigeria: Five years autopsy report. Cent Afr J Med 38:432–435, 1992.
292. Karwinski B, Svendsen E, Seim S. Pulmonary embolism and heart disease. An autopsy study. Pathol Res Pract 189:1058–1062, 1993.
293. Chan GS, Ng WK, Ng IO, Dickens P. Sudden death from massive pulmonary tumor embolism due to hepatocellular carcinoma. Forensic Sci Int 108:215–221, 2000.
294. Idir M, Oysel N, Guibaud JP, Labouyrie E, Roudaut R. Fragmentation of a right atrial myxoma presenting as a pulmonary embolism. J Am Soc Echocardiogr 13:61–63, 2000.
295. Skalidis EI, Parthenakis FI, Zacharis EA, Datseris GE, Vardas PE. Pulmonary tumor embolism from primary cardiac B-cell lymphoma. Chest 116:1489–1490, 1999.
296. Brandt SE, Zeegers WS, Ceelen TL. Fatal pulmonary fat embolism after dorsal spinal fusion. Eur Spine J 7:426–428, 1998.
297. Michalodimitrakis M, Tsatsakis A. Massive pulmonary embolism by liver tissue. Med Sci Law 38:85–87, 1998.
298. Schreck RI, Manion WL, Kambin P, Sohn M. Nucleus pulposus pulmonary embolism. A case report. Spine 20:2463–2466, 1995.
299. Luchi ME, Asherson RA, Lahita RG. Primary idiopathic pulmonary hypertension complicated by pulmonary arterial thrombosis. Association with antiphos-

pholipid antibodies. Arthritis Rheum 35:700–705, 1992.
300. Barbas CS, de Carvalho CR, Delmonte VC, et al. Behçet's disease: A rare case of simultaneous pulmonary and cerebral involvement. Am J Med 85:576–578, 1988.
301. Raz I, Okon E, Chajek-Shaul T. Pulmonary manifestations in Behçet's syndrome. Chest 95:585–589, 1989.
302. Naschitz JE, Zuckerman E, Sharif D, Croitoru S, Sabo E, Abinader EG. Case report: Extensive pulmonary and aortic thrombosis and ectasia. Am J Med Sci 310:34–37, 1995.
303. Roche-Bayard P, Rossi R, Mann JM, Cordier JF, Delahaye JP. Left pulmonary artery thrombosis in chlorpromazine-induced lupus. Chest 98:1545, 1990.
304. Connors AF, Jr., Castele RJ, Farhat NZ, Tomashefski JF, Jr. Complications of right heart catheterization. A prospective autopsy study. Chest 88:567–572, 1985.
305. Yamada I, Numano F, Suzuki S. Takayasu arteritis: Evaluation with MR imaging. Radiology 188:89–94, 1993.
306. Doyle L, McWilliam L, Hasleton PS. Giant cell arteritis with pulmonary involvement. Br J Dis Chest 82:88–92, 1988.
307. Chassagne P, Gligorov J, Dominique S. Pulmonary artery obstruction and giant cell arteritis. Ann Intern Med 122:732, 1995.
308. Butto F, Lucas RV, Jr., Edwards JE. Pulmonary arterial aneurysm. A pathologic study of five cases. Chest 91:237–241, 1987.
309. Hamuryudan V, Yurdakul S, Moral F, et al. Pulmonary arterial aneurysms in Behçet's syndrome: A report of 24 cases. Br J Rheumatol 33:48–51, 1994.
310. Jerray M, Benzarti M, Rouatbi N. Possible Behçet's disease revealed by pulmonary aneurysms. Chest 99:1282–1284, 1991.
311. Numan F, Islak C, Berkmen T, Tuzun H, Cokyuksel O. Behçet disease: Pulmonary arterial involvement in 15 cases. Radiology 192:465–468, 1994.
312. Barbour DJ, Roberts WC. Aneurysm of the pulmonary trunk unassociated with intracardiac or great vessel left-to-right shunting. Am J Cardiol 59:192–194, 1987.
313. Karak P, Dimick R, Hamrick KM, Schwartzberg M, Saddekni S. Immediate transcatheter embolization of Swan–Ganz catheter-induced pulmonary artery pseudoaneurysm. Chest 111:1450–1452, 1997.
314. Fukai I, Masaoka A, Yamakawa Y, et al. Rupture of congenital peripheral pulmonary aneurysm. Ann Thorac Surg 59:528–530, 1995.
315. Hankins GD, Brekken AL, Davis LM. Maternal death secondary to a dissecting aneurysm of the pulmonary artery. Obstet Gynecol 65:45S–48S, 1985.
316. Steingrub J, Detore A, Teres D. Spontaneous rupture of pulmonary artery. Crit Care Med 15:270–271, 1987.
317. Coard KC, Martin MP. Ruptured saccular pulmonary artery aneurysm associated with persistent ductus arteriosus. Arch Pathol Lab Med 116:159–161, 1992.
318. Masuda S, Ishii T, Asuwa N, Ishikawa Y, Kiguchi H, Uchiyama T. Concurrent pulmonary arterial dissection and saccular aneurysm associated with primary pulmonary hypertension. Arch Pathol Lab Med 120:309–312, 1996.

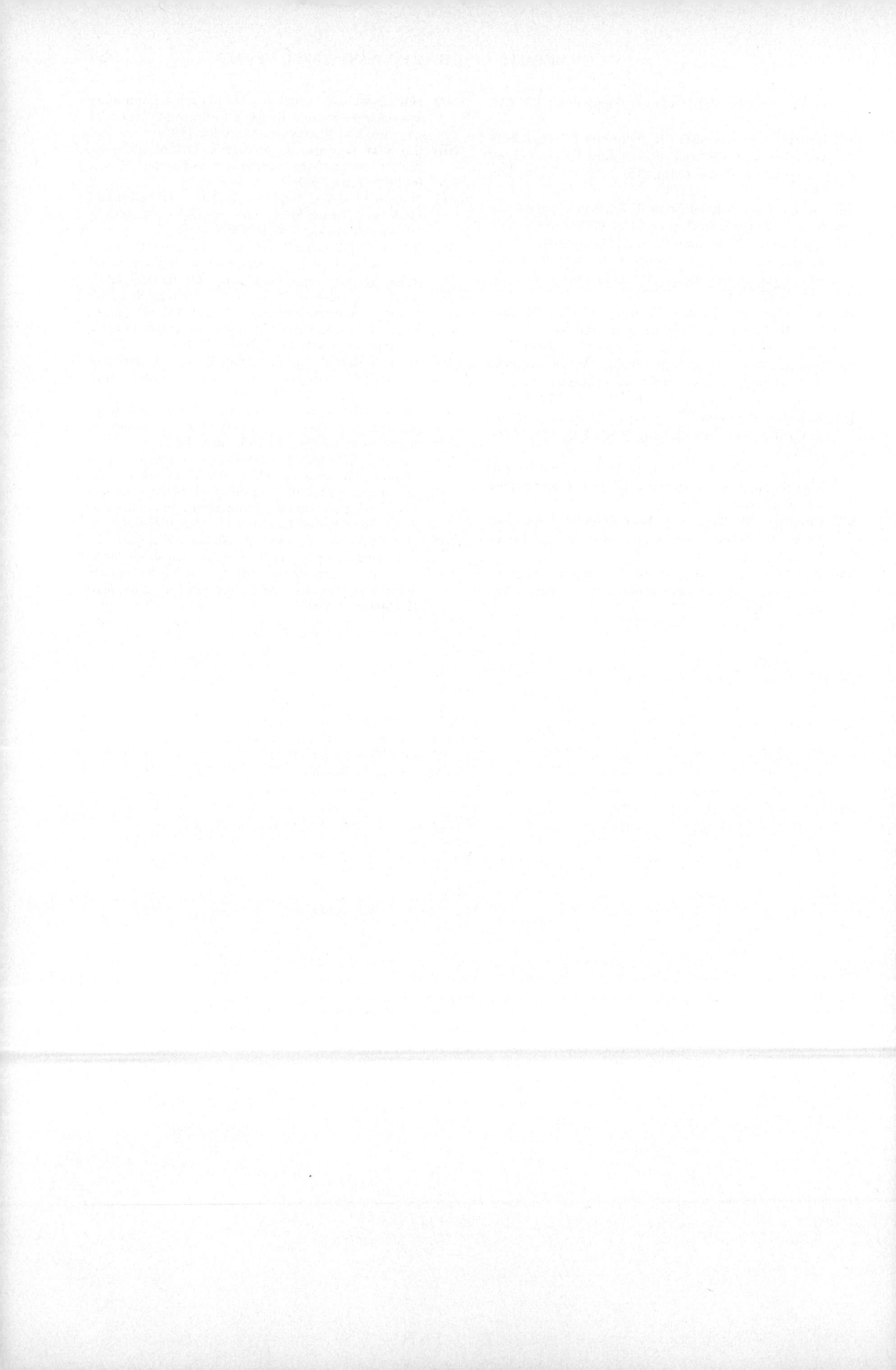

Index

Note: Page numbers followed by the letter f refer to figures and those followed by t refer to tables.

VIRMANI

ISBN 0-7216-8165-4